MOSBY'S COMPREHENSIVE REVIEW

for the Canadian PN Exam

MOSBY'S COMPREHENSIVE REVIEW

for the Canadian PN Exam

Karen Katsademas, RN, BScN, MN
Fanshawe College, London, ON

Marianne Langille, RN, BScN, MEd
Fanshawe College, London, ON

ELSEVIER

Library of Congress Control Number: 2018964893

VP Education Content: Kevonne Holloway
Content Strategist (Acquisitions): Roberta A. Spinosa-Millman
Developmental Editor: Kathleen Nahm/Theresa Fitzgerald
Publishing Services Manager: Shereen Jameel
Project Manager: Umarani Natarajan
Copy Editor: Claudia Forgas
Book Designer: Margaret Reid
Typesetting and Assembly: Toppan Best-set Premedia Ltd

4   5   6   7   8   9

Printed in India

ELSEVIER

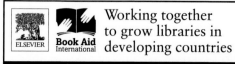

Working together
to grow libraries in
developing countries

www.elsevier.com • www.bookaid.org

For my family

Karen Katsademas

To my husband, Roy, and children, Leanne, Patrick, and Justin, for their support and encouragement

Marianne Langille

CONTENTS

DETAILED CONTENTS

Mosby's Comprehensive Review for the Canadian PN Exam 2019 has been designed to provide a rapid reference with easily obtainable information for the student who is preparing for the Canadian Practical Nurse Registration Examination (CPNRE). It is uniquely Canadian, with content created specifically for the Canadian market. Expert contributors from across Canada have joined with editors to ensure that the text reflects current Canadian nursing practice and trends. The content, based on the blueprint for the CPNRE, is a refresher of learned knowledge, with a focus on the role of the practical nurse, health promotion, professional practice, preventive and primary health care, teaching–learning, nursing judgement, and critical thinking. Gerontological considerations, evidence-informed practice, community focus, and non-traditional settings are included, as appropriate. Appendices include the CPNRE Competencies, Medical Terminology, Abbreviations, Common Laboratory and Diagnostic Tests, and Mathematical Formulae.

Beyond requiring a broad knowledge of nursing theory, students also need to feel confident tackling the particular types of questions found in the CPNRE. For many, it is not a lack of nursing knowledge that affects their performance on the examination but difficulties in applying their knowledge in the exam situation. Chapters that introduce and describe the examination and that offer tips for mastering multiple-choice questions provide valuable guidelines. Each chapter in this comprehensive review includes practice questions representative of those found on the CPNRE and authored within the framework of practical nursing practice in Canada. These questions provide the student with an opportunity to apply learned knowledge to the test situation, particularly at the critical thinking and application cognitive levels. In addition to the practice questions that appear in the chapters, two practice exams are included at the end of the book. Questions have been authored by nursing experts in the field of exam preparation and referenced to established resources. Answers and rationales for the practice exams are also provided.

ACKNOWLEDGEMENTS

We would like to acknowledge and thank the following individuals for their time, support, and expertise in the preparation of this text: Roberta Spinosa-Millman, Kathleen Nahm, and Kelly Skelton of Elsevier, and Lorie Ranieri, for her nursing expertise in contributing to the maternal–newborn and pediatric nursing chapters. We would like to acknowledge and thank Claudia Forgas for her expertise and guidance with the copy editing of the text.

We would also like to recognize the contribution of Janice Marshall-Henty, Cheryl Sams, and Jonathon Bradshaw, authors of *Mosby's Comprehensive Review for the Canadian RN Exam*, along with its numerous contributors. Their original work served as a foundation for our writing and set a standard of excellence we conscientiously followed.

LIST OF CONTRIBUTOR AND REVIEWERS

Lorie Ranieri, RN, BScN, BEd
Fanshawe College
London, ON
(Chapter 9: Maternal–Newborn Nursing,
Chapter10: Pediatric Nursing, Practice Exam
Book One and Two)

REVIEWERS

Mary DeLong, RN, BN, MScN
Nursing Instructor
School of Health and Wellness, Nursing Department
Bow Valley College
Calgary, AB

Sharon Demers, RN, BN, CAE, CCNE
Instructor
Practical Nursing
Assiniboine Community College
Winnipeg, MB

Julian Faulkner, MN, RN
Professor Practical Nursing
Health, Wellness and Sciences
Georgian College, Barrie Campus
Barrie, ON

Staci Gillespie, LPN, IDP
LPN, NBCC Instructor
Practical Nurse
New Brunswick Community College (NBCC)
Miramichi, NB

Monica Gordon, LPN
Licensed Practical Nurse
Health and Wellness
Portage College
Cold Lake, AB

Claudette McDonald, MN, RN
Practical Nursing Faculty
Nova Scotia Community College
Alton, NS

Kari Dawn Ubels, CD, HBScN, RN
Associate Chair of Practical Nurse Curriculum
Faculty of Health and Community Studies
NorQuest College
Edmonton, AB

Roxanne Williams, RN, BScN, M.Ed., PSS
Manager, Practical Nursing Program
Health and Human Services
Nova Scotia Community College
Halifax, NS

Introduction

BACKGROUND TO THE CANADIAN PRACTICAL NURSE REGISTRATION EXAMINATION

To practise as a practical nurse in Canada, you must be registered, or licensed. A component of the registration is successful completion of the Canadian Practical Nurse Registration Examination (CPNRE). The examination, offered in English and French, is the same for all practical nursing applicants across Canada with the exception of Quebec. The CPNRE is developed by practical nurse educators, clinicians, and administrators from across Canada with the assistance of Yardstick Assessment Strategies Inc. To write the exam, you must have completed an approved practical nursing program or have foreign qualifications that have been assessed as being equivalent to a Canadian nursing education. The exam is computer-based except in Newfoundland and Labrador and the Yukon, which offer a paper-based format. There are several exam windows per year. Applicants may choose from a number of secure test centres in more than 100 cities and towns in Canada. The computer-based examination is delivered in Pearson VUE's network of proctored test centres across Canada. To search for Pearson VUE test centres, visit http://www.pearsonvue.com/cpnre/. If you pass the exam in your home province or territory and meet all other requirements for registration, you qualify to apply for registration in all jurisdictions (with the exception of Quebec).

Questions on the CPNRE are designed to evaluate the knowledge of an entry-level practical nurse who has just finished his or her education. Nursing specialties are not tested. Testable material is applicable to all Canadian settings: large cities, small towns, the East Coast or West Coast, community clinics, acute care hospitals, as well as nontraditional settings. When writing the examination, you need to be able to answer based on the knowledge, skills, and behaviours of a model nurse, not just based on what you or your colleagues might have experienced in a particular setting.

The examination is based on a specific blueprint, or framework. Individual questions were authored by a team of nursing experts from across Canada, and all are referenced to at least two published or reliable on-line resources. All questions were tested experimentally and analyzed statistically to determine their suitability for inclusion in the examination.

A complex scoring system is used to mark the exam, but essentially you receive a mark for all correct responses. Marks are not deducted for incorrect answers. The results of the examination are reported as "Pass" or "Fail." Students who are about to write the examination often worry, "What happens if I fail?" With proper preparation, including management of "test stress," this should not happen. If you do not pass the first time you write the CPNRE, you may rewrite the exam. All provinces and territories allow a candidate to write the exam a total of three times.

MOSBY'S COMPREHENSIVE REVIEW

Mosby's Comprehensive Review for the Canadian PN Exam is designed to provide a rapid reference with easily obtainable information for the student who is preparing for the CPNRE. It is the only comprehensive review text that contains content specific to the Canadian examination. Each chapter is a refresher of previously learned knowledge that provides need-to-know information focused on nursing judgement, actions, critical thinking, and the role of the practical nurse. Necessary medical terminology, relevant math formulae, and common laboratory and diagnostic tests are included as appendices at the end of the text.

Chapter 2 presents a description of the CPNRE so that you may become familiar with the format of the test and the types of questions it includes. Tips for studying and taking the multiple-choice examination are provided. Each subsequent chapter contains a review of a major clinical area, followed by questions that test the practical nurse's knowledge of principles and theories underlying nursing care in a range of different situations and settings. Rationales for correct answers for these practice questions are provided, as are the latest competencies and identification of question taxonomies.

In addition, this text includes two practice examinations that are similar in format and content to the CPNRE. These practice exams give you the opportunity to apply your knowledge to the particular types of questions you will experience in the CPNRE. You can choose to write an entire exam to mimic true test conditions or to answer particular sections or questions.

After you have answered the questions, review the correct answers and rationales for each item. Analyze your mistakes. Were there knowledge gaps? Did you misread the question?

Did you assume information that wasn't given in the question? Did you misunderstand what the question meant? Identify the frequency with which you made particular errors and use this information as a reference database for further study. Perhaps you need to review certain topics, practise your math skills, or increase your reading comprehension.

Do not attempt to memorize any of the information from the practice questions or to use any of the questions to study content. All test items on the CPNRE are secure and have never been published; questions in this text will *not* be on the CPNRE.

Remember, you are not expected to get a perfect score. If you correctly answer about 65% of the practice questions in this text, you are likely to succeed on the actual CPNRE.

BIBLIOGRAPHY

Assessment Strategies Inc. (2016). *The Canadian Practical Nurse Registration Examination (CPNRE) prep guide* (5th ed.). Ottawa: Author.

Assessment Strategies Inc. (2017). *Canadian Practical Nurse Registration Examination blueprint*. Ottawa: Author.

Marshall-Henty, J., & Bradshaw, J. (2011). *Mosby's prep guide for the Canadian RN exam* (2nd ed.). Toronto: Mosby.

WEB SITE

- **Canadian Practical Nurse Registration Examination (CPNRE)** (http://cpnre.ca): This site includes information about the CPNRE.

Tips for Writing the CPNRE

DESCRIPTION OF THE EXAMINATION AND TEST-TAKING TIPS

The Canadian Practical Nurse Registration Examination (CPNRE) consists of 165–170 questions, including experimental questions that are not counted toward your examination score. Some of the experimental questions may be in a format other than multiple choice. An experimental question is one that has not been statistically validated and is undergoing trial evaluation with exam candidates. You will not know which questions are the experimental questions, so answer all questions as though they count toward your grade. The writing time for the exam is 4 hours.

Multiple-Choice Questions

The multiple-choice test items are written as either case-based or independent questions. Case-based questions present a healthcare scenario along with approximately three to five questions related to the scenario. Independent, or stand-alone, questions contain all the information necessary to answer the question. In the CPNRE, 30–50% of the questions are case-based.

Each multiple-choice question is made up of two components. The part that asks the question or poses a problem is called the *stem*. The alternatives from which you are asked to select the best answer are called the *options*. There are four options, and *only one* of the options is the correct answer. The other three options are called *distractors*. Distractors may seem to be reasonable answers but are, in fact, incorrect or incomplete. All questions are worth one mark. Marks are not deducted for wrong answers.

Sample Question

While receiving a blood transfusion, Mr. Ryan develops chills and a headache. What would be the nurse's initial action?

1. Notify the physician stat.
2. Stop the transfusion immediately.
3. Cover Mr. Ryan with a blanket and administer ordered acetaminophen (Tylenol).
4. Slow the blood flow to keep the vein open.

The correct answer is 2. Mr. Ryan is experiencing a transfusion reaction. Thus, the blood infusion must be stopped immediately.

Examination Blueprint

The CPNRE is written according to a blueprint that includes competencies; levels of cognitive ability called *taxonomies*; and the variables of client type, client age, client diversity, and work environment. It is not organized into sections on maternal–newborn nursing, medical–surgical nursing, pediatric nursing, mental health nursing, and so on.

Competencies

Competencies include knowledge, skills, behaviours, and clinical judgements that a practical nurse is expected to demonstrate in order to provide safe, professional care. In the exam, competencies are applied to various health situations and clients. For example, what are the safety hazards for the mental health client, the infant, or the older adult? How do you prevent the spread of infection in a hospital, in a daycare centre, or to an immunocompromised client? Practical nurses learn these competencies in their education programs. There are 85 competencies in three categories. See Appendix A for a complete list of the CPNRE competencies.

Competency categories
Professional, ethical, and legal practice

Practical nurses are responsible for providing safe, competent, compassionate and ethical nursing care while developing and maintaining a therapeutic nurse–client relationship. Professional standards and ethics provide direction for practical nurses to uphold the highest quality of care. The practical nurse maintains autonomy and is accountable to the public, the client, the employer, the profession, colleagues and one's self. (Assessment Strategies Inc., 2017, p. 5)

Approximately one-quarter of the questions on the exam (20–30%) concern professional, ethical, and legal practice.
Sample Competency and Related Sample Question:
- PR-9—adhere to legal requirements regarding documentation.

Sample Question

Mrs. Leung was found by the nurse at 0100 hours lying on the floor beside her bed. What should the nurse document in the health record?

---

1. Mrs. Leung fell out of bed at 0100.
2. At 0100 hours, Mrs. Leung was found by the nurse on the floor beside her bed.
3. Mrs. Leung got out of bed at 0100 hours, slipped, and fell on the floor.
4. Mrs. Leung apparently fell out of bed at approximately 0100 hours.

The correct answer is 2. This notation provides factual and objective documentation about the practical nurse's observation.

Foundations of practice

As a member of the health-care team, practical nurses are integral in the assessment, nursing diagnosis, planning, implementation, evaluation and documentation of nursing care. Using critical inquiry, practical nurses formulate clinical decisions based on evidence. Practical nurses promote, support and advocate for client self-determination to achieve optimum health outcomes. (Assessment Strategies Inc., 2017, p. 5)

Over half of the questions (55–65%) relate to this competency.
Sample Competency and Related Sample Question:
• FP-8—engage in safe infusion therapy practices.

Sample Question
The physician order reads, "IV TKVO." What does this mean?
1. Intravenous infusion rate of 10 mL per hour
2. Intravenous infusion rate of 15 mL per hour
3. Intravenous to be locked with saline
4. Intravenous rate that will maintain the patency of the infusion

The correct answer is 4. *TKVO* means "to keep vein open."

Collaborative practice

Practical nurses work collaboratively while maintaining autonomy within their legislated scope of practice and individual competence. They recognize that collaborative practice is guided by shared values and accountability, a common purpose, care outcomes, mutual respect and effective communication. ... The practical nurse demonstrates leadership while fostering continued growth of self and others to meet the challenges of the evolving health-care system. (Assessment Strategies Inc., 2017, p. 5)

Nearly one-quarter of the questions on the exam (10–20%) relate to collaborative practice.
Sample Competency and Related Sample Question:
• CP-3—demonstrate leadership in collaborative practice.

Sample Question
The practical nurse checks on a client who was admitted to the hospital with pneumonia. He has been coughing profusely and has required nasotracheal suctioning. He has an intravenous infusion of antibiotics. He is febrile. Which of the following tasks may the practical nurse delegate to the support worker assigned to the client today?
1. Assessing vital signs
2. Changing intravenous dressing
3. Nasotracheal suctioning
4. Administering a bed bath

The correct answer is 4. The practical nurse may delegate this task to the support worker.

Taxonomies of Questions

To test your thinking abilities, questions are written at different cognitive levels: knowledge/comprehension, application, and critical thinking. Knowing the percentage of questions on the exam pertaining to each cognitive level will help guide your studying.

Knowledge and Comprehension

The knowledge/comprehension level requires recollection of facts. For these types of questions, you are required to define, identify, or select remembered information. Knowledge questions require basic memorization. A maximum of 10% of the questions on the CPNRE are of the knowledge/comprehension type.

Sample Question
Which of the following is an adverse effect of digoxin?
1. Tachycardia
2. Bradycardia
3. Diarrhea
4. Urticaria

The answer is 2, bradycardia. To answer this question correctly, you need to have memorized the adverse effects of digoxin and the terms *tachycardia* and *bradycardia*.

Application

The application level of the intellectual process requires not only knowing and understanding information but also being able to apply it to a new situation. This level includes modifying, manipulating, or adapting information when providing client care. A minimum of 55% of the questions on the CPNRE are application-based.

Sample Question
Before taking Mr. Singh's vital signs, the nurse asks him if he is taking any medications. He answers, "Digoxin every morning and Tylenol in the evening." Which of the following vital sign changes might the practical nurse anticipate?

1. Increased blood pressure to 140/85 mm Hg
2. Decreased pulse to 53 beats per minute
3. Decreased respiratory rate to 10 breaths per minute
4. Increased temperature to 38.5°C

   The answer is 2, decreased pulse. This question requires knowledge about several drugs, interpretation of vital signs, and application of this information to a particular client.

Critical Thinking

Critical-thinking questions require the most complex level of cognitive function. They ask you to analyze, evaluate, problem-solve, or interpret data from a variety of sources before you respond to them. This often involves prioritizing practical nursing actions. Many refer to critical-thinking questions as "tricky" or "unfair" because the options may all be correct, but only one option is considered the most important or comprehensive response. A minimum of 35% of the questions on the CPNRE are critical-thinking questions.

Sample Question

Mr. Singh has asthma and is experiencing acute shortness of breath and wheezing. What should the nurse do first?
1. Administer his ordered "rescue inhaler"
2. Administer his ordered combination inhaled drugs
3. Notify the physician
4. Encourage increased fluid intake

   The answer is 1, administer his rescue inhaler. All the options could be correct, but administering the rescue inhaler is the first thing the practical nurse should do. Consider the nursing process: validate your data.

Other Blueprint Variables

Client Type

In the CPNRE, a *client* is defined as an individual (or their designated representative), family, and group (Assessment Strategies Inc., 2017).

Client Age

Questions reflect the statistical representation of Canadians in relation to age, from birth to older adult.

Client Diversity

"Items will be included that measure awareness, sensitivity and respect for diversity, without introducing stereotypes" (Assessment Strategies Inc., 2017, p. 8). Because Canada comprises a variety of cultural backgrounds, the CPNRE integrates sensitivity and respect for diverse beliefs and values. It does not specifically test knowledge of individual cultures, other than that of Indigenous* people in Canada.

---

*The CPNRE uses the term *Aboriginal.* However, this book uses Indigenous, which has become the predominant term used in reference to the First Peoples of Canada since Canada's full endorsement of the 2007 United Nations Declaration on the Rights of Indigenous Peoples (UNDRIP) in May 2016.

Work Environment

"Practical nurses work in a variety of practice settings and contexts where health care is delivered. As a result, the work environment is *only* specified where necessary" (Assessment Strategies Inc., 2017, p. 24).

STUDY AND EXAMINATION TIPS

Although you may be academically well prepared to write the CPNRE, strategies for studying, stress management, and test-taking will increase your chances of success and help alleviate test anxiety.

Study Tips

It is easy to become overwhelmed as you prepare to study for the CPNRE. Remember, though, that you know a lot more than you think you do. While studying is crucial, much learning is not a conscious activity. The first key to developing successful study strategies is to be realistic. Identify where you have incomplete knowledge or the need to refresh your learning.

Keep in mind that most of the questions on the exam do not merely test recalled facts, so you should try to understand the material that you read, rather than memorize it. The focus of your studies should be on principles of care and nursing interventions within a particular health situation; that is, What should the nurse do or say?

Because the exam will likely include approximately one or two questions per competency, make sure you do not get bogged down in one particular content area. For example, there may be only one competency related to assessment and monitoring of central venous catheters (CVCs), so you should not spend too much time studying CVCs.

One of the best strategies for learning is to form a study group. Self-testing and peer testing have proven to be the most effective methods for consolidating material. Have each member of the group choose a topic to teach the other members. This way, you stimulate discussion and get different perspectives on the subjects, which will help you in understanding and remembering them. If you are unable to participate in a study group, try teaching yourself the information. Rephrase or reword the written information to aid in understanding rather than memorizing.

Repetition works well for many people. If you are having trouble remembering some knowledge material, it may help to record it so that you can play it aloud while performing other activities.

Schedule your studying. Start reviewing content several months prior to the exam so that you do not feel rushed or panicked at the volume of material you need to learn. Cramming or "all-nighters" may be useful for memorizing facts, but the CPNRE is an exam that requires problem-solving based on a comprehensive knowledge base. It is better to think through and analyze the material, make judgements, and determine how the subject relates to nursing. By performing these analytical and reflective processes, you are more likely to commit the information to long-term memory, which is much more reliable than your short-term memory.

To remember the strategies for studying, you can use the initialism PQRS, which stands for *p*lanning, *q*uestions practice, *r*epetition, and *s*elf- and peer testing.

While you study, remember to stay hydrated, eat sensibly, build in exercise breaks, and get plenty of sleep. It is also important to pursue other activities and not be involved solely in study. Research has shown that both sleep and "time out," in the form of exercise, social activities, or nutrition breaks, help consolidate learned information.

Managing Test Stress

"If I take one more multiple-choice test, I think I may become physically ill. I won't be able to help myself. Can't they think of any other way of assessing how much we know?"

The student quoted above is setting himself up for failure because of his negativity toward the format of the test.

It is perfectly normal to feel nervous and anxious about the CPNRE. You have worked hard to be successful in your nursing program, and now all that effort comes down to passing a 4-hour exam. As you prepare for the CPNRE, empower yourself by developing a positive mental attitude. Henry Ford said, "Whether you think you can or think you can't … you're right." Challenge your negative thoughts! Do not let them guide you.

Stress Management Tips

Become active and positive about your learning and your preparation. The more actively you plan and prepare, the more likely you will be successful. The following tips will help you manage stress:

- Try to avoid fellow students who feel overly anxious about the exam. Anxiety is like a communicable disease. You can catch it.
- Use the power of positive thinking. Build up your self-confidence by repeating to yourself, "I am well prepared. I will pass this exam."
- Practise yoga or other forms of exercise; they are great stress relievers.
- Try aromatherapy—lavender works well to promote relaxation. Sometimes just the smell will help you remember to relax and breathe.
- Eat a well-balanced diet, and get plenty of rest.
  ### The evening before the examination

  "The night before a test, I can't sleep. Then I worry because I can't sleep. Then I can't sleep because I'm worrying that I'm worried that I can't sleep. By morning, I'm glad to get out of bed just to stop the terrible racket in my head."

The evening before the exam, organize your clothes and exam supplies. Make sure you know the location of the exam and have arranged your transportation to the exam.

Then be nice to yourself. Do something you enjoy and get a good night's sleep. Information is processed during sleep, so sleep will help you retain what you have studied. Last-minute cramming may have aided you in past test situations, but it is helpful only for memorizing facts. It actually decreases your ability to problem-solve the application and critical-thinking types of questions that are on the CPNRE.

The day of the examination. Eat a healthy breakfast of protein and complex carbohydrates. If you absolutely cannot eat, try drinking a sports electrolyte solution. Although you need to be adequately hydrated, do not drink too many fluids or cups of coffee. Dress in comfortable clothes, preferably in layers, so that you can add or take off articles depending on the temperature of the exam room. If possible, try to make time for light exercise, even if it is walking the last few blocks to the exam centre.

Plan to arrive at the test location at least 30 minutes ahead of the exam start time. This cushion will allow you time to relax, visit with friends, and prepare yourself mentally. However, avoid talking about the exam with your friends, as conversations about it will only make you more anxious. Arriving early also gives you time for that last-minute washroom trip—stress is a potent diuretic. When you sit down in the exam room, make a conscious effort to relax and continue your positive thinking.

During the examination. Remember to keep that positive focus during the exam. Repeat to yourself: "I know this information, and I can answer these questions. I will pass the exam." Reading and keeping focused is essential. Take mini "brain breaks" by performing relaxation exercises in your seat, such as slow deep breaths, shoulder shrugs, neck rolls, and arm and leg rotations.

After the examination. After the exam, you will likely feel a sense of relief that it is over, but you may also feel the need to review questions in your head and discuss answers with your peers. Try not to dwell on this activity for too long. These post-mortems can bring you down. Remember, you have probably done better than you think!

Tips for Writing Multiple-Choice Exams

Listed below are some tips for completing the multiple-choice questions particular to the CPNRE:

A. Read and listen to the exam instructions carefully.

B. Plan your time and pace yourself. Although it is important not to speed through questions, do not spend more than 1–1.5 minutes on any question (Assessment Strategies Inc., 2016). Keep track of time. You should answer approximately 25–30 questions in each half-hour.

C. Do not spend a lot of time on one question if you do not know the answer. If you are stuck on a question, leave it and return to it later. Go on to a question that you find easy. The feeling of success will give you confidence.

D. Reading comprehension is crucial to success. Read the stem of each question carefully and make sure that you understand exactly what it asks. One of the most common test-taking errors is misreading the question. In the CPNRE, important words are not highlighted, so you should identify words such as *initial* or *most important* or *priority*. Take special note of any negatives such as *never* or *except*.

Sample Question

The nurse discovers that Ms. Chang has received twice the dose of an ordered medication. What is the most important initial action for the nurse to perform?
1. Complete an incident report.
2. Notify the ordering physician.
3. Assess Ms. Chang for adverse effects of the overdose.
4. Report the error to the nurse administrator.

E. Because the majority of the questions are either at the application or critical-thinking cognitive levels, you must be prepared to problem-solve *every* question. There are no rules for answering questions. Each question must be approached with a view to solving the problem based on your nursing judgement in this particular situation.

F. Try to answer the question before looking at the multiple-choice options.

G. Read all the options before choosing one. Do not immediately assume that a response is correct without looking at all the other options; another answer may be *more correct* than the one you choose first.

H. Read each option carefully, mentally crossing out the options you know are incorrect. Choose the best option out of the ones remaining.

I. Some questions that appear to be trick questions may, in reality, measure your ability to think critically. If you believe all the options are correct, choose the one that is most comprehensive, makes the most common sense, or is the most professional answer.

Sample Question

Which of the following is most important when performing a preoperative assessment?
1. Physical assessment
2. Cardiac assessment
3. Assessment of vital signs
4. Auscultation of breath sounds
   All options are valid, but answer 1 is the most inclusive.

J. To choose the most important nursing action when all of the answers appear to be correct, use the following guidelines:
   • Read the situation and question very carefully.
   • In many cases, consider the mnemonic *ABC* (*a*irway, *b*reathing, *c*irculation).
   • Remember the nursing process: collect and validate information before acting.
   • Consider safety—for the client and for yourself.
   • Choose an action that can be completed quickly and safely, almost at the same time as other actions.
   • Do not necessarily look for fancy answers.
   • Choose simple, common-sense, safe actions.
   • Choose the sickest, most unstable client as the priority.

K. A common error students make is choosing a response that might have been applicable in a specific client situation that they have experienced. Always answer according to "textbook," or standard, nursing principles.

L. Answer as you believe the perfect "textbook nurse" would answer.

M. Do not assume any information that is not given. Choose your answer based only on information in the question asked.

N. Do not panic if you have never heard of a particular disease or client situation. Apply general nursing principles to each question—you may be able to answer the question by doing so. Candidates for the exam come from various academic backgrounds, and curricula are not identical in all colleges. You are not expected to know all the answers, nor are you expected to write a perfect exam!

Sample Question

Ms. Townsend is suffering from Hick's asymmetrical dementia. Which of the following activities would be appropriate for her condition?
1. Vigorous exercise
2. Competitive games
3. Social stimulation in group activities
4. Solitary reading
   Hick's asymmetrical dementia is a fictitious disorder. The care needs for a client with dementia are fundamental, so the correct response is answer 3. This is a "trick question" for the purpose of illustration. The CPNRE, however, contains no trick questions.

O. Your first answer choice is usually correct. You may have learned some information subconsciously, and your first impression is often an automatic response to what you have learned. Do not second-guess yourself unless you are absolutely sure that you have misunderstood the question or provided a wrong answer.

P. Select answers that are therapeutic, show respect, involve the client in care, and focus on nursing judgement rather than hospital rules or orders from other health team members.

Sample Question

Jessica tells the practical nurse, "I am tired of waiting for you to brush my hair. You're never here when I want you." Which of the following responses is the most appropriate for the practical nurse to give?
1. "I'm sorry you've had to wait. I'll get your hairbrush out for you and be back in 15 minutes to do your hair."
2. "That's not fair. I spent my lunch break with you yesterday."
3. "Jeremy down the hall is really sick, and he needs me more than you do right now."
4. "I'm doing my best, but I have a really busy assignment today."
   Option 1 acknowledges the client's feelings, shows respect, and provides a clear, factual response.

Sample Question

Ms. Steele asks the practical nurse when she can start eating after bowel surgery. What is the most appropriate response for the practical nurse to give?
1. "You'll have to ask the doctor."
2. "Tell me about your appetite."
3. "You'll likely start on clear fluids once bowel sounds can be heard."
4. "I'll have the dietitian consult with you about the most nutritious postsurgery menus."

Option 3 involves nursing judgement and directly answers the client's question.

Q. Most questions will ask about actions that are based on nursing judgement rather than physician's orders. However, some questions may test your knowledge of the scope of nursing practice and have as a correct response "contact the doctor." Examples of such situations include unclear or illegible orders, a specific request from a client, deteriorating client condition, and a client emergency.

R. In the case of communication questions, answers that demonstrate the practical nurse asking the client open-ended questions are most often correct.

Sample Question

Which of the following would elicit the best information from Mr. Loates about his pain?
1. "Do you have severe pain?"
2. "Do you have any pain?"
3. "Is your pain throbbing or stabbing?"
4. "Describe your pain to me."

Option 4 is open-ended—that is, it requires the client to give more than a one- or two-word answer. Phrasing questions in an open-ended fashion is a key component of therapeutic nursing communication.

S. Do not choose an answer because you have seen that question before and think you recall the answer. Questions on the exam may look similar to ones you have encountered during practice but will not be exactly the same. Therefore, the answer may also not be the same.

T. There is no pattern to the assigned answers. Do not change an answer because you have had too many answers in the same position.

U. If all else fails, guess. Never leave a question unanswered. You have at least a 25% chance of getting it correct.

Tips for Guessing

1. If two of the options are similar except for one or two words, choose one of those.
   Example:
   Take the apical pulse
   Take the radial pulse
2. If two options have opposite meanings, choose one of those.
   Example:
   Vasodilation
   Vasoconstriction
3. If two quantities or mathematical calculations are similar, choose one of those.
   Example:
   0.14 mL
   0.014 mL

V. When you have finished the exam, be sure to check your scanning card against each of the questions to make sure that you have coded your answers correctly. Make sure the scanning card contains no marks other than those designating the options you have selected.

W. Answering 165–170 questions can be boring, stressful, and tiring. You may find yourself becoming confused about what information relates to the question. Throughout the exam, take a mini-exercise break every 20 minutes; sip water, do neck rolls, and flex your arms and legs.

X. Do not panic if someone leaves when you have completed only 20 questions. Most "early leavers" do not do better than exam writers who use the entire allotted time.

SUMMARY

Preparing for the examination well in advance, ensuring comprehensive content review, following the test-taking tips, developing your reading comprehension, and maintaining a positive outlook will equip you with the necessary abilities to be successful in the CPNRE.

REFERENCES

Assessment Strategies Inc. (2016). *The Canadian Practical Nurse Registration Examination (CPNRE) prep guide* (5th ed.). Ottawa: Author.

Assessment Strategies Inc. (2017). *Canadian Practical Nurse Registration Examination blueprint*. Ottawa: Author.

BIBLIOGRAPHY

Canadian Nurses Association. (2010). *Blueprint for the Canadian Registered Nurse Examination: June 2010–May 2015* (3rd ed.). Ottawa: Author.

Canadian Nurses Association. (2010). *The Canadian Registered Nurse Examination prep guide* (5th ed.). Ottawa: Author.

Dickson, K. (2015). Learner success: Mastering exam anxiety (Athabasca University). Retrieved from http://www.athabascau.ca/counselling/exam_anxiety.php.

Eyles, M. (2014). *Mosby's comprehensive review of practical nursing for the NCLEX-PN examination* (17th ed.). St. Louis: Mosby.

Hanoski, T. (2018). Exam anxiety. Retrieved from https://drthanoski.com/exam-anxiety.

Learning Skills Services (University of Western Ontario). (2017). Managing test anxiety. Retrieved from https://www.uwo.ca/sdc/learning/selfhelp/skill_building_handouts/PDFs/Exams%20

-%20Preparing,%20Writing,%20and%20Beyond/Managing %20Test%20Anxiety.pdf.

Learning Skills Services (University of Western Ontario). (2017). Writing multiple-choice tests. Retrieved from https://www .uwo.ca/sdc/learning/selfhelp/skill_building_handouts/PDFs/ Exams%20-%20Preparing,%20Writing,%20and%20Beyond/ Writing%20Multiple.pdf.

Marshall-Henty, J., & Bradshaw, J. (2011). *Mosby's prep guide for the Canadian RN exam* (2nd ed.). Toronto: Elsevier Canada.

Nugent, P. M., Green, J. S., Hellmer Saul, M. A., et al. (2012). *Mosby's comprehensive review of nursing for the NCLEX-RN examination* (20th ed.). St. Louis: Mosby.

Nugent, P. M., & Vitale, B. A. (2004). *Fundamentals success: A course review applying critical thinking to test taking.* Philadelphia: F.A. Davis.

WEB SITES

- **Association for Applied Psychophysiology and Biofeedback** (http://www.aapb.org): This site contains information and resources concerning biofeedback and its benefits.
- **How Successful Students Prepare for Tests** (http://capone .mtsu.edu/studskl/sucstu.html): This Middle Tennessee State University site provides useful tips about how to learn material and prepare for examinations.
- **Medical Mnemonics** (http://www.medicalmnemonics.com): This site lists mnemonics that can help students memorize information related to specific topics in anatomy and pathology.

3

Professional Practice and the Nurse–Client Relationship

Practical nurses in Canada are major contributors to and an essential part of the healthcare system. Changes in healthcare delivery have occurred in healthcare organizations over the past years to meet the changing needs of client populations and the healthcare system. Practical nurses are adapting to these changes to provide a highly competent workforce caring for stable clients in acute and long-term care, as well as in community and mental healthcare settings. Practical nurses are valuable members of the healthcare team in providing quality client care.

An understanding of the unique and overlapping scopes of practice within nursing and how nursing teams function effectively contributes to safe, competent care and quality outcomes for clients. Nursing care delivery models are based on principles of collaboration and partnership, allowing for optimal teamwork, respect, and knowledge sharing.

The Canadian Council for Practical Nurse Regulators (CCPNR, 2013b) outlines the practice expectations of licensed practical nurses/registered practical nurses (LPNs/RPNs) across Canada. Practical nurses are expected to uphold a code of ethics, meet standards of practice, and have the required skills, abilities, and entry-to-practice competencies that ensure consistently safe and competent care. The practical nurse provides care to the individual, family, group, community, and larger populations. The scope of practice of a practical nurse depends on the complexity of knowledge, critical thinking, and judgement required in the practice environment.

REGULATION AND LICENSING OF NURSING IN CANADA

In Canada, nursing is a profession that is self-regulated and consists of different groups of nurses. These groups are as follows (Canadian Institute for Health Information [CIHI], 2017):

- Registered practical nurses (RPNs) in Ontario or licensed practical nurses (LPNs) in the rest of Canada
- Registered nurses (RNs)
- Registered psychiatric nurses (RPNs) who practise only in British Columbia, Alberta, Saskatchewan, Manitoba, and Yukon
- Nurse practitioners (NPs)

Provincial and territorial regulatory bodies are responsible for the licensing and registration of all nurses in Canada. These regulatory bodies are responsible for defining the scope of practice, standards of practice, and codes of ethics that nurses must meet in their particular jurisdiction. Self-regulation also means that the regulator or licensing organization is responsible for disciplining nurses who do not meet the established standards of practice (Potter, Perry, Stockert, et al., 2019, pp. 102 and 1423).

Nursing Legislation

Nursing practice acts and health professions acts regulate the registration and licensing of nurses, describe continuing competency requirements and any restricted or controlled acts, and explain discipline procedures for the profession. Nursing practice acts have been revised across the country to reflect the growing autonomy and expanding roles of the nurse. The legislative acts exist primarily to protect the public in terms of health, safety, and welfare. Most provinces and territories provide a registration certificate, while others provide a licence. Legislation also provides title protection for nurses. Using the titles RN, LPN, RPN, and, in some provinces and territories, NP is limited to only those nurses who are authorized to do so by their legislative and regulatory bodies.

Practical Nursing Scope of Practice

In Canada, the practical nurse's scope of practice is determined by legislation and regulatory and licensure requirements (CIHI, 2017). Standards of nursing practice define the expectation for practical nurses in various practice settings and situations, and generally guide nursing practice.

Practical nurses must be able to practise entry-level competencies using knowledge, skill, and judgement. The practical nurse is determined to be competent if he or she successfully completes an approved Canadian practical nursing educational program (or an equivalent non-Canadian nursing program) and passes the Canadian Practical Nurse Registration Examination (CPNRE). On the last point, the only exception is Quebec, which administers its own nursing examination through its regulatory body (Potter et al., 2019). Internationally prepared nurses must meet specific regulatory requirements, including passing a registration examination and meeting academic standards, to be eligible to become a practical nurse (Potter et al., 2019).

Reciprocity between provinces and territories may allow qualifying practical nurses to practise in different provinces and territories. This reciprocity becomes available once the practical nurse has completed the registration process. Practical nurses in most provinces are required to write a jurisprudence examination before becoming registered. The jurisprudence examination assesses an applicant's knowledge and understanding of the laws, regulations, bylaws, practice standards, and guidelines that govern the practice of nursing (visit the web site of your jurisdiction's regulatory body for more information on the jurisprudence examination).

A regulatory body is mandated by the province or territory to set minimum entry-to-practice requirements to promote public safety and professional accountability. Jurisdictions typically include the following entry-to-practice requirements for practical nursing:

- Graduation from an approved postsecondary program for practical nursing
- A clear criminal record check
- Knowledge of the nursing process (assessment, planning, implementing, and evaluating nursing care) for clients of differing ages
- Ability to work independently as well as collaboratively with other healthcare providers in more acute, unpredictable situations
- Ability to work with a range of clients: individuals, families, groups, and (if need be) communities
- Understanding of and ability to apply ethical practice standards
- Ability to collaborate and communicate with others, including the client and other healthcare providers
- Ability to be accountable and responsible for one's own actions
- Ability to work within the scope of practice
- Willingness to learn on an ongoing basis
- Ability to cope with change (Potter et al., 2019)

EDUCATION

For the practical nurse, the entry-level educational requirement in Canadian jurisdictions is a 2-year diploma program (Potter et al., 2019). Many academic institutions in Canada are beginning to offer pathways that bridge practical nursing and registered nursing programs. Practical nurses have many opportunities to further their education through certification in specialty areas such as operating room technique and management, geriatric nursing, dialysis, women's health, and mental health (Potter et al., 2019). It is important that practical nurses continually update their knowledge and skills. In today's rapidly changing healthcare workplace, there are frequent advances in research, technology, and practice. It is essential for practical nurses to be lifelong learners and to expand their knowledge base as well as keep current with practice standards.

PRACTICE ENVIRONMENTS

Practical nurses work in a multitude of practice environments across Canada. Practice environments range from chronic care to acute care, and they include nontraditional settings such as businesses and governmental organizations. Most practical nurses work in long-term/geriatric care, rehabilitation, acute care, and community health. Practical nurses may also be employed as administrators, educators, and researchers.

Long-Term Care Facilities and Rehabilitation Centres

Long-term care facilities employ the majority of practical nurses in Canada (CIHI, 2017, p. 4). Long-term care facilities are mostly residential. They provide nursing care for individuals with chronic illnesses who require 24-hour nursing care and support services for individuals who cannot care for themselves at home but do not require hospital care. The facilities also provide respite care. Geriatric care will depend on the individual's health status and care requirements.

Rehabilitation centres focus on helping clients become as independent as possible so that they can take care of their own needs. Practical nurses work as part of an extensive healthcare team that plans clients' rehabilitation and their return to the community. These clients may have a chronic illness or may have experienced an acute illness.

Acute Care Facilities

Acute care settings have clients with complex, multisystem conditions who have many healthcare needs. Practical nurses in these settings must possess a wide variety of technical skills and must meet the physical and psychological needs of these acutely ill clients and their families.

Community and Other Settings

Many community practical nurses are involved in important roles such as performing health assessments and direct care to clients or groups (e.g., families that need parenting skills) within a community setting. The scope of community nursing practice includes population-focused health promotion, protection, maintenance, and restoration. The term *community nursing* is broad and encompasses public health nursing, community health nursing, and community-based nursing.

In recent years, clients are being sent home earlier from acute care facilities. This trend has increased the need for community-based practical nurses. The required nursing services are more complex because the level of care needed in these community populations is increasingly acute. This acuity is in part due to the earlier discharges from hospitals. However, in addition, more clients are being cared for at home rather than being admitted to long-term care facilities. For example, practical nurses now require the skills to provide home care for clients with tracheostomies, central venous lines, and home dialysis.

NURSING ROLES

The Role of the Practical Nurse

Most provinces now have two categories of nurses: (a) registered nurses (including nurse practitioners) and (b) practical nurses. The title of a practical nurse is "registered practical nurse" (RPN) in Ontario and "licensed practical nurse" (LPN) in the rest of the provinces and territories. Most jurisdictions recognize that practical nursing is a separate category within the wider field of professional nursing. Most jurisdictions also recognize that practical nurses and RNs learn approximately the same body of nursing knowledge. RNs study this content in more detail and over a longer period of time, while practical nurses study for a shorter period, resulting in more focused knowledge (Potter et al., 2019).

Practical nurses may work independently or they may work collaboratively with RNs. "While specific scopes of practice may differ among jurisdictions, it is common to find that as the complexity and unpredictability of the patient's condition and risk of negative outcomes increase, practical nurses will need more collaboration and support from RNs" (Potter et al., 2019, p. 1419).

The Role of the Registered Nurse

For the RN, the entry-level educational requirement is a 4-year baccalaureate degree in nursing, with the exception of Quebec, which accepts a 3-year college diploma. Many nurses go on to further their education and study for a master's or doctoral degree in nursing or other disciplines. A master's degree in nursing is necessary for nurses seeking positions as clinical nurse specialists, nurse practitioners, nurse administrators, or nurse educators. RNs are caregivers, client and family advocates, clinical educators, administrators, professors, and researchers, and fulfill many other roles.

The Role of the Unregulated Care Provider

"Unregulated care providers (UCPs) are healthcare providers who perform clearly identified services under the direction and supervision of a client, family member, regulated healthcare provider, or employer" (Sorrentino, Remmert, & Wilk, 2018, p. 11). UCPs are not licensed under law in a jurisdiction. There are many other titles for this role, such as *resident care aide*, *personal support worker*, or *nursing attendant*. These support workers are usually employees of a facility or an agency and are bound to perform in their role as per the terms of their employment agreement. Registered/licensed staff working with these individuals must be aware of the role expectations set by the employer for this category of worker and of the level of competence of the individual worker. Registered/licensed staff are not accountable for the care provided by the support worker (Sorrentino et al., 2018).

NURSING PRACTICE AND THE LAW

It is important for practical nurses to know the legal parameters they work within to protect their clients' rights as well as their own. They need to know the specific nursing laws of the jurisdiction in which they practise and be familiar with the federal *Canada Health Act* (1985), which applies to health care across Canada. Provincial and territorial legislatures create laws that apply only to their jurisdiction. For example, *The Nursing Act* in Ontario describes the boundaries of nursing practice within this province only. Provincial and territorial laws also give authority to their nursing regulatory bodies (Potter et al., 2019).

Nursing regulatory bodies are responsible to the public. Their mandate is to ensure that the nursing care delivered to the public is safe and competent and meets standards of care and a code of ethics. In addition, regulatory bodies set nursing examinations and grant registration or licensure.

These regulatory bodies also can revoke or suspend a practical nurse's licence if a practical nurse violates the parameters of the registration statute. An investigation of public complaints or misconduct is carried out by the regulatory body, and a hearing may be held. The practical nurse must be informed of the charges. Further legal action may occur if the practical nurse's registration is revoked or removed from the jurisdiction's register and there are criminal or civil wrongs (Potter et al., 2019).

Most healthcare organizations are accredited by Accreditation Canada. The accreditation requires that these organizations have clear, written nursing policies and procedures that meet the standards of care and guide a practical nurse's practice. If a charge of negligence is brought against an individual nurse that results in a lawsuit, the practical nurse's actions and practice are compared with the organization's standards of care and the provincial or territorial nursing standards of practice. If an organizational policy violates the jurisdictional standards of practice, then the organizational policy is overridden by law. It is the practical nurse's responsibility to know the jurisdictional law and standards of practice (Potter et al., 2019).

Legal Liability

A tort is "a civil wrong committed against a person or property" (Potter et al., 2019, p. 103); it excludes breach of contract (Duhaime, n.d.). A tort is not a criminal act, but if it is serious enough, a practical nurse may be charged with a criminal offence. Most lawsuits involving practical nurses are for negligence or malpractice, which comes under the "unintentional" classification. The terms *negligence* and *malpractice* are sometimes used interchangeably (Irvine, Osborne, & Shariff, 2013).

Intentional Torts

Intentional torts are deliberate actions that violate another's rights and include assault, battery, invasion of privacy, and false imprisonment (Duhaime, n.d.):

- Assault is a physical or verbal threat that creates apprehension or a fear of being harmed. No contact is necessary. For example, if a practical nurse threatens to start an intravenous (IV) line without a client's consent, then the practical nurse could be sued for assault. Consent would negate the possibility of a lawsuit (Fridman, 2012; Irvine et al., 2013).
- Battery is intentional physical contact with an individual without that person's consent. The contact may not necessarily be harmful but may be offensive (Fridman, 2012; Osborne, 2015; Potter et al., 2019). If the practical nurse started the IV line without consent, the practical nurse could be sued for battery.
- Invasion of privacy protects the client's rights to be free from intrusion into his or her private affairs. For example,

a practical nurse would be liable if the practical nurse released confidential information about a client to an unauthorized individual without the client's consent.

- False imprisonment is intended to protect an individual's freedom and basic rights. For example, a practical nurse may be liable if the practical nurse prevents a client from leaving a healthcare agency voluntarily. Also, a practical nurse who uses restraints (chemical or physical) inappropriately may be considered liable (Potter et al., 2019).

Unintentional Torts

Negligence is a failure to take the care that a reasonable nurse in similar circumstances would have taken (Canadian Nurses Protective Society [CNPS], 2004). Negligence can be considered a liable act if it causes injury, even if there was no intent. Practical nurses are negligent if they do not meet the standards of practice that are set by their regulatory body and cause injury to the client because of a lack of nursing care or prevention of injury (Potter et al., 2019). Usually, the courts consider negligence to be the failure to use that degree of skill or learning ordinarily used under the same or similar circumstances by other nursing professionals (Potter et al., 2019). In order for a practical nurse to be found negligent, the court must have evidence that the practical nurse:

- *Did not meet the duty of care*, a term meaning that the client relies on the practical nurse's professional skills and knowledge and the nurse has a legal duty to take reasonable care.
- *Breached the standard of care*, meaning that the court will determine what constituted reasonable nursing care in the circumstances.
- *Caused foreseeable harm through a breach in the standard of care*, meaning that the client was actually harmed. It must be proven that the practical nurse's negligent act caused the harm (Osborne, 2015).

Practical nurses are accountable for their own actions. An agency may also be found jointly liable with the practical nurse if the agency does not ensure that standards of nursing practice are being met in its facility. Common negligent acts are listed in Box 3.1.

Criminal Prosecution

Practical nurses may be reported to the police if involvement in criminal activity is suspected. The police may investigate, and charges will be laid under the *Criminal Code of Canada* if there is sufficient evidence. Nurses are interviewed by the investigators, and a formal statement will be requested. Any information given by the practical nurse can be used as evidence in the trial proceedings. Therefore, it is important for a practical nurse to consult with a criminal lawyer before giving any statement or answering questions (CNPS, 1999).

Some examples of criminal activities that nurses could be charged with include the following:

- Theft of narcotics
- Theft of client or agency property
- Assisted suicide
- Criminal negligence

> ### BOX 3.1 Common Negligent Acts
>
> - Medication errors that result in injury to patients
> - Intravenous therapy errors that result in infiltrations or phlebitis
> - Burns caused by equipment, bathing, or spills of hot liquids and foods
> - Falls resulting in injury to patients
> - Failure to use aseptic technique as required
> - Errors in sponge, instrument, or needle counts in surgical cases
> - Failure to give a report, or giving an incomplete report, to an incoming shift of healthcare staff
> - Failure to monitor a patient's condition adequately
> - Failure to notify a physician of a significant change in a patient's status
> - Failure to properly delegate or supervise

From Potter, P., Perry, A., Stockert, P., et al. (2019). *Canadian fundamentals of nursing* (6th ed., p. 104, Box 8.1). Milton, ON: Elsevier.

- Battery by threatening or inflicting bodily harm
- Sexual assault

NURSING PROFESSIONAL PRACTICE

Practical Nursing Accountability

Practical nurses are responsible and accountable for their decisions and actions. Accountability is one of the professional practice competencies for practical nurses. Principles of accountability for practical nurses include:

- Practical nurses are responsible and accountable for their decisions and actions.
- Practical nurses engage in self-reflection and continuous learning to maintain and enhance competence.
- Practical nurses are accountable and responsible for assessing their individual fitness to practice.
- Practical nurses demonstrate and apply knowledge of the distinction between ethical responsibilities and legal rights (CCPNR, 2013b).

Ethical Nursing Practice

Ethics is "the moral principles or values that guide people when they decide what is right and what is wrong" (Potter et al., 2019, p. 1419). Nursing regulatory bodies are tasked with establishing and upholding a code of ethics. A code of ethics provides nurses with guidance on ethical standards, decision making, behaviour, and relationships. Most codes of ethics for practical nurses promote the following values:

- Being accountable for one's actions
- Upholding the patient's rights to privacy and confidentiality
- Providing care that maintains the patient's dignity
- Demonstrating respect for the patient at all times
- Promoting integrity by providing safe, competent, and ethical nursing care
- Evaluating one's work and maintaining competency (Potter et al., 2019, p. 1419)

NURSING PROFESSIONAL RELATIONSHIPS AND COMMUNICATION

The Therapeutic Nurse–Client Relationship

The nurse–client relationship is central to nursing. A professional relationship is created through the nurse's application of knowledge, communication theory, understanding of human behaviour, and commitment to ethical behaviour. Helping relationships are at the foundation of clinical nursing practice. The practical nurse is considered the helper and interacts with the client in consideration of the client's unique health needs, human responses, and patterns of living (Potter et al., 2019). The key points in this relationship are as follows:

- The relationship is based on trust, respect, empathy, and professional intimacy and requires the appropriate use of power.
- The purpose of the relationship is to meet the needs of the client.
- Practical nurses establish, maintain, re-establish, and terminate relationships with clients.
- Practical nurses use a client-centred care approach to ensure that all professional behaviours and actions meet the therapeutic needs of the client.
- Practical nurses are responsible for effectively establishing and maintaining the boundaries in the relationship.
- Practical nurses protect the client from harm by ensuring that abuse is prevented or stopped and reported (Potter et al., 2019).

The nurse–client relationship goes through a series of developmental phases. The four phases are pre-interaction, orientation, working, and termination:

1. The *pre-interaction phase* begins before the practical nurse meets the client and may involve accessing information about the client, a diagnosis, or a procedure. It includes identifying a suitable setting and anticipation of the client's needs, issues, or concerns.
2. The *orientation phase* involves the meeting of the practical nurse and the client. This stage begins with a social exchange and expands to include decision making regarding the client's goals, the role of both the client and the practical nurse in facilitating fulfillment of the goals, and the expected length of the relationship.
3. The *working phase* consists of the practical nurse and the client working together to facilitate the accomplishment of the client's goals. It is important for the practical nurse to use therapeutic communication skills to encourage the client to self-explore and take action to meet his or her goals.
4. The *termination phase* is a time to evaluate the achievement of goals and for the practical nurse and the client to separate and make the transition whereby the client or another caregiver assumes responsibility for the care (Potter et al., 2019).

Communication

It is critical that practical nurses develop and use effective communication skills to facilitate optimum relationship building. Communication is an ongoing, dynamic, and multidimensional process that consists of a variety of interactions between a sender and a receiver. The referent (e.g., a message, perception, or sound) motivates a person to share information with another person. The sender encodes a message, the content of the communication, and sends it to a receiver (through a particular channel), who decodes the message. The message may be influenced by many factors, including the environment in which the communication occurs, and interpersonal variables, such as the educational, developmental, or cultural background that each individual brings to the communication. Feedback is the message returned by the receiver. For effective communication, both the sender and the receiver need to be sensitive and open to each other's message. In the nurse–client relationship, the practical nurse needs to take primary responsibility for ensuring that communication is open, purposeful, and therapeutic. Fig. 3.1 illustrates the concepts in active communication.

Practical nurses use a wide range of effective communication strategies and interpersonal skills to guide their interactions with clients and with all members of the interprofessional team. They must have an awareness of cultural factors that influence communication. Practical nurses plan and provide care by recognizing and respecting the diversity of different cultures. Positive interpersonal communication is vital for creating a positive therapeutic environment and includes the following:

- The use of warmth and genuineness as the nurse ensures confidentiality, connects with clients, and demonstrates respect for spiritual, psychological, and physical aspects of care

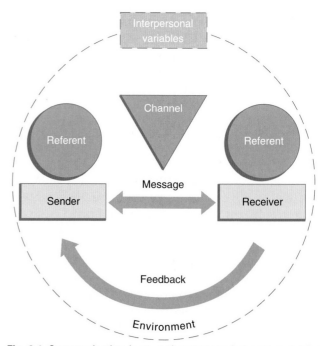

Fig. 3.1 Communication is an active process between a sender and a receiver. (From Potter, P., Perry, A., Stockert, P., et al. [2019]. *Canadian fundamentals of nursing* [6th ed., p. 245, Figure 17-1]. Milton, ON: Elsevier.)

- Being respectful of clients and other members of the inter-professional team
- Being empathetic to the client experience
- Using self-disclosure appropriately

Communication involves the use of verbal and non-verbal means. Verbal communication includes the spoken word, and non-verbal communication includes factors such as tone, rate, and volume of the voice, as well as facial expression, mannerisms, and appearance. When delivering or receiving communication, it is important to consider both the verbal and non-verbal aspects of the message.

A key factor associated with communication is the use of effective listening skills. Listening is an active process that involves paying attention to both verbal and the non-verbal cues and is required by the practical nurse when interacting with clients, other nurses, and members of the interprofessional team.

Conflict Resolution

The healthcare team is composed of many different people. Each team member has a different background and brings his or her own professional knowledge, expertise, values, beliefs, and goals into the workplace. Sometimes, differences between people can lead to conflict and disagreements.

Conflict occurs at four levels:
- Intrapersonal conflict that occurs within the individual
- Interpersonal conflict that occurs between two or more individuals
- Intragroup conflict that occurs within a group
- Intergroup conflict that occurs between two or more groups, departments, or organizations

Many factors contribute to conflict, such as unclear roles and responsibilities, limited resources, unresolved prior conflicts, and ineffective communication. It is important to resolve conflicts when they occur.

Effective conflict resolution begins with an acknowledgement that there is a conflict and that it needs to be positively addressed. Collaboration is the best approach to conflict resolution. It satisfies the interests of most parties because it requires that they work together to find a common solution. Collaboration involves the use of active listening and defining a clear agreement to resolve the conflict.

Practice Standard Documentation

Accurate documentation by practical nurses is an important standard of care from a legal as well as an ethical perspective. Practical nurses document important details of client care on the client health record. Accurate and detailed documentation improves client outcomes because the healthcare team can better plan care, improve assessment, and evaluate the effectiveness of care interventions. Verbal documentation such as verbal physician's orders should be avoided except in specific—usually emergency—situations because of the increased risk of error or misinterpretation. People who have the authority to write orders, including physicians and NPs, need to sign any verbal order they made as soon as possible after the event. Individual healthcare facilities have telephone communication policies in place to facilitate this process. Practical nurses should refer to agency policy for issues relating to late entries, correcting errors, or completing an omission. Late entries are often documented by writing the current date and time in the next available space and writing "late entry for [date and shift]" (Potter et al., 2019).

Documentation is important in all other aspects of nursing practice as well. Documentation formats have changed; electronic records and fax transmissions are replacing paper records. Electronic and fax records must also be kept confidential. Confidentiality of health records is integral to documentation, accountability, and nurses' ethical standards.

From a legal and ethical perspective, practical nurses must keep all client information confidential and can only release the information with the written consent of the client or authorized designate, such as a guardian or someone who has power of attorney/power of care. Clients or other authorized designates and other members of the specific client's healthcare team can access and read the client health record. Individual healthcare facilities all have a system in place and specific policies to ensure that client confidentiality is maintained. The College of Nurses of Ontario (CNO) practice standards regarding documentation stress the importance of maintaining confidentiality of client health information, including passwords or information required to access the client health record. Nurses are not allowed to share their password to access the electronic health record (EHR) with anyone else and must log off the EHR when not using it.

Practical nurses must understand and adhere to policies, standards, and legislation related to confidentiality when using the EHR. Only access information for which you have a professional need to provide care (CNO, 2017). "Maintaining the confidentiality of medical records is an essential responsibility of all members of the healthcare team" (Potter et al., 2019, p. 238). It is important to safeguard any information regarding personal health information as well. Do not leave such information around for unauthorized people to view. You must destroy anything that is printed when the print information is no longer required. Most agencies have shredders or locked receptacles for shredding or later incineration (Potter et al., 2019).

Some institutions have a prescribed order entry. The prescriber enters an order directly into the computer, which avoids need for the transcription of orders. Computer interfaces transfer the order to the medication administration record (MAR), the pharmacy record, and the automated dispensing system (Potter et al., 2019). Practical nurses are accountable to determine whether the medication ordered is the correct medication. Administering medications requires knowledge and skill to prevent medication errors.

Accreditation Canada has developed key criteria for providing good documentation. Documentation should include information that is factual, accurate, complete, and current and complies with the standards of Accreditation Canada (Potter et al., 2019), as outlined below:

- Documentation should include factual records that contain descriptive and objective information.
- It should be accurate, with exact measurements, the agency's approved abbreviations, correct spelling, date and time, and the recorder's name and role, such as "Cheryl Sams, LPN [or RPN]," which confirms that the nursing care has been delivered.
- Current records need to be recorded with timed entries on a regular basis and always as soon as possible in the following instances:
  - When vital signs are monitored
  - Preparation for tests or surgeries
  - Change in client status and who was notified of the change
  - Admission, transfer, discharge, or death of a client
  - Treatment for a sudden change in status
- It should be organized, with the information presented in a logical order.
- It must comply with standards set by the Accreditation Canada as well as jurisdictional legislation and regulatory bodies.

Each healthcare facility also has its own policies that need to be followed to ensure consistency and complete information recording. Some examples include the following:

- Subjective-objective-assessment-plan (SOAP)
- Problem-intervention-evaluation (PIE), which can be added to the SOAP format
- Narrative notes that describe the nursing care delivered and the client's response
- Focus charting, which includes *d*ata (subjective and objective), *a*ction, or nursing interventions, and *r*esponse from the client (DAR)
- Charting by exception (CBE) systems, in which the practical nurse only records abnormal findings and trends in clinical care (Potter et al., 2019)

Table 3.1 describes the legal guidelines for information recording.

The change-of-shift report is very important in settings where one nurse takes over care responsibilities from another nurse. The communication about the client's condition is only a small part of the report. The change-of-shift report needs to be concise but comprehensive so that the nurse starting the new shift will be able to provide a level of continuity of care. However, the change-of-shift report is not a part of the legal permanent client health record. Table 3.2 provides a comparison of do's and don'ts of the change-of-shift report. SBAR (*S*ituation, *B*ackground, *A*ssessment, and *R*ecommendation) is one example of a communication tool that enables information to be transferred accurately between nurses. It uses a simple, structured framework that allows nurses to produce hand-off reports that are standardized and clear. Effective communication is a vital factor in the delivery of safe, quality client care. It also helps provide continuity of care among nurses (Potter et al., 2019). Box. 3.2 describes the Identification, Situation, Background, Assessment, Recommendation, Repeat back (I-SBAR-R) technique, a reformulation of SBAR, that is used in many different reporting situations.

BOX 3.2   The Identification, Situation, Background, Assessment, Recommendation, Repeat Back (I-SBAR-R) Technique

When calling the physician, follow the I-SBAR-R process as follows:

Identification: Who is calling and who are you calling about?
- Identify yourself and your role
- Identify the unit, the patient, and the room number

Situation: What is the situation you are calling about?
- Briefly state the problem: What it is, when it started, and the severity

Background: Provide background information as necessary related to the situation, including the following:
- The admitting diagnosis, date of admission, and pertinent medical history
- List of current medications, allergies, intravenous fluids, and laboratory tests
- Laboratory results (date and time each test was performed and results of previous tests for comparison)
- Other clinical information
- Code status

Assessment: What is your assessment of the situation? Examples include the following:
- Most recent vital signs
- Changes in vital signs or assessment from previous assessments

Recommendation: What is your recommendation, or what do you think needs to be done? Examples include the following:
- Patient to be admitted or transferred
- New medication or further tests
- Patient to be seen now
- Orders to be changed

Repeat back:
- Repeat back orders that have been given
- Clarify any questions

From Potter, A., Perry, A., Stockert, P., et al. (2019). *Canadian fundamentals of nursing* (6th ed., p. 248, Table 15-9). Milton, ON: Elsevier. Adapted from Joint Commission on Accreditation of Healthcare Organizations. (2005, February). The SBAR technique: Improves communication, enhances patient safety. *Joint Commission Perspectives on Patient Safety, 5*(2), 2; Enlow, M., Shanks, L., Guhde, J., et al. (2010). Incorporating interprofessional communication skills (ISBARR) into an undergraduate nursing curriculum. *Nurse Educator, 35*(4), 176–180; and Grbach, W., Struth, D., & Vincent, I. (2008). *Reformulating SBAR to "I-SBAR-R."* Chapel Hill, NC: Quality and Safety Education for Nurses. Retrieved from http://qsen.org/reformulating-sbar-to-i-sbar-r/.

CONSENT

Ethical Implications

Consent to treatment is a very important aspect of ethical care. It is critical that clients are fully informed and fully understand the implications of the treatment before authorizing the care, whether via signed consent or verbal consent. Practical nurses assist and support client participation in making decisions about their health and well-being when

TABLE 3.1   Legal Guidelines for Documentation

Guidelines for Electronic and Written Documentation	Rationale	Correct Action
Do not document retaliatory or critical comments about a patient or care provided by another healthcare provider. Do not enter personal opinions.	Statements can be used as evidence for nonprofessional behaviour or poor quality of care.	Enter only objective and factual descriptions of a patient's behaviour or the actions of another healthcare provider. Quote all patient statements.
Correct all errors promptly.	Errors in recording can lead to errors in treatment or may imply an attempt to mislead or hide evidence.	Avoid rushing to complete documentation; be sure that information is accurate and complete.
Record all facts.	Record must be accurate, factual, and objective.	Be certain entry is factual and thorough. A person reading your documentation needs to be able to determine that a patient received adequate care.
Document as close as prudently possible to the time of the event.	Most accurate method of recalling details. Details can be lost and discrepancies can arise the longer the wait to the documentation of the event.	Document as soon after the event as possible to ensure accuracy.
If an order is questioned, record that clarification was sought.	If you perform an order known to be incorrect, you are just as liable for prosecution as the prescriber is.	Do not record "physician made error"; instead, chart that "Dr. Wong was called to clarify order for analgesic." Include the date and time of phone call, whom you spoke with, and the outcome.
Document only for yourself.	You are accountable for information you enter into a patient's record.	Never enter documentation for someone else. Check agency policy for circumstances when a third party may document for another nurse (e.g., designated recorder for emergency situations).
Avoid using generalized, empty phrases such as "status unchanged" or "had good day."	This type of documentation is subjective and does not reflect patient assessment.	Use complete, concise descriptions of assessments and care so that documentation is objective and factual.
Begin each entry with the date and time and end with your signature and credentials.	Ensures that the correct sequence of events is recorded; signature documents who is accountable for care delivered.	Do not wait until end of shift to record important changes that occurred several hours earlier; sign each entry according to agency policy (e.g., Mei Lin, LPN).
Avoid "precharting" (documenting an entry before performing a treatment or an assessment or before giving a medication).	Invites error and thus endangers the health and safety of the patient; it is also illegal and can constitute falsification of healthcare records.	Document during or immediately after giving care or after administering a medication.
Protect the security of your password for computer documentation.	Maintains security and confidentiality.	Once logged into a computer, do not leave computer screen unattended. Log out when you leave the computer. Make sure the computer screen is not accessible for public viewing.

Guidelines Specific to Written Documentation	Rationale	Correct Action
Do not erase, apply correction fluid to, or scratch out errors made while recording.	Charting becomes illegible: It may appear as if you were attempting to hide information or deface record.	Draw a single line through error; write "error" above it, and sign your name or initials and date it. Then record note correctly.
Do not leave blank spaces or lines in a written nurse's progress notes.	Allows another person to add incorrect information in open space.	Chart consecutively, line by line; if space is left, draw a line horizontally through it and place your signature and credentials at the end.
Record all entries legibly and in black ink. Do not use felt-tip pens or erasable ink.	Illegible entries can be misinterpreted, thereby causing errors and lawsuits; ink from felt-tip pens can smudge or run when wet and may destroy documentation; erasures are not permitted in clinical documentation; black ink is more legible when records are photocopied or scanned.	Never use pencil to document in a written clinical record. Never erase entries or use correction fluid. To indicate an error in written documentation, place a single line through the inaccurate information and write your signature with credentials at the end of the text that has been crossed out.

From Potter, A., Perry, A., Stockert, P., et al. (2019). *Canadian fundamentals of nursing* (6th ed., p. 235, Table 15.1). Milton, ON: Elsevier.

TABLE 3.2 Do's and Don'ts for Change-of-Shift Reports

Do's	Don'ts
Do provide only essential background information about patient (i.e., name, sex, age, physician's diagnosis, and medical history).	Don't review all routine care procedures or tasks (e.g., bathing, scheduled changes).
Do identify patient's nursing diagnoses or healthcare problems and their related causes.	Don't review all biographical information already available in written form.
Do describe objective measurements or observations about patient's condition and response to health problem, and emphasize recent changes.	Don't use critical comments about patient's behaviour, such as "Mrs. Wills is so demanding."
Do share significant information about family members as it relates to patient's problems.	Don't make assumptions about relationships between family members.
Do continuously review ongoing discharge plan (e.g., need for resources, patient's level of preparation to go home).	Don't wait until near discharge to discuss the plan.
Do relay to staff significant changes in the way therapies are given (e.g., different position for pain relief, new medication).	Don't describe basic steps of a procedure.
Do describe instructions given in teaching plan and patient's response.	Don't explain detailed content unless staff members ask for clarification.
Do evaluate results of nursing or medical care measures (e.g., effect of back rub or analgesic administration), and describe results specifically.	Don't simply describe results as "good" or "poor."
Do be clear about priorities to which incoming staff must attend.	Don't force incoming staff to guess what to do first.

From Potter, P., Perry, A., Stockert, P., et al. (2019). *Canadian fundamentals of nursing* (6th ed., p. 247, Table 15.4). Milton, ON: Elsevier.

factors reduce their capacity for making decisions, in accordance with applicable legislation and regulation (CCPNR, 2013a, 2013b).

CCPNR provides guidance to practical nurses on the ethical responsibilities affecting informed consent. According to the CCPNR code of ethics, LPNs:

2.1 Respect the right and responsibility of clients to be informed and make decisions about their health care.
2.1.1 Respect and support client choices.
2.1.2 Assist and support client participation in making decisions about their health and well-being when factors reduce their capacity for making decisions, in accordance with applicable legislation and regulation.
2.1.3 Respect and adhere to the jurisdictional legislation on capacity assessment and substitute decision-making when the client is incapable of consent.
2.1.4 Consider with other healthcare professionals and substitute decision-makers the best interests of the client and any previously known wishes or advanced directives that apply in situations where the client is incapable of consent.
2.6 Provide care to each client recognizing their individuality and their right to choice. (CCPNR, 2013a, p. 5)

Legal Implications

There are also legal implications in relation to informed consent. Clients must fully understand the implications of the consent and receive full disclosure on all the risks, benefits, alternatives, and consequences of refusal of treatment or care (Black, 2009). The legal obligation falls to the physician or healthcare provider to disclose the information in such a way that the client can understand all the information that is being delivered. The consent form must specify the details of the procedure, including the name of the person who is performing the procedure. The person who will perform the

procedure should obtain consent from the client. It is essential to remember that except in emergency situations, failure to obtain consent for treatment (whether written or verbal) could result in a lawsuit with charges of battery.

Practical nurses cannot obtain informed consent for surgery because they do not perform surgery. The same is true for other procedures that require consent that will not be performed by the practical nurse. It is the physician's responsibility to obtain consent for the procedure if he or she will be performing the procedure. Practical nurses may sign as witnesses to the client's written consent, proving that the client appears to be mentally competent and confirming the identity of the signature and that the client signed voluntarily, although some agency policies may not support this practice. The practical nurse should ask the client if he or she understands the procedure before the consent is witnessed. If there is a suspicion that the client does not understand, the physician needs to inform the client further. If a client refuses to provide consent, the practical nurse needs to explore and determine the reason for refusal and discuss it with the healthcare team.

Currently, practical nurses rarely require written consent from a client to perform a particular procedure. However, they must obtain verbal consent before starting the procedure. Doing so ensures that the client understands the care goals and reduces the risk that a battery lawsuit could occur against the practical nurse (Keatings & Smith, 2010). Consent can be verbal, written, or implicit. For example, if a client lifts up a leg for the practical nurse to provide wound care, then it is implicit that the client is giving consent.

If the client is unable to understand the nature of the consent, then a substitute decision maker with the appropriate authority will need to provide consent for care, which may involve signing a consent form. The substitute decision maker may receive the authority by proxy or power of attorney/power of care or may be appointed through court guardianship. Clients with mental health issues or older adults may still have the ability to provide informed consent and to refuse treatment unless the court has ruled that they are legally incompetent to make personal healthcare decisions (Keatings & Smith, 2010).

RESTRAINTS

Restraints are physical, chemical, or a restricted environment. There has been much controversy over the past few years concerning the risks and benefits of restraints. The ethical question of consent for restraints has also arisen, as well as the possible liability issues of lack of consent. The ideal situation is not to use restraints, but it may be necessary for clients, particularly those with mental illness, who are at risk of harming themselves or others. Statistics clearly indicate that personal injuries are higher when a client is restrained (Potter et al., 2019).

Clients have been asphyxiated by physical restraints. Other complications from the use of restraints include pressure ulcers, constipation, pneumonia, urinary and fecal incontinence, and urinary retention. There is also the issue of the anxiety and fear experienced by clients under restraint, as well as the impact on the client's self-esteem (Potter et al., 2019). A policy of least restraint is the usual agency approach, which ensures that all care alternatives have been attempted prior to restraint. It is important for practical nurses to know the restraint policies of their agencies and the legal implications of these.

If restraints are used, practical nurses need to check the restraints and the client's condition frequently to make sure that the client's circulation is not impaired and that no other injuries or potential risks are present. It is always recommended that practical nurses try alternative methods of intervention to address difficult behaviour, such as frequent toileting to reduce agitation or utilizing a "sitter."

PALLIATIVE CARE APPROACH AND RESUSCITATION GUIDELINES

Advance Directives and the Palliative Care Approach

One of the most important roles that practical nurses have is to work with and support clients and families as they make difficult end-of-life decisions. This is a complex issue that presents many legal and ethical dilemmas as well as nursing practice implications. A joint position statement by the Canadian Nurses Association (CNA), Canadian Hospice Palliative Care Association (CHPCA), and Canadian Hospice Palliative Care Nurses Group (CHPC-NG) (CNA, CHPCA, & CHPC-NG, 2015) provides guidance on the role of the nurse in palliative care. The joint position statement defines the nursing responsibilities that ensure that client autonomy is promoted and that the individual who is considering the palliative approach to care is fully informed and has the right to be an active participant in his or her own care. This client (or the substitute decision maker) should express his or her healthcare needs and personal values of health before making end-of-life directives. The joint position statement states that the palliative care approach objective is "to help people live well until death, across the lifespan, in all practice settings" (CNA, CHPCA, & CHPC-NG, 2015, p. 1). It also states that nurses "advocate for high-quality palliative and end-of-life care that is accessible to all Canadians and is provided in a setting of choice that best suits their care needs" (CNA, CHPCA, & CHPC-NG, 2015, p. 1). The palliative care approach promotes person-centred care in which illness, caregiving needs, and dying are in accordance with the client's and supporting family's desires and wishes. Respecting the client's goals for health care is paramount to ensuring high-quality palliative care.

Self-determinism is particularly important in end-of-life planning and advance directives (CNPS, 2006). Clients do have the right to refuse life-sustaining measures. Advance care planning can help guide end-of-life care to ensure clients' wishes are honoured. Planning requires ongoing, open communication and documentation among the client, family, and healthcare providers. It can be initiated at any time along the client's health continuum (CNA, CHPCA, & CHPC-NG, 2015).

In Canada, "advance directives ... are legal documents in which a person states specific wishes about future health care, treatment, and personal care. An advance directive is used when a person can no longer make decisions or express personal wishes. Every province and territory has legislation about advance directive" (Sorrentino et al., 2018, p. 1069).

Two types of advance directives are available to Canadians. An instructional advance directive (also called a *living will*) provides direction on the levels of health intervention a client wishes to receive if he or she were to become incapacitated and unable to make healthcare decisions. It typically includes client directives on whether the client wants to have cardiopulmonary resuscitation (CPR) administered, to be admitted to a Critical Care Unit, to be transferred to another agency, to receive tube feeding, or to receive blood transfusions (CNA, 2017a; CNA, CHPCA, & CHPC-NG, 2015). The second type of advance directive is a power of attorney, which names a capable person with legal authority (substitute decision maker) to make healthcare treatment decisions for an individual in the event that the individual becomes incapacitated.

Clients can revise their advance directives at any time (CNA, CHPCA, & CHPC-NG, 2015). Advance directives are still evolving in terms of their legal status, and there are some differences across the provinces and territories. Provincial and territorial legislation is not uniform across Canada, so each jurisdiction has its own guidelines related to substitute decision-making and instructional directives for treatment and care. Practical nurses need to know the legalities and regulations associated with advance directives as well as the nursing role responsibilities for their individual jurisdictions.

Medical Assistance in Dying (MAID)

Nurses continue to play an important role in providing person-centred end-of-life care in palliative care, natural death, and medical assistance in dying (MAID) (CNA, 2017b, p. 3). Nurses provide much of the care for clients who are at the end of their life. The CNA has defined palliative care as providing active, compassionate, and supportive care of the dying (CNA, CHPCA, & CHPC-NG, 2015).

The CNA (2017b) developed a framework to help nurses understand changes in the federal law that now allows MAID in Canada under certain circumstances and within defined regulatory standards. Bill C-14 came into effect on June 17, 2016, and amended the *Criminal Code* in relation to MAID. Under Bill C-14, an individual who meets all the eligibility requirements may receive MAID. See Box 3.3 for eligibility criteria for MAID. "The law developed safeguards for the clients and offers protection to healthcare providers who provide medical assistance in dying, along with people who assist in the process in accordance to the law" (CNA, 2017b, p. 7). Section 241.1 of the act defines MAID as follows:

> (a) the administering by a medical practitioner or nurse practitioner of a substance to a person, at their request, that causes their death; or
>
> (b) the prescribing or providing by a medical practitioner or nurse practitioner of a substance to a person, at their request, so that they may self-administer the substance and in doing so cause their own death (CNA, 2017b, p. 7)

The CNA framework outlines resources for all nurses involved in end-of-life care decision making and care around MAID (CNA, 2017b, p. 4). It is important for practical nurses to refer to the associated policies and guidelines in their jurisdiction and consult with their regulatory body and employer for specific instructions. Policies must be consistent with the law. Before assisting with MAID, the practical nurse should confirm that the legal conditions for MAID have been established.

Practical nurses can provide nursing care and skills such as the insertion of an IV line that will deliver the medication that will cause death of the client. Practical nurses require a doctor's order for the IV insertion. An NP or a physician is the only person who can administer any required medications for MAID. They cannot delegate any of their roles to the practical nurse.

Practical nurses can assist in the education of clients regarding MAID. When providing information to a client or family on MAID, the practical nurse must ensure that he or she does not advise or persuade the client in any way to choose MAID. The decision to take medication to end the client's life must be the client's own decision, with no encouragement or counselling from the nurse.

The practical nurse has the right to conscientiously object to participate in MAID and transfer the care to another nurse who is agreeable to providing care for the client. A conscientious objector is to provide holistic nursing care to the client that is not connected to MAID until a replacement nurse is found. At no time is the nurse to discuss their own personal beliefs or feelings regarding MAID to the client.

Determining the eligibility of a client for MAID is not the responsibility of a practical nurse. This falls under the scope of practice of the NP or physician along with obtaining informed consent. However, practical nurses do provide bereavement care to the family of the person receiving MAID (CNA, 2017b, pp. 9–18).

Caring for the palliative population requires palliative education to provide high-quality palliative care and adequate pain control. Practical nurses help decrease suffering and support a dignified and peaceful death. They make an important contribution to the healthcare team in the provision of palliative and end-of-life care. As well, they encompass the ethical principles of the CCPNR code of ethics so that they understand their role and responsibility when providing safe, competent, and ethical end-of-life care to clients undergoing MAID.

Cardiopulmonary Resuscitation

CPR is the standard treatment for respiratory or cardiac arrest in many healthcare facilities. CPR is commonly performed as it has the potential to revive clients. Because CPR is considered a treatment, client consent may be required before initiating the resuscitation, although emergency situations are unique (CNPS, 2006).

When a capable client does not want to have CPR performed, the refusal must be documented in the client health record. This refusal is often documented by the physician. Some provincial or territorial legislation allows practical nurses to accept the refusal for CPR and document the refusal in the client's health record as Do Not Resuscitate (DNR). If the client is legally capable of making decisions, then the family cannot overrule the client's treatment or care wishes.

BOX 3.3 Who Is Eligible for Medical Assistance in Dying?

In order to be eligible for medical assistance in dying, a person must meet **all** of the following criteria:

- The person must be eligible for health services funded by the federal government, or a province or territory.
  - Generally, visitors to Canada are not eligible for medical assistance in dying.
- The person must be at least 18 years old and mentally competent. This means being capable of making healthcare decisions for his or herself.
- The person has a grievous and irremediable medical condition.
- The person has made a voluntary request for medical assistance in dying that is not the result of outside pressure or influence.
- The person has given informed consent to receive medical assistance in dying.

Adapted from Government of Canada. (2018). Medical assistance in dying. Retrieved from https://www.canada.ca/en/health-canada/services/medical-assistance-dying.html#a2

Healthcare facilities should have DNR policies in place that guide the healthcare team in the decision-making process surrounding the DNR issue.

Physicians often write "Do Not Resuscitate," "DNR," or "No Code" orders for a client who is not expected to recover. Such an order means that the client will not be resuscitated and is allowed to die in peace and with dignity. The orders are written after consulting with the client and family. The family, or proxy, in consultation with the physician, makes the decision about the DNR order if the client is not mentally able. Some people prepare an advance directive that contains DNR order. (Sorrentino et al., 2018, pp. 1069–1070)

Jurisdictions and agencies have different sets of resuscitation protocols from legal and regulatory bodies. DNR orders are necessary in some jurisdictions, and in others, CPR requires consent. It is essential that practical nurses know the protocols in their jurisdictions.

It is the responsibility of the healthcare team to discuss the potential care requirements with the client and his or her family, including providing CPR, and together to devise a comprehensive plan of treatment. This plan needs to be documented in the client health record. Healthcare providers do not have to provide CPR if it will not benefit the client. CPR may, in fact, be harmful in some situations by increasing pain and suffering and prolonging the dying process. The plan of care must include the client's current condition and the expectation for the future condition. The plan must be based on current best practices and treatment goals. The client must consent to the treatment plan. If the client requests CPR and the healthcare team does not think that CPR will benefit the client, then the healthcare team must discuss this decision with the client and his or her family. Variations of the DNR can allow for partial resuscitation in accordance with the client's request. The DNR can be suspended at any time and then reinstated when the client would like it reordered (CNPS, 2006).

The regulatory body of the practical nurse's jurisdiction determines the standards of care for resuscitation. For example, the CNO practice standard of resuscitation is based on ethical values of nursing, including the following (CNO, 2009):

- Respect for the client's well-being
- Client choice
- Privacy and confidentiality
- Respect for life
- Maintaining commitments
- Truthfulness and fairness

Practical nurses play an important role in making certain that the client's wishes are identified and communicated clearly to the healthcare team. In addition, practical nurses must encourage the client to be the decision maker in the treatment plan, document communication about end-of-life and resuscitation concerns in the health record, review the resuscitation wishes, advocate on behalf of the client, and implement the client's wishes (CNA, CHPCA, & CHPC-NG, 2015, p. 5). It is critical that practical nurses

discuss the presence of advance directives and meet the legislation requirements of their jurisdiction. It is important that practical nurses follow the capable client's wishes whether or not there is a written order on the client's health record.

Practical nurses are expected to be competent in providing CPR if required for their role. Some healthcare facilities require a formal credential such as Health Care Provider and Automated External Defibrillator (AED) certification.

MEDICATION ADMINISTRATION

Medication administration is an important role for practical nurses. Medication is used for a variety of purposes, including diagnosis, treatment, cure, relief, or prevention of health problems. Practical nurses give medications in many practice settings with many nursing responsibilities. Practical nurses are responsible for delivering medication accurately and safely to the client, teaching the client about the medication, and evaluating the effect of the medication on the client (Potter et al., 2019).

Implications for Administering Medications

The scope of practice of practical nurses is determined by legislative acts at the federal and provincial/territorial levels. Practical nurses must know their own jurisdictional laws that affect drug administration. In addition, practical nurses must be aware of their own practice agencies' drug policies before they administer medications. They must have the knowledge, skill, and judgement before they give drugs. This knowledge is particularly necessary in the case of controlled substances that are regulated by law. Violations of the *Narcotic Control Act* may lead to a loss of nursing licence or registration, fines, or imprisonment (Potter et al., 2019).

Medication Actions

There are many variables in how medications act and their types of actions. There are factors other than the characteristics of the drug that affect the medication actions. For example, individuals react very differently to drugs and may not react the same way to successive doses. It is very important for practical nurses to understand all the effects of the medications on individuals so that drug impact can be evaluated. Types of medication effects are listed below:

- Therapeutic effect is the expected or predicted physiological response from the medication and is the desired outcome.
- Side effects are unintended, secondary effects that a medication predictably will cause. The side effects can be harmless or can harm the individual.
- Toxic effects can develop after taking a drug for a long time or when the level of a medication increases in the blood because of impaired metabolism and drug clearance. Toxic effects can be lethal depending on the drug action.
- Adverse effects are generally severe, negative responses to medication that were unexpected and not seen during drug testing. These effects should be reported to the Health

Products and Food Branch of the federal government. Reporting is voluntary.

- Idiosyncratic reactions are unpredictable and occur when an individual overreacts to a medication or has a different reaction from the norm.
- Allergic reactions are unpredictable responses to a medication after repeated doses. The drug is perceived by the body as an allergen, causing a release of antibodies. The reaction can be mild or severe and cause an anaphylactic reaction leading to airway obstruction from swelling of the larynx and pharynx, severe wheezing, and shortness of breath. Urticaria, angioedema, and the delayed action of a rash and fever are other possible symptoms. Allergic reactions can be life-threatening, particularly when the individual becomes hypotensive from vasodilation.
- Medication interactions can occur when one medication potentiates (increases) or decreases the action of another. This commonly occurs when several medications are taken. Two drugs can have a synergistic effect, and the drugs together cause more of a drug effect than if they had been given separately (Potter et al., 2019).

Medication Dose Responses

After a medication is taken, it breaks down in the body and is absorbed, distributed, metabolized, and excreted. The individual's metabolism, weight, gender, and body size affect the drug response. Many drugs take some time to be absorbed, with the exception of IV medications, which are absorbed directly into the bloodstream. It is important that the drug is kept at a constant level in the blood—one within the therapeutic range between the peak high (the highest serum concentration) and a trough low. The therapeutic level prevents toxicity and resultant damage to the body. In order to keep the medication at a therapeutic level, the practical nurse needs to administer the drug at regular times throughout the day. With IV infusions, the peak concentration occurs quickly, but the serum level also begins to fall immediately. It is important for the practical nurse to teach the client to take the drugs on the prescribed schedule to maximize their effect. Refer to Fig. 3.2 to see a picture of the different forms of oral medication.

Nursing Roles in Medication Administration

Practical nurses must have the knowledge necessary to administer and evaluate medications effectively. This knowledge comes from the life sciences and includes an understanding of pharmacokinetics (the study of drug concentrations), human growth and development, human anatomy, nutrition, and mathematics. In addition to the knowledge, practical nurses and employers need to assess practical nurses' ability to carry out their roles relating to medications competently and safely in each situation. Practical nurses need the knowledge, skill, and judgement to independently meet the medication standard of practice. Practical nurses must also hold the competencies and resources to provide interventions during an adverse drug event. The practical nurse needs a working knowledge of the medication action.

Fig. 3.2 Forms of oral medications. *Top row:* Uniquely shaped tablet, capsule, scored tablet. *Bottom row:* Gelatin-coated liquid, extended-release capsule, enteric-coated tablet. (From Potter, P., Perry, A., Stockert, P., et al. [2019]. *Canadian fundamentals of nursing* [6th ed., p. 728, Figure 34-1]. Milton, ON: Elsevier.)

A critical role for nursing in medication administration is client teaching. The practical nurse needs to assess the client's ability to safely administer his or her own medication. The situations can be complex, and the practical nurse needs to be able to assess for client attitude, knowledge, physical and mental status, and responses.

In order to accurately and safely administer medications, practical nurses must learn to use the "10 rights" to ensure accuracy. These rights are as follows:

- Right medication
- Right dose
- Right client (see Fig. 3.3)
- Right route
- Right time and frequency
- Right documentation
- Right reason
- Right to refuse
- Right client education
- Right evaluation

A practical nurse meets the medication standard of practice by doing the following:

- Verifying that the prescription is complete and accurate or following up with the prescriber to get a complete prescription
- Assessing the appropriateness of the drug as prescribed for the client in the particular situation
- Not implementing or giving a medication order that is incomplete, illegible, or misinterpreted, and following up with the prescriber
- Considering the medication when scheduling dosing times, if not specified
- Knowing the trade and generic medication names
- Knowing the accepted abbreviations for their agency
- Processing the prescription as written or computerized physician order entry and not substituting generic or therapeutic interchanges

Fig. 3.3 Before administering any medication, the nurse checks the bar code on the client's bracelet and on the medication packet. (From Williams, P. [2018]. *deWit's Fundamental concepts and skills for nursing* [5th ed., p. 640, Figure 33.4]. St. Louis: Elsevier.)

- Making any necessary changes to the medication administration record (MAR or eMAR) to record the medication name
- Requesting written orders or computerized physician order entries when the prescriber is present and avoiding the use of verbal orders except in emergencies
- Repeating verbal or telephone orders in their entirety for accuracy and documenting them in the health record
- Assessing if the medication is ordered appropriately for that particular situation
- Retaining faxed and printed e-mail orders and refusing unsecured e-mail orders
- Consulting with colleagues and presenting a clear, evidence-informed rationale explaining their concerns is a must if nurses disagree with a medication order. The nurses then present their concerns to the prescriber, discuss the situation with their immediate nursing authority if the concern is unresolved, and contact the prescriber for more discussion. If the concern is still unresolved, then they must contact a higher nursing authority and inform the prescriber. Next, nurses document their concerns in the health record and fill out an unusual occurrence form or incident report.

Routes of Medication Administration

The route of the medication is prescribed according to the medication properties and desired effect on the client's condition. The practical nurse collaborates with the prescriber to decide on the best route. The medication administration routes are as follows:

- Oral medications are given by mouth. This is the most common and easiest route and has the slowest and most prolonged effect.
- Sublingual medications are placed under the tongue and absorbed. This medication should not be swallowed.
- Buccal route medications are placed against the mucous membrane of the cheek until the solid medication dissolves. They should not be swallowed or chewed.

- Parenteral medications are injected into body tissues. The four main sites are intradermal, subcutaneous (only for volumes of 0.5–1 mL), intramuscular (for volumes of up to 3 mL), and IV. Other sites for injections into body cavities include epidural, intrathecal, intraosseous, intraperitoneal, intrapleural, and intra-arterial. Additional education would be needed to administer medications at these extra sites and may be beyond the scope of practice of the practical nurse.
- Topical medications are applied by spreading them on the skin, applying moist dressings, soaking body parts in a solution, flushing the affected part, or giving medicated baths. The effects can be systemic if the client's skin is thin or broken down, if the concentration is too high, or if contact with the skin is prolonged. Transdermal discs or patches can also be used. Instilling drops or ointment to the mucous membranes can also be done.
- The inhalation route can be used to administer medications through nasal passages, orally, by endotracheal tube, or via a tracheostomy.
- Using the intraocular route involves inserting a medication directly into the client's eye.
- Ear installation involves placing a solution into the ear canal for product dissolving and absorption.
- Intravaginal or intra-anal medications (suppositories) are inserted into the anal or vaginal cavities and melt when they reach body temperature, releasing the medication for absorption (Potter et al., 2019).

NURSING ISSUES AND TRENDS

The Nursing Process

A practical nurse uses the nursing process to guide, plan, organize, provide, and evaluate nursing care. A practical nurse must use the nursing process in combination with an ability to think critically and the ability to synthesize relevant knowledge, clinical experiences, and standards of practice. Fig. 3.4 outlines critical thinking and the nursing assessment process.

Assessment

Assessment is a collection of personal, socio-cultural, physiological, and psychological health status data, as well as general information. It is a determination of current health status from the physical assessment.

Analysis

Analysis is a classification of data: screening, organizing, and grouping significant, related information. It is also a definition of a client's problem: determining an appropriate nursing diagnosis that is a definitive statement of the client's actual or potential difficulties, concerns, or deficits that can be altered through nursing interventions.

Planning

Planning involves the client, family or significant others, and practical nurse, who collaborates with the appropriate health team members to formulate the plan. Planning also

KNOWLEDGE
Underlying disease process
Normal growth and development
Normal physiology and psychology
Normal assessment findings
Health promotion
Assessment skills
Communication skills

EXPERIENCE
Previous client care experience
Validation of assessment findings
Observation of assessment
techniques

NURSING PROCESS

Assessment

Evaluation

Diagnosis

Implementation

Planning

STANDARDS
CNA
Specialty standards of practice
Intellectual standards of
measurement

QUALITIES
Perseverance
Fairness
Integrity
Confidence
Creativity

Fig. 3.4 Critical thinking and the assessment process. *CNA,* Canadian Nurses Association. (From Potter, P., Perry, A., Stockert, P., et al. [2019]. *Canadian fundamentals of nursing* [6th ed., p. 189, Figure 13-2]. Milton, ON: Elsevier.)

establishes client outcomes. Outcomes are expected changes in the client's behaviour, activity, or physical state. Outcomes must be objective, realistic, and measurable and include a realistic period for accomplishment.

Implementation

Implementation is the actual administration of the planned care.

Evaluation, Outcome, and Revision of Care

If an outcome is not reached in the specified time, the client is reassessed. Reordering of priorities may be necessary because the process of evaluation is ongoing.

Evidence-Informed Practice and Best Practice Guidelines

Evidence-informed practice is the systematic application of the best available evidence to decision making in relation to clinical management and policy setting. Practical nurses are using evidence-informed practice as they manage the need for efficiency and improved client outcomes along with increasing demands for accountability.

Best Practice Guidelines (BPGs) are evidence-informed tools that when implemented improve client, practical nurse, and organizational outcomes. These guidelines are systematically developed statements, based on the best available evidence, that assist practical nurses to make decisions about appropriate care. Goals for using BPGs include the following:
- Improved client care
- Reduction in the variation in care
- Transfer of research evidence into practice

- Assistance with clinical decision making
- Reduction of cost

Advocacy

All practical nurses are expected to take on advocacy roles within the Canadian healthcare system. They are expected to advocate for the best health interest for their clients and families and to advocate for the client's wishes and expectations, especially when clients are unable to express their needs clearly.

Practical nurses advocate for organizational or system changes that will improve quality care for clients. When practical nurses advocate, they give their clients a voice. When done correctly, advocacy leads to empowered clients. Empowered clients ask questions to gain a better understanding of all the options available within their plan of care. Practical nurses are expected to be client advocates within all practice areas and within the healthcare team.

Political Activism

Practical nurses may become politically active within their profession and communities. Political activism is usually seen as nurses advocating for the Canadian public in general or involving themselves in current healthcare issues that clients are experiencing (e.g., access to services).

Political activities can include lobbying all levels of government to introduce policies, laws, and regulations that benefit the health of Canadians, such as increased funding for community care or cancer treatment centres.

A practical nurse's involvement in nursing organizations is based on the province or territory in which the practical nurse is employed as well as individual choice. In all cases, if the individual is employed as a practical nurse, he or she must be a member of the appropriate nursing regulatory body (e.g., CNO). In addition, in most provinces or territories, the practical nurse must also join the professional nursing association. In those situations, the regulatory body and professional association are one entity (such as the College of Licensed Practical Nurses of Manitoba). The regulatory function, whether part of the professional association or not, involves registering or licensing individuals to the profession, setting standards of practice, and disciplining nurses who do not meet the standards (Potter et al., 2019). When the regulatory body is separate from the nursing professional association, the individual practical nurse has the choice to join or not join the professional nursing association (such as the Registered Practical Nurses Association of Ontario). The regulatory body registers the practical nurse and has a mandate of public protection. The professional association represents the nursing profession and promotes the role and use of practical nurses in the healthcare system.

Labour organizations (often termed *unions*) are separate from both the professional association and the regulatory organization. Unions assist practical nurses with workplace issues, including the application and interpretation of labour laws and health and safety issues. When a practical nurse is employed by an organization that has an established union contract, the practical nurse must then pay associated fees to the union. Membership in the union is voluntary, but payment of union fees becomes mandatory.

PRACTICE QUESTIONS

Case 1

A nurse educator has revised the hospital's orientation program in anticipation of the hospital orientating many new graduate practical nurses within the next 3 months. The nurse educator decides to use sample client health records to highlight areas of professional practice. He conducts his first education session with the new graduates.

Questions 1–5 refer to this case.

1. During the documentation session, one of the new practical nurses asks what abbreviations can be used within the client's health record. What abbreviations should the practical nurse use?
   1. Abbreviations learned in nursing school
   2. Abbreviations that have been approved by the Canadian Nurses Association
   3. Abbreviations that have been approved by the hospital
   4. Abbreviations that are in common use on specific units within the hospital
2. Which of the following statements is the most accurate information with regard to client consent?
   1. Practical nurses are responsible for ensuring that clients sign all consent forms on the health record.
   2. The healthcare provider proposing the procedure requiring written consent is the person who must ensure that written client consent is obtained.
   3. Verbal consent for an operative procedure is acceptable, and signed consents are not always necessary.
   4. When a client is admitted to the hospital, the client signs a written consent that covers all treatments.
3. In the sample client's health record, the new graduate practical nurses discover that a nurse has written "Verbal Order, acetaminophen (Tylenol), 325 mg, PO, prn, for pain." There is no evidence that this was an emergency situation. Which of the following describes best practice in relation to verbal medication orders?
   1. Verbal orders are to be avoided, except in an emergency situation.

2. Practical nurses should follow the same practice for verbal orders as for telephone orders.
3. Verbal orders should never be accepted, including in emergency situations.
4. Only registered nurses may receive verbal orders for medications from a physician.
4. The new graduate practical nurses review a variety of orders on the sample health records. Which of the following is a correct medication order?
   1. Acetaminophen 325 mg PO for pain
   2. Acetaminophen 325–650 mg PO for pain q4–6h prn
   3. Acetaminophen 325–650 mg PO for pain as needed
   4. Acetaminophen 325 or 650 mg q4–6h prn
5. During the orientation, the nurse educator explains that the hospital uses evidence-informed practice to guide clinical decision making. Which of the following statements best describes evidence-informed practice?
   1. An opportunity to obtain funding from the government
   2. An opportunity to transfer research findings into practice
   3. A chance for professionals to trial untested research findings
   4. A way to promote enhanced assessment skills

Case 2

A manager of home care nurses has noticed over the past 3 months a lack of clarity about the roles of the team members, poor team morale, increasing negative communication, and team conflict. The manager decides to support her staff by providing an education session.

Questions 6–9 refer to this case.

6. One of the new team members is a nurse practitioner (NP). How should the manager describe the level of education for the NP?
   1. A nurse who has specialty certification from the Canadian Nurses Association

2. A nurse who has taken a special interest course in a unique field

3. A nurse who has an undergraduate degree in a discipline other than nursing

4. A nurse educated at the master's level with a specialization in a particular practice area

7. The manager is preparing the education session for her staff group. Which of the following is true in relation to the teaching and learning process?

1. It is important to use the same approach with all types of learners.

2. It is better to introduce all new knowledge instead of connecting it to previously learned knowledge.

3. Learning occurs best when the individual has an identified need to learn.

4. It is always best to deliver education quickly and at the same time of day.

8. The manager explains that effective interpersonal communication with clients and team members includes which of the following?

1. The use of "you" statements when interacting with clients and colleagues

2. The use of warmth and genuineness in interactions

3. The use of questions that elicit single-word responses in order to promote efficient communication

4. The use of frequent self-disclosure to ensure that others will share your point of view

9. In situations in which a team conflict has arisen, what would be the best statement by the manager to her staff?

1. "We should put aside our differences and work together as a team."

2. "I think we should employ a conflict-resolution specialist to help us."

3. "Let's have a discussion about what we can agree is expected team behaviour."

4. "These are the guidelines for team behaviour in this agency."

Case 3

A practical nurse works in a long-term care facility where many of the residents experience acute agitation.

Questions 10–12 refer to this case.

10. The facility follows a "least-restraint policy." What is the most important consideration with a "least-restraint policy"?

1. That a family conference is organized prior to the implementation of a restraint

2. That all possible alternative interventions have been exhausted before a restraint is implemented

3. That the client has no manifestations of delirium or dementia

4. That the client has signed consent for the application of restraints

11. The practical nurse charts the behaviour of a client. Which of the following statements would be the most appropriate documentation?

1. "The client was agitated today."

2. "The client was confused this morning."

3. "The client was shaking his fist at the practical nurse at 1100 hours."

4. "The client was behaving inappropriately during the evening shift."

12. The practical nurse consults the provincial or territorial standards of nursing practice when contemplating the use of restraints. What is the most important purpose for using standards of nursing practice?

1. Standards will help the practical nurse make decisions about ongoing learning needs.

2. Standards will act as a guide to the practical nurse's clinical decision making.

3. Standards will help the practical nurse in malpractice situations.

4. Standards will guide the practical nurse to be aware of protection of personal health, safety, and welfare.

Case 4

A practical nurse has immigrated to Canada from Poland. She received her nursing education in Poland and is now studying for the Canadian Practical Nurse Registration Examination (CPNRE). She has discovered many differences in terms and meaning between nursing practice in Canada and nursing practice in Poland.

Questions 13–15 refer to this case.

13. The practical nurse knows she must be able to articulate the differences and similarities between various nursing organizations. The mandate of nursing regulatory organizations is which of the following?

1. Protection of the public

2. Protection of nurses

3. Protection of nursing employers

4. Protection of all regulated healthcare providers

14. The practical nurse is trying to distinguish the difference between standards of nursing practice and the nursing Best Practice Guidelines. What are the Best Practice Guidelines?

1. Classifications that assist in the analysis and grouping of data

2. Advance directives that clearly indicate the client's wishes and needs

3. Tools based on proven criteria that improve client, nurse, and organizational outcomes

4. Policies that guide compassionate care and ethical nursing decisions

15. The practical nurse has noticed the term *DNR* in one of the sample questions in the exam preparatory book. What does DNR mean?

1. Do not perform cardiopulmonary resuscitation

2. Do not administer cardiac compressions

3. Do not perform any life-saving actions

4. Do not perform any form of resuscitation that has not been agreed upon by the client or substitute decision maker

Independent Questions

Questions 16–30 do not refer to a particular case.

16. Which member of the interprofessional team would be a beneficial resource for the practical nurse to consult with regarding her client who has difficulty communicating and eating after a cerebrovascular accident?
    1. Physiotherapist
    2. Speech-language pathologist
    3. Dietitian
    4. Social worker

17. Meaghan, age 17 years, attends a community eating-disorder support group. Meaghan was hospitalized last year for anorexia nervosa, and she continues to restrict her diet to 700 calories per day. Meaghan stated at today's meeting that she is 3 months pregnant. The public health nurse, who facilitates the support group, is concerned about Meaghan and the fetus. Which of the following actions should the nurse take?
    1. Call the family physician and notify him of the pregnancy.
    2. Call Meaghan's parents and notify them of the pregnancy.
    3. Obtain Meaghan's consent to contact the physician.
    4. Contact Children's Aid Society after the baby is born and explain the situation.

18. A practical nurse is temporarily employed in a family physician's office while the regular practical nurse is on vacation. The physician has left a note for the temporary practical nurse to complete a referral to a gynecologist for a client requesting a therapeutic abortion. The practical nurse has strong religious values against abortion, and she was unaware that working with clients requesting abortions would be part of her role in the office. What is the best action for the practical nurse?
    1. Leave a note for the physician indicating that she refuses to make the referral for an abortion.
    2. Complete the referral to the gynecologist as part of her obligation to provide care for the client in the absence of the regular office practical nurse.
    3. Notify the physician that she will not be working in the office after today's shift.
    4. Tell the client that the usual practical nurse will make the referral when she returns from vacation next week.

19. A practical nurse working her first evening shift as the "in-charge" practical nurse in a long-term care facility hears an unregulated care provider (UCP) tell a client: "If you don't stay quiet in your bed while I help this other resident, I won't feed you your supper." What would be the priority action for the practical nurse?
    1. Ask the resident to repeat what the UCP stated.
    2. Make sure that the UCP is not assigned to that resident when future resident assignments are developed.
    3. Remove the UCP from the client situation and report the incident to the nurse manager the next morning.
    4. Determine whether the UCP needs help with the residents.

20. A resident in a long-term care facility tells the practical nurse that his leg hurts from the fall he had an hour ago. The practical nurse was unaware of the fall and obtains details about the fall from the unregulated care provider (UCP) who cared for the resident at the time of the fall. Which statement related to accountability is correct?
    1. The practical nurse is accountable in all situations for the actions of the UCP.
    2. The practical nurse is not accountable for the actions of the UCP because she was on her lunch break at the time of the fall.
    3. The practical nurse is accountable for the resident's fall because the practical nurse was the only registered/licensed staff on duty at the time of the fall.
    4. The practical nurse is not accountable for the care or actions of the UCP.

21. A practical nurse has been asked by his manager to work an extra 4 hours after his 12-hour shift because three nurses have called in sick. The practical nurse has worked four 12-hour shifts consecutively. He admits he is tired and not sure whether he is too fatigued to work the extra 4 hours. Which of the following is the most appropriate?
    1. The practical nurse cannot refuse to work the additional 4 hours as his manager has made the request and there are no other replacements.
    2. The practical nurse has no obligation to work the additional 4 hours, and he should report his decision to his union representative.
    3. The practical nurse must be offered time and a half for the extra 4 hours.
    4. The practical nurse's first priority in deciding to work the extra 4 hours is whether he is competent to provide safe care.

22. Brandon, age 42, has Lou Gehrig's disease. He is married and has two school-aged children. He has consented to have Medical Assistance in Dying (MAID). What is the practical nurse's role in providing MAID in accordance with the law?
    1. Inserting an IV line (with a doctor's order) that will be used to administer medication that will cause the death of the client
    2. Administering medication through the IV line that will cause the death of the client
    3. Advising the client that MAID is the best way to die without any pain or discomfort
    4. Providing post-mortem care to the client but not bereavement care to the family. Only the nurse practitioner or physician can provide bereavement care.

23. A second-year practical nursing student obtains an apical heart rate of 140 bpm on Cara, a 6-year-old child. The student practical nurse assumes that she has made an error in counting the beats. She did not take any action in relation to her findings, and she did not report the elevated heart rate to anyone. Who is responsible for this error in care?
    1. The student practical nurse because she did not report the heart rate or take any action

2. The staff nurse working with the student practical nurse because she should have asked about the heart rate
3. The student practical nurse's clinical instructor because she knows the student practical nurse's strengths and weaknesses
4. The clinical instructor, student practical nurse, and staff nurse are all equally responsible

24. A client is ordered 325 mg of acetylsalicylic acid (ASA) prn for headache. The practical nurse is aware that this client is also receiving warfarin (Coumadin). Which of the following is the most appropriate action to be taken by the practical nurse?
   1. Contact the doctor for clarification of the orders.
   2. Ask the client if he has taken Aspirin before while also taking Coumadin.
   3. Contact the pharmacist about the potential drug interaction.
   4. Consult with nursing colleagues about whether to give the ASA to the client.

25. A second-year practical nursing student has asked his preceptor about the use of restraints. Which of the following is not considered a restraint category?
   1. Chemical
   2. Physical
   3. Hazardous
   4. Environmental

26. A student practical nurse has forgotten her computer password. She asks a staff nurse to share her password in order to access a client's chart. What should the staff nurse do?
   1. Share the password since the student practical nurse provided direct client care.
   2. Ask the student practical nurse to write the care on a piece of paper, and the staff nurse will enter it later.
   3. Do not share the password and direct the student practical nurse to the policy on retrieving forgotten passwords.
   4. Explain the situation to the charge nurse, who will locate a password.

27. A client is ordered venlafaxine (Effexor) for depression. The client refuses to take the medication, stating that it causes headaches. What should the practical nurse do?

   1. Do not give the medication because the client has withdrawn her consent.
   2. Tell the charge nurse the situation to see if she can convince the client to take the medication.
   3. Administer the medication because the client has been diagnosed with depression.
   4. Insist that the client take the medication but tell her she will give her Tylenol for the headache.

28. In a hospital setting, what is the priority practice by a practical nurse to ensure administration of the correct medication to the correct client?
   1. Check each client's identification bracelet.
   2. Address each client by his or her last name prior to administering the medication.
   3. Check each client's health card or hospital identification card.
   4. Check the names that are posted above the client's bed or attached to the bottom of the bed.

29. The practical nurse is not able to read the obstetrician's handwriting for postpartum orders for a client. The obstetrician has returned to her office outside the hospital. What should the practical nurse do?
   1. Ask the client what her obstetrician ordered for postpartum pain relief
   2. Contact the obstetrician for clarification of the orders
   3. Ask the unit clerk for clarification of the obstetrician's handwriting
   4. Consult other postpartum charts for this obstetrician to compare similar orders

30. In which of the following situations would the practical nurse use a code of ethics to guide practice?
   1. A practical nurse needs information on how to reposition a client after hip replacement
   2. An informal caregiver and neighbour is curious and asks for details about the client's care
   3. A unit coordinator does not allow practical nurses to work to their full scope of practice on the surgical unit
   4. A practical nurse has not worked previously with unregulated care provider (UCPs) and requires assistance on how best to delegate tasks to UCPs

REFERENCES

Black, H.C. (2009). *Black's law dictionary* (10th ed.). St. Paul, MN: West Publishing.

Canada Health Act, RSC 1985, c C-6.

Canadian Council for Practical Nurse Regulators. (2013a). *Code of ethics for licensed practical nurses in Canada.* n.p.: Author. Retrieved from http://www.ccpnr.ca/wp-content/uploads/2013/09/IJLPN-CE-Final.pdf.

Canadian Council for Practical Nurse Regulators. (2013b). *Standards of practice for licensed practical nurses in Canada.* n.p.: Author. Retrieved from https://www.clpna.com/wp-content/uploads/2013/02/doc_CCPNR_CLPNA_Standards_of _Practice.pdf.

Canadian Institute for Health Information. (2017). *Regulated nurses, 2016.* Ottawa: Author. Retrieved from https://secure .cihi.ca/free_products/regulated-nurses-2016-report-en -web.pdf.

Canadian Nurses Association. (2017a). *Code of ethics for registered nurses.* Ottawa: Author. Retrieved from https://cna-aiic.ca/en/ nursing-practice/nursing-ethics.

Canadian Nurses Association. (2017b). *National nursing framework: On medical assistance in dying in Canada.* Ottawa: Author. Retrieved from https://cna-aiic.ca/~/media/cna/page-content/ pdf-en/cna-national-nursing-framework-on-maid.pdf?la=en.

Canadian Nurses Association, The Canadian Hospice Palliative Care Association, & The Canadian Hospice Palliative Care Nurses Group. (2015). Joint position statement: The palliative approach to care and the role of the nurse. Retrieved from https://www.cna-aiic.ca/~/media/cna/page-content/pdf-en/the-palliative-approach-to-care-and-the-role-of-the-nurse_e.pdf.

Canadian Nurses Protective Society. (1999). Legal risks in nursing. *InfoLAW, 8*(1).

Canadian Nurses Protective Society. (2004). Negligence: When would a nurse face an allegation of negligence? *InfoLAW, 3*(1).

Canadian Nurses Protective Society. (2006). Consent for CPR. *InfoLAW, 15*(2). Retrieved from https://www.cnps.ca/upload-files/pdf_english/cpr.pdf.

College of Nurses of Ontario. (2009). *Guiding decisions about end-of-life care, 2009*. Toronto: Author. Retrieved from http://nsmhpcn.ca/wp-content/uploads/2014/11/CNO-Guiding-Decisions-about-End-of-Life-Care.pdf.

College of Nurses of Ontario. (2017). *Practice standard: Medication*. Toronto: Author. Retrieved from http://www.cno.org/globalassets/docs/prac/41007_medication.pdf.

Duhaime, L. (n.d.). Tort. *Duhaime's legal dictionary*. Retrieved from http://www.duhaime.org/LegalDictionary/T/Tort.aspx.

Fridman, G. (2012). *Introduction to the Canadian law of torts* (3rd ed.). Markham, ON: LexisNexis Canada.

Government of Canada. (2018). Medical assistance in dying. Retrieved from https://www.canada.ca/en/health-canada/services/medical-assistance-dying.html#a2.

Irvine, J., Osborne, P., & Shariff, M. (2013). *Canadian medical law* (4th ed.). Toronto: Carswell.

Keatings, M., & Smith, O. (2010). *Ethical and legal issues in Canadian nursing* (3rd ed.). Toronto: Elsevier Canada.

Osborne, P.H. (2015). *Essentials of Canadian law: The law of torts* (5th ed.). Toronto: Irwin Law.

Potter, P., Perry, A., Stockert, P., et al. (2019). *Canadian fundamentals of nursing* (6th ed.). Milton, ON: Elsevier.

Sorrentino, S., Remmert, L., & Wilk, M. (2018). *Mosby's Canadian textbook for the support worker* (4th ed.). Toronto: Elsevier.

Williams, P. (2018). *deWit's Fundamental concepts and skills for nursing* (5th ed.). St. Louis: Elsevier.

BIBLIOGRAPHY

Balzer Riley, J. (2017). *Communication in nursing* (8th ed.). Philadelphia: Mosby.

College of Nurses of Ontario. (2006). *Practice standard: Therapeutic nurse–client relationship*. Toronto: Author. Retrieved from http://www.cno.org/globalassets/docs/prac/41033_therapeutic.pdf.

College of Nurses of Ontario. (2009). *Practice guideline: Culturally sensitive care*. Toronto: Author. Retrieved from http://www.cno.org/globalassets/docs/prac/41040_culturallysens.pdf.

College of Nurses of Ontario. (2014). *Practice guideline: RN and RPN practice: The client, the nurse and the environment*. Toronto: Author. Retrieved from http://www.cno.org/globalassets/docs/prac/41062.pdf.

College of Nurses of Ontario. (2017). *Practice standard: Documentation: Revised 2008*. Toronto: Author. Retrieved from http://www.cno.org/globalassets/docs/prac/41001_documentation.pdf.

Stein-Parbury, J. (2018). *Patient & person: Interpersonal skills in nursing* (6th ed.). Chatswood, Australia: Elsevier.

WEB SITES

- **Association of New Brunswick Licensed Practical Nurses** (http://www.anblpn.ca): This site contains links to information on all aspects of being an LPN professional in New Brunswick.
- **Canadian Council for Practical Nurse Regulators** (http://ccpnr.ca): This site contains information on the four standards of practice that govern the ethical principles of all LPNs/RPNs as well as the legal and professional expectations of LPN/RPNs.
- **Canadian Nurses Association: CNA Code of Ethics for Registered Nurses** (http://www.cna-nurses.ca/cna/documents/pdf/publications/Code_of_Ethics_2008_e.pdf): This document serves as a foundation for nurses' ethical practice.
- **College of Licensed Practical Nurses of Alberta** (http://www.clpna.com): This site contains links to information on all aspects of being an LPN professional in Alberta.
- **College of Licensed Practical Nurses of British Columbia** (http://www.clpnbc.org): This site contains links to information on all aspects of being an LPN professional in British Columbia.
- **College of Licensed Practical Nurses of Manitoba** (http://www.clpnm.ca): This site contains links to information on all aspects of being an LPN professional in Manitoba.
- **College of Licensed Practical Nurses of Newfoundland and Labrador** (http://www.clpnnl.ca): This site contains links to information on all aspects of being an LPN professional in Newfoundland and Labrador.
- **College of Licensed Practical Nurses of Nova Scotia** (http://www.clpnns.ca): This site contains links to information on all aspects of being an LPN professional in Nova Scotia.
- **College of Licensed Practical Nurses of Prince Edward Island** (https://clpnpei.ca): This site contains links to information on all aspects of being an LPN professional in Prince Edward Island.
- **College of Nurses of Ontario** (http://www.cno.org): This site contains links to information related to all aspects of being a registered practical nursing professional in Ontario.
- **Ordre des infirmières et infirmiers auxiliaires du Québec** (http://www.oiiaq.org): This site contains links to information on all aspects of being an LPN professional in Quebec.
- **Registered Practical Nurses Association of Ontario** (http://www.rpnao.org): This site contains information on the professional association representing the voice of practical nurses in Ontario.
- **Saskatchewan Association of Licensed Practical Nurses** (http://www.salpn.com): This site contains links to information on all aspects of being an LPN professional in Saskatchewan.

Health Assessment Across the Lifespan

Health assessment is the collection of information about an individual's well-being. The information can come from a variety of sources; there is verbal information from the person or the person's family; there is physical information that the practical nurse obtains through inspection, palpation, and auscultation; and there is laboratory testing. All of these and any other sources of information are gathered to assist the practitioner to obtain a complete picture of the individual's well-being.

For the purpose of easy access, this chapter is divided into site-specific sections. Normally, the practical nurse must consider the person as a whole rather than as the sum of many individual parts. However, this chapter focuses on one system or area at a time. One of the arts of nursing is to paint the whole picture once all the parts are known. Imagine an artist's palette; the areas of information are the colours on the palette, and the care for the client will be determined once the picture has been painted.

As a member of the healthcare team, it is imperative that the practical nurse assess the client and that the assessment be recorded. The practical nurse must believe what she or he hears and report it, especially if it is abnormal. The practical nurse, especially the novice practical nurse, must not second-guess and ignore the findings due to feelings of doubt. If you are in doubt, report the findings and ask a more experienced member of the team to verify them.

The most important aspect of health assessment is the history. Not only is *what* is said important, but *how* it is said is also key. The role of the practical nurse is to get the whole story by asking pertinent questions and steering the conversation in a way that is productive and time-efficient. The physical examination will confirm or refute the story and assist the practical nurse in obtaining the information needed to help make the diagnosis. Whether the result is a nursing diagnosis or a medical diagnosis, the story is a vital component.

INTERVIEWING SKILLS AND HISTORY-TAKING

Communication Techniques

To take a history, or to listen to a history, the practical nurse must use a variety of question types, as summarized in Table 4.1.

How the practical nurse responds to the answers can be as important as the questions themselves. Table 4.2 provides a number of responses, descriptors, and examples.

It is not just the spoken word of an interview that can give you the complete story. It is important to observe the client's posture, eye contact, facial expressions, voice, language, the use of touch, and any gestures. All of these factors enhance the depth and meaning of the spoken word. Table 4.3 gives examples of positive and negative non-verbal behaviours of the interviewer.

A complete history can take up to an hour or even longer to obtain, which is not always practical even at the best of times. The practical nurse must therefore decide what information is a priority in a shortened amount of time. Over the course of caring for the client, the practical nurse can continue to ask questions and listen to the whole story. Another reason to do a complete history is to find out any areas of concern in which health teaching and health promotion would be beneficial.

It is not always possible for the history to come from the client. For an infant or young child, the history will come from the child's caregiver (parent, grandparent, or guardian). In the case of an adult who is comatose or too ill to engage in conversation, the information may come from a spouse, a child, or a friend. Understand that information gathered in these circumstances is modified by the person relaying it. Watch the child closely for non-verbal communication. Be inclusive and call the person by name. Now you must build up a therapeutic relationship not just with the client but also with the provider of information.

Interviewing adolescents can present its challenges. Teens want to be considered as adults but can revert to wanting a parent close by, especially when they are in a stressful situation. Certain information will not be shared unless a good trusting relationship has been built, which may happen only if the parent is not present. Not all adolescents are the same. Levels of maturity, understanding, and the ability to express oneself can range widely. Starting with the easiest questions can be helpful, and when there is a greater sense of trust, the more sensitive questions can be broached.

Interviewing the older adult can be a much slower process. Giving the client more time to answer will decrease the potential for frustration and stress. Open-ended questions might take longer to answer because they may cover a lengthy life history. If the client has a deficit in short-term memory,

TABLE 4.1   Communication Techniques

Type of Question	Description of Question	Examples
Open-ended questions	• They are good at the beginning of the interview. • They can lead to a lot of information. • Questions are unbiased. • The practical nurse to be an active and interested listener and encourage the story; for example, using "Tell me more" promotes more information. • They can lead clients to go off on many tangents.	"How are you feeling today?" "Tell me about your health concerns." "Why have you come to the clinic today?"
Closed or direct questions	• They are good for specific details. • They are useful to fill in the gaps from the open-ended response. • They can be used to expedite the interview. • Practical nurses should ask one question at a time only. • Practical nurses should use culturally appropriate language. • Client answers are quite often "yes" or "no."	"Do you have any drug allergies?" "Do you get short of breath climbing a flight of stairs?" "When was the last time you ate anything?"

TABLE 4.2   Examples of Responses and Descriptors

Response	Description of Response	Examples
Facilitation	• It encourages further information. • It shows an interest in the information being shared, which will promote storytelling.	Practical nurse: "Yes" Nodding your head Good eye contact "Mm-hmm" or "Uh-huh" "Go on, I'm listening."
Silence	• It is useful after open-ended questions. • Maintain good eye contact. • Try not to interrupt. • Watch the client for non-verbal clues.	
Reflection	• Repeat part of what the client said to allow him or her to expand on it. • Expand on an important concept. • Specifically focus on an emotional aspect of what the client has said.	Client: "I don't understand how to do it. I feel so scared." Practical nurse: "You feel scared?" Client: "I suffered from this last year and now it's back." Practical nurse: "You had this last year?"
Empathy	• It gives the client a sense of feeling understood. • It can promote the therapeutic relationship. • It gives the green light to the client to talk about his or her thoughts and feelings.	Practical nurse: "This is probably very scary for you to go through." "I can imagine that if that happened to me I would also be scared, frightened, upset … " etc. "I can understand how frustrating this must be for you."
Clarification	• Seek clarification when you do not understand what the client is saying or when you think that what he or she is saying can be interpreted in more than one way. • Use information the client has shared as a point of clarification. Are you on the right track?	Client: "My job is very heavy." Practical nurse: "You do a lot of heavy lifting in your job?" Practical nurse: "Let me get this straight: the pain occurs only in the morning, you get relief when you drink three cups of coffee, and the pain does not return until the following morning. Is that correct?" Client: "Yes, that's right."
Confrontation Interpretation Explanation Summary	• Leave these responses to the end and use as a wrap-up of the interview. • If you do not agree with something that the client has said, question him or her on it. • Using interpretation helps the client identify with an emotion or explanation as to why something has happened. • Using explanation literally explains the why and what of some notion. • Using summarizing can clarify the issues, put them into sequence, restate your client's perceptions and your own, and validate the information with the client.	Practical nurse: "You say that you are okay with being in the hospital, but you seem to be so sad and worried." "Do you realize that every time you come to the emergency department with abdominal pain, your mother-in-law is visiting from out of town?" "You must drink the CT dye so that the X-ray will be clear for the doctor to interpret."

TABLE 4.3 Non-Verbal Behaviours of the Interviewer

Positive	Negative
Professional appearance is appropriate to the context	Appearance objectionable to patient
Equal-status seating	Standing
Close proximity to patient	Sitting behind desk, far away, turned away
Relaxed open posture	Tense posture
Leaning slightly toward patient	Slouched back
Occasional facilitating gestures	Critical or distracting gestures: pointing finger, clenched fist, finger tapping, foot swinging, looking at watch
Facial animation, interest	Bland expression, yawning, tight mouth
Appropriate smiling	Frowning, lip biting
Appropriate eye contact	Shifty, avoiding eye contact, focusing on notes, computer screen, iPad, etc.
Moderate tone of voice	Strident, high-pitched tone
Moderate rate of speech	Rate too slow or too fast
Appropriate use and consent of touch, depending on the context	Too frequent or inappropriate touch. Touch without consent of patient and/or patient's caregiver

From Jarvis, C., Browne, A. J., MacDonald-Jenkins, J., et al. (2018). *Physical examination & health assessment* (3rd Cdn. ed., p. 54, Table 4.2). Toronto: Saunders.

the practical nurse will need to rely on the family members to fill in the gaps.

If a client has a hearing deficit, sit directly in front of the client. Speak clearly and loudly enough for the client to hear and understand what you are saying.

If the deficit is significant, make sure that the person is wearing hearing aids if appropriate or that a sign-language interpreter is available.

If there is a language barrier, if possible, use an interpreter who is not a family member. The family member might not translate all the information, thinking that he or she is protecting the client from difficult information.

If the client starts to cry during the interview process, let the person cry. Crying is an important expression of grief and release. Do not move on to another topic to avoid the painful issue. Offer a tissue and perhaps a hand on the shoulder, if this is culturally acceptable.

Be careful if you sense a threat of violence. Practical nurses can be very vulnerable in the workplace to clients who are under the influence of drugs and alcohol or who are very angry. Recognizing these factors and positioning yourself accordingly can prevent possible physical abuse that might be directed at you. Do not stay in a closed room alone with such a client. Always make sure that other members of the healthcare team can see you. If you suspect there is a potential for violence, protect yourself, do not take any risks, and think of safety first. Talk calmly and quietly; do not raise your voice and argue with the client. Verbal abuse from clients or toward clients is also not acceptable. Practical nurses must make it known that they are health professionals and must be treated accordingly.

Cross-cultural issues in client care can be a learning experience for both parties but can also be a deterrent to complete care. Be careful to try to understand cultural differences. What are the codes of behaviour? Who can be touched or not, and who can be in a room without a chaperone? If there is a language barrier, such differences might be more difficult to interpret. What are the client's perceptions of healthcare workers, the system, and the treatments? In order to build a trusting therapeutic relationship with clients from some cultures, you may have to divulge some information about yourself, too. It is best to start the interview process formally. Stand to greet the client, let him or her know how you would like to be referred to, and elicit the same from them. Keep a good distance apart; 1.5–3 metres is acceptable. Be tolerant of different cultural beliefs and adjust your questions and responses accordingly.

The Complete Health History

A complete history includes many aspects. Keep in mind who is providing the information, which may be the client, a parent, the spouse, a friend, or someone else. If the client is very ill or if it is an emergency situation, stress will be an added factor in the presentation of the story. The following is a list of the different areas of information to be collected:

- Biographical data
- Reason for seeking care
- Present health or history of the present illness
- Past history
- Family history
- Review of all systems
- Functional assessment or activities of daily living

If there is pain, further information is needed. Use the mnemonic "PQRSTU" (Jarvis, Browne, MacDonald-Jenkins, et al., 2018) to explore all areas:

P: Provocative: What starts the pain? What makes it worse? What makes it better?

Q: Quality of the pain: Neuropathic or nociceptive? How does it feel?

R: Region or Radiation: Where is the pain? Does it spread?

S: Severity scale: On a scale of 0–10, where 0 is no pain and 10 is the most severe pain that you can imagine, where is your pain?

T: Timing: When did the pain start? How often does the pain occur, and how long does it last?

U: Understanding client's perception of the problem. What do you think that it means?

Keep in mind any cultural differences. If the client is not native to Canada, determine when he or she arrived, the country or region of origin, and the conditions in that location. Are there any religious considerations that would affect blood-product transfusions, dietary options, the need for clergy, or perhaps the necessity of a chaperone during an examination?

If the client is an infant, include details of pre- and postnatal health and labour and delivery. Also ask about the developmental history. It is challenging at times to get a complete history from adolescents. Keep in mind that it is important to include a psychological assessment as adolescents can be very vulnerable to depression and suicide.

The Mental Status Examination

A person's mental status is defined as his or her emotional and cognitive function assessed through behaviour. By assessing mental status first, the practical nurse can establish a baseline, and reassessment can monitor any changes, especially in response to the stress of illness and feeling of being unwell. Serious health problems such as alcoholism, renal failure, diabetes, liver disease, or brain disease might alter the mental assessment. Various medications can also alter the assessment, as will lower educational levels.

It is difficult to assess mental status in a child, but the older the child, the easier it is as the cerebral cortex matures and the attention span increases with age. Assessing the older adult client often takes longer because the client may need more time to answer the questions, and there may also be recent memory loss. As well as memory loss, sensory losses of sight and hearing can cause frustration, social isolation, and apathy. The older adult client might also have experienced a number of losses, such as loved ones, friends, job, income, or health, giving rise to an added risk of depression and despair.

The behaviour assessment should include the following factors:

- Consciousness
- Language
- Mood affect
- Orientation
- Attention
- Memory
- Abstract reasoning
- Thought process
- Thought content
- Perceptions

For the average client, the mental assessment can be incorporated into the rest of the health history. The four main headings are *appearance*, *behaviour*, *cognition*, and *thought*

process (ABCT) (Jarvis et al., 2018). The Mini-Mental State Examination (MMSE) can be performed if a more thorough assessment is needed (Folstein, Folstein, & McHugh, 1975).

ASSESSMENT TECHNIQUES

The practical nurse uses the following techniques when objectively assessing the client:

- Inspection
- Palpation
- Auscultation

The techniques are performed in order with the exception of the examination of the abdomen, when auscultation is done immediately after inspection. Note that percussion is part of the assessment technique but is not a required competency of the entry-level practical nurse.

The Technique of Inspection

Inspection is the most powerful of all the technical skills. It yields the most data because the practical nurse's physical examination is guided by the observation of any abnormalities. The inspection starts as soon as the practitioner sees the person and continues throughout the whole encounter. Practical nurses must learn to be astute in the art of looking. It is very difficult at first not to touch the client. So just stand back and observe. Perform a general body scan. Watch for behaviour, as well as generalized symmetry. Then move on to more specific observations.

The Technique of Palpation

Palpation is the art of touching the body to assess the skin and the underlying organs, as well as any abnormalities. The sense of touch can be used to feel texture; temperature; moisture; vibration; pulsation; swelling; rigidity; spasticity; organ location; crepitations; the presence of any lumps, bumps, or lesions; or the presence of any pain or tenderness.

Generally, the pads of the fingertips are used. Make sure that your hands are warm. Be careful not to poke the skin but to gently rub the fingertips in a circular motion. Palpation should feel good to the client and should be soothing and relaxed. If there is a painful area, palpate it last. If the client is very ticklish, place the client's hand on the skin first, put your hand on next, ask the client to start palpating, and then gently slide the client's hand out. Start with light palpation and progress to deep palpation where appropriate.

The dorsa of the hands are used for assessing temperature and moisture. The skin on the back of the hand is thinner and more sensitive. The base of the fingers or the ulnar edge of the hand is used to detect vibrations. Bimanual palpation is the use of both hands at the same time.

The Technique of Auscultation

Auscultation is listening to body sounds through a stethoscope. The earpieces should be comfortable and directed toward the nose. As you bend your head to listen, the earpieces should make a perfect seal with the natural curvature of the ear canal. There are two parts to the stethoscope, the diaphragm and the bell. The diaphragm is used to listen to high-pitched sounds, such as bowel, respiratory, or heart sounds, whereas the bell is useful for hearing low-pitched sounds, such as heart murmurs or bruits. The bell must be placed on the skin very lightly, and the diaphragm should be pressed firmly down on the skin. Clean the stethoscope with an alcohol wipe between uses as it can become a vector for cross-contamination. The neck of the stethoscope should be 30–35 cm in length. The noise in the surrounding areas should be minimal. If the client's chest is particularly hairy, wet the hair to avoid mistaking it for "crackles" in the lungs. The sounds are more accurate if listened to over bare skin and not over clothes.

The General Survey

At your first encounter with the client, start your general survey. Establish that the airway is clear, that the client is breathing, and that there is circulation. Throughout the general survey, establish that appearance, behaviour, cognition, and thought processes are all intact.

Physical appearance: Does the client look his or her stated age? Is the client oriented to time, place, and person? Is the sexual development appropriate for the client's age and gender? Do a general scan of the colour and condition of the skin. Are there any signs of acute distress?

Body structure: Check height and weight. Are these the expected values? Look at body symmetry and posture. How comfortable is the client sitting or lying down? Is the body proportionate?

Mobility: Assess gait if possible. Note the range of motion of the limbs and joints.

Vital signs: Take the pulse, respiratory rate, blood pressure, temperature, and oxygen saturation and assess for pain.

For infants, measure the circumference of the head and the length of the body.

HEAD AND NECK WITH REGIONAL LYMPHATICS ASSESSMENT

The Anatomy and Landmarks of the Head and Neck

Keep in mind that there are two halves to the body: the left and the right. Remember to examine both sides of the body and always assess for symmetry. The symmetry is not perfect, but, for the most part, it is very close.

The skull is composed of cranial bones; sutures separate the frontal, temporal, parietal, and occipital bones. At birth, the sutures have not approximated completely to allow room for the brain to grow. The areas where they have not joined together are called *fontanelles*. The posterior fontanelle closes within the first 2 months of birth, and the frontal fontanelle closes sometime between 9 months and 2 years of age.

There are 14 facial bones, and the head sits upon the vertebrae of the cervical spine. The first vertebra, C1, is located at the base of the spine and is called the *atlas*; the second, C2, is called the *axis*. The cervical vertebrae continue down to C7,

which is called the *vertebra prominens*. The prominens is highly palpable when the neck is flexed forward as it has a long spinous process.

Many muscles control the face and facial expressions. The motor component to cranial nerve VII, or the facial nerve, innervates most of the muscles. Cranial nerve V, the trigeminal nerve, controls the movement of the masseter muscles—which assist in talking and chewing—from the mandible and the temporomandibular joint. The sensory component of the trigeminal nerve is responsible for feeling light touch along the areas controlled by the three sections of the nerve: the forehead, the cheek, and the chin. The sensory component of the facial nerve is taste on the anterior two-thirds of the tongue.

The pulsation of the temporal artery can be felt anterior to the ear. This artery supplies blood and nutrients to the face and head.

Salivary glands protect the teeth and mucosa by rinsing them and aid digestion by containing enzymes to start the digestive process and providing lubrication for the food bolus. The parotid gland is located anterior to and slightly below the tragus of the ear on either side of the face. The submandibular gland is located at the angle of the jaw and below the mandible. The sublingual glands are under the tongue at the front of the mouth. None of the glands are normally palpable.

The muscles of the neck are the sternomastoid, the trapezius, and the omohyoid. They are innervated by cranial nerve XI, the spinal accessory nerve. These muscles are responsible for holding the head up and providing the range of motion of the head. At the base of the neck is the clavicle. Down along the neck there are a variety of structures: the hyoid bone, the thyroid cartilage, the cricoid cartilage, the trachea, and the manubrium at the bottom.

The thyroid gland is an endocrine gland that synthesizes and secretes thyroxine (T_4) and triiodothyronine (T_3), hormones that regulate cellular metabolism and growth. The thyroid gland is also responsible for calcitonin, which regulates the amount of calcium in the bloodstream and stimulates growth. The gland has two lobes and should be smooth, without lumps or bumps. The cricoid cartilage is just above the thyroid.

The Anatomy and Landmarks of the Regional Lymphatic System

The lymphatic system plays a vital role in the body. It is responsible for cleaning the blood, returning fluid to the blood from the tissues, and fighting infection. The lymph nodes that are situated along the pathways of the lymphatic system filter bacteria and foreign particles from the lymph fluid. If there is an infection, the lymph nodes become swollen and sore. If they become cancerous, they are fixed, nontender, and firm.

Subjective Data Specific to the Head and Neck

*Questions specific to the older adult

- Are you experiencing any headaches? If yes, describe the headache.

- What types of stress do you have in your life?
- What coping strategies have you been using?
- Are you taking any medications?
- Do you have any allergies?
- Have you had a recent head injury?
- Did you lose consciousness?
* **Do you have any illnesses now, such as diabetes or lung or heart disease?**
* **Are you experiencing vertigo or dizziness? If yes, does it interfere with your daily routine?**
- Do you have any neck pain?
* **Have you noticed any decrease in the range of motion of your neck? If yes, does it restrict your ability to do your daily activities or work?**
- Have you had any trouble breathing?
- Have you had any trouble swallowing?
- Do you smoke? If so, how many cigarettes per day and for how many years?
- How often do you drink alcohol?
- Have you noticed any lumps or bumps in your neck?
- Have you had a cold recently?
- Have you ever had surgery to the head or neck region?
- If the client is an infant, ask the adult: Were there any difficulties with the pregnancy, labour, or delivery? Has your baby been following a normal growth pattern?

Objective Data Specific to the Head and Neck

- Inspect and palpate the head and hair. Look at and feel the head for redness, swelling, lumps, bumps, and lesions. Check the hair for texture and the presence of lice. The eggs are white ovals that stick to the hair strands and will not brush off easily. They come off individually when they are pulled off with fingernails, as opposed to dandruff, which will flake off or blow off the hair quite easily. The nits are black and can jump around the head. They tend to migrate to the base of the hair at the back of the neck and around the posterior of the ears. They can be very irritating to the skin.
- Palpating the head should be relaxing to the client. At every opportunity, make the examination process a relaxing and calm one for the client and for you.
- For an infant, measure the circumference of the head. Assess for any tenderness over any of the cranial bones.
- Palpate the temporal artery pulse.
- Palpate the temporomandibular joint (TMJ), assessing for tenderness, cracking, or crepitus. Test for range of movement, as well as smooth movement when the mouth is opened.
- Test the movement of the mandible against resistance for strength.
- Inspect the face, looking at the skin condition, facial expressions, and symmetry. Note any tics or fasciculation.
- Inspect and palpate the neck. Assess for symmetry and that the trachea is midline.
- Look for the client's ability to perform voluntary head movements. Perform a series of range-of-motion exercises with the neck and assess for strength using movement against resistance. With an infant, assess the head posture and control. By 4 months, an infant should have head control.
- Using the fingertips and creeping down the skin, not poking it, feel for all the lymph nodes in the neck. If there is a palpable node, note its size and consistency and feel for tenderness. Check both sides simultaneously for symmetry.

EYE ASSESSMENT

Landmarks of the Eye

- Palpebral fissures are the space between the upper and lower eyelids. When the eye is closed, the eyelids approximate with no distance between them. When open, the eye is partially covered to the upper part of the iris by the upper eyelid.
- The limbus is where the sclera and cornea come together.
- The canthus can be found where the eyelids meet in the corners of the eye. The lateral (outer) canthus is toward the ear, and the medial (inner) canthus is toward the nose. At the inner canthus is the caruncle, a fleshy area that contains sebaceous glands.
- The upper lids contain Meibomian glands within the tarsal plate. The tarsal plates contain connective tissue that gives the eyelid its shape. In the older adult, the connective tissue loses elasticity, thus not maintaining the eyelid's shape. The Meibomian glands secrete an oily substance that lubricates the eye, prevents the tears from overflowing, and maintains a good seal when the eyes are closed.
- The palpebral conjunctiva is a thin mucous membrane. It lines the inside of the eyelids and is clear with many blood vessels. The bulbar conjunctiva covers the eyeball, overlying the sclera. The bulbar conjunctiva merges with the cornea at the limbus, where the cornea covers and protects the iris and pupil.
- The lacrimal apparatus provides protection to the eye by providing an irrigation system to keep the cornea and the conjunctiva moist and lubricated. Tears form in the lacrimal gland and wash over the eyes. The tears drain out of the eye through the puncta at the inner canthus into the lacrimal sac and down the lacrimal duct into the inferior meatus and turbinates of the nose.
- Eye movement is controlled by six extraocular muscles attached to the eye and the orbit. The muscles provide straight and rotary movement. The muscles of the eyes are coordinated so that the eyes move in a parallel fashion (called *conjugate movement*). This movement is important as the brain can only perceive one image at a time. Cranial nerves III, IV, and VI (oculomotor, trochlear, and abducens) innervate the muscles of the eye to produce various movements.

The Internal Anatomy of the Eye

The outer layer of the eye is called the *sclera*. It is made up of a white fibrous tissue and should have a smooth consistency. It serves as a protective shield and is continuous with the transparent cornea that protects the iris and pupil.

The cornea bends (refracts) the incoming light rays, which are then directed back to the retina. The cornea is very sensitive to touch. The corneal reflex is tested by touching the cornea with a wisp of cotton. If the reflex is normal, the fifth cranial nerve (the trigeminal nerve) sends a message to the brain and cranial nerve VII sends a message to the eye to blink.

The eye's middle layer consists of the choroid, iris, pupil, lens, and anterior and posterior chambers. The choroid protects the retina by supplying blood to it and by decreasing the amount of light that reflects internally. Anteriorly, it is continuous with the muscle of the ciliary body, which controls the thickness of the lens. The muscle fibres in the iris contract, or dilate, the pupil to vary the amount of light admitted into the eye. This is called the *papillary reflex.* A direct reflex occurs when the light is shone into the eye; a consensual light reflex is the constriction of the contralateral pupil—in other words, when the light is shone into one eye, the pupil of the other eye also constricts. Accommodation occurs when the pupils constrict to help the eye to focus on close objects. The lens lies posterior to the pupil. It flattens to see distant objects and bulges to see close objects. After the age of 40 years, a person's lens starts to lose elasticity and the ability to see close objects diminishes; this is called *presbyopia.* By 70 years of age, the lens begins to thicken due to a clumping of proteins and yellow deposits called *nuclear stenosis* or *senile cataract.*

The posterior chamber contains the aqueous humour. It provides nutrients and removes waste products to the surrounding tissues. The anterior chamber, which sits between the cornea and the lens and iris, allows the outflow of the aqueous humour. Intraocular pressure measures the balance between the amount of aqueous humour produced and the resistance to its outflow. Increased intraocular pressure, or glaucoma, increases with age and is three to six times more likely to occur in people of African descent.

The inner retinal layer is responsible for changing the waves of light into nerve impulses. When you are looking through an ophthalmoscope, the optic disc, where the optic nerve lies, is located toward the nose. The disc is yellow-orange to pink, is oval to round in shape, and is where fibres from the retina converge to form the optic nerve. The physiological cup inside the optic disc is a brighter yellow than the disc and is the location of the entrance and exit of the retinal blood vessels. The blood vessels drain through the cup. The macula is grey in colour and is responsible for central vision. Through an ophthalmoscope, it can be located by looking toward the ear. It is at the macula that the sharpest vision can be seen. Age can decrease the effectiveness of the macula, decreasing central vision. The retinal vessels converge into the optic disc. The arteries are redder and smaller than the veins. The background of the fundus depends on the person's skin colour. Generally, it has a reddish-orange hue.

Subjective Data Specific to the Eye

- Do you have any difficulty with your vision?
- Have you noticed any difficulty reading or seeing close objects?
- Do you have any difficulty with night vision?
- Do you have any pain in your eyes?
- Do you see double?
- Have you ever had "crossed eyes"?
- Do you have any redness or swelling in your eyes?
- Do you have any discharge or watering in your eyes?
- Do your eyes feel dry or burning?
- Do you have any past history of eye problems?
- Do you have any past history of glaucoma?
- When was the last time you were checked for glaucoma?
- Do you have any family history of glaucoma?
- Do you use glasses or contacts? If yes, do they work well for you?
- When was your last eye examination?
- Were you given a prescription for glasses?
- Have you ever had any surgery on your eyes?
- Do you take any medications or drops for your eyes?

Objective Data Specific to the Eye

- Test for vision. Test the function of cranial nerve II, the optic nerve.
- Use a Snellen eye chart. The person should stand 20 feet away from a 20-foot chart or 10 feet from a 10-foot chart, cover one eye with a shield, and read the letters aloud, starting from left to right, top to bottom. Ask the person not to use a hand to cover the eye as this can compress the eyeball and distort its vision. The client should read the lowest line that he or she can without making more than two mistakes. Switch to the other eye, this time asking the person to read from right to left. Reading glasses must be removed, but glasses with corrective lenses for distance should stay on. Normal vision is 20/20; in other words, the person can read at 20 feet what a person with normal vision can read at 20 feet. The numerator is the distance from the client to the chart, and the denominator is the distance from which a person with normal vision can read the same line.
- For children who do not know the alphabet or for those who cannot read English letters, use a picture chart or an E chart.
- Newborn infants can be tested for visual acuity using light perception. The infant should blink when you shine a light into the eyes.
- To test for presbyopia, use the Jaegar chart. The person should hold the card 35 cm away from the eye and be able to read it. Test each eye separately.
- Test visual fields for peripheral vision loss. The confrontation test is a broad or gross examination of peripheral vision. Stand 2 feet from the client and at his or her level. Cover your right eye and the client's left eye with opaque cards. Tell the client to look straight at your uncovered eye. Wiggle your finger and move it slowly from the periphery into the centre between you and the client. Assuming that your own peripheral vision is good, the client should see the finger at the same time you do. Then switch to the other eye.
- Test cranial nerves III, IV, and VI (oculomotor, trochlear, and abducens).

- Test the corneal light reflex (Hirschberg test). Shine a light from a distance of 12 inches into the client's eyes and ask him or her to look straight ahead. There should be a symmetrical reflection of the light in both eyes. If not, then perform the cover test.
- The cover test: Ask the person to look forward and stare at your nose. Cover one eye while the person is staring; the other eye should maintain the stare and not jump around to fixate again. Repeat the test with the other eye.
- Diagnostic position test (the six fields of gaze): Direct the client to follow the movement of your outstretched finger with his or her eyes and without moving the head. Move your finger to the left superior oblique, left lateral, left inferior oblique, right superior oblique, right lateral, and right inferior oblique, returning to the centre each time. The eyes should move in a parallel fashion. Watch for any shaking of the eyeball (nystagmus). It is not abnormal to see it at the far lateral point.

Inspect the External Eye

- Eyebrows, eyelashes: Observe for hair distribution and the presence of scaling or lice.
- Eyelids: Observe for lid lag. The upper eyelid should cover the upper area of the iris. The lashes should approximate when closed. The skin should be without lumps, bumps, redness, or lesions.
- Eyeballs: The eyeballs should not be sunken in or protruding.
- Conjunctiva and sclera: Ask the client to look up; pull the lower lids down and inspect the conjunctiva for colour (very red may be infection, pallor may be anemia), lumps, bumps, or lesions. The sclera should be china white without lesions. In people of African descent, you may find brown macules and yellow fat deposits.
- Lacrimal apparatus: Note that the eyes are glossy and well lubricated without excess tearing. Press with your thumbs on the lacrimal gland and sac and assess for tenderness, redness, blocked ducts, and swelling.
- Cornea and lens: Shine a light on the cornea from the side and assess for any scratches or opacities.
- Iris and pupil: Note the size, shape, and equality of the pupils. Anisocoria (two different pupil sizes) occurs in 5% of the population. Test for direct and consensual pupillary light reflex. In a darkened area, shine a light into one eye and note the constriction of the pupil of that eye and the consensual constriction of that of the other eye. Repeat the test with the other eye.
- Accommodation: Ask the client to look at a distant object. The pupils will dilate. Then quickly get the client to focus on a close object. The pupils will constrict, and the eyeballs will converge. Record the findings as PERRLA: *P*upils *E*qual, *R*ound, *R*eact to *L*ight, and *A*ccommodation.

EAR ASSESSMENT

The ear is a sensory organ responsible for hearing and equilibrium. Cranial nerve VIII, the acoustic nerve, is responsible for the sense of hearing. There are three parts to the ear: the outer or external, middle, and inner ear. Behind the ear is a bony prominence called the *mastoid process*. In Fig. 4.1, the three parts of the ear are illustrated.

The Anatomy and Landmarks of the Ear
The External or Outer Ear

The outer ear consists of the auricle, the external auditory canal, and the tympanic membrane. The auricle, or pinna, consists of cartilage and skin. The tragus is the projection of skin-covered cartilage that is proximal to the opening (meatus) to the external canal. Sound waves enter the ear through the meatus and travel through the external canal. In the adult ear, the canal has a slight S-shape.

Cerumen (wax) is produced by small glands that line the canal. The cerumen is necessary to lubricate the canal and to protect it from foreign material. It is yellow and sticky. The wax is naturally excreted from the ear through the mechanisms of chewing and talking. Some people make more cerumen than the average person. The use of cotton swabs to clean out the cerumen is poor practice as the swab can impact, or compress, the cerumen, causing a buildup and blockage in the canal. It is better to dissolve excessive cerumen with a few drops of olive oil in the ear at night, sealed with a small cotton ball at the meatus.

At the end of the external canal is the tympanic membrane. Commonly known as the *eardrum*, the tympanic membrane is the dividing line between the external and middle ear. It is translucent and pearly grey in colour. It is possible to see parts of the malleus bone (umbo, manubrium, and short process) through the membrane of the middle ear. The tympanic membrane will bulge out into the external canal if there is an excess of fluid or exudate in the middle ear. If there is an infection in the middle ear, the membrane will be a red colour. A blockage of the tympanic membrane with either fluid or exudate will impair hearing. For the young child, when language development is so important, a decrease in hearing can be very detrimental.

The Middle Ear

The middle ear consists of the small ear bones and is a small cavity filled with air. The middle ear has three functions: protection of the inner ear from loud sound by reducing the amplitude; conducting sound waves through the vibration of the three little bones (malleus, incus, and stapes) to the inner ear through the oval window; and maintaining equalization of pressure on either side of the membrane using the eustachian tube. The eustachian tube connects the middle ear to the nasopharynx. The eustachian tube is shorter and straighter in infants and small children, giving rise to an increased risk of middle-ear infections in that population.

The Inner Ear

The inner ear consists of the bony labyrinth that contains the vestibule and the semicircular canals. The cochlea, which is the central hearing apparatus, is also present in the inner

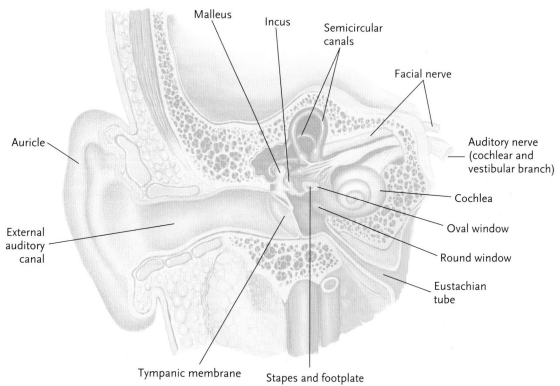

Fig. 4.1 Anatomy of the ear. (From Seidel, H. M., Ball, J. W., Dains, J. E., et al. [2011]. *Mosby's guide to physical examination* [7th ed., p. 298, Figure 12-2]. St. Louis: Mosby.)

ear. The sensory organs for hearing and equilibrium are within the inner ear.

Sound vibrations continue from the middle ear into the inner ear and into the cochlea. Basilar membranes vibrate depending on the frequency of the sound. Along the basilar membrane are receptor hair cells of the organ of Corti. As the hairs bend, the vibration is transformed into electrical impulses that cranial nerve VIII (the acoustic nerve) can transmit to the brainstem. In the cortex, the sound is interpreted.

Hearing can be divided into two types: conductive hearing, through both air and bone, and sensorineural hearing. Conductive hearing loss is a mechanical dysfunction in the outer or middle ear. It might be a blockage in the canal or, in the adult, a hardening of the footplate of the stapes so that it becomes fixed and cannot vibrate. In the older adult, the cilia lining the ear canal can become coarse and stiff, decreasing the conduction of sound waves through the canal.

Sensorineural hearing loss occurs when there is gradual nerve degeneration of the acoustic nerve. This starts at approximately 50 years of age and gets progressively worse. At 70 years of age, the transmission time for the sound to travel to the brain slows, which decreases the reaction time for older adults.

There can also be a mixed hearing loss. This loss is a combination of conductive and sensorineural hearing loss.

Subjective Data Specific to the Ear

- Do you have any pain in your ear?
- Do you have a history of ear infections, recent or as a child?
- Have you noticed that your child is having any difficulty hearing or is talking unusually loudly?
- Have you ever had surgery on your ear?
- Do you have any discharge coming out of your ear? If so, what colour is it? Does it have an odour?
- Do you have any trouble hearing? If so, is this new for you?
- Do you experience any excess noise at home, at work, or during leisure activities?
- Do you notice any ringing in your ear?
- Have you ever taken a drug called CISplatin (Platinol AQ)?
- Are you taking any medication?
- Do you have any allergies?
- Are you experiencing any vertigo or dizziness?
- Do you feel as if the room is spinning around or that you are spinning around?
- When was your last hearing test?
- Do you wear any hearing aids?

Objective Data Specific to the Ear
Inspect and Palpate the Outer Ear

- Assess the size, shape, and position of the ears. They should be symmetrical and positioned in line with the eye from the top of the ear. Inspect and palpate the skin for colour, lumps, bumps, or lesions. Note the edge of the helix for basal cell carcinoma.
- Assess the ear for tenderness: Press on the tragus to test for possible otitis media and wiggle the auricle for possible otitis externa. Palpate the mastoid process for any tenderness.

Tests for Hearing Acuity

There are three tests for hearing acuity: the whispered voice test, Weber test, and Rinne test. These are all crude tests, and, if positive, the client will have to be seen for more thorough tests.

- The whispered voice test: Ask the client to repeat after you two-syllable words that you whisper 30–60 cm from one ear while the other ear is occluded. Repeat with the other ear. A whisper is a high-pitched sound. The inability to hear it shows some high-tone loss.
- Weber test: Hit the tuning fork, taking care to hold it at the base of the handle, and place it in the middle of the head. If that is not possible, place it anywhere down the midline on a bone, such as on the forehead or chin. The sound should be heard by the client equilaterally in both ears. If there is lateralization of the sound, then the ear that hears the sound more loudly may have conductive or sensorineural loss.
- Rinne test: This test compares bone conduction with air conduction. Air conduction should take twice as long as bone conduction. To test bone conduction, hit the tuning fork, place the base onto the client's mastoid process, and say, "Can you hear this? (Yes!) Tell me when you cannot hear it anymore," and then start counting. When the client cannot hear it, place the tip of the tuning fork to the opening of the ear canal to test air conduction. Do this quickly and avoid touching the hair or skin of the client. Repeat the same question and count again. The air conduction count should be twice as long as the bone conduction count.

Testing for Balance

The Romberg test is used to assess for altered equilibrium.

- Ask the client to stand with arms at his or her sides and close his or her eyes for 20 seconds. Stand close to the client in case he or she loses balance. The Romberg test also assesses the function of the cerebellum.

NOSE, MOUTH, AND THROAT ASSESSMENT

Anatomy and Landmarks of the Nose

The nose is the beginning of the airway. It has several functions apart from being a distinguishing feature on a person's face. The nose is rich in blood supply so that it can warm up the outside air before the air travels into the lungs. The hairs in the nose trap and filter large airborne particles, and the mucosal lining traps fine airborne particles before they travel into the lungs. With age, the nasal hairs can become coarse and stiff and not filter as well.

The nasal cavity is split down the centre by the nasal septum. Kiesselbach's plexus is in the anterior of the septum. It is very rich in blood supply and is the most common area for nosebleeds. The septum can be misaligned in some people, making it difficult to breathe from one nare or the other. Along the walls of each nasal cavity lie the turbinates. The sinuses and nasolacrimal duct drain into the turbinates.

The olfactory receptors are spread across the upper area of the cavity and along the upper third of the septum. The receptors merge into cranial nerve I, the olfactory nerve, which is responsible for smell. Without the sense of smell, it is difficult to taste. Over time, the number of receptors can decrease, reducing the sense of smell.

Paranasal sinuses are located in the cranium. They are air-filled spaces that aerate the head, keeping it light. When they get filled with mucus, the head feels heavy. The sinus ducts are in the nose and can get blocked, increasing the chance of sinusitis.

There are four sets of sinuses. The ethmoid sinuses are behind the orbits, and the sphenoid sinuses are deep within the sphenoid bone. These are not possible to examine without medical imaging. The maxillary sinuses, which are behind the upper cheeks under the orbits, and the frontal sinuses, which are above the medial aspect of the eyebrow, are easier to access. The frontal and maxillary sinuses are not present at birth but grow from the age of 6–8 years. The sphenoid sinus, although present at birth, does not grow until after puberty.

Anatomy and Landmarks of the Mouth

The mouth is also an opening for the respiratory system, but more importantly, it is the opening to and the beginning of the digestive system. Within the mouth are the tongue, gums (gingiva), buccal and lingual mucosa, teeth, and salivary glands. The lips frame the opening of the mouth.

The roof of the mouth is divided into the hard palate (anterior) and the soft palate. The uvula hangs from the soft palate at the back of the mouth. In the infant, the lip or palate might not have approximated, leaving a cleft, a condition more common in people of Asian and Indigenous descent, up to 50% of whom have a bony ridge, called the *torsus palatinus*, that runs along the hard palate.

The tongue is a mass of muscle tissue that has the ability to move and change shape. It helps in speech, chewing, swallowing, and cleaning the teeth. The taste buds are embedded into the tongue. The frenulum is a midline fold of tissue that joins the bottom of the tongue to the floor of the mouth. When children start to talk, it is noticeable if the frenulum is too short. This tongue-tied situation usually corrects itself, or the frenulum may need to be clipped to loosen it.

Over a lifetime, humans develop two sets of teeth. The first set contains 20 teeth that start to erupt between 6 months and 2½ years and fall out between 6 and 12 years. They are replaced by 32 permanent teeth. With age, teeth or gums that are not well cared for may develop tooth decay or gingivitis, which can lead to tooth loss. Bone resorption may also occur. Without teeth, the older adult may experience changes in nutrition because of an inability to chew properly.

The salivary glands provide lubrication to the mouth, which is very important in speech, cleaning the teeth, and digestion. There are three sets of salivary glands. The largest are the parotid glands. The parotid glands can be found in the cheeks, anterior to and slightly below the tragus of the ears. The duct of this gland, Stensen's duct, can be found on the upper outer area of the buccal mucosa. The submandibular gland can be found where the mandible and upper jaw meet. The opening, Wharton's duct, is on either side of the frenulum. The sublingual gland is on the anterior floor of the mouth and has many openings beside it.

Anatomy and Landmarks of the Throat

Behind the mouth and the nose is the pharynx, or the throat. It is divided into the nasopharynx behind the nose, where the eustachian tubes drain and the adenoids are located, and the oropharynx, which is continuous with the mouth and contains the tonsils.

Subjective Data Specific to the Nose, Mouth, and Throat

- Are you experiencing any discharge from the nose?
- Do you get colds often? Are you experiencing any pain in the sinus area?
- Do you get nosebleeds often?
- Do you have any allergies?
- Are you taking any medications?
- Have you ever had any trauma to the nose, mouth, or throat?
- Have you ever had any surgery to the nose, mouth, or throat?
- Have you had any change in smell or taste?
- Do you have any sores in your mouth?
- Do you have a sore throat? If yes, do you have any cold symptoms?
- Do your gums bleed?
- Has there been any change to your voice?
- Do you have any difficulty swallowing?
- Is your mouth unusually dry? Do you smoke or drink alcohol? When was your last visit to the dentist?
- How often do you brush your teeth?
- Do you have any dentures or removable teeth?
- Do you grind your teeth?

Objective Data Specific to the Nose, Mouth, and Throat

Inspect and Palpate the Nose

- Inspect the nose for symmetry and to see if it is without deviation. Inspect the skin for any lumps, bumps, or lesions. Check patency by getting the client to close one nostril and breathe through the other. Repeat with the other nostril.
- Test cranial nerve I: Ask the client to close one nostril again and to close the eyes while you introduce something for the client to smell. Ask the client to identify the scent. Repeat with the other nostril and another scent.
- Inspect the nasal cavity with a speculum and a light source. Look at the turbinates. If the client has a cold, the turbinates will be reddened, and if the client has allergies, the turbinates will have a grey-lavender hue. In some clients, the turbinates will look corroded, particularly if the client has been using cocaine. Other causes of corrosion include the overuse of decongestants, foreign objects in the nose,

or nasal trauma. Note any deviation or holes in the septum, foreign bodies, polyps, swelling, or discharge.

Inspect and Palpate the Sinuses, Mouth, and Throat

- Palpate or gently tap over the sinus areas and assess for pain.
- Inspect the lips inside and out. Note any cracking, swelling, or lesions. In infants, it is normal to see a sucking tubercle caused by the friction of sucking on the breast or bottle.
- Inspect the teeth for any large caries; check for signs of bone resorption, gingivitis, or missing teeth and observe the gum line and buccal and lingual mucosa. In small children, assess for "baby bottle syndrome," in which the front teeth have been destroyed by the baby sucking on sugary fluid such as juice or sugar water. With a glove on, palpate the mucosa for lumps, bumps, and lesions. Assess the salivary ducts.
- Check cranial nerves IX and X, the glossopharyngeal and vagus nerves. Using a tongue depressor and light source, ask the client to say "Ahhh" and watch for the soft palate and the uvula to move up and back in the mouth. Then move the tongue depressor back quickly to elicit a gag response.
- Inspect the tonsils for closeness to each other and for exudate. Rate the tonsils 1+ = visible, 2+ = halfway between the tonsillar pillars and the uvula, 3+ = touching the uvula, or 4+ = touching each other.
- Test cranial nerve XII, the hypoglossal nerve. Ask the client to say "light," "tight," and "dynamite" to assess for the client's lingual speech. Instruct the client to push the tongue into the cheek against the resistance of your hand outside on the face to check tongue strength. Repeat on the other side. Ask the client to stick out the tongue and inspect it for fissures, colour, and symmetry.

RESPIRATORY ASSESSMENT

Anatomy and Landmarks of the Thorax and Lungs

The function of the respiratory system is to provide a gas exchange that supplies oxygen to the body for energy production and that removes carbon dioxide. It also maintains an acid–base equilibrium of the arterial blood. In addition, respiration helps to regulate the heat of the body, although less so in humans than in animals.

The thoracic cage is composed of the clavicle, sternum, ribs, scapulae, and vertebrae. The floor of the thoracic cage is the diaphragm. The function of the thoracic cage is to give shape to the body and to protect the organs found within, such as the lungs, heart, and liver. The chest is larger in people of European and African descent than in people of Asian and Indigenous descent.

The anterior landmarks include the clavicle on either side at the top. Between the clavicles is the top of the sternum, the manubrium. Just below the manubrium, where the sternum joins, is the manubriosternal notch, or angle of Louis. The notch protrudes slightly and is the landmark for the second rib and where the trachea bifurcates. The sternum, or breast bone, is connected to the first seven of the 12 pairs of ribs. The costal angle should be 90°. This is the angle between the costal margins; the xiphoid process is in the middle.

The posterior landmarks include the seven cervical vertebrae, the vertebra prominens, the scapulae—where the inferior border is at the level of the eighth rib—and the thoracic vertebrae. The spinous processes stick out, making it easier to count them. The twelfth, or floating, rib is not present on the anterior side. See Fig. 4.2 for illustrations of the anterior cage and the posterior thoracic cage.

It is important to imagine and understand the landmark lines on the thoracic cage. They are as follows:

- Midsternal line—the line along the sternum
- Midclavicular line—a vertical line down from the middle of the clavicle
- Anterior axillary line—a vertical line down from the anterior axillary fold
- Posterior axillary line—a vertical line down from the posterior axillary fold
- Midaxillary line—a vertical line from the apex of the axilla

A   **Anterior view**

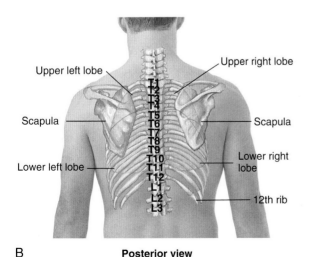

B   **Posterior view**

Fig. 4.2 Anatomy of the thoracic cage. **A,** Anterior view; **B,** Posterior view. (From Wilson, S. F., & Giddens, J. F. [2017]. *Health assessment for nursing practice* [6th ed., p. 183, Fig. 11-3]. St. Louis: Elsevier.)

The lung borders. Looking from the anterior, the apex of each lung is 3 cm above the clavicle. From an anterior perspective, the upper right lobe extends down to the fourth rib at the sternum and the fifth rib at the anterior axillary line. The right middle lobe extends from the fourth rib at the sternum and the fifth rib at the anterior axillary line down to the sixth rib at the midclavicular line. The right lower lobe extends from the fifth rib at the anterior axillary line down to the sixth rib at the midclavicular line and to the seventh rib at the anterior axillary line.

From a posterior perspective, the right and left upper lobes start at the level of cervical vertebra C7 and down to thoracic vertebra 10 (T10) on inspiration and T12 on expiration.

The pleurae. There is a thin, slippery layer lining the chest wall and diaphragm called the *parietal pleura* and one lining the outside of the lungs called the *visceral pleura*. Between these linings is a very small amount of lubricating fluid to help the lungs move smoothly and noiselessly with the movement of respiration. There is normally vacuum pressure between these two layers. Any additional fluid or air between these pleural layers will compromise the expansion of the lungs and hence air exchange.

Air enters the mouth or nose and travels down the trachea, which bifurcates just below the sternal angle, and into the bronchioles, the alveolar ducts and sacs, and, finally, the alveoli. Gas exchange occurs in the alveoli. These are protected from debris by the bronchi, which have goblet cells that secrete mucus to trap debris and cilia that move the debris upward, where it can then be swallowed or coughed out of the mouth.

The control of respiration occurs in the respiratory centre in the brainstem, specifically in the pons and medulla. The need for respirations is guided by an increase in carbon dioxide in the blood and less so by a decrease in oxygen.

With each inspiration, the diaphragm moves down, causing a slight negative pressure relative to the atmosphere outside the body, which results in air rushing in to fill the vacuum. Expiration is more passive.

In infants, the rib cage is more elastic; this increases the work of breathing when the chest is recoiling and re-expanding during episodes of respiratory distress.

In the older adult, there can be calcification of the costal cartilage and a loss of elasticity of the lung tissue, decreasing its ability to recoil. There is also a decrease in the number of alveoli, causing an equivalent decrease in gas exchange. This leaves the older adult at a higher risk for infection, a weakened cough reflex, increased secretions, and dyspnea on exertion.

Subjective Data Specific to the Thorax and Lungs

- Do you have a cough? If so, does a change in position change the cough? If you have a cough, is the cough productive? If so, what colour is the sputum?
- Are you experiencing any shortness of breath? Can you walk up a flight of stairs without having to stop in the middle? Do you have any chest wall pain?
- Do you have any pain on breathing?

- Have you had problems with your respiratory system in the past? Was it chronic or acute?
- Do you smoke? What do you smoke? How many per day and for how many years?
- Are there any environmental irritants at work or home that can affect your breathing?
- When was your last chest X-ray, tuberculosis test, and influenza or pneumonia vaccine?

Objective Data Specific to the Thorax and Lungs

Inspection of the Anterior Chest

- Assess the level of consciousness.
- Note the size and configuration of the chest. The anterior–posterior measurement should be half the length of the transverse.
- Note the musculature of the neck and chest. Is the client using the accessory muscles or the muscles of the intercostal spaces to assist in breathing? Examine the skin for colour, texture, temperature, moisture, lumps, bumps, or lesions; observe the facial expression and the use of pursed lips to breathe. Inspect the downward slope of the ribs and the presence of a 45° costal margin angle from the ribs to the xiphoid process. Check the respiratory rate, depth, and ease.

Palpation of the Anterior Chest

- Palpate the anterior chest wall for skin temperature, moisture, texture, turgor, lumps, bumps, tenderness, or pain.
- Symmetrical chest expansion: With your hands shaped like a butterfly, rest them on the chest along the costal margins, capture a bit of skin and fat in the middle of the chest at the xiphoid process with your thumbs, and ask the client to breathe. The chest wall should move symmetrically, your thumbs should move an equal distance apart, and the fold of fat and skin should flatten.
- Assess for tactile fremitus, which is a palpable vibration, by asking the client to say "99" every time you move your hand. You can use either the ulnar edge of the hand or the bottom of the fingers on the palm to assess for vibration. Place your hands symmetrically at the area just above the clavicle and move down the chest at 5-cm intervals. You should feel vibration at the top, and it should diminish quickly as you test further down the chest wall.

Auscultation of the Anterior Chest

- Auscultate the lungs. Say to the client, "Every time that I move my stethoscope, I would like you to take a breath." This will give you control over the examination, and you will be able to hear the complete breath sound. Follow the same pattern as that for percussion.
- Listen to the complete breath sound—a complete inspiration and expiration—as a wheeze might only be audible at the end of the expiration. There should be tracheal breath sounds over the trachea, bronchovesicular sounds over the bronchi, and vesicular sounds over the rest of the chest.
- Listen for abnormal or adventitious sounds, including wheezing, stridor, crackles, and pleural friction.

- If the breath sounds are abnormal, then assess voice sounds. Bronchophony, egophony, and whispered pectoriloquy are examples of voice sounds.

Inspection of the Posterior Chest

- Inspect the posterior chest.
- Assess the curvature of the spine. Ask the client to bend over at the waist and look at the scapulae. Are the scapulae symmetrical?
- Is the client using the accessory muscles or the muscles of the intercostal spaces to assist in breathing?
- Examine the skin for colour, texture, temperature, moisture, lumps, bumps, or lesions. Carefully inspect the skin for the presence of moles. The client might not be aware of these, and they should be monitored for any change in size, shape, and appearance.

Palpation of the Posterior Chest

- Palpate the posterior chest wall for skin temperature, moisture, texture, turgor, lumps, bumps, tenderness, or pain.
- Palpate for symmetrical chest expansion: With your hands shaped like a butterfly, rest your hands on the chest along the costal margins at the level of T10, capture a bit of skin and fat in the middle of the back with your thumbs, and ask the client to breathe. The chest wall should move symmetrically, your thumbs should move apart an equal distance, and the fold of fat and skin should flatten.
- Assess for tactile fremitus by asking the client to say "99" every time you move your hand. You can use either the ulnar edge of the hand or the bottom of the fingers on the palm to assess for vibration. Place your hands symmetrically at the area of the vertebral prominens, C7, and move down the chest in 5-cm intervals. You should feel vibration at the top, and it should diminish quickly as you test further down the back. Increased vibration can mean a density of some kind, such as a tumour.

Auscultation of the Posterior Chest

- Auscultate the lung tissue on the back. There should be bronchovesicular sounds from C7 to T5 in the centre of the back. The sounds over the rest of the lungs should be vesicular sounds. Listen for any abnormal or adventitious sounds.

ANATOMY AND LANDMARKS OF THE BREASTS AND REGIONAL LYMPHATICS

The breasts, or mammary glands, can be found anterior to the pectoralis major muscles and the serratus muscles in both males and females. They lie between the second and the sixth ribs, the sternum medially, and the tail of Spence and midaxillary line laterally.

For females, the breasts serve as part of the reproductive system. Their function is to produce milk for the newborn. The nipple is just below the centre of the breast, and around it is the areola, a darker pigmented area. Within the areola are

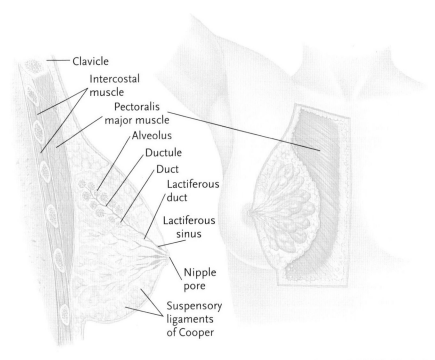

Fig. 4.3 Anatomy of the breast. (From Seidel, H. M., Ball, J. W., Dains, J. E., et al. [2011]. *Mosby's guide to physical examination* [7th ed., p. 457, Figure 16-1]. St. Louis: Mosby.)

Montgomery's glands, which lubricate the areola during lactation.

Internally, the breasts are composed of glandular tissue, fibrous tissue, and adipose tissue. The glandular tissue produces the milk in lobules, and it is excreted through a series of ducts. The fibrous tissue, including Cooper's ligaments, supports the breast tissue and attaches it to the chest wall. Cooper's ligaments contract with the presence of cancer, causing a dimpling effect on the skin. With age, the elasticity of these ligaments decreases and with it the support of the breast. An illustration of the anatomy of the breast is shown in Fig. 4.3.

There is an extensive network of lymph nodes and vessels around the breast area. There are four groups of nodes: the central axillary nodes, the pectoral nodes, the subscapular nodes, and the lateral nodes.

Breast cancer is the second cause of cancer death in women. Early detection and treatment can decrease the mortality rate. The risk factors for breast cancer are as follows: increase in age, nulliparous, not breastfeeding, increased fat in the diet, postmenopausal hormone therapy, family history of breast cancer, a positive *BRCA1* or *BRCA2* blood test, and a first child born after age 30.

Subjective Data Specific to the Breasts and Regional Lymphatics

*Specific questions for the older woman
^Specific questions for the adolescent girl

- Do you have any pain in the breast area?
- Have you noticed any discharge from your nipple?
- Have you noticed any lumps in your breast or under your arm?

- Have you noticed any swelling in one or both of your breasts?
- Have you noticed any skin changes to your breast, such as a rash or an "orange-skin" appearance?
- Has there been any recent trauma to either of your breasts?
- Do you have any history of breast disease?
- When did you experience menarche?
* **When did you start menopause?**
* **Have you taken hormone replacement therapy?**
- How many pregnancies or live births have you had?
- Did you breastfeed your children? If yes, for how long?
- Do you have any family history of breast disease?
- Did you ever have surgery to your breast or underarm?
- Do you perform breast self-examination? If yes, how often?
* **When was your last mammogram?**
^ **Have you noticed any change in your breasts?**
^ **Is there anyone you can talk to about the changes in your body?**

Objective Data Specific to the Breasts and Regional Lymphatics
Inspection of the Breast and Lymphatics
- Note the general appearance of the breasts.
- Inspect for symmetry and symmetrical movement. Ask the client to raise her arms sideways, in front, and above her head. Ask the client to place her hands together and squeeze the chest muscles. Assess for any pulling or dimpling of the skin. Inspect the skin for the look of peau d'orange ("orange-peel" skin).
- Inspect the skin for areas of redness, lumps, bumps, or lesions.

- Inspect the nipple for colour, discharge, and the presence of a supernumerary nipple (extra nipple).

Palpation of the Breast and Lymphatics

- Palpate the axilla for lymph nodes. Rest the client's right forearm on your right forearm and hold the elbow with your right hand. You now have full manoeuvrability of the right arm. Move it up, down, and side to side while palpating the right axilla with your left hand. Repeat the examination on the other side. You do not want the muscles to be taut, as a tight muscle will prevent the subtle palpation of the underlying lymph nodes. Imagine dividing the breast tissue into a pattern such as the spokes of a wheel. With the pads of your fingertips and in a circular motion, palpate throughout the entire breast. Do not poke at the tissue; a breast lump might be very difficult to feel, and poking it will only push it deeper.
- Repeat the palpation with the woman lying down. Raise her arm over her head and assess the axilla again. If you find a lump, assess the size, texture, shape, position, and whether or not it is tender.
- Gently squeeze the nipple and look for any discharge.
- For the male client, inspect and palpate the breast and assess for signs of gynecomastia.

HEART AND NECK VESSEL ASSESSMENT

Anatomy and Landmarks of the Heart

The heart is a mechanical pump that pumps blood through two different circulations: the pulmonary circulation and the systemic circulation. The pulmonary circulation brings blood to the lungs via the pulmonary arteries. Here gas exchange occurs, oxygenating the blood and ridding the body of carbon dioxide. The pulmonary circulation then returns the oxygen-rich blood to the heart via the pulmonary veins. At this point, the systemic circulation takes the oxygen-rich blood and pumps it around the body via the systemic arteries. The blood leaves the heart via the aorta and returns to the heart via the systemic veins, entering the inferior and superior vena cava and re-entering the pulmonary circulation. The cycle is continuous.

The heart is upside down, with the apex at the bottom. It can be found at the fifth intercostal space, 7–9 cm from the midsternal border. The base of the heart, which is wider than the apex, can be found at the top of the heart by the second intercostal space. The heart is rotated slightly so that the right side is more anterior and the left side is more posterior. In an infant, the heart is more midline and assumes the adult position when the child is 6 years old.

The heart wall comprises three layers. The pericardium is the outermost and is divided into two layers with a small amount of pericardial fluid in between so that there is smooth movement of the heart muscle. The pericardium is a tough, fibrous, protective layer. The myocardium is the muscle of the heart. The endocardium is the inner lining of the heart chambers (ventricles and atria) and the valves. There are four chambers in the heart: two ventricles and two atria. Valves divide the chambers so that there is no backflow of the blood. The right atrioventricular (AV) valve is the tricuspid valve and the left is the mitral valve. The AV valves open during the diastole so the ventricles can fill. The systole occurs when the pulmonic and aortic valves (semilunar valves) open to allow the blood to be pumped out of the heart. An illustration of the heart anatomy is shown in Fig. 4.4.

The first heart sound, S_1, occurs with the closure of the AV valves. This sound can be heard loudest using the diaphragm of the stethoscope over the apex of the heart. The second sound, S_2, occurs at the end of systole, when the semilunar valves close, and can be heard best at the base of the heart. The S_3 sound is an abnormal sound that occurs with vibration at ventricular filling and can be heard immediately after S_2. S_4 occurs just before S_1 when there is resistance to the ventricles accepting the blood from the atrium.

A murmur is the sound of turbulent blood flow through the valves of the heart. This can happen from increased speed of the blood through the heart from, for example, exercise, a decrease in blood viscosity, structural defects in the valves, or structural defects on the wall of the chambers.

The heart has its own conduction system. The pacemaker is the sinoatrial node that is located near the superior vena cava and starts the conduction. It is then passed on over the atria to the AV node that is low in the atrial septum. After waiting for the atria to contract, the electrical current then moves on to the bundle of histidine (His) and then over the ventricles.

Anatomy and Landmarks of the Neck Vessels

The neck vessels include the two carotid arteries that supply the brain with blood. They are considered central arteries as they are the closest to the heart. The pulsation of the carotid artery can be found at the space between the sternomastoid muscle and the trachea. Each side should be palpated separately as you do not want to cut off all blood supply to the brain.

The jugular veins bring unoxygenated blood to the heart via the superior vena cava. If they flutter or oscillate, the jugular vein pulsations may indicate a problem with the pumping efficiency of the right side of the heart. The right external jugular vein can be seen lateral to the sternomastoid muscle, just above the clavicle, and is the easiest of the jugular veins to see.

Risk factors for heart disease and stroke are smoking, high blood pressure, obesity, sedentary lifestyle, diabetes, high serum cholesterol, and stress. Adults of African descent have a higher risk of heart disease and stroke than any other group.

Subjective Data Specific to the Heart and Neck Vessels

*Specific questions for the older woman
  ^Specific questions concerning the child
- Do you experience any chest pain?
- Do you take nitroglycerine pills?
- Do you have any shortness of breath?
- How many pillows do you use at night to sleep?
- Do you have a cough? Is the cough worse at night?

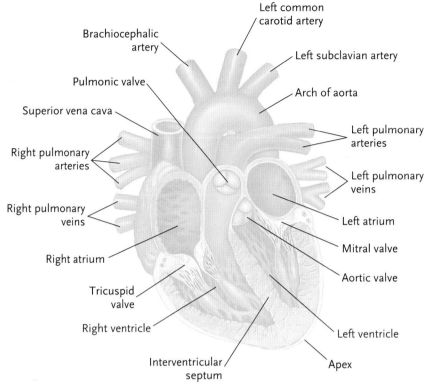

Fig. 4.4 Anatomy of the heart. (From Seidel, H. M., Ball, J. W., Dains, J. E., et al. [2011]. *Mosby's guide to physical examination* [7th ed., p. 386, Figure 14-10]. St. Louis: Mosby.)

- Do you get tired easily?
- Have you or your family noticed any change in your skin colour?
- Have you noticed any puffiness around your eyes or in your feet and ankles?
- How many times do you wake up in the middle of the night to urinate?
- Do you or any family members have a history of heart disease?
- ∧ **Were the pregnancy, labour, and delivery normal?**
- ∧ **Does the baby turn blue when feeding?**
- ∧ **Have you noticed any growth or mobility problems?**
- ∧ **Is the child able to participate in regular activities and sports at school?**
- ∧ **Does the child have frequent nosebleeds?**
- ∧ **Has the child complained of unexplained joint or bone pain?**
- ∧ **Does the child have an increased number of colds or streptococcal infections?**
- * **Do you have any lung disease?**
- * **Do you have to climb stairs at home? Can you manage climbing them?**
- Cardiac risk factors:
  - Please describe your normal daily diet.
  - Do you smoke? What, how many, and for how long?
  - Do you drink alcohol? How much, how often, and for how long?
  - Do you exercise? How often, what type of exercise, and for how long?

- Do you take any cardiac drugs or birth control pills? Which ones, for how long, and how much do you take?

Objective Data Specific to the Heart and Neck Vessels

Explain to the client that you are going to listen to the heart in many places and that they should not become alarmed if you are listening for a long time. Take the client's blood pressure. If you suspect orthostatic hypotension, take the blood pressure when the client is lying down and again quickly when the client sits up. Note any fall in pressure between the two positions.

Palpation of the Neck Vessels

- Palpate the carotid arteries; assess the amplitude, strength, and contour of the pulse.

Inspection of the Precordium

- Inspect the anterior chest. Look for any heaves or bulges.
- Find the apical pulse at the fifth intercostal space, mid-clavicular line. If you cannot see the apical pulse, palpate it. If that is difficult, ask the client to lie on his or her left side or to sit up and lean forward so that the heart moves closer to the chest wall and palpate again.
- Palpate the skin for lumps, bumps, lesions, and tenderness or pain.

Auscultation of the Precordium

- With the diaphragm of the stethoscope, auscultate the aortic valve at the second right intercostal space, the pulmonic valve at the second left intercostal space, the tricuspid valve at the left lower sternal border, the mitral valve at the fifth intercostal space midclavicular line, and Erb's point, located at the fourth intercostal space.

- Listen to the normal heart sounds, S_1 at the tricuspid and mitral valve region and S_2 at the aortic and pulmonic valves, and for the abnormal sounds, S_3 and S_4.
- Listen to the apical pulse for 1 minute.
- Feel the carotid pulse while listening to the S_1 sounds. They should match in rhythm and rate.

PERIPHERAL VASCULAR AND LYMPHATIC SYSTEMS ASSESSMENT

Anatomy and Landmarks of the Peripheral Vascular and Lymphatic Systems

The peripheral vascular system is made up of the blood vessels that travel away from and toward the heart. The lymphatic system runs parallel to the circulatory system. The arteries in the blood provide the tissues with oxygen and nutrients, and the veins act as a transport for the unoxygenated blood to go back to the heart and lungs to start the cycle again.

The arteries will have a pulse as the blood flows in a wave-like pattern with the recoil and expansion of the vessel. The pulse areas are brachial, ulnar, radial, femoral, popliteal, posterior tibialis, and dorsalis pedis.

Ischemia is the lack of blood flow to the tissues. It is usually caused by a blockage in the artery. When the client exercises and the tissues need a greater supply of oxygen and nutrients, more pain will occur from the ischemia. If the blockage is complete, the distal cells will die.

There are two sets of veins: the deep veins and the superficial veins. In addition, the perforators are small veins that join these two types together. As long as the deep veins are working well, the superficial, saphenous, veins can be removed safely.

The skeletal muscles assist in pushing the blood back to the heart by contracting and relaxing. There are also valves that prevent the backflow of the blood.

In the older adult, the veins and arteries may occlude partially or fully due to atherosclerosis or arteriosclerosis. Prolonged bed rest, long airplane flights or sitting, cancer, and the birth control pill increase the risk of a deep vein thrombosis, which, if it breaks off, can lead to a myocardial infarction or a stroke.

The lymphatic system runs alongside the blood system. It is responsible for returning the excess fluid and proteins from the interstitial tissues to the blood. It is also responsible for collecting waste products, supporting the immune system, and collecting lipids from the intestinal tract.

The easiest lymph nodes to feel are the cervical, axillary, epitrochlear, and inguinal. The nodes should not be enlarged. If they are, assess for mobility, firmness, tenderness, and matting. Check proximally for signs of infection. Cancerous nodes are usually firm, nontender, and fixed, and if advanced, they can be matted. The spleen, tonsils, and thymus are also part of the lymphatic immune system. It is not unusual for children to have small, shoddy nodes that are not pathological.

Subjective Data Specific to the Peripheral Vascular and Lymphatic Systems

- Have you noticed any pain in your legs, especially the calves? If yes, does it become worse when you walk?
- Has there been any swelling in your legs or arms or puffiness around your eyes? If so, is the swelling worse in the evening?
- Do you have any skin sores that have not healed in a reasonable amount of time?
- Has there been any change in the temperature or hair distribution on one of your extremities?
- Have you felt any swollen glands?
- Do you have a history of cardiac disease, diabetes, high blood pressure, or pregnancy?
- Do you smoke? If so, how much and how often?
- Are you on any medication?

Objective Data Specific to the Peripheral Vascular and Lymphatic Systems

Inspection and Palpation of the Peripheral Vascular and Lymphatic Systems

- Inspect and palpate the arms for skin colour, texture, condition, temperature, and symmetry.
- Take vital signs, including brachial, radial, and ulnar pulses.
- Assess pulses for rate, symmetry, rhythm, and amplitude.
- Inspect nails for profile sign to assess for clubbing and measure the capillary refill. It should be less than 3 seconds.
- Inspect and palpate the legs for skin colour, texture, condition, and temperature, as well as for symmetry.
- Palpate the femoral, popliteal, posterior tibial, and dorsalis pedis pulses.
- Measure the calf circumference for symmetry, and if the measurement is off by more than 1 cm, refer the client for deep vein thrombosis assessment.
- Palpate the skin for edema starting from the ankle and moving your way up the leg. If edema is present, measure the distance of the edema from the knee. Inspect the backs of the legs for varicosities, especially in pregnant women or women who have had multiple pregnancies. Inspect the skin for hair distribution. In the older adult, there may be a decrease in hair growth and peripheral pulses, and the skin can become shiny and thin. These are normal signs of aging caused by a decrease in arterial circulation.

ABDOMINAL ASSESSMENT

Anatomy and Landmarks of the Abdomen

The abdomen is a large cavity that extends from the diaphragm at the top to the pelvis at the bottom, to the vertebra and paravertebral muscles in the back, and to the lower ribs and abdominal muscles in the front.

There are four abdominal muscles, including the rectus abdominis, which is joined along the midline by the linea alba (Fig. 4.5, *A*). The umbilicus is the midpoint in the abdomen.

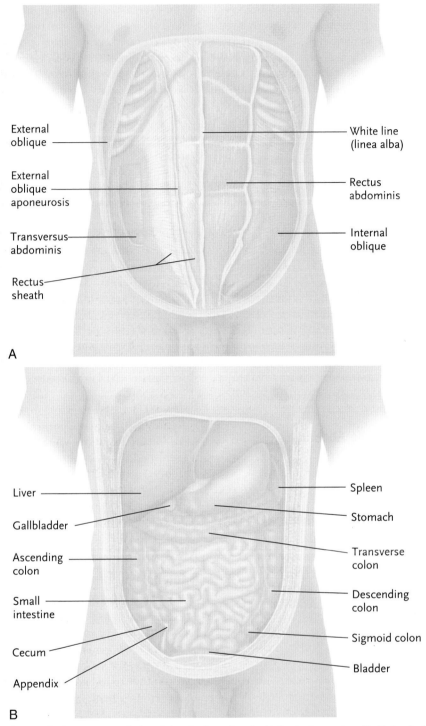

Fig. 4.5 Anatomical structures of the abdominal cavity. A, Abdominal muscles; **B,** Abdominal organs. (From Seidel, H. M., Ball, J. W., Dains, J. E., et al. [2011]. *Mosby's guide to physical examination* [7th ed., p. 485, Figure 17-1]. St. Louis: Mosby.)

It should be slightly inverted and uniform in colour with the rest of the skin. With abdominal bleeding, the blood can be seen around the umbilicus; it will have a blue circle around it called Cullen's sign. In the newborn, the umbilicus is very pronounced. The clamp and the extra tissue will turn black and fall off a few days after birth.

The contour of the abdomen varies. There are flat, round, protuberant, and scaphoid shapes. The first two are normal; the scaphoid shape can be a sign of malnutrition, and the protuberant shape can be a sign of obesity or ascites.

Within the abdominal cavity are many viscera. The solid viscera include the liver, which can be found in the upper right quadrant above the costal margin; the spleen, which should normally be posterior to the left midaxillary line parallel to the tenth rib; the pancreas, which is behind the stomach; the kidneys, which are retroperitoneal along the eleventh and twelfth ribs for the left one and slightly lower for the right; the adrenal glands, which are on top of the kidneys; the aorta, which is just left of the midline at the upper part of the abdomen and extends down to 2 cm above the umbilicus, where it bifurcates into the iliac arteries; and the ovaries and uterus, which are in the lower abdomen and pelvis. The liver decreases in size with age, especially after 80 years, even though the function remains normal, except for drug metabolism. In the newborn, the liver is normally felt 0.5–2.5 cm below the costal margin.

The hollow viscera include the stomach, which is below the diaphragm midline; the small intestine, which is in all quadrants; the large intestine (colon); the gallbladder, which is posterior to the liver at the right midclavicular line; and the bladder, which is at the top of the pelvis. In the infant, the bladder is positioned higher. The ileocecal valve, where the small intestine and the colon meet, is in the right lower quadrant.

With age, there is an increased reporting of constipation. The causes of constipation (more than three days between defecation, hard stool, straining, and the feeling of incomplete emptying) include a decrease in mobility; not enough water intake; low-residue foods; adverse effects of medication; difficulty getting to a bathroom or commode; hypothyroidism; irritable bowel syndrome; and bowel obstruction. Fig. 4.5, *B*, illustrates the abdominal organs.

Subjective Data Specific to the Abdomen

*Specific questions for the older adult
^Specific questions concerning the infant

- Has there been any change to your appetite?
- What have you eaten in the last 24 hours?
- * **Who prepares your food or buys the groceries?**
- * **Do you eat alone?**
- ^ **Does the child breastfeed?**
- ^ **Have you introduced any new foods into the child's diet?**
- Have you gained or lost weight recently?
- Do you have any difficulty swallowing?
- Are there any foods that you cannot eat?
- Are you allergic to any foods?
- Are you experiencing any abdominal pain?
- Do you have any nausea or vomiting? What are you vomiting?
- How often do you have a bowel movement?
- Has there been a recent change to your bowel movements?
- Has there been any change to the consistency of the stool?
- Do you have a history of any problems with your gastrointestinal system?
- Do you take any medications?
- Do you exercise at all? If so, what do you do and for how long?

Objective Data Specific to the Abdomen
Inspection of the Abdomen

- Inspect the abdominal shape or contour. Stand at the foot of the bed and assess the shape of the abdomen. To check for symmetry and masses, shine a light across the abdomen and see if any shadows fall on the skin.
- Inspect the skin for colour, temperature, moisture, condition, texture, scars, lumps, bumps, or lesions.
- Check the umbilicus for any sign of hernia, Cullen's sign, or infection.
- Check for any pulsation and peristalsis. It is quite common to see the pulsation of the aorta.
- What is the hair distribution like? Normally, a male will have a diamond hair pattern on the abdomen, and a female will have a triangle pattern.
- Assess the position of the client. Does the client look comfortable? What is the breathing pattern like?

Auscultation of the Abdomen

Auscultate next so that the bowel sounds are accurate. Palpation and percussion will increase the sounds.

- With the diaphragm of the stethoscope, listen for up to 5 minutes in each quadrant for the tinkling sound of gas, fluid, and stool passing through the bowels. As soon as you hear and assess the bowel sound in one quadrant, move on to the next quadrant.
- Start auscultation in the lower right quadrant, the location of the ileocecal valve, as more sounds will be there.

Palpation of the Abdomen

- Lightly palpate the abdomen and assess for pain or tenderness, temperature, moisture, lumps, or bumps. Palpate any tender areas last to decrease the amount of guarding.
- If the client is ticklish, place your hand on top of the client's, start palpating, and then gently slide the client's hand out from under yours.

MUSCULO-SKELETAL SYSTEM ASSESSMENT

Anatomy and Landmarks of the Musculo-skeletal System

The musculo-skeletal system comprises the bones, muscles, and joints. The system protects the inside core of the body and keeps the body erect. Bone marrow is produced in the bone, giving rise to the blood cells. The bones also store calcium and phosphorus. Another component to this system is movement. Most of the assessment will focus on movement.

There are many joints in the body, of which there are two types: synovial and nonsynovial joints. The nonsynovial joints are fixed, while the synovial ones are movable. In the synovial joint, there is a layer of cartilage over the opposing bones, and the joint is encased with synovial fluid lubricating it. Ligaments are attached from one bone to another, adding strength to the joint. A bursa is a small synovia-filled sac that adds protection to the bone.

Muscles make up 40–50% of the body's weight. There are three types of muscles: skeletal, smooth, and cardiac. The skeletal muscles are involved with the assessable movement of the body. The muscles are attached to the bone with tendons.

When the muscles contract, they create movement. There are many different types of movement: flexion, extension, adduction, abduction, pronation, supination, circumduction, inversion, eversion, rotation, protraction, retraction, elevation, and depression.

Subjective Data Specific to the Musculo-skeletal System

*Specific questions for the older adult
^Specific questions concerning the infant

- Are you experiencing any joint pain or stiffness?
- Have you noticed any swelling or redness around your joints?
- Do you get any cramping in your muscles?
- Do you have cramping in your calf muscles when you walk?
- Have you noticed any weakness in your muscles?
- * **Has there been any change in the weakness recently?**
- * **Do you use any aids to help you walk, such as a cane or walker?**
- Do you have any bone pain?
- Have you ever broken a bone?
- Do you have any numbness or tingling sensations?
- Have you noticed any deformities in the bone?
- ^ **Has the infant progressed in a normal growth pattern?**
- * **Have you noticed that you have stumbled or fallen more over the last few months?**
- Are you involved in any exercise program?
- Are you involved in any sports?
- Do you have any difficulty getting around or maintaining your activities of daily living?
- Have you ever had surgery on your muscles, bones, or joints?
- Do you take any medication?

Objective Data Specific to the Musculo-skeletal System

Inspection and Palpation of the Musculo-skeletal System

- Perform a general inspection of the body. Can the client walk and support the body?
- Is there a general symmetry? Is the client protecting a limb?
- Inspect each joint for redness, size and contour, and deformity.
- Inspect the muscles for symmetry, size, and tone. Inspect for curvature of the spine by asking the client to bend over. The scapulae should be even, as should the buttocks, and the spine should follow a straight line down.
- Palpate each joint for temperature, pain or tenderness, swelling, and smoothness in movement.
- Perform a range-of-motion examination for all the muscles, both upper body and lower body. Watch closely for symmetry. Note any restrictions in the movement. Measure the flexion and extension with a goniometer if

you think that there is a problem. Check the muscle strength using movement against resistance.

NEUROLOGICAL SYSTEM ASSESSMENT

Anatomy and Landmarks of the Neurological System

The Central Nervous System

The neurological system can be divided into the central system, which includes the brain and the spinal cord, and the peripheral system, which includes the 12 pairs of cranial nerves and the 31 pairs of spinal nerves.

The central nervous system is complex. The brain has two hemispheres; the right side governs the left side of the body, and the left side governs the right side of the body. It is very important to always assess both sides of the body. The four lobes that make up the brain are the frontal lobe, needed for personality, intellect, emotions, and voluntary movement; the parietal lobe, responsible for sensation; the occipital lobe, which has the visual receptors; and the temporal lobe, which is the centre for hearing. Within the temporal lobe is Wernicke's area, responsible for language comprehension. In the frontal lobe, there is Broca's area, which is responsible for motor speech.

In the aging adult, there is a progressive loss of brain functioning due to a loss of neurons. Also, the speed at which information travels along the neurons decreases with age. There may also be a decrease in the amount of blood reaching the brain, as well as an increased risk of stroke, both hemorrhagic and thrombotic. The infant's nervous system is not fully developed at birth. As myelinization occurs, the nervous response increases.

The neural pathways are split between the sensory and motor pathways. The sensory ones include the spinothalamic tract, where sensations of soft touch, hot and cold, and pain are carried to the thalamus and on to the sensory cortex for interpretation. The posterior column is responsible for the sense of position, vibration, and finely localized touch.

The motor pathways are responsible for the movement and coordination of the muscles. They include the pyramidal and extrapyramidal tracts, the cerebellum, and the upper and lower motor neurons. The cerebellum is more responsible for fine motor coordination and balance.

The Peripheral Nervous System

The peripheral nervous system includes the cranial nerves, the reflexes, and the spinal nerves. There are 12 cranial nerves that enter and exit the brain. Nerves I and II extend from the cerebrum, while III–VII extend from the brainstem and diencephalons. These are both sensory and motor nerves, some of which are responsible for both.

There are 31 pairs of spinal nerves. They enter and exit from the spinal column. There are 8 cervical (arms, neck and side of the head, and top of the chest), 12 thoracic (chest and abdomen), 5 lumbar (legs), and 5 sacral (inner thigh, ankle, and groin) nerves, and 1 coccygeal nerve.

Subjective Data Specific to the Neurological System

*Specific questions for the older adult
^Specific questions concerning the infant

- Have you been experiencing frequent headaches recently?
- Did you recently have any head injury? If yes, what part of your head was hit?
- Have you been experiencing either vertigo (a spinning sensation) or dizziness (feeling faint)?
- Have you had any seizures? If so, describe them.
- Do you have any tremors? If so, are they worse with stress?
- Have you noticed any signs of tingling or numbness (pins and needles)?
- Have you noticed any weakness?
- Do you have any problems with coordination?
- Have you noticed any difficulty with speech?
- Have you noticed any difficulty with swallowing?
- Are you taking any medication?
- Do you have any allergies?
- Are there any environmental hazards at work or home?
- * **Have you or your family noticed any change in your mental function?**
- ^ **Was the labour and delivery without difficulty?**

Objective Data Specific to the Neurological System

It is important to perform a general mental survey in the neurological examination. Include an assessment of the client's appearance, behaviour, cognition, and thought processes (ABCT).

Cranial Nerve Testing

- Olfactory (I): Sensory nerve. Check for nasal patency and introduce a scent for each nostril while the client closes the eyes and smells.
- Optic (II): Sensory nerve. Use the Snellen chart and Jaeger test chart for eye acuity and the confrontation test for peripheral vision and examine the ocular fundus and optic disc with an ophthalmoscope.
- Oculomotor (III), trochlear (IV), and abducens (VI): Motor nerves. Perform the six fields of gaze test, watching for nystagmus (normal in the far lateral gaze), and check for PERRLA with direct and consensual light reaction.
- Trigeminal (V): Sensory and motor nerve. Assess for fine touch at the areas of the three branches of the nerve: the forehead, cheek, and chin on both sides. For the motor component, test the movement of the mandible (jaw) and also its movement against resistance.
- Facial (VII): Sensory and motor nerve. Test the anterior two-thirds of the tongue for taste. For the motor component, test the movement of the face by asking the client to smile, frown, puff out the cheeks, and squeeze the eyes shut. Watch for symmetry. The corneal reflex is used to test the sensory V and motor VII; omit doing this test unless there are abnormalities in the other tests.
- Acoustic (VIII): Sensory nerve. Assess the client's hearing using the whisper test, the Weber test, and the Rinne test.
- Glossopharyngeal (IX) and vagus (X): Both sensory and motor nerves. It is not possible to test the sensory component of the glossopharyngeal nerve as it governs taste in the posterior one-third of the tongue. For the motor component, ask the client to say "Ahhh" and look in the mouth to see if the soft palate and uvula move up and back in the back of the mouth. Check the gag reflex.
- Spinal accessory (XI): Motor nerve. Check for range of motion and movement against resistance of the neck and shoulders.
- Hypoglossal (XII): Motor nerve. Check the range of motion and movement against resistance in the tongue. Ask the client to stick out the tongue and assess for any tremors and have the client repeat after you: "light," "tight," and "dynamite."

Motor, Sensory, Cerebellum, and Reflex Nerve Testing

- To test the cerebellum, ask the client to walk normally and then with a heel-to-toe tandem walk, knee bends, and Romberg test (ask the client to stand for 30 seconds with the feet together and the hands close to the sides and to close the eyes). For these tests, assess for coordination and balance. In addition, assess for fine motor coordination using rapid alternating movements. If the client cannot get out of bed, ask the client to run an ankle up and down the opposite shin.
- To assess the spinothalamic tract, use a cotton ball for soft touch and a broken tongue depressor with a sharp and dull side or, alternatively, two test tubes, one with cold water and one with hot water. For each of the tests, assess for symmetry and sensation. For soft touch, say to the client, "Every time you feel me touching you, say 'now.'" For the sensation of pain, don't follow any pattern, but apply both the sharp and dull sides of the stick and say, "Let me know if you feel sharpness or dullness when I touch you." For hot and cold, let the client feel the difference and ask the client to tell you if he or she feels hot or cold. Follow the dermatomes around the body, making sure to test the most distal areas.
- The posterior tract can be tested for vibration by striking a tuning fork and asking the client if he or she can feel the vibration as you place it on a bone of the big toes and thumbs. If not, work your way up the bony prominences until a sensation can be felt. It is normal for the older adult not to feel the vibration at the outer periphery.
- For position sensation, show the client that "up" is when you lift the finger or toe upward, and "down" is when you move the finger downward. Ask the client to close his or her eyes and say "up" or "down" with the movement. Hold the finger or toe on the outside edges rather than on the top and bottom.

- For fine touch, use stereognosis: with the client's eyes closed, place a small object in the hand and ask the client to tell you what it is. Don't forget to repeat it with the other hand. Test for graphesthesia as well: with the client's eyes closed, draw a number or a letter on the hand and ask the client to identify it. Two-point discrimination involves using two points on the skin and asking the client to tell you if one or two points can be felt. Move the points together slowly and see at what distance the client can only feel one point.
- Check for symmetry on the other side. Extinction is the test to assess if the client can identify whether or not he was touched with one or two points. With point location, you are testing to see if the client can point to where you just touched him or her. These are all testing the sensory cortex. With the older adult, these sensations likely will be reduced and delayed.
- In an infant, check the rooting, grasping, Moro, sucking, stepping, and tonic neck reflexes. There should normally be a Babinski reflex up until the infant is 2–2½ years of age.

- Motor nerves should be checked simultaneously whenever possible so that you can check for symmetry. Assess the muscles for tone, size, range of motion, and strength using movement against resistance. Watch for any involuntary movements.

MALE GENITOURINARY SYSTEM ASSESSMENT

Anatomy and Landmarks of the Male Genitourinary System

The male genitourinary system is composed of the bladder, penis, testicles, scrotum, prostate, and inguinal area. Fig. 4.6 illustrates these structures. The bladder is the storage area for urine. The urine leaves the bladder via the urethra, passing through the penis and out of the body.

The penis is a sexual organ as well as a functional organ. Sexually, it provides the transportation of the male sperm to the woman's vaginal vault. A milky alkaline fluid that protects the sperm's viability is produced in the prostate. Prostate cancer is one of the leading cancers in men. The incidence is

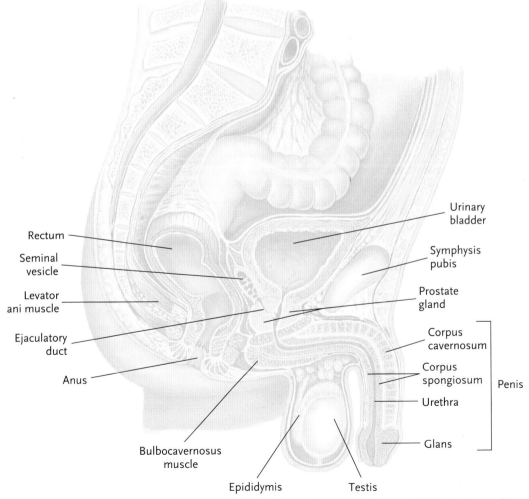

Fig. 4.6 The male pelvic organs. (From Seidel, H. M., Ball, J. W., Dains, J. E., et al. [2011]. *Mosby's guide to physical examination* [7th ed., p. 602, Figure 19-1]. St. Louis: Mosby.)

higher in men of African descent. Signs of benign prostatic hypertrophy (enlarged prostate) or cancer of the prostate are nocturia, frequency, decreased flow, urgency, and the feeling of not emptying the bladder.

The scrotum is a protective sac for the testicles. The testicles produce the sperm needed for reproduction. The cremaster muscle controls the elasticity of the scrotum. The muscle will permit the scrotum to shrink in cold conditions, drawing the testicles closer to the body, and to allow the testicles to descend in warm conditions to prevent them from overheating. It is important to check that the male infant's testicles are descended. Cancer of the testes is more likely to occur in men 17–25 years of age.

Within the inguinal area are the inguinal lymph nodes, the inguinal canal, and the femoral arteries and veins.

Subjective Data Specific to the Male Genitourinary System

*Specific questions for the older adult
   ^Specific questions concerning the infant or child

- Do you have any burning or pain when you urinate or ejaculate?
- Do you have any trouble starting to urinate?
- What colour is your urine?
- Do you have any lumps, bumps, or lesions on your penis?
- Is there any discharge coming from your penis?
- Are there any lumps or bumps that you have noticed on your testicles?
- Are you experiencing any pain in the scrotum?
- Do you do testicular self-examination?
- Are you sexually active?
- Are you having difficulty maintaining an erection?
- Do you use condoms?
- How many sexual partners have you had in the last 6 months?
- Have you been exposed to any sexually transmitted infections?
- ^ **Is the child toilet-trained?**
- ^ **Is the child holding on to his genitals and crying when he urinates?**
- ^ **Does the child have both testicles?**
- ^ **Is the child urinating a lot or constantly thirsty?**
- * **Do you have trouble with urine leaking?**
- * **How many times do you get up at night to urinate?**
- * **Do you have trouble with urgency?**
- * **How many times do you urinate during the day?**

Objective Data Specific to the Male Genitourinary System

Inspection and Palpation of the Male Genitourinary System

Inspect and palpate the penis. It should be smooth and without lesions. The foreskin should retract easily. The urethral meatus should be central in the glans. The distribution, colour, and density of the pubic hair should be normal for the client's age group and should be lice-free.

Inspect and palpate the scrotum. The scrotum skin should be free of lesions. Be careful to examine the underside of the scrotum. Gently feel the testicles for any lumps. Inspect and palpate the inguinal area. Assess the femoral pulse.

FEMALE GENITOURINARY SYSTEM ASSESSMENT

Anatomy and Landmarks of the Female Genitourinary System

The female genitourinary system is made up of the external (vulva) and internal genitalia, the bladder, the urethra, and the urethral meatus. The vulva comprises the labia majora and labia minora. These are folds of skin from the mons pubis. The clitoris is at the top of the labia majora and is highly sensitive to tactile stimulation. The urethral opening is close to the vaginal opening and not far from the anus, so it is very possible for bacteria to enter this opening, giving rise to a bladder infection.

The internal genitalia include the vaginal vault and the cervix, which is the opening to the uterus. The fallopian tubes and the ovaries extend from the uterus.

The labia of the infant at birth are quite engorged due to the presence of the mother's estrogen. The first signs of puberty usually occur between $8\frac{1}{2}$ and 13 years of age.

In the aging adult, the hormone level drops, giving rise to menopause, shrinkage and drooping of the uterus, shortening of the vagina, and decreased vaginal secretions. The internal female genitalia are illustrated in Fig. 4.7.

It is important to note that a vaccine is now available to eradicate most types of human papilloma virus (HPV), which is the major risk factor for cervical cancer.

Subjective Data Specific to the Female Genitourinary System

*Specific questions for the older adult
   ^Specific questions concerning the infant or child

- Do you have any burning or pain when you urinate?
- Do you have any trouble starting to urinate?
- What colour is your urine?
- Are there any lumps or bumps that you have noticed on the perineum?
- ^ **Is the child toilet-trained?**
- ^ **Does she cry when she urinates?**
- ^ **Is the child urinating a lot or constantly thirsty?**
- * **Do you have trouble with urine leaking?**
- * **How many times do you get up at night to urinate?**
- * **Do you have trouble with urgency?**
- * **How many times do you urinate during the day?**
- Do you or your sexual partners use condoms?
- How many sexual partners have you had in the last 6 months?
- Have you been exposed to any sexually transmitted infections?
- How old were you at menarche?
- How many times have you been pregnant?

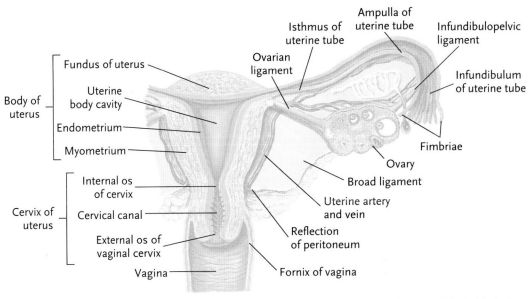

Fig. 4.7 The internal female genitalia. (From Seidel, H. M., Ball, J. W., Dains, J. E., et al. [2011]. *Mosby's guide to physical examination* [7th ed., p. 538, Figure 18-4]. St. Louis: Mosby.)

- How old were you at the first pregnancy?
- How many live births have you had?
- How many abortions have you had?
- What was the date of your last menstrual period?
* **When did you start menopause?**
* **Do you experience any pain or bleeding during or after intercourse?**
- Do you experience any bleeding between your periods?
* **Does sneezing or laughing cause you to urinate?**

Objective Data Specific to the Female Genitourinary System

- Place the client in the lithotomy position and examine the external genitalia.
- Inspect the pubic hair for distribution and lice; the skin for colour and the presence of any lumps, bumps, or lesions; the urethral meatus for position and condition; and the vaginal opening and the anus for discharge.

PRACTICE QUESTIONS

Case 1

A registered practical nurse is newly employed in a retirement residence. Her duties include performing annual health assessments for the residents. Mrs. Clara Sloane, 86, arrives for her health assessment with the practical nurse.

Questions 1–7 refer to this case.

1. What is the most appropriate approach for the practical nurse to use during the interview stage of the health assessment with Mrs. Sloane?
   1. Address her as Clara rather than Mrs. Sloane as older adults respond better to use of their first name.
   2. Be sure to speak loudly to Mrs. Sloane if she is hard of hearing.
   3. Adjust the pace of the interview to provide extra time for Mrs. Sloane to answer questions.
   4. Be careful not to touch Mrs. Sloane as she may be uncomfortable with this familiarity.

2. The practical nurse measures Mrs. Sloane and finds her to be 110 cm. Mrs. Sloane states that she used to be 114 cm and asks why she is now shorter. What is the primary reason older adults lose height as they age?
   1. Decreased muscle mass
   2. Thinning of the vertebral discs
   3. Many older adults develop osteoporosis
   4. Most older adults have some degree of kyphosis

3. The practical nurse takes Mrs. Sloane's blood pressure. Which of the following is true concerning blood pressure in older adults?
   1. Both systolic and diastolic pressures are decreased.
   2. Diastolic pressure increases, while systolic pressure remains the same.
   3. Blood pressure readings become variable and unstable.
   4. There is a widening pulse pressure.

4. The practical nurse performs a skin survey with Mrs. Sloane. Which of the following would be a normal finding?
   1. Acrochordons (skin tags) on her eyelids and neck
   2. Edema in her lower limbs
   3. Decreased hair on her upper lip and chin
   4. Thicker skin on the dorsa of her hands and forearms

5. The practical nurse examines Mrs. Sloane's eyes and finds a grey-white arc around the cornea. What would the practical nurse say to Mrs. Sloane about this finding?

1. "You have the beginnings of cataracts and should see an eye surgeon."
2. "These are a normal finding in your age group and will not affect vision."
3. "This is caused by thickening of your cornea and is probably causing some blurring of your vision."
4. "The discolouration in your eyes is called *xanthelasma* and is caused by high levels of cholesterol."

6. Mrs. Sloane is to receive olive oil in both ears at night for cerumen impaction. What intervention should the practical nurse perform?
   1. Application of a small cotton ball at the meatus after instillation of the ear drops
   2. Removal of coarse ear hairs
   3. Referral to an ear, nose, and throat (ENT) physician
   4. Evacuation of the cerumen using a cotton-tipped swab

7. The practical nurse is aware that in the older age group, neurological assessment is important. Which of the following results of Mrs. Sloane's neurological assessments would be of most concern to the practical nurse?
   1. Mrs. Sloane is not sure which day of the week it is today.
   2. Mrs. Sloane's Mini-Mental State Examination has declined from 27 last year to 25 today.
   3. Mrs. Sloane states that she often misplaces her hearing aid.
   4. Mrs. Sloane believes she presently lives in her former home, which she left 2 years ago.

Case 2

Ms. Perlstein delivered a healthy 3 200-g boy yesterday. The practical nurse plans to perform a health assessment with Ms. Perlstein and the baby.

Questions 8–13 refer to this case.

8. When the practical nurse enters the room, baby Perlstein is asleep. What assessment should the practical nurse first perform?
   1. Respirations
   2. Apical heart rate
   3. Temperature
   4. General appearance

9. Which of the following should the practical nurse be aware of when examining baby Perlstein?
   1. The baby should be completely naked for the entire examination.
   2. The parents should not be present as they may be distressed by the examination.
   3. She should use a soft, crooning voice.
   4. The examination is best done just before feeding.

10. Which of the following would be part of a normal respiratory assessment for neonate Perlstein?
    1. Observation of abdominal breathing
    2. Obtaining a respiratory rate of 70 breaths per minute
    3. Noting a breathing pattern that is regular, with an even rate

4. Assessing that the baby is primarily mouth-breathing rather than nose-breathing

11. The practical nurse measures the head circumference of baby Perlstein. Why is this a component of a neonatal examination?
    1. The circumference indicates the degree of moulding resulting from the birth process.
    2. It is part of the Apgar score.
    3. Variations from normal may indicate a genetic abnormality or increased intracranial pressure.
    4. Abnormalities in fontanelles are more accurately assessed.

12. How would the practical nurse best confirm a patent rectum and anus in baby Perlstein?
    1. Confirm that the passage of meconium took place within 24–48 hours after birth.
    2. Stroke the anus and note a quick contraction of the sphincter.
    3. Introduce a rectal thermometer or cotton-tipped swab into the anus.
    4. Gently insert a gloved well-lubricated fifth finger into the rectum.

13. How would the practical nurse elicit the Moro reflex from baby Perlstein?
    1. Stroke the bottom of his feet.
    2. Hold him on his back and allow his head and trunk to drop back a short distance.
    3. Perform a sharp handclap beside his ear.
    4. Hold him vertically, allowing one foot to touch a surface.

Case 3

A registered practical nurse working in the community provides health care to students at a secondary school as part of his job.

Questions 14–20 refer to this case.

14. How should the practical nurse approach health assessments and teaching with adolescents?
    1. Involve the parents, as they will be able to reinforce health teaching with their teenagers.
    2. Maintain a professional and strict attitude, as adolescents will respond positively to authority.
    3. Provide factual information about how students can manage specific problems they identify.
    4. Provide information related to future health problems, such as risk for heart disease and osteoporosis.

15. A thin 16-year-old girl, Hilary, is worried that she has not yet begun to menstruate. What question might the practical nurse ask Hilary?
    1. "Tell me about your alcohol intake."
    2. "Have any women in your family had ovarian cancer?"
    3. "What kinds and amounts of food do you eat?"
    4. "How much sleep do you get each night?"

16. Bradley, age 14, states that his friends make fun of him because he is short and still looks "like a kid." Which response by the practical nurse is the most appropriate?

1. "It is normal to be teased by your friends; don't let it worry you."
2. "You are very short for your age, so perhaps the doctor should examine you."
3. "I will show you some exercises that will help you to develop your muscles."
4. "All boys begin puberty at different ages, so you will probably grow and become more muscular when this happens."

17. Genevieve, age 13, tells the practical nurse that her parents want her assessed for scoliosis. How would the practical nurse assess whether Genevieve has scoliosis?
    1. Have her bend at the waist to inspect for asymmetry of the scapulae.
    2. Ask her to stand sideways to him so he may measure any degree of kyphosis.
    3. Tell Genevieve to rotate sideways and observe for uneven shoulder height.
    4. Observe Genevieve from the back as she climbs a flight of stairs.

18. Sheldon, age 16, says he is very pleased that he was chosen to play for the school football team. What safety-related assessment question is important for the practical nurse to ask Sheldon?
    1. "Do your parents come to watch you play?"
    2. "Are you able to manage attending your games and completing your school work?"
    3. "Are you planning to play professional football one day?"
    4. "Do you use special protective equipment?"

19. Some teachers are concerned about Warren, age 18, because he has been exhibiting labile, unusual behaviours they describe as "paranoic." They wonder if he is abusing street drugs or has a mental health disorder such as schizophrenia. The practical nurse performs a mental health examination. What might he say to Warren to best determine his thought processes and perceptions?
    1. "What are your grades like in school?"
    2. "How do you feel today?"
    3. "I am going to ask you to remember four words, and in a few minutes, I will ask you to recall them."
    4. "Do other people talk about you?"

20. The practical nurse teaches a group of students about skin care. What is the most common skin problem in adolescence?
    1. Contact dermatitis
    2. Acne
    3. Eczema
    4. Rosacea

Independent Questions

Questions 21–30 do not refer to a particular case.

21. What manifestation would indicate an abnormal finding during a health assessment?
    1. When auscultating the precordium, a third heart sound is heard.
    2. The practical nurse is able to palpate the apical pulse when the hand is placed over the precordium.
    3. On palpation of the nail capillary, refill is 2 seconds.
    4. The right calf measures 38 cm, while the left calf measures 38.7 cm.

22. Which of the following correctly outlines the sequence of events the practical nurse should follow when examining the abdomen?
    1. Inspection, auscultation, palpation
    2. Palpation, inspection, auscultation
    3. Light palpation, inspection, auscultation
    4. Inspection, palpation, auscultation

23. Which pulse would be of most concern to the practical nurse?
    1. Two-month-old infant: 110 bpm at rest
    2. Ten-year-old boy: 104 bpm after exercise
    3. Seventeen-year-old athlete: 50 bpm at rest
    4. Five-day-old infant: 70 bpm after crying

24. Which of the following would be of most concern to the practical nurse if noted in an 8-year-old child after he fell from his bike and hit his head?
    1. Nausea
    2. Memory loss for familiar surroundings and objects
    3. Swelling and aching pain at the site of injury
    4. Blood pressure changing from 100/60 to 110/70 mm Hg

25. Mrs. Sandoz tells the practical nurse her stools are a light grey to a very light brown colour. Which of the following conditions might the practical nurse suspect as the cause?
    1. Renal failure
    2. Intestinal polyps
    3. Gallbladder disease
    4. Celiac disease

26. The practical nurse is assessing Mr. Robin for possible discharge from a psychiatric facility. He must assess Mr. Robin's ability to make sound judgements and decisions. Which of the following assessment questions would best evaluate this ability?
    1. Ask Mr. Robin to explain a proverb such as "a stitch in time saves nine."
    2. Ask Mr. Robin to spell *moose* backwards.
    3. Ask Mr. Robin what action he would take if his house caught fire.
    4. Ask Mr. Robin how a train and an airplane are similar.

27. Ms. Leigh is examined in the emergency department by a practical nurse who notes on the chart "PERRLA." Which organ does this notation pertain to?
    1. Eyes
    2. Ears
    3. Mouth
    4. Lungs

28. Where would the healthcare provider place his or her hands to assess a client for the possible presence of a goitre?
    1. Over the scapulae
    2. Over the maxillary sinuses

3. Over the anterior portion of the neck
4. Over the angle of Louis

29. A practical nurse is employed in an Inuit community. Many adolescent men live on the reserve. What would be the most important assessment to be aware of in this population?
   1. Risk for suicide
   2. Risk for type 2 diabetes
   3. Risk for cardiovascular disease
   4. Risk for tuberculosis

30. Ms. Martin is a pregnant woman who comes to the clinic for her first prenatal appointment. Protocol in the clinic is that every woman is screened for intimate partner violence. How would the practical nurse best introduce the topic to Ms. Martin?
   1. "Since you have been pregnant, has your partner ever physically hurt you?"
   2. "Have you ever been the victim of intimate partner violence?"
   3. "It is clinic policy to ask if you are in an abusive relationship."
   4. "Because domestic violence is so prevalent in our society, we ask all women about any experience with abuse."

REFERENCES

Folstein, M. F., Folstein, S. E., & McHugh, P. R. (1975). Mini-mental state: A practical method for grading the cognitive state of clients for the clinician. *Journal of Psychiatric Research*, 12(3), 189–198.

Jarvis, C., Browne, A. J., MacDonald-Jenkins, J., et al. (2018). *Physical examination & health assessment* (3rd Cdn). Toronto: Saunders.

Seidel, H. M., Ball, J. W., Dains, J. E., et al. (2011). *Mosby's guide to physical examination* (7th ed.). St. Louis: Mosby.

Wilson, S. F., & Giddens, J. F. (2017). *Health assessment for nursing practice* (6th ed.). St. Louis: Elsevier.

BIBLIOGRAPHY

Doerflinger, D. M. (2016). Mental status assessment of older adults: The Mini-Cog. Retrieved from https://consultgeri.org/try-this/general-assessment/issue-3.1.

Flaherty, E. (2007). Pain assessment for older adults. Retrieved from https://consultgeri.org/try-this/general-assessment/issue-7.

Hartford Institute for Geriatric Nursing. (2008). Try this: Best practices in nursing care to older adults series. Retrieved from https://consultgeri.org/tools.

Registered Nurses' Association of Ontario. (2004). Nursing Best Practice Guideline: Assessment and management of venous leg ulcers [includes a 2007 supplement]. Retrieved from http://rnao.ca/bpg/guidelines/assessment-and-management-venous-leg-ulcers.

Registered Nurses' Association of Ontario. (2008). *Nursing Best Practice Guideline: Oral health: Nursing assessment and interventions*. Toronto: Author. Retrieved from http://rnao.ca/bpg/guidelines/oral-health-nursing-assessment-and-intervention.

Registered Nurses' Association of Ontario. (2013). *Nursing Best Practice Guideline: Assessment and management of foot ulcers for people with diabetes* (2nd ed.). Toronto: Author. Retrieved from http://rnao.ca/bpg/guidelines/assessment-and-management-foot-ulcers-people-diabetes-second-edition.

Registered Nurses' Association of Ontario. (2013). *Nursing Best Practice Guideline: Assessment and management of pain* (3rd ed.). Toronto: Author. Retrieved from http://rnao.ca/bpg/guidelines/assessment-and-management-pain.

Registered Nurses' Association of Ontario. (2016). *Delirium, dementia, and depression in older adults: Assessment and care* (2nd ed.). Toronto: Author. Retrieved from http://rnao.ca/bpg/guidelines/assessment-and-care-older-adults-delirium-dementia-and-depression.

WEB SITES

- **College of Licensed Practical Nurses of Alberta** (http://www.clpna.com): This site contains links to information on all aspects of being a licensed practical nurse (LPN) professional in Alberta.
- **College of Licensed Practical Nurses of British Columbia** (http://www.clpnbc.org): This site contains links to information on all aspects of being an LPN professional in British Columbia.
- **College of Nurses of Ontario** (http://www.cno.org): This site contains links to information on all aspects of being a registered practical nursing professional in Ontario.
- **College of Nurses of Ontario: Registration Information** (http://www.cno.org/en/become-a-nurse/): This site contains information on how to become a registered practical nurse in Ontario.
- **Registered Practical Nursing Association of Ontario** (http://www.rpnao.org): This site contains information on the professional association representing the voice of practical nurses in Ontario.
- **Saskatchewan Association of Licensed Practical Nurses** (http://www.clpnm.ca): This site contains links to information on all aspects of being an LPN professional in Saskatchewan.

Health and Wellness

According to every theory of nursing, and every nursing practice act in Canada, health promotion is considered an essential role for practical nurses. However, how we define health and what we consider to be priorities for health promotion have varied across time, cultures, and geography. In Canada today, there is growing recognition that health promotion involves promoting health for individuals or families (changing the person) as well as promoting changes in the community and population that result in healthier environments (changing the world). This chapter provides an overview of health, determinants of health, health promotion strategies involving individual and family action, and population health initiatives that aim to foster healthy environments in Canada.

GUIDING PHILOSOPHIES FOR HEALTH AND WELLNESS

A Definition of Health

Each individual and family has its own definition of health. The same is true for groups of people, communities, and populations. A very important goal of practical nursing is to help individuals and groups achieve their optimum level of health and wellness. Numerous definitions of health continue to influence how practical nurses attain this goal within the Canadian healthcare system. Some common conceptualizations of health that currently inform practical nursing practice are as follows:

- An individual's perception of health is multidimensional and is based on a myriad of interacting parts of the human experience. The interconnected parts include physical, mental, social, and spiritual health (Pender, Murdaugh, & Parsons, 2015).
- Health is "a state of complete physical, mental, and social well-being, not merely the absence of disease or infirmity" (World Health Organization [WHO], 1986).
- Health is a balance of "biopsychological, spiritual, cultural and environmental dimensions. In a holistic view of health, an assessment is not complete unless it involves individuals, families, and communities in which individuals live and function" (Pender et al., 2015, p. 22).
- Health is also a "product of reciprocal interactions between individuals and their environments" (McMurray & Clendon, 2015, p. 5).

Determinants of Health

Informed by studies on the factors influencing health, Health Canada has delineated 12 key determinants of health (Public Health Agency of Canada [PHAC], 2013; see Table 5.1). Each determinant interacts with and has an impact on the others. Our understanding of these determinants continues to evolve, and so too does our work in addressing and influencing them (Hales & Lauzon, 2018; Potter, Perry, Stockert, et al., 2019).

Historical Approaches to Health

In the West during modern times, there have been three main approaches to health that influence the structure of our healthcare services. These approaches offer a useful framework for examining the evolution of health orientations in Canada (Laverack, 2004; Potter et al., 2019).

Medical Approach

The medical approach has historically been the most prevalent in our healthcare system and remains the most common. In terms of health and wellness, the medical approach encourages healthcare providers to focus on disease prevention among high-risk groups. This approach is commonly considered "top down" and is directed by what some consider "expert" knowledge of the risks for disease.

The Behavioural, or Lifestyle, Approach

The behavioural, or lifestyle, approach includes health teaching and awareness campaigns that help to change individual health behaviours and lifestyles. This approach became popular in the 1970s with the help of the 1974 LaLonde Report (LaLonde, 1974), a federal government report that recognized the health and economic limitations to the medical model and hospital-based care.

The Socio-Environmental Approach

The socio-environmental approach became popular in the 1980s when a new concept of health emerged that accounted for the structural influences (poverty and appropriate housing) on health behaviours (Potter et al., 2019). It was then that we began to understand and articulate the broad determinants of health and the interrelationships among them. More recently, practical nurses have begun to build on this approach by using a socio-ecological model to guide their work. A socio-ecological model of health offers a critical framework for understanding the system of interrelated

TABLE 5.1 Determinants of Health

Health Determinants	Description
Income and social status	Greatest influence on health status, behaviours, and the use of healthcare services. Lower-income Canadians have poorer health with more chronic illness and earlier death than higher-income Canadians, regardless of age, gender, culture, race, or residence.
Social support networks	Social contacts and support networks are linked with better health by providing emotional support, caregiving, and improved management of adversity.
Education and literacy	Higher education improves a person's state of health. Education increases opportunities for earning higher incomes and improves problem-solving capacity and access to health information.
Employment/working conditions	Unemployment or employment that is stressful or unsafe is linked to poorer health. Income, social contacts, and emotional health are all affected by the workplace.
Social environments	Community, region, province, and country provide resource-sharing and social networks, which create safety nets and improve overall health for their community members.
Physical environments	Environmental contaminants in the air, soil, water, and food can cause poor health, such as respiratory conditions or other serious illnesses. Environments in the built community can impact on health in many ways, such as poor air quality and unsafe building codes.
Personal health practices and coping skills	This segment refers to those measures that individuals can do themselves to promote their own health and manage challenges. Self-sufficiency and making healthy choices will optimize their level of health.
Healthy child development	What happens to a child during the growing years will impact on the child's long-term health and the development of chronic illnesses; for example, low-birth-weight infants have almost twice the incidence of lifelong diseases.
Biology and genetic endowment	Genetics play an important role in individuals' health status. Genetic predisposition to certain conditions, as well as environmental interrelationships, puts certain individuals at risk for specific diseases.
Health services	Available health services have a direct impact on individuals', families', groups', and communities' ability to prevent disease and adequately treat secondary conditions. There are still inequities in terms of accessibility to these essential services; for example, urban populations with increased access to health services have better morbidity and mortality rates than rural populations with less access.
Gender	Gender refers to differences in biologics, roles in society, personalities, attitudes, values, and socio-economic position. These differences have a direct bearing on health. A gender-specific predisposition for certain disease states and treatment programs exists as well.
Culture	There are health risks related to cultural and ethnic backgrounds that affect an individual and family. Culturally specific lifestyles may influence health choices. Socio-economic status has a major influence on health. For example, access and health care may be difficult for new immigrants who don't know the language and how to enter and manoeuvre within the healthcare system. It is essential that culturally appropriate care be available.

Adapted from Public Health Agency of Canada. (2013). What makes Canadians healthy or unhealthy? Retrieved from https://www.canada.ca/en/public-health/services/health-promotion/population-health/what-determines-health/what-makes-canadians-healthy-unhealthy.html. Reproduced with the permission of the Minister of Health.

socio-cultural, political, and physical environmental influences on health (Best, Stokols, Green, et al., 2003; Golden, McLeroy, Green, et al., 2015; Stanhope, Lancaster, Jakubec, et al., 2017).

Defining Health Promotion and Disease and Injury Prevention

Health promotion and disease and injury prevention in nursing build on our conceptualizations of and approaches to health.

Health Promotion

Health promotion is most often defined in the following ways:

- It is "the process of enabling people to increase control over, and to improve, their health" (WHO, 1986). It involves helping people optimize their sense of well-being

and health potential. It entails helping people make lifestyle changes and is considered a combination of educational and ecological supports for actions and conditions of living conducive to health (Pender et al., 2015).

- "It is about enabling and empowering people, communities, and societies to take charge of their own health and quality of life. It covers a wide range of social and environmental interventions that are designed to benefit and protect individual people's health and quality of life by addressing and preventing the root causes of ill health, not just focusing on treatment and cure. The three key elements of health promotion are good governance for health, health literacy, and healthy cities" (WHO, 2016).

- It emphasizes "the importance of interventions to prevent disease and promote well-being rather than relying upon remedial action to treat damaging effects" (Laverack, 2004, p. 5).

From a socio-ecological perspective, health promotion is more effective if the individual as well as the organizational, community, and policy levels are targeted (Golden et al., 2015; Hales & Lauzon, 2018; McMurray & Clendon, 2015; Pender et al., 2015; Potter et al., 2019).

The 1986 Ottawa Charter for Health Promotion highlights the significance of health promotion activities that extend beyond the individual level to address the context and the resources needed to promote the health of community members (WHO, 1986). The Ottawa charter outlines five main strategies for health promotion (depicted in Fig. 5.1):

- Building healthy public policy through intersectoral collaborations. This strategy recognizes that collaboration among multiple sectors, such as education, industry, justice, health, and recreation, is critical to developing policies that influence health.
- Creating supportive environments through physical and social resources. This involves engaging people in creating healthy physical and social environments in their homes, organizations, and communities.
- Strengthening community action. This means that community members should be involved in sharing health-related information and capitalizing on one another's strengths and resources to foster health within their communities.

- Developing personal skills through community-based education. This involves creating opportunities for the development of the knowledge and skills necessary for people to promote their own health as well as the health of their families and communities.
- Reorienting health services. This strategy means that health services should reflect the health promotion needs of the community and should be designed and operationalized with the involvement of citizens, practitioners, and decision makers from multiple sectors.

Stanhope and colleagues (2017) provide an illustration of how the Ottawa charter can inform interventions for the prevention of the human papilloma virus for an aggregate population of females (Fig. 5.2).

Disease and Injury Prevention

Disease prevention is also commonly referred to as *health protection*. It involves helping people reduce their risks for disease, detect disease early, or maintain optimal functioning while living with disease (Pender et al., 2015; Potter et al., 2019). Examples include screening for disease (e.g., breast self-examination and mammography), health education for behavioural change (e.g., self-care activities for clients with diabetes), and environmental intervention (e.g., ensuring that fecal occult blood tests for the early detection of colon cancer are available at local pharmacies).

Fig. 5.1 The Ottawa Charter for Health Promotion. (From World Health Organization. [1986]. The Ottawa Charter for Health Promotion. Retrieved from http://www.who.int/healthpromotion/conferences/previous/ottawa/en/index4.html.)

e.g.: Support community action to obtain available human papilloma virus (HPV) vaccine and establish an HPV program.

e.g.: Boards of Education can ensure that HPV vaccine information is included in the school curriculum.

e.g.: Communities can provide opportunities for HPV testing, HPV counselling, and administration of the HPV vaccine and ensure that all opportunities are available and accessible.

e.g.: Social marketing campaigns can heighten public awareness of the importance and availability of the HPV vaccine.

Fig. 5.2 The population health promotion model applied to a female aggregate. (From Stanhope, M., Lancaster, J., Jakubec, S., et al. [2017]. *Community health nursing in Canada* [3rd ed., p. 110, Figure 4.3]. Toronto: Elsevier. Reproduced with the permission of the Minister of Health, 2012. Adapted from Health Canada. [2001]. Population health promotion: An integrated model of population health and health promotion.)

According to Pender et al. (2015), to promote health, one must first assess how health is defined by the individual, family, or community and then identify realistic strategies to achieve desired health goals. Individual health cannot be separated from the health of the family, community, nation, and world. A shift to this broader perspective of health facilitates development of proactive policies to improve the health of all.

Measures of health need to encompass the complexity of health. They should characterize health by conditions that define its presence rather than its absence; identify a spectrum of health states; and reflect a lifespan developmental perspective. In addition, the social determinants of health must be taken into consideration when measuring the health of individuals and communities.

There are three main levels of prevention that distinguish nursing initiatives aimed at optimizing health and well-being, and preventing disease and injury (McMurray & Clendon, 2015). These levels of prevention are as follows:

- Primary prevention—Activities that promote health and reduce risks for disease and injury. Example: Promoting healthy nutrition, rest, and physical activity by educating community members at a local health fair.
- Secondary prevention—Early detection of disease or steps taken to recover from disease and injury. Example: Screening for skin cancer during regular client assessments.
- Tertiary prevention—Maintaining an optimal level of health while living with disease and injury. Example: Creating exercise programs for women with osteoarthritis.

As Edelman and Kudzma (2018) note, "the levels of prevention operate on a continuum but may overlap in practice. The nurse must clearly understand the goals of each level to intervene effectively in keeping people healthy" (p. 9).

Sometimes the terms *upstream*, *midstream*, and *downstream* are used to describe primary, secondary, and tertiary prevention interventions (Fig. 5.3). In primary prevention, upstream interventions are aimed at preventing the development of health problems before there are risks to health. In secondary prevention, midstream interventions focus on enhancing health by minimizing (low to moderate) risks to health. Tertiary prevention entails working downstream where health problems and concerns are evident.

Socio-Ecological System

Health promotion and disease and injury prevention occur at multiple levels within the socio-ecological system and require a combination of health education, advocacy and community development, as well as political activity and policy change in the social, workplace, and community environments (McMurray & Clendon, 2015).

Health education example:
- Client teaching and learning about healthy eating, healthy relationships, and physical activity (individual level)

Advocacy and community development examples:
- Collaborating with colleagues from multiple sectors to advocate for changes in hospital discharge teaching practice
- Collaborating with community health boards to advocate for the development of safe walking trails
- To enable "walk-to-school" programs that encourage accessible outdoor physical activity for children (organizational and community levels)

Political activity and policy change in the social, workplace, and community environments examples:
- Involvement in hospital committees to change the organization's smoking regulations
- Reformulating protocols for preoperative teaching (policy level)

Facilitating Learning Is Integral to Nursing

Health promotion inevitably involves facilitating learning. All nursing practice acts in Canada call upon practical nurses to be health teachers and client educators. Understanding how to teach needs to be guided by an understanding of how people learn. Teaching in professional practical nursing involves knowledge of content (information shared by a practical nurse is current, comprehensive, and evidence-informed) and process (communicating in ways that clients can understand and be enabled to learn).

Multilevel health promotion

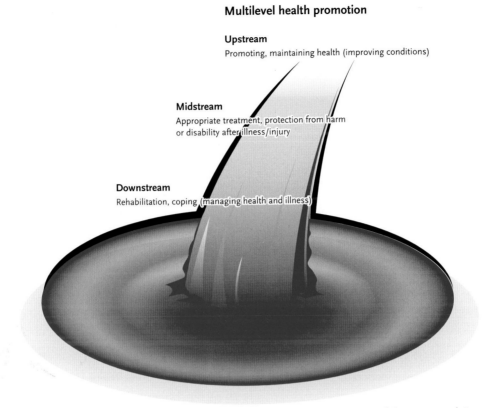

Upstream
Promoting, maintaining health (improving conditions)

Midstream
Appropriate treatment, protection from harm
or disability after illness/injury

Downstream
Rehabilitation, coping (managing health and illness)

Fig. 5.3 Primary, secondary, and tertiary prevention: upstream, midstream, and downstream interventions. (From McMurray, A., & Clendon, J. [2015]. *Community health and wellness: Primary health care in practice* [5th ed., p. 75, Figure 4.4]. Sydney: Elsevier.)

Adults typically learn more successfully when they are encouraged to use past experiences to solve problems. Practical nurses and adult clients should collaborate on educational topics and goals. They should develop care plans that reflect what clients feel is important regarding their own health and well-being. Needs or issues that are important to the adult should be addressed early in the teaching–learning process. Ultimately, adults must accept responsibility for changing their own behaviours (Potter et al., 2019). "People cannot achieve their fullest health potential unless they are able to take control of those things which determine their health" (WHO, 1986).

According to McMurray and Clendon (2015):

Heath education facilitates empowerment by showing people where to access appropriate, relevant information on health, and how to use it to build health capacity…. The approach of knowledge plus capacity is the "new health education," which is orientated towards empowerment rather than persuasion. When health education is delivered in an empowering way, knowledge nurtures the self-esteem and self-confidence that is essential for developing health literacy. (p. 70)

Key Teaching and Learning Theories Relevant to Nursing
Paolo Freire's Theory of Community Empowerment, 1970.
Education is never neutral, and in participatory community education, community members must be involved in naming their own problems and proposing their own solutions

(Freire, 1970). "Health education is an integral strategy in promoting community health. The process begins by building the knowledge base, then working with community members to identify strengths, weaknesses, assets, inequities, vulnerabilities or other aspects of community life that may impinge on health" (McMurray & Clendon, 2015, p. 69).

Freire's theory of community empowerment can be applied to health education involving social action—efforts to change a whole community rather than one person at a time. A community empowerment approach also seeks to give voice to those affected by forces of oppression—including poverty, racism, and violence—which have such devastating effects on health.

Prochaska and DiClemente's Model of Planned Behaviour Change, 1998
Prochaska and DiClemente developed a transtheoretical model of behaviour change (DiClemente & Prochaska, 1998). This model describes behaviour change and involves the following stages:
- Precontemplation—There is little conscious intent to change, as well as resistance or defensiveness.
- Contemplation—The person experiences ambivalence but is more serious about changing a behaviour.
- Preparation—There are preliminary healthy behaviour attempts and conscious planning for change.
- Action—The person lives the plan.

- Maintenance—The individual employs relapse prevention strategies.

In recent years, a sixth stage entitled *relapse* has been added to describe the process of changing health-related behaviours, such as returning to an unhealthy diet or returning to substance abuse (Svensson, Miller, & Hurd, 2016).

This model has been used to explain the process of changing behaviours that are most resistant to change, such as addictions, diet, weight control, or sexual behaviour related to HIV control (DiClemente & Prochaska, 1998). In addition, nurse practitioners apply this model in the management of treatment-resistant major depression (Svensson, Miller, & Hurd, 2016).

Alfred Bandura's Social Cognitive Theory, 1977. Human health is a social matter, not just an individual one. This theory proposes that self-efficacy beliefs operate together with goals, outcome expectations, and perceived environmental facilitators and impediments in regulating human motivation, behaviour, and well-being (Bandura, 2004). The theory holds that people with high self-efficacy (the belief that "I can do it") can accomplish what they set out to learn or to do. Practical nurses can help clients to develop the following sources of self-efficacy (Bandura, 2004):

- Personal mastery—Developing awareness of past successes in similar situations
- Vicarious experiences—Observing role models, recognizing what has worked for others
- Verbal persuasion—Encouragement, receiving information, having questions answered
- Physiological feedback—Evidence of positive bodily changes

Bandura's theory has been utilized, for example, in enhancing self-efficacy for optimized client outcome through the theory of symptom self-management (Hoffman, 2013) and breastfeeding support (Baker, Weideman, & Facello, 2015).

Nola Pender's Health Promotion Model, 2006. Nola Pender's health promotion model integrates knowledge from nursing with the behavioural sciences to explore motivations for health-promoting behaviours and how healthcare providers can promote such behaviours in the persons they serve. Her model includes the following ideas (Pender, Murdaugh, & Parsons, 2006):

- Persons have the capacity for reflective self-awareness, including assessment of their own abilities.
- Persons commit to engaging in behaviours from which they anticipate deriving personally valued benefits.
- Perceived barriers can constrain commitment to health-promoting actions.
- Greater perceived self-efficacy results in fewer perceived barriers to a health behaviour.
- Persons can modify thoughts and emotions and their environment to create incentives for health actions.
- Families, peers, and healthcare providers are important sources of influence that can increase or decrease commitment to and engagement in health-promoting behaviour.

Pender's model is based on the concept of the human capacity for reflection, change, and action.

HEALTH CARE IN CANADA: POLITICAL, SOCIAL, AND ECONOMIC CONSIDERATIONS

Funding Health Care

- Publicly funded care: Universal coverage for Canadians that includes all medically necessary hospital and physician services that are funded by medicare, a national health insurance system, and governed by the *Canada Health Act*. The principles of the *Canada Health Act* are universality, accessibility, portability, comprehensiveness, and public administration (Government of Canada, 2016a).
- Privately funded care: Supplemental health services that are usually purchased from a for-profit organization as extended health coverage, either through an employer or through a policy (such as private hospital rooms, workplace drug and dental plans, and private MRI clinics).
- Voluntary services: Non-profit organizations provide financial support and services for the prevention and detection of illness and for specific health problems (e.g., the Heart and Stroke Foundation of Canada, Diabetes Canada, and Canadian Red Cross).

The Organization of the Healthcare System

It is the responsibility of the provinces and territories to manage, organize, and deliver healthcare services. The federal government described medicare as a set of 13 interlocking provincial and territorial health insurance plans, all of which have commonalities and basic standards of coverage (Government of Canada, 2016a). The federal government also plays a role in healthcare administration.

Levels of Care

There are five levels of health care: promotive, preventive, curative (diagnosis and treatment), rehabilitative, and supportive.

- Health promotion services and activities are designed to enable people to increase their control over, and improve, their health (e.g., the promotion of self-esteem in children and adolescents, advocacy for healthy public policy) (WHO, 1986).
- Disease and injury prevention services are designed to reduce risk factors for disease and injury (including screening, immunization, and support groups).
- Diagnosis and treatment services provide diagnosis and treatment of an existing healthcare problem. Care provided at this level can be labelled as primary, secondary, or tertiary and is described below (Potter et al., 2019):
  - Primary care is the first contact a person makes with the healthcare system, which leads to diagnosis and management of the person's actual or potential health problem.
  - Secondary care involves the provision of a specialized medical service by a medical specialist in his or her office, clinic, or hospital. The client has developed recognizable signs and symptoms that have been diagnosed or require a further diagnostic workup.

- Tertiary care is specialized consultative care, usually on referral from primary or secondary medical care providers, provided by specialists working in a setting that has personnel and facilities for diagnosing and treating complicated health problems.
- Rehabilitation helps clients attain their optimal level of physical, mental, social, and vocational functioning. Rehabilitation generally occurs after a physical or mental illness, injury, or chemical addiction and focuses on improving quality of life while promoting independence and self-care (Potter et al., 2019).
- Supportive care services are provided over prolonged periods of time to clients who are disabled, who are not functioning independently, or who have a terminal illness (Potter et al., 2019). Types of supportive care include palliative and respite care.

Settings for Healthcare Delivery
Institutional Sector

Institutional sector refers to hospitals, long-term care facilities, psychiatric facilities, and rehabilitation centres that provide services to inpatients as well as outpatients (Potter et al., 2019).

- Hospitals generally specialize in providing care over a short period of time for the purpose of diagnosis and treatment of healthcare problems (acute care). Examples of services within a hospital include emergency and diagnostic services, general inpatient services, Critical Care Units (CCUs), outpatient services, surgical intervention, and rehabilitation facilities.
- Long-term care facilities provide accommodations for clients who require the delivery of 24-hour, on-site, supervised care, including professional health services, personal care, and services such as meals, laundry, and housekeeping (Potter et al., 2019).
- Psychiatric facilities are located in hospitals, independent outpatient clinics, or mental health clinics and provide inpatient and outpatient care for clients with mental health disorders and or those who are experiencing emotional crisis (Halter, Pollard, & Jacubec, 2019; Potter et al., 2019).
- Rehabilitation centres provide on-site therapy and training to clients with the purpose of minimizing the client's dependence on care (Potter et al., 2019).

Community Sector

- There has been a shift from institution-based care to community-based care, although community-based care is not guaranteed public funding as hospital-based care has been.
- With a focus on primary and secondary care, this sector provides services for clients that are available where clients live, work, and learn (Potter et al., 2019).
- This sector provides surveillance and monitoring of the environment and the health of the community through the public sector.
- This sector provides specialized services that meet specific client needs (such as food banks or meals on wheels).

- Focus is generally on health promotion and illness prevention as well as palliative and restorative care (Potter et al., 2019).
- Common community settings include public health departments, physicians' offices, community health centres, assisted living facilities, home care, adult daycare centres, community and voluntary agencies, palliative and respite care services, and parish nursing.

Challenges to the Healthcare System

Two of the main challenges to the Canadian healthcare system are the increasing cost of care and problems with providing equal and accessible care for all Canadians (Potter et al., 2019).

Cost of Health Services

Many factors have caused an increase in health expenditures, including new and improved technology, new pharmaceuticals, an increase in chronic and age-related diseases, an aging population, women becoming pregnant later in life, and expectations of the healthcare consumer (Canadian Institute for Health Information [CIHI], 2016), as well as salary increases for healthcare providers.

Equality and Access

There continue to be issues with accessibility to healthcare services, including the following (Potter et al., 2019):

- Low-income Canadians experience unequal access to those factors that determine health, such as nutritious food and safe shelter, and therefore commonly have poorer health. Also, while hospital and physician services are available to all under the terms of the *Canada Health Act*, services such as pharmacy, dental, and vision care often involve private-pay or private-insurance systems and hence are available only to those with the means to pay for them.
- Many experts believe that medicare can only be saved by privatizing certain services within the healthcare system.
- A shortage of nurses and physicians is compromising accessibility of healthcare services.

Canada as a Diverse Society

Approximately 20% of Canada's population has been born outside the country (Statistics Canada, 2016). Increasingly, immigrants to Canada are from Asian countries, including the Middle East. In 1971, 12% of immigrants to Canada were Asian and 61% were European; between 2006 and 2011, 57% of immigrants to Canada were Asian and 14% were European. Since 1999, immigration has now outpaced the natural birth rate, accounting for an estimated 66% of all population growth (Potter et al., 2019; Statistics Canada, 2017).

Culture and Health

Culture has a direct impact on health and on health behaviours, including the following (Potter et al., 2019):

- Specific health problems
- Biological response to treatments

- Birth rites
- Death rites
- Dietary beliefs and practices
- Time orientation
- Attitude toward older adults
- Personal space
- Gender roles
- Social roles
- Attitude toward the healthcare system
- Beliefs about illness and treatments

Providing Culturally Competent Care

According to the Canadian Council for Practical Nurse Regulators (CCPNR) principle "Responsibility to the Public," licensed practical nurses must "respect the rights of all individuals regardless of their diverse values, beliefs and cultures" (CCPNR, 2013, p. 4). In addition, the College of Nurses of Ontario (CNO) issued its *Culturally Sensitive Care* document, which emphasizes that nurses recognize their culture, the client's culture, and how both cultures influence the nurse–client relationship (CNO, 2009, p. 3). The goal of culturally competent care is for nurses to provide care and services appropriate to clients' cultural characteristics. Clients include individuals, families, groups, or populations. Practical nurses need to value diversity, to know about the cultural mores and traditions of the population they serve, and to be sensitive to these when they are caring for clients (CNO, 2009). In order to provide culturally sensitive care, it is important for practical nurses to do the following:

- Identify their own cultural beliefs and values and assess how they may differ from the client's beliefs and how they may influence nursing care
- Research information about the client's cultural background
- Assess the client's health behaviours and methods of communication
- Avoid stereotyping, generalizations, and assumptions
- Work with the individual client to develop the most culturally appropriate health interventions (CNO, 2009; Potter et al., 2019).

Reforms in the Canadian Healthcare System

Two national reports, the Kirby Report, *The Health of Canadians* (Kirby, 2002), and the Romanow Report, *The Future of Health Care in Canada* (Romanow, 2002), have provided recommendations for reforming health care in Canada. One important recommendation includes improving and expanding primary health care (PHC).

Primary Health Care

PHC is described as the key to healthcare reform and sustainability. It is a philosophy and model for improving health that focuses on preventing illness and promoting health (Potter et al., 2019). PHC is based on a social justice approach (equal access for all) and addresses the factors in a person's social, economic, and physical environment that make them ill. Building community capacity for sustainable health is the main goal of PHC (McMurray & Clendon, 2015). The six principles of PHC are accessibility, community participation, health promotion, appropriate skills and technology, intersectoral co-operation, and cultural sensitivity (McMurray & Clendon, 2015). The principles are interconnected.

Accessibility. As practical nurses, it is important to address social justice issues at all levels, from global health to individual healthcare needs. Inequalities in access to health care exist, and population health is strongly influenced by the social determinants of health. Nurses living and working in a community have the skills and knowledge to improve health for that community and to work with others for social justice to bring about equity. Health services are available to all Canadians, regardless of location and economic status. The WHO (2008) have reported that there is widening gap in access to health services, even in highly developed countries, between men and women, different cultures, Indigenous and non-Indigenous people, and urban and rural or remote locations. Barriers to the ability of individuals to access health care include unemployment, lack of education and health literacy, age, gender, functional capacity, and cultural or language difficulties. Barriers to community capacity include geographical features that isolate people from services or opportunities, civil conflict, and lack of structures and services (McMurray & Clendon, 2015).

Community participation. Clients participate in making decisions about their own health, and they can identify health needs in the community as well as strategies to address those needs. Community partnerships are empowering: "they enhance capacity for developing social capital with mutual trust and reciprocity as well as co-operative networks for better health" (McMurray & Clendon, 2015, p. 15). The focus of community partnerships is the achievement of better health, equity, justice, and good governance in health services. However, achieving these outcomes requires the political will to support good health for all community members (McMurray & Clendon, 2015).

Health promotion. Encouraging community capacity through comprehensive promotion of health for the entire community is essential. At the local level, strategies may involve instituting measures to ensure healthy lunches or access to workplace-based health services. At the global level, health promotion is being aware of problems of other countries and making sure their health issues are understood and publicized. Health promotion actions may include creating daycare centres for older adults to prevent them from being socially isolated, or working with new parents to ensure they have the information and support systems they need (McMurray & Clendon, 2015).

Appropriate skills and technology. Appropriate skills and technology include methods of care, service delivery, procedures, and equipment that are socially acceptable and affordable. PHC emphasizes the right care for the right person or community at the right time to maximize efficiency and equity, rather than the most expensive technologies for all communities (McMurray & Clendon, 2015).

Intersectoral co-operation. Intersectoral co-operation requires that all sectors—including government, community, and health—be committed to meeting the needs of Canadians. Ultimately, it requires that health, disability services, transportation, education, environment, and other sectors work together to respond to all the social determinants of health. Collaborative alliances encourage efficient and effective use of resources (e.g., a team of specialists from different sectors working together to ensure the long-term continuity and success of a health initiative) (McMurray & Clendon, 2015).

Cultural sensitivity. Cultural sensitivity refers to being aware of your own and others' cultural beliefs, values, and knowledge and how these shape health and wellness decisions. It means being responsive to the way an individual or group's cultural mores and lifestyle habits shape health and health behaviours. It requires cultural literacy that is developed through openness to people's interpretation of their cultural identity and how their expressions of culture shape their behaviour. It also requires attention to the way language is used to describe different members of a culture. It is important to be careful to assess people's needs from their perspective to avoid jumping to conclusions (McMurray & Clendon, 2015). Cultural safety refers to "exploring, reflecting on, and understanding one's own culture and how it relates to other cultures. Understanding and accepting oneself and one's own beliefs and culture is therefore the starting point for culturally safe and sensitive practice, to ensure that no one culture has dominance over another culture" (McMurray & Clendon, 2015, p. 15).

Community Health Nursing

Changes in the healthcare system (including increased health spending, technology and medical advances, and client involvement in healthcare) have created a situation whereby clients are receiving care in their homes and communities.

- Goals for community health nursing include keeping individuals healthy, providing in-home care to those who are sick and disabled, encouraging participation in care, and cost containment. The community health nursing focus is broad, emphasizing both the community's health and direct care to subpopulations within the community (Potter et al., 2019).
- Community health nursing is a specialty nursing practice that may be carried out in a variety of settings. Examples of community health practice areas include public health nursing, home health nursing, occupational health nursing, parish nursing, street or outreach nursing, and telenurse and outpost nursing. Street nurses are typically registered nurses. However, a practical nurse may work in a homeless shelter. Refer to Table 5.2.
- Community health nurses (CHNs) promote and protect the health of individuals, families, groups, and communities. Public health policy and initiative programs that coordinate care are usually managed by a registered nurse (RN). CHNs will collaborate with other healthcare providers on the team, such as the practical nurse caring for the client (Potter et al., 2019).
- CHNs must complete community assessments in order to promote client (individual, family, group, community) health and identify needs for health policy, program development, and services (Potter et al., 2019). The three components of a community that should be assessed by the CHN include structure or locale, the people, and the social systems (Potter et al., 2019).

HEALTH PROMOTION AND DISEASE AND INJURY PREVENTION: PRACTICE FOCUS

Nutrition and Healthy Eating

Categories of Nutrients

Six nutrients are necessary for body processes and function. These nutrients are water, carbohydrates, proteins, fats, vitamins, and minerals and are described below (Potter et al., 2019):

Water.
- Water makes up 60–70% of body weight.
- Water acts as a solvent for metabolic processes.
- Daily losses are through urine, feces, respiration, and perspiration; losses increase with exercise, hot weather, and fever.
- Adult intake should be approximately 1 500 mL per day to survive, including fluid and solid food sources. About 2 000 to 2 500 mL of fluid per day is needed for normal fluid balance.

Carbohydrates.
- The diet should provide approximately 55% of energy in the form of carbohydrates, the major source of energy for the body.
- Sources are primarily plants and include simple forms (sugars) and complex forms (starches).
- Complex carbohydrates are the preferred energy source.
- Fibre is an indigestible form of complex carbohydrate and is thought to be an important dietary factor in the prevention of some diseases.

Proteins.
- Approximately 20% of the diet should come from proteins.
- Proteins are necessary for tissue growth, maintenance, and repair; synthesis of hormones and enzymes; composition of DNA; acid–base balance; blood clotting; and other metabolic processes.
- Complete proteins contain all the essential amino acids and come primarily from animals and seafood.
- Incomplete proteins are found in lentils, nuts, grains, soya, and peas.
- Vegetarians must ensure that they include appropriate ratios and combinations of plant proteins in order to obtain all necessary amino acids.

Fats.
- The diet should include no more than 25–30% fat and no more than 10% as saturated fat.

TABLE 5.2   Examples of Community Health Nursing Practice Areas

Community Health Nurses	Definition	Practice Settings	Client Group	Educational Preparation	Examples of Roles and Activities	Funding
Public health nurse (PHN)	A nurse who uses knowledge of nursing, social sciences, and public health sciences for the promotion and protection of health and for the prevention of disease among populations	• Community groups • Community health centres • Workplaces • Street clinics • Schools • Outpost settings • Homes	• Population • Aggregates and groups • Community • Families • Individuals	Baccalaureate degree in nursing or registered or licensed practical nurse (RPN or LPN)*	• Health promotion • Disease prevention • Client advocacy • Education • Direct care in clinics	Provincial and municipal governments funding
Home health nurse (HHN)	A nurse who uses knowledge and skills to provide direct care and treatment for individuals to maintain and restore health or palliation during illness	• Client's home • Schools • Clinics • Workplaces • Transition services (from hospital to home) • Older adults' housing programs • Shelter or safe house programs	• Individuals • Families • Caregivers	Registered nurse (RN) or RPN or LPN*	• Direct client care • Disease prevention • Health promotion with individual clients	Public or private funding
Occupational health nurse (OHN)	A nurse who specializes in workplace health and safety, health promotion, disease prevention, and rehabilitation for workers	• Workplaces	• Employees (individuals or groups)	RN with certificate in occupational health	• Direct care • Assessment of the workplace • Education of employees on health and safety issues	Employer
Parish nurse	A nurse who serves the health and wellness needs of faith community members	• Clients' homes • Places of worship • Hospitals	• Individuals • Families • Groups	RN	• Health promotion • Health counsellor • Liaison • Health advocate • Integrator of faith and health	Religious or faith community funding
Primary health care nurse practitioner (PHCNP)	A nurse with advanced-practice education, which allows for an expanded role, such as diagnosing episodic illnesses, prescribing medication, and ordering diagnostic tests	• Community health centres • Clinics • Physicians' offices • Emergency departments in hospitals • Nursing stations • Long-term care facilities	• Individuals • Families • Groups • Communities	Baccalaureate degree in nursing, minimum of postbaccalaureate diploma with licensing in Extended Class (EC)	• Direct care (i.e., health assessment, diagnosis, and treatment of episodic illness) • Health promotion • Disease prevention • Community development and planning	Public or private funding

Role	Description	Setting	Population/Focus	Credential	Activities	Funding
Outpost nurse	A nurse who works in an outpost or rural setting that is often geographically separated from face-to-face physician contact	• Nursing stations • Clients' homes • Community	• Individuals • Families • Groups • Rural communities	RN	• Direct care • Health promotion • Liaison with other healthcare providers • Referral	Provincial or federal funding
Military nurse	A nurse and nursing officer who is employed by the Canadian Armed Forces Health Services	• Military hospitals • Military outpatient centres • Civilian tertiary care facilities • Military operational units	• Individuals • Families	Baccalaureate degree in nursing	• Direct client care • Disease prevention • Occupational health care • Environmental health care	Federal funding
Forensic nurse	A nurse who has completed continuing education programs in the area of forensic science	• Sexual assault treatment settings, often in hospital emergency departments	• Adults and children who are victims of acute sexual assault or survivors of intimate-partner violence	RN or registered psychiatric nurse	• Direct care for collection of physical evidence • Providing crisis response, such as counselling and referral	Provincial funding
Telenurse	A nurse who provides nursing service over the telephone	• Community agencies	• Individuals • Families • Caregivers	RN	• Telephone advice • Telehealth network (live video links for nurse-led telehealth clinics)	Provincial funding provided to private companies
Corrections nurse	A nurse who works in a correctional facility	• Correctional facilities	• Inmates (individuals, groups) • Correctional facility staff	RN	• Direct care • Health promotion • Disease prevention • Inmate advocate • Crisis intervention	Provincial or federal funding
Nurse entrepreneur	A nurse who is self-employed in the provision of nursing services	• Home • Variety of workplace settings	• Individuals • Families • Groups • Communities	RN or RPN or LPN*	• Direct client care as contracted • Consultant • Advocate • Health promotion • Disease prevention	Private funding
Street or outreach nurse	A nurse who serves the health and wellness needs of marginalized populations living on the streets	• Community streets	• Individuals • Families • Communities	RN	• Direct client care (i.e., wound care; drug overdose treatment) • Disease prevention • Health promotion • Client advocate • Political activist	Provincial or municipal funding

*Some Canadian provinces and territories designate registered practical nurses (RPNs) or licensed practical nurses (LPNs) to work in some settings such as home health nursing and public health nursing. Note: In some provinces, RPN refers to *registered psychiatric nurse*; however, in this table, the abbreviation designates *registered practical nurse*.

From Stanhope, M., Lancaster, J., Jakubec, S., et al. (2017). *Community health nursing in Canada* (3rd ed., pp. 20–22, Table 1.4). Toronto: Elsevier.

- Fats or lipids are necessary as an energy source; for insulation, hormone production, vitamin absorption, nerve conduction; as a component of cell walls; and for padding and insulation of organs and the body.
- Saturated fats, found primarily in animal products, have been implicated in cardiovascular disease, cancers, and obesity.
- Unsaturated fats from plant sources (such as olive oil and flaxseed oil) are considered healthier.
- Omega-3 fatty acids from oily fish sources are believed to decrease levels of low-density lipoproteins and are recommended as part of the weekly diet.
- Plant-based unsaturated fats that have been hydrogenated to a solid form are called *trans fats*; these fats, found in solid margarines, baked goods, and table spreads, have health risks similar to those of saturated fats.

Vitamins.

- Vitamins are elements obtained through dietary intake that are necessary for normal metabolism.
- Vitamins found in fresh foods are preferable to synthetic supplements.
- Vitamins are classified as water soluble (B complex and C) and fat soluble (A, D, E, K); fat-soluble vitamins can be stored by the body and are not easily destroyed in cooking or storage; water-soluble vitamins are not stored in the body and are easily lost in cooking.
- Vitamins A, C, and E and beta-carotene may act as antioxidants, neutralizing free radicals that cause oxidative damage to cells.

Minerals. Minerals are inorganic elements essential to the body as catalysts in biochemical reactions. Minerals become part of the structure of the body and enzymes (Hales & Lauzon, 2018). For example:

- Iron becomes attached to a protein globin to form hemoglobin, which enhances oxygen-carrying capacity. It plays a part in energy formation.
- Calcium is a component of bones and teeth and is needed for muscle and nerve activity and blood clotting.
- Potassium is needed to maintain fluid balance and acid–base balance in body cells. It is needed for muscle and nerve activity.
- Sodium is needed to maintain fluid balance and acid–base activity in body cells. It is critical for nerve-impulse transmission.
- Chloride aids in digestion and is needed to maintain fluid balance and acid–base balance in body cells.
- Phosphorous is a component of bone and teeth formation. It plays a part in energy formation and is needed to maintain cell membranes.
- Magnesium is a component of bones and teeth and is needed for nerve activity, energy, and protein formation. It plays a part in the immune function.
- Zinc is part of protein reproduction. It is a component of insulin and activates many enzymes. It helps transport vitamin A.
- Fluoride is a component of bones and teeth (enamel). It confers decay resistance in teeth.
- Iodine is a component of thyroid hormones that helps regulate energy production and growth (Hales & Lauzon, 2018, pp. 119–120).

Eating well helps us live and feel well. Sensible eating can provide energy for our daily tasks and protect us from many chronic illnesses, such as diabetes, obesity, and cardiovascular disease. It may even contribute to longevity (Hales & Lauzon, 2018). A number of interrelated determinants of healthy eating influence the overall well-being of individuals and the community. These determinants include physiological state; food preferences; nutritional knowledge; perceptions of healthy eating; influence of family and friends; physical, social, and economic influences; and healthy public policy (Potter et al., 2019). Promoting good nutrition is a critical concern in prevention and health promotion and an important dimension in competent self-care. Cultural and ethnic backgrounds influence eating behaviour and must be accounted for in changing eating patterns. The individual, family, and community must all be part of nutritional interventions. Research has substantiated the complexity of factors that determine eating behaviours, and all of these determinants must be part of a strategy for successful change to occur (Pender et al., 2015).

Determinants of Healthy Eating

- Physiological state: Physiological development or deterioration at both ends of the lifespan (childhood and older adult) affects eating behaviour.
- Food preferences: Food preference may be individual in nature or affected by social and cultural norms.
- Nutritional knowledge: The amount of nutritional knowledge affects healthy eating choices in adults but has not been demonstrated to affect children and adolescents.
- Perceptions of healthy eating: Perceptions of healthy eating are influenced by current dietary guidelines and cultural influences.
- Psychological factors: Psychological factors shown to affect food choices include self-esteem, body image, chronic dieting, mood, and focus of attention.
- Interpersonal influences: Family, peers, and feelings of social isolation affect patterns of healthy eating.
- Physical environment: This determines the availability of food and access to that food, such as the proximity of supermarkets.
- Social environment: Social status and culture often influence food choice; for example, Canadian society devalues preparation of food in the home and favours takeout and quick meals from the freezer.
- Economic environment: Eating behaviours are influenced by corporate-driven economic interests.
- Healthy public policy: Policies define what is considered relevant and influence our food choices, such as through the subsidization of low-energy, nutrient-dense foods.

Eating Well With Canada's Food Guide

The purpose of *Eating Well with Canada's Food Guide* (Fig. 5.4) is to assist people in making food choices that promote health and prevent nutrition-related disease (Health Canada, 2011). It does not prescribe a particular dietary pattern but promotes desirable ways of eating (Potter et al., 2019). The food guide provides special recommendations for children, women of child-bearing age, and adults over the age of 50 (Hales & Lauzon, 2018). *Eating Well with Canada's Food Guide: First Nations, Inuit and Métis* is also available to assist Indigenous people in incorporating traditional food choices into their diet (Health Canada, 2007). *Eating Well with Canada's Food Guide* is also available in 12 languages: English, French, Arabic, Chinese, Farsi (Persian), Korean, Punjabi, Russian, Spanish, Tagalog, Tamil, and Urdu.

- Children: Children should be provided with small meals and snacks throughout the day; foods that contain fat should not be restricted as fat provides a source of calories required for growth; children learn eating behaviours from adults, who serve as important role models.
- Women of child-bearing age: Women who are planning on getting pregnant should consider taking a supplement of 0.4 mg of folic acid each day, in addition to the amount of folate found in a healthy diet. Neural tube defects can appear within the first month of a pregnancy, so health experts recommend starting the supplement as soon as birth control is stopped (Hales & Lauzon, 2018).

Fig. 5.4 Eating Well with Canada's Food Guide. (Extract from Health Canada. [2011]. *Eating well with Canada's food guide*. Ottawa: Author. Retrieved from http://www.hc-sc.gc.ca/fn-an/food-guide -aliment/index_e.html. Reproduced with permission of the Minister of Public Works and Government Services Canada.)

- Women who are pregnant: Extra calories are required during pregnancy and lactation; an extra 2–3 food guide servings are recommended each day.
- Adults over the age of 50: Vitamin D requirements increase at age 50 (to 400 IU) and then again at age 70 (to 600 IU). Vitamin D intake is associated with health benefits that include improved muscle strength, higher bone mineral density, reduced fracture rates, reduced rates of falling, and improved mobility.

Physical Activity

The importance of regular exercise is becoming increasingly clear as more research studies are done. The impact of physical activity on health is listed below.

- Regular physical exercise promotes health and well-being from a physical perspective as well as a psychological one.
- Exercise increases respiratory capacity, improves digestion and fat metabolism, strengthens bones, improves joint flexibility, improves circulation, improves mood, reduces psychological symptoms, reduces the risk of heart disease, lowers body fat and reduces weight, and increases muscle strength and tone (Hales & Lauzon, 2018).
- Physical inactivity is an important public health concern for Canadians of all ages. The WHO has identified it as the fourth leading risk factor for global mortality and linked it to a number of chronic diseases, including cardiovascular disease, cancer, and diabetes (Government of Canada, 2017). Other health risks of inactivity include premature death, obesity, high blood pressure, osteoporosis, stroke, depression, and colon cancer (Hales & Lauzon, 2018).
- C lients should be assessed by a physician before starting an exercise program.
- The amount of physical activity required on a daily basis is directly correlated to the intensity of the workout (Hales & Lauzon, 2018).
- The three types of activities required to keep the body healthy are endurance exercises, flexibility activities, and strength activities (Hales & Lauzon, 2018).
- Adults should engage in 30 minutes of moderate-intensity physical activity 5 days per week. The recommendation is for 150 minutes of moderate-to-vigorous physical activity each week, in bouts of 10 minutes or more (Government of Canada, 2017; Hales & Lauzon, 2018).
- Over half of Canadian children are not active enough for optimal growth and development. Lack of exercise among children is a major contributor to weight gain and obesity (Government of Canada, 2017).
- Benefits of regular physical activity for older adults include continued independent living, reduced risk of falls, improved quality of life, improved balance and posture, and prevention of bone loss (Hales & Lauzon, 2018).

Rest and Sleep

Rest and sleep are as important to health as proper nutrition and exercise (Hales & Lauzon, 2018).

- Sleep promotes tissue repair and recovery of body systems and is essential for cognitive and emotional function.

- Sleep is governed by an individual's sleep–wake cycles, or circadian rhythms; circadian rhythms are influential in controlling the pattern of major biological functions such as body temperature, heart rate, blood pressure, hormone and electrolyte secretions, and sensory acuity.
- Circadian rhythms are affected by light, temperature, and social factors (such as shift work).
- All people have individual sleep–wake cycles; hospital routines rarely take these into consideration.
- Although individual needs vary, most people require approximately 7–9 hours of sleep per night.
- Any disruption in the sleep–wake cycle may lead to suppressed immunity, decreased tissue repair, impaired judgement, irritability, decreased appetite, and weight loss; some accidents are believed to result from sleep deprivation, which leads to distortion of sensory perceptions. Chronic sleep deprivation may cause weight gain by altering metabolism and by stimulating excess stress hormones. It also reduces the levels of hormones that regulate appetite, which may encourage more eating (Hales & Lauzon, 2018).
- Sleep cycles are categorized as non–rapid eye movement (non-REM) and REM; non-REM stage 4 is the deepest level of sleep and is believed to be important for physical restoration; heart rate and respirations are decreased in stage 4.
- REM sleep is important for psychological restoration; dreaming occurs most often in this stage; heart rate and respirations increase in REM sleep.

Sleep Disturbances

- Changes in sleep habits and rituals may alter the ability to sleep (including shift workers and hospital clients).
- Stress or anxiety may cause loss of sleep and less time spent in REM sleep.
- Large or spicy meals before bedtime, as well as caffeine and alcohol, may cause difficulty in sleeping.
- Excessive environmental stimulation and noise will interfere with sleep (as in CCU psychosis).
- Technology devices (smartphones, computers, tablets, television) have been implicated as a potential factor in adolescent sleep deprivation. The use of technology and the number of devices used in the hour before sleep were significantly associated with problems in daytime function, increased frequency of waking too early, waking unrefreshed, and daytime sleepiness (Johansson, Petrisko, & Chasens, 2016).
- Discomfort and illness may cause difficulties in falling or staying asleep (such as pain, respiratory difficulty, restless leg syndrome).
- Enuresis (bedwetting) and nocturia (urination during the night) disrupt the sleep cycle.
- Side effects from medications, both prescription and over the counter (OTC), may lead to insomnia and disturbances in the sleep cycle; overuse of sedatives may lead to insomnia and sleep-cycle disturbances.

Sleep Abnormalities

- Insomnia is difficulty falling asleep or staying asleep; it may be temporary or chronic.
- Hypersomnia is too much sleep and may be caused by a physical illness or depression.
- Narcolepsy is brief, uncontrollable episodes of sleep that last from a few seconds to 30 minutes.
- Somnambulism (sleepwalking) is most common in children.
- Sleep apnea—pauses in breathing lasting over 10 seconds—is most commonly caused by upper-airway obstruction due to relaxed muscles in the oral cavity; it occurs most often in overweight, middle-aged men and postmenopausal women; loud snoring and excessive daytime sleepiness are manifestations of sleep apnea.

A Healthy Environment

The socio-ecological model of health described in the first section provides the theoretical basis for practical nurses to address individual needs as well as the social and physical environment in an effort to create conditions that support and facilitate healthy behaviours and lifestyles. More and more research is suggesting that our economic and social environment has a greater effect on our health than do advances in medicine (McMurray & Clendon, 2015).

Practical nurses strive to promote and restore the health of individuals with an understanding that the health of individuals is inescapably tied to the health of their families, communities, and societies (Pender et al., 2015). The social environment must be taken into account in health promotion and disease and injury prevention, and be addressed in combination with health education. McMurray and Clendon (2015) noted that "the community itself is the center of care, and members of the community are empowered by knowledge and the expectation that they will be full participants in health decision-making" (p. 92).

Social Environment

The social environment is a critical determinant of health (see Table 5.1), and researchers contend that it is as influential on health as healthy eating or physical activity (PHAC, 2013). According to McMurray and Clendon (2015), "when the social environment is supportive, creating a climate of trust and mutual respect, people are more likely to be *empowered*, in control of their life, and therefore their health" (p. 7). To effect changes in the social environment, practical nurses can do the following:

- Involve families in their own care
- Connect clients and families to appropriate resources in the community (support groups, family resource centres, community kitchens)
- Help strengthen the social environment

A healthy social environment is created through regulations and policies that foster cohesive, safe communities with supportive social networks and resources. To be effective and sustainable, these regulations and policies must be developed, enacted, and evaluated jointly by multiple sectors (e.g., education, housing, environment, health, justice) and community members themselves. Examples of how a healthy social environment might be created include the following:

- Example 1—In targeting smoking behaviours, practical nurses raise awareness of the effects of smoking and strategies for cessation, and address the social environment by advocating for no-smoking regulations in public places and for controls on media advertisements and the accessibility of tobacco.
- Example 2—In a community faced with high levels of crime, practical nurses educate youths and their families on minimizing risky behaviours. Practical nurses work with other sectors to identify high-risk areas within the community and to improve policing and supervision of those areas. Safe and accessible recreational opportunities for youth are also developed.

Physical Environment

The physical environment is an important determinant of health as well (PHAC, 2013). Factors such as contaminants in the indoor and outdoor environment influence health. These contaminants, whether transmitted through air, water, food, or soil, can cause cancer, birth defects, or respiratory illness (Canadian Nurses Association [CNA], 2005; PHAC, 2013).

Research indicates that 5–10% of cancers are linked to environmental contaminants (Canadian Cancer Society, 2017; CNA, 2005). Children are particularly at risk for adverse effects due to the immaturity of their metabolism and limited physiological ability to detoxify and excrete chemicals. They inhale more air in proportion to their body weight, are closer to the ground where toxins may exist, and are more apt to put things in their mouths (CNA, 2017; Edelman & Kudzma, 2018). Those living in poverty are also disproportionately affected by environmental contaminants (Hales & Lauzon, 2018) because "[t]heir burden of physical, chemical and biological exposure is greater (e.g., living close to factories or expressways, and in older buildings that may have lead paint or asbestos insulation); and … they have less access to resources that help mitigate the negative effects of this exposure (e.g., nutritious food and high quality medical care)" (CNA, 2005, p. 4).

Practical nurses have a responsibility to address environmental health problems through their care for clients, families, and communities. Box 5.1 presents CNA (2017) recommendations on the role of nurses in environmental health.

The CNA's position statement on environmental health begins as follows: "The environment is an important determinant of health and has a profound impact on why some people are healthy and others are not. There is a role for every nurse to promote and support actions to optimize the health of the environment because of the link to human health" (CNA, 2017, p. 1).

Through a combination of health education and awareness campaigns, as well as ongoing changes to regulations and policy, practical nurses need to help reduce harmful exposure

---

BOX 5.1   Nurses and Environmental Health

The role of nurses in environmental health includes:

- Assessing and communicating risks of environmental hazards to individuals, families and communities
- Educating patients, families and communities about environmental health and how to address key environmental health issues
- Showing leadership in personal practices that support and reduce harm to the environment
- Collaborating with interdisciplinary colleagues to identify and mitigate environmental health risks in practice environments
- Advocating for policies that protect health by preventing exposure to those hazards and promoting sustainability
- Producing nursing science, including interdisciplinary research, related to environmental health issues
- Promoting the development of natural and built environments that support health

From Canadian Nurses Association. (2017). Position statement: Nurses and environmental health (pp. 1–2). Retrieved from https://www.cna-aiic.ca/~/media/cna/page-content/pdf-en/nurses-and-environmental-health-position-statement.pdf?la=en

---

to environmental contaminants such as air pollutants (indoor and outdoor), pesticides, polluted water, lead, and radon. Examples of how this might be accomplished include the following:

- Example 1—Providing health education to clients, families, schools, and communities on issues such as avoiding harmful exposure to pesticides and chemicals
- Example 2—Working with community health boards or groups to change pesticide bylaws or working with hospital-based teams to improve air quality and hospital recycling programs

In conjunction with interventions aimed at limiting contaminant exposure, practical nurses need to use the ample (yet often underutilized) evidence that suggests that interacting with natural environments (in the form of gardens, plants, and animals) can have many positive spiritual, physical, and mental effects (Burton, 2012; Finlay, Franke, McKay, et al., 2015; Mensah, Andres, Perera, et al., 2016) and can influence behaviours that then help to protect and sustain the health of the planet. Two examples follow; see Table 5.3 for additional examples.

- Example 1—Providing health education to clients and families about the health benefits of interacting with nature as well as ways to engage with the natural environment to promote their health, such as encouraging outdoor physical activity in green spaces
- Example 2—Working with hospital "green teams" to redesign hospital spaces that incorporate more green plants, gardens, and window access to natural spaces. Green teams strive to create environmentally responsive healthcare settings and sectors (Petros & Georgi, 2011).

TABLE 5.3   Examples of Multilevel Health Promotion and Disease Prevention Initiatives

System Level	Intervention
Individual level	• Health education in schools focused on healthy eating and physical activity • Health teaching with clients and families on healthy eating, physical activity, and benefits of engaging with nature • Linking clients and families to community resources and programs that support healthy living behaviours
Organizational and policy levels	• School-curriculum changes (e.g., increasing the frequency of physical education classes and banning school sales of chocolate bars and pop) • Increasing the availability of healthy foods in school and university cafeterias and vending machines • Redesigning community-based recreational areas to improve access to playgrounds and natural spaces that provide settings for physical activity • Creating community and nature-based walking trails that enable walk-to-school programs

Promoting Client Safety

The Concept of Safety Promotion and Injury Prevention

Injuries, a leading cause of disability and death, are usually preventable. Practical nurses can integrate discussions of safety promotion and injury prevention into all healthcare encounters, particularly with more vulnerable populations, such as children, youth, and older adults. Injury prevention requires both client education and collective action to build safer environments.

Promoting Infant Safety

Most infant injuries happen in the home and are attributed to lapses in caregiver attention, the presence of household hazards, and enhanced mobility of older infants as they develop. Accidental falls are the leading cause of infant injury in Canada. Other common infant injuries include lacerations, burns, poisonings, and choking (Hockenberry & Wilson, 2015). Approaches to reduce the risk of injury in infants include the following:

- Install smoke alarms and check them every month.
- Ensure that baby equipment, including second-hand equipment, meets Canadian safety standards, such as rear-facing infant car seats. See specific car seat safety regulations in Chapter 10.
- Keep small objects such as buttons or coins out of babies' reach. Do not feed candy, nuts, popcorn, grapes, or hotdogs to a baby, as these can cause choking.
- Avoid ribbons and ties on baby clothes and toys.

- Keep one hand on the baby at all times during care such as diaper changes. Babies can easily roll off beds and change tables.
- Do not use baby walkers with wheels.
- Know that microwaved food can be very hot on the inside while the outside is cool and can burn a baby. Stir and check the temperature before feeding.
- Always test bath water first. Hot bath water can burn a baby.
- Put the baby on his or her back to sleep.
  - Develop strategies to support sleep safety principles for all sleep at all times of the day and night. Provide health teaching to parents regarding sudden unexpected infant death (SUID) and the importance of not co-sleeping with the infant on noninfant surfaces such as the parents' bed, a couch, or another child's bed (Hockenberry & Wilson, 2015).
- Keep medicines, cleaning products, alcohol, tobacco products, and cosmetics out of reach. The most common form of poisoning involves unintentional ingestion of medicines (Edelman & Kudzma, 2018).

Safety Promotion With Children and Youth

Injuries are the leading cause of death and disability among children and adolescents (Canadian Institute of Child Health [CICH], 2001; CICH, Safe Kids Canada, & Safe Start, 2012). Leading forms of injuries include motor vehicle occupant and pedestrian accidents, drowning, and residential fires (Hockenberry & Wilson, 2015; Yanchar, Warda, & Fuselli, 2016). Approaches to reduce the risk of injury in childhood and adolescence include the following:

- Teach children to swim and always maintain supervision around water.
- Teach children how to cross streets and parking lots.
- Teach children to not handle or eat items found in the street or grass.
- Teach children to not accept gifts from or go with strangers.
- Teach the safe use of equipment for play and work. Promote the use of sports helmets.
- Never allow children access to firearms.
- Encourage teens to enroll in driver education.
- Encourage teens to wear their seat belt and to avoid driving under the influence of drugs or alcohol or riding with someone who is under the influence (Edelman & Kudzma, 2018).
- Teach safe use of the Internet:
  - School educators can reinforce to youth the dangers of mobile technology while crossing the street, walking on the sidewalk, cycling, or driving a vehicle.
  - New public safety initiatives can be created, such as phone apps to prevent texting and driving; mass media campaigns promoting the awareness of one's actions while texting, cycling, or driving; and policy and law enforcement initiatives to address dangerous texting behaviours (Stavrinos, Pope, Shen, et al., 2018).

- Implement traffic calming measures, such as speed bumps to reduce speeding and aggressive driving on residential streets.
- Create more bike lanes or paths on roads.
- Change the design of products such as toys and sports equipment used by children.
- Ensure that there are padded dashboards and shatterproof windows in automobiles.
- Children should wear a seat belt or be in an age-appropriate booster seat as needed; older children should ride with a restraint system and in the back seat until age 12.
- Subsidize the costs of safety equipment such as bicycle helmets so that these items are affordable (Letovsky, Rowe, Friedman, et al., 2015).
- Provide health teaching and counselling on safer sex practices.

For more information on pediatric safety, refer to Chapter 10.

Safety Promotion With Older Adults

Falls are the leading cause of injuries among older adults (Potter et al., 2019). Approaches to reduce the risk of falls include the following:

- Ensure that stairs are of uniform size, treaded, and well lit.
- Install grab rails near the toilet and tub.
- Secure all mats and carpets so they do not skid.
- Promote the wearing of skid-free footwear.
- Remove clutter.
- Provide close supervision of confused clients.
- Lock beds and wheelchairs when transferring clients.
- Use alternatives to restraints (relaxation techniques, scheduled toileting, instituting scheduled walking and ambulation routines). Restraints do not prevent falls or injury and may actually increase the severity of injury (Potter et al., 2019).

Understanding the Concept of Sexual Health

Sexual health is evidenced in the free and responsible expressions of sexual capabilities that foster harmonious personal and social wellness, enriching individual and social life. It is not merely the absence of dysfunction, disease, or infirmity (Pan American Health Organization [PAHO] & WHO, 2000; WHO, 2015). Sexual health requires a positive and respectful approach to sexuality and sexual relations—one that is free of coercion, discrimination, and violence (WHO, 2015).

Components of Sexuality

Components of sexuality include the following:

- Sex—A multidimensional biological construct that encompasses anatomy, physiology, genes, and hormones, which together create a human "package" that affects how we are labelled.
- Gender—A social construct that is culturally based and historically specific and is constantly changing. Gender refers to the socially prescribed and experienced dimensions of "femaleness" and "maleness."
- Gender roles—The behavioural norms applied to males and females in societies, which influence individuals'

everyday actions, expectations, and experiences. In some cultures, these are sharply defined; in other cultures, the lines between male and female gender roles may be more blurred.

- Gender identity—How one sees one's own gender: as male, female, or some combination, such as androgynous, intersex, or transgender (Hales & Lauzon, 2018; Potter et al., 2019).
- Sexual orientation—The predominant gender preference of a person's sexual attraction over time. Examples include heterosexuality, homosexuality, and bisexuality (Potter et al., 2019).

Sexual Behaviours

Sexually healthy behaviours include the appreciation of one's own body; interacting with both genders in respectful ways; expressing love and intimacy in appropriate ways; avoiding exploitative or manipulative relationships; identifying and living according to one's values; effective communication with family, peers, and partners; making informed choices about family options and lifestyles; seeking prenatal and reproductive health care; avoiding contracting or transmitting a sexually transmitted infection (STI); and preventing sexual abuse (Hales & Lauzon, 2018; Sexuality Information and Education Council of the United States, 2008).

The Practical Nurse's Role in Sexual Health Promotion

- Promoting positive sexual health is essential for all healthcare providers, including practical nurses. Sexuality impacts all areas of life and human development. Growing concerns about epidemics of STIs, the impact of sexual violence on health, and sexual dysfunction also require that practical nurses understand the prevention of disease.
- Sensitivity is essential as practical nurses strive to explore and better understand clients' experiences of sexuality in health and illness. There are many different sexual cultural norms, and these norms influence attitudes toward sexual practices. The PLISSIT model may serve practical nurses to assess and intervene sensitively in matters related to sexual health and well-being (Potter et al., 2019):
  - *Permission*—Allowing the client to share concerns, experiences, and ask questions
  - *Limited Information*—Giving the client basic information on sexuality and sexual functioning
  - *Specific Suggestions*—Making specific suggestions regarding a sexual concern or issue
  - *Intensive Therapy*—Providing referral to intensive therapy; the level of intervention depends on your experience and knowledge. Examples of interventions include referral to a qualified practitioner such as a social worker or sexuality counsellor (Potter et al., 2019).

All practical nurses should be able to encourage clients to discuss matters related to sexual health and to give limited information and specific suggestions as entry-level competencies, depending on their own scope of knowledge. It is important for practical nurses to examine their own attitudes toward sexuality and be comfortable with different types of sexuality so that they can approach clients in an ethical, professional, and nonjudgemental way.

Alterations in sexual health include infertility; sexual dysfunction (including dyspareunia, lack of libido, erectile dysfunction); STIs; lack of comfort with sexual orientation, gender identity, or gender role; body image disturbance; sexual deviation; and sexual abuse (Hales & Lauzon, 2018; Potter et al., 2019).

Promoting Mental Wellness and Stress Management
Emotions and Health

- Negative emotions, such as depression, anxiety, anger, or hostility, trigger neuroendocrine and immune responses, which, in turn, promote the development of a range of chronic health problems such as cardiovascular disease, certain cancers, osteoporosis, type 2 diabetes, prolonged infection, and decreased wound healing (Hales & Lauzon, 2018; Potter et al., 2019).
- The "fight or flight" response to stress has been described in the literature for over 60 years. The response is a general arousal of the sympathetic nervous system, which causes increasing heart and respiratory rates, decreased intestinal perfusion and motility, increased alertness, increased blood pressure, and increased blood sugar levels.
- More recently, there was an investigation of the "tend and befriend" response, which claims that the hormone involved in the biobehaviour of nurturance and affiliation, oxytocin, causes some women experiencing stress to nurture one another rather than to run or fight and that this response is more common among women (Taylor, Klein, Lewis, et al., 2000).

Coping

Coping is defined as a person's effort to manage psychological stress. Coping involves some combination of problem-focused and emotion-focused strategies (Lazarus, 1999). For example, gathering information about a stressor focuses on the problem and what to do about it; resisting learning about a condition is a way of regulating unpleasant emotions. "The broaden and build theory of positive emotions suggest that positive emotions have the ability to fuel resilience directly, as well indirectly by promoting adaptive coping and demoting maladaptive coping strategies" (Gloria & Steinhardt, 2016). Coping approaches vary among individuals and in different situations and times.

Emotional Intelligence

Emotional intelligence allows an individual to have self-awareness and to give and receive love. Psychologist Daniel Goleman describes emotional intelligence as involving the following five components (Hales & Lauzon, 2018):

- Self-awareness
- Altruism
- Personal motivation
- Empathy
- The ability to love and be loved

Approaches to Stress Management

Approaches to stress management include intrapersonal, interpersonal, and spiritual approaches, including the following (Hales & Lauzon, 2018):
- Connecting with others, developing support systems
- Regular exercise
- Obtaining sufficient sleep
- Learning time-management techniques
- Using guided imagery and visualization
- Practising progressive muscle relaxation
- Obtaining assertiveness training
- Journal writing
- Maintaining a clear separation between work and home life
- Maintaining humour, laughter
- Learning to accept, respect, and love oneself; letting intuition be a guide
- Stretching oneself—learning something new in order to grow
- Helping others
- Practising prayer, meditation, experiences in nature
- Seeking treatment in crisis and in mental illness

Complementary and Alternative Therapies
Canadian Context

Interest and involvement in complementary and alternative medicine (CAM) is a fast-growing trend in Canada. A nation of immigrants, we represent the world's cultures coming together, and the WHO estimates that 80% of the world's population and more than 70% of Canadians use medicines that would be considered alternatives to conventional North American medicines (PHAC, 2008; Potter et al., 2019; WHO, 2013). There has been a growing awareness of the limits of conventional medicine and a rise in requests for holistic care that treats the client's mind, body, and spirit. The WHO published *WHO Traditional Medicine Strategy: 2014–2023* to advance the potential use of alternative healthcare traditions in safe and effective ways and to help countries regulate medicines and make them safer and more accessible to their populations (Hales & Lauzon, 2018; Potter et al., 2019).

Key Terms Related to Complementary and Alternative Therapies

- *Complementary therapies* are those therapies used in addition to conventional treatment. An example would be the use of aromatherapy to lessen postsurgical anxiety.
- *Alternative therapies*, while they may include similar methods, are primarily intended to replace conventional therapies. An example would be the use of a special diet to treat cancer rather than the chemotherapy recommended by a doctor trained in conventional medicine (National Center for Complementary and Integrative Health [NCCIH], 2016).
- *Integrative therapies* involve building bridges between complementary and mainstream medicine and developing clinical approaches that encourage mainstream and

complementary practitioners to work together in the client's best interest (NCCIH, 2016).

Categories of CAM

- Alternative medical systems, such as homeopathy, naturopathy, Ayurvedic medicine from India, and traditional Chinese medicine
- Mind–body interventions, such as meditation, prayer, and art, music, or dance therapy
- Biologically based therapies, such as the use of herbs, foods, and vitamins
- Manipulative and body-based therapies, such as massage and chiropractic
- Indigenous healing, which incorporates a holistic concept of health. The four aspects of health are spiritual, emotional, intellectual, and physical. A weakness in any of these areas causes a person to become unbalanced. Healing circles, sweat lodges, traditional medicine, and the use of medicine wheels and healing ceremonies are some of the approaches that are used to support the health and well-being of Indigenous people (Hales & Lauzon, 2018).
- Energy therapies, which include biofield therapies such as Qigong, Reiki, and Therapeutic Touch and bioelectromagnetic-based therapies (e.g., the use of pulsating magnetic fields) (NCCIH, 2016)

Benefits, Risks, Controversies, and Nursing Responsibilities

CAM holds much promise. Considerable research has found great efficacy in some CAM therapies, particularly in promoting relaxation and in pain relief, thereby strengthening the immune response in health and illness. More and more complementary therapies have become integrated into "traditional" approaches; for example, registered nurses certified in Therapeutic Touch are applying this practice with ventilated clients in CCUs. Oncology nurses practise imagery in talking children through cancer procedures. Clients are asking practical nurses for massage and aromatherapy and about herbal remedies not found in any Canadian textbooks. Many complementary therapies would seem to fall naturally into the practice of nursing (NCCIH, 2016), as practical nurses are called upon to promote holistic health, prevent disease, and provide care in episodic or chronic illness.

CAM also involves controversy. Some methods are unsupported by research, and some may involve harm and risk (NCCIH, 2016). For example, herbal remedies are not standardized, and some may be toxic or interact with other medicines a person may be using. Many practitioners of CAM remain unlicensed and unregulated. Without regulation, one can call oneself a practitioner or therapist with substandard or insufficient educational preparation or supervision. Without adherence to a professional code of ethics, practitioners may exploit frightened or uninformed people for personal or financial gain. "In Canada, training standards have been set by governing organizations for specific alternative health practices. Among these licensed therapies, training standard are not necessarily 'standards.' They do vary widely from province to province/territory. There is no uniform regulation system for alternative medicine in Canada" (Hales & Lauzon, 2018, p. 365).

Professional guidelines for nurses' involvement in CAM are evolving. In 2014, for example, the CNO cautioned nurses to be careful in designating a particular therapy as "nursing" and associating it with nurses' work (CNO, 2014). For example, the use of Therapeutic Touch, imagery, hypnotherapy, meditation, prayer, and art therapy by practical nurses can fall within conventional nursing practice if practical nurses are adequately prepared in their practice. With any therapy—conventional or otherwise—practical nurses are called upon to provide ethical care, promoting genuine and voluntary consent free of duress, fraud, or misrepresentation and to ensure that sufficient information is given about the nature and expected benefits of a treatment, its side effects, consequences of refusal, and possible alternatives (CNO, 2014).

Immunization

The objectives of immunization programs are to prevent, control, eliminate, or eradicate vaccine-preventable diseases by directly protecting vaccine recipients and indirectly protecting vulnerable individuals who may not respond to vaccines or for whom vaccines may be contraindicated (Government of Canada, 2016b). Immunization enables the immune system to build up resistance to disease. Vaccines contain small amounts of viruses or bacteria that are dead (inactivated), weakened (live attenuated), or purified (subunit) components (Potter et al., 2019). Vaccines prompt the immune system to produce antibodies that will attack the virus or bacteria to prevent disease. The immune system stores the information about how to produce those antibodies and responds if there is exposure to that same virus or bacteria in the future (Hales & Lauzon, 2018). The Canadian Immunization Guide provides up-to-date information on the use of vaccines in Canada. It includes specific recommendations for certain population groups, including children and adults (Government of Canada, 2018). Table 5.4 details the immunization schedule for adults (over 18). Recommended schedules for children and adolescents are provided in Chapter 10.

Vaccination and Risk Communication

Practical nurses must be knowledgeable not only in the principles and practices of immunization but also in risk communication as public concerns about safety continue to mount. The Government of Canada has described four principles of effective communication that healthcare providers can use in their daily practice (Government of Canada, 2016b):

- Clearly communicate current knowledge using an evidence-informed approach: Have a wide variety of information formats that are tailored to different languages and levels of education. Take into account what the client knows and the information requested. Make the

TABLE 5.4   Adult Immunization Schedule—Recommendation for Routine Immunization in Healthy Adults at Low Risk*

Vaccine	Dosing Schedule (When No Record or Unclear History of Immunization)	Booster Schedule (After Primary Series Completed)
Tetanus and diphtheria given as Td, and pertussis given as Tdap	Doses 1 and 2 are given 4–8 weeks apart, and dose 3 is given at 6–12 months later; one of the doses should be given as Tdap for pertussis protection.	Td booster is given every 10 years; adults not previously immunized with tetanus vaccine should receive 1 dose of Tdap as part of booster.
Measles, mumps, and rubella given as MMR	One dose for adults born in or after 1970 without a history of measles or those individuals without evidence of immunity to rubella or mumps; a second dose for selected groups. Individuals born before 1970 are considered immune. Rubella-susceptible adults are given 1 dose. If vaccine is indicated, pregnant women should be immunized after delivery.	Not routinely required.
Varicella	Doses 1 and 2 are given at least 4 weeks apart for susceptible adults (with no history of natural disease or seronegativity). Susceptible adults up to and including 49 years of age are given 2 doses. If only 1 dose was previously received, a second dose should be provided. Known seronegative adults 50 years of age and older are given 2 doses (routine testing not advised).	Not currently recommended.
Herpes zoster (shingles)	Individuals 60 years of age and older are given 1 dose. Individuals 50–59 years of age may be given 1 dose.	
Human papillomavirus (HPV)	Women up to and including 26 years of age are given bivalent (HPV2) or quadrivalent (HPV4) or non-avalent (HPV9) vaccine. Men up to and including 26 years of age are given HPV4 or HPV9 vaccine.	
Influenza	Annually	
Meningococcal conjugate	Adults up to and including 24 years of age not immunized in adolescence are given 1 dose.	
Pertussis	One dose of acellular pertussis-containing vaccine is given in adulthood. Adults who will be in close contact with young infants should be immunized as early as possible.	
Pneumococcal polysaccharide 23-valent	Individuals 65 years of age and older are given 1 dose.	
Polio	Primary series for previous unimmunized adults is given when a primary series of tetanus toxoid- and diphtheria toxoid-containing vaccine is being given or with routine tetanus toxoid- and diphtheria toxoid-containing vaccine booster doses.	

*It is important to check schedules frequently for updates.
From Government of Canada. (2018). Canadian immunization guide (Immunization of adults). Retrieved from https://www.canada.ca/en/public-health/services/publications/healthy-living/canadian-immunization-guide-part-3-vaccination-specific-populations/page-2-immunization-of-adults.html#p3c1t1.

most of each opportunity to present information on vaccines and immunizations: Clarify commonly held misconceptions, encourage the client to ask questions, and provide appropriate resources based on evidence.
- Respect differences of opinion about immunization: Understand the underlying reasons for a client's refusal of a vaccine and the strength of his or her position.
- Represent the risks and benefits of vaccines fairly and openly: Compare the known risks associated with the vaccine with the risks associated with the vaccine-preventable infection.
- Adopt a client-centred approach: All clients have input into their decision to vaccinate and retain responsibility for their own health or the health of their children.

Workplace Safety for Nurses
Infection Control
- Practical nurses provide intimate bodily care to others, including those with infectious diseases.
- Hand hygiene before and after any client contact is essential to reducing transmission. Routine practices apply to blood, semen, and vaginal secretions; cerebrospinal,

synovial, pleural, peritoneal, pericardial, and amniotic fluids; and any items or surfaces (such as laundry, dressings, floors, and tabletops) in contact with them. Protective barriers such as gloves, gowns, masks, and protective eyewear can reduce the risk of exposure.

- Take caution with the use and disposal of needles, scalpel blades, and other sharps. Never recap a used needle. Use special puncture-resistant containers for sharps.
- Adhere to public health recommendations for the immunization of healthcare workers.
- Additional isolation precautions may be necessary for airborne infections or those involving droplets, such as the use of gowns, masks, and reverse airflow engineering systems (Potter et al., 2019).

For further information about infection control related to specific diseases, refer to Chapter 6.

Safe Client Handling

Healthcare workers experience musculo-skeletal disorders at a rate exceeding the rate of workers in construction, mining, and manufacturing (Kurowski, Gore, Roberts, et al., 2017). These disorders are associated with excessive back and shoulder loading due to lifting heavy loads during manual client handling or the required use of awkward postures during client care (Kurowski et al., 2017). Training in good body mechanics has been shown to be insufficient in reducing back injuries among nurses. Evidence supports the use of mechanical lifts and transfer devices to reduce musculo-skeletal injuries among healthcare workers. "Reduction of injuries among nursing home staff is plausibly attributed to the introduction of sufficient mechanical lifting equipment for all residents who need it, along with the training in its uses, and regular battery charging" (Kurowski et al., 2017).

Preventing Workplace Violence

- The Canadian Centre for Occupational Health and Safety (CCOHS) defines workplace violence as "any act in which a person is abused, threatened, intimidated, or assaulted, degraded, or humiliated in his or her employment" (CCOHS, 2017).
- Nurses work with the public, including unstable or volatile clients. Nurses have access to narcotics. Most nurses are women. Concern is growing about violent incidents in the healthcare workplace, including concern about the tolerance of violence as "part of the job" (International Council of Nurses [ICN], 2017).

  The ICN "supports the development of policies that reflect a 'zero tolerance' of violence of any form from any source, including nurses themselves, in any workplace" (ICN, 2017). Furthermore, if quality client care is to be provided, nurses must be ensured a safe work environment and respectful treatment.

  - The ICN (2017) recommends the following:
    - Promoting comfort and reducing client frustration in healthcare settings
    - Instituting programs such as the Nonviolent Crisis Prevention program, which is available to help practical nurses learn respectful, noninvasive methods for de-escalating anger and safely managing disruptive and assaultive behaviour through behaviour management while still protecting the therapeutic relationship with those in their care (Crisis Prevention Institute [CPI], 2012)
    - Ensuring that staff are not alone in emergency and other high-risk settings
    - Installing and maintaining alarm systems, wearing panic alarm badges
    - Liaising with local police and reporting all incidents of violence

Reducing the Risk of Heart Disease and Cancer
Leading Causes of Morbidity and Mortality in Canada

The leading causes of morbidity and mortality among adults in Canada are cardiovascular disease and cancer. As with other diseases, the incidence is higher among low-income Canadians (Health Canada, 2001). This group is a vulnerable population that is more likely than middle-income Canadians to have poor nutrition and to experience higher levels of stress. Practical nurses can contribute toward building healthier communities and to educating clients about modifying controllable risk factors.

Forms of cardiovascular disease include coronary artery disease, myocardial infarction (heart attack), and cerebral vascular accidents (CVAs, or stroke). Common forms of cancer include lung cancer in both men and women and breast cancer in women.

Risk Factors for Cardiovascular Disease

The risk factors for developing cardiovascular disease are as follows:
- A sedentary lifestyle
- Tobacco use
- Obesity
- High levels of blood fats (cholesterol, high-density lipoproteins, triglycerides)
- Diabetes mellitus
- Negative emotions, such as anxiety, depression, and anger
- Illegal drug use (cocaine, amphetamines, hallucinogens, heroin)
- Heredity
- African descent
- Male gender if under age 45
- Older age

Prevention

- Primary prevention of cardiovascular disease involves modification of any of the above risk factors that are within one's control: eating a balanced diet, avoiding illicit drugs and tobacco products, and maintaining a normal body weight.
- Secondary prevention of cardiovascular disease includes screening for hypertension, elevated blood glucose levels, and blood fat levels. With medical advice, certain medications, such as statins and Aspirin, may also limit the progression of cardiovascular disease (Hales & Lauzon, 2018).

Reducing Risk Factors for Cancer

- Minimize exposure to carcinogens in the environment.
- Cigarette smoke is a leading cause of lung cancer. Efforts to reduce or eliminate tobacco use involve smoking prevention and cessation programs.
- Promote cancer-smart nutrition: diets high in antioxidant-rich fruits and vegetables; reducing dietary fats; avoiding smoked, cured, and barbecued meats; and maintaining a healthy body weight (Hales & Lauzon, 2018).
- Risk factors for breast cancer include female gender; advancing age; menarche prior to age 12; combined estrogen–progesterone hormone replacement therapy; and heavy use of alcohol (Hales & Lauzon, 2018). However, 70% of women diagnosed with breast cancer have no known risks other than being female (Canadian Cancer Society, 2011). Having a first child in one's teens or twenties (Hales & Lauzon, 2018) and breastfeeding at any age do provide some protection from breast cancer.
- Skin cancers are malignancies that most often develop due to chronic or sporadic but intense overexposure to both natural and artificial sources of ultraviolet (UV) light. Most are preventable (Shih, Carter, Heward, et al., 2017). Fair skin colouring, freckling tendency, high nevi count, a family history of skin cancer, and childhood sun-exposure history influence an individual's risk for skin cancer (Hales & Lauzon, 2018). At one time, scientists thought exposure to the B range of ultraviolet light (UVB), the wavelength of light responsible for sunburn, posed the greatest danger for skin cancer. However, longer wavelength UVA, which penetrates deeper into the skin, also plays a major role in skin cancers (Hales & Lauzon, 2018). Artificial tanning is a multi-billion-dollar industry frequented by increasing numbers of teenaged girls and young women—and contributing to rising rates of skin cancer. Commercial advertising promotes sunscreens as effective for "safe tanning." However, several studies have concluded that a safe tan is not possible as DNA damage is required to initiate tanning, and the DNA damage intermediate that promotes the tanning pathway is identical to the intermediate seen in carcinogenesis. Therefore, the DNA damage incurred during the tanning process outweighs any photoprotective benefit of sunscreen. While sunscreens help prevent sunburn, they do not show preventive activity against basal cell carcinomas and melanoma (Friedman, English, & Ferris, 2015).
- Best-practice sun protection involves precautions to avoid overexposure to the sun. Do not use indoor sunlamps, tanning parlours, or tanning pills. Inform clients who are on medications that make the skin more sensitive to the sun (oral contraceptives, antibiotics, antihypertensives, anti-inflammatories, immunosuppressives) to take extra precautions when spending time in the sun. Inform parents to protect their children from the sun (Potter et al., 2019).

In their role as health educators, practical nurses have a responsibility to disseminate knowledge about cancer prevention, to help enable people to choose positive health behaviours, and to contribute to reducing our "ecological footprint" in our own workplaces. Ecological changes that reduce the emission of carcinogens (such as toxic wastes and pesticides) into the air, water, and soil we share involve collective action in our communities and nations and a commitment to planetary health.

Program Evaluation

Evaluation processes are critical entry-level competencies required of registered practical nurses. In health promotion practice, evaluation is essential to assessing, improving, and sustaining effective behavioural and environmental interventions that help to promote the health of individuals, families, and communities (Pender et al., 2015). Evaluation data, such as findings from a research study, can be used to advocate for policy change and to acquire funding to support the continuation and development of health promotion initiatives.

Evaluation should be ongoing throughout the design and implementation of health promotion interventions and programs. Process and outcome evaluations are two types of evaluations aimed at understanding the effectiveness of the content, approach, and results of the health promotion interventions. Process evaluations most often target health teaching content and delivery and are therefore helpful in improving the design and implementation of the interventions. On the other hand, outcome evaluations help us to understand the effects of our interventions on health. Outcome evaluations help to pinpoint what health-related changes have occurred as a result of the health promotion intervention (Pender et al., 2015).

For example, process evaluation might entail effectively evaluating health promotion teaching interventions with a group of clients recovering from a myocardial infarction may involve having these same people evaluate the content of what was covered, the teaching style, and the usability of the pamphlets provided. Outcome evaluations of these same interventions could be delineated by tracking the rates of readmission for cardiac-related problems.

PRACTICE QUESTIONS

Case 1

The Canadian Nurses Association has recommended that practical nurses be involved in efforts to promote more environmentally responsible health care. A practical nurse is involved in her hospital's green team. The green team's goals are to improve the hospital's recycling practices, reduce energy use, and promote more environmentally preferable healthcare products.

Questions 1–3 refer to this case.

1. The practical nurse understands that both the energy used and the waste produced by the health sector significantly contribute to which of the following?

1. Global climate change and emissions of dioxins
2. Landfill runoff
3. Contamination of indoor air
4. The development of wind energy alternatives

2. The green team understands that the support of all hospital staff, healthcare consumers, and community administrators is critical to designing and implementing effective, sustainable disease and injury prevention initiatives. This process is best referred to as which of the following?
   1. Conflict resolution
   2. Advocacy and community building
   3. Focus-group planning
   4. Community promotion

3. How would the practical nurse and the green team best increase environmentally responsible behaviours within their agency?
   1. Meet with administrators to outline required policy changes.
   2. Assess all clients for exposure to environmental contaminants.
   3. Implement educational sessions on environmentally responsible health care.
   4. Promote environmentally friendly products in the hospital gift store.

Case 2

A practical nurse visits a shelter for the homeless in a large Canadian city. Many clients have substance abuse problems and malnutrition. All fall into the low-income bracket.

Questions 4–7 refer to this case.

4. The practical nurse approaches the local food bank to ask for donations. What types of foods would be most appropriate for clients?
   1. Calorie-rich
   2. Nutrient-rich
   3. Inexpensive
   4. Canned

5. The practical nurse is committed to improving the health of the clients in the shelter. What strategy has the greatest chance of sustaining improved health for the homeless?
   1. Treatment of addictions
   2. Stable housing
   3. Treatment of chronic illnesses
   4. Improved nutrition

6. There is an outbreak of tuberculosis at the shelter. What is the best action by the practical nurse to ensure that the affected clients comply with their medication regimen?
   1. Arrange for the affected individuals to be admitted to hospital.
   2. Provide directly observed therapy (DOT).
   3. Administer the drugs in a sustained-release formula.
   4. Select drugs that have the lowest incidence of side effects.

7. Many of the practical nurse's clients have chronic open and infected wounds. What is the most likely reason for these lesions to be chronic?

1. Frequent reinjury to wounds not adequately cleaned
2. Inadequate clothes and footwear to protect the skin
3. Close association with others who have infected sores
4. Poor wound healing due to protein–calorie malnutrition

Case 3

A registered practical nurse at City Hospital is a certified Reiki therapist. A client, Olga, has asked the practical nurse to practice Reiki on her as she recovers from breast cancer. The practical nurse is well informed and experienced with Reiki in her native Germany. City Hospital policies support the practical nurse in performing complementary therapies at work.

Questions 8 and 9 refer to this case.

8. What is the practical nurse's responsibility in this situation?
   1. Therapies such as Reiki are controversial, and the practical nurse must not practise Reiki in an accredited hospital.
   2. The practical nurse may practise Reiki within her role as a certified Reiki therapist, as she is fully competent, and Olga has made an informed and legitimate request.
   3. The practical nurse may practise Reiki at City Hospital, but only after her assigned shift and not as part of her practical nursing duties.
   4. The practical nurse may practice Reiki, but only after Olga is discharged from hospital.

9. Reiki is considered to be a complementary therapy. What is the definition of *complementary therapy*?
   1. A therapy that is used in conjunction with traditional Western medicine
   2. A therapy that is used instead of traditional Western medicine
   3. A therapy that is considered to be homeopathic
   4. A therapy that uses only natural methods for treatment

Case 4

Mrs. Broadfoot, age 42, is admitted to a large hospital from her remote northern community. She is experiencing complications from her type 2 diabetes, including kidney failure and peripheral vascular disease. Mrs. Broadfoot is an Indigenous person.

Questions 10–13 refer to this case.

10. What should the practical nurse consider first when developing a plan of care to recognize Mrs. Broadfoot's cultural beliefs and practices?
    1. Include recognized Indigenous cultural factors.
    2. Value Mrs. Broadfoot's individually expressed wishes.
    3. Interview Mrs. Broadfoot's family for culturally specific guidelines.
    4. Refer to the unit procedure for creating care plans for Indigenous people.

11. During morning care, the practical nurse begins a dialogue with Mrs. Broadfoot about her illness. Mrs. Broadfoot is often silent during this interaction. What is the most likely reason for Mrs. Broadfoot's silence?

1. She does not understand English.
2. She is too tired and weak to speak.
3. She is in denial about her health and does not wish to speak about it.
4. She is using a culturally common form of communication.

12. The practical nurse reviews the laboratory results and discovers Mrs. Broadfoot has a low hemoglobin indicating she is anemic. Which of the following foods would be best included in Mrs. Broadfoot's diet?
    1. Beef liver
    2. Tofu
    3. Spinach
    4. Fortified cereals

13. Mrs. Broadfoot has a sudden and unexpected myocardial infarction. Her family is notified but is not able to arrive by plane before she dies. What should the practical nurse do prior to performing a post-mortem care for Mrs. Broadfoot?
    1. Leave Mrs. Broadfoot in her bed so the family may view the body.
    2. Ensure that there is consent for autopsy.
    3. Avoid touching the body until the traditional shaman has provided permission.
    4. Identify cultural death rites that should be respected.

Independent Questions

Questions 14–31 do not refer to a particular case.

14. Ms. Nguyen is ready for discharge home after giving birth to a healthy baby girl. Which of the following safety instructions should be given to all families with infants?
    1. Infants should be positioned on their backs to sleep.
    2. Infants should be positioned on their bellies to sleep.
    3. Infants should be prohibited from co-sleeping with their mothers.
    4. Infants should be bundled up in hats and booties when they sleep.

15. Which of the following is an example of primary prevention?
    1. Annual Papanicolaou (PAP) smears
    2. Megavitamin therapy as a complementary therapy while receiving chemotherapy
    3. Removal of an inflamed appendix before it ruptures
    4. Remaining out of direct sunlight when working outdoors in summertime

16. What is the leading cause of preventable child mortality and morbidity in Canada?
    1. Cancer
    2. Asthma
    3. Injuries
    4. Congenital anomalies

17. Various types of pediatric disease are the result of exposure to contaminants in the indoor and outdoor environment. These health problems include which of the following?
    1. Respiratory diseases
    2. Type 1 diabetes
    3. Juvenile arthritis
    4. Irritable bowel syndrome

18. Mr. Jones, age 60, is admitted to the hospital following a stroke. Mr. Jones weighs 132 kg and has limited mobility. The practical nurse plans to assist Mr. Jones to move from his bed to sit in a special chair. What is the safest way for the practical nurse to move Mr. Jones?
    1. Implement good body mechanics during the transfer from bed to chair.
    2. Assign two personal support workers to move him from bed to his chair.
    3. Use a mechanical lift with the assistance of another healthcare provider.
    4. Explain the procedure carefully to Mr. Jones to ensure he stands using the support aid.

19. At the antenatal clinic, a practical nurse interviews Ms. Capelas, who is nine weeks pregnant. Ms. Capelas tells the practical nurse she has been experiencing a lot of nausea but finds that chewing on crystallized ginger root alleviates the nausea. The practical nurse should do which of the following?
    1. Tell Ms. Capelas to take only medications prescribed by a medical doctor.
    2. Inform Ms. Capelas that there is no scientific basis for this and that she is likely experiencing a placebo effect.
    3. Review current research about ginger as an antiemetic and share this information with Ms. Capelas.
    4. Caution Ms. Capelas that no drugs or home remedies are safe in the first trimester of pregnancy while the baby's organs are forming.

20. Mr. Drosinsky has had nerve-sparing surgery for prostate cancer. The practical nurse includes sexuality in his post-operative health teaching. Which of the following sentences would best introduce the topic?
    1. "I know that you are concerned about achieving an erection after prostate surgery."
    2. "Are you in a sexual relationship now?"
    3. "Many men feel concerned about their sexuality after prostate surgery."
    4. "You are lucky that with nerve-sparing surgery, you will not experience sexual difficulties."

21. Carmen, age 6, has been determined to be obese for her age and height. Of the following, which is the most likely to have been the major factor leading to her obesity?
    1. She does not participate in school sports.
    2. She eats a lot of fast foods.
    3. She watches a lot of TV.
    4. Her parents are obese.

22. What is the most effective diet to achieve sustained weight loss?
    1. A low-fat diet.
    2. A low-carbohydrate diet.
    3. A low-calorie diet.
    4. A Canada food guide diet with reduced portions.

23. Ms. Blanche has been advised by a nutritionist to increase her intake of vitamin D to 1 000 international units (IU). How would Ms. Blanche best achieve this?
   1. Increase the amount of time she spends in the sunshine to at least one hour each day.
   2. Increase her intake of milk.
   3. Take a vitamin D supplement.
   4. Eat a fortified ready-to-eat cereal each morning.

24. The parents of children at Humber Valley Public School are concerned that sexuality is to be included in the Grade 5 health curriculum. The school's practical nurse makes a presentation about the sexual health component of the curriculum at a parent–teacher meeting. She explains which of the following concerning children and sexuality?
   1. All people, regardless of age, are sexual beings.
   2. It is best for children to learn the correct facts about sexuality at school rather than from family or friends.
   3. A discussion about sexuality will prepare them for sexual intercourse.
   4. In Canadian culture, society values children learning about sexuality at an early age.

25. Brendan, age 17, talks to the practical nurse at the student health centre at the university he attends. He tells the practical nurse that he frequently feels too tired to attend classes. What would be the first question the practical nurse would ask Brendan?
   1. "How many hours of sleep do you get each night?"
   2. "What time do you go to bed every night?"
   3. "What time do you get up in the morning?"
   4. "Do you have any health problems that would interfere with sleeping?"

26. The practical nurse visits Mr. and Mrs. Wales, a retired couple in their 80s. The Waleses are fairly active but feel they are not as strong as they used to be, and both experience occasional moments of unsteadiness. The practical nurse performs an environmental assessment of their home. Of the following, what would be the most important assistive device to arrange for Mr. and Mrs. Wales?
   1. Walkers
   2. Grab bars in the bathtub
   3. Blocks under the chair and sofa
   4. A hand-held shower attachment

27. Which of the following would be the best heart-healthy lunch menu?
   1. Purchased chicken soup and a bagel
   2. Delicatessen luncheon meat sandwich and a Caesar salad
   3. Purchased bran muffin and cheddar cheese slices
   4. Grilled chicken, lettuce, and tomato sandwich on whole-grain bread

28. The Collins family regularly visits their mother, age 95, who is in a long-term care facility. What is the most important advice for the practical nurse to provide the family when they visit in order to protect their mother from a communicable disease?
   1. Do not visit if they feel sick.
   2. Use the alcohol gel hand wash located outside her room before entering.
   3. Do not bring children younger than 5 years old to visit.
   4. If they have to cough or sneeze while visiting, they should use a disposable tissue.

29. Ms. Price is a single mother who works part-time at a fast-food outlet. She has three children. Her youngest child, Kyle, has just been prescribed three different medications by the doctor for his asthma, in addition to an over-the-counter antihistamine for his allergies. What would be important for the practical nurse to say to Ms. Price related to Kyle's treatment?
   1. "These medications are expensive. Do you have concerns or questions for me regarding the prescribed medications?"
   2. "Kyle really needs these medications. You must be sure you buy them and give them to him as directed."
   3. "If you can't afford all these medications, don't give Kyle the antihistamine."
   4. "There are generic forms of these medications. I will change the prescription to the less expensive forms of the drugs."

30. The mother of a 5-year-old child asks the practical nurse how best to teach her child to cross a street safely. How would the practical nurse respond?
   1. Buy him a computer game about road safety for children.
   2. Reward the child every time he crosses the street in an approved manner.
   3. Talk to the child daily about the rules of crossing the road.
   4. Provide role-modelling and practise street safety.

31. A practical nurse works in a street clinic. Many of the clients at the clinic are intravenous drug users. On a visit to the clinic washroom one day, the practical nurse finds several used syringes and needles. What initial action should the practical nurse take?
   1. Contact the police and municipal authorities.
   2. Place a puncture-proof sharps container in the bathroom.
   3. Wear protective clothing and dispose of needles in a puncture-proof container.
   4. Ask the client whom the nurse suspects left the needles and syringes to dispose of them.

REFERENCES

Baker, A., Weideman, Y., & Facello, D. (2015). Increasing hospital breastfeeding rates through online education for staff registered nurses. *Clinical Lactation*, 6(1), 24–34. Retrieved from https://doi.org/10.1891/2158-0782.6.1.24.

Bandura, A. (2004). Health promotion by social cognitive means. *Health Education and Behavior*, 31(2), 143.

Best, A., Stokols, D., Green, L. W., et al. (2003). An integrative framework for community partnering to translate theory into effective health promotion strategy. *American Journal of Health Promotion*, 18(2), 168–176.

Burton, E. (2012). Streets ahead? The role of the built environment in healthy aging. *Perspectives in Public Health*, 132(4), 161–162. doi:10.1177/1757913912449570.

Canadian Cancer Society. (2011). Causes of breast cancer. Retrieved from http://www.cancer.ca/Canada-wide/About%20cancer/Types%20of%20cancer/Causes%20of%20breast%20cancer.aspx?sc_lang=en.

Canadian Cancer Society. (2017). Harmful substances and environmental risks. Retrieved from http://www.cancer.ca/en/prevention-and-screening/be-aware/harmful-substances-and-environmental-risks/?region=mb.

Canadian Centre for Occupational Health and Safety. (2017). Violence/bullying. Retrieved from https://ccohs.ca/topics/wellness/violence/.

Canadian Council for Practical Nurse Regulators. (2013). *Standards of practice for licensed practical nurses in Canada.* n.p.: Author. Retrieved from https://www.clpna.com/wp-content/uploads/2013/02/doc_CCPNR_CLPNA_Standards_of_Practice.pdf.

Canadian Institute for Health Information. (2016). *National health expenditure trends, 1975–2016.* Ottawa: Author. Retrieved from https://www.cihi.ca/sites/default/files/document/nhex-trends-narrative-report_2016_en.pdf.

Canadian Institute of Child Health. (2001). *The health of Canada's children: A CICH profile: Pocket guide.* Ottawa: Author. Retrieved from http://www.cich.ca/PDFFiles/ProfilePocketGuide.pdf.

Canadian Institute of Child Health, Safe Kids Canada, & Safe Start. (2012). *Fact sheets: Keep your kids safe.* Ottawa: Author.

Canadian Nurses Association. (2005). CNA backgrounder: The ecosystem, the natural environment, and health and nursing: A summary of the issues. Retrieved from https://www.cna-aiic.ca/~/media/cna/page-content/pdf-en/bg4_the_ecosystem_e.pdf?la=en.

Canadian Nurses Association. (2017). Position statement: Nurses and environmental health. Retrieved from https://www.cna-aiic.ca/~/media/cna/page-content/pdf-en/nurses-and-environmental-health-position-statement.pdf?la=en.

College of Nurses of Ontario. (2009). *Practice guideline: Culturally sensitive care.* Toronto: Author. Retrieved from http://www.cno.org/globalassets/docs/prac/41040_culturallysens.pdf.

College of Nurses of Ontario. (2014). *Practice guideline: Complementary therapies.* Toronto: Author. Retrieved from https://www.cno.org/globalassets/docs/prac/41021_comptherapies.pdf.

Crisis Prevention Institute. (2012). About CPI. Retrieved from http://www.crisisprevention.com/about/history.html.

DiClemente, C. C., & Prochaska, J. O. (1998). Toward a comprehensive, transtheoretical model of change: Stages of change and addictive behaviors. In W. R. Miller & N. Heather (Eds.), *Treating addictive behaviours* (2nd ed., pp. 3–24). New York: Plenum.

Edelman, C., & Kudzma, E. (2018). *Health promotion throughout the life span* (9th ed.). St. Louis: Elsevier.

Finlay, J., Franke, T., McKay, H., et al. (2015). Therapeutic landscapes and well-being in later life: Impacts of blue and green spaces for older adults. *Health & Place*, 34, 97–106. Retrieved from https://doi.org/10.1016/j.healthplace.2015.05.001.

Freire, P. (1970). *Pedagogy of the oppressed.* New York: Continuum.

Friedman, B., English, J., & Ferris, L. (2015). Indoor tanning, skin cancer and the young female patient: A review of the literature. *Journal of Pediatric and Adolescent Gynecology*, 28(4), 275–283. Retrieved from http://dx.doi.org/10.1016/j.jpag.2014.07.015.

Gloria, C., & Steinhardt, M. (2016). Relationships among positive emotions, coping, resilience and mental health. *Stress and Health*, 32(2), 145–156. doi:10.1002/smi.2589.

Golden, S., McLeroy, K., Green, L., et al. (2015). Upending the social ecological model to guide health promotion efforts toward policy and environmental change. *Health Education and Behavior*, 42(1), 1–24. Retrieved from http://journals.sagepub.com/doi/full/10.1177/1090198115575098.

Government of Canada. (2016a). Canada's health care system. Retrieved from https://www.canada.ca/en/health-canada/services/canada-health-care-system.html.

Government of Canada. (2016b). Communicating effectively about immunization. Principles of effective communication. Retrieved from https://www.canada.ca/en/public-health/services/publications/healthy-living/canadian-immunization-guide-part-1-key-immunization-information/page-5-communicating-effectively-immunization.html#p1c4a2.

Government of Canada. (2017). How healthy are Canadians? Physical inactivity. Retrieved from https://www.canada.ca/en/public-health/services/publications/healthy-living/how-healthy-canadians.html#s3-1-2.

Government of Canada. (2018). Canadian immunization guide. Retrieved from https://www.canada.ca/en/public-health/services/publications/healthy-living/canadian-immunization-guide-part-1-key-immunization-information.html.

Hales, D., & Lauzon, L. (2018). *An invitation to health* (5th Cdn. ed.). Toronto: Nelson.

Halter, M. J., Pollard, C. L., & Jacubec, S. L. (2019). *Varcarolis' Canadian psychiatric mental health nursing: A clinical approach* (2nd Cdn. ed.). Milton, ON: Elsevier Canada.

Health Canada. (2001). Population health promotion: An integrated model of population health and health promotion. Retrieved from http://www.phac-aspc.gc.ca/ph-sp/php-psp/php3-eng.php.

Health Canada. (2007). *Eating well with Canada's food guide: First nations, Inuit and métis.* Ottawa: Author. Retrieved from https://www.canada.ca/content/dam/hc-sc/migration/hc-sc/fn-an/alt_formats/fnihb-dgspni/pdf/pubs/fnim-pnim/2007_fnim-pnim_food-guide-aliment-eng.pdf.

Health Canada. (2011). *Eating well with Canada's food guide.* Ottawa: Author. Retrieved from http://www.hc-sc.gc.ca/fn-an/food-guide-aliment/index_e.html.

Hockenberry, M., & Wilson, D. (2015). *Wong's nursing care of infants and children* (10th ed.). St. Louis: Elsevier/Mosby.

Hoffman, A. (2013). Enhancing self-efficacy for optimized patient outcomes through the theory of symptom self-management. *Cancer Nursing*, 38(1), E16–E26. Retrieved from http://doi.org/10.1097/NCC.0b013e31824a730a.

International Council of Nurses. (2017). *Position statement: Prevention and management of workplace violence.* Geneva, Switzerland: Author. Retrieved from http://www.icn.ch/images/stories/documents/publications/position_statements/ICN_PS_Prevention_and_management_of_workplace_violence.pdf.

Johansson, A., Petrisko, M., & Chasens, E. (2016). Adolescent sleep and the impact of technology use before sleep on daytime function. *Journal of Pediatric Nursing*, 31(5), 498–504. Retrieved from https://www.ncbi.nlm.nih.gov/pmc/articles/PMC5026973/.

Kirby, M. (2002). *Vol. 6: Recommendations for reform. The health of canadians—the federal role.* Ottawa: The Standing Senate Committee on Social Affairs, Science and Technology.

Kurowski, A., Gore, R., Roberts, Y., et al. (2017). Injury rates before and after the implementation of a safe resident handling program in the long term care sector. *Safety Science*, 92, 217–224. Retrieved from http://dx.doi.org/10.1016/j.ssci.2016.10.012.

LaLonde, M. (1974). *A new perspective on the health of Canadians. A working document*. Ottawa: Government of Canada. Retrieved from http://www.phac-aspc.gc.ca/ph-sp/pdf/perspect-eng.pdf.

Laverack, G. (2004). *Health promotion practice: Power and empowerment*. London, UK: Sage.

Lazarus, R. (1999). *Stress and emotion: A new synthesis*. New York: Springer.

Letovsky, E., Rowe, B., Friedman, S., et al. (2015). Improving bicycle safety in Canada. *Canadian Journal of Emergency Medicine*, 17(3), 323–327. Retrieved from https://doi.org/10.2310/8000.2014.201402.

McMurray, A., & Clendon, J. (2015). *Community health and wellness: Primary health care in practice* (5th ed.). Sydney, Australia: Elsevier.

Mensah, C., Andres, L., Perera, U., et al. (2016). Enhancing quality of life through the lens of green spaces: A systematic review approach. *International Journal of Wellbeing*, 6(1), 142–163. doi:10.5502/ijw.v6i1.445.

National Center for Complementary and Integrative Health. (2016). Complementary, alternative, or integrative health: What's in a name? Retrieved from https://nccih.nih.gov/health/integrative-health#cvsa.

Pan American Health Organization, & World Health Organization. (2000). *Promotion of sexual health: Recommendations for action*. Geneva, Switzerland: World Health Organization.

Pender, N., Murdaugh, C., & Parsons, M. (2006). *Health promotion in nursing practice* (5th ed.). Upper Saddle River, NJ: Pearson Prentice Hall.

Pender, N., Murdaugh, C., & Parsons, M. (2015). *Health promotion in nursing practice* (7th ed.). Upper Saddle River, NJ: Pearson Education, Inc.

Petros, A., & Georgi, J. (2011). Landscape preference evaluation for hospital environmental design. *Journal of Environmental Protection*, 2, 639–647. doi:10.4236/jep.2011.25073.

Potter, P., Perry, A., Stockert, P., et al. (2019). *Canadian fundamentals of nursing* (6th ed.). Milton, ON: Elsevier.

Public Health Agency of Canada. (2008). Complementary and alternative health. Retrieved from http://www.phac-aspc.gc.ca/chn-rcs/cah-acps-eng.php.

Public Health Agency of Canada. (2013). What determines health? Determinants of health: What makes Canadians healthy or unhealthy? Retrieved from https://www.canada.ca/en/public-health/services/health-promotion/population-health/what-determines-health/what-makes-canadians-healthy-unhealthy.html.

Romanow, R. J. (2002). *Building on values: The future of health care in Canada—final report*. Ottawa: Commission on the Future of Health Care in Canada.

Sexuality Information and Education Council of the United States. (2008). *Human development*. Washington, DC: Author. Retrieved from http://www.sexedlibrary.org/index.cfm?pageId=723.

Shih, S., Carter, R., Heward, S., et al. (2017). Skin cancer has a large impact on our public hospitals but prevention programs continue to demonstrate strong economic credentials. *Australian and New Zealand Journal of Public Health*, 41(4), 371–376. doi:10.1111/1753-6405.12679.

Stanhope, M., Lancaster, J., Jakubec, S., et al. (2017). *Community health nursing in Canada* (3rd ed.). Toronto: Elsevier.

Statistics Canada. (2016). Immigration and ethnocultural diversity in Canada. Retrieved from http://www12.statcan.gc.ca/nhs-enm/2011/as-sa/99-010-x/99-010-x2011001-eng.cfm.

Statistics Canada. (2017). Population growth: Migration increase overtakes natural increase. Retrieved from http://www.statcan.gc.ca/pub/11-630-x/11-630-x2014001-eng.htm.

Stavrinos, D., Pope, C., Shen, J., et al. (2018). Distracted walking, bicycling and driving; Systematic review and meta-analysis of mobile technology and youth crash risk. *Child Development*, 89(1), 118–128. Retrieved from http://onlinelibrary.wiley.com/doi/10.1111/cdev.12827/full.

Svensson, T., Miller, L., & Hurd, C. (2016). Expanding the nurse practitioner role in treatment resistant major depression. *Journal of Hospital & Medical Management*. Retrieved from http://hospital-medical-management.imedpub.com/expanding-the-nurse-practitioner-role-in-treatment-resistant-major-depression.php?aid=9302.

Taylor, S. E., Klein, L. C., Lewis, B. P., et al. (2000). Biobehavioral responses to stress in females: Tend-and-befriend, not fight-or-flight. *Psychological Review*, 107(3), 411–429.

World Health Organization. (1986). The Ottawa charter for health promotion. Retrieved from http://www.who.int/healthpromotion/conferences/previous/ottawa/en/index4.html.

World Health Organization. (2008). The world health report 2008—primary health care (Now more than ever). Retrieved from http://www.who.int/whr/2008/en/.

World Health Organization. (2013). *WHO traditional medicine strategy 2014–2023*. Geneva, Switzerland: Author. Retrieved from http://apps.who.int/iris/bitstream/10665/92455/1/9789241506090_eng.pdf.

World Health Organization. (2015). Sexual health, human rights and the law. Retrieved from http://apps.who.int/iris/bitstream/10665/175556/1/9789241564984_eng.pdf?ua=1.

World Health Organization. (2016). *What is health promotion?* Author. Retrieved from http://www.who.int/features/qa/health-promotion/en/.

Yanchar, N., Warda, L., & Fuselli, P. (2016). Child and youth injury prevention: A public health approach. *Canadian Paediatric Society*, 17(9), 511. Retrieved from https://www.ncbi.nlm.nih.gov/pmc/articles/PMC5026973/.

BIBLIOGRAPHY

Bandura, A. (1977). *Social learning theory*. Englewood Cliffs, NJ: Prentice Hall.

Canadian Cancer Society. (2018). What is breast cancer? Retrieved from http://www.cancer.ca/en/cancer-information/cancer-type/breast/breast-cancer/?region=on.

DiClemente, C. C. (2007). The transtheoretical model of intentional behaviour change. *Drugs and Alcohol Today*, 7(1), 29–33.

Edwards, N. (1999). Population health: Determinants and interventions. *Canadian Journal of Public Health*, 90(1), 10–11.

Health Canada. (2004). What is long-term facilities-based care? Retrieved from https://www.canada.ca/en/health-canada/services/home-continuing-care/long-term-facilities-based-care.html.

Registered Nurses' Association of Ontario. (2018). Environmental determinants of health. Retrieved from http://rnao.ca/policy/projects/environmental-determinants-health.

WEB SITES

- **Canada Communicable Disease Report (CCDR)** (https://www
.canada.ca/en/public-health/services/reports-publications/canad
a-communicable-disease-report-ccdr.html): This government
journal provides information on the prevention and control of
emerging and persistent infectious diseases. It publishes
surveillance reports, outbreak reports, original research, rapid
communications, advisory committee statements.
- **Dietary Reference Intakes Tables** (http://www.hc-sc.gc.ca/
fn-an/nutrition/reference/table/index_e.html#rvm): This Health
Canada site contains information about daily requirements for
different nutrients.
- **Eating Well with Canada's Food Guide** (https://www.canada.ca/
en/health-canada/services/canada-food-guides.html): This site
includes links to the latest version of the food guide for the
general population as well as the food guide for First
Nations people, Inuit, and Métis; translated versions of the
food guide; and a wealth of other links pertaining to nutrition
in Canada.
- **Joint Position Statement on Environmentally Responsible
Activity in the Health-Care Sector by the Canadian Nurses
Association and Canadian Medical Association** (https://
www.cna-aiic.ca/~/media/cna/page-content/pdf-en/jps99
_environmental_e.pdf?la=en): This joint statement advocates
for environmental awareness and environmentally sound
conduct on the part of health care providers.
- **Natural and Non-prescription Health Products Directorate**
(https://www.canada.ca/en/health-canada/services/
drugs-health-products/natural-non-prescription.html): This
Health Canada site provides information on natural health
products for consumers and the industry.

Nursing Fundamentals and Clinical Skills

Practical nurses need a strong knowledge base that is rooted in the best evidence in order to provide high-quality and safe care to clients in the healthcare setting. This chapter provides a review of the fundamental knowledge that underlies all nursing care and the clinical skills that are needed to enact this care.

VITAL SIGNS

Body Temperature

Body temperature represents the balance between heat produced and heat lost by the body. Acceptable body temperatures range from 36–38°C, but there is not one temperature that is normal for all people. The average oral or tympanic temperature is 37°C for a healthy adult and 36°C for an older adult. Rectal temperatures are 0.5°C higher (37.5°C) and axillary temperatures are 0.5°C lower (36.5°C) than oral temperatures (Potter, Perry, Stockert, et al., 2019).

Core and Surface Temperatures

- Core temperatures (temperatures of the deep tissues) are relatively constant. Examples include rectal, tympanic, esophageal, pulmonary artery, and urinary bladder temperatures.
- Surface temperatures fluctuate depending on blood flow to the skin and environmental conditions. Examples include skin, axillary, and oral temperatures.

Temperature Measurement Sites

The temperature measurement sites used routinely are the mouth, rectum, axilla, and tympanic membrane. It is the practical nurse's responsibility to choose the safest and most accurate site for a particular client. Listed next are some advantages and disadvantages of the commonly used sites (Potter et al., 2019).

Oral temperature. Oral temperatures reflect rapid fluctuations in the core temperature. They cannot be used in infants, small children, or confused, unco-operative, or unconscious clients. It is also necessary to wait 20–30 minutes before taking an oral temperature if the client has smoked or ingested hot or cold liquids or foods.

Rectal temperature. Rectal temperatures are the preferred method of measurement in young children who cannot use oral thermometers, but they should not be used for newborns due to the risk of anal perforation. Some disadvantages are that rectal temperatures may lag behind a core temperature during rapid temperature changes, and they require privacy and the use of a lubricant.

Axillary temperature. Axillary temperature is the safest site to measure temperatures in newborns. Disadvantages include a longer measurement time and a lag behind core temperature during rapid temperature changes.

Tympanic membrane temperature. The tympanic membrane is an easily accessible site that provides a core temperature quickly; however, it has greater variability in results than other core temperature methods due to user variability. Inconsistencies regarding the accuracy of tympanic membrane temperature (TMT) measurements in determining fever in infants and small children have been reported in the literature (Hockenberry & Wilson, 2015).

Pulse

The *pulse* is the "bounding of arterial blood flow that is palpable at various points on the body" (Potter et al., 2019, p. 542). Any artery can be used for checking the pulse, but the radial and carotid arteries are most commonly used as they are easily palpable. The carotid pulse is commonly used in emergency situations.

Common Pulse Rate Assessment Sites

The radial and apical locations are the most common sites for pulse rate assessment in adults.

Radial pulse. Assessment of the radial pulse includes measurement of the rate (60–100 beats per minute in adults), rhythm (regular or irregular), strength or force (bounding, strong, weak, or thready), and equality (assessing radial pulses in both arms). If the pulse is regular, the practical nurse counts the pulse rate for 30 seconds and multiplies by 2. If the pulse is irregular, the nurse counts the pulse rate for 1 full minute.

Apical pulse. The apical pulse is measured with a stethoscope. It is located at the fifth intercostal space at the left midclavicular line. The apical rate is used to count the heart rate in infants and young children where the heart rates are very rapid and difficult to palpate and count accurately at a peripheral site. The apical site is also used to auscultate heart sounds when an abnormal peripheral pulse is palpated.

Key Terms Related to Pulse

- *Bradycardia* is a heart rate below 60 beats per minute in an adult.

- *Tachycardia* is a heart rate above 100 beats per minute in an adult.
- *Dysrhythmia* is an irregular or abnormal rhythm.
- *Sinus arrhythmia* is a normal increase in heart rate associated with inspiration. It is more common in children but often found in adults.
- *Pulse deficit* is the difference between the apical and radial pulse rates. It is frequently associated with an abnormal rhythm and is a result of ineffective heart contractions where the pulse wave is not transmitted to the periphery (Potter et al., 2019). Apical and radial rates are assessed at the same time by two practical nurses to determine the presence of a pulse deficit.

Respirations

Respiration is "the mechanism that the body uses to exchange gases between the atmosphere and the blood and between the blood and the cells" (Potter et al., 2019, p. 549).

Assessment of Respirations

Accurate measurement of respirations requires observation and palpation of chest wall movement. A complete assessment includes assessment of respiratory rate (12–20 breaths per minute in adults), depth (deep, normal, or shallow), and rhythm (regular or irregular). The practical nurse counts respirations for 30 seconds if respirations are normal and for 1 full minute if abnormalities are suspected.

Key Terms Related to Alterations in Adult Breathing Patterns

- *Bradypnea* is regular but slow breathing at a rate of less than 12 breaths per minute (Potter et al., 2019).
- *Tachypnea* is regular but rapid breathing at a rate of greater than 20 breaths per minute (Potter et al., 2019).
- *Hyperpnea* is laboured, deep respirations at a rate of greater than 20 breaths per minute. It occurs normally with exercise (Potter et al., 2019).
- *Apnea* is the temporary cessation of breathing and then resume. Persistent cessation results in respiratory arrest (Potter et al., 2019).
- *Dyspnea* is shortness of breath resulting in laboured or difficult breathing (Potter et al., 2019).
- *Orthopnea* is an abnormal condition in which a person must sit or stand to breathe deeply or comfortably. Assessment includes noting the number of pillows used by the client. Clients with orthopnea also report sleeping in recliners (Mosby, 2013).

Pulse Oximetry

Pulse oximetry is the indirect measure of arterial oxygen saturation. The pulse oximeter measures pulse oxygen saturation (SpO_2), which is a reliable estimate of SaO_2 (the percentage of hemoglobin that is bound with oxygen in the arteries or the percentage of saturation of hemoglobin) (Potter et al., 2019). It is usually between 95–100%. Pulse oximetry is less accurate at saturations less than 70%. Some factors that affect accurate readings include peripheral vascular disease, hypothermia,

hypotension, peripheral edema, jaundice, and the presence of nail polish (Potter et al., 2019).

Blood Pressure

Blood pressure (BP) is the force of the blood under pressure pushing on the walls of an artery (Jarvis, Browne, MacDonald-Jenkins, et al., 2019). BP depends on the cardiac output (CO) and peripheral vascular resistance (PVR). BP is a good indicator of cardiovascular health.

Measurement of BP

- *BP* is recorded in millimetres of mercury (mm Hg) as the systolic over the diastolic reading (e.g., 120/80). Optimal BP is less than 120/80.
- *Systolic BP* is the peak of maximum pressure when the left ventricle contracts and ejects blood under high pressure into the aorta.
- *Diastolic pressure* is the minimum pressure (resting pressure) exerted on the arterial walls when the ventricles relax.
- *Pulse pressure* is the difference between the systolic and diastolic pressures. For a BP of 130/90, the pulse pressure is 40 mm Hg.

Korotkoff sounds. *Korotkoff sounds* are the sounds of blood flow auscultated during BP measurement. There are five sounds; the first sound (onset of clear rhythmic tapping) and the last sound (disappearance of sound) are used for the systolic and diastolic BP readings in adolescents and adults (Jarvis et al., 2019).

Auscultatory gap. The *auscultatory gap* is the temporary disappearance of Korotkoff sounds during auscultation of BP. It typically occurs between the first and second Korotkoff sounds and may range from 10–40 mm Hg. It is more common in clients with hypertension or older adults. It can cause underestimation of systolic BP or overestimation of diastolic BP (Jarvis et al., 2019; Potter et al., 2019).

Nursing considerations related to measurement of BP.
- Verify BP in both arms initially to compare and collect baseline data.
- Lower extremities (e.g., the popliteal artery behind the knee) can be used if the arms are not accessible.
- Choose a cuff with a bladder size matched to the size of the arm. For BP measurements by auscultation, the bladder width should be close to 40% of arm circumference and bladder length should cover 80–100% of arm circumference (Hypertension Canada, 2017; Potter et al., 2019).
- Avoid applying the BP cuff to an arm with intravenous (IV) therapy, an arteriovenous shunt or fistula, breast or axillary surgery, a cast, or a bulky bandage.

Hypertension

Hypertension is persistently elevated BP and is often asymptomatic. It is the result of thickening and loss of elasticity of arterial walls. Hypertension is present when diastolic readings are greater than 90 mm Hg and systolic readings are greater than 140 mm Hg. The diagnosis of high normal BP is a diastolic reading between 85–89 mm Hg and systolic BP between 130–139 mm Hg. The diagnosis of high normal BP or hypertension is made on the basis of two or more BP readings on consecutive visits (Hypertension Canada, 2017; Potter et al., 2019).

Hypotension

Hypotension occurs when the systolic BP falls to 90 mm Hg or below (Potter et al., 2019). This can be a normal BP for some adults, but it is often associated with illness. Possible causes of low BP include pregnancy, medications (particularly drugs used to treat high BP), heart or endocrine problems, dehydration, severe blood loss, severe infection (septicemia), allergic reaction (anaphylaxis), or nutritional deficiencies.

Orthostatic Hypotension

Orthostatic hypotension, or *postural hypotension*, occurs when a person with BP within the normal range develops symptoms as well as low BP when moving to an upright position. Symptoms include fainting, weakness, or lightheadedness, as well as a drop in BP and a rise in pulse rate. Clients at risk for orthostatic hypotension include clients with dehydration, anemia, recent blood loss, prolonged immobility, or new medications, such as antihypertensives. To assess for orthostatic hypotension, the nurse records BP and pulse (P) with the client supine, sitting, and standing (Potter et al., 2019).

INFECTION PREVENTION AND CONTROL

Infectious Process

Infection is the invasion of the body by pathogens (disease-producing organisms) and the reaction of the tissues to their presence and to the toxins generated by them. Signs and symptoms of infection may be local or systemic.

- Areas of localized infection may exhibit redness, swelling, and warmth or heat due to inflammation. Other symptoms may include discharge or exudate and pain or tenderness at the site.
- Systemic infections cause more generalized symptoms, such as fever, fatigue, and malaise. Other symptoms include enlargement of lymph nodes in the involved area, loss of appetite, nausea, or vomiting.
- Infections in older adults may not present typically as older adults tend to have lower body temperatures, decreased pain sensation, and a reduced immune response to infection. They may have advanced infection before it is identified.

Chain of Infection

The development of an infection occurs in a cycle that depends on the presence of all of the following six elements: infectious agent, reservoir, portal of exit, mode of transmission, portal of entry, and susceptible host (Potter et al., 2019). Healthcare workers follow infection prevention and control practices to break the links in this chain so that infections will not develop.

1. *Infectious agent (pathogen):* an invading organism (such as a bacterium, virus, fungus, or protozoan)

2. *Reservoir:* an environment in which a pathogen can survive and may or may not multiply; the human body is the most common reservoir
3. *Portal of exit:* a mode of escape from the reservoir (e.g., the mouth, nose, rectal, vaginal, urethra opening, or respiratory or gastro-intestinal tract)
4. *Mode of transmission:* the method by which a pathogen is transmitted to a new host (direct or indirect contact, airborne, food, and so on)
5. *Portal of entry:* the means by which the pathogen enters a new host (such as via the respiratory tract or through broken skin or mucous membranes)
6. *Susceptible host:* susceptibility depends on the individual degree of resistance to a pathogen

Nosocomial or Healthcare–Associated Infections

Healthcare–associated infections (HAIs) are infections acquired after admission to a hospital or another healthcare agency that were not present or incubating at the time of admission. Clients most susceptible are children and older adults and individuals with severe underlying illness, a weak immune system, poor nutritional status, or loss of skin integrity. Clients in intensive care settings are most susceptible due to the necessity for many invasive lines (including vascular access devices and urinary catheters) and the heavy use of antibiotics.

Medical and Surgical Asepsis
Medical Asepsis

Medical asepsis (clean technique) refers to procedures used to reduce and prevent the spread of micro-organisms. Common examples include hand hygiene, using clean disposable gloves to prevent direct contact with blood or body fluids, and cleaning the environment and equipment routinely (Potter et al., 2019).

Surgical Asepsis

Surgical asepsis (sterile technique) includes all procedures used to eliminate all micro-organisms, including pathogens and spores, from an object or area. Examples of surgical asepsis include (a) procedures in which the client's skin is punctured (such as IV insertion or injections); (b) nonintact skin due to injury or surgery; and (c) insertion of catheters or surgical instruments into sterile body cavities (urinary catheterization, peritoneal dialysis catheters, and so on) (Potter et al., 2019).

Key principles of surgical asepsis.
- A sterile object remains sterile only when touched by another sterile object.
- Only sterile objects may be placed on a sterile field.
- A sterile object or field out of the range of vision or an object held below a person's waist is considered contaminated.
- A sterile object or field becomes contaminated by prolonged exposure to airborne micro-organisms.
- When a sterile surface comes in contact with a wet, contaminated surface, the sterile object or field becomes contaminated by micro-organisms drawn from above or below by capillary action.

- Fluid flows in the direction of gravity.
- The edges of a sterile field or container are considered to be unsterile.
- Qualities such as conscientiousness or an "infection-control conscience," vigilance, and honesty are very important in maintaining surgical asepsis (Lewis, Bucher, Heitkemper, et al., 2014).

Infection Prevention and Control Guidelines

The risk of transmitting infection in the hospital is high, so healthcare workers must follow strict infection-control guidelines to prevent and control the spread of infection. Guidelines consist of two tiers: one tier of precautions to be followed for the care of all clients, called *routine practices*, and a second tier called *additional precautions* to be used to contain or isolate pathogens in one area.

Routine Practices

Routine practices (called *standard precautions* by the U.S. Centers for Disease Control and Prevention [CDC]) are infection-control precautions designed for the care of "all clients in any setting regardless of their diagnosis or presumed infectiousness" (Potter et al., 2019, p. 705). Routine practices "apply when a healthcare worker is or potentially may be exposed to (a) blood; (b) all body fluids, secretions, and excretions except sweat; (c) nonintact skin; or (d) mucous membranes" (Potter et al., 2019, p. 705). Routine practices include hand hygiene; use of personal protective equipment (PPE) such as gloves, masks, eye protection, face protection, or gowns; proper disposal of sharps; routine cleaning of client equipment; waste disposal; care of laundry; and routine environmental cleaning. A key element of routine practices is "to assess the risk of transmission of microorganisms before any interaction with patients/clients/residents" and then to decide on risk reduction strategies (Canadian Committee on Antibiotic Resistance, 2007, p. 12).

Additional Precautions

Additional precautions (called *transmission-based precautions* by the CDC) are designed to contain pathogens in one area, usually the client's room, so they are also called *isolation precautions*. These precautions are in addition to routine practices. There are three categories of precautions (airborne, droplet, and contact), and the category that is used depends on how a particular pathogen is spread.

Airborne precautions. Airborne precautions are used for known or suspected infections caused by microbes transmitted by airborne droplets, such as measles, chicken pox (varicella), disseminated varicella zoster, and tuberculosis (TB). Barrier protection used with airborne precautions includes (a) a private negative-pressure room (door closed) and (b) a respiratory device (such as an N-95 respirator mask if the client has TB or when the client has the other conditions mentioned and the healthcare worker is not immune). A mask is also placed on the client if it is necessary for the client to leave the room (Potter et al., 2019).

Droplet precautions. Droplet precautions are used for known or suspected infections caused by microbes transmitted by droplets produced by coughing, sneezing, or talking. Examples include diphtheria, rubella, influenza, pertussis, mumps, mycoplasmal or meningococcal pneumonia, scarlet fever, and sepsis. Barrier protection with droplet precautions includes (a) using a private room or cohorting clients (room door must be closed) and (b) using a mask (Lewis et al., 2019; Potter et al., 2019).

Contact precautions. Contact precautions are used for known or suspected infections caused by direct or indirect contact, such as colonization or infection with antibiotic-resistant organisms (AROs); major wound infections; respiratory infections such as respiratory syncytial virus (RSV); enteric infections such as *Clostridium difficile*; skin infections such as herpes simplex, impetigo, pediculosis, and scabies; and eye infections such as conjunctivitis. Barrier protection with contact precautions includes (a) using a private room or cohorting clients (the door can be open) and (b) using gloves and a mask when in contact with the client (Lewis et al., 2019; Potter et al., 2019).

Hand Hygiene

Hand hygiene is the practice of removing or killing pathogens on the hands and maintaining good skin integrity (Ontario Agency for Health Protection and Promotion [Public Health Ontario], Provincial Infectious Diseases Advisory Committee [Ontario Agency for Health Protection and Promotion], 2014; Potter et al., 2019). Hand hygiene consists of the use of alcohol-based hand rubs or handwashing and is the most important method of preventing HAIs.

Alcohol-based hand rubs. Alcohol-based hand rubs or alcohol hand antiseptics are the gold standard for hand hygiene. They are quicker, easier, and more effective than handwashing if used correctly.

Handwashing. Handwashing must be performed when hands are visibly soiled. The mechanical action of washing, rinsing, and drying hands removes pathogens (Ontario Agency for Health Protection and Promotion, 2014; Potter et al., 2014). Hands need to be washed with soap and water for 40–60 seconds with special attention to areas that are frequently missed, such as around the nails, the thumb area, and between the fingers. If the hands are visibly soiled, more time may be required to wash the hands. To determine when and what type of hand hygiene to perform is based on: the type of procedure or activity performed, the amount of time with the contaminated object or client, the degree or amount of contamination that will occur with the contact, and the susceptibility of the client or the health care worker to infection (Potter et al., 2019).

Personal Protective Equipment

Personal protective equipment (PPE) is clothing or equipment worn by healthcare providers for their protection. The use of PPE is part of routine practices when the nurse is likely to be in contact with blood, body fluids, mucous membranes, nonintact skin, body tissues, or contaminated equipment or surfaces (Potter et al., 2019). PPE includes the use of any or all of the following: masks, gloves, gowns, face protection, or eye protection. The choice of PPE is also dependent on the situation, procedure, or type of additional precautions required.

Multidrug-Resistant Organisms

Multidrug-resistant organisms (MDROs), also known as *AROs* or "superbugs," are "microorganisms, predominantly bacteria, that are resistant to one or more classes of antimicrobial agents" (CDC, 2006). The two most common are MRSA (methicillin-resistant *Staphylococcus aureus*) and VRE (vancomycin-resistant *Enterococcus*). During the last few decades, MDROs in hospitals have been increasing at alarming rates. Options for treating clients with these infections are extremely limited. Increased lengths of stay in hospital, costs, and mortality are associated with MDROs (CDC, 2006). There is strong evidence to suggest that MDROs are carried from client to client via the hands of healthcare providers (Duckro, Blom, Lyle, et al., 2005).

Community-associated MRSA. MRSA infections that are acquired by persons who have not been hospitalized within the last year or undergone a medical procedure such as dialysis or surgery are known as *community-associated MRSA infections*. "Staph" or MRSA infections in the community are on the rise and usually manifest as skin infections (pimples and boils) in otherwise healthy people (CDC, 2016).

MEDICATION ADMINISTRATION

The administration of medications is one of the primary responsibilities of practical nurses. It is important for practical nurses to have knowledge about the actions and effects of the medications that they give to clients. To safely and accurately administer medications, practical nurses also need knowledge about pharmacological concepts, human anatomy, growth and development, pathophysiology, psychology, nutrition, and mathematics (Potter et al., 2019).

Pharmacological Concepts
Drug Names

A drug has several different names, including a chemical, a generic, and a trade name:

1. The chemical name is a description of the medication's composition and molecular structure. This name is rarely used in clinical practice. An example of a chemical name is acetylsalicylic acid (Potter et al., 2019).
2. The generic or nonproprietary name is the first manufacturer's name for the drug, and this name is protected by law. It is the official name that is listed in the *Compendium of Pharmaceuticals and Specialties* (CPS) and *Canadian Formulary* (CF). An example of a generic name is Aspirin (Potter et al., 2019).
3. The trade name, brand name, or proprietary name denotes the marketing name that the manufacturer uses to sell a medication. The trade name has a trademark (™) symbol beside it (as in Tempra™ or Motrin™), indicating that the name is trademarked (Potter et al., 2019).

Classification

Each drug can be categorized in one or more subcategories called *classifications*. Drugs that affect the body in similar ways are in the same classification. Drug classification indicates "the effect of the medication on a body system, the symptoms the medication relieves, or the medication's desired effects" (Potter et al., 2019, p. 728). Drugs can be in more than one classification if they have several different types of therapeutic effects, such as Aspirin, which is an analgesic, an antipyretic, and an anti-inflammatory. Other examples of drug classifications include antibiotics and antihypertensives.

Systems of Medication Administration
Metric System

The metric system involves decimals and uses divisions and multiples of 10. The basic units are metre (length), litre (volume), and gram (weight). Most countries, including Canada, use metric as their standard of measurement.

- Common metric abbreviations for volume include L (litre) and mm (millimetre).
- Common metric abbreviations for weight include kg (kilogram); g (gram); mg (milligram); and mcg (microgram).

Household Measurements

Prescriptions to be self-administered at home are often written in household measures. Examples include cups, teaspoons, or pints for volume and ounces and pounds for weight.

Conversions and Calculations

Conversion between metric units. To convert larger to smaller, multiply by 1 000 or move the decimal point three places to the right. For example, to convert 1 g to milligrams, multiply by 1 000 ($1 \times 1 000 = 1 000$ mg). To convert smaller to larger, divide by 1 000 or move the decimal point three places to the left. For example, to convert 500 mL to litres, divide by 1 000 or move the decimal point three places to the left ($500 \div 1 000 = 0.5$ L).

Conversions between systems. The practical nurse may find it necessary to convert weights or volumes from one system to another. Metric units may need to be converted to household measurements for home administration. The nurse must know or refer to an equivalence table in this case. For example, if the client is to take 10 mL of brompheniramine-PPA (Dimetapp) elixir at home, the nurse must know that 1 teaspoon (tsp) equals 5 mL and that 10 mL = 2 tsp. Common conversions include the following:

2.2 lb. = 1 kg; 1 tbsp = 15 mL; and 1 tsp = 5 mL.

Dose calculations. There are several methods of calculating medication doses. The following formula is useful for either solid or liquid doses:

Example using the formula:

$$\frac{\text{Dose Ordered}}{\text{Dose on Hand}} \times \text{Amount on Hand} = \text{Amount to Administer}$$

The doctor has ordered 4 mg of morphine to be given subcutaneously. The morphine is available in 10 mg/mL ampoules. Using the formula, the amount to administer would be 0.4 mL (4 mg ÷ 10 mg × 1 mL = 0.4 mL).

Routes of Medication Administration

Oral Route

The oral route is convenient and easy, but it has a slower onset of action. This route is avoided when the client has gastro-intestinal alterations such as vomiting or reduced intestinal motility or has had gastro-intestinal surgery.

- Sublingual tablets are designed for rapid absorption when placed under the tongue.
- Buccal administration involves placing the solid medication in the mouth and against the mucous membranes of the cheek until the medication dissolves.
- Enteric-coated tablets and sustained-released capsules delay absorption until the medication reaches the small intestine, so these medications cannot be crushed.
- Liquid medications in quantities of less than 10 mL should be measured in an oral syringe for accuracy.
- If possible, tablets and capsules should be swallowed with 60–100 mL of fluid.

Parenteral Route

Parenteral administration is the injection of a medication into body tissues. There are four routes: intradermal (ID), subcutaneous, intramuscular (IM), and IV.

Intradermal route. *ID injection* refers to injection into the dermis, just under the epidermis. It is used for the tuberculin skin test or allergy testing. The most common site is the inner forearm. The bevel of the needle is pointing up during the injection so that medication is less likely to be deposited into tissues below the dermis. It is given at a 5–15-degree angle. A small bleb (resembling a mosquito bite) appears. The area should not be massaged.

Subcutaneous route. *Subcutaneous (subcut) injections* involve injecting medication into the loose connective tissue under the dermis at a 45–90-degree angle. Absorption of medication is slower via this route than via IM sites because adipose tissue is not very vascular. The most common sites are the outer posterior aspects of the upper arms, the abdomen, and the anterior aspects of the thighs. Only 0.5–1 mL should be given subcutaneously as subcutaneous injections can be painful. Injecting into a blood vessel during subcutaneous injections is very rare, so aspiration is not necessary. Pinch the skin before injection to elevate the skin and subcutaneous tissue above the muscle.

Subcutaneous medications requiring special consideration.
- Insulin injection sites for diabetes should be rotated, with no one site being used again for one month to avoid the development of hard lumps and fat deposits. Clients with diabetes who inject insulin should practise intrasite rotation (rotating injection sites within the same body part) to provide greater consistency in the absorption of insulin.
- Injections of heparin and its derivative, low-molecular-weight heparin (LMWH), are best given in the abdomen.

To prevent bruising, these injection sites should not be massaged.

IM route. *IM injections* are administered directly into the muscle at a 90-degree angle. This route provides fast absorption due to the greater vascularity of muscle. The muscle can also tolerate more viscous or irritating substances. From 1–3 mL can be given intramuscularly, depending on the site. The skin is pulled taut at the site to ensure that the medication is injected into the muscle. IM injections are associated with more risks, and it is important that bony landmarks are used for landmarking all IM sites. The common IM injection sites are the ventrogluteal, dorsogluteal, vastus lateralis, and deltoid muscles.

Ventrogluteal site. The ventrogluteal muscle is the safest site and the preferred site for adults and children over 7–12 months of age. It is free of major nerves and blood vessels and has easily palpable bony landmarks. The bony landmarks are the anterior superior iliac spine (ASIS) and the trochanter. The heel of the hand is placed over the greater trochanter with the thumb toward the groin and the fingers toward the client's head. The index finger (on the ASIS), the middle finger (on the iliac crest in the direction of the buttock), and the iliac crest form the injection site triangle (Fig. 6.1).

Dorsogluteal site. The dorsogluteal muscle was the traditional site for IM injections but is no longer recommended. Bony landmarks are the greater trochanter and the posterior superior iliac crest (PSIC). There is risk of damage to the sciatic nerve as well as risk of injecting into the thicker subcutaneous tissue rather than the muscle in the area. The exact location of the sciatic nerve varies from one person to another. If the needle hits the sciatic nerve, the client may experience permanent or partial paralysis of the involved leg.

Vastus lateralis site. The vastus lateralis muscle is a site commonly used with infants and young children but may be used with adults as well. It is the preferred site for infants under 12 months receiving immunizations (Potter et al., 2019). The muscle is located on the anterior–lateral aspect of the thigh. Bony landmarks are the trochanter and the knee. The site for injection is the middle third of the muscle, a

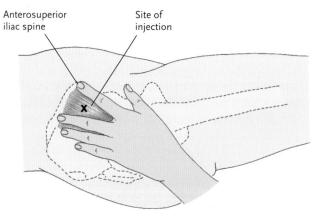

Fig. 6.1 Landmarks for the ventrogluteal site. (From Potter, P., Perry, A., Stockert, P., et al. [2019]. *Canadian fundamentals of nursing* [6th ed., p. 793, Figure 34-24A]. Milton, ON: Elsevier.)

handbreadth below the trochanter and a handbreadth above the knee (Fig. 6.2).

Deltoid site. The deltoid muscle is an easily accessible site but is not well developed in all clients. This site should be used only for small medication volumes (less than 1 mL), when giving immunizations, or when other sites are not accessible (Potter et al., 2019). This site is not without risks as the axillary, radial, brachial, and ulnar nerves, as well as the brachial artery, lie in close proximity. The bony landmark used is the acromion process. The injection site is 3–5 cm below the acromion process (Fig. 6.3).

IV route. *IV injections* are administered directly into a vein. Medications are rapidly absorbed, and adverse reactions can happen immediately.

General principles for preparing parenteral injections.

- When using a vial, inject air equal to the amount of medication that needs to be withdrawn into the vial to prevent negative pressure and to help with aspiration.
- When using an ampoule, tap the neck to force medication into the ampoule. Protect your fingers with an unopened alcohol wipe or a small gauze pad when snapping off the top of the ampoule.
- Change the needle after drawing up medication from an ampoule or vial.
- Use the appropriate-length needle to make sure the medication is deposited where it is intended to go.
- Aspirate for blood when administering IM injections. If blood is present, discard the syringe and medication and repeat the entire procedure.
- Inject medication slowly at a rate of 1 mL per 10 seconds to decrease pain and allow time for dispersion.
- The Z-track method is recommended for highly irritating substances given by IM injection, and there is some evidence that all injections should be given this way. Z-track injections seal medications into muscle tissue and minimize local skin irritation. The skin and overlying subcutaneous tissues are pulled laterally prior to the injection, the needle is left in place for 10 seconds, and the skin is released after the injection. This leaves a zigzag path that seals the needle path and locks the medication in the muscle.
- Never recap needles. Use a one-handed scoop technique if it is absolutely necessary to recap.
- Use safety-engineered needles or needleless systems to eliminate the risk of needle-stick injuries. Some syringes are designed with a sheath or guard that encloses the needle after it is withdrawn from the skin to eliminate the possibility of a needle-stick injury (Potter et al., 2019). Several provinces in Canada have mandatory regulations for safety-engineered devices under their occupational health and safety acts.

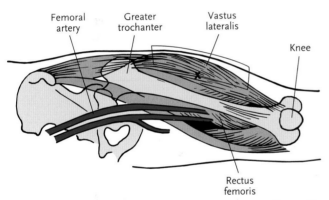

Fig. 6.2 Landmarks for the vastus lateralis site. (From Potter, P., Perry, A., Stockert, P., et al. [2019]. *Canadian fundamentals of nursing* [6th ed., p. 793, Figure 34-25A]. Milton, ON: Elsevier.)

Skin Route

Topical medications. Topical medications are applied to the skin by painting them, spreading them over an area, applying a moist dressing, soaking body parts in a solution, or giving medicated baths. These medications generally have local effects.

Transdermal medications. Transdermal medications have a systemic effect because they are applied topically via a transdermal disc or patch (such as nitroglycerine, scopolamine, or estrogen) that secures the medication to the skin and stays in place for 1–7 days (Potter et al., 2019). The old transdermal patch must be removed before applying the new patch, and it is important to use gloves for application of the new patch to prevent accidental absorption of the medication through the practical nurse's skin.

Mucous membrane medications.

Eyes. Medications for eyes are available in the form of eye drops or eye ointments. Have the client look up before administering ophthalmic medications. Expose the lower conjunctiva. If using drops, place them in the lower conjunctiva near the outer canthus. If using ointment, squeeze a ribbon of ointment into the lower conjunctiva, moving from the inner to the outer canthus. Do not touch the eye with the bottle or tube. Have the client blink a few times to disperse the medication.

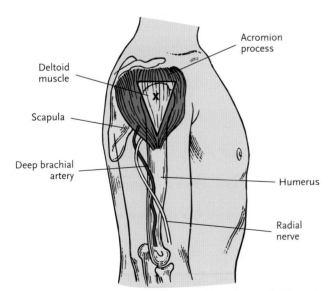

Fig. 6.3 Landmarks for the deltoid site. (From Potter, P., Perry, A., Stockert, P., et al. [2019]. *Canadian fundamentals of nursing* [6th ed., p. 794, Figure 34-26A]. Milton, ON: Elsevier.)

Ears. Otic medications are available in the form of ear drops or irrigations. If the client is supine, ask him or her to turn onto the unaffected side to aid gravitational flow. If he or she is sitting, tilt the client's head toward the unaffected side. Straighten the ear canal by pulling the pinna up and back for adults or down and back for infants and children under 3 years. Have the client remain on his or her side for 2–3 minutes to allow the medication to reach the inner ear canal. Apply gentle massage or pressure to the tragus of the ear with your finger unless contraindicated due to pain (Potter et al., 2019).

Nose. Nasal medications are available in atomizers or in drops. Clients should blow their noses first to clear any mucus. The client should be positioned with the head tilted back to aid in gravitational flow. The atomizer is squeezed quickly and firmly, or the correct number of drops is instilled in each nostril.

Vagina. Vaginal medications are available as liquid douches, creams, foam, jellies, suppositories, or tablets. The client should void prior to receiving vaginal medication. The client should be in the dorsal recumbent position with hips and knees flexed if possible. The applicator or suppository may need to be lubricated with a water-soluble lubricant. The labia are separated, and the applicator is inserted approximately 5–7.5 cm (angled downward and back).

Rectum. Rectal medications are available in the form of suppositories. The client is positioned in a left Sims' position. The suppository is lubricated with a water-soluble lubricant and inserted approximately 10 cm (past the internal anal sphincter) toward the wall of the rectum in the direction of the umbilicus. The client is encouraged to hold the suppository as long as possible for the medication to be effective.

Inhalation. Inhalants are available primarily in the form of metered-dose inhalers (MDIs) or dry powder inhalers (DPIs). They are designed to produce local effects such as bronchodilation. An MDI delivers a premeasured amount of medication with each push of the canister. A spacer may be used with an MDI for the client who is having difficulty coordinating all the steps involved in self-administration. DPIs hold dry powdered medication and create an aerosol when the client inhales.

Abbreviations

Abbreviations that are used in communicating the dosage administration schedule appear in Table 6.1.

Error-Prone Abbreviations, Symbols, and Dose Designations

The practical nurse should avoid unusual abbreviations and symbols and should always be familiar with the agency-approved abbreviation policy in the place of employment. Many abbreviations, symbols, and dose designations are frequently misinterpreted and have been involved in harmful medication errors (Table 6.2) and should never be used in communicating medical information.

TABLE 6.1 Common Dosage Administration Schedule Abbreviations

Abbreviation	Meaning
AC or ac	Before meals
ad lib	As desired
at bedtime	At bedtime (do not use abbreviation)
bid, BID	Twice a day
daily or every day	Daily (do not use abbreviation)
PC or pc	After meals
prn	Whenever there is a need
Qam	Every morning
qh	Every hour
q2h	Every 2 hours
qid, QID	Four times a day
STAT	Give immediately
tid, TID	Three times a day

Adapted from Potter, P., Perry, A., Stockert, P., et al. (2019). *Canadian fundamentals of nursing* (6th ed., p. 733, Table 34.3). Milton, ON: Elsevier.

TABLE 6.2 Error-Prone Abbreviations, Symbols, and Dose Designations

Term	Intended Meaning	Misinterpretation	Correction
µg	microgram	Mistaken as "mg"	Use "mcg"
U or u	Unit	Mistaken as number 0 or 4 (e.g., 4U seen as "40" or 4u seen as "44")	Use "unit"
OD or od	Once daily	Mistaken as "right eye" (OD: oculus dexter)	Use "daily"
q.d. or QD	Every day	Mistaken as q.i.d. (four times daily)	Use "daily"
SC, SQ, sub q	Subcutaneous	SC mistaken as SL (sublingual); SQ mistaken as "5 every"	Use "subcut" or "subcutaneously"
Trailing zero after decimal point (e.g., 1.0 mg)	1 mg	Mistaken as 10 mg if decimal point not seen	Do not use trailing zeros
"Naked" decimal point (e.g., .5 mg)	0.5 mg	Mistaken as 5 mg if decimal point not seen	Use zero before a decimal point when the dose is less than a whole unit

Adapted from Institute for Safe Medication Practices. (2017b). List of error-prone abbreviations. Retrieved from https://www.ismp.org/recommendations/error-prone-abbreviations-list.

Nursing Standards for Administration of Medication: the "10 Rights"

To administer medications safely and effectively in all practice settings, the practical nurse needs to be aware of provincial legislation and regulation as well as practice standards. Administering a medication requires knowledge, skill, and judgement. To ensure safe medication administration, the practical nurse needs to be aware of the following "10 rights" of medication administration.

Right Medication (Drug)

- Administer only the drugs that you prepare. Do not leave medications unattended. The practical nurse who administers the drug is responsible if there is an error.
- Perform three checks to compare the label on the medication package to the medication administration record (MAR). The three checks occur before removing the medication from the drawer or shelf, as the medication ordered is removed from the container or drawer, and before returning the container to the storage area (or before opening at the client's bedside for unit-dose medications).
- Compare any inconsistencies with the original doctor's orders. Compare the MAR or computer order with the prescriber's written order.
- Listen to the client's concerns if the client states that the medication is different.
- Know both the generic and the trade name for the medication. Consult the pharmacist if you are unsure of a medication.

Right Dose

- Know the customary dose and appropriateness for different ages and sizes. Consult a reference book or pharmacist if uncertain.
- Ensure that all calculated doses or "high-alert medications" are checked by another registered nurse (RN). Make sure that double-checking is truly independent. High-alert drugs are drugs that have a high incidence of medication errors associated with their administration. Double-checking alone will not always be the most practical strategy for error-reduction for some medication. Other special safeguards should be implemented to reduce the risk of errors. Strategies may involve standardizing orders; storage; preparation; administration of these drugs; improving access to information about the drugs; limiting access to special high-alert medications; and automated or independent double-checking. Some examples of high-alert drugs are insulin, morphine, hydromorphone (Dilaudid), and heparin (Institute for Safe Medication Practices [ISMP], 2017a).
- Understand that pill cutters should be used to split pills, and crushing devices should be used to crush pills. Enteric-coated pills or sustained-release capsules cannot be crushed or split.

Right Client

- Use two unique client identifiers to identify your client. For example, check the MAR against the client's identification bracelet and ask the client to state his or her full name.
- Acquire a new identification bracelet for the client if one is missing, illegible, or incorrect.

Right Route

- Contact the prescriber if the route is not specified.
- Prepare injections from preparations designated "for injectable use only."
- Use special oral syringes (not compatible with IV tubing) for oral medications.

Right Time and Frequency

- Ensure that all routinely ordered medications are given within 60 minutes of the times for which they are ordered (i.e., 30 minutes before or after the prescribed time).
- Understand why a medication is ordered for certain times of the day and whether the times can be altered. For example, a medication is ordered every 8 hours around the clock to maintain a therapeutic blood level in comparison with a medication ordered tid and meant to be given only during the hours the client is awake.
- Exercise clinical judgement in determining the proper time for administration of certain medications, such as prn medications.

Right Documentation

- Chart the time administered as well as the site for injections with your signature.
- After the client takes the medication, complete the MAR according to the agency policy to verify that the medication was administered as ordered. Chart preadministration data such as BP, pulse, or blood glucose level.
- Chart the effectiveness of certain medications, such as prn medications (such as analgesics or antiemetics).

Right Reason

- Understand why the client is getting the medication and if it makes sense.

Right to Refuse

- Be aware that in order for the client to refuse a medication, they need to be fully informed about the potential consequences of the refusal.

Right Client Education

- To ensure client safety, fully inform clients and family members about the medication and the consequences of not taking it.
- Provide information about the drug being given: the reason for taking it, its action, and possible adverse effects the client may experience while taking it.

Right Evaluation

- Before medication administration, check to make sure that the order is correct and the medication is available and accessible to the client.
- Check any special assessments required before administration of the medication.
- After the medication administration, monitor the client for medication effectiveness, side effects, adverse drug reactions, and drug interactions.

Medication Administration for Older Adults

- Allow extra time for administration of medications to older adults.
- Assess functional status to see whether a client will need help in taking the medications.
- Have older clients drink a little fluid before taking oral medications to ease swallowing, and encourage them to drink 150–180 mL after medications to prevent the medication from lodging in the esophagus.
- Have clients sit up straight in bed and tuck in their chins to decrease the risk of aspiration when taking medications.
- Request liquid medications from the prescriber if the client has trouble swallowing large pills or capsules.

Medication Errors

Medication errors are preventable events associated with the prescribing, transcribing, dispensing, or administering of medications. Many medication errors are not reported. Unreported errors mean that no one can correct their cause or reduce their incidence. Errors are rarely the fault of individual healthcare providers but instead stem from failures of a complicated healthcare system. The best approach is a nonpunitive, multidisciplinary approach in which the process is targeted rather than the practitioner. This approach focuses on why an error occurred rather than blaming the person or people involved. When an error occurs, it should be acknowledged immediately and reported to the appropriate hospital personnel. Measures to counteract the effects of the error may also be necessary. Client safety is the first concern of the practical nurse. The practical nurse is also responsible for completing an incident report for the agency about the details of the incident. The practical nurse follows agency policy about disclosure to the client and client's family. See Chapter 7 for a more detailed discussion of medications.

ACTIVITY AND EXERCISE

Body Mechanics

Body mechanics are "the coordinated efforts of the musculo-skeletal and nervous systems to maintain balance, posture, and body alignment during lifting, bending, moving, and performing activities of daily living" (Potter et al., 2019, p. 833). Proper use of body mechanics will conserve energy, reduce stress and strain on body structures, increase safety for the caregiver and the client, and reduce the possibility of personal injury. Repeated lifting and forceful movements associated with care of clients can lead to work-related injury or illness, such as musculo-skeletal disorders (MSDs). The activities of lifting, transferring, and repositioning clients place healthcare workers at risk for MSDs, especially back injuries. Body mechanics training has proven ineffective in preventing job-related injuries. Many facilities found implementing "no-lift" policies and Safe Handling programs to be more effective.

Research has shown that sound ergonomics programs in healthcare facilities can lead to reductions in injuries (CDC, 2017). The use of technology such as lifting devices and the use of special algorithms for each client who needs help to move are crucial to the success of ergonomics programs. Box 6.1 presents guidelines for moving clients safely and avoiding back injuries.

Exercise

Exercise is physical activity for the purpose of toning the body, improving health, and maintaining fitness. It can also be used therapeutically to correct a deformity or restore the client's body to a maximal state of health. Activity tolerance (the kind and amount of exercise or activity that a client is able to perform) must be assessed prior to planning physical activity for clients with health problems. Some of the factors that influence activity tolerance include pain, lack of sleep, prior exercise pattern, anxiety, age, and muscular or skeletal impairments (Potter et al., 2019). See Chapter 5 for a more detailed discussion of physical activity.

BOX 6.1   Health Care Worker Guidelines for Moving Clients Safely

- Arrange for adequate assistance when moving or transferring a client.
- Use algorithms to determine the safest equipment and client-handling technique to use for each activity or movement to be completed.
- When possible, use mechanical aids such as lifts, transfer chairs or boards, or pivot devices for lifts and transfers.
- Instruct clients about moving safely and encourage them to assist as much as possible to minimize the workload for the nurse.
- Keep the spine, neck, pelvis, and feet aligned. Avoid twisting.
- Flex the knees; keep the feet wide apart to broaden the base of support.
- Position yourself close to the client (or object being lifted) to minimize the load.
- Use the stronger, larger muscles of the arms and legs rather than those of the back.
- Slide the client toward you using a draw sheet rather than pulling or lifting.
- Tighten your abdominal and gluteal muscles in preparation for a move.

Based on Potter, P., Perry, A., Stockert, P., et al. (2019). *Canadian fundamentals of nursing* (6th ed., p. 860, Table 36.2). Milton, ON: Elsevier.

CLIENT SAFETY

Restraints

Types of Restraints

- *Physical restraints* are any manual method or any physical or mechanical device, material, or piece of equipment that reduces the ability of the client to move freely. Examples include locked geriatric chairs, restrictive side rails, belts, hand mitts, sheet ties, and chest restraints.
- *Chemical restraints* are medications given to restrict or manage a client's behaviour or to restrict a client's movement that are not a standard therapy or dose for the client's condition.
- *Environmental restraints* control a client's mobility. Examples include a locked room, as in the case of clients placed in seclusion. A locked nursing unit is another form of environmental restraint that is designed to allow residents with dementia to wander freely and safely around the unit.

Use of Least Restraint

Least restraint means that all other possible interventions have been attempted before the decision is made to use a restraint. Restraints are a temporary or short-term intervention, and the least restrictive method for the shortest duration possible is chosen. The optimal goal is a restraint-free environment. Research indicates that restraints do not actually prevent falls and injury and may even increase the severity of injury. Restraints require a physician's order and are part of the client's individualized plan of care. Regularly reviewing the continued use of restraints is essential. It is important that the client and client's family or substitute decision maker are informed and involved in the plan of care as well.

Assessment of restraints. Routine assessment of a client in restraints is essential to prevent client injury. The restraint must be removed and the client checked and repositioned at regular intervals. Restraints should be tied with a quick-release tie rather than a knot. Proper placement of the restraint, skin integrity, pulses, and colour and sensation of the restrained part should be assessed every hour or according to agency policy. It is important to document this information.

Alternatives to restraints. Alternatives to restraints include low-height beds, bedside mats and hip guards, bed sensors or monitoring devices, and the presence of a family member or paid companion to stay with the client at risk.

Seizure Disorder Precautions

Seizures are sudden, transient alterations in brain function that result from excessive levels of electrical activity in the brain and lead to a sudden, violent, involuntary series of contractions of a group of muscles (Potter et al., 2019). Seizures can vary in severity, and the client may or may not lose consciousness.

Nursing Interventions

- Protect clients from traumatic injury: If they are standing or sitting, lay them on the floor, bed, or other flat surface.

If they are in hospital, make sure the bed is in the low position, flat, and the side rails are elevated and padded. Place a pillow or folded blanket under the head. Loosen restrictive clothing. Do not attempt to restrain clients but clear the area of hazards and articles that might harm them.
- Position clients for adequate ventilation and drainage of oral secretions: Clients need to be on a flat surface. Nothing should be inserted into the mouth except in the case of status epilepticus (a medical emergency in which there are continual seizures), and then an oral airway is necessary. If possible, turn clients on their side.
- Provide privacy and support following the procedure: Stay with clients, observing and timing the seizure. Immediately following the seizure, place clients in the recovery position to prevent aspiration and remain with them until they have recovered fully. Explain what happened and answer client questions. Some clients may experience postseizure confusion and may need to have explanations repeated.

HYGIENE

Bathing

During hygienic care, the practical nurse incorporates other activities, such as communication, physical assessment, skin and wound care, health teaching, assessment of self-care abilities, and range-of-motion (ROM) exercises. The practical nurse provides hygienic care according to the client's needs and preferences, taking into consideration cultural and developmental factors.

- A complete bed bath is a bath for clients who are completely dependent and require all their care to be provided by another person.
- A partial bed bath involves bathing only certain parts of the body (such as the face, hands, underarms, and perineal area) to refresh clients and because certain areas may be more prone to skin breakdown or odour if not bathed.

Guidelines for Bathing

- Provide privacy by exposing only the areas being bathed.
- Maintain safety by keeping side rails up and providing a call bell when you are away from the bedside.
- Maintain warmth by exposing only the areas being bathed and keeping bath water warm.
- Unless contraindicated, bathe limbs from distal to proximal areas (fingers to axilla) with long, firm strokes to promote circulation and venous return.
- Promote independence by encouraging the client to participate as much as possible.
- Anticipate needs by having all your equipment at hand.

Perineal Care

Special attention to perineal care is needed for clients with in-dwelling catheters, recent rectal or gynecological surgery, recent childbirth, morbid obesity, or urinary or fecal incontinence as these clients are the most at risk for infection.

In these cases, the practical nurse performs perineal care even if the client is able to do so, so that the practical nurse may assess the perineal area for skin breakdown or infection and is able to clean the area thoroughly.

Nail and Foot Care

Clients with diabetes mellitus or peripheral vascular disease require special nail and foot care as they are at risk of complications such as infection due to poor circulation, especially in their feet. Diabetics also have reduced sensation to the feet. The practical nurse should not trim the nails of a client with impaired lower extremity circulation before checking agency policy to see if a physician's order is necessary.

Foot Care Guidelines for High-Risk Clients

- Inspect feet daily and do not walk barefoot.
- People with diabetes should see a qualified healthcare provider, such as a podiatrist, for a thorough yearly foot exam.
- Wash feet daily with lukewarm water but do not soak them as that can cause maceration. Dry well and do not put cream between toes.
- Do not cut corns or calluses or use commercial removers. Consult a podiatrist.
- File the toenails straight across and square and do not use clippers or scissors. Get help to cut nails if necessary.
- Avoid crossing the legs or wearing elastic stockings and knee-high hose that can impair circulation to the lower extremities.
- Wear clean socks and stockings daily that remain dry and free of holes.
- Wear properly fitting, nonslip shoes that fully cover the feet.
- Exercise regularly to promote lower extremity circulation.
- Do not use heating pads or hot water bottles on extremities.
- Wash all cuts immediately, dry thoroughly, and treat with a mild antiseptic (Potter et al., 2019).

Oral Hygiene

Oral hygiene includes the brushing and flossing of teeth as well as care of the mouth, gums, and lips. Oral hygiene is an important practice that maintains the health of the mouth, teeth, gums, and lips; enhances comfort; and stimulates appetite.

Mouth Care for Unconscious Clients

Unconscious clients are more susceptible to drying of the mouth because they are not eating or drinking, cannot swallow oral secretions, and frequently breathe through their mouths. Oxygen therapy can also be very drying to the mouth. Proper oral hygiene reduces the incidence of pneumonia, which can be caused by Gram-negative bacteria aspirated from the mouth and into the lung (Potter et al., 2019). When giving oral hygiene, it is important to prevent the client from choking and aspiration. The client should be positioned on the side with the head turned toward the dependent side. Suction machine equipment should also be close at hand. If possible, a padded tongue blade can be used behind the back molars to separate upper and lower teeth. The mouth can be cleansed with a toothbrush or toothette moistened with water or hydrogen peroxide. A bulb syringe can be used to rinse the oral cavity; it should then be suctioned to make sure that no fluid is left in the mouth.

Stomatitis

Stomatitis is inflammation of the mouth that is caused by a variety of conditions, including viral infections, chemical irritation, radiation therapy, and chemotherapy. Gentle brushing and flossing is important. Clients with this condition should not use commercial mouthwash, drink alcohol, or smoke. Normal saline mouthwashes can be given every 2 hours if necessary, and a mild analgesic might be necessary for pain.

CARDIOPULMONARY FUNCTIONING AND OXYGENATION

Suctioning

Suctioning is the aspiration of secretions from the trachea and bronchial tree by application of negative-pressure suction. It is used to maintain a patent airway, collect sputum specimens, or stimulate a cough (Potter et al., 2019). Clients should be encouraged to cough and suctioned only when necessary, as it is uncomfortable and traumatic to the airway. Signs that the client needs to be suctioned may include one or more of the following: gurgling respirations, respiratory distress, low oxygen-saturation levels, and coarse crackles on auscultation.

Oropharyngeal and nasopharyngeal suctioning can be delegated to a practical nurse. Tracheobronchial and tracheal suctioning is a deep suction of the lower respiratory passages removing secretions from the trachea and bronchi. This skill may not be delegated to a practical nurse. Practical nurses need to check their legal scope of practice in their jurisdiction and the policies of the practical setting they are working in regarding whether they can perform this skill in collaboration with an RN (Perry, Potter, & Ostendorf, 2018).

Types of Suctioning

- Oropharyngeal and nasopharyngeal suctioning is used when the client is able to cough effectively but is unable to clear secretions by coughing or swallowing.
- Orotracheal or nasotracheal suctioning utilizes a catheter that is passed through the nose or mouth to the trachea. This route is used when the client is not able to cough and manage his or her own secretions. It is a sterile procedure.
- Tracheal suctioning is done through an artificial airway, such as an endotracheal or tracheostomy tube. Surgical asepsis is maintained for new tracheostomies and endotracheal suctioning.

Principles of Suctioning

- Suctioning should not be performed routinely but should follow a comprehensive respiratory assessment that includes chest auscultation (Perry et al., 2018).

- Lubricate the catheter with sterile normal saline, except for nasopharyngeal or nasotracheal suctioning, which requires the use of a water-soluble lubricant.
- Insert the catheter until resistance is met or the client coughs and then pull back 1 cm for tracheal suctioning (Perry et al., 2018). Insert 16 cm in adults for nasopharyngeal suctioning and 16–20 cm in adults for nasotracheal suctioning.
- Do not apply suction while inserting the catheter.
- While removing the catheter, apply suction intermittently and rotate the catheter to prevent injury to the mucosa. Do not suction longer than 10–15 seconds, as this can increase the risk of mucosal damage and hypoxemia (Perry et al., 2018).
- Wait 1–2 minutes between passes to allow the client to rest.
- It may be necessary to hyperoxygenate the client before and after suctioning by using a manual resuscitation bag, increasing the oxygen flow rate, or having the client take deep breaths, especially if the client has had signs of cardiopulmonary compromise in the past.
- Evaluate the client's response postprocedure. Suctioning can cause hypoxemia, hypotension, arrhythmias, and possible trauma to the mucosa of the lung.

Tracheostomy Care

Tracheostomy care is the removal of copious, thick, tenacious, or dried secretions from the tracheostomy tube in order to maintain a patent airway, prevent infection, and prevent irritation. Practical nurses need to check their legal scope of practice in their jurisdiction and the policies of the facility they are working in regarding whether they can perform tracheostomy care in collaboration with an RN.

Guidelines for Tracheostomy Care

- Provide tracheostomy care every 8 hours.
- Suction to remove secretions from the lumen of the tube when necessary.
- If an inner cannula is present:
  - Remove the disposable inner cannula and replace it with a new one.
  - Provide care for a nondisposable inner cannula, which involves (a) removing and placing the cannula in normal saline; (b) removing secretions from the cannula with a sterile brush; (c) rinsing the cannula with normal saline; (d) draining excess saline before inserting the cannula; and (e) locking the inner cannula in place (Perry et al., 2018; Potter et al., 2019).
  - Clean around the stoma in a circular motion from the stoma site outward with saline; moving in an outward circle pulls mucus and other contaminants from the stoma periphery (Perry et al., 2018; Potter et al., 2019).
  - Change the tracheostomy tape or ties if necessary, being careful not to dislodge the cannula and to secure the tracheostomy tube by holding the cannula in place by lightly pressing with one finger and using a double square knot. The knot should be located on the side

rather than at the back of the neck, where it would cause pressure.
  - Insert a sterile tracheostomy dressing under the ties and faceplate to absorb drainage and to prevent pressure on the clavicle (Perry et al., 2018; Potter et al., 2019).

Chest Tubes

A *chest tube* is a catheter inserted through the thorax to remove abnormal accumulations of air, fluid, or blood from the pleural space or mediastinum. The chest tube drainage system returns negative pressure to the intrapleural space. This is a skill that will require collaboration with an RN. Practical nurses need to ensure this skill is within their legal scope of practice in their jurisdiction and permitted by the policies of the facility in which they are working.

Commercial Drainage Systems

Wet suction control drainage system.
- The collection chamber collects drainage from the chest tube in a series of calibrated columns.
- The water seal chamber prevents atmospheric air from entering the pleural space. The fluid level will fluctuate with respirations until the lung is fully expanded. Continuous bubbling may indicate a leak in the chest tube system.
- If gravity drainage is insufficient, the suction control chamber is used to provide suction between 10–20 cm of water and will drain air and fluid from the chest cavity. Gentle bubbling in this section indicates that there is suction.
Dry suction control drainage system.
- The dry suction control chamber system contains no water. It provides higher suction pressure levels.
- It has a visual alert that indicates if the suction is not working. No bubbling is seen in the third chamber (Lewis et al., 2019).

See Fig. 6.4 for an example of a Pleur-evac chest drainage system.

Nursing Care of the Client With a Chest Tube

- Monitor drainage; notify the physician if drainage is greater than 100 mL per hour or if drainage becomes bright red or increases suddenly.
- Mark the chest tube drainage in the collection chamber at 1–4-hour intervals, according to hospital policy to monitor output.
- Ensure that the tubing is not kinked, all connections are secure, and there are no dependent loops.
- Maintain the drainage system below the level of the chest to prevent reflux and decrease the risk of infection.
- Maintain a sterile occlusive dressing at the insertion site to prevent an air leak.
- Turn the client frequently to promote drainage and ventilation.
- Observe for fluctuation of fluid in the water seal chamber; the level will rise on inhalation and fall on exhalation; if there are no fluctuations, either the lung has re-expanded or the chest tube is clogged (Lewis et al., 2019).

Fig. 6.4 Chest drainage system. A, Pleur-evac chest drainage system, a commercial three-chamber chest drainage device. **B,** Schematic of the drainage device. (From Ignatavicius, D. D., Workman, M. L., & Rebar, C. [2018]. *Medical-surgical nursing: Concepts for interprofessional collaborative care* [9th ed., p. 591, Figure 30-15]. St. Louis: Elsevier.)

- Monitor the suction control chamber to make sure there is gentle bubbling in the suction control chamber. Vigorous bubbling indicates an air leak, and the physician should be notified (Lewis et al., 2019).
- Encourage coughing and deep breathing every 2 hours with splinting of the chest area if necessary and encourage ROM exercises to the shoulder of the affected side. Encouraging incentive spirometry every hour while awake may help prevent atelectasis or pneumonia (Lewis et al., 2019).
- Determine agency policy regarding clamping of chest tubes. Chest tubes are rarely clamped, and a chest tube should never be clamped without a written order from a

physician. Clamping can cause a tension pneumothorax where air pressure builds up in the pleural space, collapsing the lung and creating a life-threatening emergency. A doctor may order clamping for 24 hours to evaluate for accumulation of air or fluid before discontinuing the chest tube (Lewis et al., 2019).
- If the drainage system cracks or breaks, insert the chest tube temporarily into a bottle of sterile water to maintain a water seal and then replace the drainage system.
- If the chest tube is pulled out of the chest accidentally, pinch the skin together, apply an occlusive dressing, and call the physician immediately.
- Keep a clamp, a bottle of sterile water, and a sterile occlusive dressing at the bedside at all times. Clamps are kept at the bedside for special procedures, such as changing the chest drainage system.

Oxygen Therapy

Oxygen is a drug and as such can have serious side effects, such as absorption atelectasis or oxygen toxicity. The goal of oxygen therapy is to relieve or prevent hypoxia (reduced tissue oxygenation despite adequate perfusion). Signs of worsening hypoxia include increasing tachypnea and dyspnea, skin colour changes (pale at first, then cyanotic), increasing tachycardia, hypertension, restlessness, and disorientation (Lewis et al., 2019; Potter et al., 2019).

Methods of Oxygen Delivery

Low-flow devices. Low-flow devices provide oxygen in concentrations that vary with the person's respiratory effort (Lewis et al., 2019; Potter et al., 2019). When the total ventilation exceeds the capacity of the oxygen reservoir, room air is entrained. The final concentration of oxygen delivered depends on the ventilatory demands of the client, the size of the oxygen reservoir, and the rate at which the reservoir is filled. Most methods of oxygen delivery are low-flow systems. Examples of low-flow devices are nasal cannulas, the simple face mask, and reservoir masks.

Nasal cannula. The nasal cannula (nasal prongs) is a low-flow device used for a flow rate of 1–6 L/min, providing oxygen concentrations of 24% (at 1 L/min) and 44% (at 6 L/min) (Potter et al., 2019). A flow rate above 4 L/min can be very drying for the nasal mucosa and cause irritation. The practical nurse also needs to be alert for skin breakdown over the ears and in the nares from nasal prongs that are too tight.

Oxygen masks. Oxygen masks are devices used to administer oxygen, humidity, or both. Different types of face masks are as follows:
- The simple face mask delivers 40–60% oxygen concentrations. It is used for short-term oxygen therapy or for the delivery of oxygen in an emergency (Potter et al., 2019). This mask is contraindicated for clients with carbon dioxide (CO_2) retention.
- The partial rebreather mask combines a mask and a reservoir bag. It provides an oxygen concentration of 40–70% with a minimum flow rate of 10 L/min (Potter et al., 2019).

- The non-rebreather mask provides the highest oxygen concentration of the low-flow systems. It has a mask and a reservoir bag and can deliver an oxygen concentration of 60–80%, depending on the client's ventilatory efforts. It is commonly used for the client with deteriorating respiratory status who might need to be intubated. The flow rate is 10–15 L/min to maintain the reservoir bag two-thirds full. The one-way valves on non-rebreather masks prevent expired air from flowing back into the bag. If it is deflated, the client may be breathing large amounts of exhaled CO_2 (Potter et al., 2019).

High-flow devices. High-flow devices deliver oxygen at rates above the normal inspiratory flow and maintain a fixed F_iO_2 (fraction of inspired oxygen) independent of the client's respiratory pattern (Lewis et al., 2019). The most common example is the Venturi mask, which entrains room air to achieve a consistent, precise oxygen concentration. Other examples include aerosol devices such as the face tent and the tracheostomy collar or mask.

Venturi masks. The Venturi mask, or air-entrainment mask, delivers oxygen concentrations of 24–60%, with a flow rate of 2–12 L/min (Potter et al., 2019). The Venturi mask is useful for delivering low, precise oxygen concentrations to clients with chronic obstructive pulmonary disease (COPD) (Lewis et al., 2019; Potter et al., 2019).

Oxygen Therapy for Clients With COPD

For an average adult, a high CO_2 level stimulates the brain to breathe. People with COPD and a high CO_2 level may become less sensitive to a high CO_2 level, reducing the drive to breathe. A client who has hypoxemia (a low oxygen level in the blood) and is a chronic CO_2 retainer may require a low level of oxygen delivery at 1–2 L/min. A low arterial oxygen level will stimulate a COPD client to breathe. Careful, ongoing assessment when administering oxygen therapy to COPD clients is very important (Lewis et al., 2019).

Home Oxygen Therapy

- Indications for home oxygen therapy include a partial pressure of arterial oxygen (PaO_2) of 55 mm Hg or less via arterial blood gas analysis or an SpO_2 of 88% or less via pulse oximetry on room air at rest, on exertion, or with exercise (Potter et al., 2019). This therapy improves clients' exercise tolerance and fatigue levels and may assist with the management of dyspnea.
- Home oxygen is usually delivered by nasal cannula or transtracheal oxygen (TTO); a tracheostomy collar is used in the case of the client with a permanent tracheostomy.

FLUID, ELECTROLYTE, AND ACID–BASE BALANCES

Fluid and Electrolyte Balance

- Body fluids are distributed in two compartments: one containing intracellular fluid (intracerebral fluid, or all the fluid within body cells, comprising 40% of body weight) and the other extracellular fluid (ECF) (extracerebral fluid, or all the fluid outside body cells, comprising 20% of body weight) (Potter et al., 2019).
- Body fluids are regulated by (a) fluid intake and the thirst mechanism; (b) hormonal controls such as antidiuretic hormone (ADH), aldosterone, and renin; and (c) fluid output through the kidneys, the skin, the lungs, and the gastro-intestinal system, with the kidneys being the most important in regulating fluid balance. This physiological balance is called *homeostasis* (Potter et al., 2019).
- Clients who are very young or very old as well as clients with chronic or serious illnesses are at greater risk for fluid, electrolyte, and acid–base imbalances.
- Assessment of fluid, electrolyte, and acid–base alterations includes collating data from the nursing health history and physical and behavioural assessments, as well as measuring intake and output, weighing the clients daily, and analyzing specific laboratory data, such as electrolyte results (Potter et al., 2019). See Chapter 8 for a more detailed discussion of electrolyte balance and homeostasis.

Venous Access Devices

Venous access devices (VADs) are inserted into a vein for the purpose of delivering medication or fluids directly into the bloodstream. To determine the most appropriate type of VAD, the practical nurse needs to consider the following factors: prescribed therapy, duration of therapy, physical assessment, client health history, support system and resources, device availability, and client preference (Registered Nurses' Association of Ontario [RNAO], 2004). Practical nurses need to ensure this skill is within their legal scope of practice in their jurisdiction and permitted by the policies of the facility in which they are working. In some facilities, the practical nurse with the proper training may change the peripherally inserted central catheter (PICC) line dressing, deliver medication via PICC line, and is able to remove the PICC line.

Types of VADs

Peripheral venous access devices. Peripheral venous access devices (PVADs) are designed for short-term use. There are two common types: short peripheral and midline. Short peripheral IVs are most commonly placed in the arm and are described in more detail under "Nursing Care of Clients with PVAD Infusion Therapy." Midline catheters range in length from 7.5–25 cm and lie deep in the cephalic or basilic vein with the tip not extending past the axilla. They can stay in place for up to 4 weeks (Williams, 2018).

Central venous access devices. Central venous access devices (CVADs) or central venous catheters (CVCs) are used to administer medications and solutions irritating to veins, deliver long-term therapy, and deliver rapid infusion of medications or large amounts of fluid. Figs. 6.5 to 6.7 show examples of CVADs.

With the exception of the PICC device, these catheters are inserted in the central part of the body by way of the internal jugular, subclavian, or femoral vein. All central-line devices terminate in the vena cava immediately above the right

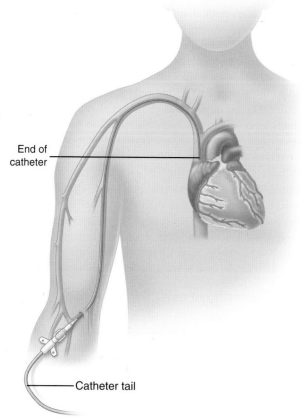

Fig. 6.5 Peripherally inserted central catheter (PICC) is placed peripherally in a vein of the upper arm with the tip resting in the superior vena cava. (From Ignatavicius, D. D., Workman, M. L., & Rebar, C. [2018]. *Medical-surgical nursing: Concepts for interprofessional collaborative care* [9th ed., p. 205, Figure 13-6]. St. Louis: Elsevier.)

Fig. 6.6 Tunnelled central venous catheter. Part of the catheter lies in a subcutaneous tunnel, separating the point where the catheter enters the vein from where it exits the skin. (From Ignatavicius, D. D., Workman, M. L., & Rebar, C. [2018]. *Medical-surgical nursing: Concepts for interprofessional collaborative care* [9th ed., p. 207, Figure 13-8]. St. Louis: Elsevier.)

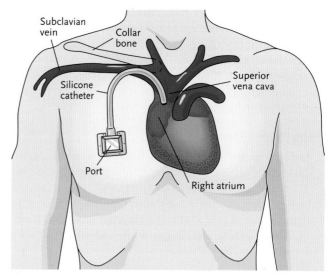

Fig. 6.7 Implanted infusion port and central venous catheter. (From Perry, A. G., Potter, P. A., & Ostendorf, W. [2018]. *Clinical nursing skills and techniques* [9th ed., p. 786, Figure 29.7]. St. Louis: Mosby.)

atrium, where blood flow is very rapid at 2 L/min. There are four types of CVADs:

- Nontunnelled catheters—They are inserted by a physician, and clients with these catheters must remain in the acute care setting. There is a high rate of infection with nontunnelled catheters because they are inserted percutaneously in areas that are warm and moist, such as the neck and groin. For this reason, they are not left in place for as long as other CVADs.
- Tunnelled catheters (e.g., Hickman catheters)—They are inserted in the operating room under a local anaesthetic and can be left in for years. They are hard to disguise and require daily care but can be cared for in the home setting.
- Implanted ports (e.g., Port-A-Caths)—They require insertion in the operating room with local anaesthesia and also can be left in place for years. They are commonly implanted in the chest.
- PICC lines—They are placed most commonly in peripheral veins, such as the basilic or cephalic veins. They are easy to insert at the bedside either by doctors or specially trained nurses. They have a low infection rate because

fewer bacterial colonies are present in the antecubital fossa (Lewis et al., 2019).

Purpose of Infusion Therapy

- To correct or prevent fluid and electrolyte imbalances
- To administer medications

- To administer blood and blood products
- To provide venous access in emergency situations
- To correct or prevent nutritional imbalances

Types of Solutions

- Isotonic solutions: They have the same osmolality as body fluids. They are used most commonly for ECF replacement; for example, 0.9% saline or normal saline (NS), 5% dextrose in water (D_5W), or lactated Ringer's solution (LR) (Potter et al., 2019).
- Hypotonic solutions: They have a lower osmolality than body fluids. These solutions cause the movement of water into cells by osmosis; for example, 0.45% saline (½ NS) (Potter et al., 2019).
- Hypertonic solutions: They have a higher osmolality than body fluids. They concentrate ECF and cause movement of water from cells into the ECF by osmosis; for example, 10% dextrose in water ($D_{10}W$) (Potter et al., 2019).

Nursing Care of Clients With PVAD Infusion Therapy

Initiation of infusion therapy.

- Common IV sites are the veins in the hand, forearm, and antecubital fossa.
- The IV infusion is started by venipuncture through the use of a butterfly (metal) needle or an over-the-needle plastic catheter.
- The IV infusion is started distally to provide the option of proceeding up the extremity if necessary later.
- The practical nurse needs to check the IV solution against the prescriber's orders for the type, amount, and percentage of solution and the rate of flow.

Regulation of infusion flow rate.

- The practical nurse must regulate the rate of infusion according to the prescriber's orders.
- The practical nurse calculates the infusion rate to prevent too slow or too rapid administration of IV fluids.
- Fluids that run by gravity are adjusted by means of a regulator or roller clamp. An electronic infusion pump can also regulate the rate that is preset by the nurse.
- For IV infusions running by gravity, the practical nurse calculates the minute flow rate or drop rate based on the drop factor of the infusion, set using this formula:

$$\frac{100\,mL \times 15\,gtt}{60\,min} = 25\,gtt/min$$

- For example, the minute flow rate or drop rate for an IV running at 100 mL/hr with a drop factor of 15 gtt/mL would be:

$$\frac{100\,mL \times 15\,gtt}{60\,min} = 25\,gtt/min$$

Maintenance of infusion therapy.

- Change the venipuncture site every 48–72 hours, the IV dressing every 72 hours, and the IV tubing every 24–72 hours (depending on agency policy).

- Be aware that incompatibilities can occur between certain solutions and medications.
- Assess the "rights" for administration of medications.
- Assess the IV site and equipment regularly for complications.

Intermittent Venous Access or Saline Locks

Saline locks are used when intravascular access is desired for intermittent administration of medications by IV bolus (push) or IV piggyback (secondary administration of medications). It allows the client to be free from an IV line except when medication must be given, and it allows emergency IV access if necessary. Patency is maintained by periodic flushing with 1–3 mL of NS (depending on agency policy).

Complications of infusion therapy. Common complications of infusion therapy are infiltration, phlebitis (inflammation of the vein), infection, fluid (circulatory) overload, and bleeding or bruising at the site.

Blood Transfusions

Purpose of Blood Transfusions

- To restore blood volume after hemorrhage, surgery, or trauma
- To restore the oxygen-carrying capacity of the blood and to increase hemoglobin levels in severe anemias
- To replace specific blood components, such as clotting factors, platelets, or albumin

Nursing Care of Clients Receiving a Blood Transfusion

- Check your agency policy and your legal scope of practice with regard to blood transfusions. Some jurisdictions may prohibit the practical nurse from initiating blood products but will allow monitoring of a stable client.
- Check that the blood or blood components have been typed and cross-matched, indicating that the blood of the donor and the recipient are compatible.
- Know that blood should never be administered straight from the refrigerator and should be returned to the blood bank fridge if not used immediately.
- Take baseline vital signs (including temperature) pre-administration and frequently throughout administration (check agency policy).
- Know that an IV with NS infusing through a blood administration set with a special filter is used to start the infusion.
- Maintain standard precautions/routine practices when handling blood and IV equipment.
- Know that the client needs to sign a blood administration consent form in many agencies.
- Know that before beginning the infusion, two RNs or one RN and one practical nurse (see agency policy) verify the blood type, Rh factor, client and blood numbers, and expiration date of the blood.
- Invert the container gently to suspend the red blood cells within the plasma.
- Stay with the client for the first 15 minutes, as that is when a reaction most often occurs.
- Observe for signs of a hemolytic reaction, which generally occur early in the transfusion (within the first 5–15

minutes). Signs include shivering, headache, lower back pain, increased pulse and respiratory rate, hemoglobinuria, oliguria, and hypotension (Lewis et al., 2019).

- Observe for signs of a febrile reaction (usually within 30 minutes). Signs include shaking, headache, elevated temperature, back pain, confusion, and hematemesis (Lewis et al., 2019).
- Observe for signs of an allergic reaction, such as hives, wheezing, pruritis, and joint pain (Lewis et al., 2019).
- If any reaction occurs, stop the infusion immediately and maintain patency of the IV with NS; monitor vital signs as often as every 5 minutes; notify the physician; stay with the client; and prepare to administer emergency drugs and to perform cardiopulmonary resuscitation if necessary. A urine sample may be needed to determine the presence of hemoglobin as a result of RBC hemolysis. Save the blood container, tubing, attached labels, and transfusion record and return them to the laboratory.

PAIN AND COMFORT

The International Association for the Study of Pain defined *pain* as "an unpleasant sensory and emotional experience associated with actual or potential tissue damage, or described in terms of such damage" (International Association of Pain, 2017). Pain is subjective, and the client's self-report about pain is key to effective management. Pain is unique and individualized for each person. The process between an injury and perceiving pain involves four steps: transduction, transmission, modulation, and perception.

Types of Pain

Nociceptive and Neuropathic Pain

Pain is categorized as nociceptive, neuropathic, or both, according to underlying pathology. Nociceptive pain is caused by damage to somatic or visceral tissue. Examples include pain from a surgical incision, a broken leg, arthritis, or angina (Lewis et al., 2014). Neuropathic pain is caused by damage to nerve cells or changes in spinal cord processing and is described as burning, shooting, or stabbing. This type can be difficult to treat. Examples include phantom limb pain and diabetic neuropathy (Lewis et al., 2019).

Acute and Persistent Pain

Acute pain usually has a sudden onset and diminishes over time as healing occurs. Examples include postoperative pain, labour pain, or angina. Persistent pain persists beyond the normal time for healing. It can be disabling and is often accompanied by depression and anxiety.

Pain Scales

Descriptive scales are an objective means of measuring pain intensity. Various scales can be used for adults and children to rate pain before and after interventions. The most common one used with adults is the numeric rating scale, with which clients rate their pain on a scale of 0–10 (0 being no pain; 10 being the most severe pain ever experienced). Pain should be rated before and after administration of analgesics. For clients who are unable to respond to other pain intensity scales, a series of faces ranging from "smiling" to "crying" can be used. These scales can be used in a variety of client populations, including young children and older adults (Lewis et al., 2019).

Best Practices for Pain Control

- Practice guidelines are available that recommend systematic ways of using analgesics. One example is the pain relief ladder developed by the World Health Organization (WHO) for cancer pain relief in adults. The WHO treatment plan emphasizes that different drugs are administered, depending on the severity of pain. The three-step ladder approach is used to determine the severity of the pain: step 1: nonopioids are administered for mild pain; step 2: mild opioids are administered as necessary for mild to moderate pain; step 3: strong opioids are administered for moderate to severe pain. If pain persists or increases, drugs from the next higher step are used to control the pain. The steps are not meant to be sequential if someone has moderate to severe pain: for this person, the analgesics given would be the stronger analgesics listed in steps 2 and 3 (Lewis et al., 2019). The WHO has developed a two-step approach to the pharmacological treatment of persisting pain in children as well (World Health Organization [WHO], 2012).
- "Advocate for the most effective dosing schedule, considering the medication(s) duration of onset, effect(s) and half-life. The optimal analgesia dose is one that effectively relieves pain with minimum adverse effects" (RNAO, 2013, p. 34). Current best practice suggests that only one long-acting opioid at a given time is ordered for management of continuous moderate to severe pain. Examples of long-acting oral opioids are morphine sulphate controlled-release tablets (MS Contin) and morphine sulphate extended-release capsule (M-Eslon).
- It is important to give breakthrough medication doses as necessary and to consider adjuvant therapies and treatments.
- Patient-controlled analgesia (PCA) is an infusion pump that is programmed for dose and time intervals, allowing clients to control analgesic administration without overdose. The PCA pump can be IV, subcutaneous, intrathecal, transdermal, or epidural and is a good short-term option for postoperative pain. PCA offers a number of benefits. PCA empowers clients to have some control over their pain, which helps alleviate anxiety and medication use. Because clients are active participants in their care, they can medicate themselves when the pain starts. Pain relief allows clients to ambulate earlier, and, as a result, they have fewer pulmonary problems. Use of PCAs promotes healing, which leads to faster recovery and shorter hospital stays (Potter et al., 2019; Williams, 2018). The RN usually has the primary responsibility for PCAs and epidural pumps. The practical nurse may be required to monitor or assist with the pump. It is important to monitor the IV site and assess for side effects of the medication (Williams, 2018). The practical nurse needs to check with the agency regarding the scope of practice for PCA pumps.

Nonpharmacological Methods of Pain Relief

These methods can be used alone or in combination with pharmacological methods. Examples include progressive relaxation, guided imagery, biofeedback, transcutaneous electrical nerve stimulation (TENS), music therapy, acupressure, massage, and the application of heat or cold.

NUTRITION

Nutrients are the elements necessary for body processes and functions. A balanced diet with carbohydrates, fats, proteins, vitamins, and minerals provides the essential nutrients to carry out the body's normal physiological functioning.

- Carbohydrates are the main source of energy in the diet.
- Proteins are made from amino acids and are essential for the growth, maintenance, and repair of body tissue.
- Fats (lipids) are the most calorie-dense nutrient and are composed of triglycerides and fatty acids. They provide a concentrated source and stored form of energy.
- Vitamins facilitate metabolism of proteins, fats, and carbohydrates and are essential for normal metabolism. Vitamin content is usually highest in fresh foods that are used quickly and exposed minimally to cooking, storage, preparation, and processing.
- Fat-soluble vitamins A, D, E, and K can be stored in the body and are not easily destroyed by cooking or storage.
- Water-soluble vitamins (B complex and C) are not stored in the body, are easily destroyed by cooking, and can be excreted in the urine.
- Vitamin K is important in the production of prothrombin (necessary for the coagulation of blood).
- Vitamin C functions in the production of collagen, which is important in wound healing.
- Vitamin A is important in the maintenance of eyesight and epithelial linings.
- Minerals are essential to the body as catalysts in biochemical reactions. Examples include calcium, chloride, magnesium, phosphorus, potassium, sodium, iron, and zinc (Potter et al., 2019).

Eating Well With Canada's Food Guide

Eating Well with Canada's Food Guide helps clients to make appropriate nutritional choices from the four basic food groups: vegetables and fruit; grain products; milk and alternatives; and meat and alternatives (Health Canada, 2011). In the guide, the different sizes of the arcs in the rainbow represent the proportion of each of the four food groups that is recommended for healthy eating. The vegetables and fruit food group is the most prominent arc, emphasizing the important role these foods play.

The guide's recommendations are based on age and gender. Guidelines for dietary change advocate reducing the intake of fats, saturated fats, sodium, refined sugar, and cholesterol and increasing the intake of complex carbohydrates and fibre. See Fig. 5.4 in Chapter 5 for an extract from *Eating Well with Canada's Food Guide*.

Therapeutic Diets

A *therapeutic diet* is a diet intended to treat disease or help to manage a medical condition. See Table 6.3 for types of therapeutic diets, indications for use of these diets, and foods permitted on the diets.

Enteral Nutrition

Enteral nutrition (EN) refers to the delivery of liquid nutrients into the gastro-intestinal tract via a tube. EN is used when the client cannot ingest food but can still digest and absorb nutrients.

Types of Feeding Tubes

- Nasogastric (NG) tubes are inserted through the nose to the stomach (see the section "Bowel Elimination" for more details).
- Nasoenteral, or small-bore, feeding tubes (such as Dobbhoff tubes) are placed through the nose into the stomach and then moved into the duodenum. Placement is checked by radiography prior to commencing tube feedings.
  Surgically placed feeding tubes.
- A gastrostomy tube (G-tube) is placed directly into the stomach through the abdominal wall and sutured in place.
- A jejunostomy tube (J-tube) is inserted directly into the jejunum for clients with pathological conditions of the upper gastro-intestinal tract.
  Feeding tubes inserted by endoscopy. In this procedure, the stomach or the jejunum is punctured during a laparotomy or an endoscopy procedure that does not require a general anaesthetic. The two types are PEG (percutaneous endoscopic gastrostomy) and PEJ (percutaneous endoscopic jejunostomy).

Nursing Care of Clients With EN

- Ensure that the head of the bed is elevated 30–45 degrees at all times to prevent regurgitation of feedings and aspiration into the lungs.
- Monitor the client for abdominal distension and check the residual contents of the stomach regularly to see whether the client is tolerating the feeds. Aspirate all stomach contents (residual), measure the amount, and return the contents to the stomach if the residual is less than 100–150 mL (depending on agency policy). If the residual volume is more than 150 mL, it indicates delayed gastric emptying, which places the client at a higher risk of aspiration, and the feeds should be withheld.
- Check placement of the tube by (a) aspirating the gastric contents and checking the pH of any gastric fluids, and (b) X-ray examination. Do not rely on the auscultation method to differentiate between gastric and respiratory placement or to differentiate between gastric and small bowel placement. To verify whether a feeding tube has sustained the proper position, mark the exit site of the feeding tube during the initial radiograph and observe for any changes in the external tube length during feedings. If a significant increase in the external length is observed, use

TABLE 6.3 Therapeutic Diets

Type of Diet	Uses of Diet	Foods Permitted
Clear fluids	Often a postoperative diet, also used for diarrhea or initial feeding after complete bowel rest	Broth, coffee, tea, carbonated beverages, clear fruit juices, Popsicles, Jell-O
Thickened fluids	Used for clients who have dysphagia (difficulty swallowing) and are at risk for aspiration	Any liquid can be thickened with thickening agents
Full fluids	Can be used after clear fluids following surgery. Also for clients who are unable to chew or swallow.	Clear fluids, plus smooth-textured dairy products, puddings and custards, refined cooked cereals, ice cream, and all fruit juices
Pureed	Can be used for client with dental problems or problems swallowing or chewing	All of the above, with the addition of scrambled eggs, pureed meats, vegetables, fruits, mashed potatoes and gravy
Mechanical soft	Can be used for client with dental problems, problems swallowing or chewing, and mouth ulcerations	All of the above, with the addition of foods such as ground or finely diced meats, flaked fish, cheese, rice, potatoes, cooked vegetables, bananas, soups, etc.
High fibre	Can be used for clients with constipation or to prevent constipation	Addition of fresh uncooked fruits, steamed vegetables, bran, oatmeal, and dried fruits
Low sodium	For control of hypertension (no added salt [NAS]) and to reduce edema in clients with heart failure	Can vary from NAS to severe sodium restrictions
Low cholesterol	Used for clients with high cholesterol levels	Restrictions on foods high in cholesterol, such as eggs, regular cheese and ice cream, organ meats, fried food, and fast food
Diabetic	Used for diabetic clients	Clients with diabetes follow a healthy diet recommended for the general population as outlined in *Eating Well with Canada's Food Guide*. In hospitals, the meals are often labelled "diabetic" or "no added sugar" to indicate that the meal plan follows Diabetes Canada's current nutritional guidelines for diabetics.
Regular		No restrictions

Adapted from Potter, P., Perry, A., Stockert, P., et al. (2019). *Canadian fundamentals of nursing* (6th ed., p. 1127, Box 42.9). Milton, ON: Elsevier.

other bedside tests to help determine whether the tube has become dislocated. When in doubt, obtain a radiograph to determine tube location (Lewis et al., 2019, Potter et al., 2019).

- Assess bowel sounds; if absent, withhold feeds and notify the physician.
- Feeding pumps may be used for continuous feeds.
- For bolus feeds (300–400 mL of formula every 3–6 hours), leave the client in the high Fowler's position for 30 minutes after feeding.
- Change the feeding container and tubing every 24 hours to prevent bacterial growth.
- Do not hang more than 4 hours' worth of formula to prevent bacterial growth.
- Flush with 30–60 mL of water (according to agency policy) with an irrigation syringe after feeding.
- With feeding tubes, "monitor fingerstick blood glucose levels every 6 hours until maximum administration rate is reached and maintained for 24 hours" (Potter et al., 2019, p. 1145).

Complications of EN

Complications of EN include aspiration, diarrhea, vomiting, abdominal distension, and clogging of the feeding tube.

Parenteral Nutrition

Parenteral nutrition (PN) is a form of specialized nutrition support in which nutrients are provided intravenously to provide a positive nitrogen balance. PN can be administered in the home as well as the hospital. Practical nurses need to ensure administering PN is within their legal scope of practice in their jurisdiction and permitted by the policies of the facility in which they are working.

Types of PN

Total PN is a nutritionally adequate hypertonic solution consisting of glucose, electrolytes, and other nutrients administered through a CVAD site.

- Peripheral parenteral nutrition (PPN) can be used for clients who are experiencing mild or moderate malnutrition for up to weeks as long as the formula has a final dextrose concentration of 5–10% and an amino acid content of 3%. Often PPN is administered through a PICC line (Perry et al., 2018).
- Total parenteral nutrition or central parenteral nutrition (TPN/CPN) is administration of carbohydrates in the form of dextrose, fats in special emulsified form, proteins in the form of amino acids, vitamins, minerals, and water.

High-osmolality solutions (25% dextrose) are administered in conjunction with 5–10% amino acids, electrolytes, minerals, and vitamins. TPN/CPN is administered via a central line (usually the superior vena cava) (Lewis et al., 2019; Potter et al., 2019). CPN using concentrated dextrose solutions should not be infused into a peripheral IV or midline catheter because of the increased risk for phlebitis (Perry et al., 2018).

- Intralipid therapy is an infusion of 10–20% fat emulsion that provides essential fatty acids. It is usually administered at the same time as PPN or TPN. It can be administered alone through a separate peripheral catheter, through a CVAD, by Y-connector tubing, or as an admixture to TPN solution (Potter et al., 2019).
- Total nutrient admixture (TNA) is a combination of dextrose, amino acids, and lipids in one container. TNA is administered over 24 hours through a central line (Potter et al., 2019).

Indications for PN

Indications for initiation of PN include a nonfunctional gastro-intestinal tract (e.g., following bowel surgery; trauma to the head, neck, or abdomen; intestinal obstruction; chemotherapy; or radiation therapy); extended bowel rest (e.g., due to inflammatory bowel disease, severe diarrhea, or pancreatitis); or preoperative TPN (such as in the case of severe malnutrition or preoperative bowel rest).

Nursing care of clients with PN.

- Infuse TPN through a large vein, such as the subclavian, due to the high osmolarity of the solution. Registered nurses with specialized training insert PICC lines that are started in a vein of the forearm or upper arm and threaded into the subclavian vein or superior vena cava. Physicians may insert the catheter in the superior vena cava (Potter et al., 2019).
- Ensure proper placement of the line after insertion and prior to starting TPN. Placement should be confirmed by X-ray, as accidental pneumothorax can occur during insertion.
- Regulate flow carefully using an infusion pump. Rapid infusion can cause movement of fluid into the intravascular compartment, causing dehydration, circulatory overload, and hyperglycemia (Perry et al., 2018). Slow infusion can result in hypoglycemia as the body adapts to the high osmolarity by secreting more insulin; for this reason, therapy is never terminated abruptly (Perry et al., 2018).
- Use aseptic technique when handling the infusion and IV tubing or when changing dressings. Check agency policy regarding the frequency of tubing change (usually every 24 hours) and dressing change (usually every 48 hours).
- Use an in-line filter to remove crystals from the TPN solution.
- Record daily weights and monitor blood glucose levels frequently.
- Check laboratory reports daily (glucose, creatinine, blood urea nitrogen, and electrolytes); also check serum lipids and liver function if lipids are administered (Perry et al., 2018).
- Monitor temperature every 4 hours, as infection is the most common TPN complication; obtain cultures of blood, urine, and sputum (according to agency policy) to rule out other sources of infection if the client develops a fever (Perry et al., 2018).

URINARY ELIMINATION

Key Terms Related to Urinary Elimination

- *Anuria* is the absence of urine formation.
- *Diuresis* is the passage of large amounts of urine.
- *Dysuria* is painful or difficult urination.
- *Frequency* is voiding at frequent intervals (less than 2-hour intervals) or voiding more than eight times in 24 hours.
- *Hematuria* is the presence of blood in the urine.
- *Nocturia* is excessive or frequent urination after going to bed.
- *Oliguria* is urine output of less than 400 mL/day.
- *Polyuria* is voiding large amounts of urine (Potter et al., 2019).

Altered Urinary Elimination
Urinary Retention

Urinary retention is the marked accumulation of urine in the bladder as a result of the inability of the bladder to empty. Retention can occur in the postoperative period due to the effect of the anaesthetic. Prolonged retention can lead to stasis of urine in the bladder and increased risk of a urinary tract infection (UTI). Signs and symptoms of retention include any of the following: frequent voiding of small amounts, absence of urine output with palpable tender bladder, dull sound on percussion, sensation of bladder fullness, abdominal discomfort, restlessness, diaphoresis, and dribbling.

Urinary Tract Infection

UTI is the most common HAI due to the frequency of urinary catheterizations. If left untreated, UTIs can spread to the kidneys, causing kidney infection and eventually kidney damage. Signs and symptoms include any of the following: dysuria; fever; chills; frequency; urgency; hematuria; and concentrated, cloudy (possibly foul-smelling) urine (Potter et al., 2019).

Urinary Incontinence

Urinary incontinence is the loss of control over micturition. It may present as any of the following types (RNAO, 2005):

- Transient—loss of urine outside of or affecting the urinary system that resolves when the underlying cause(s), such as acute confusion or UTI, are treated
- Urge—involuntary passage of urine after a strong sense of urgency to void, for example, with alcohol or caffeine ingestion or a UTI
- Stress—leakage of small volumes of urine caused by a sudden increase in intra-abdominal pressure, such as during coughing or sneezing

- Mixed—having features of both stress and urge incontinence
- Functional—involuntary, unpredictable passage of urine in a client with an intact urinary and nervous system, as in the case when an older adult with bladder control is unable to reach the toilet
- Overflow—voluntary or involuntary loss of a small amount of urine (20–30 mL) from an overdistended bladder (as in the case of diabetics or spinal cord injury clients)
- Reflex—involuntary loss of urine occurring at somewhat predictable intervals
- Total—continuous and unpredictable loss of urine

Urinary Diversions

Urinary diversions divert the flow of urine from the kidneys directly to the abdominal surface via a urinary stoma. The diversion can be permanent or temporary and either continent or incontinent.

Maintaining Normal Urinary Elimination

- Promote fluid intake of 1500–2000 mL daily for the average adult and an increased intake for clients at risk of UTI and renal calculi, as well as clients with catheters.
- Maintain normal voiding habits. Void every 3–4 hours to maintain a normal bladder capacity (400–500 mL) and to avoid urinary stasis.

Measuring Intake and Output

- Fluid intake should equal output. Intake is considered all dietary items that are fluid at room temperature as well as IV fluids, including blood. Output is urine, vomitus, suction drainage, bleeding, and insensible loss, such as sweating.
- Normal urine output is 60 mL/hr or 1500 mL/day. Urine outputs below 30 mL/hr (0.5 mL/kg/hr) for more than 2 hours in an adult should be reported. Also, urine outputs over 2000 to 2500 mL daily (polyuria) should be reported to a physician (Potter et al., 2019).
- Daily weights are the single most important indicator of fluid status. Clients should be weighed daily on the same weigh scale at the same time after voiding.

Urine Testing and Specimen Collection

Urine samples can be random (routine urinalysis), clean-catch or midstream (culture and sensitivity), or sterile (culture and sensitivity). For midstream urine specimens, the client cleans the perineum with an antiseptic solution, initiates urination to cleanse the meatus, and then urinates into a sterile specimen container. Some tests require 24-hour collection of urine, such as the creatinine clearance test. The urine is collected in a special collection container that may have a preservative added.

Catheterization and Catheter Care

Intermittent Catheterization

A straight single-lumen catheter is introduced to empty the bladder and removed after the bladder is drained. Indications for use include relief of bladder distension and obtaining a sterile urine specimen.

In-Dwelling Catheterization (Retention or Foley Catheterization)

A catheter with an inflatable balloon is inserted into the bladder on a short- or long-term basis. Indications for use include prostate enlargement, measuring urine output in critically ill clients, or ulcers or wounds irritated by contact with urine.

Catheterization for Residual Urine

Catheterization for residual urine involves inserting a catheter after a client voids to check for the amount of urine remaining in the bladder. The bladder normally holds less than 50 mL after voiding. If the volume of urine (residual volume) is greater than 100 mL, the catheter may be left in situ. Portable bladder scanners offer a noninvasive means of assessing postvoid residual volumes (Potter et al., 2019).

Catheter Care

- Keep the urinary drainage bag below the level of the bladder to prevent reflux, which can lead to UTIs.
- Secure the catheter to the client's inner thigh or abdomen with a strip of non-allergenic tape or (or multipurpose tube holders with a Velcro strap) to reduce the pressure on the urethra and the possibility of tissue injury.
- Keep the drainage tubing coiled on the bed to aid gravity drainage.
- Do not open a closed system unless absolutely necessary, to lessen the chance of UTIs.
- Perform catheter care twice daily with soap and water to cleanse the urinary meatus and encrustations on the catheter and after a bowel movement in order to reduce infections.
- Empty the drainage bag every 8 hours and record the amount, colour, odour, and consistency of urinary drainage.
- Change the urinary catheter bag and catheter regularly according to agency policy.
- Remove the catheter as soon as clinically possible to prevent UTIs.

Bladder Irrigation

Closed and open catheter or bladder irrigations are irrigations or flushes used to maintain the patency of in-dwelling catheters or to wash out the bladder and treat local infections.

BOWEL ELIMINATION

Common Bowel Elimination Challenges

- Constipation usually involves infrequent bowel movements, difficult defecation, inability to defecate at will, and hard feces (Potter et al., 2019). It can also involve abdominal distension and pain and pressure in the rectum.
- Fecal impaction is a condition in which a collection of hardened feces cannot be expelled from the rectum. The common sign is inability to pass stool for several days.

Impaction should be suspected if there is a continuous oozing of diarrhea (liquid feces from higher in the bowel is seeping around the impaction).

- Diarrhea is the passage of liquid feces and an increase in the number of stools. The greatest danger from diarrhea is fluid and electrolyte imbalance.
- Fecal incontinence is the inability to control the passage of feces and gas. Skin breakdown can occur after repeated contact with liquid stool.
- Flatulence is excessive gas in the stomach and intestine. Reduction in gastro-intestinal motility, resulting from opiates, general anaesthetics, abdominal surgery, or immobilization, can cause abdominal distension due to flatulence.
- Hemorrhoids (internal and external) are dilated, engorged veins in the rectal area (either external or internal). They can make defecation painful.

Bowel Diversions

Bowel diversions divert the feces from the bowel directly to the abdominal surface. Surgical openings can be created in the ileum (ileostomy) or colon (colostomy) to create an artificial opening called a *stoma*. The location of the ostomy determines the consistency of the stool, with the ileostomy having more frequent liquid stools and the colostomy resulting in more solid formed stool. Proper selection and maintenance of an ostomy pouching system is important to prevent damage to the skin around the stoma.

Promoting Regular or Normal Defecation

- Understand that foods high in fibre and an increased fluid intake keep feces soft.
- Provide clients with as much privacy as possible. Lack of privacy may cause the client to ignore the urge to defecate.
- Provide clients with a position as close to normal as possible for defecation (such as on a commode chair) and give them enough time.
- Be aware of the client's normal routine and when defecation is most likely to occur, for example, 1 hour after a meal. Establishing a specific time for defecation may help to prevent constipation.
- Regular exercise within the client's physical ability is important in stimulating peristalsis and a regular bowel routine.
- Know that warm fluids and certain juices (prune) can stimulate bowel motility.

Enemas

Enemas are an instillation of a solution into the rectum and sigmoid colon. They stimulate peristalsis and initiate defection. They are commonly used for relief of constipation but can also deliver medications that have a local effect on the rectal mucosa. The most common types of enemas are cleansing and oil retention. Enemas may also be used in preparing for diagnostic tests or for performing diagnostic tests of the bowel or rectum, such as barium enemas.

Types of Enemas

- Cleansing enemas include tap water, NS, low-volume hypertonic (Fleet), and soap suds.
- Oil retention enemas lubricate the rectum and colon. The feces become softer and easier to pass. The client is advised to hold the enema for 30 minutes to 3 hours.

Nursing Care of Clients Receiving an Enema

- Explain the procedure to the client and ensure privacy.
- Explain how long the client must retain the enema.
- Place the client in the left Sims' position.
- Ensure that the rectal tube attached to the enema bag is lubricated and inserted 7–10 cm into the rectum.
- Ensure that the client has access to a bathroom, commode, or bedpan.
- Observe and record the amount and consistency of the return from the enema.

Digital Removal of Stool

Digital removal of stool is used when the client has a fecal impaction. The practical nurse breaks up the fecal mass with a finger and removes it in sections. This procedure can be painful, can damage the rectal mucosa, and can cause vagal stimulation (resulting in reflex slowing of the heart rate). In some agencies, a physician's order is necessary to remove a fecal impaction. Vital signs should be checked before and after the procedure.

Nasogastric Tubes

Nasogastric (NG) tubes are pliable tubes inserted through the nasopharynx and into the stomach. Commonly used types are Levin or Salem sump NG tubes. Practical nurses need to check their legal scope of practice in their jurisdiction and the policies of the facility they are working in regarding whether they can insert NG tubes or care for NG tubes.

Purposes of NG Tubes

- Decompression: removal of secretions from the gastro-intestinal tract for the prevention and relief of abdominal distension
- Feeding or gavage: instillation of liquid nutritional supplements into the stomach for clients unable to swallow
- Compression: internal application of pressure by means of an inflated balloon to prevent internal esophageal or gastro-intestinal hemorrhage
- Lavage: irrigation of the stomach for active bleeding, poisoning, or gastric dilation.

Insertion of an NG Tube

- Place the client in the high Fowler's position.
- Measure from the tip of the nose to the earlobe to the xiphoid process to determine the length of insertion.
- Lubricate 7.5 cm with water-soluble lubricant.
- Instruct the client to bend the head forward to close the epiglottis.

- Insert the tube into the patent nostril and advance it backward into the nasopharynx.
- Have the client dry swallow or sip on water (if allowed) and advance the tube as the client swallows to the predetermined length.
- If the client experiences respiratory distress (coughing or choking), remove the tube and resume the procedure when the client has recovered.
- Tape the tube in place and confirm placement of the tube.

Assessment of Tube Placement

- The most reliable method to check placement is by radiography.
- Tube placement is assessed every 4 hours and before administering medications or feedings.
- The most reliable method to assess tube placement at the bedside is to aspirate gastric contents and test the gastric pH. Gastric pH should be less than 4. Intestinal aspirates are greater than 4, and respiratory aspirates are greater than 5.5.
- Auscultation is not considered a reliable method for the identification of tube placement because a tube inadvertently placed in the lungs, pharynx, or esophagus can transmit a sound similar to that of air entering the stomach (Potter et al., 2019).
- Irrigation of an NG tube is gentle instillation of 30–50 mL of water or NS (check agency policy) to check and maintain patency of the NG tube. Check placement of the tube prior to irrigating. A doctor's order may be required to irrigate the NG tube of gastric surgery clients.

Medication Administration via an NG Tube

- Crush medications or open capsules (if allowed) or use liquid forms.
- Dissolve medication in 10–30 mL of warm water and draw up into a 60-mL syringe.
- Check placement of the NG tube as well as residual volume in the stomach.
- Flush the NG tube with 30 mL of water (check agency policy).
- Instill medication into the tube.
- Flush the NG tube with 30–60 mL of water (check agency policy).
- Clamp the tube for 30–60 minutes if the client is on intermittent suction (check agency policy).

Considerations Relating to the Older Adult

- Constipation can be a common complaint in older adults due to a combination of impaired general health, use of medication, decreased motility, and physical activity.

MOBILITY AND IMMOBILITY

Mobility refers to the ability to move easily and independently. Certain illnesses, surgery, pain, and aging can impair mobility temporarily or permanently. It is important to know the hazards of immobility and how to prevent them as well as how to care for clients who are immobile.

Systemic Effects of Immobility

When there is an alteration in mobility, each body system is at risk for impairment. Some of the changes that can happen—the "hazards of immobility"—are as follows:

- Metabolic changes include a lowered metabolic rate, a negative nitrogen balance, anorexia (loss of appetite), and a negative calcium balance (calcium is lost from bones).
- Respiratory changes include shallow respirations and decreased vital capacity, pooling of respiratory secretions, atelectasis (collapse of alveoli), and hypostatic pneumonia (inflammation of the lung from stasis or pooling of secretions).
- Cardiovascular changes include diminished cardiac reserve, increased use of the Valsalva manoeuvre (such as when the client holds his or her breath to change position in bed), orthostatic hypotension, and venous dilation and stasis, which can cause edema and deep vein thrombosis (DVT).
- Musculo-skeletal changes include disuse osteoporosis, disuse atrophy, contractures, foot drop (foot permanently fixed in plantar flexion), and external hip rotation.
- Urinary elimination changes include urinary stasis, urinary calculi, urinary retention, and urinary infection.
- Gastro-intestinal system changes include constipation and decreased peristalsis.
- Integumentary changes include less skin turgor (elasticity) and possible skin breakdown, as well as the formation of pressure sores or ulcers (Lewis et al., 2019; Potter et al., 2019).

Positioning and Body Alignment

- Immobile clients need to be repositioned at least every 2 hours or more frequently if there are reddened skin areas. The 30-degree lateral position is best as it does not put direct pressure on the trochanter.
- Clients should be placed in a variety of positions to prevent pressure areas. Different bed positions used include Fowler's; supine (dorsal) recumbent; prone (face down); side-lying (lateral); and Sims' (semiprone).
- Limbs need to be anatomically aligned in a slightly flexed position. Bony surfaces should not touch; for example, a pillow is often placed between knees. Trochanter rolls can be used to prevent external hip rotation, footboards to prevent foot drop, and hand–wrist or foot–ankle splints to keep the joints anatomically aligned.

Range-of-Motion Exercises

- ROM exercises can be active (the client is able to move all joints through their ROM unassisted) or passive (the client is unable to move some or all of the joints independently, and the practical nurse assists certain or all joints through their ROM).
- Exercises should begin as soon as possible, as joints begin to stiffen within 24 hours of loss of movement in an

extremity or joint (Potter et al., 2014). It is best to schedule them at specific times, such as during the bath.

- Each joint movement is repeated five times during each session. No force is exerted.

Moving and Transferring Clients Safely

A thorough assessment must be made prior to moving or positioning a client. The client needs to be assessed for the degree of exertion permitted, capabilities such as mobility and strength, comprehension, pain level, weight, and presence of orthostatic hypotension. The practical nurse must also assess his or her own strength and ability to move the client and how much assistance is available from other healthcare providers or if mechanical lifts are available. Finally, the practical nurse must assess the environment to make sure the transfer can be done safely.

- Consider the client's abilities and disabilities when deciding appropriate transfer technique and the need for assistive devices; for example, for hemiplegia, place the wheelchair on the side opposite the affected extremities; for paraplegia, the client may use a trapeze, slide board, or wheelchair with a removable arm.
- Use the principles of body mechanics (see Box 6.1).

WOUND CARE

Types of Wounds

- Acute wounds, such as surgical wounds, follow the normal healing process in a predictable and timely fashion.
- Chronic wounds, such as pressure injuries, do not heal easily, and the normal reparative process is interrupted.

Types of Wound Healing
Primary Intention

Wounds that heal by primary intention have little or no tissue loss, have well-approximated wound margins, and heal quickly. Two examples are a clean surgical wound or a paper cut.

Secondary Intention

Wounds that heal by secondary intention have loss of tissue, such as second- or third-degree burns, or pressure injuries, and there is no approximation of the wound edges. Healing and granulation take place from the edges inward and from the base of the wound to the top. The wound is left open and takes longer to heal (Potter et al., 2019).

Tertiary Intention

Tertiary Intention (delayed primary intention) healing occurs with postponing suturing of a wound in which two layers of granulation tissue are sutured together. The wound is left open until the infection is resolved (Lewis et al., 2019).

Complications of Wound Healing

- Hemorrhage or bleeding from the wound may occur externally or internally.
- Wound infection is the second most common HAI. Signs of wound infection may include any of the following: pain

and tenderness at the site, erythema, edema, inflammation of wound edges, purulent drainage, warmth of tissues at the site, fever or chills, elevated white blood cell (WBC) count, and delayed healing (Potter et al., 2019).

- Dehiscence is the partial or total separation of the wound layers (Potter et al., 2019). It usually occurs at 3–11 days postinjury or surgery. It most commonly involves surgical wounds of the abdomen and can occur after a vigorous bout of coughing or straining. A strategy to prevent dehiscence is to provide support to the area, such as using a pillow as a splint when the client is coughing.
- Evisceration is protrusion of the abdominal organs through the wound opening. This is a medical emergency and requires surgical intervention. The practical nurse should cover the organs with sterile saline-soaked towels, keep the client NPO (nil per os, or nothing by mouth), and monitor for signs and symptoms of shock.
- A fistula is an "abnormal passage between two organs or between an organ and the outside of the body" (Potter et al., 2019, p. 1309). It is the result of infection, poor wound healing, or a complication of diseases such as Crohn's disease.

Types of Wound Drainage

Wound drainage can be serous (clear and watery), purulent (thick green, yellow, or brown and containing pus cells), serosanguineous (thin, watery, and blood-tinged), or sanguineous (bloody).

Wound Assessment

Wound assessment includes observing wound appearance (size, location, stage of healing, approximation, and condition of skin around the wound); the character and amount of drainage; the presence and amount of drainage from drains such as the Penrose, Hemovac, or Jackson-Pratt; and the presence of sutures, staples, or packing. Wound assessment may also involve palpating the wound for warmth, tenderness, hardness, or pain and may require collection of a wound culture if the wound appears infected.

Pressure (Ulcers) Injuries

The term *pressure injury* replaces the term *pressure ulcer* in the National Pressure Ulcer Advisory Panel Pressure Injury Staging System (National Pressure Ulcer Advisory Panel [NPUAP], 2016). The new term is considered to better describe pressure injuries to both intact and ulcerated skin.

A pressure injury is localized damage to the skin and/or underlying soft tissue, usually over a bony prominence or related to a medical or other device. The injury can present as intact skin or an open ulcer and may be painful. The injury occurs as a consequence of intense and/or prolonged pressure or pressure in combination with shear (NPUAP, 2016; Potter et al., 2019). Pressure is the main source of pressure injuries, and they often develop over a bony prominence when tissue is compressed between the bone and a hard surface such as a bed or chair. The following are other factors that work with pressure to cause skin damage and necrosis:

- Friction is when two surfaces are rubbed against each other. For example, dragging a client across the sheets can cause an abrasion.
- Shear is the parallel force that happens when the skin and underlying subcutaneous tissue are pulled taut, obstructing capillary blood flow and causing tissue necrosis in the deep tissue layers. Shear occurs when the client is moved incorrectly; for example, when he or she is dragged instead of lifted clear of the mattress, or when the head of the bed is elevated above 30 degrees for long periods of time, causing the client to slide down in bed.
- Moisture caused by wound discharge, excess diaphoresis, or incontinence can be a factor leading to skin breakdown.

Risk Assessment for Pressure Injuries

Identify at-risk clients early by using a validated risk-assessment tool such as the Braden Scale. The Braden Scale measures sensory perception, moisture, activity, mobility, nutrition, and friction and shear. The scale needs to be used preventively (on admission) and consistently (daily in high-risk clients). As soon as a client is identified to be at risk for developing pressure injuries, prevention strategies should be started.

Staging System for Pressure Injuries

Pressure injuries are described according to the following stages:
- Suspected deep tissue injury—A purple or maroon localized area of discoloured intact skin or blood-filled blister, caused by damage to the underlying soft tissue from pressure or shear, or both.
- Stage I pressure injury—Intact skin with nonblanchable redness of a localized area, usually over a bony prominence. Darkly pigmented skin may not have visible blanching, but its colour may differ from that of the surrounding skin. The area may be painful, firm, warm, or cooler as compared with adjacent tissue.
- Stage II pressure injury—Partial-thickness loss of dermis presenting as a shallow open ulcer with a red-pink wound bed, without slough. It may also present as an intact, an open, or a ruptured serum-filled blister.
- Stage III pressure injury—Full-thickness tissue loss. Subcutaneous fat may be visible, but bone, tendon, or muscle is not exposed. Slough may be present. It may include undermining or tunnelling. The depth of a stage III pressure injury varies by anatomical location.
- Stage IV pressure injury—Full-thickness tissue loss with exposed bone, tendon, or muscle. Slough or eschar may be present on some parts of the wound bed. Often it includes tunnelling and undermining. The depth of a stage IV pressure injury varies by anatomical location.
- Unstageable pressure injury—Full-thickness tissue loss in which the base of the injury is covered in slough, eschar, or both. *Slough* is a viscous yellow layer that often covers the wound. *Eschar* is thick, dry, black, necrotic tissue covering a wound (NPUAP, 2016; Potter et al., 2019).

Prevention of Pressure Injuries

- Reposition clients every 2 hours or more if they are high risk. Encourage clients with some independent mobility to shift their weight every 15 minutes when sitting.
- Inspect the condition of the client's skin at least daily, and examine bony prominences carefully. Nonblanchable erythema or discoloration of the skin may indicate early signs of tissue injury.
- Keep linens dry to prevent maceration of skin and wrinkle-free to prevent pressure.
- Position the client in a 30-degree lateral position to either side to avoid pressure on the trochanter.
- Do not massage over bony prominences or reddened areas.
- Avoid elevating the head of the bed to more than 30 degrees, as that increases the shearing force.
- Use support surfaces (pressure redistribution devices), such as pressure-reducing and pressure-relieving mattresses, for at-risk clients. A pressure-reducing mattress reduces the interface pressure (the pressure between the body and the support surface) but not below the capillary-closing pressure (Potter et al., 2019). A pressure-relieving mattress relieves the interface pressure below the capillary-closing pressure, which is 32 mm Hg (Potter et al., 2019).
- Promote a diet that is high in protein and calories and ensure adequate hydration. Assess teeth or dentures; ensure good mouth care.
- Keep skin clean and well hydrated.

Treatment of Pressure Injuries

- Perform a comprehensive assessment of the pressure injury, including staging, measurement of size (depth, width, and length), character and amount of exudate, wound bed characteristics, pain, condition of surrounding skin, and evidence of tunnelling or undermining (Potter et al., 2019).
- Determine the need for local wound care by assessing the wound bed for debris, infection, and moisture balance. If slough is present, the wound may need to be irrigated, debrided, or both.
- Wound debridement removes necrotic material that interferes with healing. There are different methods of debridement, such as surgical or sharp, autolytic, enzymatic, or mechanical. Mechanical debridement (also called a *wet-to-dry dressing*) is no longer recommended as it is not selective and can damage new granulating tissue (Potter et al., 2019).
- Moist interactive wound healing involves keeping the wound bed moist and warm and not disturbing it too much by changing the dressing. A moist, interactive wound healing environment results in faster healing, better tissue quality, and reduced pain (Potter et al., 2019).
- Negative pressure wound therapy (NPWT) is a device that assists in wound closure by applying localized negative pressure to draw the edges of a wound together (Lewis et al., 2019; Potter et al., 2019). It can be used with both acute, traumatic, dehiscence, and chronic wounds. It

removes fluid from the area surrounding the wound and can accelerate healing.

Applying Dry Dressings

- The purpose of dressings is to protect the wound from contamination, aid hemostasis, absorb drainage, and promote a moist healing environment.
- Wounds are commonly cleansed with NS, which is not toxic to cells.
- The wound or incision should be cleansed from the least contaminated area (the wound or incision) to the most contaminated (the surrounding skin).
- Acute wounds usually require aseptic dressing techniques, while chronic wounds may require only clean dressing techniques.
- It is important to observe the character, colour, amount, and odour of drainage on the dressing and the appearance of the wound, as well as the skin around the wound.

Applying an Elastic Bandage

- An elastic bandage is used to create pressure over a body part, to immobilize a body part, to support a wound, to reduce or minimize edema, to secure a splint, or to secure dressings.
- The bandage is applied from distal to proximal to promote venous return.
- Assess distal circulation when the bandage is first applied and every 4 hours afterward. Check the limb distally for colour, warmth, sensation, and movement. Palpate and compare pulses bilaterally and check capillary refill.

SENSORY ALTERATIONS

Sensory deficits are losses in the normal function of sensory reception and perception, such as vision or hearing impairments. Aging most commonly results in a gradual decline of acuity in all senses. Clients who are immobilized or isolated are at risk for sensory alterations.

Sensory Deprivation

Sensory deprivation is the result of inadequate sensory stimuli (either in quality or quantity). Sensory deprivation can be the result of (a) reduced sensory input, as in the case of vision or hearing impairment; (b) the elimination of order or meaning from input, for example, exposure to strange environments; or (c) restriction in the environment, as when a client is confined to bed rest or receives reduced cues or no variation in cues from the environment. When clients are placed in isolation, a decrease in stimuli can occur (Potter et al., 2019).

Sensory Overload

Sensory overload occurs when clients receive multiple sensory stimuli and cannot disregard or filter out some stimuli. Their tolerance to sensory overload may vary depending on many factors, such as level of fatigue, attitude, or state of well-being (physical, mental, and emotional). It may lead to delirium, a serious condition experienced by clients with sensory

alterations. Providing calendars, clocks, diming lights, family support, and clear communication can help prevent sensory overload and delirium (Potter et al., 2019).

CARE OF SURGICAL CLIENTS

Preoperative Surgical Phase

Informed Consent

The surgeon is responsible for obtaining the client's informed consent for surgery before sedation is given.

Minors require a parent or guardian to sign the consent.

Nutrition

When the client is going to have general anaesthesia, solid foods and liquids are usually withheld after midnight the night before surgery to avoid the possibility of vomiting and subsequent aspiration during surgery. Protocols may vary if the client is having local anaesthesia or the surgery is scheduled for late in the day. Varying NPO protocols exist; the NPO protocol of each surgical facility should be followed (Lewis et al., 2014). An IV line may be initiated prior to surgery or in the operating room.

Elimination

An enema or laxative may be ordered for clients having intestinal or abdominal surgery. The client should void immediately before surgery, or the insertion of a Foley catheter may be ordered.

Care of Surgical Site

The surgical site may be scrubbed with an antiseptic soap the night before surgery, or the client may be required to take a chlorhexidine shower and scrub the night before and the morning of the surgery. Shaving the skin is no longer recommended because it causes microscopic cuts. Hair is removed only if it interferes with surgery, and clippers instead of razors are used for hair removal.

Preoperative Teaching

The client needs to be informed before surgery about what to expect postoperatively. Teaching involves topics such as pain relief and use of the PCA pump, postoperative breathing exercises and the use of the incentive spirometer, foot and leg exercises, and instructions about invasive lines or devices to be expected after surgery (such as chest tubes, Foley catheter, drains, and NG tubes).

Psychological Preparation

Monitor the client's anxiety level and provide support as needed. Answer any of the client's questions or concerns or those of the client's family.

Preoperative Medication

Most clients will be told to take their routine cardiac, antihypertensive, and asthma medications on the day of surgery, but there is no routine protocol. If the medications are oral, they are taken with a minimal amount of water. Eye drops are often ordered preoperatively for clients undergoing cataract or other eye surgery. IV antibiotics are often given as prophylaxis against infection for orthopaedic, cardiac, and gastro-intestinal surgery clients. Sedatives are occasionally ordered, and it is important that the consent is signed before the client receives sedatives or narcotics.

Preoperative Checklist

The preoperative checklist needs to be reviewed thoroughly before the client is transferred to surgery. The client needs to be wearing an identification bracelet. The practical nurse needs to check the chart for recorded allergies, signed consent forms for surgery and blood transfusions, or both; a complete history and physical examination; routine blood work results (including urinalysis, electrolytes, and complete blood count); electrocardiogram and chest X-ray results; and blood cross and type results, if ordered. All jewellery, makeup, nail polish, dentures, and prostheses need to be removed. All valuables should be given to family members or locked away for safekeeping. The practical nurse needs to document when the client last ate or drank, when the client last voided, if the client was given preoperative medication, and a current set of baseline vital signs.

Intraoperative Surgical Phase

The circulating nurse is an RN. His or her responsibilities include verifying the client's identification bracelet with the chart and the client's verbal response, as well as reviewing the chart for completeness and confirming the operative procedure and operative site. The primary focus of the intraoperative phase is to prevent injury and complications related to anaesthesia, surgery, positioning, and equipment used. The circulating nurse acts as the client's advocate during the intraoperative phase. The scrub nurse maintains a sterile field during the procedure, hands the surgeon sterile instruments and supplies, and counts sponges, needles, and instruments during and after the surgery. In many Canadian institutions, a trained practical nurse performs the scrubbing function (Lewis et al., 2014). The circulating nurse positions the client on the operating room table, drapes the client, assists the anaesthetist to intubate, assists the surgeon and scrub nurse to don sterile attire, and maintains complete and accurate written records.

Postoperative Surgical Phase
Immediate Postoperative Stage

The immediate postoperative stage is the period from 1–4 hours after surgery in the postanaesthesia care unit (PACU).

Respiratory status. The respiratory status may be depressed as a result of anaesthesia. Maintain a patent airway until the gag reflex returns. Position the client on his or her side to prevent aspiration and the accumulation of secretions. Monitor heart rate and rhythm, symmetry of chest movement, breath sounds, pulse oximeter readings, and colour. Administer oxygen as ordered and suction as needed to remove secretions.

Circulatory status. The circulatory status may be compromised by anaesthesia and immobility during surgery. Monitor the heart rate and rhythm as well as BP at least every 15 minutes while in the postanaesthesia care unit. Monitor peripheral circulation by noting the colour, temperature, capillary refill, and presence of pulses. Monitor for hemorrhage by watching for hypotension and observing and measuring wound drainage.

Neurological status. The client's neurological status may be affected by preoperative and anaesthetic agents that depress the central nervous system. Monitor the client's level of consciousness and responses to stimuli. Monitor blink and gag reflexes. Monitor for loss or return of sensation or movement when specific areas have been surgically treated. Reorient the client to time, place, and situation and call the client by name. Answer questions simply and reassure the client.

Wound care. Note the location of the wound and the colour, odour, amount, and consistency of drainage. Circle drainage on the dressing to assess the extent of bleeding over time. Reinforce postoperative dressings as the first dressing change is often done by the surgeon.

Care of drains and tubes. Maintain the patency of all tubing. Attach to suction when ordered. Monitor drain output to assess for hemorrhage.

Fluid and electrolyte needs. Maintain IV therapy as ordered. Record intake and output accurately.

Comfort needs. Assess the client's level of pain on the 0–10 scale. Medicate as ordered to reduce pain and increase postoperative compliance with coughing, deep breathing, and activity. Splinting at the surgical site may decrease discomfort when coughing. Instruct the client in the use of PCA.

Care of clients with regional anaesthesia. Regional anaesthesia causes the loss of sensation to an area of the body. No loss of consciousness occurs, but the client may receive sedation. Examples include nerve blocks and spinal or epidural anaesthesia. For both spinal and epidural anaesthesia, the client must be observed closely for signs of autonomic nervous system blockade, signalled by hypotension, bradycardia, nausea, and vomiting (Lewis et al., 2019). If the block or level of anaesthesia rises (in other words, if spinal anaesthesia migrates up the spinal cord), breathing may be affected (Lewis et al., 2019). Burns and other trauma can also occur on the parts of the body affected by the anaesthesia without the client feeling it, so it is important to monitor the position of the extremities and the condition of the skin frequently (Potter et al., 2019).

Postoperative Convalescence Stage

The postoperative convalescence stage varies again, depending on the extent of surgery and clients recovery process. For ambulatory clients, convalescence may occur at home. For hospitalized clients, it may occur in the hospital for one or more days.

Respiratory status. Continue to monitor vital signs every 2–4 hours according to agency policy using the same assessments from the immediate postoperative stage. Encourage coughing and deep breathing and incentive spirometer every 1–2 hours.

Circulatory status. Continue to monitor circulatory status as described above every 2–4 hours, according to agency policy. Use antiembolism or elastic stockings, if prescribed, to promote venous return.

Musculo-skeletal status. Encourage progressive ambulation, starting with leg-dangling at the bedside as soon as possible and following doctors' orders. If the client is unable to ambulate, reposition him or her in bed every 2 hours.

Gastro-intestinal status. Monitor intake and output. Administer frequent mouth care. Assess for bowel sounds in all four quadrants. When oral fluids are permitted, start with ice chips and water. The client advances from clear fluids to a full diet when bowel sounds are heard. Monitor the client for flatus and encourage ambulation.

Renal status. Monitor urine output, which should be greater than 30 mL/hr (0.5 mL/kg/hr). Clients without Foley catheters should void at least 200 mL within 6–8 hours postoperatively.

Wound care. Assess the surgical site and drains and maintain an intact, dry dressing. Monitor the amount of drainage from drains and the incision. Reinforce dressing as needed.

The assessments from the postoperative convalescence stage continue, but less frequently. Continue to encourage ambulation to promote peristalsis and the passage of flatus. Continue to increase ambulation to regain muscle strength. Change the dressing as needed using aseptic technique and assess the incision and drainage. Monitor for signs and symptoms of infection by checking for pain, redness, and swelling at the incision site, fever, or an elevated WBC.

Postoperative Complications

Respiratory complications such as pneumonia and atelectasis are the most common. Other postoperative complications include hypoxia, pulmonary embolism, hemorrhage, shock, thrombophlebitis (inflammation of a vein accompanied by clot formation), urinary retention, constipation, and paralytic ileus (loss of the forward flow of intestinal contents as a result of anaesthetic medications or manipulation of the bowel during surgery, wound infection, wound dehiscence, or wound evisceration).

Postoperative Exercises
Respiratory Exercises

Deep breathing. The client is instructed to take 10 slow deep breaths every hour during the postoperative period until mobile. Diaphragmatic and pursed-lip breathing are examples of different methods of deep breathing.

Use of incentive spirometer. Incentive spirometry (IS) is a way to encourage deep breathing in clients by providing visual feedback about their inspiratory volume. It is used to prevent or treat atelectasis in the postoperative client and should be used hourly while awake. IS is used in many practice settings, but research does not support its benefit over other methods, such as coughing, deep breathing, and ambulation (Potter et al., 2019).

Controlled coughing. The client is in the upright position and takes two slow, deep breaths, inhaling through the nose and out through the mouth. On the third intake of breath, the client holds to a count of three and gives two to three consecutive coughs without inhaling between coughs.

Leg Exercises

Leg exercises should be performed at least every 2 hours for five successive times while awake. They include foot circles, alternating dorsiflexion and plantar flexion of both feet, quadriceps (thigh) setting, and hip and knee movements.

PALLIATIVE CARE

Palliative care is supportive care or treatment that relieves or reduces the severity of symptoms rather than providing a cure. Palliative care is designed for individuals and family members who are living with a life-threatening illness, often at an advanced stage (Government of Canada, 2016). It is a philosophy of total care with the aim of relieving suffering, emphasizing dignity, and improving the quality of living and dying, from diagnosis to the end of life and bereavement. Care is provided by a multidisciplinary team that consists of many care providers, such as nurses, physicians, social workers, chaplains, volunteers, pharmacists, physiotherapists, occupational therapists, and alternative therapists, such as massage therapists. Palliative care occurs in many settings, including hospitals, long-term care facilities, hospices, and clients' homes. Client and family needs are the focus of any interventions. Refer to Chapter 3 for more on the palliative care approach.

PRACTICE QUESTIONS

Case 1

A new graduate practical nurse is working a 12-hour day shift on a complex medicine unit. She has four clients assigned to her care.

Questions 1–6 refer to this case.

1. The practical nurse knows that it is important to take accurate blood pressure measurements because many of her clients are on antihypertensive medications. Which of the following statements is correct about measurement of blood pressure?

1. All older adults have an auscultatory gap.
2. Normal pulse pressure, or the difference between systolic and diastolic pressures, is 50–60 mm Hg.
3. Orthostatic hypotension is measured by recording blood pressure and pulse with the client sitting.
4. An auscultatory gap can cause underestimation of systolic blood pressure or overestimation of diastolic blood pressure.

2. Mrs. Lucas, 88 years old, has been febrile for several days due to a severe kidney infection. The physician asks the

practical nurse to check a core temperature for the next set of vital signs. Which of the following temperature sites can the practical nurse use to check a core temperature?

1. Rectal
2. Oral
3. Axillary
4. Skin

3. Mr. Hamas, age 55, requires an elastic wrap applied to his left ankle this morning for a sprained ankle injury. One hour after the practical nurse applied the elastic wrap around his left foot, he complained of severe discomfort and tingling in the foot. Which action should the practical nurse take?

1. Reassure the client that the pain is a direct result of the sprain ankle injury.
2. Administer an analgesia for the pain in the left foot.
3. Assess the circulation, sensation, and movement in the left foot.
4. Elevate the foot on a pillow to decrease the swelling.

4. The practical nurse accidentally sustains a needle-stick injury after giving Mr. Hamas his injection. What could have prevented this injury?

1. Giving the injection quickly and putting the needle directly into the sharps container
2. Using safety-engineered needles to reduce the risk of needle-stick injuries
3. Advocating for oral rather than parenteral administration of medications
4. Wearing gloves when giving the injection

5. Mr. Aboud, 24 years old, has an intravenous (IV) order for 1 000 mL of normal saline to run over 8 hours. The IV is started at 1100 hours, and 600 mL is left in the bag at 1500 hours. What adjustment in the flow rate must the practical nurse make to ensure that the solution is infused no earlier or later than 1900 hours as ordered?

1. Regulate the IV flow rate to 75 mL/hr
2. Regulate the IV flow rate to 100 mL/hr
3. Regulate the IV flow rate to 125 mL/hr
4. Regulate the IV flow rate to 150 mL/hr

6. Mrs. Roman, 77, has heart failure and a history of angina. The practical nurse must apply a transdermal patch of nitroglycerine at 0800 hours. Which of the following statements about transdermal medications is correct?

1. They may be applied to any area of the body, regardless of hair distribution as this does not interfere with absorption.
2. Transdermal medications are applied to the skin by patch or disc and stay in place for 7 days.
3. Removal of the old patch or disc prior to applying the new medication is recommended but not mandatory as all the medication has been absorbed from the old patch.
4. Transdermal medications can be absorbed through the skin of the nurse's hands in the process of applying the medication to Mrs. Roman.

Case 2

Mrs. Gupta, age 55, has had a total hysterectomy. She has an intravenous drip of normal saline infusing at 100 mL/hr.

Questions 7–12 refer to this case.

7. Mrs. Gupta has just returned from surgery. Her vital signs are blood pressure 88/60, pulse 74, respiratory rate 16, and oxygen saturation 95%. What is the first priority for the practical nurse after taking these vital signs?

1. Ask Mrs. Gupta how she is feeling and review the health record for baseline vital signs.
2. Call the doctor to report the vital signs.
3. Increase the intravenous rate to 125 mL/hr as Mrs. Gupta is probably dehydrated.
4. Position Mrs. Gupta in a modified Trendelenburg position.

8. After surgery, Mrs. Gupta is started on a clear fluid diet until bowel sounds return. Which of the following foods are permitted on a clear fluid diet?

1. Porridge, broth, apple juice
2. Cream soup, ice cream, orange juice
3. Broth, Popsicles, orange juice
4. Tea, Jell-O, apple juice

9. Postoperatively, Mrs. Gupta develops a paralytic ileus. What is the most likely reason for this postoperative complication?

1. She did not ambulate soon enough after surgery.
2. She should have eaten a full diet after surgery to stimulate peristalsis.
3. She is experiencing the effects of the anaesthetic and the manipulation of the bowel.
4. She did not receive a rectal suppository to stimulate peristalsis on the first day after her surgery.

10. The practical nurse helps Mrs. Gupta wash her legs. She removes the elastic (TED) stockings and notices that one calf is larger than the other. What should the practical nurse do next?

1. Examine the calf carefully and ask Mrs. Gupta if she has any pain.
2. Put the TED stocking back on her leg and elevate her leg.
3. Measure the calf with a tape measure and call the doctor immediately.
4. Wash her leg and ask her to exercise that leg a bit more to reduce the swelling.

11. Mrs. Gupta vomits 600 mL of bile-coloured fluid. After consulting with the physician, the practical nurse inserts a nasogastric tube to decompress the stomach. Which of the following is correct with regard to insertion of a nasogastric tube?

1. Measure from the tip of the nose to the xiphoid process prior to inserting the tube.
2. Have the client swallow as much water as possible during the insertion to close the epiglottis.
3. The placement of the nasogastric tube must be confirmed by radiography.
4. A reliable method of testing the correct placement of the tube is aspirating gastric contents and testing pH.

12. In addition to her primary intravenous (IV), an IV infusion of normal saline with 20 mmol KCl is ordered to replace Mrs. Gupta's nasogastric losses. What is the drop rate for her replacement IV if 640 mL must infuse over the next 8 hours and the drop factor is 15?
    1. 80 mL/hr
    2. 100 mL/hr
    3. 20 gtt/min
    4. 25 gtt/min

Case 3

Ms. Abbey, a 20-year-old malnourished woman, requires surgery for her Crohn's disease. The healthcare team decides to start her on total parenteral nutrition (TPN) prior to surgery. This is the practical nurse's first time caring for a client with TPN.
Questions 13–15 refer to this case.

13. What important nursing consideration does the practical nurse need to know when managing Ms. Abbey's TPN?
    1. All intravascular delivery system components up to the hub are changed weekly to prevent infection.
    2. Serum glucose levels and weights are checked weekly.
    3. TPN requires daily temperatures, as infection is the most common complication of TPN.
    4. Speeding up or slowing the infusion rate is contraindicated.
14. Ms. Abbey has a fever of 39°C. The practical nurse gives her an antipyretic and notifies the physician. What orders might the practical nurse anticipate?
    1. Isolate the client for possible septicemia.
    2. Collect blood, urine, and sputum cultures to isolate the cause of infection.
    3. Hold the TPN until blood cultures are clear of pathogens.
    4. Run dextrose 10% via the central line until the cause of the infection is discovered.
15. Ms. Abbey's dressing for her subclavian central line is changed using strict aseptic technique to prevent infection. Which of the following actions by the practical nurse would compromise the principles of surgical asepsis during this dressing change?
    1. The normal saline cap drops onto the floor after the nurse pours the saline onto her tray.
    2. The practical nurse discards the disposable gloves used to remove the old dressing prior to opening her sterile tray.
    3. The practical nurse uses a hand sanitizer for 15 seconds prior to starting the dressing change.
    4. The normal saline was opened previously, and there is no date and time on it.

Case 4

Mr. Roustas, 42 years old, has a spinal cord injury. He is isolated for a methicillin-resistant *Staphylococcus aureus* (MRSA) infection of a decubitus (injury) on his coccyx. He had the pressure injury on admission to the hospital but acquired the infection postadmission. He is in a private room. The sign on his door says "Isolation Precautions."

Questions 16–19 refer to this case.

16. Mr. Roustas has a healthcare–associated infection (HAI, or nosocomial infection). Which of the following would be the most significant factor in his susceptibility to HAI?
    1. Administration of antibiotics
    2. Diagnosis of spinal cord injury
    3. Age
    4. Skin breakdown
17. The practical nurse wears a mask, a gown, and gloves when caring for Mr. Roustas. What is the principal mode of transmission of an antibiotic-resistant organism such as MRSA?
    1. A colonized or infected healthcare worker
    2. Transfer from client to client on the hands of hospital personnel
    3. Environmental contamination
    4. Droplet transmission
18. Mr. Roustas is receiving vancomycin (Vancocin) intravenously for his wound infection. The practical nurse observes redness around the intravenous site, and Mr. Roustas is complaining that the site is painful. What corrective action should the practical nurse take?
    1. Slow the rate of infusion.
    2. Change the site of the infusion.
    3. Notify the physician.
    4. Stop the infusion for at least 24 hours.
19. Mr. Roustas has his pressure injury debrided by the skin care nurse. His dressing is changed daily after debridement. The practical nurse irrigates the wound with normal saline and packs it with saline-soaked gauze to promote moist, interactive wound healing. What is the benefit of moist, interactive wound healing?
    1. It can be used with iodine, which is an effective antimicrobial agent.
    2. It promotes faster healing and better tissue quality.
    3. It requires fewer supplies and equipment.
    4. There is less incidence of bacterial invasion of the wound.

Independent Questions

Questions 20–40 do not refer to a particular case.

20. A practical nurse enters a client's room and finds the client having laboured, dyspneic breathing with audible wheezes. The client appears very anxious and restless. On auscultating her chest, the practical nurse hears crackles in both lower lobes of the lungs posteriorly. What initial actions should the practical nurse take in this situation?
    1. Chart her findings and report to the nurse team leader.
    2. Encourage the client to deep breathe and cough.
    3. Elevate the head of the bed and administer oxygen.
    4. Go to the nurses' station and call the physician.
21. A postoperative client reports sensations of prickling and itchiness around his abdominal incision site after the initial dressing change. How should the practical nurse proceed?
    1. Administer the client analgesia for the prickling and itchiness sensation.

2. Remove the dressing and assess the skin area around the incision.

3. Inform the client that this is a normal sensation to feel after the surgery.

4. Notify the doctor of his complaints of prickling and itchiness around the incision.

22. What is the most effective method for the practical nurse to validate the effectiveness of pain relief with most clients?

    1. Ask clients to rate their pain verbally from mild to severe.

    2. Monitor their facial expressions before and after administration of analgesics.

    3. Monitor their vital signs in response to analgesics given.

    4. Ask clients to rate pain using a numeric rating scale before and after analgesics.

23. A community practical nurse is training a family member to care for her 92-year-old mother who has diabetes. What should the practical nurse teach the family member about foot care for her mother?

    1. Soak both feet daily for less than 15 minutes.

    2. File the mother's toenails straight across and square.

    3. Inspect the mother's feet at least twice a month for problems.

    4. Keep the mother's feet warm with heavy socks and a hot water bottle.

24. How does the practical nurse know when to suction a client with a tracheostomy tube?

    1. The client is coughing up copious amounts of sputum from the tracheostomy.

    2. The client tells the practical nurse when suctioning is necessary.

    3. The doctor specifies how often to suction in the orders.

    4. The practical nurse bases her decision on assessment data heard on lung auscultation.

25. Mrs. DeLuca, 34 years old, gave birth to her third child 6 hours ago and would like to be discharged. She has not urinated since the birth. On palpation, the practical nurse determines a full bladder, and the bladder scanner indicates 1 000 mL of urine in her bladder. What should the practical nurse do?

    1. Have her sit in a warm bath to see if she can void in the bathtub.

    2. Insert an intermittent catheter and drain the bladder.

    3. Let her go home, as Mrs. DeLuca feels she will be able to void in the privacy of her own home.

    4. Insert an in-dwelling catheter for 24 hours so that her bladder will remain empty and her uterus will involute normally.

26. A nursing instructor is teaching her first-year practical nursing students the difference between medical and surgical asepsis. Which of the following would the teacher use as an example of medical asepsis?

    1. Inserting a urinary catheter for postoperative urinary retention

    2. Changing an abdominal dressing for the first time after surgery

    3. Cleaning the hospital environment and equipment routinely

    4. Giving an intramuscular injection in the ventrogluteal region

27. A practical nurse finds a client who has fallen in his room and is bleeding from a head injury to the temporal region of the forehead. Why does the practical nurse put on personal protective equipment (PPE)?

    1. To reduce his exposure to bloodborne microorganisms

    2. To prevent the client from acquiring a healthcare–associated infection

    3. To protect himself from potentially infectious substances

    4. To protect both himself and his client

28. Omotayo, 1 month old, is receiving ampicillin (Ampicin) every 6 hours. The hospital formulary indicates that a safe dose is 200–400 mg/kg/day. What is the recommended dosage range for Omotayo, who weighs 11 pounds?

    1. 11 000–44 000 mg/day

    2. 1 100–4 400 mg/day

    3. 1 000–2 000 mg/day

    4. 1 000–2 000 mg/dose

29. Which of the following is correct regarding subcutaneous injections?

    1. Hold the skin taut at the site of the injection to compress the subcutaneous tissue.

    2. All subcutaneous injection sites can be massaged, with the exception of those for insulin.

    3. Best practice is not to aspirate for all subcutaneous injections, except for heparin.

    4. Aspiration is not necessary, as it is rare to inject into a blood vessel.

30. Mr. Valencia, 83 years old, is confused after his hip-replacement surgery and has been trying to get out of bed when the family is not present. His family wants him to be restrained so he does not injure himself. What should the practical nurse explain to the family?

    1. "Restraining your father will only make him more agitated."

    2. "We do not restrain clients anymore, as it is against the law."

    3. "Would it be possible to have a family member stay with him until he is less confused?"

    4. "Would you like me to call the doctor to get an order for restraints for your father?"

31. Mrs. Parsons has stomatitis as a result of recent chemotherapy. The practical nurse knows that Mrs. Parsons understands the oral hygiene instructions given by the practical nurse when she makes which of the following comments?

    1. "I don't brush my teeth every day, but when I do, I use my ordinary toothbrush."

    2. "I use diluted Listerine mouthwash every 4 hours. It stings, so I know it is working."

3. "Rinsing my mouth with normal saline every 2 hours has helped me tremendously."

4. "I never need analgesics. If my mouth is too painful, I just do not brush or rinse for a day or two and the pain passes."

32. Mr. Pelletier returns from surgery with chest tubes in place. What should the practical nurse say to Mr. Pelletier concerning his chest tubes?
    1. "You have chest tubes to remove abnormal accumulations of fluid from inside your lungs."
    2. "You need to turn in bed frequently to promote drainage from the pleural space and improve lung expansion."
    3. "Your chest tubes will be clamped every time you get out of bed to prevent a leak from developing in the drainage system."
    4. "The chest tube drainage system should remain at the level of the chest at all times."

33. Mr. Singh requires a blood transfusion. Which of the following statements is correct about blood administration?
    1. The practical nurse stays with the client for the first 5 minutes, as this is when reactions are most likely to occur.
    2. Two registered nurses or a registered nurse and a practical nurse are required to check the client's blood bag, chart, and ID band prior to administration of the blood product.
    3. Vital signs must be checked before and after blood administration and during administration if there are any untoward reactions.
    4. Signs of a febrile reaction are hives, wheezing, pruritus, and joint pain.

34. A practical nurse works in a long-term care facility. In a rush to complete the 1000 hour medications, the practical nurse gives Mr. Smith the wrong medication. What is the practical nurse's first responsibility?
    1. Disclose the incident to Mr. Smith and his family.
    2. Inform the unit manager and prescriber of the medication error.
    3. Complete an incident report for the agency about the details of the incident.
    4. Assess Mr. Smith to ensure that he is not in immediate danger.

35. What are the responsibilities of a practical nurse who is caring for a client in wrist restraints?
    1. Remove the restraints and arrange for a paid sitter as soon as possible.
    2. Make sure that the restraints are tied tightly and secured with a knot.
    3. Check skin integrity, pulses, colour, and sensation of the restrained part as often as every 1–2 hours.
    4. Ensure that the physician reorders the wrist restraints on a weekly basis.

36. A practical nurse working in a community clinic sees many older clients. Which of the following facts does the practical nurse need to be aware of when treating older clients?

1. Normal temperature for an older adult is 36.5°C orally.
2. The older adult might have an advanced infection before it is identified.
3. The older adult has increased sensitivity to pain sensation.
4. The constipation common in older clients is primarily due to polypharmacy.

37. Mr. and Mrs. McNamara ask the practical nurse for advice about caring for their 24-year-old son, who has been newly diagnosed with a seizure disorder. What will the practical nurse teach them about care of their son during a seizure?
    1. Restrain him gently until the seizure passes.
    2. Use a padded tongue blade to prevent damage to his tongue during the seizure.
    3. Put him in a side-lying position as soon as the seizure starts.
    4. Loosen restrictive clothing and clear the area of hazards and articles that might harm him.

38. Mrs. Hathaway, age 98 years, is admitted to an acute care hospital from a long-term care facility. The practical nurse documents the Braden Scale score on her chart shortly after she arrives on the unit. What is the main purpose of the Braden Scale?
    1. To identify clients at risk for pressure injury early
    2. To identify interventions that can be implemented to treat pressure injuries
    3. To measure friction- and shear-related skin problems on admission to the hospital
    4. To identify preventive measures to reduce the incidence of pressure injuries

39. Mr. Ciavallo, age 57 years, has been diagnosed with lung cancer and is scheduled for resection of his right lung tomorrow. What will the practical nurse teach him about what to expect with his postoperative care?
    1. "You will have incentive spirometry at least four times daily to prevent atelectasis."
    2. "Leg exercises will be carried out every 2 hours while you are awake."
    3. "Vigorous coughing will be necessary to expectorate excess sputum."
    4. "There will be a right-sided chest tube, and you will be on bed rest until it is removed."

40. Mrs. Lin, age 45 years, has end-stage breast cancer with metastases to her lungs and brain. Her family and the palliative care team are caring for her at home. Which of the following best describes palliative care for Mrs. Lin?
    1. Mrs. Lin will be kept comfortable and free from pain.
    2. Enteral feeds will be started to prevent starvation and malnutrition.
    3. Interventions will be focused only on the needs of Mrs. Lin.
    4. Services by the team terminate at the death of Mrs. Lin.

REFERENCES

Canadian Committee on Antibiotic Resistance. (2007). *Infection prevention and control best practices for long term care, home and community care including health care offices and ambulatory clinics.* Vancouver: Author. Retrieved from http://www.ccar-ccra.com/english/pdfs/IPC-BestPractices-June2007.pdf.

Centers for Disease Control and Prevention. (2006). Management of multidrug-resistant organisms in healthcare settings. Retrieved from https://www.cdc.gov/infectioncontrol/guidelines/mdro/background.html.

Centers for Disease Control and Prevention. (2016). The National Institute for Occupational Safety and Health (NIOSH): MRSA and the workplace. Retrieved from https://www.cdc.gov/niosh/topics/mrsa/.

Centers for Disease Control and Prevention. (2017). The National Institute for Occupational Safety and Health (NIOSH): Safe patient handling and mobility. Retrieved from https://www.cdc.gov/niosh/topics/safepatient/default.html.

Duckro, A. N., Blom, D. W., Lyle, E. A., et al. (2005). Transfer of vancomycin-resistant *enterococci* via health care worker hands. *Archives of Internal Medicine, 165*(3), 302–307.

Government of Canada. (2016). Palliative care. Retrieved from https://www.canada.ca/en/health-canada/services/palliative-care.html.

Health Canada. (2011). *Eating well with Canada's food guide.* Ottawa: Author. Retrieved from http://www.hc-sc.gc.ca/fn-an/food-guide-aliment/index_e.html.

Hockenberry, M., & Wilson, D. (2015). *Wong's nursing care of infants and children* (10th ed.). St. Louis: Elsevier/Mosby.

Hypertension Canada. (2017). Measuring blood pressure. Retrieved from http://guidelines.hypertension.ca/diagnosis-assessment/measuring-blood-pressure/.

Ignatavicius, D. D., Workman, M. L., & Rebar, C. (2018). *Medical-surgical nursing: Concepts for interprofessional collaborative care* (9th ed.). St. Louis: Elsevier.

Institute for Safe Medication Practices. (2017a). High-alert medications in long-term Care (LTC) settings. Retrieved from https://www.ismp.org/recommendations/high-alert-medications-long-term-care-list.

Institute for Safe Medication Practices. (2017b). List of error-prone abbreviations. Retrieved from https://www.ismp.org/recommendations/error-prone-abbreviations-list.

International Association for the Study of Pain. (2017). IASP terminology. Retrieved from http://www.iasp-pain.org/Education/Content.aspx?ItemNumber=1698.

Jarvis, C., Browne, A. J., MacDonald-Jenkins, J., et al. (2019). *Physical examination and health assessment* (3rd Cdn. ed.). Toronto: Saunders/Elsevier.

Lewis, S. L., Bucher, L., Heitkemper, M. M., et al. (2014). *Medical-surgical nursing in Canada: Assessment and management of clinical problems* (3rd ed.). Toronto: Elsevier/Mosby.

Lewis, S. M., Bucher, L., Heitkemper, M. M., et al. (2019). *Medical-surgical nursing in Canada: Assessment and management of clinical problems* (4th Cdn. ed.). Milton, ON: Elsevier.

Mosby. (2013). *Mosby's dictionary of medicine, nursing, and health professions* (9th ed.). St. Louis: Elsevier/Mosby.

National Pressure Ulcer Advisory Panel. (2016). NPUAP announces a change in terminology from pressure ulcer to pressure injury and updates the stages of pressure injury [Press release]. Retrieved from http://www.npuap.org/national-pressure-ulcer-advisory-panel-npuap-announces-a-change-in-terminology-from-pressure-ulcer-to-pressure-injury-and-updates-the-stages-of-pressure-injury/.

Ontario Agency for Health Protection and Promotion (Public Health Ontario), Provincial Infectious Diseases Advisory Committee. (2014). *Best practices for hand hygiene in all health care settings* (4th ed.). Toronto: Queen's Printer for Ontario. Retrieved from http://www.publichealthontario.ca/en/eRepository/2010-12%20BP%20Hand%20Hygiene.pdf.

Perry, A. G., Potter, P. A., & Ostendorf, W. (2018). *Clinical nursing skills and techniques* (9th ed.). St. Louis: Mosby.

Potter, P. A., Perry, A. G., Ross-Kerr, J. C., et al. (2014). *Canadian fundamentals of nursing* (5th ed.). Toronto: Elsevier/Mosby.

Potter, P., Perry, A., Stockert, P., et al. (2019). *Canadian fundamentals of nursing* (6th ed.). Milton, ON: Elsevier.

Registered Nurses' Association of Ontario. (2004). *Nursing best practice guideline: Assessment and device selection for vascular access* (includes revised 2008 supplement). Toronto: Author. Retrieved from http://rnao.ca/sites/rnao-ca/files/Assessment_and_Device_Selection_for_Vascular_Access.pdf.

Registered Nurses' Association of Ontario. (2005). *Nursing best practice guideline: Promoting continence using prompted voiding* (includes revised 2011 supplement). Toronto: Author. Retrieved from http://rnao.ca/sites/rnao-ca/files/Promoting_Continence_Using_Prompted_Voiding.pdf.

Registered Nurses' Association of Ontario. (2013). *Clinical best practice guidelines: assessment and management of pain* (3rd ed., p. 34). Toronto: Author. Retrieved from https://rnao.ca/sites/rnao-ca/files/AssessAndManagementOfPain2014.pdf.

Williams, P. (2018). *Dewit's fundamental concepts and skills for nursing* (5th ed.). St. Louis: Elsevier.

World Health Organization. (2012). *Pharmacological treatment of persisting pain in children with medical illnesses.* Geneva, Switzerland: Author. Retrieved from http://apps.who.int/iris/bitstream/10665/44540/1/9789241548120_Guidelines.pdf.

BIBLIOGRAPHY

College of Nurses of Ontario. (2017). *Practice standard: Medication.* Toronto: Author. Retrieved from http://www.cno.org/globalassets/docs/prac/41007_medication.pdf.

National Pressure Ulcer Advisory Panel. (2016). Pressure injury prevention points. Retrieved from http://www.npuap.org/wp-content/uploads/2016/04/Pressure-Injury-Prevention-Points-.

Registered Nurses' Association of Ontario. (2005). *Nursing best practice guideline: Care and maintenance to reduce vascular access complications* (includes revised 2008 supplement). Toronto: Author. Retrieved from http://rnao.ca/sites/rnao-ca/files/Care_and_Maintenance_to_Reduce_Vascular_Access_Complications.pdf.

Registered Nurses' Association of Ontario. (2005). *Nursing best practice guideline: Prevention of constipation in the older adult population* (includes revised 2011 supplement). Toronto: Author. Retrieved from http://rnao.ca/sites/rnao-ca/files/Prevention_of_Constipation_in_the_Older_Adult_Population.pdf.

Registered Nurses' Association of Ontario. (2005). *Nursing best practice guideline: Risk assessment and prevention of pressure ulcers* (includes revised 2011 supplement). Retrieved from http://rnao.ca/sites/rnao-ca/files/Risk_Assessment_and_Prevention_of_Pressure_Ulcers.pdf.

Registered Nurses' Association of Ontario. (2016). *Clinical best practice guidelines: Assessment and management of pressure injuries for the interprofessional team* (3rd ed.). Toronto: Author. Retrieved from http://rnao.ca/sites/rnao-ca/files/PI_BPG_FINAL_WEB_June_10_2016.pdf.

WEB SITES

- **Guidelines for Licensed Practical Nurses in Nova Scotia: The Professional Practice Series: Medication Administration (2013)** (http://www.clpnns.ca/wp-content/uploads/2013/04/Medication-Administration-Final1.pdf): This site provides practice guidelines for safe medication administration from the College of Licensed Practical Nurses of Nova Scotia (CLPNNS). The guidelines outline the licensed practical nurse's accountability in specific practice contexts. They reflect relevant legislation and are designed to help licensed practical nurses understand their responsibilities and legal obligations so that they can make safe and ethical nursing decisions.

- **Institute for Safe Medication Practices Canada** (http://www.ismp-canada.org): This site provides information and research about common medication errors, factors that can potentially lead to medication errors, and methods by which to mitigate these factors.

- **Public Health Ontario: Just Clean Your Hands** (http://www.publichealthontario.ca/en/BrowseByTopic/InfectiousDiseases/JustCleanYourHands/Pages/Just-Clean-Your-Hands.aspx): This site provides information on hand hygiene. It reviews clinical situations in which hand hygiene is important and links to other educational resources on this subject.

- **Public Health Ontario: Infection Prevention and Control (On-line Learning)** (https://www.publichealthontario.ca/en/LearningAndDevelopment/OnlineLearning/InfectiousDiseases/Pages/default.aspx): This site provides information and on-line learning modules on infection prevention and control for health care providers.

Pharmacology and Nursing Practice

A major component within the scope of practice of practical nurses practising in Canada is the administration of medications and the care of clients receiving those medications. There is a legal responsibility on the part of the practical nurse to ensure a sound knowledge base of pharmacology. Practical nurses must master the physical skill of administering medications to their clients. They are also responsible for the specific nursing interventions required in the administration of medications.

The nursing implications relating to the administration of medications are derived from a thorough understanding of the medications being administered and their actions, effects, side effects (both desirable and undesirable), contraindications, and normal dosage ranges. Only by being aware of the nature of medications, by making the appropriate assessments, and by initiating the appropriate actions prior to, during, and after the administration of medications can the practical nurse exercise professional responsibility and ensure the safe care of the client.

PHARMACOLOGY

Pharmacology is the study of drugs (chemicals) and how they affect living cells, the nature of those drugs, their biological activity on living cells, and their fate once they are absorbed into the body.

Sources of Drugs

There are many sources of drugs that are natural or synthetic products or a combination of both. Some of these sources are as follows:
- Plants (e.g., heroin and digitalis)
- Soil (e.g., Kaopectate, which includes clay)
- Animals (e.g., insulin and conjugated estrogen [Premarin])
- Minerals (e.g., iron)
- Synthesis in a laboratory provides better standardization of chemical characteristics: more consistency of effects and a reduction in the potential for allergic reactions
- Semisynthesis—Naturally occurring substances are chemically modified to produce a drug (includes many antibiotics and some human insulins)
- Biotechnology—Drugs are produced through the manipulation of DNA and RNA and cloning (includes human insulin such as Humulin and Novolin and hepatitis B vaccine).

Routes of Administration of Medications

The route of administration depends on the characteristics of the drug, the characteristics of the client, and the desired responses. The route also affects the action, absorption, and distribution of drugs.

See Table 7.1 for a comparison of different drug routes and absorption times.

Naming of Drugs
Chemical Name

This name describes the specific molecular structure and chemical composition of a drug and is used mainly by researchers (e.g., 6-chloro-3,4-dihydro-2H-1,2,4-benzothiadiazine-7-sulfonamide 1,1-dioxide).

Generic (Nonproprietary) Name

The generic name is the one commonly used by health professionals that is created when a drug is ready to be marketed, for example, hydrochlorothiazide.

Brand/Trade (Proprietary or Trademark) Name

This name is owned by the manufacturer and can be created as soon as a generic name has been approved. The choice of name is motivated by marketing considerations (e.g., HydroDIURIL).

Combination drugs. These are drugs made up of a combination of two or more active drugs in a single tablet with complementary modes of action. They provide an additive, therapeutic effect with the possibility of decreasing side effects and increasing client adherence, and they reduce the number of prescriptions and administrative costs. For example, atorvastatin–amlodipine is a combination of two drugs, an anticholesterolemic and an antihypertensive agent, and treats two different major risk factors for coronary heart disease.

CANADIAN DRUG LEGISLATION
Food and Drugs Act, 1985

Health Canada administers the *Food and Drugs Act*. In the act, a *drug* is defined as any substance or mixture of substances manufactured, sold, or represented for use in
(a) the diagnosis, treatment, mitigation, or prevention of disease, disorder, or abnormal physical state, or its symptoms, in human beings or animals,

TABLE 7.1 Drug Administration Routes and Absorption Rates

Drug Administration Route	Absorption Rate
1. Intravenous (IV)	• It has the most rapid and effective absorption and action.
2. Intramuscular (IM)	• Certain preparations can produce drug action in a few minutes, and others have a slower action.
3. Subcutaneous (SC)	• It is slower than IM, but faster than oral.
4. Oral (PO)	• Absorption action is slower than the injectable routes that bypass the digestive system. • Drugs with the fastest absorption rates are liquids, elixirs, and syrups. • Drugs with the slowest absorption rates include enteric-coated tablets. • Drugs undergo "first-pass" effects.
5. Topical (Top) (skin and mucous membranes)	• Absorption and action vary according to drug form and application site. • It is the slowest route of absorption for systemic applications compared with other parenteral routes.

(b) restoring, correcting, or modifying organic functions in human beings or animals, or

(c) disinfection in premises in which food is manufactured, prepared, or kept.

The purpose of the law is to

- Govern the distribution and use of drugs in Canada
- Protect the consumer from unsafe drugs
- Investigate discrepancies
- Monitor the advertising and sale of drugs for treatment, prevention, and cure
- Divide drugs into specific categories, depending on the classification of the drug

Controlled Drugs and Substances Act, 1996

The *Controlled Drugs and Substances Act* (CDSA) outlines the legal control of addictive and habituating drugs and provides extensive regulation and control over their possession, manufacture, sale, and distribution. Controlled substances require a specific type of prescribing and more stringent recording and record keeping.

The Government of Canada's (2015) Drug Product Database assigns drugs to one or more of the following schedules, based on the *Food and Drug Regulations*, and the CDSA:

- Prescription (prescription drugs included in the Prescription Drug List)
- Prescription Recommended (drugs that are recommended to be listed on the Prescription Drug List)
- Schedule G (control drugs)
- Schedule G (*Controlled Drugs and Substances Act* [CDSA] III)
- Schedule G (CDSA IV)

- Schedule C (drugs listed in Schedule C of the *Food and Drugs Act*, for example, radiopharmaceutical drugs)
- Schedule D (drugs listed in Schedule D of the *Food and Drugs Act*, i.e., biological products)
- Narcotic (*Narcotic Control Act*)
- Narcotic (CDSA I)
- Narcotic (CDSA II)
- Targeted (CDSA IV)
- CDSA Recommended—Undergoing Regulatory Amendment to add this new substance to Controlled Drugs Substances Act
- OTC (over-the-counter drugs that do not appear on a schedule or are not recommended to appear on any schedule)
- Ethical: a drug that, in accordance with Federal Legislation, does not require a prescription, but that is generally prescribed by a medical practitioner. Ethical products are unscheduled nonprescription professional use products (e.g., hemodialysis solutions) and a few emergency use products (e.g., nitroglycerine)

PHARMACODYNAMICS

The term *pharmacodynamics* describes the action of drugs on target cells and the changes that occur in body fluids as a result of the action of these drugs. The pharmacological effects of a drug on the body can be described as the local or systemic therapeutic effects, or both, as well as any side effects and any toxic effects.

Types of Action

Most drugs combine with receptor sites on cells and are characterized by their mechanism of action upon those cells:

- Agonist—A drug that binds to a receptor, producing a biochemical response
- Antagonist—A drug that binds to a receptor, preventing an agonist from binding to that receptor, which results in no agonist biochemical response

Factors That Affect Drug Action

- Drug dosage
- Route of administration
- Individual characteristics (age, gender, race or ethnicity, pathological condition)
- Drug–diet interaction
- Drug interactions
- Use of herbal and dietary supplements
- Genetic makeup

Drug Interactions

- Potentiation (synergism): There is interaction between two drugs with the result that the overall effect is greater than if the drugs are given separately.
- Displacement: The effects of one drug are increased when its normal binding site on plasma protein within the blood is inhibited by another drug, thereby promoting more immediate action of the first drug.

• Antidotal effect: The toxic effects of one drug are reduced by a second drug that takes up the receptor sites of the first drug, thereby preventing a biochemical response.

Nonpharmacological Effects of a Drug on the Body

• Allergic reaction: An undesirable reaction to a drug (of protein origin) that is regarded by the body as an allergen; occurs after the second or subsequent dose of the drug
• Anaphylaxis: A severe, acute, systemic reaction to an allergen, causing massive vasodilation, dyspnea, and shock and requiring immediate emergency care
• Idiosyncratic reaction: An unexpected response to a drug by a specific client; commonly the result of genetic factors that cause the client to respond differently
• Teratogenic reaction: A reaction to a drug that may produce congenital defects if taken by a woman who is pregnant, such as thalidomide, which produced deformed limbs
• Drug tolerance: Resistance of the body to the action of a drug as a result of adaptation as a result of overuse; higher dosages are required in order to produce the desired effects
• Physical dependence: Dependence on a drug resulting in the body requiring a continuous supply in order to function normally; undesirable physical manifestations result if the drug is withdrawn
• Psychological dependence: A psychological dependence on the drug, where there is an overwhelming and uncontrollable desire for the drug that forces continued usage

PHARMACOKINETICS

Pharmacokinetics refers to how the body manages a drug: its absorption, distribution, metabolism (biotransformation), and excretion.

Absorption

Absorption is the process that occurs from the time a drug enters the body until the time it enters the bloodstream. Factors that affect the absorption of a drug include the following:

• Size of the drug molecules
• Properties of the drug (such as lipophilic)
• Environmental temperature
• Membrane thickness
• Surface area of body
• Blood supply at absorption site
• Route of administration
• Presence of food or other drugs in the gastro-intestinal (GI) tract
• Drug formulation (such as enteric or slow release)
• Bioavailability—How much of the drug actually enters the bloodstream to exert its effects on body cells; the route of administration is a major determinant
• Presence of disease

Distribution

Distribution is the transport of drug molecules within the body. Factors that affect the distribution of a drug include the following:

• Blood circulation
• Plasma protein binding (drug inactivated temporarily while bound to the protein)
• Anatomical barrier (such as the blood–brain or blood–placental barrier)
• Presence of disease (such as peripheral vascular disease)
• Lipid solubility
• Storage in body tissues (the drug is inactive while in the storage site, such as in adipose tissue)

Metabolism

An individual's metabolism determines how drugs are biotransformed by the body into simple, active, or inactive metabolites. For example:

• Lipid-soluble drugs are converted to water-soluble forms to be excreted by the kidney, which is achieved by enzyme systems in the liver, kidney, lungs, GI tract, red blood cells, and plasma mucosa.
• Toxic waste products can be produced if biotransformation is extremely rapid.
• Slow biotransformations result in lower drug dosages to cells.
• Factors that affect biotransformation include the following:
  • Immaturity of organs (infants)
  • Degeneration of organs (older adults)
  • Reduced circulation
  • A diet low in protein
  • Drugs that antagonized enzyme action
  • Disease (cirrhosis of liver)
  • Genetic factors

Excretion

• Elimination of a drug from the body
• Requires an adequately functioning cardiovascular system, kidneys, GI tract, lungs, and skin
• Prior to administering drugs, an assessment of adequate organ functioning needs to be made

DRUGS THAT AFFECT THE CENTRAL NERVOUS SYSTEM

Numerous classifications of drugs affect the nervous system. In general, there are two actions a drug can exert on the nervous system—stimulation or depression. Fig. 7.1 shows the drug classifications and their therapeutic actions and effects on either the central nervous system (CNS) or the autonomic nervous system (ANS).

Analgesic Agents

Analgesics are used to relieve pain without causing loss of consciousness. There are two classifications of analgesics: opioids, prescribed for the treatment of severe pain, and

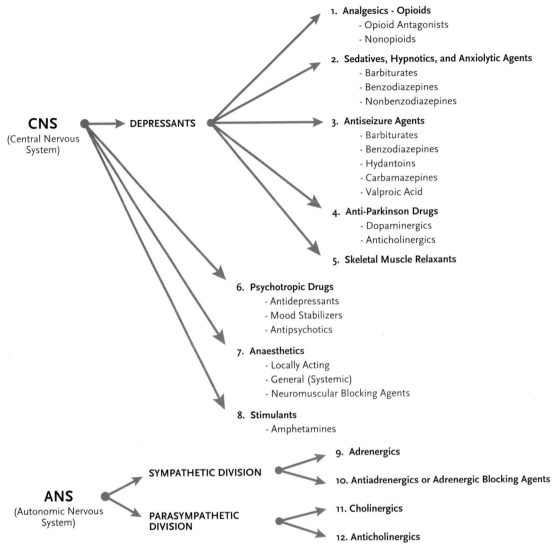

Fig. 7.1 Drugs that affect the nervous system.

nonopiate preparations, used for milder or more moderate pain. Many nonopioid preparations have both antipyretic and anti-inflammatory effects. The choice of analgesic will depend on the effectiveness of an agent, the route of administration to be used, the duration of action of the drug, the duration of the therapy, potential drug interactions (particularly if the client is receiving other depressant medications), and hypersensitivities that the client may have.

Although opioid analgesics are primarily prescribed for the treatment of pain, other therapeutic uses of specific types of opioid analgesics, such as codeine, include treatment to suppress a dry cough and severe diarrhea.

Opioid Analgesics

These are morphinelike substances that may be natural, derived from opium, or synthesized in the laboratory. These substances:

- Are controlled under the CDSA
- Are associated with a high risk of dependence

- Are prescribed for treatment of moderate to severe pain, such as pain originating from visceral sources, such as surgery, myocardial infarction (MI), colic, and cancer pain
- Inhibit the release of substance P in the central and peripheral nerves, resulting in interference with the transmission of sensory nerve impulses to the brain from peripheral tissues
- Enhance the release of naturally occurring opioid-type chemicals within the body (enkephalin, dynorphins, and endorphins)
- Include effects such as the suppression of the CNS, preventing the sensation of pain within the CNS (the substantia gelatinosa, spinal cord, brainstem, reticular formation, thalamus, and limbic system)
- Modify the perception of pain
- Include additional actions and effects of opioids, such as the following:
  - Suppression of the cough reflex
  - Suppression of GI motility
  - Stimulation of the vomiting centre

TABLE 7.2 **Common Opioid Analgesics**	
Opioid Analgesics	**Routes of Administration**
Morphine sulphate	PO, IM, epidural, intrathecal, IV
Codeine phosphate	PO, IM, SC
Fentanyl (Duragesic)	IM, IV, transdermal
Hydromorphone (Dilaudid)	IM, SC, IV, SUPP
Meperidine (Demerol)	IM, IV, SC, PO
Methadone (Metadol)	PO (not recommended for children)
Oxycodone (Oxyneo, others)	PO (not recommended for children under 12)
Tramadol and acetaminophen (Tramacet)	PO (not recommended for children)

IM, intramuscular; *IV*, intravenous; *PO*, by mouth; *SC*, subcutaneous; *SUPP*, suppository.

Common opioid analgesics. Common opioid analgesics are listed in Table 7.2.

Analgesic dosages. It is important to refer to a potency chart to ensure the correct dosage when changing the route of administration of an opioid. For example, 10 mg of morphine sulphate by intramuscular (IM) injection equals 30 mg morphine sulphate orally.

Adverse effects of opioid analgesics.
- Tolerance, physiological and psychological dependence (addiction)
- Nausea, vomiting, and constipation
- CNS depression, which may lead to respiratory depression
- Weakness, sedation
- Euphoria, disorientation, and hallucinations (particularly in older adults)

Contraindications of opioid analgesics.
- Allergy
- Respiratory insufficiency (such as asthma)
- Elevated intracranial pressure
- Pregnancy

Nursing Considerations Relating to Opioid Analgesics

- Assess client need.
- Ask the client about his or her perception of the degree of pain; medication should be administered prior to the pain becoming too severe.
- Assess the client's history of opioid use.
- Check for the time of the last dosage.
- Assess the previous client response and adverse effects; antiemetics may be administered at the same time to avoid nausea and vomiting.
- Assess respiratory rate, depth, and rhythm prior to administration. Withhold the medication and report if respiration is less than 10 breaths per minute and shallow; an opioid blocker may be required.
- Frequently assess the client's vital signs, level of consciousness, alertness, and cognitive ability during therapy.

- Facilitate the effects of the analgesic administered by promoting an environment of rest, relaxation, peace and quiet, and physical comfort.
- Coughing exercises, deep breathing, and frequent moving help maintain normal functioning.
- Maintain careful documentation of administration of opioids, noting frequency. Observe for signs of dependence; opioids require frequent reordering by a physician or prescriber to minimize overuse and abuse.
- Monitor the client's intake and urine output for possible dehydration and urinary retention.
- Monitor bowel sounds and bowel functioning for signs of constipation.
- When educating clients, include knowledge relating to the nature of drug and usage, particularly in home use.
- Due to possible drowsiness, caution clients taking opioids at home to avoid situations requiring rapid reactions, including driving a car, the operation of dangerous machinery, and smoking.
- Advise that care should be taken around the concurrent use of other CNS depressants, such as alcohol.

Agonist–Antagonist Agents

Agonist–antagonist combination drugs are narcotics with a narcotic antagonist added. They have the potency of an agonist but a lower potential for abuse than pure agonists and are commonly used to treat moderate to severe pain in clients with renal colic, burns, and cancer or as preoperative medication. Examples include the following:
- Buprenorphine (Belbuca)
- Butorphanol (PMS-Butorphanol)
- Nalbuphine (Nubain)
- Pentazocine (Talwin)

Adverse effects of agonist–antagonists are similar to those of opioid agonists.

Opioid Antagonists

These drugs block the receptor sites of opioid analgesics or displace opiates occupying receptor sites.
- They act as an antidote to opioid agonists and agonist–antagonists.
- They are used to relieve CNS and respiratory depression caused by an overdose of opioid analgesics.
- Naloxone hydrochloride (Narcan) used in the treatment of opioid overdoses.
- Naltrexone (ReVia) maintains an opiate-free state in clients addicted to opiates.

Nonopioid Analgesics (Antipyretic/Anti-Inflammatory Agents)

These analgesics relieve mild to moderate pain, fever, and the inflammatory response. Common nonopioid analgesics are listed in Table 7.3.

Uses for nonopioid analgesics (antipyretics, non-steroidal anti-inflammatory drugs [NSAIDs]) are as follows:
- Pain associated with muscles, joints, and connective tissue

TABLE 7.3 Common Nonopioid Analgesics

Classification	Action	Therapeutic Effects	Adverse Effects
Acetylsalicylic Acid (e.g., Aspirin)	• Inhibits prostaglandin synthesis by binding to both forms of cyclo-oxygenase (COX-1 and COX-2)	• Mild analgesia • Antipyretic • Anti-inflammatory • Anticoagulant	• Gastro-intestinal irritation • Tinnitus • Allergic reactions • Bleeding • Drowsiness, weakness, and dizziness
Acetaminophen (e.g., Tylenol)	• Inhibits prostaglandin synthesis in central nervous system	• Mild analgesia • Antipyretic	• Liver and renal damage; not recommended for use in severe liver disease • Drowsiness, weakness, and dizziness
Ibuprofen (e.g., Advil, Motrin)	• Inhibits prostaglandin synthesis by binding to both forms of cyclo-oxygenase (COX-1 and COX-2)	• Mild analgesia • Antipyretic • Anti-inflammatory	• Drowsiness, weakness, and dizziness
Celecoxib (e.g., Celebrex)	• Inhibits prostaglandin synthesis by binding cyclo-oxygenase (COX-2)	• Mild analgesia • Antipyretic • Anti-inflammatory	• Allergic reactions • Drowsiness, weakness, and dizziness
Naproxen (e.g., Naprosyn)	• Inhibits prostaglandin synthesis by binding cyclo-oxygenase (COX-2)	• Mild analgesia • Antipyretic • Anti-inflammatory	• Drowsiness, weakness, and dizziness

• Treatment of pain and inflammation associated with osteoarthritis (OA) and rheumatoid arthritis (RA) and rheumatic fever
• Fever
• Dysmenorrheal pain (especially ibuprofen [Advil])
• Headache
Nursing considerations relating to nonopioid analgesics (antipyretics, NSAIDs).
• Monitor clients for bleeding and petechiae (ASA [Aspirin]).
• Administer analgesics with food to reduce gastric irritation.
Advise self-medicating clients:
• Do not to exceed the recommended dosage and frequency.
• Avoid ASA if there is a history of gastric discomfort or bleeding tendency.
• Avoid activities that require alertness (driving) due to the sedating effects.
• Avoid other CNS depressants, such as alcohol.
• Seek medical attention if pain or fever persists for greater than 48–72 hours.

Sedatives, Hypnotics, and Anxiolytics

Classifications of sedatives, hypnotics, and anxiolytics include barbiturates, benzodiazepines, and nonbenzodiazepines. Irrespective of the classification of individual drugs, each has a calming, relaxing effect on the body by depressing CNS activity. Many of these drugs are strongly controlled, requiring a prescription; however, mild-acting drugs may be purchased over the counter (OTC). Certain drugs may be used for sedation and relief of anxiety in low dosages, and in high doses, they would be prescribed to produce sleep.
Sedatives:
• Decrease the functional activity of the brain and response to stimuli without producing sleep

• Produce general CNS depression
• Are used to relax clients prior to procedures and for extreme anxiety
Hypnotics:
• Are used to produce extreme sedation and sleep
• Act on the reticular activation system (RAS) to block the brain's response to incoming stimuli
• Are used to treat insomnia
• May be prescription drugs or OTC
Sedative–hypnotics:
• Produce sedative or hypnotic effects, depending on the dose administered
Anxiolytics:
• Are prescribed to produce relief of anxiety and panic disorder

Classifications of Sedatives, Hypnotics, and Anxiolytics

Benzodiazepines. These drugs act in the limbic and reticular activating systems to make gamma-aminobutyric acid (GABA), an inhibitory neurotransmitter, more effective.
Uses of benzodiazepines:
• To prevent mild to severe anxiety (including panic disorder) and insomnia
• To induce sleep
• For skeletal muscle relaxation
• As preoperative medication
Common benzodiazepines and their uses and dosages are outlined in Table 7.4.
Adverse effects of benzodiazepines:
• Headache
• Drowsiness
• Blurred vision
• Benzodiazepines (contraindicated for pregnancy and lactation and severe respiratory, kidney, or liver disorders)

TABLE 7.4   Common Benzodiazepines

Drug	Normal Dosage	Common Use
Alprazolam (Xanax)	0.25–0.5 mg tid PO	Anxiety and panic attacks
Diazepam (Valium)	2–10 mg bid PO	Mild anxiety
	2–10 mg IM/IV	Muscle relaxant
Flurazepam	15–30 mg at bedtime, PO	Insomnia
Triazolam	125–500 mcg at bedtime, PO	Insomnia
Chlordiazepoxide HCl	PO/IM/IV 5–25 mg tid/qid	Mild to severe anxiety
Lorazepam (Ativan)	2–6 mg per day PO	Anxiety; sedation
Oxazepam	10–30 mg tid/qid PO	Anxiety

bid, twice a day; *IM*, intramuscular; *IV*, intravenous; *PO*, by mouth; *qid*, four times a day; *tid*, three times a day.

TABLE 7.5   Common Nonbenzodiazepines

Drug	Dosage	Uses
Zolpidem tartrate (Sublinox)	5–10 mg at bedtime, SL	Insomnia
Zoplicone (Imovane)	5–7.5 mg at bedtime, PO	Insomnia
Diphenhydramine (Sleep-Eze)	50 mg at bedtime, PO	Antihistamine, mild hypnotic
Hydroxyzine (Atarax)	25–100 mg tid to qid per day 100 mg, IM	Sedative, anxiolytic
Sertraline (Zoloft)	50 mg daily PO	Anxiety and stress disorder

IM, intramuscular; *PO*, by mouth; *qid*, four times a day; *SL*, sublingual.

Common Nonbenzodiazepine Sedatives, Hypnotics, and Anxiolytics

Common uses and dosages of nonbenzodiazepines are outlined in Table 7.5.

Barbiturates

Barbiturates, derivatives of barbituric acid, act by inhibiting the conduction of nerve impulses within the CNS by promoting the inhibitory activity of GABA. They are less commonly used now for the treatment of anxiety, as sedatives, and for insomnia due to their side effects and strong addictive properties. The benzodiazepines and nonbenzodiazepines are the treatment of choice for these problems.

Barbiturates in common use today are as follows:
- Phenobarbital, a long-acting barbiturate, is used primarily as an anticonvulsant in conjunction with other anticonvulsants.
- Pentobarbital, a short-acting barbiturate, is used primarily as a preoperative sedative.

Nursing Considerations Relating to Sedatives, Hypnotics, and Anxiolytics

- Perform a careful assessment prior to administration, including vital signs, level of consciousness, other drugs being taken, health history, and any allergies.
- Instruct clients to avoid the concurrent use of these drugs with other CNS depressants (including alcohol).
- Take all precautions relating to drowsiness, dizziness, reduced awareness, and loss of coordination.
- Ensure that safety measures due to CNS depression are initiated to reduce the risk of injury.
- Assess clients for adverse effects and observations charted and reported.

- Teach and caution clients at home about the following:
  - The risks of overuse, misuse, and dependence
  - The avoidance of dangerous behaviours, such as smoking
  - That these drugs should be restricted to short-term use only

Antiseizure Agents

Epilepsy is not a single disorder but a collection of conditions characterized by the sudden discharge of excessive electrical energy by brain cells. The goal of therapy is to effectively limit this uncontrolled firing of neurons and to control the spread of impulses. To achieve this goal, each client's treatment is based on the type of seizure he or she experiences.

The choice of drug therapy is dependent on the proper classification of the type of seizure. This classification is based on the client's clinical symptoms and electroencephalographic (EEG) pattern.

Types of Antiseizure Agents

Barbiturates. Barbiturates such as phenobarbital act to inhibit the conduction of nerve impulses within the CNS by promoting the inhibitory activity of GABA. This reduces the abnormal electrical activity within the brain that is causing seizure activity. Phenobarbital is the drug of choice for treating children with tonic–clonic seizures.

Benzodiazepines. Benzodiazepines such as diazepam (Valium) and clonazepam (Rivotril) increase the GABA effect to inhibit neuron firing, thereby reducing abnormal electrical activity.

Hydantoins. The hydantoin class acts on the cell membrane of neurons in the cortex of the brain to stabilize nerve membranes, thus reducing voltage frequency and the spread of electrical discharges. Phenytoin (Dilantin) is the drug of choice for treating adults' tonic–clonic seizures.

Carbamazepines. Carbamazepine (Tegretol), lamotrigine (Lamictal), and gabapentin (Neurontin) increase GABA activity and block sodium and calcium channels, thus reducing the nerve action potential. They are used for tonic–clonic and simple partial seizures.

Valproic acid. Valproic acid (Depakene) increases the GABA effect, resulting in decreased electrical activity. It is used to treat absence, mixed, and complex seizures.

Adverse Effects of Antiseizure Medications

- Epigastric pain
- Nausea and vomiting
- Drowsiness
- Bradycardia
- Hypotension

Nursing Considerations Relating to Antiseizure Medications

- Prior to administration, perform a complete assessment of past and present health history for allergies, drug interactions, adverse effects experienced, and kidney, liver, and heart disease, and take vital signs.
- Teach clients that the drug should be given at the same time each day.
- Advise clients that food should be eaten to avoid GI irritation, nausea, and vomiting.
- Inform clients of possible drowsiness that may occur initially.
- Caution clients to avoid taking antacids at the same time as medication.
- Caution clients about abruptly stopping medication.
- Advise clients to report any undesirable effects immediately.
- Advise clients to avoid other CNS depressants, such as alcohol.
- Perform an assessment of therapeutic blood levels for clients on long-term therapy.
- Perform liver function tests on a regular basis.
- Educate clients about the use of a MedicAlert bracelet as a protective measure.

Anti–Parkinson's Disease Agents

Anti-Parkinson's pharmacotherapy is aimed at increasing or enhancing the action of dopamine in the brain (using dopaminergic agents) and inhibiting the action of acetylcholine (Ach) (with anticholinergic agents) for the purpose of restoring the balance between dopamine and Ach.

Dopaminergic Agents

These drugs increase the effects of dopamine at receptor sites in the substantia nigra. Since dopamine cannot cross the blood–brain barrier, drugs that act like dopamine or increase dopamine concentration are used.

- Levodopa (L-dopa) crosses the blood–brain barrier, where it is converted to dopamine. Large amounts are broken down to dopamine prior to passing through the blood–brain barrier and into the CNS. Levodopa given alone requires a high dosage to produce the desired effects.
- Carbidopa inhibits the breakdown of levodopa outside the CNS, allowing greater amounts of levodopa to enter the CNS. This effect results in a lower dosage requirement. Commonly, a levodopa–carbidopa combination drug is administered.
- Amantadine (Dom-Amantadine) increases dopamine release and blocks the reuptake of dopamine into the presynaptic neuron.
- Selegiline (Apo-Selegiline) decreases the breakdown of dopamine by monoamine oxidase B (MAO-B) inhibitors. (Monoamine oxidase is an enzyme that breaks down neurotransmitters.)
- Entacapone decreases the breakdown of dopamine by COMT (catechol O-methyltransferase, the enzyme that breaks down levodopa).

Adverse effects of dopaminergic agents.

- Nausea and vomiting
- Orthostatic hypotension
- Palpitations
- Dizziness
- Nervousness and agitation
- Muscle irritability

The beneficial effects of dopaminergic drugs are not seen until a few weeks after treatment begins. Vitamin B_6 facilitates the breakdown of levodopa, reducing levels outside the CNS and limiting the amount of dopamine reaching the brain.

Anticholinergic Drugs

These drugs oppose the effect of Ach at the receptor sites in the substantia nigra and corpus striatum, thus helping restore chemical balance in the area. They also help alleviate the tremors and rigidity associated with Parkinson's disease. Examples include benztropine and trihexyphenidyl.

Adverse effects of anticholinergic drugs.

- Drowsiness
- Confusion
- Constipation
- Dry mouth
- Urinary retention
- Pupillary dilation

Nursing Considerations Relating to Anti-Parkinson's Drugs

- Prior to administration, perform an assessment of health history for CNS, GI, and urinary functioning and psychological state, such as swallowing, voiding patterns, constipation, peptic ulcer disease, prostate enlargement, depression, and so on, to identify possible contraindications or cautions.
- Administer following meals and at bedtime with a full glass of water.
- Encourage regular mouth care due to drying effects.
- Advise clients to avoid foods high in vitamin B_6 (such as spinach, bananas, liver, and sweet potato).

- Teach the importance of ingesting foods high in fibre to maintain regular GI functioning and avoid constipation.
- Teach clients that entacapone will produce a brownish discoloration of the urine that is normal.
- Observe for and chart desired and adverse effects experienced by clients.
- Encourage clients to report any undesirable effects that are experienced.

Skeletal Muscle Relaxants

Skeletal muscle relaxants depress the CNS by blocking nerve impulses that cause muscle tone and contraction. The primary use is for the treatment of muscle spasm. The majority of muscle relaxants act on the CNS by depressing the system and indirectly relaxing the muscles. However, a few act directly by depressing the contraction of muscle fibres (such as dantrolene).

- Baclofen (Lioresal) is used to treat the spasticity of multiple sclerosis (MS) and spinal cord injury.
- Dantrolene (Dantrium) inhibits muscle contraction, relieving muscle spasticity and malignant hypertension. (The safety of these drugs for children 12 years and under has not been established.)
- Diazepam (Valium) is used for muscle spasm and inflammation.
- Methocarbamol (Robaxin) is used for muscle spasm and inflammation.

Nursing Considerations Relating to Muscle Relaxants

- Use all safety precautions relating to drugs that produce CNS depression.
- Teach clients about avoiding dangerous activities that require alertness and quick reflexes.

Psychotropic Drugs

Psychotropic drugs are used to treat clients who have lost the ability to cope with the normal activities of daily living due to changes in their mental state. An inability to cope with normal day-to-day functions can be the result of depression, changes in personality and mood, or psychotic behaviour. The three categories of drugs include antidepressants, mood stabilizers, and antipsychotics.

Antidepressants

Depression has no known external cause. It is theorized to be the result of decreased levels of the neurotransmitters norepinephrine (NE), dopamine, or serotonin in key areas of the brain. Older drugs, such as the tricyclic antidepressants (TCAs) and monoamine oxidase inhibitors (MAOIs), as well as newer drugs, such as the selective serotonin reuptake inhibitors (SSRIs), share the following characteristics:

- Relieve depression
- Must be taken for 2–4 weeks before depression symptoms improve
- Can be administered by mouth (PO)
- Are metabolized by cytochrome enzyme P-450 in the liver

Classifications of antidepressants.
Tricyclic antidepressants (TCAs)
- TCAs reduce the uptake of serotonin and NE into nerves by inhibiting the presynaptic uptake; this, in turn, leads to increased levels in the synaptic cleft.
- Adverse effects of TCAs include the following:
  - Sedation
  - Sleep disturbances
  - Fatigue
  - Hallucination
  - Visual disturbances
  - Tremors
  - GI problems
  - Cardiac dysrhythmias
- Examples include imipramine, used to treat depression and childhood enuresis; amitriptyline (Elavil), used to treat depression; and clomipramine (Anafranil), used to treat obsessive–compulsive disorder (OCD).

Monoamine oxidase inhibitors (MAOIs)
- They are rarely prescribed today because of the requirement that clients have a specific diet free of tyramine, which produces drug toxicity.
- Examples are phenelzine (Nardil) and tranylcypromine (Parnate).

Selective serotonin reuptake inhibitors (SSRIs)
- The newest group of antidepressants
- Block the uptake of serotonin with little to no effect on NE; an increase in levels in the synaptic cleft promotes nerve impulse transmission and results in an antidepressant effect
- Examples include the following:
  - Fluoxetine (Prozac)—For treatment of depression, OCD, and bulimia nervosa
  - Fluvoxamine (Luvox)—For depression
  - Paroxetine (Paxil)—For depression, OCD, and generalized anxiety disorder
  - Sertraline (Zoloft)—For depression, OCD, and panic attacks
  - Citalopram (Celexa)—For depression
- Adverse effects of SSRIs include the following:
  - Fewer adverse effects are produced than with TCAs; however, because they bind significantly to plasma protein (with a half-life of 24–72 hours), accumulation within the body can occur when taken over a protracted period.
  - Anxiety
  - Dizziness
  - Seizures
  - GI effects
  - Must be used with caution in children and older adults

Mood Stabilizers

Lithium carbonate and lithium citrate, plus two lithium salts, are available for treatment and prevention of manic episodes. Lithium salts appear to alter sodium transport at nerve endings, inhibiting cyclic adenosine monophosphate (AMP) formation in nerve cells and enhancing the uptake of NE and serotonin by nerve cells.

Lithium is not metabolized by the body and is entirely excreted by the kidneys; therefore, renal function assessment is necessary prior to treatment. Cardiac and thyroid status should also be assessed prior to treatment due to the drug's potential adverse effects on these organs.

Sodium levels can affect the reabsorption of lithium; therefore, electrolyte levels should also be monitored. Lithium has a narrow therapeutic index. Early signs of lithium toxicity include gastrointestinal discomfort, drowsiness, muscle weakness, tremors, unsteadiness, and lack of coordination. Examples of mood stabilizers include:

- Olanzapine (Zyprexa)—Used to treat mania and schizophrenia
- Carbamazepine (Tegretol)—Used to treat bipolar disorder (also an anticonvulsant)
- Valproic acid (Depakene)—Used to treat bipolar disorder (also an anticonvulsant)

Nursing Considerations Relating to Antidepressants or Mood-Stabilizing Drugs

- Do a careful assessment of the client's history of receiving antidepressant drugs.
- Assess for blood dyscrasias (such as leukopenia) and liver functioning.
- Monitor for extrapyramidal symptoms (EPSs) and cardiac dysrhythmias.
- Monitor the behaviour of clients with a history of suicidal attempts.
- Monitor vital signs: blood pressure (BP), pulse, and respiratory rates initially.
  Client teaching points:
- Understand that desirable effects may take several weeks to be established.
- Take the medication as prescribed and avoid missing or doubling dosages.
- Take the medication with food to avoid GI irritation.
- Understand the adverse effects of CNS stimulation.
- Report to a doctor if adverse effects are experienced.
- Do not discontinue prescribed medication independently.
- Avoid taking other CNS-affecting drugs, such as alcohol, coffee, or tobacco.
- Avoid exposure to direct sunlight and use sunscreen and protective clothing.

Antipsychotic Drugs

Neuroleptics or major tranquilizers are antipsychotic drugs. They are designed to bind to dopamine receptors and block the action of dopamine. These drugs are used primarily in the treatment of schizophrenia but may also be used to treat psychotic symptoms brought about by head injury, tumour, stroke, and other disorders.

Phenothiazines. This is the largest group of antipsychotic drugs and includes chlorpromazine (Largactil PO, IM), a prototype drug used in treating adults, older adults, and children.

Major side effects include sedation, extrapyramidal reactions, and moderate to high hypotension.

Thioxanthenes. These drugs cause fewer sedative and hypotensive effects than the phenothiazines but cause extrapyramidal effects. An example is thiothixene (Navane).

Atypical agents.
- These agents block both dopamine and serotonin receptors in the brain and relieve negative and positive symptoms of psychosis.
- Clozapine (Clozaril) is used as a second line of treatment for clients who do not respond well to the typical drugs.
- Risperidone (Risperdal) may be used as the first agent in the management of schizophrenia and inappropriate behaviour associated with dementia.

Nursing Considerations Relating to Antipsychotic Drugs

- Perform an assessment of clients' history of receiving antipsychotic drugs.
- Monitor for EPSs and cardiac dysrhythmias.
- Monitor the behaviour of clients with a history of suicide attempts.
- Monitor vital signs, including BP, pulse, and respiratory rates (e.g., assess for postural hypotension).
- Monitor blood count and liver function.
  Client teaching points:
- Understand that beneficial effects may take several weeks to become evident.
- Take the medication as prescribed and avoid missing or doubling dosages.
- Understand the adverse effects of CNS stimulation.
- Report to a doctor if adverse effects are experienced and not discontinue prescribed medication independently.
- Avoid taking other CNS-affecting drugs, such as alcohol or coffee.
- Wear sunscreen and protective clothing when outdoors or in direct sunlight.
- Take the drugs with food or milk to avoid gastric problems.
- Understand the possible sexual irregularities, such as enlargement of the breasts or menstrual irregularities.

Anaesthetics

Anaesthetics depress the CNS, producing loss of sensation. In the case of a local anaesthetic, the loss of sensation is to a particular area of the body; with a general anaesthetic, the result is loss of consciousness. The overall action of an anaesthetic is suppression of nerve impulse conduction, causing loss of sensation. The primary purpose is to desensitize the client to pain.

Local Anaesthetics

Drugs in this classification are primarily used to eliminate sensation to a specific region to prevent discomfort. Dental surgery commonly uses local anaesthesia. It is also used to alleviate the discomfort of certain hospital procedures, such as the suturing of wounds, the insertion of certain therapeutic devices, and during certain diagnostic procedures. Clients need to be cautioned to protect the anaesthetized area until normal sensation returns to avoid injury or damage. A common local anaesthetic is lidocaine (Xylocaine).

General Anaesthetics

These preparations produce loss of consciousness, skeletal muscle relaxation, and suppression of reflexes. Deep general anaesthetics will depress respirations; thus, the client will require respiratory support. General anaesthetics are used most commonly for the performance of surgical procedures.

Commonly, a combination of anaesthetics is used: an intravenous (IV) short-acting CNS depressant to induce unconsciousness, followed by an anaesthetic gas to maintain unconsciousness for the duration of the surgical procedure. The administration of general anaesthetic drugs is carried out by an anaesthesiologist, who is responsible for the client's normal vital functioning during surgical procedures.

Central Nervous System Stimulants

CNS stimulants are used to enhance nervous system activity. CNS stimulants can elevate mood, decrease perception of fatigue, increase alertness, decrease appetite, and improve motor function. Stimulants may be used improperly to maintain alertness in order to avoid sleep. One stimulant commonly used to maintain general alertness is caffeine. However, some CNS stimulants have the potential to produce tolerance and severe physiological and psychological dependence when used continuously. As a result, many are classified as controlled substances.

The main CNS stimulants in use today are the amphetamines, including dextroamphetamine (Dexedrine), amphetamine sulphate (Adderall XR), and methylphenidate HCl (Ritalin). These agents are prescribed primarily for the treatment of narcolepsy and attention-deficit/hyperactivity disorder (ADHD). They act by increasing the amount of neurotransmitters and dopamine—and possibly serotonin—in the system to promote mood elevation, increase alertness, and prolong wakefulness.

Nursing Considerations Relating to CNS Stimulants

- Perform a careful physical and mental health history, including other medications being taken and any self-medication with herbal remedies, such as ginseng.
- Observe for adverse effects relating to overstimulation of the CNS.
- Check for cardiovascular system effects, mental hyperactivity, and insomnia; report adverse effects immediately to a physician.
- Alert clients to the dangers of overuse and abuse.
- Instruct clients to take only the dosage and frequency prescribed.

DRUGS THAT AFFECT THE AUTONOMIC NERVOUS SYSTEM

The four categories of drugs that affect the functioning of this division of the nervous system can stimulate or suppress the sympathetic and the parasympathetic branches. An easy way to learn the general effects produced by each of the four groups of drugs is to recall the actions of the two systems and the effects they produce on the body. The following drugs will, in general, mimic these effects.

Adrenergic Agonists (Sympathomimetic) Drugs

Drugs belonging to this category stimulate the sympathetic nervous system. Many adrenergic drugs are used as emergency agents for treating cardiac arrest and cardiovascular collapse. Adrenergic agonists can stimulate both alpha adrenergic receptors (alpha agonists) and beta adrenergic receptors (beta agonists) of the ANS. The action of these agonists mimics the actions of the sympathetic nervous system and the neurotransmitters NE and epinephrine, producing varied effects, including increased cardiac contractions, increased heart rate, bronchodilation, decreased gastric motility, decreased intraocular pressure, and pupil dilation.

Vasoactive agents that influence blood vessels.
- Dopamine: Used to treat hypotension and shock
- Epinephrine (adrenaline): Used to treat allergic reactions, cardiac arrest, hypotension and shock, bronchodilation, and cardiac stimulation
- Norepinephrine (Levophed): Used to treat hypotension and shock

Adrenergic agents used to treat asthma and bronchitis. These agents produce bronchodilation:
- Salbutamol (Ventolin)
- Epinephrine (adrenaline)
- Isoproterenol HCl

Adrenergic agents that suppress appetite. Appetite suppressants include dextroamphetamine (Dexedrine).

Adrenergic agents used in treating glaucoma. These agents reduce intraocular pressure and dilate the pupil. They include tetrahydrozoline (Murine, Visine).

Adrenergic agents used as nasal decongestants. A common decongestant is pseudoephedrine (Sudafed).

Adrenergic Blocking Agents (Sympatholytic) Drugs

Adrenergic blocking agents inhibit or block the responses of adrenergic neurotransmitters at alpha and beta adrenergic receptor sites. In general, they block the action of the sympathetic nervous system.

Alpha blockers cause a decrease in BP and are used in treating headaches, hypertension, and peripheral vascular diseases. These agents promote blood flow to vasoconstricted areas. Examples include doxazosin (Cardura) and prazosin (Minipress).

Beta blockers also cause a decrease in BP. These agents decrease the heart rate and force of contraction, which decreases the load on the heart. Examples include the following:
- Propranolol
- Metoprolol
- Atenolol (Tenormin)
- Sotalol
- Timolol (Timoptic)

Cholinergic (Parasympathomimetic) Drugs

In general, cholinergic drugs imitate the parasympathetic nervous system. Cholinergic drugs have limited use. Their primary uses are in the treatment of urinary retention and GI disturbances. Their actions mimic the neurotransmitter Ach. Examples include the following:

- Bethanechol chloride (Duvoid)—Prescribed for the treatment of urinary retention
- Pyridostigmine (Mestinon) and neostigmine (Prostigmin)—Stimulate skeletal muscle contraction and are used in the treatment of myasthenia gravis. (These drugs are indirect-acting cholinergic agonists that react chemically with acetylcholinesterase (Ach-ase) in the synaptic cleft to prevent the breakdown of Ach.)
- Rivastigmine (Exelon)—Alzheimer's disease is associated with decreased Ach levels in the brain, and certain cholinergic agents can be employed to block Ach-ase.

Adverse Effects of Cholinergic Drugs

As previously stated, by recalling the effects of the parasympathetic nervous system, the adverse effects of cholinergic drugs can be identified. Pulmonary secretions, bronchospasm, respiratory depression, and respiratory paralysis are some of the potentially life-threatening adverse effects. Atropine sulphate should be close at hand to reverse the cholinergic effect in the event that a client experiences a cholinergic crisis. Also, prior to administering cholinergic agents, nurses should ensure that intubation equipment is readily available should respiratory depression or arrest occur.

Anticholinergic (Parasympatholytic) Drugs

These agents act by blocking Ach receptors. Their pharmacological action results in pupil dilation, decreased lacrimation, increased heart rate, decreased GI motility, decreased salivation, and suppression of other physiological functions associated with Ach activity. Examples include the following:

- Atropine sulphate—This agent may be used as a preoperative drug to decrease GI and respiratory secretions. Atropine sulphate crosses the blood–brain barrier and in a sufficiently large dose will act as a stimulant. At toxic dose levels, it causes CNS depression.
- Hyoscine (Buscopan)—This agent has both anticholinergic and antispasmodic effects. It is usually prescribed for GI spasms in irritable bowel syndrome and bladder spasms in clients with biliary or renal colic.
- Benztropine, biperiden, and ethopropazine (Parsitan)—These agents are used to treat the cholinergic disorder in Parkinson's disease.
- Flavoxate and oxybutynin—These agents are used for hyperactive urinary bladders.
  Since antacids decrease the therapeutic effects of anticholinergic agents, the following precautions should be taken:
- Drugs should be administered at least 1 hour apart.
- Clients should be warned about undertaking activities that cause perspiration since anticholinergic agents inhibit perspiration, making clients susceptible to heat stroke.
- Clients should also be cautioned against using OTC drugs with antihistamine and drinking alcoholic beverages.

Nursing Considerations Relating to Sympathomimetic Drugs

- Maintain awareness of sympathetic and parasympathetic nervous system effects on the body.
- Be aware that observations relating to sympathomimetics include tachycardia, elevation in BP, hyperactivity, sleeplessness, dry mouth, and pupillary dilation.
- Be aware that observations relating to sympatholytics will include bradycardia, decreased BP, sedation, weakness, lethargy, and dizziness.
- Be aware that observations relating to parasympathomimetics will include bradycardia, hypotension, bronchoconstriction, increased salivation, perspiration, abdominal cramps, dizziness, and pupillary constriction.
- Be aware that observations relating to parasympathetic blockers include tachycardia, restlessness, confusion, pupillary dilation, blurred vision, urinary retention, dry mouth, and constipation.
- Monitor vital signs carefully.
- Promote a relaxing environment for clients on stimulant classifications of ANS drugs.
- Provide mouth care for dry mouth.
- Teach clients to report adverse effects.
- Caution clients on depressant classifications of ANS drugs about safety precautions, particularly driving or operating dangerous machinery.
- Advise clients taking anticholinergics that these drugs may cause sensitivity to light due to pupillary dilation; use of sunglasses and avoidance of bright lights should be encouraged.
- Advise clients taking sympathomimetics and anticholinergics that these drugs may cause urinary retention; teach clients to report urination problems.

DRUGS THAT AFFECT THE CARDIOVASCULAR SYSTEM

Drugs that affect the cardiovascular system are outlined in Fig. 7.2.

Agents Affecting Blood Coagulation

Two overall classifications of drugs affect blood coagulation: agents that inhibit blood coagulation and those that promote it. Classes of drugs that inhibit abnormal coagulation of blood (clot formation) may be divided into three general classifications: anticoagulants, antiplatelet agents, and thrombolytics. Agents that promote blood coagulation (to prevent abnormal blood loss) are called *fibrinolytics*.

Preliminary Tests

Before and during the administration of agents that affect the clotting of blood, a number of blood tests are used to assess

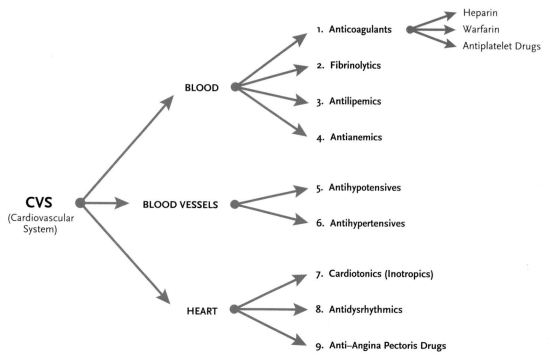

Fig. 7.2 Drugs that affect the cardiovascular system.

the clotting processes within the body. These include the following (normal values are given in parentheses):

- Platelet count—(150 000–400 000 mm³)
- Hemoglobin (Hgb)—(male: 140–180 g/L; female: 120–160 g/L)
- Hematocrit (Hct)—(male: 42–52%; female: 37–47%)
- Prothrombin time (PT)—(11–12.5 seconds)
- Partial thromboplastin time (PTT)—(60–70 seconds)
- Activated partial thromboplastin time (aPTT)—(30–40 seconds)
- International normalized ratio (INR)—0.81–1.2

For clients taking heparin, the aPTT or PTT is used to monitor the prescribed therapeutic range. For clients taking oral anticoagulants, PT or INR is used to monitor the prescribed therapeutic range.

Anticoagulants (Coagulation-Modifying Agents)

Anticoagulants prevent the formation of clots by inhibiting certain clotting factors and platelets. They are only given prophylactically as they have no direct effect on a blood clot that has already formed.

Common uses.
- Myocardial infarction (MI)
- Unstable angina pectoris
- Atrial fibrillation
- Emboli (pulmonary emboli)
- In-dwelling devices (pacemakers, mechanical valves)
- Pelvic surgeries (prostatectomy)

Primary anticoagulants prescribed.

Heparin
- Heparin is commonly prescribed during the acute stage of a condition requiring anticoagulant therapy.

- Heparin activates antithrombin 3, causing neutralization of thrombin and inhibition of clot formation.
- Onset of action following subcutaneous (SC) injection is 20–60 minutes; duration of action is approximately 8–12 hours.
- Dosage is based on PTT or aPTT; therapeutic range is 1.5–2.5 times normal.

Warfarin (Coumadin)
- Warfarin is commonly prescribed after the acute stage of a condition requiring anticoagulant therapy to maintain therapeutic blood levels of anticoagulation.
- Warfarin interferes with production of vitamin K (necessary for clotting of blood). Vitamin K is necessary for the production of clotting factors 2, 7, 9, and 10.
- Onset of action is 2–7 days.
- Dosage is based on the PT and INR; the desirable therapeutic range is 1.5–2.5 times normal.

Antiplatelet drugs
- These drugs interfere with the ability of platelets to aggregate during the process of blood clotting.
- Antiplatelet drugs are commonly prescribed to prevent arterial thrombosis and where a thromboembolism disorder exists, as in the prevention and management of conditions such as MI, cerebrovascular accident, and transient ischemic attacks.
- Bleeding time and PT are used to monitor the therapeutic effects of drugs.

Examples include the following:
- Acetylsalicylic acid (Aspirin)
- Ticlopidine (Ticlid)
- Clopidogrel (Plavix)

Adverse effects of anticoagulant drugs (coagulation-modifying agents).
- Hemorrhage: Indicated by occult blood in stool, melena stool, petechia, bruising, bleeding from gums
- Gastric ulceration (ASA)

Nursing Considerations Relating to Anticoagulant Drugs (Coagulation-Modifying Agents)
- Observe for signs of hemorrhage, such as hematuria or black stool, and report.
- Administer oral medications with food to avoid gastric irritation.
- Administer SC heparin to avoid local bruising. Use a half-inch needle, do not aspirate the plunger, inject into the deep fatty tissue of the abdomen, withdraw carefully, and apply pressure to the site for several minutes; do not massage the site.
- Monitor blood tests for the degree of anticoagulation and report if abnormal for therapeutic dose.
- Use elastic stockings to promote circulation.
- Teach clients to exercise legs to promote circulation and prevent clot formation.
- Teach clients to avoid positions that impede blood circulation, such as dangling or crossing the legs or wearing restricting clothing.
- Maintain proper hydration to avoid hemoconcentration.
- Caution clients to avoid activities that may cause trauma or increase the tendency to bleed, including the following:
  - Contact sports and other potentially risky activities
  - Vigorous teeth-brushing or using a coarse-bristled toothbrush
- Remind clients to report abnormal bruising or unusual bleeding.
- Caution clients to avoid food high in vitamin K.
- Caution clients to avoid taking ASA if taking other anticoagulants.
- Instruct clients to take oral medications, particularly ASA, with food.
- Ensure that when a client is changed from heparin to a warfarin preparation, the client will remain on the heparin until the warfarin preparation achieves therapeutic levels in the blood.
- Carefully monitor PPT, aPPT (heparin), and PT and INR (warfarin) during therapy and when the client is changed from a parenteral to an oral preparation.

Fibrinolytic (Thrombolytic) Agents
- These agents act by converting plasminogen to plasmin (an enzyme that breaks down the fibrin in clots that have formed).
- Early initiation of therapy is required immediately after the condition develops to be effective.
- They are prescribed to act on clots that have formed in coronary artery occlusion (MI), pulmonary embolus, cerebral emboli (stroke), and deep vein thrombosis (DVT).
- They are administered by IV infusion.

- Clients receiving fibrinolytic drugs require care in the Critical Care Unit during therapy.

Reverse anticoagulant agents. These agents are used when an overdose of anticoagulant has occurred. Examples include the following:
- Protamine sulphate—Used in the case of heparin overdose; neutralizes heparin activity
- Vitamin K—Used for a warfarin overdose

Antilipemics (Agents Used to Treat Dyslipidemia)
Antilipemic drugs are used to reduce lipid levels when dietary measures, weight loss, and exercise have been unsuccessful. Indication for treatment includes elevated plasma cholesterol, triglyceride, and low-density lipoprotein (LDL) levels.

Preliminary Tests
The following are the normal ranges for preliminary levels.
- Cholesterol: <5.0 mmol/L
- Triglycerides: Male 0.45–1.81 mmol/L, female 0.40-1.52 mmol/L
- LDL: <2.59 mmol/L

The choice of treatment depends on which type of lipid is elevated.

Bile Acid Sequestrants
These preparations combine with the bile acids in the intestine to form a nonabsorbable complex that is then excreted in the feces. This lack of reabsorption of bile forces the liver cells to metabolize cholesterol to produce more bile acids, thus reducing LDLs and total cholesterol levels. An example is cholestyramine resin (Questran).

HMG-CoA Reductase Inhibitors (Statins)
This is the most widely used classification of antilipemics in the treatment of dyslipidemia. Statins block the formation of cellular cholesterol, causing a reduction in blood LDL and total cholesterol within weeks. Examples include the following:
- Lovastatin
- Atorvastatin (Lipitor)
- Pravastatin (Pravachol)
- Simvastatin (Zocor)

Fibric Acids
These acids stimulate the breakdown and reduction in synthesis of very-low-density lipoproteins (VLDLs). Therapeutic effects include the lowering of VLDLs, the reduction of triglycerides, and the increase of high-density lipoprotein (HDL) levels. Examples include fenofibrate and gemfibrozil.

Niacin (Vitamin B₃)
Niacin acts on liver cells to inhibit LDL and triglyceride production. It may be prescribed in combination with other antihyperlipidemic drugs.

Adverse Effects of Antilipemics
- The reduction of fat-soluble vitamins due to bile salts reducing their absorption

TABLE 7.6   Nutritional Deficiency Anemia Drug Treatments

Preparation	Uses	Adverse Effects	Nursing Considerations
Iron • Ferrous fumarate • Ferrous gluconate • Ferrous sulphate	• Iron deficiency anemia	• Gastro-intestinal irritation • Discoloration of tooth enamel • Black stool • Drug allergy	• Oral preparations: give with food • Liquid preparations: drink with straw • IM: deep IM, Z-track technique to reduce tissue irritation
Folic Acid • Folvite	• Pregnancy • Megaloblastic anemia • Tropical sprue • Pernicious anemia	• Rare • Discoloration of urine • Possible allergy	• Take with food
Vitamin B$_{12}$ • Cyanocobalamin		In large doses: • Diarrhea • Pruritis • Hypokalemia	• Take with food • Usually required for life

IM, intramuscular.

• The formation of gallstones (fibric acid preparations disturb the fat level of the blood)
• The effects of statins are usually mild; however, they should be used with caution in clients with liver and kidney impairment.
• Headache
• GI disturbances—Nausea, vomiting, distension, irritation, diarrhea, or constipation
• Myopathy (muscle aches)—Uncommon but significant (with statins)
• Flushing, skin rash, and itchiness (with niacin)
• Jaundice
• Antilipemics are contraindicated in liver and kidney disease.

Nursing Considerations Relating to Antilipemics

Client teaching points:
• Take the medication as prescribed (this point should be stressed).
• Promptly comply with laboratory requests and physician appointments.
• Report side effects to a physician (myopathy with statins, jaundice).
• Change dietary habits; reduce fat intake.
• Supplement fat-soluble vitamins (A, D, E, K).
• Increase dietary fibre and fluid intake.
• Understand the importance of moderate exercise and weight reduction.
• Do not discontinue medications without consulting with a physician.
• Understand that mild side effects usually dissipate after medication is established within the body.
• Do not take statins with grapefruit juice.
• Ensure that medication is taken with or without meals, according to the preparation.

Antianemics

There are many different classifications of anemia with differing causes, manifestations, and origins. Regardless of the type of anemia, the end result is a decrease in the concentration of circulating red blood cells or a low hemoglobin level.

Anemias result from a deficiency of nutrients necessary for the development of healthy red blood cells and hemoglobin (such as iron deficiency anemia (iron), fetal damage in pregnancy (folic acid deficiency), or pernicious anemia (vitamin B$_{12}$ deficiency), or an abnormality of the bone marrow that produces the cells, such as marrow destruction as a result of radiation, or genetic deviation, such as sickle cell anemia or thalassemia. Refer to Table 7.6, which outlines the medications used to treat nutritional deficiency anemia.

Nutritional Deficiency Anemia

Nursing considerations relating to antianemics. When the client takes dietary supplements for the treatment of nutritional deficiency anemia, the practical nurse should do the following:
• Teach the client to take prescribed medications as required to maintain optimal blood levels.
• Encourage the client not to discontinue medication without consultation with a physician.
• Observe the client for adverse effects and measures.
• Encourage the client to take medication in the method prescribed.
• Encourage the client to use natural dietary sources to complement prescribed medication.
• Teach the client not to break or crush preparations into a powder (many are coated to reduce irritation).

Antihypotensive Agents

These agents are used to treat low BP and circulatory shock and to re-establish effective circulation and BP. Sympathomimetic drugs are the most common classification of drugs used for the treatment of the above conditions and are effective in an emergency situation.

Classifications of Antihypotensive Agents

Table 7.7 summarizes the classifications and actions of antihypotensive agents.

TABLE 7.7 Classifications of Antihypotensive Agents

Type	Drug	Action
Alpha Adrenergic Agents	• Norepinephrine (noradrenaline) • Phenylephrine (Neosynephrine)	• Causes constriction of vascular smooth muscle, resulting in increased peripheral vascular resistance and increased BP
Beta Adrenergic Agents	• Dobutamine (Dobutrex) • Isoproterenol (Isuprel)	• Increases myocardial contractility and heart rate, resulting in increased BP
Alpha and Beta Adrenergic Agents	• Dopamine HCl • Epinephrine (adrenaline)	• Causes constriction of vascular smooth muscle and stimulates cardiac contractility • Increases blood flow to kidneys, preventing renal shutdown (dopamine) • Bronchodilation

BP, blood pressure; *HCl*, hydrochloric acid.

TABLE 7.8 Classifications of Antihypertensive Agents

Type	Drug	Action
Diuretics (thiazide, loop, potassium sparing)	• Hydrochlorothiazide • Furosemide (Lasix) • Spironolactone (Aldactone)	• Reduce circulating and interstitial fluid → reduce peripheral vascular resistance → ↓ BP
ACE inhibitors	• Captopril • Enalapril (Vasotec) • Ramipril (Altace)	• Block enzyme that converts angiotensin I to angiotensin II → vasodilation → decrease peripheral vascular resistance → ↓ BP
Alpha adrenergic blockers	• Doxazosin (Cardura) (alpha$_1$) • Terazosin (alpha$_1$) • Clonidine (alpha$_2$)	• Block stimulation of alpha adrenergic receptors in blood → vasodilation → decrease peripheral vascular resistance → ↓ BP
Beta adrenergic blockers	• Atenolol (Tenormin) • Metoprolol • Propranolol	• Block beta adrenergic receptors within heart muscle → reduce strength and rate of cardiac contraction → decrease peripheral resistance → ↓ BP
Calcium channel blockers	• Nifedipine (Adalat) • Diltiazem (Cardizem) • Verapamil (Isoptin)	• Prevent the action of calcium at receptor sites, inhibiting smooth muscle contraction → vasodilation → decrease peripheral vascular resistance → ↓ BP
Centrally acting antihypertensives	• Clonidine • Methyldopa	• Stimulate the brain to modify the action of the sympathetic nervous system → reduce strength of cardiac activity and inhibit vasoconstriction → decrease peripheral vascular resistance → ↓ BP
Vasodilators	• Hydralazine (Apresoline) • Minoxidil (Rogaine)	• Produce vasodilation by acting directly on the arterial smooth muscle → decrease peripheral vascular resistance → ↓ BP

ACE, angiotensin-converting enzyme; *BP*, blood pressure.

Dopamine and epinephrine are the most commonly used agents for shock and hypotension.

Antihypertensive Agents

Antihypertensive agents are usually prescribed for clients when diet, exercise, and other measures designed to reduce BP have failed to lower BP to a level that does not pose a health risk to the cardiovascular and renal systems. In general, to reduce BP, antihypertensive drugs either reduce blood volume (such as diuretics) or cause dilation of blood vessels (i.e., they reduce peripheral resistance).

Treatment for hypertension depends on the severity of the disorder. Antihypertensive therapy for mild to moderate hypertension usually begins with a single medication, such as a thiazide diuretic. In the presence of moderate hypertension, in some clients, it may be necessary to give a combination of two drugs (e.g., a thiazide diuretic in addition to one of a beta blocker, an angiotensin-converting enzyme [ACE] inhibitor, a vasodilator, a centrally acting antihypertensive agent, or an alpha blocker). For severe hypertension, a combination of drugs designed specifically for the client will be prescribed.

Classifications of Antihypertensive Agents

Table 7.8 summarizes the classifications and actions of antihypertensive agents.

Adverse Effects of Antihypertensive Agents

Adverse effects vary according to the category of drug prescribed. In general, adverse effects most commonly experienced are the result of vasodilation and reduced cardiac action, including the following:

- Hypokalemia (diuretics, such as thiazides)
- Muscle cramps (loop diuretics)
- Lightheadedness, dizziness, weakness, lethargy
- Orthostatic hypotension
- Dehydration (diuretics)
- Urticaria (thiazide and loop)
- Photosensitivity (thiazide and loop)

- Headache (vasodilating effects)
- Gynecomastia (potassium sparing in men)
- Erectile dysfunction (thiazide)
- Menstrual irregularities (potassium sparing in women)

Nursing Considerations Relating to Antihypertensive Agents

- Observe for adverse effects related to specific medication prescribed (such as dehydration or electrolyte imbalance).
- Monitor vital signs—BP and pulse—lying and standing. Client teaching points:
- Understand the dangers of uncontrolled hypertension.
- Report adverse effects that may occur initially.
- Do not suddenly stop taking the prescribed medication.
- Take the medication as prescribed.
- Do not double up if a dose is missed.
- Take care when ambulating due to postural hypotension.
- Avoid very hot showers or baths due to vasodilating effects and dizziness that could result.
- Ensure proper hydration; avoid becoming dehydrated, monitor fluid intake.
- Avoid excess alcohol use, since it is vasodilating and the effects produced interfere with drug metabolism and cause dehydration.
- Monitor and report signs of swelling of lower extremities.
- Keep physician and laboratory appointments for reassessments.
- Understand the importance of the following:
  - Weight reduction
  - Balanced diet (restrict salt intake; potassium supplementation if on diuretics)
  - Stress reduction
  - Adequate rest

Agents Used to Treat Heart Failure

A variety of treatment regimens exist for the management of heart failure. The following classifications of drugs may be prescribed to promote more effective cardiovascular functioning.

Vasodilators

Vasodilators decrease the workload of the heart and include ACE inhibitors, nitrates, and angiotensin II receptor blockers (used if ACE inhibitors are not tolerated well).

Diuretics

These drugs increase urine output and decrease sodium levels in the body. They are commonly used in combination with other medications to treat heart failure and include thiazides and furosemide.

Beta Adrenergic Agonists

These agonists stimulate sympathetic nervous system activity to increase calcium flow into the cardiac muscle, resulting in increased contractility. Examples include dobutamine hydrochloride.

Cardiotonic (Inotropic) Drugs

This class of drug is widely used in the treatment of heart failure. These drugs act by increasing the strength of cardiac contraction (positive inotropic effect), which results in increased cardiac output. The drug also slows the rate of cardiac contraction (negative chronotropic effect), leading to more effective heart action, an increase in renal output, and a decrease in renin release results.

Cardiac glycosides.

- They have a narrow therapeutic index.
- They are excreted from the body by the kidney (renal impairment may cause accumulation, leading to toxic levels).
- Dosages should be adjusted to prevent blood levels from becoming toxic.
- Examples include digitalis preparations, such as digoxin (Lanoxin).

Symptoms of digitalis toxicity.

- Drowsiness, weakness, dizziness
- Confusion
- GI upset—Nausea, vomiting, diarrhea
- Visual disturbances (yellow-green distortion)
- Bradycardia or tachycardia
- Heart block

Digitalization.   When a client is initially started on a digitalis preparation, a higher than normal dosage of the drug is commonly given to establish therapeutic levels as quickly as possible. The subsequent (maintenance) dosage is established to maintain the therapeutic level in the blood following the initial high dose. Careful monitoring of blood levels is undertaken to avoid possible toxicity and to establish the most effective maintenance dosage.

Nursing considerations: Implications relating to digoxin.

- Assess for adverse or toxic effects, reporting and charting immediately.
- Do not administer digoxin concurrently with the following drugs:
  - Antacids, which reduce absorption
  - Antimicrobial agents and calcium preparations, which may promote toxicity
- Monitor digoxin serum levels throughout treatment to detect toxic levels.
- Following each administration of the drug, be aware that charting should include indicating the apical heart rate at the time of administration.
- If the apical pulse rate is erratic, below 60 beats per minute in adults (less than 90 beats per minute in infants), or above 100–120 beats per minute, withhold the digoxin and report for additional assessment by the physician.
- Monitor clients with hypokalemia, hypothyroidism, and acute MI more frequently for toxic effects.
- Know that the antidote for severe toxicity is digoxin immune fab (Digibind), which inactivates digoxin by drawing the drug from the tissues and binding to it.

Client teaching points:

- Monitor for adverse effects, such as visual changes (colour perception).
- Monitor heart rate (teach the client how to do so).
- Report concerns regarding the effects of the drug.
- Eat food high in potassium (due to loss through urine).
- Avoid taking several medications if a drug interaction may occur.
- Do not to take a double dose if a dose is missed.

Phosphodiesterase Inhibitors (PDIs)

- PDIs produce an inotropic effect on the heart as well as dilating arteries and veins.
- They increase the force of contractility of the heart muscles and decrease pre- and afterload on the heart.
- PDIs are administered intravenously.
- An example is milrinone.
- Potential adverse effects of PDI administration include hypotension and dysrhythmias.
- Clients must be evaluated for BP, cardiac rhythm and rate, and cardiac output during and for several hours following administration.

Antidysrhythmic Drugs

Antidysrhythmics are drugs used to treat dysrhythmias, to slow conduction of electrical impulses in the heart, to reduce spontaneous depolarization of myocardial cells, or to prolong the effective refractory period.

The Vaughan Williams classification of antidysrhythmic drugs, which is based on the effect that agents produce on action potential in the heart, list four classes of agents:

Class I: Sodium channel blockers (e.g., quinidine, disopyramide, or procainamide)

Class II: Beta blockers (e.g., sotalol or propranolol)

Class III: Potassium channel blockers (such as amiodarone, bretylium, and ibutilide)

Class IV: Calcium channel blockers (such as diltiazem [Cardizem] and verapamil [Isoptin SR])

Other Drug Classifications

- Atropine for bradyarrhythmias
- Digoxin for atrial fibrillation

These drugs, regardless of class, cause depression of the normal heart function.

Adverse Effects

- Quinidine can result in disturbed hearing, giddiness, and impaired vision (cinchonism).
- Amiodarone can accumulate in tissue, causing photosensitivity rashes and lung problems.
- See the section "Symptoms of Digitalis Toxicity."

Precautions

For quinidine:

- Monitor for toxicity.
- Caution about diet that alkalinizes the urine.

- Monitor for therapeutic range: 2–6 mcg/mL; toxicity results when levels exceed 8 mcg/mL.

Anti–Angina Pectoris Drugs

Anti-angina medications are prescribed to relieve angina pain and reduce the frequency of angina attacks. The drug helps restore oxygen supply to the heart by improving blood supply to the myocardium. This is accomplished by dilating coronary blood vessels, which, in turn, increase blood supply to the heart, relieving the hypoxia in myocardial cells.

Classifications of Drugs Used to Treat Angina Pectoris

Nitrates. Nitrates act by relaxing vascular smooth muscle, which dilates coronary blood vessels and increases blood flow to the myocardium. Examples are nitroglycerine (Nitrostat) and isosorbide mononitrate.

Calcium channel blockers. These drugs act by relaxing vascular smooth muscle, which dilates the coronary blood vessels and increases blood flow to the myocardium. Examples include amlodipine (Norvasc), diltiazem (Cardizem), and nifedipine (Adalet).

Beta adrenergic blockers. Beta adrenergic blockers act to help reduce the risk of angina by decreasing the influence of the sympathetic nervous system on stimulating the myocardium, resulting in decreased cardiac output, reduced oxygen demand, and lower BP. Examples are propranolol, atenolol (Tenormin), and nadolol.

Adverse Effects of Anti–Angina Pectoris Medications

- Headache
- Flushing of skin
- Dizziness, weakness, and fainting

Nursing Considerations Relating to Anti–Angina Pectoris Medications

- Oral preparations and patches are used for the prevention of anginal attacks.
- Sprays and sublingual preparations are used for acute attacks.
- For treatment of acute anginal pain, the sublingual dose range for nitrate is 0.3–0.6 mg. The dose of nitrate may be repeated twice at 5-minute intervals. If the pain persists, the client should seek medical attention immediately as the potential for MI exists.

  Clients should be taught the following:
- Techniques for administration
- To recognize adverse effects and report
- To rest while taking medication during an anginal attack
- To avoid swallowing for several minutes when administering sublingual preparations
- To store sublingual medications in a dry, cool, dark place
- To carry medication at all times
- To note and observe expiratory dates and replace
- That sublingual spray preparations should not be frozen, and prior to administration, priming of the pump is required

- That patches applied to the skin should be stored in a dry environment and applied to an area of skin without hair, the old patch is removed and the skin is cleansed, and the new patch is applied to a different area; apply at the same time each day
- To take oral preparations on an empty stomach
- To avoid developing tolerance by removing the nitroglycerine patch for 8 hours overnight

DRUGS THAT AFFECT THE GASTRO-INTESTINAL SYSTEM

Drugs that affect the GI system are outlined in Fig. 7.3.

There are four common disorders of the GI system for which drugs are frequently prescribed: constipation, diarrhea, hyperacidity, and nausea and vomiting. Some of these disorders may be treated using OTC preparations, but for clients with serious conditions or those in institutions, the healthcare provider may prescribe the appropriate medication.

Laxatives

In this group, drugs are used to speed the passage of intestinal contents through the GI tract. They may be administered to prevent or relieve constipation (most common use), to prepare a client for lower GI tract procedures, to reduce the strain of defecation in clients with cardiovascular disease or hemorrhoids, to remove ingested toxic substances, or as treatment for parasitic infestations or other such conditions.

Classifications of Laxatives

Table 7.9 outlines the different classifications of laxatives, their actions, and their uses.

Adverse Effects Relating to the Use of Laxatives

- Diarrhea
- Abdominal cramps (can occur with the rapid-acting stimulant and saline laxatives and irritating stimulant laxative classifications)
- Flatulence
- Tolerance
- Bowel impaction or obstruction (with bulk-forming preparations)
- Electrolyte imbalances (with saline laxatives)

Nursing Considerations Relating to Laxatives

- Assess client need; evaluate record of bowel movements.
- Know that contraindications include bowel surgery and bowel diseases.
- Observe and record therapeutic effects and adverse effects.
- Ambulate client as soon as possible, since exercise promotes bowel action.
- Push fluids if not contraindicated.

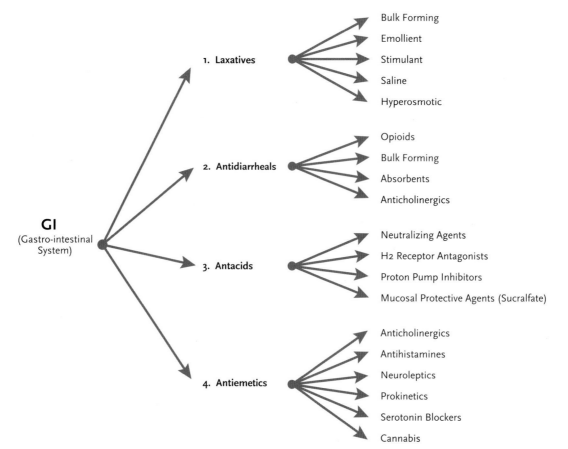

Fig. 7.3 Drugs that affect the gastro-intestinal system.

TABLE 7.9 Classifications of Laxatives

Type of Laxative	Action	Uses
Bulk-Forming Laxative • Psyllium (Metamucil)	• Acts by absorbing water into intestine → increases bulk and distends bowel → reflex bowel activity (peristalsis)	• Slow-acting (12–48 hours) • Long-term therapy for chronic constipation
Stimulant Laxative • Bisacodyl (Dulcolax)	• Irritates or stimulates the nerve plexus in the mucosa of small intestine and colon → increasing peristalsis	• Rapid evacuation of bowel for diagnostic tests • Acute constipation
Saline Laxative • Magnesium citrate (Citro-Mag) • Magnesium hydroxide (Milk of Magnesia)	• Draws water into the bowel by osmotic action → watery stool and distended bowel → stimulates stretch receptors → stimulates peristalsis	• Bowel cleansing • Acute constipation • Rapid onset
Emollient Laxative (Stool Softener) • Docusate sodium (Colace) • Mineral oil	• Detergentlike action that lowers surface tension of gastro-intestinal fluids → water and fat absorbed into stool and increased peristalsis • Lubricates bowel for easier passage of stool	• Mild, gentle relief of constipation • Prevention of constipation
Hyperosmotic Laxative • Lactulose (Apo-Lactulose) • Polyethylene glycol (Miralax)	• Produces a hyperosmolar environment in bowel → draws water from intestinal lining into bowel → distension of bowel with added water → stimulation of peristalsis	• Relieves acute constipation • Bowel preparation for diagnostic and surgical procedures • Very cleansing

TABLE 7.10 Classifications of Antidiarrheals

Classification	Action	Uses
Opioids • Codeine sulphate • Loperamide (Imodium) • Diphenoxylate + atropine (Lomotil)	• Suppress gastro-intestinal (GI) smooth muscle activity → ↓ GI motility, prolonging transit time → absorption of fluid and nutrients • Analgesic effect	• Acute diarrhea • Not usually recommended for diarrhea caused by infections as infectious agents may be retained within the bowel
Bulk-Forming Agents • Psyllium (Metamucil)	• Absorb water from large intestine → increase bulk → stool becomes less watery	• Symptomatic treatment of diarrhea
Absorbents • Bismuth subsalicylate (Pepto-Bismol) • Kaolin-pectin (Kaopectate)	• Absorb irritants and coat lining of the intestinal tract → inhibit irritation of the lining of intestines and absorb toxic substances for excretion in feces	• Diarrhea associated with intestinal infections and chronic bowel diseases, such as diverticulitis and ulcerative colitis
Anticholinergics • Belladonna	• Suppress parasympathetic nervous system activity of the intestinal tract → suppress peristalsis → reduce spasm and speed of passage of intestinal contents	• Require prescription; administered in conjunction with opioid preparation • Diarrhea associated with irritable and inflammatory bowel conditions

- Provide a relaxed, unrushed, and private area for defecation. Client teaching points:
- Follow the directions indicated on the medication container (e.g., take with the full glass of water; take before bedtime).
- Increase fluid intake throughout the day if not contraindicated.
- Increase fibre in the diet.
- Reduce constipating foods in the diet.
- Increase exercise.
- Avoid overuse of medications as tolerance can develop.
- If possible, use milder classifications such as stool softeners or bulk-forming laxatives.
- Avoid overuse of bulk-forming laxatives, which can interfere with absorption of other medications and cause distension and possible obstruction.
- Do not take prescribed medication if abdominal pain or nausea and vomiting are present.

Antidiarrheal Agents

Usually, the medication prescribed to treat diarrhea is given to treat the unpleasant symptoms or the underlying cause of the diarrhea. Some medications may be purchased without prescription and are available on pharmacy shelves or OTC, whereas others require a prescription because of the classification of the drug or the severity of the condition to be treated (such as opiate-related drugs).

Four general classifications of agents are used for the treatment of diarrhea: opioids, bulk-forming agents, absorbents, and anticholinergics. The type of drug prescribed depends on the cause and severity of the diarrhea.

Classifications of Antidiarrheals

Table 7.10 outlines the different classifications of antidiarrheals, their actions, and their uses.

Adverse Effects Related to Antidiarrheal Agents

· Constipation
· Nausea and vomiting
· Dependency (with opioids)
· Sedation, drowsiness, weakness, lethargy (with opioids)
· Urinary retention (with atropine preparations and opioids)
· Clotting disorders (with bismuth preparations)
· Allergic reactions

Nursing Considerations Relating to Antidiarrheal Agents

· Assess the client's history relating to the diarrhea and established bowel patterns.
· Identify possible causes of the diarrhea.
· Adhere to established guidelines for administration of a specific preparation, such as the time to administer.
· Assess for contraindications.
· Increase fluid intake while diarrhea persists to prevent dehydration; monitor for electrolyte imbalances.
· Monitor client's intake and output.
  Client teaching points:
· Follow administration directives, including the correct dosage and when to take the medication.
· Increase fluid intake to replace lost fluids.
· Monitor effects relating to relief of diarrhea.
· Maintain a record of the frequency and consistency of stools until normal bowel patterns resume.
· See a doctor immediately if diarrhea persists, manifestations increase in severity, or adverse effects develop (child: 24 hours; adult 2–3 days, depending on severity).
· Avoid irritating, gaseous foods that stimulate the bowel, such as cabbage, high-fibre foods, or psyllium fibre.
· Monitor weight for possible fluid deficits.
· Avoid overuse of opioid preparations due to possible development of dependence.
· Try to identify causes of the diarrhea for possible avoidance of a recurrence of the problem.
· Understand that sometimes the diarrhea facilitates removal of undesirable substances from the body and antidiarrheals are not always necessary.
· Understand that bismuth preparations darken the stool and that this is no cause for alarm.

Antacid Agents

Antacids form a large group of prescription and OTC drugs used to reduce the hyperacidity of the stomach. Certain alkaline drugs can directly neutralize the hydrochloric acid (HCl) secreted into the stomach (such as aluminum, magnesium, and calcium-containing drugs). Additives include simethicone, which reduces gaseous buildup and distension, and alginic acid, which protects the gastric lining and reduces the risk of acid reflux into the esophagus. Other classifications inhibit the production or release of HCl, which results in a reduction in the amount of HCl in the stomach, thereby relieving gastric irritation.

These drugs are used for the treatment of conditions such as mild gastritis, which is caused by indigestion and eating foods that cause "heartburn," gastroesophageal reflux disease (GERD), peptic ulcer disease, and hypersecretion disorders. A prescription for certain preparations may also be used as a preventive of stress ulcers caused by extreme traumatic events, such as extensive burns. The particular type of preparation prescribed is directed toward treating the specific condition.

Aluminum preparations may produce constipation, while magnesium preparations produce diarrhea; therefore, most products on the market today are a combination of products. Calcium preparations are fast-acting but are less commonly used due to the risk of developing renal calculi, acid rebound, and hypercalcemia. Sodium bicarbonate is fast and effective but highly soluble, resulting in absorption and the potential development of metabolic alkalosis.

Classification of Antacids

Table 7.11 outlines the different classifications of antacids, their actions, their uses, and adverse effects.

General Adverse Effects of Antacid Preparations

· Contraindicated in severe renal failure and GI obstruction
· Contraindicated in pregnancy and lactation; crosses barriers to infant

Nursing Considerations Relating to Antacid Preparations

· Administer at times indicated (such as after meals [pc], at bedtime, with food, for 4–6 weeks, and so on). However, sometimes clients may be prescribed low dosages of medication for extended periods.
· Observe for desired effects and adverse effects (such as constipation or diarrhea).
· Observe for occult blood or melena stool.
  Client teaching points:
· Take the medication according to the directions on the label.
· Avoid overuse or long-term use.
· See a physician if manifestations continue or if the medication is taken beyond the suggested duration.
· Reduce possible causes of irritation or ulcer formation, such as stress.
· Avoid alcohol and smoking.
· Administer with a full glass of fluid to ensure absorption.
· Take frequent small meals to maintain food within the stomach.
· Avoid irritating foods or foods that stimulate acid production.
· Remain sitting up for 1–2 hours following a meal to reduce the risk of acid reflux.
· Monitor bowel movements for constipation, diarrhea, or black stool.

Antiemetics

Antiemetics are agents used to prevent and treat nausea and vomiting. Conditions that precipitate nausea, vomiting, or both include GI irritation, infections occurring in many

TABLE 7.11 Classifications of Antacids

Classification	Action	Uses	Adverse Effects
Neutralizing Agents • Aluminum Products (Amphogel) • Calcium Products (Tums, Rolaids) • Combination Products (Gelucil, Maalox, Diovol, Gaviscon)	• Neutralized HCl in the stomach (e.g., AlOH + HCl → AlCl + H_2O) • Alginic acid—coating action of the stomach • Simethicone is added to some of these agents as an antiflatulent as it inhibits gas formation	• Treatment of acute irritation and inflammation of esophageal and gastric lining due to ingestion of certain foods and gastric reflux • Available in chewable tablets, powders, and liquid preparations • All preparations are available OTC	• Constipation (aluminum and calcium preparations) • Renal calculi (calcium preparations) • Systemic metabolic alkalosis (sodium bicarbonate) • Acid rebound hyperacidity (calcium preparations)
H_2 Receptor Antagonists • Cimetidine (Tagamet) • Ranitidine (Zantac) • Famotidine (Pepcid)	• Inhibit histamine stimulation of H_2 receptors within the parietal cells to produce HCl → reduce HCl secretion → reduce gastric acidity	• Peptic ulcer disease • GERD • Stress ulcers • Zollinger—Ellison syndrome*	• Lethargy, confusion (H_2 receptor antagonists) • Gynecomastia and erectile dysfunction (cimetidine) • Suppression of metabolic activities of the liver (cimetidine)
Proton Pump Inhibitors • Lansoprazole (Prevacid) (for *Helicobacter pylori* infections) • Omeprazole (Losec)	• Irreversibly bind to H^+/K^+ ATPase in parietal cells, preventing the movement of H^+ out of parietal cells → lowering HCl	• Erosive esophagitis • GERD • Active duodenal ulcers (short-term therapy) • Gastric hypersecretory conditions (Zollinger—Ellison syndrome*)	• GI infections due to decreased acid production (H_2 receptor antagonists, proton pump inhibitors)
Mucosal Protective Agents • Sucralfate (Sulcrate) • Bismuth	• Locally combine with HCl and proteins at ulcer site to form a thick paste that covers and sticks to the ulcer site → protect ulcer to allow for healing • Bismuth appears to stimulate prostaglandin and bicarbonate production	• Active peptic ulcers • Stress ulcers • Esophageal irritation	• Allergic reactions • Urticaria • Nausea • Constipation • Dry mouth

*Zollinger–Ellison syndrome: nonendocrine pancreatic tumours that secrete gastrin, which in turn stimulates parietal cells within the lining of the stomach to secrete HCl and pepsin, resulting in the development of peptic ulcers.
ATPase, adenosine triphosphatase; *GERD*, gastroesophageal reflux disease; *H^+*, hydrogen; *HCl*, hydrochloric acid; *K^+*, potassium; *OTC*, over the counter.

parts of the body (such as the brain), metabolic imbalances, severe pain, stress, fear and horror, motion imbalances that originate from the semicircular canals of the ear, or radiation therapy and drug toxicity within the body, such as the vomiting associated with chemotherapeutic agents for cancer.

Antiemetic agents suppress impulses travelling to the vomiting centre within the medulla oblongata of the brain to relieve the manifestation of nausea and vomiting.

Classification of Antiemetics

Table 7.12 outlines the different classifications of antiemetics, their actions, and their uses.

Adverse Effects Relating to Antiemetics
- Drowsiness, dizziness, weakness
- Orthostatic hypotension
- Visual disturbances (blurred vision)
- Dry mouth
- Urinary retention (with antihistamines, anticholinergics)
- Diarrhea (with prokinetics)

Nursing Considerations Relating to Antiemetics
- Administer medication as ordered: dose, route, and time, such as before meals (ac), IV, IM, half an hour prior to nausea-producing treatment or event.
- Monitor and record effects and adverse effects.
- Implement safety precautions due to potential for drowsiness.
- Predict potential for vomiting and administer medication prior to occurrence.
- Withhold fluids until nausea is relieved.
- Offer fluids when nausea has been relieved, initially in small amounts.
- Monitor intake and output to maintain positive balance.
- Promote rest and relaxation when nausea occurs.

TABLE 7.12   Classifications of Antiemetics

Classifications	Action	Uses
Antihistamines • Dimenhydrinate (Gravol) • Anticholinergics • Scopolamine	• Block Ach receptors in vestibular region and reticular formation → impulses blocked from stimulating chemoreceptor trigger zone (CTZ) → CTZ prevented from stimulating the vomiting centre	• Prevention and treatment of nausea and vomiting due to motion sickness
Neuroleptics • Prochlorperazine (Stemetil) • Promethazine (Phenergan)	• Block dopamine receptors in CTZ → CTZ prevented from stimulating the vomiting centre	• Prevention and treatment of nausea associated with inner ear disorders
Serotonin Blockers • Granisetron (Apo-Granisetron)	• Inhibit stimulating effect of serotonin at receptor sites in gastro-intestinal (GI) tract and CTZ → CTZ prevented from stimulating the vomiting centre	• Prevention and treatment of vomiting associated with chemotherapy
Prokinetic Agents • Metoclopramide (Apo-Metoclop)	• Stimulate release of Ach in GI tract → speed gastric emptying → decrease nausea and vomiting relating to gastric retention and distension • Block dopamine in CTZ	• Prevention and treatment of nausea and vomiting relating to gastric distension • Prevention and treatment of vomiting relating to migraine headache, chemotherapy, hiatus hernia
Cannabis	• Depresses reticular formation, thalamus, and cerebral cortex → reduces sensitivity → reduces nausea and vomiting	• Prevention and treatment of nausea associated with chemotherapy • Prevention and treatment of nausea and anorexia associated with HIV/AIDS

Ach, acetylcholine.

- Ensure that tissues and a kidney basin are available when the client is experiencing nausea.
- Provide mouth care during acute episodes of nausea and vomiting.
  Client teaching points:
- Take medications prior to nausea-producing event, such as motion sickness.
- Avoid activities that require constant alertness (such as driving) when taking antiemetics.
- See a physician if the nausea and vomiting persists beyond 24 hours.
- Avoid food and situations that cause nausea and vomiting.
- Avoid activity and promote rest when nauseated.
- After nausea has subsided, initially take small amounts of clear fluids to determine tolerance.
- Recognize specific adverse effects of the classification of drug taken; report adverse effects.

DRUGS THAT AFFECT THE RESPIRATORY SYSTEM

Drugs that affect the respiratory system are outlined in Fig. 7.4.

Several classifications of drugs are used to relieve disorders of the respiratory tract. These medications can relieve cough (antitussives), promote the removal of excess secretions from the respiratory passageways (expectorants, decongestants, and mucolytics), or facilitate the dilation of the respiratory passageways (antihistamines, corticosteroids, and bronchodilators).

Antitussives

The classification of medications prescribed for the treatment of a cough depends on whether the cough is productive or dry. Productive coughs are usually treated with expectorants and mucolytics, while dry coughs are treated with antitussives.

Antitussives (cough suppressants) are prescribed to decrease the intensity and frequency of the cough without obstructing the elimination of tracheobronchial phlegm. Since the cough reflex is required to clear the upper respiratory tract of obstructive secretions, antitussives are commonly given in combination with expectorants to prevent the congestion of respiratory secretions within the lungs.

Classifications of Antitussives

Table 7.13 outlines the different classifications of antitussives, their actions, their characteristics, and their adverse effects.

Nursing Considerations Relating to Antitussives

- Ensure care regarding dosage and frequency.
- Observe for drowsiness and sedative effects.
  Client teaching points:
- Avoid activities that require constant alertness.
- Report excessive drowsiness or sedation, headache, fever, and chest congestion.
- Take only as directed by a prescriber or pharmacist.
- Increase fluid intake to maintain hydration and liquefy respiratory secretions.
- Take syrups undiluted.
- Avoid intake of food or fluid for half an hour after administering the medication to promote local effects of syrup on throat.

Expectorants

Expectorants liquefy mucus by stimulating the secretion of natural lubricants from glands within the respiratory tract. This effect is achieved by the following:

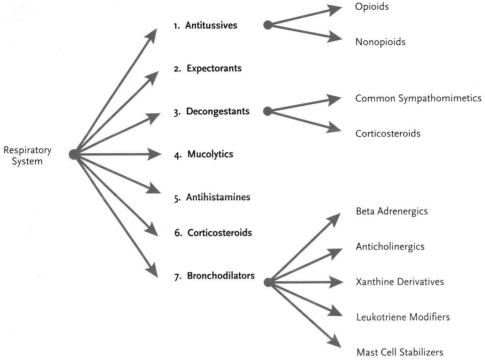

Fig. 7.4 Drugs that affect the respiratory system.

TABLE 7.13	**Classifications of Antitussives**		
Classification	**Action**	**Characteristics**	**Adverse Effects**
Opioids • Codeine • Hydrocodone (Hycodan)	• Suppress the cough centre in the medulla oblongata → suppress coughing • Suppress pain receptors → analgesic effect → ↓ cough reflex	• Low dosage reduces risk of addiction and excessive CNS depression • Commonly administered in syrup form in combination with expectorant	• Nausea and vomiting • Constipation • Weakness, dizziness
Nonopioids • Dextromethorphan (Benylin DM)	• Suppress the cough centre in the medulla oblongata → suppress coughing	• No CNS depression or analgesic effects • Commonly administered in syrup form in combination with expectorant • Available OTC	• Drowsiness • Nausea

CNS, central nervous system; *OTC,* over the counter.

- Reflex irritation of the respiratory passageways as a result of drug-induced irritation of the gastric lining, which leads to stimulation of secretions to liquefy thick mucus
- Drug-induced irritation of the linings of the respiratory passageways stimulates secretions to liquefy thick mucus.
- Ciliary action and coughing expel the liquefied phlegm from the pulmonary system.
- Use includes the treatment of productive cough (in combination with an antitussive) and inflammatory conditions of the upper respiratory tract that produce excess secretions, such as pharyngitis and the common cold.

Common Preparations

- Guaifenesin (Robitussin, Benylin E)
- Potassium iodide

Adverse Effects of Expectorant Agents

- Minimal adverse effects
- Nausea and vomiting
- GI irritation
- Iodism (potassium iodide)

Nursing Considerations Relating to Expectorants

- Increase fluid intake to assist in liquefying mucus.
- Observe for adverse effects, including those relating to antitussives.

Decongestants

Decongestants are drugs used to relieve upper airway congestion, primarily nasal, which is caused by swollen mucous membranes irritated by conditions such as allergic rhinitis and the common cold. Many of these preparations may be obtained as OTC drugs. Preparations may be oral, inhalation sprays, or nose drops.

Common Decongestant Agents

Common sympathomimetics. These products act by producing local vasoconstriction, which decreases blood flow to irritated and dilated capillaries in the mucous lining of the nasal passages and sinus cavities, widening airways for improved air entry and drainage. Examples include the following:

- Ephedrine (Vicks Vatronol)
- Oxymetazoline (Neosynephrine, Allerest, Dristan)
- Xylometazoline (Otrivin)
- Pseudoephedrine (Sudafed)—Oral

Topical corticosteroids. Corticosteroids exert an anti-inflammatory action that reduces swelling and improves air entry. Examples are as follows:

- Beclomethasone dipropionate (Beclovent)
- Budesonide (Rhinocort)
- Dexamethasone (Decadron)

Adverse effects of nasal decongestants. Usually, the dose remains topical; therefore, systemic effects are uncommon. Potential effects of sympathomimetics include the following:

- Headache
- Nervousness
- Dry mouth
- Palpitation
- Increased BP
- Urinary retention (as in prostatic hyperplasia)

Potential effects of corticosteroids include the following:

- Nasal irritation
- Nasal itchiness
- Dry mouth
- Oral fungal infections
- Cough

Nursing Considerations Relating to Decongestants

Client teaching points:

- Understand that use of decongestants is cautioned for those who have hypertension, glaucoma, or cardiac disease.
- Increase fluid intake to 2 000–3 000 mL per day, unless contraindicated.
- Take them according to label instructions.
- Ensure correct dosage and frequency.
- Avoid prolonged use of OTC medications.
- If manifestations persist for longer than 1 week, consult a physician.
- Understand that prolonged use may result in rebound congestion.
- Understand whether they are compatible with other medications.
- Monitor for adverse effects and report to a physician.
- Observe for potential adverse effects and, if they arise, discontinue the drugs and report the effects to a physician.

- Teach correct methods for effectively administering nose drops or sprays:
  - Hyperextend the neck when instilling nose drops.
  - Breathe in while instilling spray.
  - Blow the nose gently prior to administering preparation into the nose.

Mucolytics

Mucolytics are specific preparations prescribed to reduce the stickiness and viscosity of pulmonary secretions.

- Action focuses directly on the thick mucus plugs to liquefy and dissolve them, thereby promoting removal of the secretions by ciliary action, suction, postural drainage, and coughing.
- Mucolytics are prescribed for treatment of chronic bronchitis, emphysema, cystic fibrosis, and pneumonia.
- Examples include acetylcysteine (Mucomyst), inhaled by direct instillation or by nebulization, and dornase alfa, which exerts an enzyme action on thick mucus (used primarily for cystic fibrosis).

Adverse Effects of Mucolytics

- Drowsiness
- Rhinorrhea
- Bronchospasm (may occur during treatment)
- Nausea and vomiting

Nursing Considerations Relating to Mucolytics

- Assess the effectiveness of air entry prior to and after therapy.
- Follow directions regarding the preparation and administration of the product.
- Encourage increased intake of fluids to 2 000–3 000 mL per day.
- Encourage the client to cough deeply following treatment to remove secretions.
- Use suction equipment to remove excess liquefied secretions as necessary.
- Administer mouth care following treatment.

Antihistamines

Antihistamines are used to treat a variety of disorders that result in an increase in capillary permeability, constriction of smooth muscle, and increased respiratory secretions. These effects result in swelling and obstruction of respiratory passageways and can occur with allergies.

These drugs act by opposing the action of histamine at the H_1 receptor sites, which leads to a decrease in capillary permeability, the relaxation of bronchial smooth muscle, and reduced secretions, resulting in more open passageways, reduced swelling, and, therefore, improved air entry.

Common Antihistamine Agents

First-generation preparations include the following:

- Diphenhydramine (Benadryl)
- Chlorpheniramine (Chlor-Tripolon)
- Promethazine (Phenergan)

Second-generation preparations include the following:
- Loratadine (Claritin)
- Fexofenadine (Allegra)

Adverse Effects of Antihistamines

Effects vary depending on the preparation; second-generation preparations do not have as sedating an effect as those of the first generation. Possible effects include the following:
- Drowsiness
- Known drug allergies
- Dry mouth
- Urinary retention
- Dizziness, weakness, feeling faint
- Nervousness
- Nausea, vomiting
- Constipation or diarrhea
- Cardiac dysrhythmias, palpitations
- Headache
- Visual disturbances

Nursing Considerations Relating to Antihistamines

- Observe for desired effect and possible side effects.
- Note safety precautions relating to preparations with sedating effects and take caution with activities requiring constant attention.
  Client teaching points:
- Follow directions on dosage and frequency.
- Administer with meals to avoid gastric discomfort.
- Suck candies to relieve dryness in the mouth.
- Report to a physician if manifestations of the condition persist.
- Understand that weakness and drowsiness may occur.
- Consult with a physician before taking sedating products such as alcohol, sleeping pills, analgesics, and so on, which increase drowsiness and weakness.
- Report any unusual adverse effects to a physician.

Corticosteroids

Corticosteroids exert their anti-inflammatory action on the respiratory passageways by suppressing airway inflammation, thereby reducing swelling within the bronchioles, as well as by decreasing mucus production, resulting in less airway obstruction.

These desirable effects are produced by inhibiting the production of histamine, which results in reduced capillary permeability and decreased production of tissue chemicals that cause inflammation. This leads to the suppression of the movement of protein, fluid, and blood cells into interstitial spaces, also reducing swelling and inflammation; corticosteroids also facilitate the action of beta$_2$ adrenergic agonists by increasing the sensitivity of their adrenergic receptors. This classification of drug is commonly prescribed for the treatment of asthma and any other conditions that cause bronchoconstriction.

Corticosteroids may be administered by inhalation, orally, or intravenously. They are not generally effective in relieving acute episodes. The drugs require several hours to produce their desirable effects.

Common Corticosteroid Agents

- Budesonide (Pulmicort) (inhalation)
- Fluticasone (Flovent) (inhalation)
- Hydrocortisone (Solu-Cortef) (IV)
- Prednisone (oral)

Adverse Effects of Corticosteroids

- Gastric irritation
- Hypertension
- Dry mouth
- Cough
- Oral fungal infections
- Adrenal failure at high doses (with systemic doses)
- Fluid retention

Nursing Considerations Relating to Corticosteroids

- Administer oral preparations with meals.
- Observe for desirable and adverse effects (optimal effects may take hours to days).
- Caution against prolonged use and abrupt stoppage of medication due to possible adrenal shutdown.
- Instruct clients to use inhalers as directed and only when necessary; they should avoid overuse.
- Have clients rinse their mouths following each treatment to prevent the development of infection.
- Teach clients to administer the corticosteroid inhaler approximately 15 minutes to half an hour following the use of other inhalers, such as bronchodilators.
- Instruct clients to shake the inhaler prior to administration.
  Client teaching points:
- Employ the proper method for use of inhalers.
- Rest until relief of manifestations is achieved.
- Identify and avoid conditions that promote bronchoconstriction.
- Watch for possible adverse effects and report.
- Employ good mouth care to prevent oral infections.
- Drink plenty of fluids if not contraindicated.
- Do not suddenly discontinue a regularly prescribed oral preparation.
- Understand that medications require a slow "weaning" process when discontinuing.

Bronchodilators

Bronchodilators are used in the treatment of airway-obstructive diseases such as asthma. These agents relax the smooth muscles of the tracheobronchial tree, causing dilation of bronchioles and alveolar ducts, thereby decreasing the resistance to airflow.

Preparations are available in inhalation, oral, and IV forms. Inhalation and IV administration are used to treat acute attacks of bronchoconstriction; oral preparations are used for long-term prevention.

Inhalers

Inhalers or puffers release a small dose of medication into the lungs when discharged. They act topically on the lungs and require smaller doses than medications taken enterally.

Nebulizers

These devices pump compressed air through a solution of the drug, producing a fine mist that can be inhaled through a face mask.

Inhaled corticosteroids are used to prevent and treat asthma. This route reduces the need for oral corticosteroids as the inhaled versions have a direct, local effect on the inflammation in the respiratory system, with the result that systemic steroids are not required.

General Classifications of Bronchodilators

Table 7.14 outlines the different classifications of bronchodilators, their actions, their uses, and their adverse effects. Some bronchodilators may be used in combination with corticosteroids for added and more prolonged effects.

Nursing Considerations Relating to Bronchodilators

- Administer specific medication according to directions (such as dosage, method of administration).

TABLE 7.14 Classifications of Bronchodilators

Classification	Action	Uses	Adverse Effects
Beta Adrenergics • Salbutamol (Ventolin) • Epinephrine (Adrenalin) • Isoproterenol	• Beta adrenergic agents (mainly beta$_2$-agonists) stimulate receptors in the muscle → smooth muscle relaxation within the respiratory tract → dilation of bronchial tree	• Acute attacks and long-term treatment of asthma	• Cardiac dysrhythmias, hypertension, and hypotension • Restlessness, nervousness • Hyperactivity, tremors • Dizziness • Insomnia • Headache • Hyperglycemia • Hypokalemia
Anticholinergics • Ipratropium bromide (Atrovent)	• Anticholinergics block the action of acetylcholine (Ach) in the muscles → smooth muscle relaxation in the respiratory tract → dilation of bronchial tree	• Primarily used to prevent bronchoconstriction • Long-term treatment of asthma	• Hyperactivity • Dry mouth • Dry cough • Dizziness • Insomnia • Anxiety • Gastro-intestinal upset
Xanthine Derivatives • Aminophylline (Phyllocontin) • Theophylline (Theo-dur) • Oxtriphylline (Choledyl elixir)	• Act directly on smooth muscle of bronchi and blood vessels causing relaxation → dilation of bronchial tree • Inhibit release of slow-reacting substances of anaphylaxis (SRSA) and histamine → reduce bronchial swelling and narrowing caused by these two chemicals	• Acute attacks and long-term prevention of bronchoconstriction of asthma attacks	• Cardiac dysrhythmias and hypertension • Tachycardia • Restlessness, nervousness, hyperactivity • Insomnia • Headache • Nausea and vomiting • Gastroesophageal reflux (GERD)
Leukotriene Modifiers • Montelukast (Singulair) • Zafirlukast (Accolate)	• Act as leukotriene receptor antagonists by blocking receptors that control bronchoconstriction, vascular permeability, and mucus secretion → bronchodilation → ↓ frequency and severity of acute asthma attacks	• Long-term prevention of asthma attacks • Ineffective in the treatment of acute asthma attacks • Oral preparations	• Headache • Nausea and vomiting • Gastro-intestinal upset • Liver damage
Mast Cell Stabilizers • Cromolyn sodium • Nedocromil (Alocril)	• Act by stabilizing and reducing the response of mast cells to irritating substances → ↓ release of substances that stimulate inflammation and smooth muscle constriction → maintenance of smooth muscle relaxation • Does not produce bronchodilation	• Prevention of acute asthmatic attacks • Ineffective in alleviating existing bronchospasm • Available in inhalation form	• Dizziness • Headache • Dry cough • Throat discomfort • Nasal inflammation

- Observe for desired effects, relief of respiratory distress, and reduced respiratory rate and chart.
- Observe for adverse effects relating to sympathetic nervous system stimulants, including beta adrenergics, anticholinergics, and xanthines.
- Instruct avoidance of caffeine, smoking, and OTC medications (xanthines).
- Use cautiously with clients who have cardiac, renal, or hepatic disorders.
- Provide a quiet, relaxing environment to reduce stimulation.
- Increase intake of fluids, if not contraindicated.
- When administering medication during an acute attack of bronchoconstriction, institute measures to promote optimal air entry into the lungs, such as a high Fowler's position.
- Ensure the client has basic knowledge about the nature of the condition and the nature of the medications (e.g., dosage, time to be taken, and possible adverse effects).
  Client teaching points:
- Take the medication as prescribed by the prescriber and pharmacist.
- Identify and reduce possible triggers that produce bronchoconstriction.
- Demonstrate how to administer inhaled preparations correctly.
- Take oral medications with food.
- Try to relax and rest during acute attacks.
- Contact a physician immediately if manifestations do not resolve.
- Avoid drinking products that promote bronchoconstriction, such as caffeinated beverages.

- Receive flu vaccinations each year to prevent respiratory manifestations.
- Obtain prescriber advice prior to use of OTC medications.

ANTIMICROBIAL AGENTS

Fig. 7.5 outlines the major antimicrobial agents.

Antimicrobial agents are used to treat a variety of forms of pathogenic organisms capable of infecting the body. In addition to bacteria and viruses, there are a variety of pathogenic fungi, protozoans, and complex, multicellular organisms, such as worms.

Antimicrobial agents have been developed to destroy organisms or groups of organisms depending on the agent's specific chemical nature and action and the nature of the organism. Diagnosis of a particular infection, and the best antimicrobial agent to prescribe for its treatment, is commonly achieved by gathering a specimen from the client for culture and sensitivity tests. The laboratory identifies the organism and its sensitivity to the various antimicrobial agents.

Antibacterial Agents

Antibiotics is the term commonly used to refer to antibacterial drugs. Agents that destroy living organisms are said to be bactericidal, while those that interfere with their development are bacteriostatic. Antibiotics are classified into broad categories based on their chemical structures—sulphonamides, penicillins, cephalosporins, macrolides, fluoroquinolones, aminoglycosides, and tetracyclines—in addition to other miscellaneous categories, and their spectrum of activity (broad spectrum or extended spectrum).

Fig. 7.5 Antimicrobial agents.

The misuse and overprescription of antibiotics have resulted in strains of bacteria resistant to traditional antibiotic therapy. Important current strains include the following:

- Methicillin-resistant *Staphylococcus aureus* (MRSA)
- Vancomycin-resistant *Enterococcus* (VRE)
- Extended-spectrum beta-lactamase-producing *E scherichia coli* (ESBL)

Classification of Antibiotics

Table 7.15 outlines the different classifications of antibiotics, their actions, their characteristics, and their adverse effects.

Antiviral Agents

Viruses can only reproduce within the cells of a host because of their simple cellular structure (they contain only DNA or RNA). Antiviral agents act by inhibiting the entry of the virus into the host cell or by acting on the virus once it has entered the cell.

Antiviral agents most commonly inhibit the virus from replicating, and with the assistance of the body's normal immune system, destruction can then occur. Antiviral agents have been developed to target either DNA-containing viruses (antiviral agents) or viruses containing RNA (antiretroviral agents).

Vaccines and immunoglobulins are probably the best preventive for specific viral diseases. Postexposure prophylaxis (PEP) may protect persons who may have had direct contact with persons with conditions such as influenza A, HIV, or hepatitis B.

Commonly Used Non-HIV Antiviral Agents

- Acyclovir (Zovirax): Herpes zoster, genital herpes
- Amantadine (Dom-Amantadine): Influenza virus

TABLE 7.15 Classifications of Antibiotics

Classification	Action	Characteristics	Adverse Effects
Penicillins ***Natural Penicillins*** • Penicillin G (IV and IM) • Penicillin V (PO) ***Amino Penicillins*** • Amoxicillin (Amoxil) ***Extended-Spectrum Penicillins*** • Piperacillin (IV, IM) ***Penicillinase-Resistant Penicillins*** • Cloxacillin sodium (Nova-Cloxin)	• Interfere with the synthesis of bacterial cell walls	• Bactericidal • Ear, nose, throat, and respiratory tract infections • Broad spectrum • Semisynthetic penicillin • Infections of the ear, nose, throat, respiratory tract, urogenital tract, and skin • Broad spectrum • *E. coli* and other pseudomonal organisms • Staphylococcal infections, except for MRSA	• Hypersensitivity (allergic reactions): urticaria, respiratory difficulty, shock • Diarrhea • Thrombophlebitis (in clients receiving IV penicillin) • Superinfections
Cephalosporins • Structurally and pharmacologically related to penicillin • Derivative of cephalosporin C, produced by fungus and synthetically altered to produce an antibiotic • Cephalexin (Apo-Cephalex)	• Interfere with bacterial cell wall synthesis and bind to penicillin-binding proteins (PBPs) in bacteria cell walls	• Semisynthetic antibiotic • Broad spectrum • Bactericidal • Use with caution as an alternative if client has penicillin allergy • Urinary tract infections (UTIs), respiratory tract infections (RTIs), abdominal infections, septicemia, meningitis, and osteomyelitis	• Diarrhea • Thrombophlebitis • Hyperkalemia • Hypernatremia • Abnormal liver and renal function tests • Secondary infections: oral thrush, genital and anal pruritus, vaginitis, and vaginal discharge • Nephrotoxicity • Antacids, iron, and H_2 receptor antagonists may inhibit absorption
Aminoglycosides • Natural antibiotics • Gentamicin • Neomycin • Streptomycin • Semisynthetic • Amikacin	• Bind to ribosomes and thereby prevent protein synthesis within the bacteria	• Bactericidal • Poorly absorbed orally • Commonly used in combination with other antibiotics • Gram-negative bacteria that cause UTIs, wounds, and septicemias • Mainstay treatment of health care–associated infection • Reserved mainly for use in life-threatening infections	• Dizziness • Headache • Skin rash • Fever • Renal failure • Hearing loss (ototoxicity) • Not favourable for long-term use

TABLE 7.15   Classifications of Antibiotics—cont'd

Classification	Action	Characteristics	Adverse Effects
Fluoroquinolones • Norfloxacin (Noroxin) • Ciprofloxacin (Cipro)	• Inhibit activity of DNA gyrase, an enzyme necessary for replication of bacterial DNA	• Bactericidal • Excellent oral absorption • Used against wide variety of Gram-negative and selective positive bacteria • UTIs, sexually transmitted infections, and RTIs	• GI problems • Headache • Dizziness • Fatigue • Insomnia • Depression • Convulsions • Fever • Blurred vision • Tinnitus • Skin problems • Antacids decrease absorption • Contraindicated with cardiac problems
Macrolides • Erythromycin (Erythrocin) • Azithromycin (Zithromax) • Clarithromycin (Biaxin)	• Inhibit protein synthesis in susceptible bacteria	• Bacteriostatic • Bactericidal in high concentrations • Respiratory and GI tract infections • Sexually transmitted infections, when penicillin, cephalosporins, and tetracycline cannot be used	• GI irritation: nausea, heartburn • Palpitations, chest pain • Headache, dizziness, vertigo • Hepatotoxicity • Skin reactions • Tinnitus, hearing loss • Interacts with rifampin and rifabutin to reduce antibiotic effect and may increase adverse GI effects
Tetracyclines • Natural tetracyclines • Tetracycline (Novo-Tetra) • Semisynthetic tetracyclines • Doxycycline	• Inhibit protein synthesis in susceptible bacteria by binding to a portion of the ribosomes and stopping bacterial growth	• Bacteriostatic • Inhibit growth of many Gram-positive and Gram-negative organisms, some protozoa • Treatment of sexually transmitted infections • Lyme disease • Rickettsia • Chlamydia • *Mycoplasma* organisms	• Do not administer with milk, antacids, or iron salts • Contraindicated in pregnancy, allergies • Tooth discoloration in children (younger than 8 years) • Superinfections • Diarrhea, nausea, abdominal cramps, vomiting • Photosensitivity • Enhance the anticoagulant effect of warfarin
Sulphonamides • Trimethoprim-sulphamethoxazole (Co-Trimoxazole)	• Prevent synthesis of folic acid required by the bacteria for proper synthesis of purines and nucleic acid	• Bacteriostatic • Treat both Gram-positive and Gram-negative bacteria • UTIs, traveller's diarrhea, acute otitis media, and acute exacerbations of chronic bronchitis in adults	• GI irritation • Rash • Photosensitivity • Renal calculi

GI, gastro-intestinal; *IM*, intramuscular; *IV*, intravenous; *MRSA*, methicillin-resistant *Staphylococcus aureus*; *PO*, by mouth.

• Famciclovir (Famvir): Herpes zoster, genital herpes
• Valganciclovir (Valcyte): Cytomegalovirus

Commonly Used Antiretroviral Agents in HIV/AIDS
• Zidovudine (Retrovir)
• Tenofovir (Viread)
• Emtricitabine (Emtriva)
• Raltegravir potassium (Isentress)

Antitubercular Agents
Tuberculosis is caused by *Mycobacterium tuberculosis*, an aerobic bacterium requiring high concentrations of oxygen in order to survive and replicate. The bacterium (tubercle bacillus) is very slow-growing and, after infecting the lungs, may become inactivated and encapsulated by fibrous tissue. Because of this slow growth, monotherapy with the usual antibiotics, such as streptomycin, does not provide effective treatment.

The treatment can be either monotherapy or combination therapy using first-line agents or second-line agents. The prescribed agent will depend on whether the goal is prevention or active treatment.

Common First-Line Agents for the Treatment of Tuberculosis
• Isoniazid (Isotamine)
• Ethambutol (Etibi)
• Rifampin (Rofact)
• Pyrazinamide (Tebrazid)

Common Second-Line Agents for the Treatment of Tuberculosis

- Amikacin sulphate
- Levofloxacin hemihydrate
- Moxifloxacin hydrochloride

Liver damage can result from long-term therapy. Clients should not drink alcohol while on therapy due to alcohol and drug interaction and resultant liver damage.

Antifungal Agents

These drugs are used in the treatment of pathogenic fungal diseases, both systemic and local. Fungal diseases vary from superficial (skin, hair, and nail infections) to systemic (histoplasmosis and opportunistic mycotic diseases, such as aspergillosis and candidiasis).

Few mycotic drugs are available because most drugs that are effective in treating mycotic infections are toxic to human cells. Human cells are similar to fungal cells.

Common Examples of Antifungal Agents

- Amphotericin B (Fungizone): Used to treat systemic infections (candidiasis and histoplasmosis)
- Nystatin (Mycostatin): Used to treat candidiasis of skin and mucous membranes
- Tolnaftate (Tinactin): Used to treat cutaneous mycosis, such as athlete's foot
- Terbinafine hydrochloride (Lamisil): Used to treat athlete's foot (tinea pedis)
- Atovaquone (Mepron): Used to treat *Pneumocystis* pneumonia
- Metronidazole (Flagyl): Used to treat vaginal fungal infections

Antiprotozoal Agents

Antimalarial Agents

These agents are prescribed for the treatment of malaria. The agents are most effective when the malaria parasite is in its nonreproductive stage after entering the human body.

Common antimalarial agents.

- Hydroxychloroquine sulphate (Apo-Hydroxyquine): Used to treat an acute attack or as a preventive
- Primaquine (Aminoquinoline): Effective against malaria in red blood cells and tissue
- Quinine sulphate: Used to treat chloroquine-resistant strains

Other Antiprotozoal Agents

Other protozoal diseases are common to tropical countries. Protozoal diseases encountered in Canada include trichomoniasis and toxoplasmosis. Treatment for these conditions includes the following:

- Atovaquone (Mepron)—Used to treat *Trichomonas* vaginitis
- Metronidazole (Flagyl)—Used to treat toxoplasmosis

Anthelmintic Agents

These agents are used for the treatment of infections caused by worms, including pinworms, tapeworms, flatworms, and roundworms. These organisms are large in size, are sometimes visible to the naked eye, and commonly infest the GI tract. Systemic infections occur with some types of worms, particularly those from the tropics. Medications focus on the specific type of worm infection.

Common Anthelmintic Agents

- Praziquantel (Biltricide)
- Mebendazole (Vermox)

Antiseptics and Disinfectants

Antiseptic Agents

Antiseptic agents may be applied locally for cleansing the skin and mucous membranes. Antiseptics inhibit microbial growth (carbolic acid is bacteriostatic) and at high concentration may kill microbes (e.g., tincture of iodine is bactericidal).

Common Antiseptics

- Chlorhexidine gluconate
- Povidone
- Benzalkonium chloride

Disinfectant Agents

Disinfectants are agents that are applied to nonanimate objects, usually to destroy micro-organisms; for example, glutaraldehyde (Cidex) has a bactericidal effect.

Common Disinfectants

- Iodine
- Hydrogen peroxide
- Formaldehyde

Nursing Considerations Relating to Antimicrobial Agents

- Perform a complete assessment of the client's history of taking antibiotics, including possible allergies, liver or renal disease, culture and sensitivity (C and S) reports, adverse effects previously experienced, and other drugs being taken.
- Take C and S specimens prior to administering the first dose of medication.
- Maintain awareness of contraindications and drug interactions with other medications being taken.
- Administer at the times indicated.
- Administer on an empty stomach if possible, with plenty of liquid.
- Administer for the length of time ordered.
- Monitor the desired effects, such as a reduction in fever or relief of manifestations.
- Monitor the client for possible allergic reactions (skin rash, shortness of breath, etc.) for at least 2 hours following administration.
- Hold medication and report if allergic reactions are observed.
- Monitor for development of superinfections.
- Observe for adverse effects, record, and report.
- Administer IM injections deep intramuscularly to reduce irritation and tissue damage.

- Administer IV preparations according to dilution ordered; monitor the drip rate carefully.
Client teaching points:
- Report any adverse effects immediately.
- Take medications at the times ordered.
- Ensure that the complete prescription is taken to avoid recurrence of infection.
- Take medication with at least one full glass of liquid.
- Wear a MedicAlert bracelet if any allergies were experienced with past antimicrobial use.
- Take medication with food if gastric manifestations occur.
- Learn about potential adverse effects relating to specific preparations, such as photosensitivity with tetracyclines (avoid exposure to sun).
- Avoid taking tetracyclines with dairy products.
- Drink plenty of liquids when taking sulpha drugs to avoid renal calculi.

DRUGS THAT AFFECT THE URINARY SYSTEM

Drugs that affect the urinary system are outlined in Fig. 7.6.

Diuretics

Diuretics are drugs or substances that increase the production and excretion of urine by inhibiting the reabsorption of sodium and water from the nephron filtrate. Various diuretics differ in their chemical structure, the region within the kidneys in which they exert their actions, and their potency. Primary uses of diuretics include the following:

- Hypertension—A reduced circulating fluid volume decreases BP.
- Heart failure—A decreased circulating fluid volume decreases the preload and afterload on the heart.
- Kidney failure—Stimulates optimal functioning of the damaged kidney and reduces retained fluid.
- Liver failure—Reduces retained fluid and wastes (ascites) by stimulating maximum functioning of the kidney.
- Increased intracranial pressure—Removes retained fluids within the brain to relieve pressure.
- For hormonal imbalances that result in the retention of fluid, such as during the premenstrual period and with corticosteroid use.

Classifications of Diuretics

Table 7.16 outlines the different classifications of diuretics, their actions, their uses, and adverse effects.

Combination Drugs

A combination diuretic is the potassium-sparing plus thiazide type, such as the following:
- Spironolactone + hydrochlorothiazide (Aldactazide)
- Triamterene + hydrochlorothiazide (Dyazide)

Nursing Considerations Relating to Diuretics

- Perform a careful assessment of the following:
  - Hydration levels
  - Blood glucose levels
  - Serum electrolyte levels: sodium (Na^+), potassium (K^+), chloride (Cl^-)
  - Vital signs
  - Urine output
  - Relief of fluid overload as manifested by edema and dyspnea
- Ensure that toilet facilities are readily available.
- Be aware that clients may require potassium supplementation based on the class of diuretic and potassium levels.
- Administer with food to avoid gastric irritation.
- Monitor intake and output to assess effects.
Client teaching points:
- Eat foods high in potassium, such as bananas and orange juice.
- Take potassium supplements as ordered with food.
- Take medication in the morning to reduce the need for nocturnal voiding and loss of sleep.
- Fluid restrictions may be necessary.
- Avoid high-sodium foods.
- Avoid beverages with diuretic effects such as caffeine and alcohol as they may produce excess effects.
- Monitor blood glucose levels carefully if taking thiazide or loop diuretics.
- Use caution when rising from a lying to a sitting position due to possible postural hypotension.
- Keep scheduled physicians' visits to monitor progress.
- Report adverse effects immediately to a physician.

Fig. 7.6 Drugs that affect the urinary system.

TABLE 7.16   Classifications of Diuretics

Classification	Action	Uses	Adverse Effects
Carbonic Anhydrase Inhibitors • Acetazolamide (Diamox) • Methazolamide (Neptazane)	• Inhibit the enzyme carbonic anhydrate from promoting the reabsorption of Na^+ from the proximal tubules → water remains in filtrate and is excreted	• Mild diuretic effect • Reduce intraocular pressure in glaucoma • Altitude sickness • Seizures (adjunct with other drugs)	• Drowsiness • Weakness • Visual disturbances • Hyperglycemia • Hypokalemia • Aplastic anemia • Crystalluria
Potent Loop Diuretics • Furosemide (Lasix)	• Block reabsorption of Na^+ and Cl^- in ascending loop of Henle → water remains in filtrate due to change in concentration gradient	• Provide potent and rapid diuresis • Heart failure • Liver failure • Renal disease • Hypertension	• Hypokalemia • Hypocalcemia • Hyperglycemia • Dizziness, headache, blurred vision • Nausea and vomiting • Abdominal pain
Osmotic Diuretics • Mannitol (Osmitrol)	• Filtered by glomerulus but are not reabsorbed → highly concentrated filtrate produced → inhibits reabsorption of water	• Produce large quantity of urine • Increased intracranial pressure • Acute renal failure • Situations requiring rapid reduction in water content (e.g., intraspinal pressure)	• Lung congestion • Seizures • Thrombophlebitis • Headache • Visual disturbances • Tachycardia
Potassium-Sparing Diuretics • Spironolactone (Aldactone) • Triamterene (Dyrenium) • Amiloride (Midamor)	• Inhibit the exchange of Na^+ and K^+ in distal tubules independent of aldosterone → water and Na^+ are excreted; K^+ is retained	• Produce a mild diuretic effect • Hyperaldosteronism • Hypertension • Heart failure	• Dizziness, headache • Hyperkalemia • Abdominal cramps • Nausea, vomiting, and diarrhea • Gynecomastia in men (with long-term use)
Thiazides and Thiazidelike Diuretics • Hydrochlorothiazide (HydroDIURIL) • Chlorothiazide (Diuril) • Metolazone (Zaroxolyn)	• Block reabsorption of Na^+, K^+, and Cl^- in distal tubules → water is retained in tubules and excreted as urine • Arteriole smooth muscle relaxation → ↓ preload and afterload in heart	• Heart failure • Liver failure • Edema due to corticosteroid use or hormonal imbalance	• Hypokalemia • Hypocalcemia • Hyperglycemia • Dizziness, headache • Muscle spasm • Abdominal pain

Cl^-, chloride; K^+, potassium; Na^+, sodium.

• Monitor weight carefully; increased weight is indicative of fluid retention.

Urinary Anaesthetics

These preparations produce relief of the discomfort produced by inflammation or infections of the bladder. They act by coating the lining of the urinary system, particularly the bladder, providing a local analgesic or anaesthetic effects; however, they have no antimicrobial properties.

• An example is phenazopyridine (Pyridium).
• It is important to inform the client that urine will become orange in colour (due to the drug's dye properties). This is normal.
• Clients should be aware of the importance of continuing the concurrent antimicrobial therapy as this medication has no antimicrobial properties.

Smooth Muscle Stimulants (Cholinergics)

Specific cholinergic drugs may be prescribed to relieve urinary retention that is nonobstructive in nature. Cholinergics act by stimulating cholinergic receptors in the bladder, resulting in the contraction of the bladder smooth muscle and micturition. An example is bethanechol (Urecholine).

• Clients should be advised of cholinergic effects.
• Adverse effects include abdominal discomfort, bronchospasm, increased salivation, abdominal cramps, hypotension, and bradycardia.
• Clients should be advised to make position changes slowly to avoid postural hypotension.

VITAMINS AND MINERALS

Vitamins and minerals are outlined in Fig. 7.7.

Vitamins

Vitamins are complex chemical nutrients present in many foods and required in small amounts by the body to facilitate metabolic processes. Of the 13 major vitamins (A, B complex, C, D, E, and K), only D is made by the body. Vitamins function as coenzymes (except the vitamin B group) and

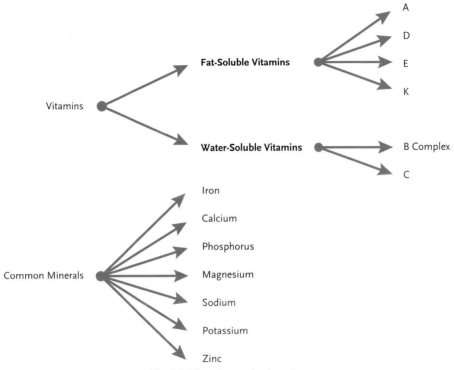

Fig. 7.7 Vitamins and minerals.

as antioxidants (A, C, and E) to neutralize free radicals in the body.

Vitamin Uses

Vitamins are prescribed as supplements for clients with symptoms of vitamin deficiency or for older adults who may be at risk for deficiencies due to restricted diets. Older adults also may have impaired bowel function and high serum cholesterol levels, both of which can affect vitamin absorption. Vitamin D is prescribed for the treatment of osteoporosis.

Vitamin Deficiencies

Deficiencies may occur if intake is lower than the body's requirement. Shortages of the water-soluble vitamins (B and C) are more likely than of the fat-soluble vitamins (A, D, E, and K) because water-soluble vitamins are not stored in the body. Deficiencies of fat-soluble vitamins may occur in the absence of bile. Vitamin K can be depleted within about 10 days.

The body may also be unable to absorb and utilize nutrients. This malabsorption may be due to diseases, such as celiac disease, which affects the absorption of fat, or a lack of the intrinsic factor necessary for the absorption of vitamin B_{12}, causing pernicious anemia. A population also may have vitamin deficiencies due to poor food choices and low income.

Table 7.17 outlines the different vitamins and their dosages, effects, and adverse effects.

Natural Sources of Vitamins

- Brewer's yeast is the best source of B-complex vitamins and many minerals and protects against vitamin D toxicity.
- Liver, beans, meat, eggs, wheat germ, yeast, and dairy products are sources of vitamins.
- Fresh fruits are rich in vitamin C.

Minerals

Minerals are essential in trace amounts for normal metabolic processes. They are usually obtained from a balanced diet. They function as structural components, helping to form healthy bones, teeth, and nails. In addition, minerals function as components of enzymes.

Other major functions for minerals include regulation of water metabolism, blood volume, cell membrane permeability, generation of nerve fibre action potentials, and maintenance of the acid–base balance. A mineral deficiency may be due to the inability to absorb minerals from the diet or a lack in the diet.

Common Mineral Agents

- Ferrous gluconate, iron dextran injection, and ferrous sulphate may be used to treat iron deficiency anemia.
- Magnesium oxide, hydroxide, and sulphate are used to prevent and treat hypomagnesia, hypertension, and convulsion associated with toxemia of pregnancy or acute nephritis in children.
- Potassium chloride (Apo-K, K-Lyte, Slow-K, Micro-K) supplement is used to prevent and treat hypokalemia.
- Sodium chloride injections are given to treat hyponatremia.
- Zinc sulphate (A, D, E, K and pediatric drops) are used to prevent and treat zinc deficiency.
- Multiple mineral electrolytes such as Pedialyte are used to prevent and treat fluid and electrolyte deficiency.

TABLE 7.17   Classifications of Vitamins

Vitamin	Therapeutic Dosage	Effects	Adverse Effects
Water-Soluble Vitamins (Cannot Be Stored by the Body)			
Vitamin B_1 (thiamine)	5–30 mg/day	• Promotes carbohydrate, aerobic metabolism, transmission of nerve impulses	• Restlessness • Pulmonary edema • Hypersensitivity
Vitamin B_2 (riboflavin)	5–30 mg/day	• Acts as catalyst in oxidation of glucose and amino acid	
Vitamin B_3 (niacin)	50–100 mg/day	• Acts as catalyst in the reactions of cholesterol and fats • Causes vasodilation and treats pellagra	• Nausea, vomiting • Flatulence • Jaundice
Vitamin B_6 (pyridoxine)	2–10 mg/day	• Promotes protein, fat, and glucose metabolism and formation of neurotransmitters • Treats neuropathy • Pyridoxine supplements are used to relieve symptoms in women with premenstrual syndrome and neuritis due to treatment with isoniazid for tuberculosis	• Paresthesia • Seizure (these effects are rare)
Vitamin B_9 (folic acid)	IM, IV 0.25–1 mg/day	• Helps in protein synthesis and erythropoiesis	• Altered sleep patterns • Irritability • Depression • Anorexia
Vitamin B_{12} (cyanocobalamin)	1 000–2 000 mcg/day	• Essential for cell growth and reproduction • Treatment for pernicious anemia	• Hypersensitivity
Vitamin C (ascorbic acid)	100–250 mg	• Antioxidant • Promotes collagen formation and tissue repair • High doses of vitamin C help prevent and treat common colds	• Rapid IV administration may lead to fainting • Overdose causes nausea, vomiting, gout attack, and renal stones
Fat-Soluble Vitamins (Can Be Stored by the Body)			
Vitamin A (retinol)	10 000–20 000 IU and up to 500 000 IU daily	• Derivates of vitamin A (retinoids) are used to treat severe acne	• Anorexia • Vomiting • Irritability • Muscle pain
Vitamin D (cholecalciferol)	400–600 IU daily	• Required for absorption and use of calcium and phosphorus by the body • Used to treat calcium deficiencies (e.g., osteoporosis)	• Dehydration • Vomiting • Decreased appetite (anorexia) • Irritability • Constipation • Fatigue
Vitamin E (tocopherol)	60–75 IU daily	• Antioxidant	• Fatigue • Nausea • Blurred vision • Diarrhea
Vitamin K (phylloquinone, menaquinones)	90 mcg daily	• Necessary for normal clotting of blood • Used to treat deficiencies resulting in bleeding, petechiae, or bruising	• Can increase coagulation in clients taking warfarin

IM, intramuscular; *IV*, intravenous.

- Calcium is used to treat deficiency and tetany in newborns.
- Phosphorus may be given to treat a deficiency, although this is rare.

Effects of Deficiency or Excess of Mineral Agents

- Hypernatremia (serum levels >145 mmol/L) causes electrolyte imbalance, nausea, and vomiting.
- Hyponatremia (serum levels <135 mmol/L) may cause nausea and abdominal cramps, as well as cerebral edema (mental deterioration).
- Hyperkalemia (serum levels >5.5 mmol/L) causes hypotension, muscle weakness, nausea, and diarrhea.
- Hypokalemia (serum levels <3.5 mmol/L) causes cardiac arrhythmias, muscle weakness, nausea, vomiting, and delayed gastric emptying.

- Hypercalcemia (serum levels >2.75 mmol/L) may cause muscle weakness and headache, even confusion and coma.
- Hypocalcemia (serum levels <2.25 mmol/L) causes tetany, seizures, mental changes, and delayed ventricular repolarization.
- Excess iron causes diarrhea or constipation, vomiting, and dark stool.
- Iron deficiency causes tachycardia, brittle nails, and glossitis.

Nursing Considerations Relating to Minerals

- Teach clients that iron should be administered with citrus or fruit juice to enhance absorption.

- When administering liquid iron preparations, have the client use a straw to avoid tooth discoloration.
- Encourage clients to take iron preparations with food to avoid gastric irritation.
- Teach clients that phosphorus capsules should not be swallowed but broken to dissolve powder in water.
- Monitor clients' sodium and potassium serum levels for desired effects and overdose effects.

PRACTICE QUESTIONS

Case 1

Mrs. Mabel Hawkins, 73 years of age, has been admitted to hospital with heart failure (HF). She is prescribed several medications, including digoxin (Lanoxin). Her condition is monitored to assess the effects of the drug therapy.

Questions 1–5 refer to this situation.

1. Mrs. Hawkins asks the practical nurse why her heart rate must be taken prior to giving her the "heart pill" (digoxin). Which of the following statements would be the practical nurse's best response?
   1. "I will make adjustments in the dosage of the drug depending on what your heart rate is."
   2. "I do not need to give you the drug if your heart rate is normal."
   3. "I will only give you half the dosage if your heart rate is less than 60 beats per minute."
   4. "I will not give the drug and report to the doctor if your heart rate is below the normal rate of 60."
2. Mrs. Hawkins is receiving the diuretic furosemide (Lasix), 40 mg by mouth daily. What is the most appropriate time of day to administer this medication?
   1. Just before bedtime
   2. Any time during the day but always at the same time in order to space the doses
   3. In the morning
   4. With food, preferably the midday meal
3. Mrs. Hawkins is ordered the potassium supplement Slow-K 600 mg twice daily. What is the purpose of administering this medication?
   1. To replace potassium losses produced by the furosemide
   2. To promote the effects of the diuretic
   3. To help facilitate nerve impulse conduction within the heart
   4. To prevent adverse effects produced by digoxin
4. Mrs. Hawkins is scheduled for discharge from the hospital. She has been prescribed nitroglycerine in the form of a dermal patch and sublingual spray. Which of the following should the practical nurse teach Mrs. Hawkins concerning the correct use of nitroglycerine dermal patches?

1. Apply a patch once a day for 1 hour to ensure that the medication gets absorbed through the skin.
2. Apply each patch daily to the same area of skin to maximize absorption.
3. Remove the old patch and cleanse the area, then apply a new patch to a different area of skin.
4. Massage the area of skin around the patch to stimulate absorption of the medication.

5. What directions should the practical nurse provide to Mrs. Hawkins regarding the use of her nitroglycerine sublingual spray when she experiences angina pectoris?
   1. Spray under the tongue at 5-minute intervals. Continue the procedure until the pain subsides.
   2. Spray under the tongue. If pain continues, spray an additional time for better absorption.
   3. Spray under the tongue. If the pain is not relieved, apply a nitroglycerine patch to the skin to help facilitate the action of the spray.
   4. Spray once under the tongue at 5-minute intervals to a maximum of three times. If the pain continues, seek medical attention.

Case 2

Leslie, a nurse educator in the diabetes clinic, is teaching new practical nurses on a medical unit about type 2 diabetes and the use of insulin. He provides client scenarios for the practical nurses and asks them to "brainstorm" answers as a group.

Questions 6 and 7 refer to this case.

6. The first client scenario involves Mr. B., a client who is taking regular and NPH insulin. Regular insulin has an onset of 30–60 minutes and a peak of 2–4 hours. NPH insulin has an onset of 1–2 hours, a peak of 6–12 hours, and a duration of action of approximately 18 hours. If Mr. B. is given a combination of regular and NPH insulin at 0730 hours, when might he require another injection of insulin?
   1. Noon
   2. Mid-morning
   3. Mid-afternoon
   4. Bedtime

7. Another client scenario concerns Ms. A., who is receiving Novolin 30/70. Novolin 30/70 is a mixture of regular insulin (onset: 0.5–1 hours, peak: 2–4 hours, duration: 5–8 hours) and isophane insulin (onset: 1–3 hours, peak: 5–8 hours, duration: up to 18 hours). The practical nurse is concerned about hypoglycemia. When would hypoglycemia most likely occur?
   1. Between 0.5–1 hours and 2–3 hours after administering the insulin
   2. Between 2–4 hours and 5–8 hours after administering the insulin
   3. Between 5–8 hours and 18 hours after administering the insulin
   4. After 18 hours following the administration of the insulin

Case 3

Robert Melnick has been experiencing gastric discomfort for several months. His physician prescribes several medications, including H_2 receptor antagonists and simethicone, to alleviate the discomfort. The practical nurse teaches Mr. Melnick about his medications.

Questions 8 and 9 refer to this case.

8. The practical nurse is not familiar with H_2 receptor antagonists and asks the pharmacist for information. What would the pharmacist explain about the action of H_2 receptor antagonists?
   1. They neutralize excess hydrochloric acid (HCl) that has been secreted into the stomach.
   2. They compete with histamine for binding sites on the surface of parietal cells and block hydrogen ion (H^+) secretion.
   3. They inhibit the secretion of the digestive enzyme pepsin into the stomach.
   4. They combine with, and convert, HCl in the stomach to a salt and water.

9. What would the practical nurse explain to Mr. Melnick about the desirable effect of simethicone for the relief of gastro-intestinal distress?
   1. It stimulates peristalsis.
   2. It reduces gas distension.
   3. It prevents diarrhea.
   4. It absorbs excess HCl.

Case 4

Francesca, a student practical nurse, has read about how overprescribing of antibiotics has led to multiple drug-resistant pathogens. She asks the practical nurse for more information about antibiotics.

Questions 10 and 11 refer to this case.

10. Francesca asks the practical nurse, "What is meant by the term 'narrow-spectrum antibiotic agent'?" Which of the following would be a correct response by the practical nurse?
    1. An antimicrobial that is effective only against bacteria
    2. An antimicrobial that has a narrow therapeutic index
    3. An antimicrobial that can only be given in very small doses because of toxicity concerns
    4. An antimicrobial that is mainly effective against a few Gram-positive or Gram-negative bacteria

11. Francesca and the practical nurse discuss the treatment of infections for which antibiotics are not useful. For which of the following conditions is antibiotic treatment not indicated?
    1. Chlamydia
    2. *E. coli* infection
    3. Gonorrhea
    4. Influenza A and B

Independent Questions

Questions 12–25 do not refer to a particular case.

12. Mr. Simmons has just developed acute renal failure. What is the safest action by the practical nurse regarding administration of his prescribed medications?
    1. Plan to administer lower doses of the medications due to the decreased ability of the kidneys to eliminate the drugs.
    2. Consider administering higher doses of the medications to promote more effective elimination of the drugs.
    3. Have his prescribed medications and doses reviewed by the prescriber and pharmacist prior to administering the drugs.
    4. Do not administer any medications that are known to be eliminated through the kidneys.

13. Which of the following nursing considerations should be addressed prior to the administration of morphine sulphate (morphine) to Mr. Shafikhani, who is experiencing pain associated with his terminal colorectal cancer?
    1. Assess the requirement for an antiemetic to be administered at the same time as the morphine to prevent nausea or vomiting, or both.
    2. Administer the lowest dose of the range of morphine that has been prescribed by the physician.
    3. Assess the client for any previous history of narcotic abuse prior to administering the medication.
    4. Withhold administering the morphine if Mr. Shafikhani's respiratory rate is less than 15 respirations per minute.

14. What should the practical nurse teach Ms. Porter about a possible adverse effect of taking an oral anticoagulant drug such as warfarin (Coumadin)?
    1. Bruising, or bleeding from her gums from hemorrhage
    2. Pain and edema in her lower legs from blood clots
    3. Shortness of breath from emboli formation
    4. Chest pain from a coronary thrombosis

15. What is the primary therapeutic goal of antilipemic therapy?
    1. To lower the serum low-density lipoprotein (LDL) cholesterol levels
    2. To lower the serum high-density lipoprotein (HDL) cholesterol levels

3. To raise the serum LDL cholesterol levels
4. To raise the serum HDL cholesterol levels

16. Mr. Michael, age 40 years, has been taking the antiadrenergic drug clonidine (Dixarit) for 5 months. His blood pressure (BP) has been normal for the last 2 months. He tells the practical nurse that he would like to stop taking the drug. What is the correct advice for the practical nurse to give him?
    1. "Since your BP is normal, you may stop the drug and watch for signs of hypertension."
    2. "You may stop the drug for a month and then return to your physician for a checkup."
    3. "You may stop the drug if you decide to exercise and restrict your salt intake."
    4. "This drug should not be stopped suddenly; let's discuss it with the prescriber."

17. Ms. Dupont has been prescribed an opioid analgesic for postoperative pain. The practical nurse checks Ms. Dupont's medical history, knowing this medication is contraindicated in which disorder?
    1. Renal insufficiency
    2. Severe chronic obstructive pulmonary disease
    3. Liver disease
    4. Diabetes mellitus

18. Ms. Stellars has osteoarthritis and has heard that cyclo-oxygenase-2 (COX-2) inhibitors such as celecoxib would be beneficial for her. She believes she may be pregnant and asks the practical nurse whether she should take celecoxib. What should the practical nurse advise?
    1. "This drug is considered to be a nonsteroidal anti-inflammatory drug (NSAID) and is safe during pregnancy."
    2. "Celecoxib may cause gastro-intestinal distress and so should be avoided during pregnancy."
    3. "Women must never take any drugs during the first 3 months of pregnancy."
    4. "COX-2 inhibitors such as celecoxib have definite risks for the fetus, so you should discuss this with your physician."

19. Ronnie, age 5 years, has been diagnosed with attention-deficit/hyperactive disorder (ADHD). His parents have resisted drug therapy, but his behavioural problems have brought them to the clinic to ask the practical nurse about "that drug that they give all the hyper kids." Which of the following medications is commonly used to treat ADHD?
    1. Chlordiazepoxide (Librium)
    2. Lithium (Carbolith)
    3. Methylphenidate (Ritalin)
    4. Phenobarbital (Luminal)

20. How would the action and effect of a drug that is metabolized by the liver be affected in a client with severe cirrhosis of the liver?
    1. The rate of the excretion of the drug will increase.
    2. The duration of the action of the drug will decrease.
    3. The action and effects of the drug on body cells will be blocked—hence no effect.
    4. The action and effects of the drug on the body will be prolonged.

21. A practical nurse works in a long-term care facility where she is the medication nurse for the residents. Which of the following factors will the practical nurse take into consideration when administering drugs to older adults?
    1. Older adults require higher dosages to compensate for degenerative changes in the liver.
    2. Older adults require more frequent dose administration because of high levels of excretion by the kidneys.
    3. Older adults require lower doses due to reduced function of body organs.
    4. With older adults, the parenteral route is preferable due to less efficient absorption from the gastro-intestinal system.

22. Which of the following classifications of drugs would be prescribed for the treatment of depression?
    1. Barbiturates
    2. Antianxiolytics
    3. Selective serotonin reuptake inhibitors (SSRIs)
    4. Cholinergic agonists

23. Why do individuals who have been treated with cortisone preparations for an extended period of time have an increased risk of developing infections?
    1. Cortisone attracts microbes into the body.
    2. Cortisone suppresses the body's normal immune response.
    3. Cortisone therapy suppresses the body's natural bacteria.
    4. Cortisone causes increased capillary permeability.

24. Which of the following medications is an antiretroviral drug used in the treatment of HIV?
    1. Raltegravir (Isentress)
    2. Valganciclovir (Valcyte)
    3. Amantadine
    4. Acyclovir (Zovirax)

25. Which of the following should be taught to a client who is taking isoniazid (INH)?
    1. Urine and saliva may be reddish-orange in colour.
    2. Avoid alcohol to limit the danger of hepatic damage.
    3. Clients will need to have weekly chest X-rays.
    4. Take with an antacid to reduce gastric distress.

REFERENCES

Food and Drugs Act, RSC, 1985, c. F-27. Retrieved from http://laws-lois.justice.gc.ca/eng/acts/f-27/page-1.html.

Government of Canada. (2015). Drug Product Database (DPD). Retrieved from https://www.canada.ca/en/health-canada/services/drugs-health-products/drug-products/drug-product-database/terminology.html.

BIBLIOGRAPHY

Canadian Pharmacists Association. (2012). *Guide to drugs in Canada* (4th ed.). Toronto: Dorling Kindersley.

Clayton, B. D., & Willihnganz, M. J. (2017). *Basic pharmacology for nurses* (17th ed.). St. Louis: Elsevier.

Cowan, M. K., & Talaro, K. P. (2006). *Microbiology: A system approach.* Toronto: McGraw-Hill.

Edmunds, M. W. (2016). *Introduction to clinical pharmacology* (8th ed.). St. Louis: Mosby.

Fortinash, K. M., & Holoday-Worret, P. A. (2012). *Psychiatric mental health nursing* (5th ed.). St. Louis: Mosby.

Karch, A. M. (2017). *Focus on nursing pharmacology* (7th ed.). Philadelphia: Wolters Kluwer.

Lilley, L. L., Harrington, S., Snyder, J. S., et al. (2017). *Pharmacology for Canadian health care practice* (3rd ed.). Toronto: Elsevier.

Nix, S. (2017). *Williams' basic nutrition & diet therapy* (15th ed.). St. Louis: Elsevier.

O'Toole, M. T. (Ed.). (2017). *Mosby's dictionary of medicine, nursing & health professions* (10th ed.). St. Louis: Elsevier.

Skidmore-Roth, L. (2017). *Mosby's drug guide for nursing students* (12th ed.). St. Louis: Elsevier.

VanMeter, K. C., & Hubert, R. J. (2016). *Microbiology for the healthcare professional* (2nd ed.). St. Louis: Elsevier.

WEB SITES

- **Canadian Pharmacists Association** (http://www.pharmacists.ca): There are many useful medication-related resources on this site, which has sections for health professionals and for the general public.
- **Health Canada: Drug Product Database** (https://www.canada.ca/en/health-canada/services/drugs-health-products/drug-products/drug-product-database.html): This site has updated drug advisories, describes the drug regulation process, and contains other information for health care providers and consumers.
- **Health Canada: Therapeutic Products Directorate** (https://www.canada.ca/en/health-canada/corporate/about-health-canada/branches-agencies/health-products-food-branch/therapeutic-products-directorate.html): The Therapeutic Products Directorate is the government body that regulates therapeutic products, including drugs, in Canada.
- **medSask** (https://medsask.usask.ca): This University of Saskatchewan site has a vast amount of resources and links concerning drugs, immunization, and health and pharmaceutical organizations.

Medical-Surgical Nursing

> In Canada, our general population is aging and more people are developing chronic illnesses and disabilities that require skilled nursing intervention. Practical nursing education requires students to synthesize and critically analyze knowledge in order to provide and promote holistic care to this growing sector of the population. With this point in mind, the following chapter provides a condensed summary of many medical and surgical topics to help students build on the knowledge and skills they will need to promote health, facilitate recovery from injury or illness, and provide support with coping with chronic illness and disability.

FLUID AND ELECTROLYTE IMBALANCES

Homeostasis

Homeostasis is the state of equilibrium in the internal environment of the body. Body fluids and electrolytes play an important role in homeostasis. Water is the primary component of body fluids and serves many functions:

- Transporting nutrients and oxygen
- Transporting waste
- Providing a medium for metabolic reactions
- Insulating and helping to regulate temperature
- Providing form and substance to body tissues
- Providing lubrication

Water accounts for 60% of body weight in an adult and 70–80% of body weight in an infant. Water content will vary with gender, body mass, and age. Fatty tissue has less water content. Insensible water loss is unavoidable, immeasurable water loss. Continuous water loss by evaporation occurs through the skin as insensible perspiration, a nonvisible form of water loss. Another example of insensible water loss is the water lost via respirations. Sensible water loss is observable and measurable, such as water lost in urine.

Electrolytes are substances that dissociate in solutions and are referred to as *ions*. Cations are positively charged electrolytes such as sodium (Na^+). Anions are negatively charged electrolytes such as chloride (Cl^-). Electrolytes help regulate water and the acid–base balance. They contribute to enzyme reactions and are essential to neuromuscular activity.

The following terms relate to the mechanisms controlling fluid and electrolyte movement:

- Diffusion and facilitated diffusion
- Active transport
- Osmosis, filtration, and osmotic pressure
- Tonicity, isotonic, hypertonic, and hypotonic
- Hypovolemia and hypervolemia
- Dehydration and edema

Fluid Shifting

Fluid in the body is divided into different compartments. See Table 8.1 for an explanation of body fluid compartments and fluid spacing.

The amount and direction of fluid movement within the capillaries are determined by the following:

- Capillary hydrostatic pressure
- Plasma osmotic pressure
- Interstitial hydrostatic pressure
- Interstitial osmotic pressure
  Edema occurs when
- Fluid shifts from the plasma to the interstitial fluid.
- There is an elevation of capillary hydrostatic pressure.
- There is a decrease in plasma osmotic pressure.
- There is elevation of interstitial osmotic pressure.
  Fluid is drawn into the plasma space when
- There is an increase in plasma osmotic pressure that causes the fluid to move from the interstitial space to the plasma.
- Osmoreceptors in the hypothalamus sense a fluid deficit or an increase in plasma osmolarity, or both, stimulating the primary regulator, thirst, and the release of antidiuretic hormone (ADH) from the posterior pituitary gland.
- The adrenal cortex releases the mineralocorticoid aldosterone, which has potent sodium-retaining and potassium-excreting capabilities.

The kidneys are the primary organs for regulating fluid and electrolyte balance. The kidneys selectively reabsorb or excrete water and electrolytes. The renal tubules are sites of actions for ADH and aldosterone. Pertaining to cardiac regulation, atrial natriuretic factor (ANF) is released by the cardiac atria in response to increased atrial pressure. ANF causes vasodilation and increased urinary excretion of sodium and water. ANF inhibits the kidneys from releasing the hormone renin.

The gastro-intestinal (GI) tract receives most of the body's water intake, but only small amounts of water are eliminated by the GI tract. About 8 L of fluid is moved in the bowel during an average day; however, only 100–200 mL is lost through feces. Insensible water loss, which occurs via vaporization from the lungs and the skin, accounts for about 900 mL per day. No electrolytes are lost with insensible water

TABLE 8.1 Body Fluid Compartments and Fluid Spacing

Body Compartment and Spacing	Description
Intracellular Fluid (ICF)	• ICF fluid is found within the cell. • ICF comprises about 42% of body weight and is about 30 L in total volume. • The most prevalent cation is potassium (K^+). • The most prevalent anion is phosphate (PO_4^-).
Extracellular fluid (ECF)	• ECF fluid is the fluid that is found between cells (called *interstitial fluid*) and in the plasma space (called *intravascular fluid*). • Interstitial fluid bathes the cells and makes up two-thirds of ECF (ECF comprises about 15% of the body's total fluid volume). • The most prevalent anion is chloride (Cl^-). • The most prevalent cation is sodium (Na^+). • Intravascular fluid makes up the last third of the ECF, which is about 5% or 3 L of the body's total fluid volume.
Transcellular fluid	• Transcellular fluid is a small but important fluid compartment and totals about 1 L. • Transcellular fluid includes cerebrospinal fluid, digestive secretions in the gastro-intestinal tract, and fluid in the pleural spaces, synovial spaces, and peritoneal spaces.
First spacing	• Distribution of fluid in ICF and ECF is within normal limits.
Second spacing	• Abnormal accumulation of fluid within the interstitial space, also known as *edema*
Third spacing	• Fluid accumulates in a part of the body where it is not easily exchanged with ECF. • Fluid shifts from the vascular space into an area where it is not available for any physiological process. • Fluid is trapped and does not participate in normal functions of the ECF. • Weight does not change as the volume is not lost but is shifted to a nonfunctioning area. • This can lead to a decrease in the volume of the intravascular space. • Damage to tissues may result from the high fluid volume within the nonfunctioning space. • Treatment focuses on treating the underlying cause of the shift of fluid by removing the fluid from the third space, replacing fluid within the intravascular space, and maintaining adequate cardiac output.

loss. However, excessive sweating could lead to the loss of both water and electrolytes.

Client History and Fluid and Electrolytes

Many conditions affect the fluid and electrolyte balance, such as diabetes or renal failure. The following conditions and topics should be discussed when taking a client history:

- Medications, such as diuretics, steroids, herbs, and total parenteral nutrition
- Abnormal fluid loss, such as vomiting, diarrhea, and polyuria
- Diet, whether prescribed or client initiated
- Present fluid intake history, including the client's ability to obtain fluids, mobility, and actual amount the client drank

Extracellular Fluid Volume Imbalances

Hypovolemia

Hypovolemia can occur with the loss of normal body fluids, such as in the case of diarrhea, hemorrhage, decreased intake, or plasma loss due to interstitial fluid shift. The cause of the hypovolemia must be identified and treated. Once this is done, replacement fluid may be given either orally or intravenously (IV) with balanced solutions, isotonic sodium chloride, or blood, depending on the cause of the hypovolemia.

Hypervolemia

Hypervolemia may result from the excessive intake of fluids, abnormal retention of fluids, or interstitial loss to plasma fluid shift. Treatment for hypervolemia will depend on the cause of the hypervolemia and may include diuretics, fluid restriction, and sodium restriction.

Nursing Management for Hypovolemia and Hypervolemia

Management of both hypovolemia and hypervolemia includes assessment and monitoring of the following:

- Strict intake and output
- Cardiovascular changes
- Respiratory changes
- Daily weights, which is the best way to monitor fluid balance over time
- Skin and mucous membranes
- Neurological status

Nursing Considerations for the Geriatric Client

Older adults are at significant risk for a fluid volume deficit, which can lead to dehydration and heat stroke. The risk is due to the following:

- The decrease in muscle mass in older adults, which leads to a decrease in total body water

- The thirst response, which can be delayed in older adults
- The skin of older adults, which has less elasticity; and sweat gland atrophy
- A decreased ability to concentrate urine and possible kidney function changes
- Changes in the cardiovascular system and GI tract

Many common problems may affect older adults that can also affect fluid balance. These problems include dehydration, constipation with laxative abuse, and hyperthermia.

Nursing Considerations for the Pediatric Client

Most of the infant's body weight, 70–80%, is made up of fluid. Therefore, infants have a larger amount of extracellular fluid (ECF), where water and electrolyte disturbances can occur more frequently and rapidly. Pediatric clients need more fluid intake and output relative to their size due to the large ECF volume and the following:

- Infants exchange more fluid across capillary membranes daily compared with adults.
- Infants have immature renal function and a greater body surface area, which together have an important effect on metabolism, heat production, and heat loss.

Infants exchange 50% of their body fluids per day, whereas adults exchange one-sixth of their fluids per day. Therefore, pediatric clients have smaller fluid reserves, and the balance can be upset more quickly. Note that an infant is less able to handle large quantities of solute-free water than an older child. Therefore, when an infant is being rehydrated, a solution with electrolytes should be used rather than plain water. Rehydration should proceed slowly with infants.

Electrolytes
Sodium

Sodium (the normal, or reference, range is 135–145 mmol/L) plays a major role in electrolyte balance. This role includes its effect on ECF volume and concentration, the generation and transmission of nerve impulses, and the acid–base balance. Sodium is readily available in a balanced diet and is normally balanced within a healthy individual by the kidneys.

Hypernatremia. Hypernatremia (>145 mmol/L) is elevated serum sodium occurring with water loss or sodium gain. It is rarely seen in people with intact thirst mechanisms. Hypernatremia is caused by hyperosmolality leading to cellular dehydration. Clinical manifestations of hypernatremia include the following:

- Thirst
- Lethargy or agitation
- Disorientation
- Hallucinations
- Seizures
- Coma

Hypernatremia can be produced by nephrogenic diabetes insipidus. Management includes treating the underlying cause, as well as giving oral fluids or an IV solution of 5% dextrose in water, or hypotonic saline. Note that it is important that sodium levels be reduced gradually to avoid cerebral edema.

Hyponatremia. Hyponatremia (<135 mmol/L), a decreased level of serum sodium, can result from a loss of sodium-containing fluids or from excess water. Clinical manifestations include the following:

- Nausea, vomiting, or both
- Anorexia
- Muscle twitching
- Diminished reflexes
- Respiratory arrest
- Headache
- Confusion
- Seizures
- Coma

If hyponatremia is caused by water excess, fluid restriction is needed. If severe symptoms occur, small amounts of IV hypertonic saline solution (3% NaCl) are given. If hyponatremia is associated with abnormal fluid loss, fluid replacement with sodium-containing solution is required.

Potassium

Potassium (3.5–5 mmol/L) is necessary for the transmission and conduction of nerve impulses, the maintenance of normal cardiac rhythm, skeletal muscle contraction, and acid–base balance. Potassium is critical to the action potential of nerves. Normal renal function is needed for the maintenance of potassium balance because the majority of potassium is excreted from the body by the kidneys. The remaining potassium is lost through the bowel and perspiration. Potassium is plentiful in the normal diet of meats, fruits—particularly citrus fruits—green vegetables, and potatoes.

Hyperkalemia. Hyperkalemia (>5 mmol/L), the condition of an excessive amount of potassium in the body, can result from renal failure, potassium-sparing diuretics, an increased intake of potassium from foods high in potassium, tissue destruction, and acidosis. Clinical manifestations can include the following:

- Muscle weakness or paralysis
- Paraesthesias of the face, tongue, feet, and hands
- Nausea
- Ventricular fibrillation or cardiac standstill
- Impaired cardiac depolarization, resulting in a slow heart rate

Management focuses on elimination of the potassium source and potassium from the body through the use of potassium-wasting diuretics, polystyrene sulfonate (Kayexalate), and dialysis. IV insulin may be administered to force potassium from ECF to intracellular fluid (ICF). IV calcium gluconate may be used to reverse the membrane effects of elevated ECF potassium.

Hypokalemia. Hypokalemia (<3.5 mmol/L) can result from the increased secretion of aldosterone, the use of loop diuretics, severe vomiting, or severe diarrhea and is associated with magnesium deficiency. Clinical manifestations include the following:

- Ventricular arrhythmias and impaired repolarization
- Muscle fatigue and weakness
- Cramps

- Decreased GI motility
- Altered airway responsiveness
- Impaired regulation of arterial blood flow
- Hyperglycemia

Management of hypokalemia focuses on replacement of the potassium, either orally or intravenously. In addition, it is important to teach preventive measures, such as eating foods containing adequate amounts of potassium or ingesting potassium supplements when dietary intake is not adequate.

Calcium

Calcium (2.25–2.75 mmol/L) is obtained through food sources. Calcium has an inverse relationship with phosphorus. The majority of calcium is stored in bones. Calcium blocks sodium transport and stabilizes cell membranes. Calcium functions include the transmission of nerve impulses, myocardial contractions, blood clotting, muscle contractions, and the formation of teeth and bones. Calcium is controlled by the parathyroid hormone (PTH). When this hormone is released, it stimulates calcium resorption from the bones. Calcitonin, secreted by the thyroid gland, inhibits the resorption of calcium from the bones. Vitamin D is needed to increase the intestinal absorption of calcium, which is excreted by the intestinal and urinary tracts.

Hypercalcemia. Hypercalcemia (>2.75 mmol/L) can result from hyperparathyroidism, malignancy, vitamin D overdose, and prolonged immobilization. Clinical manifestations of hypercalcemia include the following:
- Confusion, disorientation, and decreased memory
- Fatigue
- Decreased neuromuscular excitability, weakness, and decreased deep tendon reflexes

Management of hypercalcemia includes loop diuretics, hydration with isotonic saline, synthetic calcitonin, and client mobilization.

Hypocalcemia. Hypocalcemia (<2.25 mmol/L) can result from the decreased production of PTH, acute pancreatitis, multiple blood transfusions, alkalosis, and the decreased intake of calcium. Deficiency of vitamin D or insufficient exposure to the sun can cause reduced calcium absorption from the gut. Clinical manifestations include the following:
- Positive Trousseau's sign, which indicates neuroexcitability; a positive sign is indicated if twitching of the hands and fingers occurs when a blood pressure (BP) cuff is inflated 10 mm Hg above the systolic pressure
- A positive Chvostek's sign, which indicates neuroexcitability as well; it is indicated if tapping over the facial nerve (the area below the temple) with a finger causes muscle spasms of the mouth and cheek
- Increased neuromuscular activity; tetany
- Laryngeal stridor, dysphagia, numbness, tingling around the mouth or extremities
- Decreased myocardial contractility

Management of hypocalcemia focuses on treating the cause, replacing the calcium, and ensuring that the intake of vitamin D is adequate.

Phosphate

Phosphate (0.97–1.45 mmol/L) is the primary anion in ICF and is essential for muscle and nerve function, as well as red blood cell (RBC) formation. Along with calcium, phosphate is important in the formation of bones and teeth. It is involved in the acid–base buffering system, adenosine triphosphate (ATP) production, and cellular uptake of glucose. A normal diet, including red meat, fish, poultry, eggs, milk products, and legumes, usually is sufficient for adequate phosphate absorption. However, vitamin D is needed in the absorption of phosphate. The kidneys are the major route of excretion for phosphate.

Hyperphosphatemia. Hyperphosphatemia (>1.45 mmol/L) can result from acute or chronic renal failure, chemotherapy, excessive ingestion of milk or phosphate-containing laxatives, and large doses of vitamin D. Clinical manifestations include the following:
- Hypocalcemia
- Muscle tetany
- Deposition of calcium–phosphate crystals in skin, soft tissue, cornea, viscera, and blood vessels
- Tingling of mouth and fingertips and numbness

Management focuses on identifying and treating the underlying cause, restricting foods and fluids containing phosphorus, and ensuring adequate hydration.

Hypophosphatemia. Hypophosphatemia (<0.97 mmol/L) can result from malnourishment or malabsorption, alcohol withdrawal, and the use of phosphate-binding antacids. Clinical manifestations include the following:
- Central nervous system (CNS) depression, confusion, delirium, and seizures
- Muscle weakness and pain
- Dysrhythmias, cardiomyopathy
- Acute respiratory failure (ARF)

Management includes phosphate replacement.

Magnesium

Magnesium (0.65–1.05 mmol/L) acts directly on the myoneural junction. It is also important for normal cardiac function. About two-thirds of the body's magnesium is stored in the bones, with the remaining one-third in the ICF. The kidneys are the primary route of excretion of magnesium, helping maintain a normal balance of magnesium within the body.

Hypermagnesemia. Hypermagnesemia (>1.05 mmol/L) can result from an increased intake or ingestion of products containing magnesium when renal insufficiency or failure is present. Clinical manifestations include the following:
- Lethargy, drowsiness, somnolence
- Peripheral vasodilation, causing flushing, warm skin, decreased BP, and rhythm disturbances with possible cardiac arrest
- Impaired reflexes
- Possible respiratory arrest

Management focuses on prevention, increased fluids, and IV calcium chloride or calcium gluconate.

Hypomagnesemia. Hypomagnesemia (<0.65 mmol/L) can result from prolonged fasting or starvation, chronic alcoholism, fluid loss, prolonged parenteral nutrition without supplementation, diuretics, osmotic diuretics, or high glucose levels. Hypomagnesemia is a common clinical problem. Clinical manifestations include the following:

- Hyperactive deep tendon reflexes, tremors, and seizures
- Cardiac dysrhythmias, increased heart rate and BP
- Confusion, convulsions, and disorientation

Management focuses on replacement of magnesium orally or intravenously. To prevent hypomagnesemia from occurring, adequate dietary intake of magnesium, including green vegetables, seafood, nuts, and grains, should be encouraged. Table 8.2 summarizes the major serum electrolyte concentrations and the significance of abnormal values.

Intravenous Fluids

IV fluids are used to maintain fluid balance when oral intake is not adequate and to replace fluids and electrolytes when fluid losses have occurred and electrolytes are out of balance. The amount and type of fluid replacement depend on the client's daily maintenance requirements and on any imbalances identified through laboratory work.

IV solutions can be hypotonic, isotonic, or hypertonic. These types of IV solutions are described in Table 8.3.

Acid–Base Balance and Arterial Blood Gases
Regulating Mechanisms to Balance Acid–Base

The proper balance between the acids and bases in the human body is called *acid–base homeostasis*, in other words, the

---

TABLE 8.2 Major Serum Electrolyte Concentrations and Significance of Abnormal Values

Electrolyte	Reference Range	Significance of Abnormal Values
Sodium (Na^+)	136–145 mmol/L	*Elevated:* Hypernatremia; dehydration; kidney disease; hypercortisolism *Low:* Hyponatremia; fluid overload; liver disease; adrenal insufficiency
Potassium (K^+)	3.5–5.1 mmol/L	*Elevated:* Hyperkalemia; dehydration; kidney disease; acidosis; adrenal insufficiency; crush injuries *Low:* Hypokalemia; fluid overload; diuretic therapy; alkalosis; insulin administration; hyperaldosteronism
Calcium (Ca^{2+})	2.10–2.50 mmol/L	*Elevated:* Hypercalcemia; hyperthyroidism; hyperparathyroidism *Low:* Hypocalcemia; vitamin D deficiency; hypothyroidism; hypoparathyroidism; kidney disease; excessive intake of phosphorous-containing foods and drinks
Chloride (Cl^-)	98–106 mmol/L	*Elevated:* Hyperchloremia; metabolic acidosis; respiratory alkalosis; hypercortisolism *Low:* Hypochloremia; fluid overload; excessive vomiting or diarrhea; adrenal insufficiency; diuretic therapy
Magnesium (Mg^{2+})	0.65–1.05 mmol/L	*Elevated:* Hypermagnesemia; kidney disease; hypothyroidism; adrenal insufficiency *Low:* Hypomagnesemia; malnutrition; alcoholism; ketoacidosis

Adapted from Ignatavicius, D. D., Workman, M. L., & Rebar, C. (2018). *Medical-surgical nursing: Concepts for interprofessional collaborative care* (9th ed., p. 164, Table 11.1). St. Louis: Elsevier. Data from Pagana, K., Pagana, T., & Pagana, T. (2017). *Mosby's diagnostic and laboratory test reference* (13th ed.). St. Louis: Mosby; and Pagana, K., Pagana, T., & Pike-MacDonald, S. (2013). *Mosby's Canadian manual of diagnostic and laboratory tests* (Cdn ed.). St. Louis: Mosby.

TABLE 8.3 Intravenous Fluids

Type of Solution	Description
Hypotonic intravenous solution	- It has fewer electrolytes and solutes than plasma and therefore dilute the extracellular fluid (ECF). - Osmosis moves the fluid from ECF to intracellular fluid (ICF), hydrating the cells. - An example of a hypotonic solution is 0.45% NaCl (sodium chloride).
Isotonic intravenous solution	- It has the same tonicity as plasma. - It is given to expand ECF only. - It does not change ICF volume. - Examples of an isotonic solution are 0.9% normal saline (NS) and Ringer's lactate.
Hypertonic intravenous solution	- It contains more electrolytes or solutes than are normally found in plasma. - When intravenous (IV) hypertonic fluid is given, the osmotic pressure within the vessel increases, drawing fluid from the tissues into the vascular system, thereby decreasing fluid within the tissues and increasing fluid in the IV space. - An example of a hypertonic solution is 10% dextrose in water.

body's pH, which must be maintained within a very narrow range. Arterial blood gases (ABGs) provide information about the various concentrations of the gases dissolved in the blood before the blood is distributed to the tissues. pH is the indirect measure of hydrogen (H^+) ion concentration and measures the ratio of base bicarbonate (HCO_3^-) to acid carbon dioxide (CO_2). This ratio is normally 20 : 1. Acids give up (donate) H+ ions, and bases pick up H^+ ions. The body maintains a slightly alkaline pH of 7.34–7.45 in arterial blood.

The three regulating mechanisms to maintain acid–base homeostasis are as follows:

- Chemical buffer regulators
- Respiratory regulators
- Renal regulators

Buffer regulator system. The buffer system comprises the primary chemical regulators that act immediately. They are found in the blood and tissues and include bicarbonate, proteins, and hemoglobin.

Respiratory regulator system. The respiratory system eliminates CO_2 and water (H_2O), which, when joined, are carbonic acid (H_2CO_3), thus eliminating acid from the body through respiration. The respiratory centre within the medulla controls breathing. When the blood has too much carbonic acid in it, the respiratory centre will instruct the lungs to increase the respiratory rate in order to "blow off" the acid.

If the carbonic acid levels are low, the centre will instruct the lungs to decrease the respiratory rate in an effort to conserve carbonic acid. The respiratory regulating system works within minutes to hours to balance acid–base levels.

Renal regulator system. The renal regulator system is the most powerful of the three systems. The kidneys secrete hydrogen ions and reabsorb bicarbonate ions. This activity is increased when the pH is acidotic and decreases when the pH is alkalotic. The renal system responds within hours to days to restore acid–base homeostasis.

Interpreting Blood Gases

Normal ABG values are as follows:

pH	7.35–7.45
PaCO₂	35–45 mm Hg (respiratory component)
HCO₃⁻	21–28 mmol/L (metabolic component)
PaO₂	80–100 mm Hg
SaO₂	96–100% arterial O₂ saturation

HCO_3^-, bicarbonate; *PaCO₂*, partial pressure of carbon dioxide in arterial blood; *PaO₂*, partial pressure of oxygen in arterial blood; *SaO₂*, oxygen saturation.

When interpreting ABGs, the practical nurse must evaluate the pH and determine whether it is acidotic or alkalotic. A value under 7.35 is acidosis; a value above 7.45 is alkalosis.

If there is an abnormality in the pH, the cause must be determined. Next, the respiratory component must be evaluated. If there is a high level of CO_2, above 45 mm Hg, this indicates an elevated level of carbonic acid ($H_2O + CO_2 =$

TABLE 8.4 Blood Gas Summary

Acid–Base Condition	pH Indicator	Respiratory or Metabolic Indicator
Respiratory acidosis	pH is decreased	PaCO₂ is increased
Respiratory alkalosis	pH is increased	PaCO₂ is decreased
Metabolic acidosis	pH is decreased	HCO₃⁻ is decreased
Metabolic alkalosis	pH is increased	HCO₃⁻ is increased

HCO_3^-, bicarbonate; *PaCO₂*, partial pressure of carbon dioxide in arterial blood.

H_2CO_3), and acidosis. If the level is low, below 35 mm Hg, this indicates a low level of carbonic acid (H_2CO_3) and therefore alkalosis.

The metabolic component is determined by looking at the amount of base HCO_3^-. If there is a lot of base, indicated by a reading above 28 mmol/L, then the blood is alkalotic. If there is insufficient base, indicated by a reading below 21 mmol/L, the blood would be acidotic. See the blood gas summary in Table 8.4.

If both respiratory and metabolic components match the pH, a mixed complicated disorder may be present.

The body must maintain the correct pH. The body's regulatory systems will attempt to compensate for respiratory or metabolic problems by adjusting the levels of acid or base to bring the pH back to the normal range. Compensation is evident in ABGs if the pH is normal or near normal and the partial pressure of carbon dioxide (Pco_2) or HCO_3^- is not within normal limits.

Respiratory acidosis occurs when the CO_2 is too high, causing the pH to be low (acidotic). This can be caused by hypoventilation, respiratory failure, pneumonia, pulmonary emboli, or long-standing chronic obstructive pulmonary disease (COPD).

Respiratory alkalosis occurs when the CO_2 is too low, causing the pH to rise above 7.45. It can be caused by the following:

- Hyperventilation
- Extreme anxiety
- High fever
- Sepsis
- Hypoxemia

Metabolic acidosis occurs when the HCO_3^- is low, causing the pH to fall below 7.35. It can be caused by the following:

- Anaerobic metabolism
- Lactic acidosis
- Diabetic ketoacidosis
- Anoxia
- Poisoning
- Overdose

Metabolic alkalosis occurs when the HCO_3^- is high, causing the pH to rise above 7.45. It can be caused by the following:

- Excessive vomiting
- Poisoning or overdose
- Antacid ingestion (most common)

TABLE 8.5 Acid–Base Imbalances

Common Causes	Pathophysiology	Laboratory Findings
Respiratory Acidosis Chronic obstructive pulmonary disease Barbiturate or sedative overdose Chest wall abnormality (e.g., obesity) Severe pneumonia Atelectasis Respiratory muscle weakness (e.g., Guillain-Barré syndrome) Mechanical hypoventilation	CO_2 retention from hypoventilation Compensatory response to HCO_3^- retention by kidney	↓ Plasma pH ↑ PCO_2 HCO_3^- normal (uncompensated) ↑ HCO_3^- (compensated) Urine pH <6 (compensated)
Respiratory Alkalosis Hyperventilation (caused by hypoxia, pulmonary emboli, anxiety, fear, pain, exercise, fever) Stimulated respiratory centre caused by septicemia, encephalitis, brain injury, salicylate poisoning Mechanical hyperventilation	Increased CO_2 excretion from hyperventilation Compensatory response of HCO_3^- excretion by kidney	↑ Plasma pH ↓ PCO_2 HCO_3^- normal (uncompensated) ↓ HCO_3^- (compensated) Urine pH >6 (compensated)
Metabolic Acidosis Diabetic ketoacidosis Lactic acidosis Starvation Severe diarrhea Renal tubular acidosis Renal failure Gastro-intestinal fistulas Shock	Gain of fixed acid, inability to excrete acid, or loss of base Compensatory response of CO_2 excretion by lungs	↓ Plasma pH PCO_2 normal (uncompensated) ↓ PCO_2 (compensated) ↓ HCO_3^- Urine pH <6 (compensated)
Metabolic Alkalosis Severe vomiting Excess gastric suctioning Diuretic therapy* Potassium deficit Excess $NaHCO_3$ intake Excessive mineralocorticoids	Loss of strong acid or gain of base Compensatory response of CO_2 retention by lungs	↑ Plasma pH PCO_2 normal (uncompensated) ↑ PCO_2 (compensated) ↑ HCO_3^- Urine pH >6 (compensated)

*Commonly used diuretics such as thiazides and furosemide are known to produce mild alkalosis by affecting tubular excretion of electrolytes and bicarbonate.

CO_2, carbon dioxide; HCO_3^-, bicarbonate; PCO_2, partial pressure of carbon dioxide.

From Lewis, S. M., Bucher, L., Heitkemper, M. M., et al. (2019). *Medical-surgical nursing in Canada: Assessment and management of clinical problems* (4th Cdn. ed., p. 372, Table 19.12). Milton, ON: Elsevier.

Mixed diagnoses do occur. This mixed picture occurs when the client has multiple system problems and experiences both respiratory and metabolic imbalances.

Hyperkalemia may occur in an acidotic state as the hydrogen ion drives the potassium ion out of the cell into the ECF. Once the acidosis is resolved, the hyperkalemia resolves. Acid–base imbalances are listed in Table 8.5.

IMMUNE SYSTEM DYSFUNCTION

Overview of the Immune System

The immune system has three lines of defence. Chemical and mechanical barriers such as the skin, GI tract, and mucous membranes are the first line of defence. The second line is the inflammatory response, and the third line is the immune response. The immune response is slower to develop as it is more specific and can result in permanent protection.

Central lymphoid organs include the thymus gland and bone marrow. Peripheral lymphoid organs include the tonsils; gut-, genital-, bronchial-, and skin-associated lymphoid tissues; lymph nodes; and spleen (Lewis, Bucher, Heitkemper, et al., 2019). The two immunity classifications are innate (natural) and acquired. Innate immunity is present in a person who has not been in contact with an antigen (a substance that elicits an immune response). Active acquired immunity is the consequence of an invasion of the body by foreign substances, such as microbes, and the subsequent development of antibodies and sensitized lymphocytes. Passive acquired immunity is one in which the host receives antibodies to an antigen, rather than synthesizing them, as with the immunoglobulins passed from mother to fetus.

Humoral immunity is made up of antibody-mediated immunity. This type of immunity is from antibodies that are produced in plasma (differentiated B lymphocytes [B cells]).

B lymphocytes, formed in the bone marrow, will differentiate into plasma cells when activated. These plasma cells will produce antibodies (immunoglobulins IgA, IgG, IgM, IgD, IgE) that will recognize and attack antigens. The primary immune response is seen 4–8 days after the first contact with the antigen. When the individual is exposed to the antigen a second time, a secondary antibody response occurs. This response will occur faster, is stronger, and will last longer than the primary response (Lewis et al., 2019).

Cell-mediated immunity is initiated through specific antigen recognition by T lymphocytes, or T cells. T lymphocytes develop from cells that migrate from the bone marrow to the thymus, where they differentiate. These T cells respond directly to specific targets (antigens). T cytotoxic cells attack antigens on the cell membrane of the foreign pathogens, releasing cytolytic substances that destroy the pathogen. T helper lymphocytes (CD4s) and T suppressor lymphocytes (CD8s) play a role in the regulation of cell-mediated immunity and the humoral antibody response. Natural killer cells (NK cells) are not T or B cells but are large lymphocytes that do not require prior sensitization. NK cells recognize and kill virus-infected cells, tumour cells, and transplanted grafts. Cell-mediated immunity plays an important role against pathogens that survive inside cells, as well as in tumour immunity, fungal infections, the rejection of transplanted tissues, and contact hypersensitivity reactions.

Cells involved in the immune response include mononuclear phagocytes, lymphocytes, including B lymphocytes and all forms of T lymphocytes (T cytotoxic cells, T helper cells, and T suppressor cells), and NK cells. Cytokines are soluble factors secreted by white blood cells (WBCs) and a variety of other cells in the body that act as messengers between the immune cell types.

Inflammation

Inflammation provides protection against the effects of cell injury. Regardless of the injury, the response is the same. The inflammatory agent will be diluted and neutralized, necrotic materials will be removed, and an environment will be established that supports healing and repair. The inflammatory response can be caused by heat, radiation, trauma, chemical injury, microbial injury, ischemic injury, allergens, and normal body fluids. The intensity of the response depends on the extent and severity of the injury and the health of the injured or ill person. The inflammatory response comprises a vascular response and a cellular response.

Vascular Response

After cell injury, the following vascular changes occur:
- Arterioles in the area briefly undergo transient vasoconstriction.
- Histamines and other chemicals are released from the injured cells, resulting in vasodilation.
- Vasodilation and chemical mediators increase capillary permeability, allowing fluid to move from the capillaries to the tissues.

- Initially, fluid is serous but later contains plasma proteins, primarily albumin, which exert oncotic pressure that draws additional fluid from the blood vessels.
- As the plasma protein fibrinogen leaves the blood, it is activated to form fibrin by-products of the injured cells. This fibrin strengthens a blood clot formed by platelets. The purpose of the clot is to ensnare bacteria and prevent them from spreading. The clot also serves as a frame for the healing process (Lewis et al., 2019).

Cellular Response

In the cellular response to an injury, the following events occur:
- Blood flow through capillaries in the injured area slows.
- Neutrophils are first to arrive at the injury site (at 6–12 hours), and they phagocytize (engulf) foreign material and damaged cells.
- Monocytes arrive within 3–7 days after the onset of inflammation. They transform into macrophages, which are necessary for cleaning the area so that healing can occur. Unlike neutrophils, which have a short lifespan, macrophages have a long lifespan, can multiply, and may stay in the damaged tissues for weeks.
- Lymphocytes have a primary role related to humoral and cell-mediated immunity.
- Eosinophils are active during an allergic reaction, releasing chemicals that act to control the effects of histamine and serotonin, as well as phagocytizing allergen–antibody complexes.
- Basophils carry histamine and heparin, which are released during inflammation.
- Chemical mediators include histamine, serotonin, kinins, complement components, fibrinopeptides, prostaglandins, and leukotrienes, as well as cytokines.

The complement system is the primary mediator of the inflammatory response. The most important functions of this system are increased phagocytosis, increased vascular permeability, cellular lysis, and chemotaxis.

Prostaglandins are substances that can be produced from the phospholipids of the cell membranes of most body tissues, including blood cells. Prostaglandins are powerful vasodilators that cause increased permeability. Exudates made up of fluid and leukocytes move from the circulation to the site of injury. The nature and quantity of exudates depend on the type and severity of the injury and the tissues involved (Lewis et al., 2019).

Local clinical manifestations of inflammation include the following:
- Redness
- Heat
- Pain
- Swelling
- Loss of function

Systemic clinical manifestations include the following:
- Leukocytosis with a shift to the left
- Malaise
- Nausea

Understanding Inflammation and Its Treatment

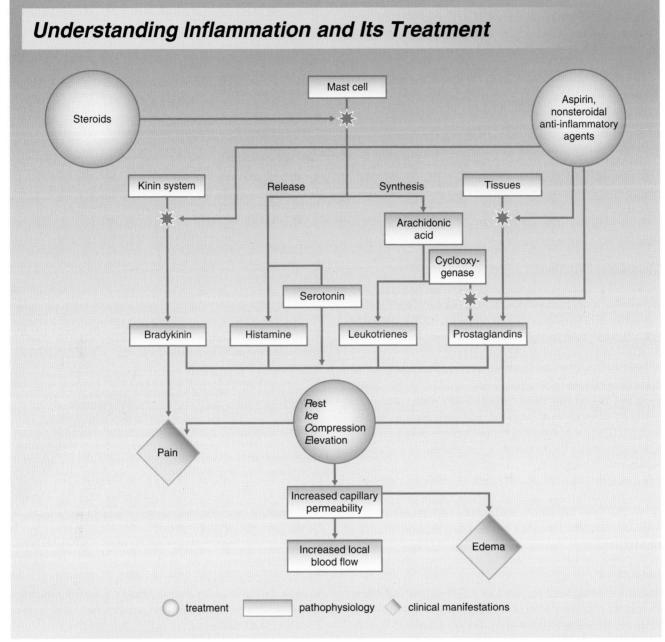

Fig. 8.1 Understanding inflammation and its treatments. (From Black, J. M., & Hawks, J. H. [2009]. *Medical-surgical nursing: Clinical management for positive outcomes* [8th ed., p. 306]. St. Louis: Saunders.)

- Anorexia
- Increased heart rate and respiratory rate
- Fever
  See Fig. 8.1 for more on inflammation and its treatment.

Human Immunodeficiency Virus Infection
Pathophysiology

Human immunodeficiency virus (HIV) is a fragile virus transmitted only through contact with blood, semen, vaginal secretions, and breast milk. The virus can be transmitted during sexual intercourse with an infected partner; through exposure to infected blood, blood products, or needles; or via pregnancy and breastfeeding.

HIV is a retrovirus that binds to specific CD4 receptor sites on the surface of the lymphocytes (also referred to as *T4 cells*) in order to enter the cell.

After the initial infection, there is intense viral replication in the blood (viremia) and widespread dissemination of HIV throughout the body. In some situations, the level of HIV remains low and may continue to remain low for many years. During this period, there may be few clinical symptoms, ranging from none at all to severe flulike symptoms. At this stage, antibodies are not being developed yet, so the client will not test positive for the virus. By the time neutralizing antibodies can be detected, HIV is thriving in the host.

HIV causes immune dysfunction by destroying CD4+ T cells (T helper cells), resulting in a high level of HIV and low CD4 counts in the blood, which are normally above 800 cells/microlitre. The client may now develop the following flulike symptoms:

- Fever
- Swollen lymph glands
- Sore throat
- Headaches
- Malaise
- Nausea
- Muscle and joint pain
- Diarrhea
- Rash

These manifestations usually occur 3 weeks into the acute phase.

Clinical Manifestations

Early chronic infection can last about 10 years and is defined as the stage at which the CD4+ T-lymphocyte counts remain above 500 cells/microlitre. In this stage, the clients often feel relatively well, with symptoms ranging from none to headache, low-grade fever, and night sweats.

Intermediate chronic infection is marked by a drop in the CD4+ T-cell count to 200–500 cells/microlitre. Earlier symptoms become worse. Fever is persistent, night sweats are excessive, diarrhea may be constant, and fatigue is severe. With the CD4 count dropping, opportunistic diseases such as oral hairy leukoplakia, *Candida* infections, and Kaposi's sarcoma may develop.

Late chronic infection, or acquired immune deficiency syndrome (AIDS), has developed when the person infected meets the case definition set out by the World Health Organization (2007). Box 8.1 outlines the diagnostic criteria for AIDS.

Diagnostics

Several screening tests are used to diagnose HIV infection, while other tests are used to assess the stage and severity of the infection. Screening tests for HIV-specific antibodies include the following:

- Enzyme immunoassay (EIA), formerly called *enzyme-linked immunosorbent assay*, is undertaken.
- If the blood is found to be positive for antibodies, the test is repeated.
- If the blood continues to test positive for antibodies, the Western blot or immunofluorescence assay test is done to confirm seropositivity from the EIA test.
- If the blood proves positive in all tests, the individual is considered to be HIV positive.

However, there is a period of up to 2 months during which antibodies may not be detected.

To monitor the stage, severity, and effectiveness of treatment of the HIV infection, CD4+ T-cell counts as well as laboratory tests measuring viral activity are done throughout the course of the infection. Viral load testing counts the number of viral particles in a sample of blood. New "rapid"

BOX 8.1   Diagnostic Criteria for AIDS

AIDS is diagnosed when an individual with HIV develops at least one of these conditions:

- HIV wasting syndrome (*wasting* is defined as a loss of 10% or more of ideal body mass)
- *Pneumocystis* pneumonia
- Recurrent bacterial pneumonia
- Chronic herpes simplex virus infection
- Esophageal candidiasis
- Extrapulmonary tuberculosis
- Kaposi's sarcoma
- Cytomegalovirus disease (other than liver, spleen, or lymph nodes)
- Central nervous system toxoplasmosis
- HIV encephalopathy
- Extrapulmonary cryptococcosis (including meningitis)
- Disseminated non-tuberculous mycobacteria infection
- Progressive multifocal leukoencephalopathy (PML)
- Chronic cryptosporidiosis
- Chronic isosporiasis
- Disseminated mycosis (coccidiomycosis or histoplasmosis)
- Recurrent non-typhoid *Salmonella* bacteremia
- Lymphoma (cerebral or B-cell non-Hodgkin's)
- Invasive cervical carcinoma
- Atypical disseminated leishmaniasis
- Symptomatic HIV-associated nephropathy
- Symptomatic HIV-associated cardiomyopathy

From World Health Organization. (2007). *WHO case definitions of HIV for surveillance and revised clinical staging and immunological classification of HIV-related disease in adults and children.* Geneva, Switzerland: Author. Retrieved from http://www.who.int/hiv/pub/guidelines/HIVstaging150307.pdf.

HIV-antibody tests are now available that provide results in 20 minutes (Lewis et al., 2019).

Therapeutics

Protocols of care change often as new knowledge about both the infection and the treatment develop. However, collaborative management of the HIV-infected person still focuses on monitoring the following:

- HIV disease progression
- Immune function
- Acute retroviral treatment
- Development of opportunistic diseases
- Symptoms
- Preventing or decreasing the complications of treatment

There is no cure for HIV. Therefore, HIV continues for the rest of the client's life, causing increasing physical disability, impaired health, and eventual death. Although there is no cure, signs and symptoms can be managed with treatment.

Primary therapy for HIV infection includes six different types of antiretroviral drugs:

- Protease inhibitors, such as tipranavir (Aptivus), indinavir (Crixivan), nelfinavir (Viracept), and atazanavir (Reyataz).
- Nucleoside reverse transcriptase inhibitors, such as zidovudine (AZT), didanosine (Videx-EC), abacavir (Ziagen), emtricitabine (Emtriva), and lamivudine (3TC)

- Nonnucleoside reverse transcriptase inhibitors, such as nevirapine (Viramune) and delavirdine (Rescriptor)
- Nucleotide reverse transcriptase inhibitors such as tenofovir disoproxil fumarate (Viread)
- Integrase inhibitors, such as dolutegravir (Tivicay) and raltegravir (Isentress)
- Fusion inhibitors, such as enfuvirtide (Fuzeon) and maraviroc (Celsentri)

These drugs are used in various combinations and are designed to suppress the viral replication process. The drugs can be toxic, and the client must be monitored for these toxicities. Other drug therapies used in AIDS include immunomodulatory drugs that are designed to boost the weakened immune system and antimicrobial and antineoplastic agents that are used to combat opportunistic infections and associated cancers.

Health promotion focuses on prevention of HIV by decreasing the risks related to sexual practices, drug use, and perinatal transmission and by encouraging abstinence or safer-sex practices.

The client with HIV/AIDS is likely to develop infections and cancers that will have an effect on his or her ability to cope psychosocially and economically. As with most chronic diseases, most of the nursing care will take place in the client's home. Family members and those people caring for a client with HIV/AIDS need to understand that the client will be anxious, fearful, and depressed at times and may develop a variety of symptoms, such as diarrhea, pain, nausea, vomiting, and fatigue, throughout the course of his or her disease. Symptom management is important.

Some clients may develop metabolic disorders, such as dyslipidemia, insulin resistance, and bone disease. The caregiver must be knowledgeable in assessing the client so that early detection and treatment can take place. Dementia often is present in the final stages of HIV.

Nursing Considerations

Assessment is important in order to identify persons at risk for HIV. Individuals should be asked if they received blood products before 1985 or shared needles, syringes, or other injection equipment with another person. They need to be asked whether they have had sexual experience with their penis, vagina, rectum, or mouth in contact with these areas of another person. Information regarding the client's history of diagnosed sexually transmitted infection is important.

Ongoing health and psychosocial assessment is paramount. Education about HIV should include what the infection is, how it is transmitted, treatment, preventing transmission, improving health, and family planning. Initially, the client may be in denial or shock, so the information needs to be repeated.

Assessment is dependent on the stage of the disease; focuses on prevention, treatment, or terminal-phase care; and must include social factors such as self-esteem, sexuality, family interactions, and finances.

The client should be encouraged to adhere to the drug regimens, to maintain a healthy lifestyle, to prevent opportunistic infections, and, most importantly, to prevent transmission to others. This plan requires developing supportive relationships, encouraging the client to maintain activity, and eventually to come to terms with issues related to living with HIV/AIDS and death and spirituality.

Dementia nursing considerations focus on safety, self-care, and helping caregivers support those activities. Prevent confusion by maintaining a consistent and familiar environment, frequent reorientation, and stress-reduction measures. Emphasis should be placed on providing support to family members and significant others, who may have difficulty dealing with the client's mental and physical deterioration (Lewis et al., 2019).

In the terminal stages of HIV, palliative care is important to provide comfort and support to the client and the family. See the section "End-of-Life Care" for further nursing considerations.

CANCER OVERVIEW

Pathophysiology

Cancer is an umbrella term for a group of disorders in which certain cells grow and multiply uncontrollably. Cancer cells are characterized by the loss of contact inhibition. They have altered recognition and adhesion and altered anchorage-dependent growth, have lost their restrictive point control, and keep on dividing. These cells do not stay put but invade other cells and are viable in blood and lymph fluid.

Cellular differentiation is normally an orderly process in which the cell progresses from a state of immaturity to a state of maturity. Malignant cells do not resemble their parent cells; they take on more of the appearance and some of the behaviours of fetal cells. The appearance of the cell and the degree of differentiation of the cell help classify the cancer. The less differentiated the cell is from the normal cell, the worse the grade of classification is. Normal cellular differentiation is illustrated in Fig. 8.2.

Proto-oncogenes are normal cellular genes that are important regulators of normal cellular processes. Mutations that alter their expression can activate them to act as oncogenes, tumour-inducing genes that promote the development of cancer. Tumour-suppressor genes help suppress the growth of tumours and render mutation inactive. Malignant tumours are able to metastasize, infiltrate, and expand; they frequently recur and have moderate to marked vascularity.

In many cases, the exact cause of cancer is unknown; however, specific factors have been implicated as causing genetic mutations. External stimuli include the following:

- Chemical carcinogens, such as tobacco smoke, arsenic, vinyl chloride benzene, exposure to viruses, and exposure to ultraviolet light
- A diet high in fat and low in fibre, which encourages the development of colon cancer
- Genetic abnormalities that affect the presence of oncogenes, proto-oncogenes, and tumour-suppressor genes

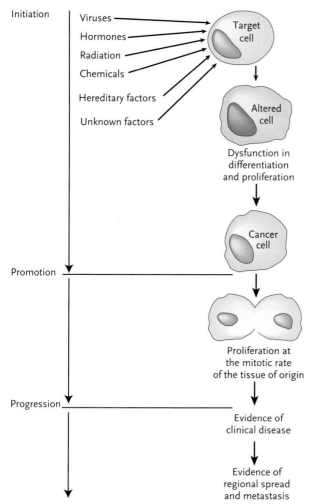

Fig. 8.2 Process of cancer development. (From Lewis, S. M., Bucher, L., Heitkemper, M. M., et al. [2019]. *Medical-surgical nursing in Canada: Assessment and management of clinical problems* [4th Cdn. ed., p. 320, Figure 18-3]. Milton, ON: Elsevier.)

- Chromosomal abnormalities, such as increased number (as in Down syndrome), deletion, translocation, and breakage of chromosomes, have been found to be present with cancer development.

Stages of cancer development. Cancer development follows a three-stage pattern: initiation, promotion, and progression.

First stage: Initiation. The first stage begins with the "initiation," when the mutation of the cell's genetic structure first occurs. Carcinogens can initiate this mutation. This is the event that causes the change in the cell. The cell is still functioning normally but has the potential to develop into a clone of a neoplastic cell (Lewis et al., 2019).

Second stage: Promotion. The promotion stage is characterized by the reversible proliferation of altered cells. A cancer cell is not a health threat unless it can divide. Lifestyle choices such as obesity, diet, and smoking can enhance promotion. If these behaviours improve, the promotion may be

reversible. If not, the initial genetic alteration proceeds to clinical cancer (Lewis et al., 2019).

Third stage: Progression. The progression stage is characterized by the increased growth rate of the tumour, as well as its invasiveness and metastasis. As progression continues, the malignant tumour will develop its own blood supply (angiogenesis). Fig. 8.2 illustrates the process of this development.

The body's immune system will attempt to reject or destroy cancer cells if they are perceived as nonself. This attempt may be inadequate, however, as the cancer cells arise from normal human cells that the immune system may perceive as self. Some cancers cells have changes on their surface, called *tumour-associated antigens* (TAAs). The response to TAAs is termed *immunological surveillance.* Lymphocytes continually check cell surfaces and detect and destroy cells with abnormalities. T cytotoxic cells, NK cells, macrophages, and B lymphocytes are involved. However, there are mechanisms by which cancer cells evade the immune system by suppressing factors that stimulate the T cells. Sometimes weak surface antigens allow cancer cells to "sneak through" surveillance. The cancer cells may develop a tolerance to the immune system. There may be a suppression of the immune response to products secreted by cancer cells, and antibodies that bind with TAAs may be blocked (Lewis et al., 2019).

Children develop different cancers than adults. Pediatric cancers are usually embryonic in origin or due to oncogenes. The child's immune system is less mature, and treatment protocols tend to be much longer than adult treatment protocols. See the section "Cancer" in Chapter 10, page 362.

Clinical Manifestations

Clinical manifestations are dependent on the type of cancer, the stage of its development, and its metastatic progression.

Diagnostics

Diagnosis involves the following:
- History and physical examination
- Blood work
- Tumour markers (oncofetal antigens)
- X-ray, computed tomography (CT), and magnetic resonance imaging (MRI)
- Ultrasonography and nuclear medicine
- Visualization via scopes
- Definitive diagnosis is done by biopsy. A biopsy of the suspected tumour is helpful only if the cancer is going to be treated.

Cancers are classified according to the following:
- Tissue of origin
- Anatomical site
- Degree of differentiation
- How closely the cancer cell resembles its parent cell

Some cancers are classified according to their receptor status, such as breast cancer; chromosomal abnormalities, including chronic myelogenous leukemia (CML), characterized by the Philadelphia chromosome; and tumour markers, such as those present in testicular cancer.

Therapeutics and Nursing Considerations

Cancer treatment goals include cure, in which the cancer is eradicated; control, in which containment of the tumour is attempted to prolong and improve quality of life; and palliation, which focuses on comfort and the relief of symptoms. Factors that determine treatment modality depend on cell type, location and size of the tumour, and extent of the disease. The physiological and psychological status of the client and his or her expressed needs must also determine treatment. Cancer treatment can involve one or more of the following:

- Surgery
- Radiation
- Chemotherapy
- Biological therapy

Surgical therapy is used to cure or control the disease process or for palliative reasons. When surgery is done, a margin of normal tissue surrounding the tumour will be removed, as well as the tumour itself. Preventive measures are used to reduce the risk of surgical seeding of the cancer cells. The usual sites of regional spread may also be removed.

Radiation therapy involves the use of high-energy particles or waves to treat the cancer. When radiation is used, many factors must be considered. The type of cell determines whether radiation will be beneficial. Malignant melanomas are not sensitive to radiation, whereas Hodgkin's disease is highly sensitive to radiation. The cycle of cell division also must be considered. Cells in the mitosis (M) and RNA synthesis (G_2) cycles are more sensitive to radiation than at other times within the cell division process. Well-oxygenated cells, as well as rapidly dividing cells, are more sensitive to radiation. The radiation breaks the chemical bonds in DNA, causing loss of the proliferative capacity. The radiologist will decide on a tumoricidal dose that can be delivered within the limits of tolerance of the surrounding tissues. Radiation is considered local therapy and will affect tissues directly radiated. Radiation can be delivered by external beam (teletherapy) or internal radiation (brachytherapy). Radiolabelled antibodies may also be used. The number of treatments will depend on the type of cancer, extent of the disease, area to be treated, dose, and fractionation, which is the administration of a course of therapeutic treatments planned as a series of fractions of the total prescribed dose. Side effects are related to damage to the normal cells in and around the treatment field. Factors affecting the development of side effects include the following:

- Tumour location
- Dose of radiation needed
- Method of delivery
- Individual factors

The destruction of the cells and the body's attempt to rid itself of the dead cells will cause fatigue. Anorexia may develop. Skin reactions may occur, and precautions should be taken in the proper care of the skin, such as using warm water, mild soap, and no antiperspirant or perfume.

The goal of chemotherapy is to reduce the number of cancer cells in the tumour site(s). Cancer cells are not sensitive to some chemotherapeutic agents when the cell is in the resting phase. Chemotherapy attacks rapidly dividing cells systemically. Because chemotherapy is systemic therapy, the side effects are different from the side effects of radiation. Some chemotherapeutic agents have known side effects, and these should be managed aggressively. Chemotherapeutic agents also have less common, unexpected toxicities, and the client should be carefully assessed to allow for early identification.

Complications of cancer include the following:

- Malnutrition
- Altered taste sensation
- Infection
- Superior vena cava syndrome
- Spinal cord compression
- Third space syndrome
- Syndrome of inappropriate antidiuretic hormone (SIADH)
- Hypercalcemia
- Tumour lysis syndrome
- Cardiac tamponade
- Carotid artery rupture

Leukemia

Pathophysiology

Leukemia is a generalized term used to describe complex cancers of the blood that affect the blood and blood-forming tissues of the bone marrow, lymph system, and spleen. Leukemia results in an accumulation of dysfunctional cells because of loss of regulation in cell division. Most leukemias result as a combination of several genetic and environmental factors, including chromosomal factors, immunological factors, viruses, and exposure to radiation or certain chemicals.

The classification of leukemia is based on the type of WBCs involved and on whether the condition is acute or chronic. Acute leukemia is characterized by the proliferation of immature cells. Chronic leukemia involves more mature forms of WBCs, and the disease onset is more gradual. Acute and chronic leukemias are classified as lymphocytic or myelogenous according to the predominant cell type (Lewis et al., 2019). The four major types of leukemia are as follows:

- Acute myelogenous leukemia (AML)
- Acute lymphocytic leukemia (ALL)
- Chronic myelogenous leukemia (CML)
- Chronic lymphocytic leukemia (CLL)

Clinical Manifestations

The clinical manifestations of leukemia will vary. Essentially, symptoms relate to problems caused by bone marrow failure and the formation of leukemic infiltrates. The leukemic cells will crowd out normal WBCs, RBCs, and platelets, causing anemia with associated fatigue, dyspnea, pallor, frequent infections and flulike symptoms, and bleeding tendencies. As the abnormal WBCs continue to accumulate, they infiltrate the client's organs, leading to splenomegaly, hepatomegaly, lymphadenopathy, bone pain, meningeal irritation, and oral lesions (Lewis et al., 2019).

Diagnostics

The definitive test for leukemia is bone marrow aspiration and biopsy, which will determine the cell type, the type of erythropoiesis, and the maturity of the leukopoietic and erythropoietic cells.

A complete blood count (CBC) will show decreased hemoglobin and hematocrit, a low platelet count, and an abnormal WBC count. A physical examination may reveal lymph node enlargement.

Therapeutics and Nursing Considerations

Treatment of the leukemia is dependent on the type. When possible, treatment will focus on achieving remission. Systemic chemotherapy is used to eradicate leukemic cells and induce remission, restoring normal bone marrow function. The type of chemotherapy will vary with the type of leukemia present. Other treatments may include the following:

- Antibiotics, antifungals, and antivirals to control infections
- Platelet transfusions to prevent bleeding
- Blood or RBC transfusions to treat the anemia
- For some clients, bone marrow transplantation

Hodgkin's Lymphoma
Pathophysiology

Hodgkin's lymphoma is a malignant lymphoma characterized by abnormal gigantic tumour cells called *Reed-Sternberg cells*, which are morphologically unique and thought to develop from immature lymphoid tissue. This lymphatic cancer initially develops in a single lymph node or chain of nodes. The disease then spreads in a predictable manner to nearby lymph tissue. If left unchecked, it will then spread to nonlymph tissue. All organs are susceptible to invasion as the disease progresses. The exact cause of Hodgkin's lymphoma is unclear, although key factors, such as infection with the Epstein–Barr virus, genetic predisposition, and exposure to occupational toxins, could be possible causes (Lewis et al., 2019).

Clinical Manifestations

The onset of Hodgkin's lymphoma is usually insidious. The initial development is most often painless enlargement of one or more lymph nodes. As the disease progresses, the client may experience the following symptoms:

- Pruritus
- Persistent fever
- Night sweats
- Fatigue
- Weight loss
- Malaise
- Headaches
- Changes in mentation
- Seizures (Lewis et al., 2019)

Diagnostics

Biopsy of the enlarged lymph nodes showing the presence of the Reed-Sternberg cell confirms the diagnosis. Other diagnostic tests should be done to rule out any infectious origin for the disease. A bone marrow biopsy will be done to identify the stage of the disease. Other tests will include a chest X-ray and a CT scan of the head, neck, chest, abdomen, and pelvis to look for possible spread of the disease.

Therapeutics and Nursing Considerations

Treatment will depend on the disease stage rather than the histological type and may include chemotherapy, radiation, or both. The prognosis for Hodgkin's lymphoma is better than for many forms of cancer or leukemia. Early-stage Hodgkin's lymphoma has a 10-year survival rate near 90%, and advanced-stage Hodgkin's lymphoma has a 10-year survival rate of more than 50% (Lewis et al., 2014).

RESPIRATORY SYSTEM DYSFUNCTION

Asthma
Pathophysiology

Asthma is a chronic reactive airway disorder that is characterized by chronic inflammation, bronchoconstriction, and bronchial hyper-responsiveness, causing increased mucus production. There is often a family history of asthma, and symptoms can occur seasonally. Asthma is commonly accompanied by nocturnal flare-ups.

Extrinsic asthma results from exposure to sensitizing agents such as pollen, animal dander, house dust, or mould. Intrinsic asthma may result from the following causes:

- Irritants
- Emotional stress
- Fatigue
- Endocrine changes
- Cold temperatures
- Exposure to noxious fumes

Other triggers of asthma include but are not limited to the following:

- Exercise
- Non-steroidal anti-inflammatory drugs (NSAIDs)
- Upper airway infections
- Food dye

The triggers initiate the inflammatory response that contributes to the airway inflammation, mucus production, and bronchoconstriction, all of which cause airway obstruction.

Clinical Manifestations

Symptoms of asthma may include the following:

- Intermittent attacks of dyspnea and wheezing
- Tightness of the chest
- Coughing that is productive of thick, clear, or yellow sputum
- Tachypnea, with the result that the client needs to use the accessory respiratory muscles to breathe
- Orthopnea, with clients sitting upright with shoulders hunched forward

Clients in severe distress may experience diaphoresis, cyanosis, pallor, and diminished breath sounds. Between attacks, the client will breathe normally.

Diagnostics

A history and physical examination revealing dyspnea, wheezing, and coughing are highly suggestive of asthma.

A chest X-ray may reveal hyperinflated lungs with air trapping during an attack. The lungs will look normal when the client is not having an attack. Pulmonary function tests are helpful in determining the extent of the client's asthma.

Therapeutics and Nursing Considerations

Treatment is usually tailored to each client and focuses on identifying and avoiding precipitating allergens and irritants. Primary drug therapy generally includes inhaled bronchodilators and steroids, either alone or in combination.

During an acute attack, respiratory function needs to be monitored closely while attempts are made to relieve the bronchoconstriction and expulsion of mucoid plugs. The client needs close supervision as he or she is likely to be frightened and needs to have constant reassurance. The nursing considerations are as follows:

- Encourage the client to sit in a semi- or high Fowler's position.
- Encourage the client to breathe using the diaphragm.
- Deliver oxygen via nasal prongs.
- Monitor for "silent chest," an indication that the client may be progressing to status asthmaticus.
- Perform a chest assessment before and after bronchodilator inhalations.
- Establish IV therapy to allow medications to be delivered quickly if necessary.
- For severe acute attacks, treatment may include IV salbutamol and hydrocortisone (Solu-Cortef).

Chronic Obstructive Pulmonary Disease
Pathophysiology

COPD is an umbrella term that refers to emphysema and chronic bronchitis, and that is characterized by airflow obstruction. COPD clients may have asthma as well. Exposure to tobacco smoke is the primary cause of COPD. Other risk factors include recurrent or chronic respiratory tract infections, allergies, and familial or hereditary factors, such as alpha-antitrypsin deficiency.

Smoking causes the following complications:
- Nicotine acts as a sympathetic nervous system (SNS) stimulant, causing vasoconstriction and increased heart rate, BP, and cardiac workload.
- Smoking decreases ciliary activity and increases proteolytic enzymes that destroy elastin and collagen and cause cellular hyperplasia. This increases the production of mucus, reduces the airway diameter, and increases the difficulty in clearing secretions.

Emphysema is an abnormal permanent enlargement of the air space distal to the terminal bronchioles accompanied by destruction of alveolar walls without obvious fibrosis. Emphysema pathology includes the following:

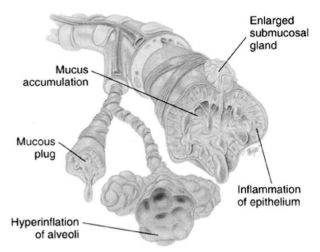

Fig. 8.3 Chronic bronchitis. (From Huether, S., Power-Kean, K., El-Hussein, M. T., et al. [2018]. *Understanding* pathophysiology [Cdn. ed., p. 709, Figure 27-11]. Milton, ON: Elsevier.)

- Hyperinflation of the alveoli
- Destruction of alveolar walls (bullae development)
- Destruction of alveolar capillary walls
- Small airway collapse (air trapping)
- Loss of lung elasticity

Chronic bronchitis is diagnosed when an individual has had a productive cough for three or more months in each of two successive years. Fig. 8.3 illustrates chronic bronchitis. Chronic bronchitis pathology includes the following:

- Hyperplasia of mucus-secreting glands in the trachea and bronchi
- An increase in the goblet cells
- Disappearance of cilia
- Chronic inflammatory changes
- Altered alveolar macrophage function
- Normal alveolar structures and capillaries

Clinical Manifestations

Clinical findings may be absent in the early stages of COPD. As the disease progresses, various symptoms develop depending on the underlying disease entity. Regardless of this underlying entity, progressive airflow obstruction will eventually lead to poor ventilation–perfusion, resulting in hypoxia. The client may experience barrel chest, cyanosis, and clubbing of the fingers and nails. Dyspnea is usually the first symptom to develop. In chronic bronchitis, cough is usually the first symptom to develop. The typical posture of persons with COPD is illustrated in Fig. 8.4. Complications may include the following:

- Polycythemia
- Acidosis
- Pulmonary hypertension
- Cor pulmonale
- Acute respiratory failure

Fig. 8.4 Typical posture of person with chronic obstructive pulmonary disease, primarily emphysema. The person tends to lean forward and uses the accessory muscles of respiration to breathe, forcing the shoulder girdle upward and causing the supraclavicular fossae to retract on inspiration.

BOX 8.2   Huff Coughing

1. The client assumes a sitting position with the neck slightly flexed, shoulders relaxed, knees flexed, forearms supported by a pillow, and, if possible, feet on the floor.
2. The client then drops the head and bends forward while using slow, pursed-lip breathing to exhale.
3. Sitting up again, the client uses diaphragmatic breathing to inhale slowly and deeply.
4. The client repeats steps 2 and 3 three to four times to facilitate the mobilization of secretions.
5. Before initiating a cough, the client should take a deep abdominal breath, bend slightly forward, and then huff cough (cough three to four times on exhalation). The client may need to support or splint his or her thorax or abdomen to achieve maximum effect.

Adapted from Lewis, S. M., Bucher, L., Heitkemper, M. M., et al. (2019). *Medical-surgical nursing in Canada: Assessment and management of clinical problems* (4th Cdn. ed., p. 679, Table 31-18). Milton, ON: Elsevier Canada.

Diagnostics

Diagnosis is based on the history and physical examination. Pulmonary function tests may show an increase in residual volume, total lung capacity, and adherence, with decreased vital capacity, diffusing capacity, and forced expiratory volumes. Blood work may show polycythemia due to the hypoxia. A chest X-ray is not diagnostic for COPD or chronic bronchitis but is often necessary to rule out other conditions.

Therapeutics and Nursing Considerations

Treatment focuses on airway expansion and airway clearance with improved gas exchange. The treatments are as follows:

- Oxygen is administered at low-flow settings to treat hypoxia.
- Antibiotics are prescribed to treat infections.
- Avoidance of smoking or air pollutants is encouraged.
- Bronchodilators are prescribed to relieve bronchospasm and facilitate mucociliary clearance.
- Steroids may be prescribed to reduce inflammation.
- Breathing techniques, such as pursed-lip breathing, are taught to control dyspnea and reduce air trapping.
- Diaphragmatic breathing, breathing using the muscles of the diaphragm rather than the accessory muscles, is also encouraged.

- Often huff coughing is taught to overcome ineffective cough patterns. Huff coughing is summarized in Box 8.2.

Nursing Considerations

Clients with severe COPD expend an increasing amount of energy doing the work of breathing. They can expend 30–50% more energy on breathing than the average person. Eating becomes an effort as a result of dyspnea. A full stomach presses up on the flattened diaphragm, causing increased dyspnea and discomfort. It is difficult for the client to eat and breathe at the same time (Lewis et al., 2019).

- The client will need to be encouraged to rest prior to eating and again after eating.
- Small, frequent meals are easier to tolerate than larger meals.
- Food that causes gas should be avoided.
- In some cases, pureed or blenderized food is easier for the client to tolerate.
- If there are no other medical conditions, the client should be encouraged to drink 3 L of fluid each day. Fluids should be offered between meals so that the client will eat a nutritious meal and then take the fluids.

COPD education focuses on the client maintaining the following:

- Effective airway clearance
- Effective gas exchange
- A balanced diet
- Adequate sleep
- Prevention of infection

In order to accomplish these, the client needs to be encouraged to be as physically active as his or her condition permits: walking each day, practising the breathing exercises, and practising energy-conserving strategies, such as assuming the tripod position (elbows supported on table and chest flexed) when tired. Relaxation techniques can be very beneficial to relieve dyspnea. Appropriate use of medications prior to an activity is helpful. Long-acting theophylline (Theolair) or a long-acting bronchodilator medication may be needed to assist the client during sleep. Oxygen therapy is frequently required for hypoxemia.

Many lifestyle changes may occur during the progression of COPD. Clients may go through the stages of grief as more and more of their normal activities may be lost (Lewis et al., 2019).

Tuberculosis
Pathophysiology

Tuberculosis (TB) is an acute or chronic infection characterized by pulmonary infiltrates and formation of granulomas with caseation, fibrosis, and cavitation. TB is caused by *Mycobacterium-tuberculosis (M. tuberculosis)*. The prevalence of TB decreased in the 1940s and 1950s but resurged after 1985, coinciding with the spread of HIV infections.

TB is more commonly found among individuals who are economically disadvantaged, homeless or living in crowded spaces, malnourished, immuno-compromised, or members of minority groups.

TB infection is spread to others via the following process:
- Droplet nuclei are released when the infected person coughs, sneezes, speaks, or sings.
- Droplets are inhaled by the recipient, and the bacilli are deposited in the lung.
- The immune system responds by sending leukocytes and macrophages to the area, ultimately resulting in encapsulation of the bacilli in the Ghon tubercle.
- At this stage, the client will demonstrate exposure to the TB bacilli via skin testing but does not have an active TB infection.
- If the tubercle and inflamed nodes rupture, the infection contaminates the surrounding tissue and may spread through the blood and lymphatic circulation to distant sites such as the kidneys, epiphyses of bone, cerebral cortex, or adrenal glands.

Clinical Manifestations
- Clients in the early stages of TB are usually asymptomatic.
- Nonspecific symptoms such as fatigue, weakness, anorexia, weight loss, night sweats, and low-grade fever may develop as TB progresses.
- The client may experience cough, productive mucopurulent sputum, and chest pain.
- Hemoptysis develops in advanced cases.

Diagnostics
Definitive diagnosis is made by the following:
- Sputum cultures and stains
- Skin testing, which detects exposure to TB but does not distinguish between exposure and infection
- Chest X-rays, which may show nodular lesions, patchy infiltrates, cavity formation, scar tissue, and calcium deposits but which cannot distinguish between active or inactive TB
- Nucleic acid amplification, a new test that gives results within hours. However, this test does not replace smears and sputum cultures.
- Interferon gamma release assays is a blood test that provides rapid results in 24 hours and is an effective diagnostic tool in certain client populations.

Purified protein derivative (PPD) of tuberculin is used primarily to detect the delayed hypersensitivity immune response of the individual. Two-step testing (the Mantoux test) is recommended for initial testing for healthcare workers. Once a two-step test has been done, follow-up testing only requires the one-step test (Lewis et al., 2019).

Therapeutics and Nursing Considerations

Prevention is very important. If the living conditions of the client cannot be changed, immunization with bacille Calmette-Guérin (BCG) may be given to prevent TB. This is commonly done in the Northwest Territories and Nunavut.

Treatment for TB includes the following:
- Antitubercular therapy usually consists of a combination of at least four drugs that are administered for at least 6 months. The five primary drugs used are isoniazid (INH), rifampin (RMP), pyrazinamide, streptomycin, and ethambutol.
- Combination therapy is used to increase the therapeutic effectiveness and decrease the development of resistant strains of *M. tuberculosis.*
- Newer drugs that are sometimes used include ciprofloxacin (Cipro), ofloxacin (Floxin), sparfloxacin (Zagam), and rifapentine (Priftin), particularly when the client develops complications from one of the earlier antitubercular agents.

The client is taught health practices such as using tissues when coughing or sneezing, discarding the tissues in appropriate garbage containers, and washing hands after each cough and sneeze. Directly observed therapy (DOT) is now being used in many overcrowded areas to help ensure that the client takes the medications as instructed for the length of time they are needed. Nonadherence is a major factor in the emergence of multidrug resistance and treatment failures (Lewis et al., 2019). Latent TB infection occurs when an individual becomes infected with *M. tuberculosis* but does not become acutely ill. INH is generally used to prevent a TB infection from developing into a clinical disease.

Acute Respiratory Distress Syndrome
Pathophysiology

Acute respiratory distress syndrome (ARDS) is a form of pulmonary edema that can lead to acute respiratory failure. ARDS results from the following:
- Increased permeability of alveolocapillary membrane, causing the alveoli to fill with fluid and resulting in severe dyspnea
- Hypoxemia refractory to supplemental oxygen

- Reduced lung compliance
- Diffuse pulmonary infiltrates
- Can result from aspiration
- Infection or sepsis
- Lung trauma
- Head injury
- Embolism
- Oxygen toxicity
- Drug overdose of barbiturates
- Blood transfusion
- Smoke or chemical inhalation
- Pancreatitis uremia
- Near-drowning

Clinical Manifestations

The client will have rapid, shallow breathing, dyspnea, hypoxemia that does not respond to supplemental oxygen, tachycardia, intercostal and suprasternal retractions, crackles, and wheezing. The client will be restless, apprehensive, and then mentally sluggish, with motor dysfunction. As ARDS progresses, it is associated with profound respiratory distress requiring endotracheal intubation and positive pressure ventilation.

Diagnostics

The history and physical examination are important where risk factors can be ascertained. The following symptoms indicate ARDS:

- Acute onset of the distress
- Bilateral pulmonary infiltrates
- Clinical absence of heart failure

Therapeutics and Nursing Considerations

Treatment focuses on correcting the underlying cause of ARDS. Aggressive supportive care is usually required. Clients with ARDS are critically ill and require close monitoring and support.

Atelectasis
Pathophysiology

Atelectasis is a condition of the lungs that may be acute or chronic and that is characterized by collapse of the alveoli. In atelectasis, a blockage impedes the passage of air to and from the alveoli. The trapped alveolar air becomes absorbed into the bloodstream, and without any replacement air, that area of the lung becomes airless and collapses.

The prognosis depends on prompt treatment, including removal of the airway obstruction, relief of hypoxia, and re-expansion of the collapsed area of the lung. Possible causes of atelectasis include the following:

- Bronchial obstruction by excessive secretions, a mucous plug, or a foreign object. This is the most common cause.
- Cancer
- Oxygen toxicity, pulmonary edema, and conditions that inhibit full lung expansion

Clinical Manifestations

Signs and symptoms are variable and may include the following:

- Cough, sputum production, and fever
- In acute atelectasis, respiratory distress is evident, and dyspnea, tachypnea, pleural pain, and central cyanosis may also be present.

Diagnostics

Decreased breath sounds and crackles during auscultation are indicators of atelectasis. A chest X-ray may be done. Pulse oximetry is usually found to be below 90%.

Therapeutics and Nursing Considerations

Strategies to prevent the development of atelectasis and to minimize or treat it by improving ventilation include the following:

- Frequent turning in bed, early ambulation, and deep-breathing exercises
- Coughing or suctioning may be needed to remove secretions that could be causing obstruction.
- Bronchodilators may be ordered to assist with removal of the secretions.
- If a pleural effusion is present, a thoracentesis may be needed to remove fluid from the lung.

Pulmonary Embolism
Pathophysiology

A pulmonary embolism (PE) is an obstruction of a pulmonary artery or a branch of the artery by a thrombus that has developed in the venous circulation or right side of the heart from blood, amniotic fluid, air, fat, bone marrow, or foreign IV material.

- The most common source of the thrombus is the deep veins of the legs.
- The thrombus breaks loose and travels as an embolus until it lodges in the pulmonary vasculature.
- This thrombus can result in complete or partial occlusion of the pulmonary arterial blood flow.
- The lung tissue distal to the embolus is ventilated but not perfused.
- This ventilation–perfusion imbalance leads to an increase in pulmonary arterial pressure. This increases the work of the heart's right ventricle to maintain pulmonary blood flow, which could lead to right-sided heart failure.

Clinical Manifestations

The severity of clinical manifestations of PE depends on the size of the emboli and the size and number of blood vessels occluded. The most common manifestations of PE are as follows:

- Anxiety and the sudden onset of unexplained dyspnea and tachypnea
- Pleuritic chest pain that often mimics angina pain
- Cough, hemoptysis, and crackles
- Fever
- Changes in mentation

A massive embolus may produce sudden collapse of the client, with shock, pallor, severe dyspnea, and crushing chest pain. The pulse is likely to be rapid and weak, and the BP will be low. Death occurs in 60% of clients with massive PE, frequently within the first hour of symptom development.

Diagnostics

Diagnosis is based on the client's history and physical examination. The following tests are done to diagnose the embolism:

- Ventilation–perfusion scan
- Pulmonary angiography
- Chest X-ray
- Electrocardiography (ECG)
- Peripheral and arterial blood studies
- Plethysmography, depending on the amount of time available

Therapeutics and Nursing Considerations

Treatment should be instituted immediately. The objectives of treatment are to prevent further growth or multiplication of thrombi in the lower extremities, to prevent embolization from the upper or lower extremities to the pulmonary vascular system, and to provide cardiopulmonary support if indicated. The following treatments may be needed:

- Oxygen by mask or nasal cannula
- Mechanical ventilation
- Thrombolytic therapy may be used to dissolve clots.
- IV anticoagulant therapy will be initiated to prevent further clots from forming.
- Pulmonary embolectomy may be done in life-threatening situations.
  Nursing care will focus on the following considerations:
- Minimizing the risk for more thrombi development
- Monitoring anticoagulation therapy and thrombolytic therapy
- Managing pain
- Managing oxygen therapy
- Relieving anxiety
- Monitoring for complications
- Educating the client and family regarding ways to prevent further thrombi formation

Pneumothorax
Pathophysiology

A *pneumothorax* is air in the pleural space. There is a resultant complete or partial collapse of a lung due to the accumulation of this air. Pneumothorax may be closed or open and, when associated with trauma, may be accompanied by hemothorax, a condition called *hemopneumothorax*. A closed pneumothorax has no associated external wound. The most common form is a spontaneous pneumothorax, which is accumulation of air in the pleural space without an apparent reason. It is caused by the following conditions:

- Rupture of small blebs on the visceral pleural space
- Trauma
- TB
- COPD

Spontaneous pneumothorax may occasionally occur in lean adolescents and young clients with no apparent precipitating cause.

An open pneumothorax occurs when air enters the pleural space through an opening in the chest wall, such as a stab or gunshot wound. A penetrating chest wound is often referred to as a *sucking chest wound*. A *tension pneumothorax* is a pneumothorax with rapid accumulation of air in the pleural space causing severely high intrapleural pressures with resultant tension on the heart and great vessels. In tension pneumothorax, air that enters the pleural space during expiration does not exit during inspiration.

Clinical Manifestations

Pneumothorax may not produce symptoms in mild cases, but in moderate to severe cases, it may produce the following symptoms:

- Profound respiratory distress
- Weak rapid pulse, pallor, jugular vein distension
- Anxiety
- Severe chest pain accompanied by tachypnea
- Asymmetrical chest wall movement
- Dyspnea, cyanosis, decreased or absent chest sounds, or hyper-resonance on the affected side

Diagnostics

Diagnosis is made from a chest X-ray revealing air in the pleural space and a possible mediastinal shift. ABGs reveal hypoxemia and respiratory alkalosis. ECG changes may be present.

Therapeutics and Nursing Considerations

Treatment depends on the cause and severity of the pneumothorax.

- In mild cases, re-expansion can be achieved using a conservative approach, with bed rest, oxygen therapy, and close monitoring of the client's vital signs.
- In more severe cases, needle aspiration of the pleural space with a large-bore needle may be required.
- The most definitive and common form of treatment is to insert a chest tube and connect it to suction (usually 20 mm Hg suction). Repeated spontaneous pneumothorax may need to be treated surgically by a partial pleurectomy, stapling, or pleurodesis to promote adherence of the pleurae to one another.

Pneumonia
Pathophysiology

Pneumonia is an acute inflammation of the lungs that commonly impairs gas exchange. The inflammatory response causes fluid or blood to fill the lung tissue, creating an excellent environment for pathogens. The invading pathogen starts changing epithelial lung cells to allow it to adhere to the cell wall. The pathogen then destroys the macrophages that travel to the site, resulting in further congestion with decreased lung ventilation.

Pneumonia is more likely to result when

- Defence mechanisms are incompetent or become overwhelmed. Pneumonia is the leading cause of death in debilitated clients.
- There are infecting pathogens, either bacterial or viral, or chemical or other irritants, such as aspirated material.
- There are predisposing factors that increase the risk of pneumonia, including chronic illness, cancer, abdominal and thoracic surgery, atelectasis, aspiration, colds, COPD, smoking, alcoholism, malnutrition, chemotherapy, radiation, and immunosuppressive therapy.
- There is onset in the community or within the first 2 days of hospitalization. This is referred to as *community-acquired pneumonia.*
- Hospital-acquired pneumonia occurs 48 hours or longer after admission.
- The abnormal entry of secretions into the lower airway causes aspiration pneumonia. There is usually a history of unconsciousness in which the gag and cough reflexes are suppressed. Gastrostomy tube feeding also carries a risk of aspiration pneumonia.

A less severe form of pneumonia is often termed "walking pneumonia." These clients often respond well to treatment at home.

Complications of pneumonia may include the following:

- Pleurisy
- Pleural effusion
- Atelectasis
- Delayed resolution
- Lung abscess
- Empyema
- Pericarditis
- Arthritis
- Meningitis
- Endocarditis

Clinical Manifestations

Clinical manifestations vary depending on the cause of the pneumonia. Symptoms may include fever, chills, tachypnea, tachycardia, dyspnea, cough with production of purulent sputum, hypoxemia, possible pleuritic chest pain, and possible confusion or stupor.

Diagnostics

Diagnosis is suspected by the history and physical examination and confirmed with a chest X-ray showing infiltrates. Blood cultures and sputum smears will define the causative agent.

Therapeutics and Nursing Considerations

Treatment focuses on clearing the infection and improving gas exchange and may include the following:

- Antibiotic therapy
- Oxygen for hypoxemia
- Analgesics for chest pain
- Antipyretics
- Influenza drugs
- Increased fluid intake
- Adequate caloric intake

Lung Cancer
Pathophysiology

Lung cancer is the leading cause of cancer-related deaths in Canada. It most commonly occurs in individuals over age 50 with a history of cigarette smoking. Smoking is responsible for 80–90% of all lung cancers. Other risk factors for the development of lung cancer include genetic predisposition and exposure to carcinogenic industrial or air pollutants, such as asbestos, uranium arsenic, chromates, radon, nickel, iron, and iron oxides.

Ninety percent of lung cancers originate from the epithelium of the bronchus, developing squamous cell carcinoma. It takes 8 to 10 years for a tumour to reach 1 cm, the smallest lesion detectable on X-ray. The lesions usually occur on segmental bronchi and the upper lobes of the lung. Pathological changes in the bronchial system result in hypersecretion of mucus, desquamation of cells, reactive hyperplasia of basal cells, and metaplasia of normal respiratory epithelium to stratified squamous cells.

Lung cancers metastasize by direct extension, blood circulation, and the lymph system. Common sites for metastatic growth include the following:

- Liver
- Brain
- Bones
- Lymph nodes
- Adrenal glands (Lewis et al., 2019)

Clinical Manifestations

Clinical manifestations appear late in the disease and depend on the type of primary lung cancer, location, degree of obstruction, and metastatic spread. The manifestations may include the following:

- Pneumonitis, persistent cough with sputum, and hemoptysis
- Chest pain
- Dyspnea
- Anorexia
- Fatigue
- Nausea and vomiting
- Hoarse voice
- Unilateral paralysis of diaphragm

Diagnostics

Diagnostic studies include a chest X-ray, which can detect a tumour 2 years before it becomes symptomatic, as well as the following:

- CT scans, MRI, and positron emission tomography (PET) to help find metastatic tumours
- Sputum specimens obtained from fibre-optic bronchoscopy, mediastinoscopy, and video-assisted thoracoscopy for cytological studies
- Biopsy of the tumour, to provide the definitive diagnosis and allow for staging of the cancer

Therapeutics and Nursing Considerations

Treatment involves combinations of surgery, radiation, and chemotherapy. However, surgery is contraindicated for small cell carcinomas. Squamous cell carcinomas, adenocarcinoma, and large cell cancer are likely treated with surgery. Radiation may be used prior to surgery to reduce the tumour size. If the tumour is nonresectable or other conditions, such as cardiac disease, exist, surgery is not an option. Radiation therapy is usually recommended for stage 1 and stage 2 lesions if surgery is contraindicated. Radiation can be used as an adjunct to surgery postoperatively.

Chemotherapy is the primary treatment for small cell lung cancer. Other therapies include biological therapy, prophylactic cranial therapy, bronchoscopic laser therapy, phototherapy, airway stenting, and cryotherapy.

Treatment focuses on providing comprehensive supportive care and client teaching to minimize complications and promote recovery from surgery, radiation, chemotherapy, or all of these. Overall goals include the following:
- Effective breathing patterns
- Adequate airway clearance
- Adequate oxygenation of tissues
- Minimal or no pain
- Providing psychological support and developing realistic attitudes toward treatment and prognosis

HEMATOLOGICAL HEALTH CHALLENGES

Anemia
Pathophysiology

Anemia is a decrease in the number of erythrocytes (RBCs), the amount of hemoglobin, or the volume of packed RBCs (hematocrit), all of which will result in a decreased amount of oxygen being delivered to the cells. Anemia is not itself a disease but rather is a clinical sign of an underlying disorder. Anemia can result from blood loss, impaired production of erythrocytes, or increased destruction of erythrocytes. The various types of anemia can be grouped according to a morphological (cellular characteristics) or an etiological (underlying cause) classification. A morphological classification gives information about the size and colour of the RBCs. Etiological classification is related to the underlying cause of the anemia.

Clinical Manifestations

Symptoms of anemia are caused by the body's response to the level of tissue hypoxia, which will depend on the severity of the anemia. When present, clinical symptoms may include the following:
- Palpitations
- Dyspnea
- Diaphoresis
- Pallor, due to reduced hemoglobin and reduced blood flow to the skin
- Jaundice, due to the increased hemolysis of RBCs, leading to increased concentrations of bilirubin
- Pruritus, due to an increased serum and skin bile salt concentration
- Cardiovascular manifestations of severe anemia result from additional attempts by the heart and lungs to provide adequate amounts of oxygen to the tissues
- Heart rate is increased in an attempt to maintain adequate cardiac output. Murmurs and bruits may develop due to the low viscosity of the blood.
- Angina, myocardial infarction (MI), and heart failure may develop due to the extreme increase in workload of the heart.
- Fatigue is common due to the increased heart rate and ineffective transportation of oxygen to the tissues.

Diagnostics

Laboratory assessment is needed to detect the type and size of RBCs as well as possible causes of the anemia. The following laboratory tests are used in the diagnosis:
- Hemoglobin, hematocrit, and reticulocyte counts
- Serum iron levels
- RBC indexes, particularly the mean corpuscular volume

Therapeutics and Nursing Considerations

Treatment of anemia is directed at correcting the cause of the anemia and maintaining adequate tissue perfusion. Oral or occasionally parenteral iron supplementation is used to replace iron. Acute interventions may include the following:
- Transfusion of blood or blood products
- Drug therapy, such as erythropoietin, vitamins, and supplements
- Oxygen therapy

Nursing considerations will be specific to the client's needs; however, all clients with anemia should be encouraged to balance rest with activity, eat a balanced diet rich in iron and folate, and be compliant with their drug therapy.

Aplastic Anemia
Pathophysiology

Aplastic anemia is a deficiency of circulating RBCs due to failure of the bone marrow to produce these cells. Stem cells in the bone marrow, or the bone marrow matrix itself, are either injured or destroyed, resulting in pancytopenia (decrease in all blood cell types). The damaged marrow is replaced by fat, resulting in bone marrow hypoplasia (decreased hematopoiesis).

Aplastic anemia may be congenital, acquired, or idiopathic. Some causes of aplastic anemia may include the following:
- Adverse drug reactions to certain medications
- Exposure to toxic agents, such as benzene, inorganic arsenic, insecticides, and radiation
- Viral or bacterial infections, such as hepatitis

Clinical Manifestations

Clinical manifestations of aplastic anemia vary with the severity of the pancytopenia. Infection, bleeding tendencies, fatigue, pallor, and dyspnea are common.

Diagnostics

Diagnosis is confirmed by laboratory studies. RBCs, WBCs, and platelets will be decreased. Morphologically, aplastic anemia is considered normocytic, normochromic anemia. A bone marrow biopsy may show hypoplasia or aplasia, with cells being replaced by fat.

Therapeutics and Nursing Considerations

Management of aplastic anemia is based on identifying and removing the causative agent (when possible) and providing supportive care. The following treatments are used:

- Blood transfusions are the mainstay of treatment. Transfusions are discontinued once the bone marrow starts producing RBCs.
- Bone marrow transplantation is the preferred treatment of aplastic anemia for clients needing constant blood transfusions.
- A splenectomy may be performed when the spleen is destroying normal RBCs.

The prognosis for aplastic anemia is poor, with a mortality rate as high as 70%. Death may result from bleeding or infection.

Sickle Cell Anemia

Sickle cell anemia is an inherited childhood disorder of autosomal recessive defects, characterized by the presence of an abnormal form of hemoglobin (called *sickle cell hemoglobin*, or HgbS) in the erythrocyte. This abnormal hemoglobin causes erythrocytes to become rigid and to take on a crescent shape in response to low oxygen levels, causing vaso-occlusive crises, and, over time, tissue hypoxia and necrosis. For more information on sickle cell anemia, see Chapter 10.

Thrombocytopenia
Pathophysiology

Thrombocytopenia is characterized by a deficiency of circulating platelets. Platelet disorders can be inherited or acquired due to decreased platelet production, increased sequestration in the spleen, or increased platelet destruction. Types of thrombocytopenia are as follows:

- Acquired thrombocytopenia may result from drugs such as NSAIDs or antibiotic chemotherapeutic agents.
- In children, idiopathic thrombocytopenia is common.
- Transient thrombocytopenia may follow a viral infection such as Epstein–Barr virus or other infections.
- Immune (idiopathic) thrombocytopenic purpura (ITP) is an autoimmune disorder with platelet destruction.
- Thrombotic thrombocytopenic purpura (TTP) is a rare disease in which thrombi occlude small vessels.

The key factor with all types of thrombocytopenia is the low platelet level: below 150×10^9/L of blood.

Clinical Manifestations

Many clients with thrombocytopenia are asymptomatic. When manifestations are present, the most common symptom is bleeding, usually noticeable only when the platelet count drops below 20 000/mL of blood. The major complication of thrombocytopenia is hemorrhage.

Diagnostics

Diagnosis is made by a laboratory test of platelets. The platelet count will be decreased. Any reduction below 150×10^9/L is termed *thrombocytopenia*.

Therapeutics and Nursing Considerations

Treatment of thrombocytopenia depends on the etiology of the decreased platelet count. The underlying cause must be treated, and treatment may include the following:

- Splenectomy for hypersplenism
- Chemotherapy for acute or chronic leukemia
- Corticosteroids to enhance vascular integrity
- Steroids, danazol (Cyclomen), or IV immune globulin for idiopathic thrombocytopenia
- Platelet transfusions for a count below 20×10^9/L
- Plasmapheresis (plasma is removed from the client and replaced with fresh frozen plasma) is the primary treatment for acute thrombocytopenia.

INGESTION, DIGESTION, ABSORPTION, AND ELIMINATION CHALLENGES
Nausea and Vomiting

Nausea is a feeling of discomfort in the epigastrium with a conscious desire to vomit. Vomiting is the forceful ejection of partially digested food and secretions (emesis) from the upper GI tract. Nausea and vomiting can occur independently but usually are closely related and treated as one problem. A client can feel nauseated and vomit in response to many conditions. Some of these conditions include the following:

- Pregnancy
- GI disorders
- Infectious diseases
- Food poisoning
- CNS disorders
- Cardiovascular disorders
- Metabolic disorders and side effects of drugs
- Other triggers of nausea may include odours, intense activity or emotional stress, or certain types of food (Lewis et al., 2019).

Clinical Manifestations

Nausea is a subjective, unpleasant, wavelike sensation the client experiences in the back of the throat, epigastrium, or abdomen. This feeling may or may not lead to the urge to vomit.

Diagnostics

Diagnosis is arrived at via a client history and physical assessment.

Therapeutics and Nursing Considerations

The goals of management are to determine and treat the underlying cause of the vomiting, remove the cause, and provide symptomatic relief. Differentiation between vomiting, regurgitation, and projectile vomiting is important. The colour and odour of the emesis can supply important information. Fecal odour and bile indicate a lower obstruction of the bowel. The colour of the emesis aids in determining whether bleeding is taking place. Many different drugs can be used to treat nausea and vomiting. The exact drug therapy will depend on the cause. IV fluids may be needed to replace fluids and electrolytes. If vomiting is continuous, a nasogastric (NG) tube may be inserted to decompress the stomach. The client will be started on clear fluids when tolerated. The client will be encouraged to drink fluids between meals rather than with meals.

Hiatus Hernia
Pathophysiology

Hiatus hernia is a protrusion of the stomach into the esophagus through an opening in the diaphragm. A sliding hiatus hernia occurs when the stomach slides through the gastroesophageal junction. A paraesophageal, or rolling, hiatus hernia occurs when the fundus or greater curvature of the stomach rolls up through the esophageal hiatus.

Many different factors may cause the development of a hiatus hernia. These include the following:
- A weakness in the muscles of the diaphragm
- Increased intra-abdominal pressure
- Obesity
- Pregnancy
- Ascites
- Tumour
- Heavy lifting
- Increasing age
- Trauma
- Poor nutrition
- Prolonged recumbent position

Potential complications of hiatus hernia are hemorrhage, obstruction, and strangulation of the hernia.

Clinical Manifestations

Clinical manifestations are similar to those of gastroesophageal reflux disease (GERD) and are as follows:
- Pyrosis, dysphagia, reflux, and discomfort are associated with position.
- Bending over may cause pain.
- Large meals may cause pain.
- Smoking and alcohol may cause pain.
- Nocturnal symptoms of heartburn are common.
- Reflux symptoms are more common with a sliding hiatus hernia, and fullness is more typical in the paraesophageal hernia.

Complications that may occur with hiatus hernia include GERD, hemorrhage from erosion, stenosis of the esophagus, ulcerations of the herniated portion of the stomach, strangulation of the hernia, and regurgitation with tracheal aspiration (Lewis et al., 2019).

Diagnostics

Diagnosis of hiatus hernia begins with the history and a physical examination as well as barium swallow X-ray, endoscopic examination, or both, looking for any protrusion of the gastric mucosa through the esophageal hiatus or abnormalities in the mucosa.

Therapeutics and Nursing Considerations

Conservative care is attempted first and may include the following:
- Lifestyle modifications similar to those for GERD
- Elevation of the head of the bed to 30 degrees
- Use of antacids and antisecretory agents such as H_2 receptor blockers
- Weight reduction if the client is overweight

Surgical treatments attempt to reduce reflux by enhancing the integrity of the lower esophageal sphincter (LES). Different types of surgery all involve "wrapping" the fundus of the stomach around the lower portion of the esophagus in order to reduce the hernia, provide acceptable LES pressure, and prevent movement of the gastroesophageal junction. Postoperative care involves the following:
- Monitoring vital signs and airway and chest sounds
- Monitoring any chest tubes and possible respiratory distress
- Monitoring an abdominal incision for infection
- Monitoring the NG tube for patency and checking the abdomen for distension
- Always assessing clients for venous thrombus following these types of surgery

Education of the client will revolve around preventing respiratory complications by deep breathing and coughing frequently. Clients should be taught to prevent gas-bloat syndrome by slowing and progressively advancing their diet. Small, frequent meals will prevent overloading of the stomach. Carbonated drinks and gas-producing foods should be avoided (Ignatavicius, Workman, & Rebar, 2018).

Esophageal Cancer
Pathophysiology

Factors predisposing to the development of esophageal cancer include the following:
- Smoking and excessive alcohol use
- A diet low in fruits, vegetables, and certain vitamins and minerals, which increases the risk
- Achalasia (peristalsis is absent in the lower two-thirds of the esophagus), which results in delayed emptying of the lower esophagus; exposure to asbestos and metal; and a history of swallowing lye

Cancer of the esophagus is caused by malignant advancement into the esophageal area. If the malignancy spreads into the submucosa, the risk for metastasis and death increases drastically. The major types of esophageal cancers are adenocarcinoma and squamous cell cancers.

Complications with esophageal cancers include the following:
- Hemorrhage that may occur if cancer erodes through the esophagus and into the aorta
- Esophageal perforation with fistula formation into the lung or trachea
- Obstruction of the esophagus

- Spread of the cancer through the lymph system; the liver and lungs are common sites of metastasis

Clinical Manifestations

Symptoms appear late in the development, usually when the esophagus is 50–60% occluded, and include progressive dysphagia, pain in the epigastric area, substernally, or in the back, which may radiate to the neck and jaw. Other common symptoms may include a sore throat, choking and hoarseness, and weight loss.

Diagnostics

Diagnostic tests used to find esophageal cancer include barium swallow with fluoroscopy, which may show a narrowing of the esophagus at the site of the tumour. Endoscopy and biopsy are needed to make a definitive diagnosis and identify the malignant cells. A CT scan and MRI may be needed to assess the extent of the disease.

Therapeutics and Nursing Considerations

Since the disease is often not diagnosed until late in its development, the prognosis is poor. Treatments include the following:

- Surgery, which may include esophagectomy, removal of part or all of the esophagus
- Esophagogastrostomy, resection of a portion of the esophagus and anastomosis of the remaining portion to the stomach
- Esophagoenterostomy, resection of a portion of the esophagus and anastomosis of a segment of colon to the remaining portion
- Chemotherapy and radiation before or after the surgery

Palliative therapy consists of restoration of the swallowing function and maintenance of nutrition and hydration. Once the client is allowed to eat, he or she must be monitored for intolerance to feeding or leakage of the food into the mediastinum. Further palliative care focuses on pain management and maintaining as normal a lifestyle as possible.

Peptic Ulcer Disease
Pathophysiology

Peptic ulcer disease includes conditions characterized by erosion of the GI mucosa in the lower esophagus, stomach and duodenum, and jejunum. The ulcer may be acute with either superficial or minimal erosion. It can be of short duration and resolve quickly when the cause is identified and removed. A chronic ulcer is of long duration, eroding through the muscular wall with the formation of fibrous tissue. Peptic ulcers develop only in the presence of an acid environment. The stomach is normally protected from autodigestion and damage by the gastric mucosal barrier. When that barrier is damaged, acid–pepsin freely enters the mucosa, and cellular inflammation and destruction occur. The precise cause of peptic ulcers is not known; however, common risk factors include the following:

- *Helicobacter pylori* infection
- The use of NSAIDs, salicylates, or steroids
- Exposure to irritants, such as alcohol, coffee, and tobacco, increases the risk of peptic ulcer development.
- Other predisposing factors include emotional stress, physical trauma, and aging.

The major complications of peptic ulcers include hemorrhage, perforation, and gastric outlet obstruction. All three complications are considered emergencies requiring prompt medical treatment.

Clinical Manifestations

Clinical manifestations are variable. Those with gastric or duodenal ulcers often do not have any pain. When pain is present, it is described as burning or cramplike and most often is located in the midepigastric region. Eating or ingesting antacids often relieves the pain.

Diagnostics

Diagnostic testing includes the following:

- An upper GI tract X-ray will show abnormalities in the mucosa.
- A barium swallow examination can diagnose gastric outlet obstruction.
- Gastric secretory studies will show hyperchlorhydria.
- An upper GI endoscopy will confirm the presence of an ulcer.
- A biopsy will help rule out cancer.
- A serological or breath urea test is done to test for the presence of *H. pylori*.
- Stool may need to be tested for occult blood.

Therapeutics and Nursing Considerations

Treatment is essentially symptomatic, with an emphasis on drug therapy and rest. The following treatments are used:

- Antacids reduce gastric acidity. Histamine-2 receptor blockers and proton pump inhibitors reduce gastric secretions in short-term therapy.
- Anticholinergics inhibit the vagus nerve effect on the parietal cells and reduce gastrin production and excessive gastric activity in duodenal ulcers.
- Sucralfate (Sulcrate), a cytoprotective drug, is used in short-term therapy and is cytoprotective of the esophagus, stomach, and duodenum.
- Antibiotic treatment may be used to reduce *H. pylori*.
- Physical rest promotes healing.
- Gastroscopy can facilitate coagulation of the bleeding site by cautery or laser therapy.
- If hemorrhage occurs, saline lavage, sclerotherapy, and angiography with vasopressin may postpone the need for surgery until the client stabilizes.

Surgery is indicated for clients with perforation or those unresponsive to conservative measures. Surgical procedures include vagotomy and pyloroplasty or distal subtotal gastrectomy.

Nutritional therapy identifies foods that cause distress, such as the following:

- Hot, spicy foods and pepper
- Alcohol
- Carbonated drinks
- Tea and coffee
- Foods high in roughage, which may irritate an inflamed mucosa

Protein is considered the best neutralizing food, but it does stimulate gastric secretions. Milk can neutralize gastric activity and contains prostaglandins and growth factors.

Diet should consist of small, dry feedings daily that are low in carbohydrates and that include a moderate amount of protein and fat. Fluids should not be taken during the meal. Clients are encouraged to rest for 30 minutes following every meal.

With an acute exacerbation when bleeding is occurring, the client often has increased pain with nausea and vomiting. The following treatment is required in this situation:

- An NG tube will be placed in the stomach with intermittent suction for 24–48 hours.
- Fluids and electrolytes will be replaced by IV infusion until the client is able to tolerate oral feedings without distress.

Management will be similar to that for upper GI bleeding. Blood, blood products, or both may be needed. The client will require the following nursing considerations:

- Careful monitoring of vital signs
- Monitoring of intake and output
- Laboratory studies
- Monitoring for signs of impending shock
- Endoscopic evaluation will reveal the degree of inflammation or bleeding as well as the location of the ulcer.

Perforation of the ulcer requires immediate action to stop spillage of gastric or duodenal contents into the peritoneal cavity and to restore blood volume. The following interventions are essential:

- An NG tube will be placed into the stomach as close to the perforation as possible.
- Circulating blood volume must be replaced.
- Packed RBCs may be needed.
- A central venous pressure line may be needed.
- An in-dwelling urinary catheter should be inserted and monitored every hour.

Surgery is not the usual method of treatment; however, it is indicated for such conditions as an intractable ulcer, history of hemorrhage, perforation, or obstruction. Surgical procedures done to treat ulcers include gastroduodenostomy (Billroth I), gastrojejunostomy (Billroth II), vagotomy, and pyloroplasty.

Postoperative complications include dumping syndrome, postprandial hypoglycemia, and bile reflux gastritis. The dumping syndrome is a direct result of surgical removal of a large portion of the stomach and pyloric sphincter. The syndrome results from the rapid emptying of gastric contents into the small bowel, which creates a fluid shift into the gut, resulting in abdominal distension. The client will feel dizzy and weak and complain of abdominal cramps.

Gastritis
Pathophysiology

Gastritis is not a disease but rather a condition of inflammation of the gastric mucosa.

- Acute gastritis is often due to eating foods contaminated with micro-organisms or food that is highly seasoned.
- Chronic gastritis is sometimes associated with autoimmune disease, such as pernicious anemia. It can also be due to benign or malignant ulcers caused by *H. pylori* bacteria.

Gastritis occurs as a result of a breakdown in the gastric mucosal barrier. In gastritis, the mucous membrane becomes edematous and hyperemic and undergoes superficial erosion. This erosion may lead to hemorrhage.

Clinical Manifestations

Acute and chronic symptoms are the same and include anorexia, nausea and vomiting, epigastric tenderness, and a feeling of fullness. Hemorrhage is particularly common with alcohol abuse.

Diagnostics

Diagnosis is often suspected with a thorough history and physical examination where ingestion of drugs and alcohol may be discussed. Definitive diagnosis is made with an endoscopic examination and biopsy of the gastric mucosa from which a histological examination will occur. Upper GI radiographic studies may be ordered.

Therapeutics and Nursing Considerations

Treatment and management revolve around removal of the precipitating cause. Initially, the client will be nothing by mouth (NPO), with possible NG insertion to remove the causative agent. The client must be monitored for dehydration, which can occur quickly. Drug therapy focuses on reducing irritation of the gastric mucosa and providing symptomatic relief. Antacids and H_2 receptor blockers such as ranitidine (Zantac) are helpful in reducing HCl secretion and in raising the pH to a more alkaline level. Nursing considerations will focus on promoting optimal nutrition, promoting fluid balance, relieving pain, and promoting self-care.

Gastroesophageal Reflux Disease
Pathophysiology

GERD refers to any clinically significant symptomatic condition of reflux of the gastric contents into the lower esophagus. There is no single cause for GERD. Predisposing factors include the following:

- Hiatus hernia
- Incompetent LES
- Decreased gastric emptying
- Pyloric stenosis

The acidic gastric secretions that reflux up into the lower esophagus result in esophageal irritation, inflammation, and corrosion.

Clinical Manifestations

Clinical manifestations include heartburn, described as a burning or tight sensation radiating to the neck. Clients with heartburn that occurs more than once a week, becomes more severe, or occurs at night and wakes the client from sleep should be investigated for GERD. Regurgitation is common and is frequently described as hot, bitter, or sour liquid coming into the mouth or throat.

Gastric symptoms may also include the following, which are related to delayed gastric emptying:

- Early satiety
- Postmeal bloating
- Nausea, vomiting

Diagnostics

Diagnosis of GERD is made by barium swallow or endoscopy to evaluate damage to the esophageal mucosa. Other tests may include biopsy with histological examination, esophageal manometric studies to monitor pH, and radionuclide tests to detect reflux and the rate of esophageal clearance.

Therapeutics and Nursing Considerations

Management focuses on lifestyle modifications and avoidance of situations that decrease LES pressure or that cause esophageal irritation. Nutritionally, clients are encouraged to avoid high-fat foods, avoid milk products at night, and avoid late-night snacking.

Drug therapy may include the following:

- H_2 receptor blockers
- Proton pump inhibitors
- Antacids
- Sucralfate
- Prokinetic drugs

If medical management is unsuccessful, fundoplication surgery (wrapping a portion of the gastric fundus around the sphincter of the esophagus) is performed. Practical nurses need to educate clients to

- Avoid factors causing reflux, such as smoking and acid-producing foods.
- Have the head of the bed elevated to about 30 degrees.
- Not lie down for two to 3 hours after eating.
- Take medications correctly.

Gastroenteritis
Pathophysiology

Gastroenteritis is an inflammation of the mucosa of the stomach and small intestine, resulting in vomiting and diarrhea. The condition usually is caused by infectious agents, such as the noroviruses and *Escherichia coli*. Most cases are self-limiting and do not require hospitalization. However, older adults and chronically ill clients may be unable to consume adequate fluids orally to compensate for fluid loss.

If the symptoms are severe, or if the client is experiencing frequent watery stools, a culture for *Clostridium difficile* should be performed.

Clinical Manifestations

Clinical manifestations include the following:

- Nausea and vomiting
- Diarrhea
- Possible fever
- Abdominal cramping and distension
- Depending on the amount of fluid that is lost, the client may experience symptoms of hypovolemia.

Diagnostics

The history and physical examination of the client are usually diagnostic. However, Gram stain of stool specimens will confirm the causative agent.

Therapeutics and Nursing Considerations

Until vomiting stops, the client should be NPO. Thereafter, the client should have bland food and fluids as tolerated. Most gastroenteritis is managed at home. If the symptoms are severe, the following treatments may be needed:

- IV replacement therapy for dehydration
- Accurate monitoring of intake and output
- Potassium supplements
- Antibiotic, antimicrobial therapy, if the causative organism is identified
- Enteric precautions

Symptomatic nursing care is given for nausea, vomiting, and diarrhea. The practical nurse should assess complaints of pain, vomiting, and diarrhea as gastroenteritis is often confused with appendicitis.

Appendicitis
Pathophysiology

Appendicitis is an inflammation of the vermiform appendix, a narrow, fingerlike appendage found just below the ileocecal valve. Inflammation of the appendix usually occurs when the lumen is obstructed by fecal material, foreign bodies, or a tumour of the cecum. This obstruction can lead to distension, venous engorgement, and the accumulation of mucus and bacteria, which can, in turn, lead to gangrene and perforation of the appendix. If the appendix ruptures or perforates, the infected contents can spill into the abdominal cavity, causing peritonitis.

Clinical Manifestations

Appendicitis typically begins with periumbilical pain, followed by anorexia, nausea, and vomiting. The pain eventually will shift to the right lower quadrant and localize at McBurney's point, with rebound tenderness and muscle guarding. The client will probably want to lie still with knees flexed. Coughing aggravates the pain.

Diagnostics

Diagnosis of appendicitis can be difficult, so although the history and physical examination are important, further tests should be done, including the following:

- Rovsing's sign may be elicited by palpating the left lower quadrant.

- WBCs will be elevated, but this is not considered diagnostic.
- An ultrasonogram or CT scan of the abdomen is often needed to confirm the diagnosis.

Therapeutics and Nursing Considerations

Appendectomy is the only effective treatment for appendicitis. If the appendix has ruptured, treatment will also include insertion of an NG tube, IV fluids and electrolytes, and administration of antibiotics. Nursing care will focus on the following:

- Pain relief
- Maintaining fluid balance
- Support to reduce anxiety
- Maintaining skin integrity
- Monitoring and managing complications that may arise

Diverticulitis
Pathophysiology

The diverticulum is a saccular outpouching of the mucosa through the muscular intestinal wall. Diverticulitis is an inflammation of the diverticular sacs, most commonly due to obstruction with fecal matter. Diverticula may occur at any point within the GI tract but are more commonly found in the sigmoid colon.

Diverticula in the sigmoid colon are thought to be associated with high luminal pressure from a deficiency in dietary fibre perhaps combined with a loss of muscle mass and collagen with the aging process. When diverticula form, the smooth muscle of the colon wall becomes thickened. Lack of dietary fibre slows transit time, and more water is absorbed from the stool, making it more difficult for it to pass through the lumen. Decreased stool size raises intraluminal pressure, thus promoting diverticula formation.

Clinical Manifestations

The majority of people with diverticulitis are asymptomatic. When symptoms are present, they usually include the following:

- Abdominal pain localized over the involved area of the colon
- Fever
- Leukocytosis
- Sometimes a palpable mass

Complications of diverticulitis include perforation with peritonitis, abscess and fistula formation, bowel obstructions, ureteral obstruction, and bleeding.

Diagnostics

Diagnostic tests include CBC, urinalysis, and fecal occult blood test, as well as X-ray of the abdomen or ultrasound/CT scan to confirm diagnosis and evaluate the severity of the condition.

Therapeutics and Nursing Considerations

In acute diverticulitis, the goal of treatment is to allow the colon to rest and the inflammation to subside. Treatments include the following:

- Ensuring the client is NPO with IV therapy to maintain fluid and electrolyte balance
- Initiating broad-spectrum antibiotic therapy
- Monitoring the client for signs of peritonitis
- Surgery is reserved for clients with complications such as abscess or obstruction.

Nursing considerations focus on maintaining normal elimination patterns, relief of pain, maintaining fluid balance, and monitoring and managing potential complications. Teaching the client that diverticular disease can be prevented by a diet high in fibre and low in fats is important.

Inflammatory Bowel Disease

Inflammatory bowel disease consists of the immunologically related disorders of Crohn's disease and ulcerative colitis. Inflammatory bowel disease is characterized by chronic, recurrent inflammation of the intestinal tract. Clinical manifestations are varied for both conditions, but these often include long periods of remission interspersed with episodes of acute inflammation. Both diseases can be debilitating. The cause of inflammatory bowel disease is unknown; however, causes may include the following:

- Infectious agents
- Autoimmune reaction
- Food allergies
- Heredity

Ulcerative Colitis
Pathophysiology

Ulcerative colitis is characterized by inflammation and ulceration of the colon and rectum. It may occur at any age but tends to peak between the ages of 15 and 25 years. It is equally prevalent in both sexes. The inflammation of ulcerative colitis usually starts in the rectum and moves in a continuous pattern toward the cecum. Ulcerative colitis is characterized by multiple ulcerations, inflammations, and shedding of the epithelium. The affected mucosa is hyperemic and edematous. The ulcerations destroy the mucosal epithelium, causing bleeding and diarrhea. This can lead to fluid and electrolyte losses, protein losses, and the development of pseudopolyps. Granulation tissue develops, and the mucosa musculature becomes thickened, shortening the colon. Intestinal complications include the following:

- Hemorrhage
- Abscess formation
- Perforation
- Toxic megacolon and colonic dilation
- Cancer

Clinical Manifestations

Clients with ulcerative colitis usually present with mild to severe acute exacerbations that occur at unpredictable intervals over many years. The major symptoms are bloody diarrhea and abdominal pain.

Diagnostics

Diagnosis of ulcerative colitis includes ruling out other diseases with similar symptoms and determining whether the client has ulcerative colitis or Crohn's disease. The following tests are done:

- CBC, serum electrolytes, and serum protein levels
- Stool will be examined for blood, pus, and mucus.
- Sigmoidoscopy and colonoscopy examination of the mucosa to look for inflammation, ulcerations, pseudopolyps, and strictures
- A double-contrast barium enema for areas of granular inflammation with ulceration

Therapeutics and Nursing Considerations

Goals of treatment include the following:

- Resting the bowel
- Control of inflammation
- Combatting infection
- Correcting malnutrition
- Alleviating stress
- Symptomatic relief and improving quality of life
- Sulfasalazines are the principal drugs of choice. They are effective in the maintenance of remission.
- Other medications that may be used are corticosteroids, 5-ASA and 4-ASA, and immunosuppressants such as azathioprine (Imuran).

Surgery is indicated if the client does not respond to medical treatment, has frequent or debilitating exacerbations, has massive bleeding or obstruction, or develops dysplasia or carcinoma. Surgical procedures include total proctocolectomy with permanent ileostomy, total proctocolectomy with continent ileostomy (Kock pouch), or total colectomy with rectal mucosal stripping and ileoanal reservoir.

Postoperatively, the practical nurse must monitor for the following:

- Stoma viability, mucocutaneous juncture, and peristomal skin integrity
- Signs of hemorrhage, abdominal abscess, small bowel obstruction, dehydration, and other complications

Diet is an important component in the treatment of ulcerative colitis. The goal is to provide adequate nutrition without exacerbating symptoms. This diet must correct and prevent malnutrition, replace fluid and electrolyte losses, and prevent weight loss. The diet should be

- High calorie
- High protein
- Low residue with vitamin and mineral supplements
  Other nursing considerations include the following:
- Maintaining normal elimination patterns
- Relieving pain
- Promoting rest
- Reducing anxiety
- Preventing skin breakdown
- Enhancing coping mechanisms

Crohn's Disease
Pathophysiology

Crohn's disease is a chronic nonspecific inflammatory bowel disorder of unknown origin that can affect any part of the GI tract from mouth to anus. Crohn's disease can occur at any age but usually presents between the ages of 15 and 30 years and affects both sexes equally.

Crohn's disease is characterized by inflammation of segments of the GI tract, and although the disease can affect any section, it is most often found in the terminal ileum. The inflammation of Crohn's disease affects all layers of the bowel wall. Eventually, deep ulcerations develop. There are also "skip lesions," in which segments of normal bowel occur between diseased portions. As the disease continues, the wall of the bowel thickens, and as strictures develop, the lumen of the bowel narrows. Severe diarrhea and malabsorption of nutrients result from the damaged bowel. Complications of Crohn's disease are similar to those of ulcerative colitis.

Clinical Manifestations

The onset of Crohn's disease is usually insidious, with non-specific complaints of the following:

- Diarrhea
- Fatigue
- Abdominal pain
- Weight loss
- Fever

Diarrhea (nonbloody) and abdominal pain are usually the symptoms that cause the client to seek medical attention. As the disease progresses, the pain may increase in severity, abdominal distension may develop, and the client may develop arthritis and finger clubbing.

Diagnostics

Diagnostic studies are similar to those needed for ulcerative colitis, including barium studies, endoscopy with biopsy, blood work, and upper GI barium swallow.

Therapeutics and Nursing Considerations

The goals of treatment revolve around controlling the inflammatory process, relieving symptoms, correcting metabolic and nutritional problems, and promoting healing of the affected area.

Treatments include the following:

- Drug therapy similar to that used with ulcerative colitis. Sulfasalazines, corticosteroids, immunosuppressive agents, metronidazole, and infliximab may be used.
- Nutritional therapy, including elemental diets; parenteral nutrition when needed; and low-residue, low-roughage, low-fat, high-calorie, and high-protein diets are recommended.

The majority of clients will eventually require surgery at least once in the course of their disease. The disease is not cured by surgery, and the recurrence rate following surgery is high.

Nursing management is similar to that required for ulcerative colitis, with frequent rest periods and skin care. Client education is very important. Teaching includes the following:

- The importance of rest and diet management
- Teaching about the medications, what they are, why they are needed, and what they will do for the client helps

clients be compliant with their medications. Clients should also be taught about possible side effects of their medications, as well as symptoms of disease recurrence.

- When to seek medical care
- The use of diversional activities to reduce stress

Colorectal Cancer

Pathophysiology

Colorectal cancer (CRC) is equally common in men and women. Nearly all CRCs are adenocarcinomas, most arising from adenomatous polyps. Tumours spread through the walls of the intestine and into the lymphatic system. Tumours commonly spread to the liver because venous blood flow from the colorectal tumour is through the portal vein.

CRC is the second leading cause of death from cancer in Canada. However, if diagnosed early, the cure rate is very high. Screening via *fecal occult blood test* (FOBT) or *fecal immunochemical test* (FIT) once a year and flexible sigmoidoscopy every 5 years beginning at age 50 are important aspects of the examination (Lewis et al., 2019).

The cause of CRC is unclear. However, risk factors for the development of CRC include the following:

- Familial tendencies
- Increasing age
- A diet high in fat and calories
- A history of inflammatory bowel disease

Clinical Manifestations

Clinical manifestations are nonspecific and may not appear until the disease is advanced. Most people with CRC have hematochezia (passage of blood through the rectum) or melena (black, tarry stools) and abdominal pain or changes in bowel habits, or both. Occult bleeding and iron deficiency anemia lead to weakness and fatigue. The signs of CRC depend on the location of the tumour.

- Left-sided lesions tend to bleed. Clients tend to alternate between constipation and diarrhea, and they tend to have narrow, ribbonlike stools.
- Right-sided lesions are usually asymptomatic or cause vague abdominal discomfort.

In later stages, findings result from extension of the cancer to adjacent organs and reflect the symptoms of advanced cancer.

Diagnostics

Diagnostic studies include family history and physical examination, distal rectal examination, colonoscopy, endorectal ultrasonography, CT scan, fecal occult blood tests, and carcinoembryonic antigen. Only a biopsy will verify the presence of CRC.

Therapeutics and Nursing Considerations

Prognosis and treatment correlate with the pathological staging of the disease. Surgery seeks to remove the cancerous tumour and adjacent tissues, as well as lymph nodes that may contain cancer cells. Chemotherapy and radiation therapy are recommended for clients with positive lymph node involvement at the time of surgery or those who have metastatic disease. Chemotherapy and radiation may be the primary treatment when the CRC is nonresectable.

- A right hemicolectomy for advanced tumours of the cecum or ascending colon may include resection of the terminal segment of the ileum, cecum, ascending colon, and right half of the transverse colon with corresponding mesentery.
- A right colectomy may be done for tumours of the proximal and middle transverse colon, which includes the resection of the transverse colon and mesentery corresponding to midcolonic vessels.
- Alternatively, the surgeon may perform segmental resection of the transverse colon and associated midcolonic vessels.
- For sigmoid colon tumours, surgery is usually limited to the sigmoid colon and mesentery.
- Upper rectum tumours usually call for anterior or low anterior resection. A newer method, using a stapler, allows resection much lower than previously possible.
- For tumours in the lower rectum, abdominoperineal resection and permanent sigmoid colostomy are usually performed.

The overall goals for the client being treated for CRC are to attain normal bowel elimination patterns, maintain quality of life appropriate for the disease progression, be free of pain, and maintain feelings of comfort and well-being.

Other nursing considerations include the following:

- Providing emotional support
- Maintaining optimal nutrition
- Providing pain relief
- Providing wound care following a surgical procedure
- Educating about colostomy care, if applicable
- Supporting a positive image

Jaundice

Pathophysiology

Jaundice results from bilirubin diffusing into tissues and giving them a yellow or greenish-yellow tinge. In the spleen, during RBC destruction, the heme is separated from the globulin. The heme further breaks down to iron and bilirubin. In the blood, bilirubin joins with albumin and travels via the blood to the liver, where it is processed and excreted in bile, urine, and feces.

Jaundice is often the first and sometimes the only symptom of liver disease. In hepatitis, it is evident in the icteric phase as hyperbilirubinemia.

The three major types of jaundice are hemolytic, hepatocellular, and obstructive jaundice.

Hemolytic jaundice. Hemolytic jaundice occurs when there is an increase in the number of RBCs destroyed, which increases the amount of bilirubin in the blood. The liver cannot handle the increased load, and the increased bilirubin remains in the blood and is not excreted in the urine or feces. Predisposing factors that may cause hemolytic jaundice are the following:

- Blood transfusions
- Anemia, especially sickle cell

- Reabsorption of extravascular blood found postoperatively or in hematomas
- Certain medications, such as chlorpromazine and penicillin

Hepatocellular jaundice. Hepatocellular jaundice develops from damaged liver cells that are unable to clear bilirubin from the blood. There is impairment of uptake, conjugation, and excretion of bilirubin. Bile salts will deposit on the skin, and the client will have yellow discoloration. Predisposing factors for hepatocellular jaundice include hepatitis, cirrhosis, and liver cancer.

Obstructive jaundice. Obstructive jaundice results from an obstruction to bile flow. Bile will back up into the liver and then into the blood. Urine will take on a deep orange colour. Stool will be light or clay coloured. Pruritus will be evident. Intrahepatic predisposing factors include the following:

- Swelling or fibrosis of the canaliculi and bile ducts in the liver
- Hepatitis
- Cirrhosis
- Tumours
- Medications

Predisposing extrahepatic factors include bile duct obstruction.

Clinical Manifestations

Body tissues including the sclera and skin become yellow or greenish-yellow tinged. The urine may be dark brown or brownish-red due to the presence of bilirubin. Depending on the cause of the jaundice, the client may experience the following symptoms:

- Loss of appetite
- Nausea
- Malaise
- Fatigue
- Weakness
- Pruritus
- Dyspepsia
- Intolerance to fatty foods

Diagnostics

The history and physical examination are important in diagnosing jaundice. Blood work including serum bilirubin, both direct and indirect, will assist in finding the cause of the jaundice. Liver function tests will give information regarding problems with the liver. Viral hepatitis testing may be needed.

Therapeutics and Nursing Considerations

Nursing management involves promoting the following:
- Acceptance of altered body image
- Control of pruritus
- Preventing skin irritation or injury
- Administering medications
- Monitoring clinical findings and laboratory data
- Providing distraction and rest

Adequate nutrition can be a challenge as the clients are often anorexic. Offering small, frequent meals of foods that the client enjoys can be beneficial. Measures to stimulate the appetite, such as mouth care and antiemetics, should be included in the nursing plan. Rest is an important factor in promoting liver cell regeneration (Lewis et al., 2019). To treat the irritating pruritus, lanolin oil or oatmeal may be added to the bath. Skin irritation and injury can be prevented by keeping nails short or wearing mitts. Antihistamines may be prescribed in some situations.

Psychological and emotional rest is as essential as physical rest. Strict bed rest may produce anxiety and extreme restlessness in some clients, which may be more damaging than reasonable ambulation (Lewis et al., 2019). Educating the family is important so they understand what is happening to the client. Family can be very instrumental in supplying diversional activities.

Cholelithiasis

Pathophysiology

Cholelithiasis refers to stones in the gallbladder. *Cholecystitis*, or inflammation of the gallbladder, is usually associated with cholelithiasis. The stones vary in size, shape, and composition and may be lodged in the neck of the gallbladder or in the cystic duct and common bile duct. Cholelithiasis may be acute or chronic. The incidence is higher in multiparous women over the age of 40 years. Sedentary lifestyle, obesity, and family tendency also are risk factors.

The actual cause of the stone is unknown. The most common gallstones are formed from cholesterol, a major component of bile. The stones may remain in the gallbladder or migrate to the cystic duct or common bile duct. They cause pain as they pass through the ducts and may lodge in the ducts and produce an obstruction. Stasis of bile in the gallbladder can lead to cholecystitis.

Clinical Manifestations

Cholelithiasis may produce severe symptoms or none at all. Severity of symptoms depends on whether the stones are stationary or mobile and whether obstruction is present. When the stones are lodged in the cystic duct, the obstruction prevents the movement of bile, so the gallbladder becomes distended, inflamed, and possibly infected. This results in biliary colic with severe upper right abdominal pain that radiates to the back or right shoulder. Other symptoms may include the following:

- Tachycardia
- Diaphoresis
- Nausea and vomiting

Pain may last up to an hour, and when it subsides, a residual tenderness in the right upper quadrant is usually felt. The attacks frequently occur 3–6 hours after a heavy meal or when the client lies down. When total obstruction occurs, symptoms related to bile blockage are manifested, including steatorrhea, pruritus, dark amber urine, a tendency to bleed, and jaundice.

Diagnostics

The following tests are used in the diagnosis:
- Ultrasonography to diagnose gallstones
- CT scan to identify ductal stones

- Endoscopic retrograde cholangiopancreatography (ERCP) allows for visualization of the gallbladder, cystic duct, common hepatic duct, and common bile duct. Bile taken during the procedure is sent for analysis to identify any possible infecting organism.
- Percutaneous transhepatic cholangiography may be used to diagnose obstructive jaundice and to locate stones within the bile ducts.
- Laboratory studies may demonstrate liver function test abnormalities, elevated serum enzymes, pancreatic enzymes, increased WBCs, elevated direct and indirect bilirubin levels, and urinary bilirubin.

Therapeutics and Nursing Considerations

Cholelithiasis is most commonly treated by means of ERCP, which will clear the stones from the biliary tree. In some cases, surgical intervention is needed. Cholecystectomy is often the preferred surgical procedure. This can be done through laparoscopic surgery, in which the gallbladder is removed through one of four tiny punctures in the abdominal wall. Clients experience minimal postoperative pain and are usually discharged home the day of surgery or the day after surgery. Nonsurgical removal of gallstones involves dissolving the gallstones, using extracorporeal shock wave lithotripsy or intracorporeal lithotripsy, but these methods have proven to be only temporary solutions. Drug therapy for gallbladder disease includes the following:

- Analgesics
- Anticholinergics
- Fat-soluble vitamins
- Bile salts
- Some pharmacological therapy can be used to dissolve small stones. This method of treatment is beneficial for clients unable to undergo surgery.

Practical nurses need to focus on the following considerations:

- Pain relief
- Improving respiratory status
- Promoting skin care
- Promoting biliary drainage
- Improving nutritional status
- Monitoring for potential complications
- Nutritional therapy for clients with cholelithiasis is a low-fat diet. If obesity is a problem, a low-calorie diet is also recommended.

Hepatitis

Pathophysiology

Hepatitis is an inflammation of the liver marked by liver cell destruction, necrosis, and autolysis. In most clients, hepatic cells eventually regenerate, with little or no residual damage. However, advanced age and serious underlying disorders make complications more likely. Prognosis is poorer if edema and hepatic encephalopathy develop. The most common cause of hepatitis is viral infection.

Viral hepatitis may be caused by one of six viruses:

- Hepatitis type A (HAV) is transmitted almost exclusively by the fecal–oral route, and outbreaks are common in areas of overcrowding and poor sanitation. Daycare centres and other institutional settings are common sources of outbreaks. The incidence is also increasing in homosexuals and in people with HIV. HAV is the most common type of hepatitis worldwide.
- Hepatitis type B (HBV) is transmitted by blood and blood products, by sexual intercourse, and through perinatal transmission.
- Hepatitis type C (HCV) is transmitted by blood and blood products as well as sexual activity with an infected partner. HCV accounts for 45% of all cases of hepatitis and is the most common liver disease in Canada. Approximately 40% of people infected with HIV also have HCV.
- Hepatitis type D (HDV) can cause an infection only if HBV is present; therefore, the routes of transmission are blood and blood products, as well as sexual intercourse with an infected partner.
- Hepatitis type E (HEV) is transmitted by the fecal–oral route.
- Hepatitis type G (HGV), also known as GB Virus C, is transmitted parenterally and sexually.

Infection with HAV or HBV provides immunity to that virus, but the client may still develop another type of viral hepatitis. Clients with HCV can be infected with another strain of hepatitis C.

Hepatitis may also be caused by cytomegalovirus (CMV), Epstein–Barr virus, the herpes virus, coxsackievirus, and the rubella virus. Despite the different causative viruses, changes in the liver are usually similar in each type of viral hepatitis.

Liver damage is mediated by cytotoxic cytokines and NK cells that cause lysis of infected hepatocytes. In hepatitis, liver cell damage results in hepatic cell necrosis. This necrosis occurs in a spotty fashion, resulting in a piecemeal appearance. Many of the cells swell and rupture, while others shrink. Inflammation then occurs with proliferation and enlargement of the Kupffer cells. Inflammation of the periportal areas may interrupt bile flow, causing jaundice. Cholestasis may occur, as well as hepatomegaly and splenomegaly. Regeneration of liver tissue normally occurs alongside the death of liver cells. The ongoing necrosis, inflammation, and regeneration distort the normal structure and may interfere with blood and bile flow. If there are no complications, the liver cells will resume their normal appearance and function. Along with the hepatic changes, there may be some systemic effects, which may include rash, angioedema, arthritis, fever, and malaise.

Thirty percent of clients with HBV and 80% of clients with HCV are asymptomatic. Most clients with hepatitis recover completely, with no complications. The mortality rate is less than 1%. Complications due to hepatitis include fulminant hepatic failure, chronic hepatitis, cirrhosis, and hepatocellular carcinoma. The characteristics of hepatitis viruses are summarized in Table 8.6.

Clinical Manifestations

The three phases of hepatitis are the preicteric phase, the icteric phase, and the posticteric phase. The preicteric phase

TABLE 8.6   Characteristics of Hepatitis Viruses

Incubation Period and Mode of Transmission	Sources of Infection	Infectivity
Hepatitis A Virus (HAV) 15–50 days (average 28) Fecal–oral route (primarily fecal contamination and oral ingestion)	Crowded conditions (e.g., day care, nursing home). Poor personal hygiene. Poor sanitation. Contaminated food, water, shellfish. Persons with subclinical infections, infected food handlers. Sexual contact with infected partner. IV drug users.	Most infectious during 2 wk before onset of symptoms. Infectious until 1–2 wk after the start of symptoms.
Hepatitis B Virus (HBV) 45–180 days (average 56–96) Percutaneous (parenteral) or permucosal exposure to blood or blood products Sexual contact Perinatal transmission	Contaminated needles, syringes, and blood products. Sexual activity with infected partner. Contact with asymptomatic carrier. Tattoos or body piercing with contaminated needles.	Before and after symptoms appear. Infectious for 4–6 mo. Carriers continue to be infectious for life.
Hepatitis C Virus (HCV) 14–180 days (average 56) Percutaneous (parenteral) or mucosal exposure to blood or blood products High-risk sexual contact Perinatal contact	Blood and blood products. Needles and syringes. Sexual activity with infected partners.	1–2 wk before symptoms appear. Continues during clinical course. 75%–85% go on to develop chronic hepatitis C and remain infectious.
Hepatitis D Virus (HDV) 2–26 wk HBV must precede HDV Chronic carriers of HBV always at risk	Same as HBV. Can cause infection only when HBV is present. Routes of transmission same as for HBV.	Blood infectious at all stages of HDV infection.
Hepatitis E Virus (HEV) 15–64 days (average 26–42 days) Fecal–oral route Outbreaks associated with contaminated water supply in developing countries	Contaminated water, poor sanitation. Found in Asia, Africa, and Mexico. Not common in United States.	Not known. May be similar to HAV.

IV, intravenous.
From Lewis, S. M., Bucher, L., Heitkemper, M. M., et al. (2019). *Medical-surgical nursing in Canada: Assessment and management of clinical problems* (4th Cdn. ed., p. 1103, Table 46.1). Milton, ON: Elsevier Canada.

is sometimes called the *intestinal phase* and may last from 1–21 days.

The *preicteric phase* is the period of maximal infectivity for HAV. This phase precedes the development of jaundice. The symptoms of this phase are as follows:

- Anorexia, nausea, and sometimes vomiting
- Abdominal discomfort, particularly the right upper quadrant
- Constipation or diarrhea
- Malaise and weight loss
  Other symptoms may include the following:
- Headache
- Low-grade fever
- Arthralgias
- Skin rashes
- A distaste for dietary protein and cigarette smoke

The *icteric phase* can last from 2–4 weeks and is characterized by jaundice. Symptoms in the icteric phase include pruritus and dark urine with light-coloured stools.

As the *posticteric phase* begins, the jaundice begins to disappear. This phase may last weeks to months, with the average being 2–4 months. Symptoms found in this phase include malaise and easy fatiguability. The disappearance of jaundice does not indicate recovery. Not all clients with viral hepatitis have jaundice; anicteric hepatitis does occur.

- In HAV, the onset of symptoms is acute, but the actual symptoms are a mild flulike manifestation.
- In HBV, the onset is insidious, and the symptoms tend to be more severe, with fewer GI symptoms.
- In HCV, the majority of clients are asymptomatic. HCV has a high rate of persistence and can induce chronic liver disease.

Diagnostics

Diagnosis of HBV will be confirmed by testing for the presence of hepatitis surface antigens and hepatitis B antibodies. These tests are as follows:

- Detection of an antibody to type A hepatitis confirms past or present infection with HAV.
- Detection of an antibody to type C hepatitis confirms a diagnosis of HCV.
- Viral load is measured by quantitative polymerase chain reaction assay and is useful in determining the need for treatment and monitoring therapy.
- The prothrombin time (PT) will be prolonged, indicating liver damage.
- Serum transaminase levels (alanine aminotransferase [ALT] and aspartate aminotransferase [AST]) will be elevated.
- Serum alkaline phosphatase will be slightly elevated.
- Serum and urine bilirubin levels are elevated.
- Serum albumin levels are low, and serum globulin levels are high.
- A liver biopsy and scan will show patchy necrosis.

Therapeutics and Nursing Considerations

There is no specific treatment for acute viral hepatitis. The following interventions are used:

- Most clients can be managed at home. Emphasis is on measures to rest the body and assist the liver in regenerating. Rest will help decrease the metabolic demands on the body and liver.
- Adequate nutrients and rest seem to be most beneficial for healing and liver cell regeneration. Dietary emphasis is on a well-balanced diet that the client can tolerate.

There is no specific drug therapy for viral hepatitis. Supportive drug therapy may include antiemetics, antihistamines, and sedatives, if needed.

Drug therapy for chronic hepatitis B is focused on decreasing the viral load, serum levels of AST and ALT, and the rate of disease progression. Alpha-interferons (Pegasys, PegIntron) and nucleoside analogues (Epovor, Hepsera) help suppress viral activity and decrease viral loads.

Drug therapy for chronic hepatitis C is directed at reducing the viral load, decreasing the progression of disease, and promoting seroconversion. Treatment includes a combination of ribavirin (Rebetol) and long-acting alpha-interferon (PegIntron).

Both hepatitis A vaccine and immune globulin are used for prevention of hepatitis A. The vaccine is used for pre-exposure prophylaxis, and the immune globulin can be used either before or after exposure. Immunization with hepatitis B vaccine is the most effective method of preventing HBV infection. For postexposure prophylaxis, the vaccine and hepatitis B immune globulin (HBIG) are used.

The diet needs to be adequate to assist hepatocytes to regenerate. The diet should be high in carbohydrates and calories. Protein may be limited if the liver is failing. Fat and sodium should be limited. Vitamin K supplements may be needed, and the client is encouraged to avoid drinking alcohol.

Cirrhosis

Pathophysiology

Cirrhosis of the liver refers to the chronic, progressive, irreversible, and widespread destruction of hepatic cells, with scar tissue (fibrosis) replacing healthy tissue. Cirrhosis can occur at any age but is more common in males between the ages of 40 and 60. Cirrhosis is the 13th leading cause of death in Canada, with alcohol ingestion being the most common cause. There are four major forms of cirrhosis:

- Alcoholic (Laennec's or portal/nutritional) cirrhosis results from malnutrition, especially protein deficiency and chronic alcohol intake. Alcohol alone has a direct hepatotoxic effect; it can produce necrosis of cells and fatty infiltrates.
- Postnecrotic cirrhosis is a complication of viral, toxic, or idiopathic hepatitis. Hepatitis C and alcohol are the two major causes of liver disease in Canada.
- Biliary cirrhosis results from bile duct disease.
- Cardiac cirrhosis is due to severe right-sided heart failure with cor pulmonale, prolonged constrictive pericarditis, and tricuspid insufficiency.
- Other forms of cirrhosis include nonspecific metabolic cirrhosis from infiltrating infections and cirrhosis due to inherited diseases such as hemochromatosis or Wilson's disease. Cirrhosis can be caused by drugs, toxins, and parasites. Non-alcoholic steatohepatitis (NASH) is found when fat builds up in the liver and eventually causes scar formation.

Pathophysiology of cirrhosis involves the destruction of hepatocytes. This hepatocyte necrosis leads to the development of scar tissue, which, in turn, disrupts blood and bile flow. This disruption then leads to an increase in pressure in the portal circulatory system, which causes portal hypertension. This hypertension damages more hepatocytes, resulting in loss of function and liver death.

Clinical Manifestations

Early manifestations of cirrhosis may be absent or minimal and then develop insidiously. These manifestations are as follows:

- Fatigue and weakness
- Decreased appetite and weight loss
- Nausea and vomiting
- Flatus
- Dull right upper quadrant discomfort due to swelling and stretching of the liver
- Possibly fever and pruritus
  Later manifestations may include the following:
- Jaundice
- Skin lesions
- Hematological problems (thrombocytopenia, anemia, leukopenia)

- Endocrine disturbances (testicular atrophy, menstrual irregularities)
- Peripheral neuropathies
- Peripheral edema
- Infections

As the liver begins to fail, the normal functions of the liver also fail.

Diagnostics

Cirrhosis is typically advanced before it is diagnosed. The following tests are done to diagnose cirrhosis:

- A liver biopsy is the definitive test to diagnose cirrhosis.
- Blood work will show abnormal liver function, impaired clotting factors, thrombocytopenia, leukopenia, and anemia, as well as electrolyte imbalances due to an increase in aldosterone and ADH.
- A liver scan will show abnormal thickening and mass.

Therapeutics and Nursing Considerations

Treatment is aimed at removing or alleviating the underlying cause of the cirrhosis, preventing further liver damage, and preventing or treating complications. Complications that may result from cirrhosis are as follows:

- Portal hypertension
- Peripheral edema
- Ascites
- Varices
- Hepatic encephalopathy
- Hepatorenal syndrome
- Fetor hepaticus

Portal hypertension can result in retention and pooling of visceral blood, which, in turn, causes congestion of adjacent viscera. The high portal venous pressure will shunt blood into the systemic circulation, causing esophageal, gastric, spleen, and rectal varices. These vessels are fragile and may rupture. Treatment for ruptured varices begins with finding the source of the bleeding and stopping it. Esophagoscopy may be done if possible to find and treat the bleeding. Gastric lavage, sclerotherapy, vasopressin injection, and an esophagogastric tamponade (Minnesota or Blakemore tube) may be used to stop the bleeding. Once stabilized, a portacaval shunt or a transjugular intrahepatic portosystemic shunt may be put in place. Fluid volume must be replaced. Vital signs must be monitored, assessing for any signs of shock.

The failing liver impairs the synthesis of albumin. With the decrease in albumin, vascular oncotic pressure decreases, resulting in peripheral edema. Ascites develop due to the decreased hepatic synthesis of albumin, increased portal vein pressure, obstructed hepatic lymph flow, and increased serum aldosterone level. Ascites may be treated with sodium restriction, diuretics, and albumin. A paracentesis may be done to remove the excess fluid. A peritoneal venous shunt (LeVeen or Denver) may be inserted to remove fluid from the peritoneum to the superior vena cava. With the removal of fluid, the BP may drop, so the practical nurse must monitor the vital signs closely. Fluid replacement may be needed.

Hepatic encephalopathy is frequently a terminal complication. It is caused by increased levels of ammonia. Classic symptoms of hepatic encephalopathy include impaired attention span, irritability and restlessness, apathy, loss of interest, lethargy, somnolence, and coma. Hepatic encephalopathy is treated by identifying the precipitating cause and treating it with antibiotics, enemas, and lactulose. Lactulose will bind with the ammonia and help evacuate it via the bowel.

Hepatorenal syndrome results from functional renal failure with advancing azotemia, oliguria, and intractable ascites. The kidneys fail due to the redistribution of blood flow from the kidneys to the periphery and visceral circulation, or as a result of hypovolemia due to ascites. Vital signs need to be monitored closely.

Fetor hepaticus is a musty, sweetish odour detected on the client's breath. The odour is due to the accumulation of digested by-products. Additional complications of cirrhosis may include exhaustion, gallstones, complications with pharmacological therapy, and pruritus.

An important role of the practical nurse is educating the client about the general management of cirrhosis, which includes rest, avoidance of alcohol and anticoagulants, managing the possible complications, and ensuring adequate and appropriate nutrition.

Pancreatitis
Pathophysiology

Pancreatitis is an inflammation of the pancreas that can be acute or chronic. The degree of inflammation varies from mild edema to severe necrosis. Pancreatitis can affect both men and women, but it is more commonly found in men. The prognosis is good when pancreatitis follows biliary disease but poor when it is a complication of alcoholism. The causes of pancreatitis are as follows:

- Alcohol is the number one cause of pancreatitis in Canada.
- Gallbladder disease is the next most common cause of pancreatitis.
- Other causes include viral infections, duodenal or peptic ulcers, pancreatic cancer, drugs such as glucocorticoids, metabolic disorders such as hyperparathyroidism and dyslipidemia, and postsurgical trauma from ERCP.

In acute pancreatitis, the inflammation that occurs is caused by premature activation of digestive enzymes, which leads to autodigestion of the surrounding tissue. The pancreatic enzymes are activated while they are still in the pancreas rather than in the small intestine, so they digest pancreatic cells, causing severe edema, interstitial hemorrhage, and necrosis, which can lead to hypotension, shock, and disseminated intravascular coagulation (DIC).

Two major complications of pancreatitis are pseudocyst and pancreatic abscess. The pseudocyst is a cavity that develops around the pancreas that is filled with necrotic products and liquid secretions. If the cyst perforates, exudate inflames the surrounding tissues, causing peritonitis, followed by scar tissue. The pseudocyst may heal by itself or require draining. A pancreatic abscess is a large fluid-containing cavity within the pancreas that results from extensive necrosis of the pancreatic cells. This abscess may become infected and perforate.

Other complications of pancreatitis include pulmonary problems such as pleural effusion, atelectasis, and pneumonia. Cardiovascular problems such as hypotension and tachycardia may occur, and the client may develop tetany due to the low calcium levels in the blood.

Clinical Manifestations

Abdominal pain unrelieved by vomiting may be the first and only symptom of mild pancreatitis. A severe attack may cause a sudden onset of extreme pain in the left upper quadrant with possible radiation to the back. The pain is often described as severe, deep, piercing, and steady. The pain is aggravated by eating or drinking alcohol and does not subside with vomiting. Other manifestations may include flushing, cyanosis, edema, nausea, vomiting, low-grade fever, leukocytosis, jaundice, hypotension, and tachycardia.

Diagnostics

Diagnosis is made through the history and physical examination. Blood work may show elevated serum amylase levels, which rules out appendicitis, acute cholecystitis, perforated ulcer, and bowel infarction. Serum lipase, glucose, and WBC levels are likely to increase, while serum calcium levels are likely to decrease. An abdominal CT scan can help distinguish between cholelithiasis and pancreatitis.

Therapeutics and Nursing Considerations

Management of pancreatitis focuses on the following:
- Pain relief
- Maintenance of circulation and fluid volume
- Decreasing pancreatic enzymes
- Analgesics, vasodilators, and antispasmodics may be given. Dopamine may be needed for hypotension.
- The client will be NPO. An NG tube will be in place to remove secretions. IV therapy will be needed to maintain fluid volume. The client will be monitored for complications. Once the client is allowed food, small, frequent meals are offered. The diet should be high in carbohydrates and protein and low in fat.

Nursing considerations will focus on the following:
- Pain relief
- Improving breathing patterns
- Improving nutritional status
- Improving skin integrity
- Monitoring and managing any complications

The practical nurse will also be involved in client teaching about discontinuing alcohol, proper nutrition and rest, and ways to improve the client's general health.

Pathophysiology of chronic pancreatitis. Chronic pancreatitis develops from repeated attacks of pancreatitis. These repeated attacks cause scarring and calcification of the pancreatic cells, which leads to the permanent and progressive destruction of the pancreas. Both exocrine and endocrine functions of the pancreas are affected. Chronic obstructive pancreatitis results from inflammation of the sphincter of Oddi and is associated with cholelithiasis. Chronic calcifying pancreatitis is alcohol-induced pancreatitis.

Clinical manifestations of chronic pancreatitis. Chronic pancreatitis manifestations include abdominal pain, usually described as a severe, heavy, gnawing feeling, burning, or cramplike pain. The client will experience malabsorption, constipation, steatorrhea, mild jaundice, and diabetes mellitus (DM).

Diagnostics for chronic pancreatitis. Diagnosis is the same as for acute pancreatitis.

Therapeutics and nursing considerations for chronic pancreatitis. Management of chronic pancreatitis focuses on prevention of attacks. During an attack, treatment is similar to that of acute pancreatitis. With chronic pancreatitis, the client needs to be taught about diet, pancreatic enzyme replacement, exogenous insulin, antacids, and cessation of alcohol intake. The client cannot tolerate fatty or rich foods. The DM is often "brittle" in response to insulin; therefore, the client may require frequent injections to control blood sugars. Client education is very important.

REGULATORY MECHANISM HEALTH CHALLENGES

Addison's Disease
Pathophysiology

Addison's disease is the most common form of adrenal insufficiency. Although Addison's disease usually results from an autoimmune disorder, it can be caused by TB, histoplasmosis, adrenal hemorrhage, cancer, lymphoma, and certain drugs. Surgical removal of the adrenal glands and abruptly stopping long-term corticosteroid therapy can also cause Addison's disease. When the cause is autoimmune, antibodies against the client's own adrenal cortex destroy the adrenal gland's ability to secrete hormones.

Clinical Manifestations

Manifestations do not tend to become apparent until about 90% of the cortex has been destroyed. Manifestations that do develop do so insidiously and may include the following:
- Progressive weakness and fatigue
- Weight loss and anorexia
- Skin hyperpigmentation (bronze colouring) is a striking feature.
- The client also may have orthostatic hypotension, a weak irregular pulse, decreased tolerance for even minor stress, poor coordination, fasting hypoglycemia, a craving for salty foods, and amenorrhea.

Diagnostics

Diagnosis is made based on clinical features and decreased serum cortisol and sodium levels. Corticotrophin, serum potassium, and blood urea nitrogen (BUN) levels are all increased. A failure of serum cortisol to rise following adrenocorticotropic hormone (ACTH) stimulation indicates primary adrenal disease.

Therapeutics and Nursing Considerations

Treatment of Addison's disease is focused on management of the underlying cause and replacement therapy.

- Hydrocortisone has both glucocorticoid and mineralocorticoid properties and is frequently used as replacement therapy.
- During periods of stress, the replacement therapy may need to be increased.
- In an adrenal crisis, the client may need prompt administration of dexamethasone, hydrocortisone, or both, and doses continue until he or she stabilizes.
- Vital signs must be monitored for signs of volume depletion and hypotension.
- Blood work needs to be monitored for altered electrolytes both before and during treatment.
- Blood glucose needs to be monitored as steroid replacement may alter insulin requirements.

  Client education regarding medication adherence is essential.

Cushing's Syndrome
Pathophysiology

Cushing's syndrome is a spectrum of clinical abnormalities caused by excess corticosteroids, particularly glucocorticoids. This adrenal hyperfunction can be caused by prolonged administration of high doses of corticosteroids, an ACTH-secreting pituitary tumour, or a cortisol-secreting neoplasm within the adrenal cortex that can be either carcinoma or adenoma.

Clinical Manifestations

Unmistakable manifestations of Cushing's syndrome include the following:

- Adiposity of the face (moon face) and neck (buffalo hump)
- Purple striae on the skin of the trunk, especially the abdomen
- Weight gain
- Muscle weakness and fatigue
- Thinning of the extremities with muscle wasting and fat mobilization
- Thin, fragile skin, ruddy complexion, hirsutism, acne, bruising, and impaired wound healing

Diagnostics

When Cushing's syndrome is suspected, a 24-hour urine collection test for free cortisol and a low-dose dexamethasone suppression test are done. If these tests are inconclusive, then a high-dose dexamethasone suppression test is done. Ultrasonography, CT scan, and angiography localize adrenal tumours. CT scan and MRI of the head help localize pituitary tumours.

Therapeutics and Nursing Considerations

The primary goal of treatment is to normalize hormone secretion. Radiation, drug therapy, or surgery may be needed to restore hormone balance and reverse Cushing's syndrome. Some examples of treatments are as follows:

- Trans-sphenoidal resection and radiation may be used for pituitary adenomas.
- Surgical removal or radiation may be used for an ectopic ACTH-secreting tumour.
- Nonendocrine corticotropin-secreting tumours require excision.
- Drug therapy with ketoconazole (Nizoral), or mitotane (Lysodren) decreases cortisol levels if symptoms persist or if the tumour is inoperable.

Before surgery, the client will require special monitoring and control of hypertension, edema, diabetes, and cardiovascular manifestations and to prevent infection. Glucocorticoid administration the morning of surgery can help prevent acute adrenal insufficiency during surgery. Nursing considerations will focus on the following:

- Decreasing risk for injury
- Decreasing risk for infection
- Encouraging rest and activity
- Promoting skin integrity
- Improving body image
- Improving thought processes
- Monitoring and managing complications

Clients with Cushing's syndrome require thorough ongoing assessment and supportive care, including emotional support, as the syndrome produces emotional lability. In some cases, sedation may be needed to help the client rest.

Hyperthyroidism
Pathophysiology

Hyperthyroidism is a clinical syndrome in which there is a sustained increase in synthesis and release of thyroid hormones by the thyroid gland. The most common form of hyperthyroidism is Graves' disease (diffuse toxic goitre), an autoimmune disease that increases T_4 (thyroxine) production, enlarges the thyroid gland (goitre), and causes multisystem changes. In Graves' disease, a thyroid-stimulating hormone (TSH) receptor autoantibody stimulates the thyroid gland to produce high concentrations of T_3 (tri-iodothyronine) and T_4. Graves' disease has also been associated with the production of several autoantibodies formed because of a defect in suppressor T-lymphocyte function.

Thyrotoxic crisis (thyroid storm) is an acute, rare condition in which all hyperthyroid manifestations are heightened. This is a life-threatening condition for which aggressive measures must be taken to prevent death.

Clinical Manifestations

Classic manifestations of Graves' disease include the following:

- A diffusely enlarged thyroid
- Nervousness and insomnia
- Hair loss
- Fatigue and muscle weakness
- Edema
- Heat intolerance
- Weight loss and increased appetite
- Splenomegaly
- Hepatomegaly

- Sweating
- Diarrhea
- Tremor
- Palpitations
- Systolic hypertension
- Arrhythmias and atrial fibrillation
- Reproductive abnormalities
- Possible exophthalmos

Treatment is aimed at reducing circulating thyroid hormone levels and treating manifestations such as high fever with antipyretics, IV therapy for fluid replacement, and elimination of stressors.

Diagnostics

Graves' disease is diagnosed by the history and physical examination and laboratory tests finding decreased TSH and increased free T_4 levels. Radioactive iodine uptake test is needed to differentiate Graves' disease from other forms of thyroiditis. A thyroid sonogram helps distinguish cystic and solid lesions. A CT scan or an MRI helps identify deep thyroid nodules.

Therapeutics and Nursing Considerations

The overall goal in the treatment of hyperthyroidism is to block the adverse effects of the thyroid hormones and stop their oversecretion. The primary forms of treatment for hyperthyroidism are as follows:
- Antithyroid drugs
- Radioactive iodine therapy
- Subtotal thyroidectomy

Choice of treatment will depend on the client's age, severity of the disease, client's present physical condition, and the client's preference.
- Propylthiouracil (Propyl-Thyracil) and methimazole (Tapazole) block thyroid hormone synthesis.
- The administration of iodine in large doses rapidly inhibits synthesis of T_3 and T_4 and blocks the release of these hormones into the circulatory system.
- Beta-adrenergic blockers are used for symptomatic relief of thyrotoxicosis that results from increased beta-adrenergic receptor stimulation caused by excess thyroid hormone.
- Radioactive iodine damages or destroys thyroid tissue, thus limiting thyroid hormone secretion. This treatment is effective but leaves the client with hypothyroidism, requiring thyroid hormone replacement therapy.
- A subtotal thyroidectomy removes a significant portion (90%) of the thyroid gland and is needed for clients who do not respond to antithyroid therapy.

Nursing considerations focus on improving nutritional status, enhancing coping measures, improving self-esteem, maintaining normal body temperatures, and monitoring and managing any complications.

Hypothyroidism
Pathophysiology

Hypothyroidism is a state of low levels of serum thyroid hormones. Hypothyroidism may result from a number of causes but is mainly caused by the following:

- A thyroidectomy
- Radiation therapy
- Chronic autoimmune thyroiditis (Hashimoto's disease)
- Inflammatory diseases, such as amyloidosis

In primary hypothyroidism, thyroid hormone production is decreased due to decreased thyroid tissue. The pituitary gland will still secrete TSH, and a goitre may develop. In secondary hypothyroidism, the pituitary fails to synthesize or secrete adequate amounts of TSH, or target tissues fail to respond to normal blood levels of the thyroid hormone. Either type may progress to myxedema (an advanced form of hypothyroidism). This condition is considered a medical emergency.

Clinical Manifestations

Clinical manifestations of hypothyroidism will vary with the severity of the condition regardless of the cause. Symptoms develop insidiously and may include the following:
- Fatigue and lethargy
- Forgetfulness
- Slow speech
- Low exercise tolerance
- Weight gain
- Bradycardia
- Anemia
- Constipation
- Cool, dry, flaky skin; dry, sparse hair; and thick, brittle nails.

Symptoms of the life-threatening myxedema include progressive personality and mental changes moving toward stupor, hypoventilation, hypoglycemia, hyponatremia, hypotension, and hypothermia.

Diagnostics

The most common and reliable laboratory tests used to evaluate thyroid function are those that measure TSH and free T_4. When TSH levels are high, the defect is in the thyroid, and when the levels are low, the defect is in the pituitary or hypothalamus.

Therapeutics and Nursing Considerations

The goal of treatment for clients with hypothyroidism is replacement of the hormones by administering synthetic levothyroxine (Synthroid, Eltroxin). The practical nurse provides the following care:
- Routinely assesses the client to see whether the medication is adequate or not.
- Encourages weight loss with a high-bulk, low-calorie diet.
- Encourages activity balanced with rest.
- Administers laxatives and stool softeners when needed.

Teach the client to watch for signs of hyperthyroidism, such as sweating, tachycardia, or rapid weight loss, and to always wear a MedicAlert bracelet or carry a MedicAlert card.

Syndrome of Inappropriate Antidiuretic Hormone
Pathophysiology

Syndrome of inappropriate antidiuretic hormone (SIADH) occurs when ADH is released despite normal or low plasma osmolarity. SIADH results from an abnormal production or sustained secretion of ADH and is characterized by fluid retention. The hyponatremia that can occur with SIADH can lead to cerebral edema. SIADH can occur due to malignant lung disease, infections, trauma, or medications that stimulate ADH release.

Clinical Manifestations

One of the chief clinical manifestations of SIADH is fluid retention; therefore, the client will gain weight and have a decreased urine output. The serum hyponatremia may cause the client to have the following symptoms as well:

- Muscle cramps, weakness, and muscle twitching
- Vomiting
- Seizures

If the hyponatremia progresses and sodium levels continue to decline, the client may experience cerebral edema, leading to lethargy, anorexia, confusion, headaches, seizure, and coma.

Diagnostics

The diagnosis of SIADH is made by simultaneous measurements of urine and serum osmolality. A serum osmolality of less than 280 mOsm/kg (280 mmol/kg) and a urine concentration greater than 100 mOsm/kg are indicative of SIADH.

Therapeutics and Nursing Considerations

Once SIADH is identified, the care is directed at the underlying cause of the condition. The immediate treatment is aimed at restoring normal fluid volume and osmolality. Fluid restriction may be all that is needed. If the hyponatremia is severe, hypertonic saline solutions may be administered cautiously as rapid administration could overload the heart.

Diabetes Insipidus
Pathophysiology

Diabetes insipidus (DI) is a group of conditions associated with a deficiency of production or secretion of ADH (vasopressin) or a decreased renal response to ADH. DI may be familial, acquired, or idiopathic.

- It can be acquired as the result of intracranial neoplastic or metastatic lesions.
- Other causes may include hypophysectomy or other neurosurgery, head trauma, infection, granulomatous disease, vascular lesions, or autoimmune disorders.

Normally, the ADH is synthesized in the hypothalamus and stored in the posterior pituitary gland. When released, ADH works on the distal and collecting tubules of the kidneys, causing water to be reabsorbed. If ADH is absent or not released, the water is excreted in the urine. As a result, the client will void copious amounts of urine.

Clinical Manifestations

The classic sign of DI is polyuria, or the passage of a large volume of urine, with amounts from 5–20 L and possibly up to 30 L/day. Polydipsia, or excessive thirst, may be present. Nocturia and fatigue are common, as well as dehydration

with weight loss, poor tissue turgor, dry mucous membranes, constipation, muscle weakness, dizziness, tachycardia, and hypotension.

Diagnostics

A complete history and physical examination are needed to diagnose DI. Baseline vital signs and weight are taken, and urine and plasma osmolalities and specific gravity of the urine tests are usually performed. A urinalysis may reveal almost colourless urine with a low osmolality and low specific gravity. A water deprivation test confirms the diagnosis. The client will be denied water for 8–16 hours. The client will be anxious and thirsty and will require reassurance and support. Vital signs will be monitored closely, and the test will be stopped if the client develops orthostatic hypotension or body weight drops by 3%.

Therapeutics and Nursing Considerations

Determining the cause of DI is critical to its treatment. Hormone replacement of ADH is needed. Care of a client with DI resulting from nephrogenic problems includes a low-sodium diet and utilizing thiazide diuretics. The thiazides are able to slow the glomerular filtration rate (GFR), allowing the kidneys to reabsorb more water in the loop of Henle and distal tubules. If this does not work, indomethacin (an anti-inflammatory) may be prescribed.

Nursing management revolves around early detection, maintenance of adequate hydration, client teaching for long-term management, and encouragement and support while the client is undergoing diagnostic studies and treatment.

Diabetes Mellitus
Pathophysiology

DM is a multisystem disease related to abnormal insulin production, impaired insulin utilization, or both. It is the leading cause of heart disease, stroke, adult blindness, and nontraumatic lower limb amputation.

Normally, insulin is produced by the beta cells in the islets of Langerhans of the pancreas. Insulin facilitates the normal glucose range of approximately 4–6 mmol/L. Insulin is a storage hormone that promotes glucose transport from the bloodstream across the cell membrane into the cytoplasm of the cell. Ingesting food stimulates the release of insulin from the pancreas into the blood. Insulin stimulates the storage of glucose as glycogen and inhibits gluconeogenesis. Insulin also enhances fat deposition in adipose tissue and increases protein synthesis. Glucagon is a hormone produced in the alpha cells of the pancreas and functions by increasing blood glucose levels.

Type 1 diabetes was formerly known as *juvenile-onset* or *insulin-dependent* diabetes. Type 1 diabetes usually affects people under the age of 30, peaking at 11–13 years, but it can affect people older than 30 years of age. Type 1 diabetes involves the progressive destruction of pancreatic beta cells. Autoantibodies cause a reduction of 80–90% of normal beta cell function before manifestations occur. The causes of type

1 diabetes may be due to genetic predisposition or exposure to a virus. Manifestations develop when the pancreas can no longer produce insulin. Symptoms tend to be rapid in onset, and the client often presents to the emergency department with ketoacidosis. Other classic symptoms include weight loss, polyuria, polydipsia, and polyphagia. Diabetic ketoacidosis (DKA) occurs in the absence of exogenous insulin. It is a life-threatening condition that results in metabolic acidosis.

Type 2 diabetes accounts for over 90% of clients with diabetes. It usually occurs in people over the age of 35; however, children are now being diagnosed with type 2 diabetes, usually due to obesity and a sedentary lifestyle. With type 2 diabetes, the pancreas continues to produce some endogenous insulin; however, the amount produced is either insufficient or is poorly utilized by the tissues. Insulin resistance is the key to type 2 diabetes, a situation in which the body does not respond to the insulin and hyperglycemia results. Some people experience glucose intolerance, in which the alteration

in the beta cells is mild. In these situations, the blood glucose levels are higher than normal but are not high enough for a diagnosis of diabetes. Inappropriate glucose production by the liver is not considered a primary factor in the development of type 2 diabetes. Insulin resistance syndrome (syndrome X) is a cluster of abnormalities that act synergistically to increase the risk of cardiovascular disease. Type 2 diabetes typically has a gradual onset; the person may go many years with undetected hyperglycemia. See Table 8.7 for further characteristics of type 1 and 2 diabetes.

Diabetes can also develop during pregnancy, when it is usually detected at 24–28 weeks of gestation. With gestational diabetes, there is an increased risk for a caesarean delivery, perinatal deaths, and neonatal complications.

Diabetes can also develop secondary to another medical condition or the treatment of a medical condition. For example, there can be abnormal blood values in a client experiencing Cushing's syndrome or as a result of the use of parenteral nutrition.

TABLE 8.7   Characteristics of Type 1 and Type 2 Diabetes Mellitus

Factor	Type 1 Diabetes Mellitus	Type 2 Diabetes Mellitus	Factor	Type 1 Diabetes Mellitus	Type 2 Diabetes Mellitus
Age at onset	More common in young people but can occur at any age	Usually ≥35 yr but can occur at any age. Incidence is increasing in children	Endogenous insulin	Minimal or absent	Possibly excessive; adequate but delayed secretion or reduced utilization; secretions diminish over time
Type of onset	Signs and symptoms abrupt, but disease process may be present for several years	Insidious; may go undiagnosed for years	Nutritional status	Thin, normal, or obese	Obese or normal
Prevalence	Accounts for 5%–10% of all types of diabetes	Accounts for 90% of all types of diabetes	Symptoms	Thirst, polyuria, polyphagia, fatigue, weight loss	Frequently none, fatigue, recurrent infections
Environmental factors	Viruses, toxins	Obesity, lack of exercise	Ketosis	Prone at onset or during insulin deficiency	Resistant except during infection or stress
Primary defect	Absent or minimal insulin production due to an autoimmune process	Insulin resistance, decreased insulin production over time, and alterations in production of adipokines	Nutritional therapy	Essential	Essential
Islet-cell antibodies	Often present at onset	Absent	Insulin	Required for all	Required for some
			Oral antihyperglycemic agents	Not indicated	Usually beneficial
			Vascular and neurological complications	Frequent	Frequent

From Lewis, S. M., Bucher, L., Heitkemper, M. M., et al. (2019). *Medical-surgical nursing in Canada: Assessment and management of clinical problems* (4th Cdn. ed., p. 1289, Table 52.1). Milton, ON: Elsevier Canada.

Clinical Manifestations

Manifestations of type 1 diabetes include classic polyuria, polydipsia, and polyphagia. The client will also experience weight loss, weakness and fatigue, and ketoacidosis. Nonspecific symptoms include fatigue, recurrent infections, prolonged wound healing, and visual changes.

Diagnostics

Diagnosis of DM is made when glycosylated hemoglobin (hemoglobin A1c) is greater than 6.5%, fasting plasma glucose is greater than 7 mmol/L, a random plasma glucose measurement is greater than 11.1 mmol/L, or a 2-hour oral glucose tolerance test (OGTT) is greater than 11.1 mmol/L when using a glucose load of 75 g. Tests used to evaluate glucose control and monitor for complications of diabetes include hemoglobin A1c, lipid profile, BUN, serum creatinine, electrolytes, and TSH. Urine can be checked for glucose and ketones.

Therapeutics and Nursing Considerations

Goals for the treatment of DM include the following:
- Reducing symptoms
- Promoting well-being
- Preventing acute complications
- Delaying the onset and progression of long-term complications

Collaborative care includes five components: education, nutrition, medications, exercise, and self-monitoring of blood glucose.

Exogenous insulin is required for type 1 diabetes. It may be prescribed for clients with type 2 diabetes who cannot control their blood glucose by other means or when the client is under stress. Human insulin is the most widely used insulin; it is cost-effective, and there is less chance of the client developing an allergic reaction. Insulin can also be derived from beef and pork.

Insulin types differ in regard to onset, peak action, and duration. Different types of insulin may be used for combination therapy. Some common types of insulin are as follows:
- Lispro is a rapid-acting insulin.
- Regular and Toronto are short-acting insulins.
- NPH and Lente are intermediate-acting insulins.
- Ultralente and Lantus are long-acting insulins.

Insulin may be administered subcutaneously. At present, insulin cannot be taken orally; however, new research is finding alternative delivery methods, including aerosol, skin patches, oral spray, and pills. Problems with insulin therapy include hypoglycemia, allergic reactions, lipodystrophy, and the Somogyi effect.

Oral agents are not insulin. These medications work to improve the mechanisms through which insulin and glucose are produced and used by the body. These medications include the following:
- Sulfonylureas, meglitinides, biguanides
- Alpha-glucosidase inhibitors
- Thiazolidinediones

- Other drugs affecting blood glucose levels are beta-adrenergic blockers, thiazide diuretics, and loop diuretics.

Nutrition and exercise in DM management. Research has shown that within the context of an overall healthy eating plan, a person with diabetes can eat the same foods as a person who does not have diabetes. The overall goal of nutrition therapy is to assist people in making changes in nutrition and exercise habits that will lead to improved metabolic control.
- A type 1 DM meal plan is based on the individual's usual food intake and is balanced with insulin and exercise patterns.
- In type 2 DM, emphasis is placed on achieving glucose, lipid, and BP goals. Calorie reduction is often needed.

Individual meal plans are developed with the assistance of a dietitian. The plan promotes a nutritional balance and does not prohibit the consumption of any one type of food. Alcohol can be included within the plan with the full understanding that alcohol is high in calories, promotes hypertriglyceridemia, and can cause severe hypoglycemia. The dietitian should provide instructions to the client and family or significant other.

Exercise is an essential part of diabetes management as it increases insulin sensitivity, lowers blood glucose levels, and decreases insulin resistance. Exercise also improves circulation and muscle tone, increases the resting metabolic rate, and alters blood lipids. The body considers exercise to be stress. In type 1 diabetes, the physiological decrease in circulating insulin that normally occurs with exercise cannot occur; therefore, clients with DM need to have small carbohydrate snacks every 30 minutes during exercise to prevent hypoglycemia. Exercise is best done after meals and should be individualized for every client. Blood glucose levels should be monitored before, during, and after exercise.

Self-monitoring of blood glucose (SMBG) enables clients to make self-management decisions regarding diet, exercise, and medications. SMBG is important for detecting episodic hyperglycemia and hypoglycemia. Client teaching is crucial. SMBG requires good visual acuity, fine motor coordination, cognitive ability, comfort with technology, willingness, and sufficient finances to pay for it.

Urine testing for glucose was a technique used before the development of SMBG. It is a less expensive technique, but it does not represent an accurate reading as the urine tested could have been in the bladder for a matter of hours. However, urine testing for ketones is essential when the client is ill.

Overall goals for the management of DM should include active participation of the client, no episodes of hypoglycemia or hyperglycemia, maintenance of normal blood glucose levels, prevention of complications, and lifestyle adjustments with minimal stress.

Acute complications of DM. Acute complications pertaining to DM are hypoglycemia, DKA, and hyperosmolar hyperglycemic non-ketotic syndrome (HHNK).

Hypoglycemia. Hypoglycemia is found in clients whose blood glucose level is abnormally below 4 mmol/L.

Hypoglycemia may be caused by too little food or too much insulin. Symptoms of hypoglycemia include the following:

- Sweating
- Trembling
- Blurred vision
- Extreme tiredness and paleness
- Headache
- Hunger
- Mood changes
- Dizziness

To treat hypoglycemia, give 10–15 g of a fast-acting simple carbohydrate, such as three to four commercially prepared glucose tabs, 120–180 mL (4–6 oz) of fruit juice or a regular soft drink, or 6–10 hard candies. The blood should be retested after 15 minutes. If the blood glucose remains low, the carbohydrate intake should be repeated. When the level goes up, the client should be given a protein with a starch. An unconscious client can be injected with 1 mg of glucagon, either subcutaneously or intramuscularly. If this is not available, a source of glucose, such as corn syrup, honey, or icing, may be placed in the client's buccal pouch. After consciousness returns, the client should be given a protein or starch snack. Hypoglycemia is preventable. Clients with diabetes should always carry a simple sugar with them and have identification confirming their diagnosis. Family and friends need to know the signs and symptoms of hypoglycemia and what they can do to assist the client.

Diabetic ketoacidosis. DKA is caused by an absence of insulin or a markedly inadequate amount. Clinical features of DKA include hyperglycemia, dehydration, and acidosis. DKA can be caused by a decreased or missed dose of insulin, an illness or infection, or undiagnosed and untreated diabetes. Clinical manifestations include the following:

- Blurred vision
- Weakness
- Headache
- Orthostatic hypotension
- Anorexia, nausea and vomiting, and abdominal pain
- Acetone breath
- Hyperventilation
- Possible mental changes

DKA is diagnosed with an elevated blood glucose, with levels varying from 14–44 mmol/L or higher. The severity of DKA is not necessarily related to the actual blood glucose level. Ketones will be found in the blood and urine, and the electrolytes may be low, normal, or high, depending on the level of dehydration.

Prevention of DKA is based on understanding the importance of food replacement during illness. A typical sick-day routine is as follows: Take insulin or oral antidiabetic agents as usual. Test blood glucose and urine for ketones every 3–4 hours. Report elevated blood glucose levels of 16 mmol/L or more or the presence of ketones in the urine to the healthcare provider. Treatment of DKA focuses on rehydration and balancing the electrolytes and pH. Clients receive potassium in the IV solution as long as they remain polyuric

and hypokalemic. The acidosis is reversed by administering insulin via an IV pump. Nursing management focuses on the following:

- Monitoring fluid and electrolyte balance
- Monitoring blood glucose levels
- Giving fluids, insulin, and other medications as ordered
- Ensuring renal function
- Monitoring for arrhythmias
- Monitoring vital signs
- Reassessing factors leading to the development of DKA

Hyperosmolar hyperglycemic non-ketotic syndrome. HHNK includes hyperglycemia, dehydration, and hyperosmolality of the plasma, with the absence of ketones in the urine. HHNK differs from DKA in that HHNK does not cause fat tissue to break down; thus, ketones will not be released. Clinical manifestations include hypotension, profound dehydration, and tachycardia, with variable neurological signs. Medical and nursing management focuses on fluid replacement, correction of electrolyte imbalances, administering IV insulin, and monitoring fluid and electrolyte balance. Insulin is not used to treat acidosis in HHNK, but it is used to treat the hyperglycemia.

Chronic complications of DM. Chronic complications of DM include microvascular and macrovascular complications and neuropathic complications. DM can cause macrovascular damage to the large blood vessels providing circulation to the brain, heart, and extremities. Dyslipidemia, hypertension, and impaired fibrinolysis have been found in uncontrolled DM.

Microvascular complications create abnormal thickening of the basement membrane in the capillaries by hyperglycemia. Hyperglycemia also disrupts platelet function.

- Retinopathy starts with small hemorrhages in the retinal capillaries. Neovascularization occurs, which can lead to proliferative retinopathy. People with DM have an increased risk of developing cataracts and open-angle glaucoma.
- Nephropathy is the leading cause of end-stage renal disease (ESRD), with the characteristic lesion being glomerulosclerosis.
- Neuropathic complications can be found in 40–50% of those with diabetes; paraesthesia, autonomic complications, and sensory disturbances are common.
- Peripheral polyneuropathy involves both neuropathy and vascular problems. The real danger for the client with this condition is that the client cannot feel pain.
- Individuals with diabetes need to watch for any signs of infection. There is a defect in the mobilization of inflammatory cells and an impairment of WBCs in phagocytosis. Persistent glycosuria encourages bladder infections. There is a delay in healing due to decreased circulation as well as protein waste leading to poor wound healing.

Pancreas transplantation is done for clients with type 1 DM who have ESRD and have had or plan to have a kidney transplantation. The pancreas transplantation eliminates the need for exogenous insulin and eliminates hypoglycemia and hyperglycemia.

REPRODUCTIVE HEALTH CHALLENGES

Breast Cancer

Pathophysiology

Breast cancer is the most diagnosed cancer in Canadian women. Genetic abnormalities account for 5–10% of breast cancers. *BRCA* gene carriers are also at risk of developing ovarian cancer. Having a first-degree relative with breast cancer increases the risk of developing breast cancer by one and a half to three times. Secondary risk factors include never giving birth, giving birth to a first child after the age of 30, prolonged hormonal stimulation, exposure to excessive ionizing radiation, and a history of endometrial, ovarian, or colon cancer.

Types of breast cancer are based on histological characteristics and growth patterns. Infiltrating ductal carcinoma is considered to be the most common form of breast cancer. The cancers generally arise from the epithelial lining of the ducts or from the epithelium of lobules. Breast cancer may be invasive or in situ. Most cancers that arise from the ducts are invasive. Factors affecting prognosis include the size of the tumour, axillary node involvement, tumour differentiation, DNA content, and estrogen and progesterone receptor status.

Ductal carcinoma in situ (DCIS) tends to be unilateral and progresses to invasive if untreated. Lobular carcinoma in situ (LCIS) appears to be more of a premalignant cancer. Women with LCIS have a greater risk of developing invasive breast cancer in the same or opposite breast.

Clinical Manifestations

Symptoms of breast cancer include the following:
- Detecting a lump or mass in the breast
- Changes in breast symmetry or size
- Changes in breast skin, such as dimpling
- Edema
- Skin ulcers
- Changes in nipples causing itching, burning, erosion, or retraction
- Skin temperature changes

The cancer often occurs in the upper outer quadrant; will present as hard, irregularly shaped, poorly delineated, and nonmobile; and will feel nontender when palpated. A serious complication of breast cancer is recurrence. Metastasis occurs primarily through lymphatic chains but can spread without invading axillary nodes.

Diagnostics

Diagnosis of breast cancer is based on biopsy and pathological evaluation of suspected tissue. Diagnostic studies used are lymph node dissection, axillary lymph node status, estrogen and progesterone receptor status, DNA content analysis, and cell proliferative indices.

Therapeutics and Nursing Considerations

Common surgical therapy involves breast conservation surgery (lumpectomy) with radiation therapy or modified radical mastectomy with or without reconstruction. Axillary node dissection is often performed regardless of treatment as it provides excellent prognostic data and helps develop further treatment.

Breast conservation surgery removes the entire tumour along with a margin of normal tissue. Radiation is delivered to the entire breast following surgery. Attempts are made to preserve as much of the breast as possible, including the nipple. A modified radical mastectomy removes the entire breast along with the axillary lymph nodes. The pectoral major muscle is preserved. This is done when the tumour is too large to excise with good margins. The client has the option of breast reconstruction.

Lymphedema, swelling caused by the localized retention of lymphatic fluid, can result from the excision or radiation of lymph nodes. This fluid can cause obstructive pressure. Lymphedema can be prevented by frequent and sustained elevation of the arms, performing arm exercises, and avoiding constrictive clothing.

The client will experience postmastectomy pain in the chest and upper arm. Tingling down the arm, numbness, and shooting or prickling pain are felt. Unbearable itching may also be present. This pain is treated with NSAIDs, antidepressants, topical lidocaine patches, EMLA (eutectic mixture of local anaesthetics) cream, and antiseizure drugs.

Radiation is employed to destroy a cancerous tumour or as a companion to surgery. The radiation will shrink the tumour to an operable size. Radiation can be used for palliative care as well.

Chemotherapy is systemic therapy designed to destroy cells that have spread undetected to distant sites, as well as to decrease the primary tumour and suppress tumour growth.

Hormonal therapy will block and destroy estrogen receptors and suppress estrogen synthesis.

Biological therapy attempts to stimulate the body's natural defences to recognize and attack cancer cells.

Mammoplasty surgically changes the size and shape of the breast for cosmetic or reconstructive reasons. Possible complications include hematoma, hemorrhage, and infection. It is often done simultaneously with or after a mastectomy. When done simultaneously, reconstruction avoids surgery after scar tissue or adhesions develop. Mammoplasty can include breast implants and tissue expansions, or a musculocutaneous flap procedure may be done. This procedure involves using the client's own tissue, usually from the back or abdomen, to repair soft tissue defects if there is insufficient muscle after a mastectomy. Nipple and areolar reconstruction can also be done.

Ovarian Cancer

Pathophysiology

Ovarian cancer, malignant neoplasm of the ovaries, has the highest mortality rate of all gynecological cancers because most women have advanced disease at diagnosis. It occurs most frequently in women between the ages of 55 and 65 years. Risk factors are as follows:

- Family history of ovarian, breast, or colon cancer
- Nulliparity; women who have never been pregnant are at greater risk
- High-fat diet
- Increased number of ovulatory cycles
- Hormone replacement therapy (HRT)
- Use of infertility drugs

Oral contraceptives, breastfeeding, multiple pregnancies, and early age at birth of a first child are associated with lower risk.

Ninety percent of ovarian cancers are epithelial carcinomas. Germ cell tumours account for 10% of ovarian cancers. Ovarian cancer can metastasize directly by shedding malignant cells that often implant in the uterus, bladder, bowel, and omentum. The cancer can also spread via the lymph system.

Clinical Manifestations

Manifestations include general abdominal discomfort, a sense of pelvic heaviness, loss of appetite, feeling of fullness, and a change in bowel habits. As the malignancy grows, there can be an increase in the abdominal girth, bowel and bladder dysfunction, persistent pelvic or abdominal pain, menstrual irregularities, and ascites.

Diagnostics

There are no screening tests at present. A yearly bimanual pelvic examination should be done. Postmenopausal women should not have palpable ovaries. An abdominal or vaginal ultrasonogram can be used to detect ovarian masses. A combination of testing for the tumour marker CA-125 (ovarian antibody) and ultrasonography is recommended in addition to the pelvic examination. CA-125 is also used to monitor the course of the disease.

Therapeutics and Nursing Considerations

Treatment usually is a total hysterectomy and bilateral salpingo-oophorectomy. Abdominal and pelvic radiation, intraperitoneal radiation, and systemic combination chemotherapy may be done after tumour-reducing surgery has been completed. Other surgical procedures include subtotal hysterectomy, panhysterectomy, simple and radical vulvectomy, vaginectomy, and radical hysterectomy. It is very important that the client and family participate in treatment decisions. Psychological support both preoperatively and postoperatively is necessary. The client will be encouraged to continue to practise cancer detection strategies postoperatively. A "second-look" procedure (laparoscopy or laparotomy) is performed a year after completion of primary treatment to confirm the absence or presence of the tumour.

Benign Prostatic Hyperplasia
Pathophysiology

Benign prostatic hyperplasia (BPH) is an enlargement of the prostate gland resulting from an increase in the number of epithelial cells and stomal tissue. It is the most common problem of the male reproductive system. It occurs in 50% of men over the age of 50. BPH does not predispose the client to the development of prostate cancer. The etiology is not really understood, but it is thought to result from endocrine changes as part of the aging process. Other theories suggest that BPH is due to the effect of chronic inflammation of the prostate gland. Research supports the theory that BPH results from a systemic hormonal (testicular androgen) alteration. As the prostate gland grows, it extends upward into the bladder and inward, narrowing the prostatic urethral channel. This obstructs urine flow.

Risk factors include family history, environment, and a diet high in zinc, butter, and margarine.

Clinical Manifestations

Symptoms usually appear gradually and include the following:
- Voiding symptoms, including a decrease in the calibre or force of the urinary stream, difficulty in initiating urination, intermittency, dribbling at the end of voiding, and incomplete bladder emptying
- Urinary frequency and urgency, dysuria, bladder pain, nocturia, and incontinence

Diagnostics

Diagnostic tests include a history and physical examination, urinalysis with culture, a prostate-specific antigen (PSA) level, serum creatinine levels, transrectal ultrasound scan (TRUS), uroflowmetry, and cystourethroscopy. A digital rectal examination should be done yearly.

Therapeutics and Nursing Considerations

The goal of treatment is to restore bladder drainage, relieve symptoms, and prevent complications. Pharmacological therapy includes finasteride (Proscar), which reduces the size of the prostate gland. Alpha blocking agents such as terazosin, doxazosin, and tamsulosin are given to constrict the prostate gland, reducing urethral pressure and improving urine flow. Improvement can be seen in 2–3 weeks. The side effects of these medications are orthostatic hypotension and dizziness. Some clients benefit from herbal therapy such as saw palmetto extract.

Invasive therapy is indicated when there is persistent residual urine in the bladder, acute urinary retention, or hydronephrosis causing decreased urine flow and discomfort. Urinary retention leaves residual urine in the bladder and creates a favourable environment for bacterial growth. Calculi may develop in the bladder due to alkalinization of residual urine. Hydronephrosis can cause renal failure. Pyelonephritis may develop, or the bladder could be damaged. Acute urinary retention is an indication for surgical removal in 25–30% of clients with BPH. Long-term catheter use is contraindicated because of the risk of infection. The choice of treatment depends on the size and location of the prostatic enlargement and the age of the client.

Transurethral resection of the prostate (TURP) removes the prostate tissue using a resectoscope inserted through the urethra. The enlarged portion of the prostate gland is then resected in small pieces.

Transurethral microwave thermotherapy (TUMT) delivers microwaves directly to the prostate in order to raise the temperature to 45°C, causing tissue death and relief of the obstruction. Postoperative urinary retention is common following the procedures. Transurethral needle ablation (TUNA) increases the temperature of the prostate tissue for localized necrosis. A low-wave frequency is used, and only the tissues that the needle touches are affected. Urinary retention, urinary tract infection (UTI), and irritative voiding symptoms may result. Laser prostatectomy delivers a beam that is used for cutting, coagulation, and vaporization of the prostatic tissue.

Goals for postoperative care include the following:
- The client is free of complications.
- The client has restored urinary control and complete bladder emptying.
- The client has satisfying sexual expression.

Clients will require teaching for adequate fluid intake, aseptic technique if using a catheter at home, medication information, and providing an opportunity to express concerns of alteration in sexual function.

Prostate Cancer
Pathophysiology
Prostate cancer is the most common cause of cancer in men, excluding skin cancer. Prostate cancers are androgen-dependent adenocarcinomas that usually develop in the outer aspect of the gland. The cancer is usually slow-growing and metastasizes in a predictable pattern. Common sites of metastasis include the lymph nodes, bone marrow, pelvis, sacrum, and lumbar spine. Risk factors include the following:
- Increasing age
- Family history
- Being of African descent
- High-fat diet
- Exposure to certain chemicals
  A history of BPH is not considered a risk factor.

Clinical Manifestations
The client is usually asymptomatic in the early stages. Eventually, symptoms similar to those with BPH develop, such as dysuria, hesitancy, dribbling, frequency, and urgency. Gross painless hematuria is the most common presenting symptom. The client may experience lumbosacral pain that radiates to the hips or legs. When these symptoms are coupled with urinary symptoms, metastasis should be considered.

Diagnostics
Diagnostic studies include a physical examination and history. A PSA blood test is likely to show elevated levels of PSA with prostatic pathology. Elevated levels of prostatic acid phosphatase (PAP) indicate prostate cancer. A direct rectal examination may find the prostate hard and enlarged with areas of indurations or nodules. A biopsy of the prostate gland is the only definitive diagnostic tool. A bone scan, CT, MRI, and TRUS are used to determine the location and extent of the spread of the cancer. Single-photon emission computed tomography (SPECT) can detect the spread of the cancer to pelvic lymph nodes.

Therapeutics and Nursing Considerations
Conservative treatment is recommended when life expectancy is less than 10 years, there is significant comorbid disease, or the cancer is a low-grade, low-stage tumour. Surgical treatment is a radical prostatectomy, in which the entire gland, seminal vesicles, and part of the bladder neck are removed. Retroperitoneal lymph node dissection is usually done for the most effective long-term survival. Complications of a radical prostatectomy include the following:
- Hemorrhage
- Urinary retention
- Infection and wound dehiscence
- Deep vein thrombosis (DVT)
- Pulmonary emboli

Sometimes nerve-sparing procedures are done to spare the nerves responsible for an erection. This type of surgery is done only when the cancer is contained in the prostate. Cryosurgery destroys cancer cells by freezing them and can be used as an initial or second-line treatment. Radiation therapy can be done by external and internal beam. External radiation is used to treat cancer confined to the prostate or the surrounding tissue. Brachytherapy includes implantation of radioactive seeds into the prostate gland. This spares the surrounding tissue and is best suited for stage A or B prostate cancers. Hormonal therapy focuses on androgen deprivation and can be used before surgery or radiation to reduce the tumour. The hormones commonly used are luteinizing hormone–releasing agonists, androgen receptor blockers, and estrogen. An orchiectomy (surgical removal of the testes) may be done in the advanced stages of prostate cancer. Chemotherapy is primarily limited to treatment for those with hormone-resistant tumours and prostate cancer in the late stages. The goal of chemotherapy is palliative.

The client is encouraged to actively participate in the therapeutic plan, which includes thorough discussion about possible sexual dysfunction.

Testicular Cancer
Testicular cancer is the most common cancer in men 15 to 35 years of age. It is a highly treatable and usually curable cancer (Day, Paul, Williams, et al., 2016).

Pathophysiology
The testicles can develop both germinal and nongerminal tumours. Germinal tumours are the most common form of testicular cancer. About half of germinal tumours are seminomas (tumours developing from sperm-producing cells of the testes). Seminomas tend to remain localized and therefore have a more favourable prognosis. Nonseminoma germinal cell tumours tend to develop earlier in the lifespan and grow quickly. Nonseminomas tend to metastasize quickly. A small percentage of testicular tumours develop in the supportive

and hormone-producing tissues or stroma. Secondary testicular tumours have metastasized from other organs. Lymphoma is the most common cause of secondary testicular cancer (Day et al., 2016).

Clinical Manifestations

A painless mass or lump gradually appears on the testicle. Testicular cancer is rarely bilateral. The client may experience heaviness in his scrotum, inguinal area, or lower abdomen. Back pain, abdominal pain, weight loss, and general weakness suggest that metastasis has already occurred.

Diagnostics

Tumour markers are substances synthesized by the tumour cells and released into the circulation in abnormal amounts. Human chorionic gonadotropin and alpha-fetoprotein are tumour markers for testicular cancer. Benign testicular tumours do not elevate the levels of these markers. The markers can also be used to evaluate the responses to therapy for testicular cancer. Effective treatment drops the level of the markers. The persistence of elevated levels of markers after orchiectomy is evidence the client has metastatic disease. Other diagnostic tests could include CT of the abdomen and chest to assess for metastasis. Lymphangiography may be ordered to assess possible spread to the lymph system. Microscopic analysis is the definitive way to determine the presence of cancer.

Therapeutics and Nursing Considerations

Treatment selection is based on cell type and the extent of the disease. An orchiectomy is performed surgically to remove the cancerous testis. The client may also undergo a radical retroperitoneal lymph node dissection. Chemotherapy and radiation therapy may be indicated for clients who are high risk for metastasis.

Issues related to body image and sexuality need to be addressed. The client will require encouragement to maintain a positive attitude during the course of his treatment. Unilateral orchiectomy and radiation will not necessarily prevent the client from fathering children. The client will be encouraged to perform testicular self-examinations (TSE).

GENITOURINARY HEALTH CHALLENGES

Urinary Tract Infections

Pathophysiology

UTIs are the second most common bacterial disease in women. Usually, the bladder and its contents are free of bacteria in the majority of healthy clients. A small minority of healthy individuals have colonizing bacteria in their bladder. This is called *asymptomatic bacteriuria* and does not justify treatment. *E. coli* is the most common pathogen causing UTIs. Clients who are immunosuppressed, have diabetes, or have undergone multiple courses of antibiotics are vulnerable to developing UTIs.

UTIs may be classified as upper and lower, depending on their location within the urinary system:

- Infections of the upper tract involve the renal parenchyma, pelvis, and ureters.
- Lower tract infections involve the lower urinary tract, bladder, and urethra.

Pyelonephritis refers to infection of the renal parenchyma and collecting system, *cystitis* indicates inflammation of the bladder wall, and *urethritis* is inflammation of the urethra. *Urosepsis* is a UTI that has spread into the systemic circulation and is a life-threatening condition requiring emergency treatment.

UTIs may also be classified as uncomplicated and complicated infections. Uncomplicated infections occur in an otherwise normal urinary tract. Complicated infections occur with coexisting conditions, such as obstruction, stones, catheters, diabetes, or neurological disease, or are recurrent infections.

The physiological and mechanical defence mechanisms that help maintain the normally sterile condition of the bladder include the actual emptying of the bladder, normal antibacterial ability of the mucosa and the urine, the uterovesical junction competence, and the peristaltic activity of the urinary tract. Alterations in any of these factors increase the risk of contracting a UTI. Organisms causing UTIs are usually introduced via the ascending route from the urethra. Less commonly, organisms can be introduced via the bloodstream or the lymphatic system. Gram-negative bacilli from the GI tract are the most common cause. Contributing factors that enhance development include urological instrumentation that allows bacteria present in the opening of the urethra to enter the urethra or bladder. Sexual intercourse promotes the "milking" of bacteria from the perineum and vagina. UTIs rarely result from the hematogenous route.

Clinical Manifestations

Symptoms of UTIs include the following:

- Dysuria, frequent urination, urgency, and suprapubic discomfort or pressure
- Urine itself may contain visible blood or sediment, giving it a cloudy appearance.
- Flank pain, chills, and fever are indicative of an upper UTI.

Diagnostics

Diagnostic studies include a urinalysis and urine for culture and sensitivity (C and S), following a complete history and physical examination of the client. Urine cultures may be obtained by clean-catch technique or catheterization or suprapubic needle aspiration. Sensitivity testing determines susceptibility to antibiotics.

Therapeutics and Nursing Considerations

Uncomplicated cystitis is treated by a short-term course of antibiotics. A complicated UTI requires a long-term treatment. Trimethoprim-sulfamethoxazole (TMP-SMX) and nitrofurantoin (Macrobid) are frequently used to treat uncomplicated or initial infections. Pyridium is an over-the-counter drug that provides soothing effects on the urinary tract mucosa. The drug stains the urine a reddish orange colour that may be mistaken for blood; however, the drug is effective in relieving discomfort. Prophylactic or suppressive antibiotics are sometimes administered to clients with repeated UTIs.

Client teaching is important to help prevent UTIs, and includes the following:

- Emptying the bladder on a regular basis and wiping the perineal area from front to back
- Avoiding constipation
- Maintaining good fluid intake

Pyelonephritis
Pathophysiology

Acute pyelonephritis is a bacterial infection of the renal pelvis, tubules, and interstitial tissue of the kidney. It usually begins with colonization and infection of the lower tract via the ascending urethral route and is frequently caused by *E. coli*, *Proteus*, *Klebsiella*, or *Enterobacter* agents. Often pre-existing factors are present, such as vesicoureteral reflux or a dysfunction of the urinary tract by obstruction, stricture, or stones. Recurring episodes lead to scarred, poorly functioning kidneys and chronic pyelonephritis.

Clinical Manifestations

Symptoms will vary from mild fatigue to sudden onset of chills, fever, vomiting, malaise, flank pain, and lower urinary tract symptoms characteristic of cystitis. Costovertebral tenderness is usually present on the affected side.

Diagnostics

Diagnostic studies such as a urinalysis will show pyuria, bacteriuria, and varying degrees of hematuria. WBC casts indicate involvement of renal parenchyma. CBC will show leukocytosis with an increase in immature bands. Ultrasonography of the urinary system helps identify anatomical abnormalities or the presence of obstructing stones. Imaging studies also are helpful to assess for impaired renal function, scarring, chronic pyelonephritis, and abscesses.

Therapeutics and Nursing Considerations

Clients with severe infections may need hospitalization for control of nausea, vomiting, and dehydration. At home, clients are encouraged to drink an adequate amount of fluids, rest to increase comfort, and take their antibiotics until the prescription has been finished.

Nephrotic Syndrome
Pathophysiology

Nephrotic syndrome is a condition characterized by marked proteinuria, hypoalbuminemia, dyslipidemia, and edema. Although nephrotic syndrome is not a disease itself, it results from a specific defect that makes the glomeruli more permeable to plasma proteins. Nephrotic syndrome usually is caused by an immune or inflammatory process. The increased glomerular permeability is responsible for a massive excretion of protein in the urine, especially albumin and immunoglobulin. This results in decreased serum protein, leading to decreased oncotic pressure with subsequent edema formation, which may include ascites and anasarca. The diminished plasma oncotic pressure also stimulates hepatic lipoprotein synthesis, which results in dyslipidemia. Fat bodies commonly appear in the urine. Because of the loss of immunoglobulins, the immune response is affected, and infections can be serious complications. Hypercoagulability with thromboembolism is potentially the most serious complication of nephrotic syndrome. The renal vein is the most common site for thrombus formation. Pulmonary emboli are also a risk.

Clinical Manifestations

Characteristic manifestations may include massive proteinuria, dyslipidemia and hypoalbuminemia, peripheral edema, possible third space shifting, foamy urine, orthostatic hypotension, malaise, and irritability.

Diagnostics

Diagnosis is made with a thorough history and physical examination. Urinalysis will reveal large quantities of protein and an increased number of hyaline, granular, and waxy, fatty casts.

Blood work shows the following:
- Increased cholesterol, phospholipid, and triglyceride levels
- Decreased albumin

Protein electrophoresis may be done to identify the type of protein lost in the urine.

Therapeutics and Nursing Considerations

Treatment aims at correction of the underlying cause if possible. Supportive treatment is aimed at protein replacement and relief of edema. Diuretics and a restricted sodium diet are ordered, with 1 g of protein per kilogram of body weight. Antibiotics may be given for infection. Some clients may need steroid medication; others may need lipid-lowering medications.

The practical nurse will pay particular attention to the relief of edema. Weigh the client daily. Accurate intake and output measurements are necessary. Abdominal girths may need to be measured. Edematous skin needs careful cleaning and care to protect it from trauma. Education regarding diet and fluid management is important.

Glomerulonephritis
Pathophysiology

Glomerulonephritis is an inflammation of glomerular capillaries caused by an immunological process. It affects both kidneys equally and can lead to renal failure. The antigen–antibody complexes can be deposited in the glomeruli, causing obstruction. The kidney tissue itself may also serve as the antigen. Inflammation occurs within the glomeruli, followed by thickening and scarring of the glomerular membrane, which decreases glomerular filtration.

Clinical Manifestations

Clinical manifestations of glomerulonephritis include varying degrees of hematuria, proteinuria, and elevated serum creatinine and BUN. Other manifestations may include some degree of hypertension and edema.

Diagnostics

Diagnosis is based on the history and physical examination along with a urinalysis, CBC, BUN, creatinine, serum albumin, complement levels, and an antistreptolysin O (ASO) titre.

Therapeutics and Nursing Considerations

In most cases, recovery is complete following rest and symptomatic treatment. This includes diuretics for fluid retention and antihypertensives if the client is hypertensive. If progressive involvement occurs, the result is destruction of renal tissue and marked renal insufficiency.

Renal Cancer
Pathophysiology

Renal cell carcinoma, also called *adenocarcinoma*, is the most common type of malignant kidney tumour. It usually starts in the proximal renal tubules. Local extension of kidney cancer into the renal vein and vena cava is common. The most common sites of metastases include the lungs, liver, and long bones. Some forms of renal carcinoma are inherited.

Clinical Manifestations

There are no characteristic early symptoms. The most common symptoms are hematuria, flank pain, and a palpable mass in the flank or abdomen. Other symptoms may be weight loss, fever, hypertension, and anemia.

Diagnostics

Diagnosis is made through the history and physical examination. An intravenous pyelogram (IVP) with nephrography or sonography is used to detect renal masses. Ultrasound helps differentiate between a tumour and a cyst. Angiography, percutaneous needle aspiration, CT scan, and MRI can also be used for diagnosis.

Therapeutics and Nursing Considerations

The treatment of renal cancer involves destruction or removal of the cancer. Radiofrequency ablation is a minimally invasive procedure that can be done to destroy the tumour. Nephrectomy (removal of a kidney) or radical nephrectomy, which is removal of the kidney, adrenal gland, surrounding fascia, part of the ureter, and draining lymph nodes, may be needed. Radiation therapy is used palliatively in inoperable cases and when there are metastases to the bone or lungs. Postoperative care focuses on the following:

- Monitoring for hemorrhage and adrenal insufficiency, which may cause hypotension
- Loss of urine output
- Changes in the level of consciousness (LOC)
- Pain management
- Fluid assessment
- Possible antibiotics and steroid replacement

The practical nurse needs to support the client and the family and share available resources with them.

Polycystic Kidney Disease
Pathophysiology

Polycystic kidney disease (PKD) is a common genetic disease. Cysts form in the renal tubules, and as they advance and increase in size, they fill the cortex and the medulla and destroy surrounding tissue by compression. The cysts are various sizes, involve both kidneys, and are filled with fluid, including blood or pus.

Clinical Manifestations

Symptoms appear when the cysts begin to enlarge. Often the first symptoms to appear are hypertension, hematuria, and feelings of heaviness in the back, side, or abdomen. On physical examination, palpable bilateral enlarged kidneys are often found. UTIs, urinary calculi, or both may be found, and chronic pain is common. The disease usually progresses to ESRD.

Diagnostics

Diagnosis is based on clinical manifestations, family history, IVP, ultrasonogram, and CT scan.

Therapeutics and Nursing Considerations

There is no specific treatment for PKD. A major aim of treatment is to prevent infections and to treat them promptly and effectively if they occur. Nephrectomy may be necessary if pain, bleeding, or infection becomes chronic. A kidney transplant may be the only cure.

Nursing management is the same as that used for the treatment and management of renal failure, namely diet modification, fluid restriction, medications, and helping the client accept the chronic disease process.

Urinary Tract Calculi
Pathophysiology

Nephrolithiasis refers to kidney stone disease. Urolithiasis (calculi) is stones in the urinary tract. Except for struvite stones, which are associated with UTI, stone disorders are more common in men than in women. The majority of clients are 20–55 years of age. Renal calculi may result from the following:

- Dehydration
- Infection
- Changes in urine pH
- Diet
- Immobilization
- Metabolic factors, such as hyperparathyroidism, cancers, and granulomatous disease

Calcium is the most common type of urolithiasis. Struvite stones are composed of magnesium, phosphate, and ammonium. Cystine and xanthine stones are associated with hereditary factors. Uric acid can also form stones. Different theories attempt to explain the development of stones in the urinary tract. One theory is that urinary constituents exceed their solubility. Keeping urine dilute reduces the risk of recurrent stone formation. Another theory is that the urinary pH affects the formation of stones. A higher pH is an environment that supports the development of calcium and phosphate stones. A lower pH supports the development of uric acid and cystine stones. Struvite stones usually form in the presence of a UTI with urea-splitting bacteria such as *Proteus* or *Klebsiella*.

Clinical Manifestations

Clinical manifestations of urinary stones occur because of the obstruction of urinary flow. Symptoms include a sudden onset of unilateral abdominal or flank pain. The type of pain is determined by the location of the stone. If the stone is not obstructing, there will not be any pain. Other symptoms include the presence of hematuria, urinary infections accompanied by fever, vomiting, nausea, and chills.

Diagnostics

Diagnosis is determined by an accurate history and physical examination. Urine pH will be checked. An X-ray of the abdomen and renal ultrasonography will reveal larger radiopaque stones. Ultrasonography can be used to identify radiopaque or radiolucent calculi in the renal pelvis, calyx, or proximal ureter. A CT scan will differentiate between a nonopaque stone and a tumour. IVP or a retrograde pyelogram localizes the degree and site of obstruction or confirms the presence of nonradiopaque stones (from cystine and uric acid). When stones are recovered, chemical analysis will be done to provide an indication of the underlying disorder.

Therapeutics and Nursing Considerations

The history and physical examination will reveal a family history of stone formation, nutritional assessment, activity pattern, a history of any prolonged illness with immobilization or dehydration, and a history of any condition or surgery involving the genitourinary or GI tract or endocrine disturbances.

Various medications are prescribed that prevent stone formation by altering urine pH, preventing excessive urinary excretion of a substance, or correcting a primary disease such as hyperparathyroidism.

Treatment for struvite stones requires control of infection. If the infection cannot be controlled, the stone will have to be surgically removed. Indications for surgical therapy include stones that are too large to pass through ureters, a client who cannot be treated medically, and a client with one kidney.

Calculi that are too large for natural passage may require surgical removal, percutaneous ultrasonic lithotripsy or extracorporeal shock wave lithotripsy (ESWL), or chemolysis.

Hematuria is common following lithotripsy procedures. Adequate fluid intake to prevent dehydration is encouraged prior to stone removal as an increase in fluids may exacerbate the colic associated with the episode. After the stone has passed, the client is encouraged to drink enough to ensure at least a 2 L output, as this will dilute concentrations of minerals. Diet modifications may be needed to help prevent further stone formation.

Nursing considerations are as follows:
- Pain management and client comfort are primary nursing responsibilities when managing a person with an obstructing stone and renal colic.
- All urine voided by the client should be strained so it can be inspected for the stone.
- Ambulation with support is encouraged to promote movement of the stone.
- Client and family teaching is necessary regarding diet and fluid intake.
- Follow-up care should be discussed with both client and family.

Renal Failure
Pathophysiology and Clinical Manifestations

Renal failure is a partial or complete impairment of renal function and is classified as acute or chronic. Acute renal failure has a rapid onset. Chronic renal failure (CRF) usually develops slowly over months or years.

Acute renal failure. ARF is a clinical syndrome characterized by a rapid loss of renal function with progressive azotemia (accumulation of nitrogenous wastes). Causes of ARF include conditions that reduce the blood flow to the kidneys, renal parenchymatous disease, and obstruction. Prerenal ARF is due to factors external to the kidney that reduce renal blood flow and lead to decreased glomerular perfusion and filtration. Prerenal causes are the most common cause of ARF and include the following:
- Hypovolemia
- Decreased cardiac output
- Decreased peripheral vascular resistance
- Vascular obstruction

Prerenal disease can lead to intrarenal disease (acute tubular necrosis) if renal ischemia is prolonged.

Intrarenal causes include the conditions that cause direct damage to the renal tissue (parenchyma), resulting in impaired nephron function. Intrarenal ARF is usually due to the following:
- Prolonged ischemia
- Nephrotoxins
- Rhabdomyolysis
- Glomerulonephritis
- Complications of diabetes on the glomerular basement membrane

Causes of postrenal ARF involve obstruction of urinary outflow. The most common causes are as follows:
- Prostate cancer and BPH
- Urinary tract calculi
- Extrarenal tumours

ARF progresses through four phases: initiation, oliguric, diuretic, and recovery.

The *initiation phase* begins at the time of the insult. This phase continues until symptoms become evident.

The *oliguric phase* reflects a reduction in the GFR that causes oliguria.

- The oliguric phase usually starts 1–7 days after the initiating event and lasts about 10–14 days.
- The longer the oliguric phase lasts, the poorer the prognosis is for complete recovery of renal function.
- Due to the decrease in urine in the oliguric phase, the client will have fluid retention.
- Fluid overload can lead to heart failure, pulmonary edema, and pericardial and pleural effusions.
- Metabolic acidosis results when the kidneys cannot synthesize ammonia, which is needed for the excretion of hydrogen ions.
- The client may exhibit Kussmaul breathing (rapid and deep) as the respiratory tract attempts to compensate and blow off carbon dioxide.
- Waste products are not eliminated and remain in the blood.
- Potassium levels rise in the blood as the kidneys are unable to eliminate potassium.
- The kidneys are unable to eliminate phosphate, so the calcium levels within the blood will drop.
- As the waste products build in the blood, the client may become anorexic and experience nausea and vomiting with bowel disturbances.
- Uremic breath may develop.
- The kidneys are unable to produce the active form of vitamin D, so absorption of calcium from the intestine is limited.
- Anemia occurs due to the kidneys' inability to produce erythropoietin.
- Hematological changes may result in GI bleeds and the development of stomatitis as the waste products damage the leukocytes, immunoglobulins, and platelets.
- Neurological changes can occur as nitrogenous waste products accumulate in the brain and other nervous tissue. Symptoms can be as mild as fatigue and difficulty concentrating or can escalate to seizures, stupor, and coma.

The *diuretic phase* begins with the gradual increase in urine output. As this phase continues, the output may be as high as 3–5 L per day or more. The diuretic phase may last 1–3 weeks or more.

- The kidneys are starting to recover their ability to excrete waste and fluid.
- During this period, the client's acid–base, electrolyte, and waste product values are beginning to normalize.
- Because of the large volume of fluid and electrolytes lost during this phase, the client must be monitored closely for hypovolemia, hypotension, hyponatremia, and hypokalemia.

The *recovery phase* begins when the GFR increases and the BUN and creatinine levels plateau.

- Although major improvements occur in the first 2 weeks of this phase, renal function may take up to 12 months to stabilize.
- Many clients who survive ARF never regain a normal GFR.

Chronic renal failure. CRF refers to the progressive, irreversible destruction of nephrons, resulting in systemic damage to all organs. The causes are as follows:

- The most common cause of CRF is uncontrolled diabetes, followed closely by uncontrolled hypertension.
- Other causes may include glomerulonephritis, renal vascular disease, pyelonephritis, and polycystic disease.

CRF is insidious; symptoms do not become evident until the GFR has dropped to 20% of its norm.

A client with CRF exhibits the following changes:

- A severely decreased GFR, with azotemia (high levels of BUN and creatinine)
- Metabolic acidosis
- Fluid retention
- Increased serum potassium, phosphate, and possibly sodium
- Decreased calcium
- Severe anemia
- Oliguria

Fig. 8.5 illustrates the manifestations of this condition. The term *uremia* refers to the entire signs and symptoms of CRF.

The final stage of CRF is ESRD. The client experiences uremic syndrome with severe metabolic acidosis and severe fluid and electrolyte imbalance. ESRD is fatal if clients do not receive dialysis or a kidney transplant.

Diagnostics

Diagnostic studies include a thorough history to determine the etiology of the failure.

Blood work shows the following:

- Elevated BUN and creatinine levels
- Elevated potassium and phosphate levels
- Acidic pH, with low levels of bicarbonate
- Hemoglobin and hematocrit

Urine specimens show the following:

- Casts, cellular debris, and decreased specific gravity, and in glomerular disease, proteinuria and urine osmolality close to serum osmolality
- The creatinine clearance test measures the GFR and is used to estimate the number of remaining functioning nephrons.
- Other studies include ultrasonography of the kidneys, renal scan, CT scan, retrograde pyelography, MRI, and plain X-ray films of the abdomen, kidneys, ureters, and bladder (KUB).

Therapeutics and Nursing Considerations

The primary goal of treatment is to find the underlying cause of the ARF and eliminate it. Management of signs and symptoms and prevention of complications are also high priorities. Assessing for adequate cardiac output is mandatory. Diuretic therapy along with volume expanders may be used to prevent fluid overload. If ARF has already been established, conservative measures may be necessary until renal function improves. Fluid intake is closely monitored. Blood work is closely

Psychological
- Anxiety
- Depression

Cardiovascular
- Hypertension
- Heart failure
- Coronary artery disease
- Pericarditis
- Peripheral artery disease

Gastro-intestinal
- Anorexia
- Nausea
- Vomiting
- Gastro-intestinal bleeding
- Gastritis

Endocrine/Reproductive
- Hyperparathyroidism
- Thyroid abnormalities
- Amenorrhea
- Erectile dysfunction

Metabolic
- Carbohydrate intolerance
- Hyperlipidemia

Hematological
- Anemia
- Bleeding
- Infection

Neurological
- Fatigue
- Headache
- Sleep disturbances
- Encephalopathy

Ocular
- Hypertensive retinopathy

Pulmonary
- Pulmonary edema
- Uremic pleuritis
- Pneumonia

Integumentary
- Pruritus
- Ecchymosis
- Dry, scaly skin

Musculo-skeletal
- Vascular and soft tissue calcifications
- Osteomalacia
- Osteitis fibrosa

Peripheral neuropathy
- Paresthesias
- Restless legs syndrome

Fig. 8.5 Clinical manifestations of chronic uremia. (From Lewis, S. M., Bucher, L., Heitkemper, M. M., et al. [2019]. *Medical-surgical nursing in Canada: Assessment and management of clinical problems* [4th Cdn. ed., p. 1209, Figure 49-3]. Milton, ON: Elsevier.)

monitored for changes in potassium, sodium, bicarbonates, phosphates, blood gases, BUN, creatinine, and calcium.

The diet will be high in carbohydrates and low in protein until the diuretic phase begins. Restriction of potassium- and sodium-containing foods will be regulated according to the levels of these electrolytes in the blood. If potassium levels rise too high, the client may be given polystyrene sulfonate (Kayexalate) to rid the body of potassium, glucose, and insulin to help move the potassium into the cells or calcium gluconate to decrease the excitability of the cell membrane. In some situations, dialysis will be initiated.

Treatment of CRF is to find the precipitating cause and treat or manage it as well as treat the consequences of the progressive condition. Once CRF has progressed to ESRD, dialysis and renal transplantation are the only options. See Fig. 8.6.

Dialysis

Dialysis is a technique in which substances move from the blood through a semipermeable membrane and into a dialysis solution (dialysate). Dialysis is used to correct fluid and electrolyte and acid–base imbalances and to remove excess waste products. The two main methods of dialysis include

hemodialysis (HD) and peritoneal dialysis (PD). In PD, the peritoneal membrane acts as a semipermeable membrane. In HD, an artificial membrane is used as the semipermeable membrane and is in contact with the client's blood. Generally, dialysis is initiated when the GFR or creatinine clearance of the client is less than 15 mL/min (normal is 100–125 mL/min); however, these criteria can vary widely in different clinical situations. Certain uremic complications indicate an immediate need for dialysis and are as follows:

- Encephalopathy
- Neuropathies
- Uncompensated metabolic acidosis
- Uncontrollable hyperkalemia
- Pericarditis
- Accelerated hypertension

The general principles of diffusion, osmosis, and ultrafiltration are involved in both forms of dialysis.

Peritoneal dialysis. With PD, a catheter is surgically placed through the anterior wall of the abdomen into the peritoneum. The catheter is sutured in place. Dialysis solutions are available commercially in 1–2 L plastic bags with glucose concentrations of 0.5%, 1.5%, 2.5%, or 4.25%. The electrolyte concentration is similar to plasma. There are two

Fig. 8.6 Concept map: End-stage renal disease. (From Ignatavicius, D. D., Workman, M. L., & Rebar, C. [2018]. *Medical-surgical nursing: Concepts for interprofessional collaborative care* [9th ed.]. St. Louis: Elsevier. Concept map by Deanne A. Blach, MSN, RN.)

forms of PD: automated peritoneal dialysis (APD) and continuous ambulatory peritoneal dialysis (CAPD), as well as three phases: the inflow, the dwell, and the drainage.

Complications pertaining to PD include the following:

- Exit site infection, peritonitis, and abdominal pain
- Outflow problems and hernias
- Lower back problems
- Bleeding
- Pulmonary complications
- Protein loss
- Carbohydrate and lipid abnormalities
- Encapsulating sclerosing peritonitis
- Loss of ultrafiltration

Peritoneal dialysis is considered effective for short-term dialysis, allowing the client more independence and ease of travelling. There are fewer dietary restrictions for clients using PD as opposed to HD.

Hemodialysis. HD requires vascular access and incorporates shunts and internal arteriovenous fistulas and grafts. The

HD dialyzers are basically long plastic cartridges that contain thousands of parallel hollow tubes or fibres.

Complications to monitor for with HD include the following:

- Hypotension
- Muscle cramps
- Loss of blood
- Hepatitis
- Sepsis
- Disequilibrium syndrome

Kidney Transplantation

Kidney transplantation is the treatment of choice for clients with ESRD and is considered extremely successful, with a high survivor rate from both cadaver and live donors. Unlike dialysis, the transplanted kidney is able to reverse many of the pathophysiological changes associated with renal failure, eliminates the dependence on dialysis, and is less expensive than dialysis after the first year following surgery.

Not all clients with ESRD are suitable for kidney transplantation. Each transplant team will have criteria that the client must meet in order to be a transplant recipient. Clients with spreading malignancies, severe cardiac disease, or chronic respiratory failure are not suitable recipients.

Histocompatibility studies will be done to identify human leukocyte antigens (HLAs) for both donors and potential recipients. Donor sources include compatible blood type cadaver donors, blood relatives, and living donors. The donor kidney will be removed (nephrectomy) either conventionally or by laparoscope. The transplanted kidney is usually placed extraperitoneally in the iliac fossa.

Emotional and psychological supports are important for both clients. Immunosuppressive drugs will be given to the recipient to prevent rejection of the new kidney. The goal of immunosuppressive therapy is to adequately suppress the immune response to prevent rejection while maintaining sufficient immunity to prevent overwhelming infection. Postoperative care for the donor is similar to care for laparoscopic nephrectomy, with close monitoring of remaining renal function. The recipient will be monitored closely for fluid and electrolyte balances.

Rejection of the kidney by the recipient is the antibody-mediated humoral reaction to the new organ. Hyperacute rejection may occur within minutes to hours of the transplant. Acute rejection can occur days to months after the transplant. Chronic rejection is a process that occurs over months to years and is irreversible.

Complications following transplantation include the following:
- Infection
- Cardiovascular disease
- Malignancies
- Recurrence of original renal disease
- Steroid-related complications

HEALTH CHALLENGES RELATED TO MOVEMENT AND COORDINATION

Headache

Pathophysiology and Clinical Manifestations

Headaches (cephalalgia) are thought to be the most common type of pain experienced by humans. Headaches are classified as either primary, with no identifiable cause, or secondary, with an underlying cause. Primary classifications of headaches include tension-type, migraine, and cluster headaches.

The tension-type headache is the most common type, in which the client experiences bilateral feelings of pressure around the head caused by irritation of the pain-sensitive structures of the brain. There is no prodrome (symptom indicative of an approaching disease). Tension-type headaches have at least two of the following characteristics:
- The sensation of pressure or tightness
- Mild to moderate severity
- Bilateral location

- Worsening with physical activity
- Sensitivity to light (photophobia) or sound (phonophobia)

Diagnostics

To diagnose tension-type headaches, a careful history and physical examination, including a neurological examination, are needed. Routine laboratory studies may be done. CT of the sinuses, MRI, angiography, and electromyography (EMG) may be performed.

Migraine Headaches

Pathophysiology and Clinical Manifestations

Migraine headaches are characterized by unilateral or bilateral throbbing pain caused by vasodilation of the dural blood vessels that then stimulate the trigeminal nerve pain pathway. Neuropeptides are released, which make the vasodilation worse. There is usually a family history of migraine headaches. The onset is usually in childhood or adolescence.

Migraine headaches may be preceded by an aura (sensation occurring before a disorder) and prodrome by days or hours. The prodrome can include psychic disturbances, GI upset, and changes in fluid balance.

The headache itself may be triggered by the following:
- Stress
- Excitement
- Bright lights
- Menstruation
- Alcohol
- Certain foods

Migraine headaches are subdivided into migraine with aura and migraine without aura. A classic symptom of an aura is flashing lights in one quadrant of the visual field (scintillating scotomata).

Migraine without aura involves at least one of the following: nausea and vomiting, photophobia, and phonophobia. Migraine without aura is the most common type of migraine.

Symptoms of a migraine with or without an aura are as follows:
- Generalized edema
- Irritability
- Pallor
- Nausea and vomiting
- Sweating

Clients may seek shelter from noise, light, odours, people, or other stressors. They feel a steady, throbbing pain synchronous with the pulse.

Diagnostics

Diagnostic tests are the same as those for tension headaches.

Cluster Headaches

Pathophysiology and Clinical Manifestations

Cluster headaches are thought to be variants of migraine headaches and are characterized by repeated headaches that occur for weeks or months at a time, followed by periods of remission. Cluster headaches are considered one of the most severe forms of head pain. The etiology of cluster headaches is unknown. The pathophysiology of cluster headaches is similar to that of migraine headaches; however, the triggers are different in that cluster headaches can be triggered by alcohol, nicotine, and histamines.

Clinical manifestations of cluster headaches include the following:

- Severe unilateral orbital, supraorbital, or temporal pain
- Associated symptoms, including nasal congestion, lacrimation, rhinorrhea, and forehead and facial swelling

Cluster headaches do not cause nausea and vomiting. The onset of the headache is usually abrupt, without prodrome. It commonly occurs at night and may recur several times a day for several days. The pain is described as deep, steady, and penetrating but not throbbing. Clients with cluster headaches often pace the floor, cry out, and avoid being touched by others.

Diagnostics

Diagnostic tests are the same as those for tension headaches.

Therapeutics and Nursing Considerations

Drug treatments for headaches are as follows:

- Tension-type headache medications may include non-narcotic analgesics used alone or in combination with a sedative, muscle relaxant, tranquilizer, or codeine.
- Migraine headache drugs focus on terminating or decreasing the symptoms.
- ASA (Aspirin) or acetaminophen (Tylenol) may be effective for mild forms of the headache.
- Other medications may include serotonin receptor agonists, alpha- and beta-adrenergic blockers, tricyclic antidepressants, ergot derivatives, calcium channel blockers, and antiseizure drugs.
- Cluster headaches are treated with alpha-adrenergic blockers and vasoconstrictors. An acute treatment for cluster headaches is inhalation of 100% oxygen delivered at a rate of 7–9 L per minute for 15–20 minutes.

Overuse of analgesics can lead to chronic daily headache or drug-induced headache.

Client and family teaching regarding the medication regimen, nonpharmacological management, and stress-reduction techniques can be very helpful. Alternative therapy such as heat or cold applications, acupuncture, or hypnosis has been found to be beneficial for many clients.

Head Injury
Pathophysiology

Head injury is any trauma to the scalp, skull, or brain. Head trauma includes an alteration in consciousness, no matter how brief. There are many causes of head injury, such as firearm-related injuries, motor vehicle accidents, falls, assaults, sports-related injuries, and recreational accidents. There is a high potential for a poor outcome when the head is injured. Not all brain damage is evident at the time of the event.

Scalp lacerations are the most minor type of head trauma. The scalp is very vascular and therefore can bleed profusely.

Trauma can result in an abrasion, contusion, laceration, or hematoma. The major complication from a scalp laceration is infection.

Skull fractures may be linear, comminuted, depressed or compound, closed or open. The type and severity of a skull fracture depend on the velocity, momentum, and direction of the injuring agent and the site of impact. The force of the damaging impact could be due to the mechanism of acceleration or deceleration. Specific manifestations of a skull fracture are generally associated with the location of the injury. The major potential complications of skull fractures are as follows:

- Intracranial infections
- Hematomas
- Meningeal and brain tissue damage

Minor head trauma includes concussions and postconcussion syndrome. A concussion involves a change in the LOC. Major head traumas are contusions and lacerations that involve severe brain trauma. Contusions are bruising of brain tissue most commonly found at the site of impact (coup injury) or in the line opposite the site of impact (contrecoup injury). Lacerations involve the actual tearing of the cortical surface vessels, which may lead to secondary hemorrhage and cerebral edema and inflammation. Intracerebral hemorrhage can be associated with cerebral laceration. The prognosis is generally poor for the person with a large intracerebral hemorrhage.

When major head trauma occurs, many delayed or secondary responses can be seen, including the following:

- Hemorrhage and hematoma formation
- Seizures
- Cerebral edema

Complications of head trauma include an epidural, subdural, or intracerebral hematoma. An epidural hematoma results from bleeding between the dura and the inner surface of the skull. Laceration of the middle meningeal artery is the usual cause, and as such, the hematoma develops rapidly and requires immediate control of the bleeding and evacuation of the blood in the epidural space.

Subdural hematomas occur from bleeding between the dura mater and arachnoid layer of the meningeal covering of the brain and are usually venous in origin and much slower to develop into a mass large enough to produce symptoms. The accumulation of clots puts pressure on the brain surface and eventually displaces brain tissue.

An intracerebral hematoma can be due to a hemorrhagic stroke or ruptured aneurysm.

Clinical Manifestations

Signs of a concussion may include a brief disruption in LOC, amnesia, and headache. Symptoms are generally of short duration. The postconcussion syndrome can occur anywhere from 2 weeks to 2 months after the head injury and involves the following:

- A persistent headache
- Lethargy
- Personality and behaviour changes

With acute subdural hematoma, the client exhibits the following signs within 48 hours of the injury:

- Appears drowsy and confused
- Ipsilateral pupil dilates and becomes fixed

With a subacute subdural hematoma, symptoms take longer to appear, between 2 to 14 days after the injury.

- Failure to regain consciousness may be an indicator.

Chronic subdural hematomas develop over weeks or months after a seemingly minor head injury. The damaged area is filled with fluid rather than blood clots, and symptoms tend to be less acute.

Diagnostics

Diagnosis of a head injury includes the history and physical examination. A CT scan is considered the best diagnostic test to determine craniocerebral trauma. MRI, PET, cervical spine and skull X-ray series, and the Glasgow Coma Scale (GCS) are also used.

Therapeutics and Nursing Considerations

Care for the client with head trauma focuses on the following:

- Monitoring the neurological status and using the GCS
- Observing for cerebrospinal fluid (CSF) leak

The overall goals are to maintain adequate cerebral perfusion; to keep the client normothermic and free from pain, discomfort, and infection; and to attain maximal cognitive, motor, and sensory function. In some situations, craniotomy, craniectomy, cranioplasty, or burr-hole surgery is done to remove the hematoma.

Nursing considerations will focus on the following:

- Promoting good air entry
- Controlling intracranial pressure (ICP)
- Maintaining temperature control
- Monitoring fluid and electrolyte balance
- Preventing infection
- Assisting the client to resume normal activities
- Providing emotional support to the client and the family

Inflammatory Brain Disorders

Bacteria, viruses, fungi, and chemicals can cause inflammatory brain disorders. Meningitis, encephalitis, and brain abscesses are among the most frequently occurring CNS infections. During an infection, infectious agents can enter the bloodstream. Once the organisms reach the brain, the CSF in the subarachnoid spaces and the pia-arachnoid membrane may become infected. The infection spreads quickly through the meninges and can invade the ventricles. This infectious process can cause serious long-term neurological deficits.

Bacterial Meningitis

Pathophysiology, Clinical Manifestations, and Diagnostics. Bacterial meningitis is a medical emergency with a high mortality rate. The inflammatory response increases CSF production and ICP. The major bacteria associated with bacterial meningitis are Streptococcus pneumoniae and Neisseria meningitidis.

Symptoms include fever, severe headache, nausea and vomiting, positive Kernig sign, positive Brudzinski sign, photophobia, decreased LOC, and signs of increased ICP. Seizures occur in 20% of all cases. The headache becomes progressively worse. Vomiting and irritability may accompany the worsening headache. Delirium and complete disorientation may develop quickly.

Rapid diagnosis is done by history and physical examination. A blood culture, lumbar puncture, and analysis of CSF are done. A head X-ray, CT scanning, and MRI may be done.

Therapeutics and nursing considerations. Antibiotic therapy is initiated after all necessary specimens are collected. The antibiotic needs to be able to cross the blood–brain barrier to be effective. The client is cared for while in a comfortable position in a darkened room to help prevent hallucinations. Pain medication is administered as needed. The client must be observed and treated for any neurological problems, such as seizures. Antipyretics should be given as needed. Hydration must be monitored and small, frequent meals offered. Aseptic technique must be utilized at all times. Progressive range-of-motion (ROM) exercises are required, and client activity should be increased as tolerated. The nursing considerations for all of the following inflammatory brain disorders are similar to those for bacterial meningitis.

Viral Meningitis

Pathophysiology, clinical manifestations, and diagnostics. Viral meningitis is most commonly caused by enterovirus, arbovirus, HIV, or herpes simplex virus (HSV). Viral meningitis, also known as *aseptic meningitis*, usually presents with a headache, fever, photophobia, myalgias, and a stiff neck. Diagnosis is done by the history and physical examination and a lumbar puncture with cultures done on CSF. In viral meningitis, the CSF will show lymphocytosis, but no organisms will be present in Gram stains or acid-fast smears.

Therapeutics and nursing considerations. Symptomatic management with full recovery should be expected. The nursing considerations for viral meningitis are similar to those for bacterial meningitis.

Encephalitis

Pathophysiology, clinical manifestations, and diagnostics. Encephalitis is an acute inflammation of the brain that can be fatal. It can be caused by a number of viruses, including West Nile virus. Ticks or mosquitoes can transmit epidemic encephalitis. Advanced age is a risk factor for developing encephalitis. Most cases have mild flulike symptoms in addition to nonspecific symptoms, such as the following:

- Fever and headache
- Nausea and vomiting
- Stiff neck
- Declining LOC

Signs appear 2–3 days postinfection and may vary from minimal alterations to coma. Abnormalities in brain function are common in encephalitis. Diagnosis is done by the history and physical examination, MRI, PET, and tests for the IgM antibody to West Nile virus in CSF. Diagnosis between meningitis and encephalitis is based on brain function.

Therapeutics and nursing considerations. The treatment for encephalitis may include diuretics, corticosteroids, acyclovir (Zovirax), vidarabine (Vira-A) for HSV infection, and antiseizure drugs. Mosquito control may be used as a preventive measure. The nursing considerations for encephalitis are similar to those for bacterial meningitis.

Brain Abscess

Pathophysiology, clinical manifestations, and diagnostics. Brain abscess is a purulent infection of the brain with an accumulation of pus within brain tissue. The infection may be due to an ear, tooth, mastoid, or sinus infection; skull fracture; brain trauma or surgery; or a complication of meningitis. *Streptococcus* and *Staphylococcus aureus* are the causative agents. The client will present with headache, fever, and nausea and vomiting and may show signs of increased ICP. The symptoms will reflect the local area of abscess. CT and MRI will be used for diagnosis.

Therapeutics and nursing considerations. Antimicrobial therapy is the primary treatment, as well as symptomatic treatment for any manifestation. The abscess may need to be drained or removed. If the abscess is left untreated, the client will not survive. The nursing considerations for brain abscesses are similar to those for bacterial meningitis.

Multiple Sclerosis
Pathophysiology

Multiple sclerosis (MS) is a chronic, progressive, degenerative neuromuscular disease that is characterized by inflammation of the white matter of the CNS. The disease usually affects young to middle-aged adults, with onset between 15–50 years of age. Women are affected more than men. The cause is unknown; however, it may be related to infectious, immunological, and genetic factors. Other autoimmune theories include the possibility that autosensitization occurring in response to an antigen on the myelin membrane or a cell-mediated immune reaction triggers the demyelination process. There is no cause-and-effect relationship between a pathogenetic agent and MS. Possible precipitating factors include the following:

- Infection
- Physical injury
- Emotional stress
- Excessive fatigue
- Pregnancy
- Poor state of health

The disease process consists of loss of myelin, disappearance of oligodendrocytes, and proliferation of astrocytes. Changes result in plaque formation, with plaques scattered throughout the CNS. Initially, the myelin sheaths of the neurons in the brain and spinal cord are attacked, but the nerve fibre is not affected. Clients may complain of noticeable impairment of function. Myelin can regenerate and symptoms disappear, resulting in remission, or myelin can be replaced by glial scar tissue. Nerve impulses slow down without myelin. With the destruction of axons, impulses are totally blocked, resulting in permanent loss of nerve function.

Clinical Manifestations

Vague symptoms can occur intermittently over months and years. The disease may not be diagnosed until long after the onset of the first symptom. Symptoms of MS are characterized by chronic, progressive deterioration in some clients, with remissions and exacerbations in others. Common signs and symptoms of MS include the following:

- Motor manifestations, which may include weakness or feelings of heaviness in the legs, paralysis of limbs, diplopia, hyper-reflexia and spasticity of muscles, and sensory, cerebellar, and neurobehavioural problems.
- Sensory manifestations can include numbness and tingling, blurred vision, vertigo, and tinnitus.
- Cerebellar manifestations include nystagmus, ataxia, dysarthria, and dysphagia.
- Neurobehavioural manifestations may include emotional lability.
- Other symptoms may include bowel and bladder dysfunction, optic neuritis, and fatigue. Sexual dysfunction can also occur with MS.

Diagnostics

Diagnosis is based primarily on the history, clinical manifestations, and the presence of multiple lesions over time as measured by an MRI. Laboratory tests will show an increase in activated T4 lymphocytes and IgG content.

Therapeutics and Nursing Considerations

The goal of treatment is to maintain the client's independence for as long as possible. Drug therapy for the treatment of MS includes the following:

- Corticosteroids, which are used to treat acute exacerbations by reducing edema and inflammation at the site of demyelination
- Immunosuppressive therapy is beneficial in clients with progressive relapsing, secondary-progressive, and primary-progressive types of MS.
- Immunomodulators include interferon-beta 1b (Betaseron), interferon-beta-1a (Avonex), glatiramer (Copaxone), natalizumab (Antegren), and mitoxantrone (Novantrone).
- Antispasmodics, CNS stimulants, anticholinergics, tricyclic antidepressants, and antiseizure medications may also be prescribed.

Surgical interventions, such as a neurectomy, rhizotomy, or cordotomy, or dorsal column electrical stimulation may be required if spasticity is not controlled with antispasmodics. Neurological dysfunction sometimes improves with physical therapy and speech therapy. Nutritional therapy prescribes a high-protein diet with supplementary vitamins. Clients will be encouraged to balance rest with activities and maintain optimal nutrition.

As the condition progresses, symptomatic treatment and assistance will be needed. Support groups for MS have been very beneficial for clients and their families.

Parkinson's Disease
Pathophysiology

Parkinson's disease is a disease of the basal ganglia characterized by slowing down in the initiation and execution of movement (bradykinesia), increased muscle tone (rigidity), tremor at rest, and impaired postural reflexes. The diagnosis of Parkinson's increases with age, with the peak onset being in the sixth decade. Parkinson's is more common in men than in women and is caused by the following conditions:

- Onset of Parkinson's before age 50 is usually due to a genetic defect.
- In many cases, the cause of Parkinson's is unknown.
- Some cases are caused by exposure to toxins from drugs and chemicals that destroy the cells in the substantia nigra of the brain.
- Other causes of Parkinson's include hydrocephalus, hypoxia, infections, stroke, tumour, and trauma.

Parkinson's affects the extrapyramidal system, which influences movement. A dopamine deficiency occurs in the basal ganglia. Reduction of dopamine in the corpus striatum upsets the normal balance between the dopamine (inhibitor) and acetylcholine (excitatory) neurotransmitters. Symptoms occur when affected brain cells can no longer perform their normal inhibitory function within the CNS.

Clinical Manifestations

Symptoms of the disease do not occur until 80% of neurons in the substantia nigra are lost. The classic triad of manifestations includes tremor, rigidity, and bradykinesia.

- Insidious tremor begins in the fingers (unilateral pill-roll tremor). The tremor is more prominent at rest and is aggravated by emotional stress or increased concentration.
- Rigidity is caused by sustained muscle contraction and consequently elicits complaints of soreness and feeling tired and achy. Rigidity inhibits the alternating contraction and relaxation in opposing muscle groups, slowing movement. The rigidity may be uniform or jerky (cogwheel rigidity). The client may have difficulty walking, with the gait lacking normal parallel motion. Bradykinesia (slow and delayed movement) is particularly evident.
- Other symptoms include a high-pitched, monotone voice, drooling, a masklike facial expression, slow, slurred speech, and dysphagia.

Complications of Parkinson's are caused by progressive deterioration and the negative impact this deterioration may have on the client. For example, dysphagia can lead to malnutrition. Dementia occurs in up to 40% of clients with Parkinson's.

Diagnostics

There are no specific tests for diagnosing Parkinson's. Diagnosis is based solely on the history and clinical features. A firm diagnosis can be made when at least two of the three classic symptoms are present. The ultimate confirmation of the disease is a positive response to antiparkinsonian drugs.

Therapeutics and Nursing Considerations

The drug therapy is aimed at correcting imbalances of neurotransmitters within the CNS. These drugs either enhance the release or supply of dopamine or antagonize or block the effects of acetylcholine. The drug treatments are as follows:

- Levodopa with carbidopa (Sinemet) is often the first drug used. Levodopa is a precursor of dopamine and can cross the blood–brain barrier. It is converted to dopamine in the basal ganglia. Carbidopa inhibits an enzyme that breaks down levodopa before it reaches the brain. The effect of Sinemet could wear off after a few years of therapy.
- Anticholinergics may be used in the management of Parkinson's.
- Antihistamines and antiviral agents are also used.
- As Parkinson's progresses, a combination therapy is often required.

Surgical procedures are aimed at relieving symptoms in clients who are usually unresponsive to drug therapy. Ablation therapy has largely been replaced by deep brain stimulation, which involves placing electrodes in the thalamus, globus pallidus, or subthalamic nucleus. Both ablation and deep brain stimulation procedures work by reducing the increased neuronal activity produced by the dopamine depletion.

Transplantation of fetal neural tissue into the basal ganglia provides dopamine-producing cells in the brains of clients with Parkinson's. This type of therapy is still experimental.

Since malnutrition and constipation can cause serious consequences, adequate nutrition is essential. Clients with dysphagia and bradykinesia need food that is easily chewed and swallowed. The client needs adequate roughage. Small, frequent meals are best to prevent fatigue. Ample time must be allowed for the client to eat and not become frustrated. Levodopa can be impaired by protein ingestion.

The goals of treatment focus on maximizing neurological function and maintaining independence in activities of daily living for as long as possible. Optimizing psychosocial well-being is very important.

Spinal Cord Injury
Pathophysiology

Spinal cord injuries (SCIs) are most common in young people between the ages of 15 and 25 years and occur much more frequently in males. The causes of this injury include motor vehicle accidents, falls, violence, and sports injuries. Types of SCI include cord concussion, in which the cord is severely jarred, as in a sports injury. There may be cord contusion, in which compression of the cord results in bleeding into the cord, causing bruising and edema. The extent of the damage will depend on the severity of the inflammatory response. Cord laceration, in which there is an actual tear in the cord, results in permanent injury as the neurons of the CNS do not regenerate. Cord transection, either complete or incomplete, results in loss of neurological function below the site of the injury.

The extent of the neurological damage caused by an SCI results from the primary injury, which is the actual physical disruption of an axon, and the secondary injury damage due to ischemia, hypoxia, microhemorrhage, and edema. Secondary injury occurs over time; therefore, a prognosis of recovery is more accurate 72 hours after the initial injury. The secondary injury refers to the ongoing progressive damage that occurs after the initial injury. This ongoing injury can be due to free radical formation, uncontrolled calcium influx, ischemia, lipid peroxidation, or some combination of these.

Spinal shock can last days to months and is characterized by the following:
- Decreased reflexes
- Loss of sensation
- Flaccid paralysis below the level of injury, which is experienced by 50% of people with acute SCI (Lewis et al., 2019)

The six syndromes associated with incomplete cord lesions are summarized in Table 8.8.

Spinal shock is manifested by the following:
- Decreased reflexes
- Loss of sensation
- Flaccid paralysis below the level of injury

These symptoms may last days to months and may mask postneurological function. In clients with spinal injuries at T6 or higher, return of the reflexes once spinal shock has been resolved may trigger the development of autonomic dysreflexia, which is a massive uncompensated cardiovascular reaction mediated by the SNS. Autonomic dysreflexia is life-threatening and usually occurs in response to visceral stimulation once the spinal shock is resolved. A distended bladder or rectum is the most common precipitating cause of autonomic dysreflexia. Manifestations of autonomic dysreflexia include the following:

- Extreme hypertension
- Blurred vision
- Throbbing headache
- Marked diaphoresis and flushed skin
- Piloerection
- Nasal congestion
- Nausea
- Anxiety (Lewis et al., 2019)

Clinical Manifestations

Clinical manifestations are generally a direct result of trauma. The manifestations are related to the level and degree of injury. With the incomplete lesion, there will be a mixture of symptoms.

A higher injury will have more serious manifestations. Sensory function closely parallels motor function at all levels. Disturbances of respiratory function in injuries below T6 are minimal. The following manifestations are common for upper-level injuries:

- Hypoventilation can be a serious complication with a cervical spine injury. Mechanical ventilation is required. Atelectasis and pneumonia can easily develop, and the client may require an artificial airway.
- An injury above the T6 level greatly decreases the influence of the SNS, resulting in bradycardia, peripheral vasodilation, and hypotension.
- With spinal cord lesions, the client may experience urinary retention and bladder distension and may need an in-dwelling catheter.

When lesions involve lower motor neurons, flaccid muscle weakness or paralysis, loss of reflex activity, and atrophy of the involved muscles are usually evident. Any lesion that destroys or interferes with upper motor neurons initially results in muscle flaccidity and hyporeflexia. Gradually, the reflex arcs become reactive. Voluntary muscle function is lost, but hyper-reflexia of all cord segments occurs, with increased muscle tone and spasticity. Pressure sores can

TABLE 8.8	Incomplete Cord Lesion Syndromes
Syndrome	**Cause and Results**
Central cord syndrome	• Damage is to the central spinal cord, with the client experiencing motor weakness and sensory loss in both upper and lower extremities.
Anterior cord syndrome	• Damage is to the anterior spinal artery, resulting in motor paralysis and loss of pain and temperature sensation below the level of injury. • Position, vibration, and touch sensations remain intact.
Brown-Seguard syndrome	• Typically, it results from a penetrating injury involving half of the spinal cord. • Loss of motor function, position, and vibratory sense occur on the same side as the injury, with contralateral loss of pain and temperature sensation.
Posterior cord syndrome	• This syndrome is the least common of the six spinal cord lesions; it involves damage to the posterior spinal artery, resulting in loss of proprioception. • Pain, temperature sensation, and motor function below the site of the lesion will be intact.
Conus medullaris syndrome and Cauda equina syndrome	• Damage is to the very lowest portion of the spinal cord (conus) and lumbar and sacral roots (cauda equina). • These types of syndromes result in lower motor neuron injury with flaccid paralysis of the bowel and bladder and loss of sexual function.

develop. Temperature regulation can be problematic as the client will have a decreased ability to sweat or shiver. Loss of body weight is common. DVT is common, with pulmonary embolism being one of the leading causes of death in clients with SCIs.

Diagnostics

SCIs are initially diagnosed on the basis of the presenting clinical manifestations. Diagnostic studies include complete spine films, CT scans, and MRIs.

Therapeutics and Nursing Considerations

The initial goals focus on sustaining life and preventing further cord damage. As the client's condition stabilizes, retraining takes place. The client:
- Will require a balanced diet with adequate calories and dietary fibre.
- May require an in-dwelling catheter or intermittent catheterization to regularly and completely empty the bladder to avoid UTIs.
- Will require a bowel training program.
- Will require monitoring of the environment to maintain proper body temperature.
- Will require respiratory rehabilitation, which may include a diaphragmatic pacemaker, ventilator care, assisted coughing, incentive spirometry, and deep-breathing exercises.

Sexuality is an important issue for all individuals who experience SCI. Reflexogenic erection is possible with upper motor neuron lesions. Drugs, vacuum devices, or surgery for erectile dysfunction may be done. Women usually remain fertile; however, uterine contractions are not felt, and menses may cease for up to 6 months following injury. Open discussion with the client and partner is essential.

Grief and depression should be anticipated. The client may regress at different stages of recovery. Wide fluctuations of emotion should be expected. Mourning is normal and must be allowed. Assistance to obtain control during the anger phase is difficult but helpful. Above all, promotion of independence is critical.

Osteomyelitis
Pathophysiology

Osteomyelitis is a severe infection of the bone, bone marrow, and surrounding soft tissue. The most common infection micro-organisms are *S. aureus*, *Staphylococcus epidermis*, *E. coli*, and *M. tuberculosis*. Osteomyelitis is usually a bloodborne disease that affects rapidly growing children.

Common sites of infection include the lower end of the femur and the upper ends of the tibia, humerus, and radius. In adults, the most common sites are the pelvis and vertebrae. The infection causes tissue necrosis, breakdown of bone structure, and decalcification.

Acute osteomyelitis refers to an infection of less than 1 month in duration. Chronic osteomyelitis is rare and is characterized by multiple draining sinus tracts and metastatic lesions.

Clinical Manifestations

Clinical manifestations are both systemic and local and include the following:
- Fever
- Night sweats
- Chills
- Restlessness
- Nausea
- Malaise
- Constant bone pain that is unrelieved by rest and worsens with activity
- Swelling, tenderness, and warmth at the infection site
- Restricted movement of the affected part and possible drainage from the sinus tracts (later sign) with chronic osteomyelitis

Long-term and rare complications of osteomyelitis include septicemia, septic arthritis, pathological fractures, squamous cell carcinoma, and amyloidosis.

Diagnostics

Diagnostic studies include a bone or soft tissue biopsy, blood or wound cultures, or both; elevated WBC and erythrocyte sedimentation rate (ESR); bone scans; MRI; and CT.

Therapeutics and Nursing Considerations

Vigorous and prolonged IV antibiotic therapy is the treatment of choice for acute osteomyelitis as long as bone ischemia has not yet occurred. Cultures or bone biopsy should be done prior to drug therapy. If antibiotic therapy is delayed, surgical debridement and decompression are often needed. Clients are discharged to home care with IV antibiotics delivered via a central venous catheter or peripherally inserted central catheter (PICC).

Surgical treatment includes the removal of the poorly vascularized tissue and dead bone. Antibiotic-impregnated polymethylmethacrylate bead chains may be implanted at this time to aid in combatting the infection. After debridement, the wound may be closed and a suction irrigation system is inserted. Intermittent or constant irrigation of the affected bone with antibiotics may also be initiated. Protection of the limb or surgical site with casts or braces is frequently done.

Hyperbaric oxygen therapy of 100% oxygen may be administered in chronic osteomyelitis. Amputation of the extremity may be necessary to preserve life and improve quality of life.

Upon discharge, family members need to know their role in monitoring the client's health. Key points of client and family education include the following:
- Family members should be aware that symptoms of bone pain, fever, swelling, and restricted limb movement should be reported immediately.
- Immobilization may be indicated to decrease pain, and excessive manipulation should be avoided.
- Pain assessment and interventions need to be taught.
- Instructions concerning wound care with sterile management and frequent changes of open wound dressings, if present, are needed.

- The family needs to understand the infection is not contagious.
- Heat application and activities such as exercise should be avoided.
- Uninvolved joints and muscles should continue to be exercised.
- Care and management of the venous access device are needed, as well as instruction about antibiotic administration.
- The importance of continuing to take the antibiotics even after the symptoms have subsided needs to be strongly impressed upon the family.

The family should be advised that periodic home nursing visits will provide support and help reduce anxiety.

Osteoporosis
Pathophysiology

Osteoporosis is a chronic, progressive, metabolic bone disease characterized by low bone mass and structural deterioration of bone tissue. The rate of bone resorption accelerates as the rate of bone formation decelerates, resulting in decreased bone mass and the bones becoming porous and brittle. Osteoporosis occurs more frequently in the spine, hips, and wrists. Risk factors for developing osteoporosis include the following:

- Female gender
- Family history
- Being of European or Asian descent
- Being of small stature
- Excess alcohol intake
- Cigarette smoking
- Early menopause
- Anorexia
- Liver disease
- Oophorectomy
- Sedentary lifestyle
- Insufficient calcium intake
- Long-term use of corticosteroids

Clinical Manifestations

Osteoporosis is often referred to as the "silent disease" because there are no symptoms. Later manifestations include fractures, back pain, kyphosis, and loss of height.

Diagnostics

Diagnosis includes a history and physical examination as well as a bone mineral density test, quantitative ultrasonography, and dual-energy X-ray absorptiometry.

Therapeutics and Nursing Considerations

Treatment focuses on proper nutrition, with calcium supplements, exercise, medications, and prevention of fractures. The following treatments are recommended:

- Taking supplemental vitamin D
- Increasing nutritional intake of good sources of calcium, including milk and milk products, green leafy vegetables, seafood, almonds, and hazelnuts
- Encouraging exercise to build up and maintain bone mass
- Advising quitting smoking and cutting down on alcohol intake to decrease bone loss
- Drug therapy may include the following:
  - HRT and calcitonin to inhibit osteoclastic activity
  - Bisphosphonates to inhibit osteoclast-mediated bone resorption
  - Selective estrogen receptor modulators, such as Evista, may be ordered, as well as Forteo, which contains recombinant PTH.

Nursing plays an important role in health promotion and teaching how to optimize bone health and prevent osteoporosis.

Fibromyalgia Syndrome
Pathophysiology

Fibromyalgia syndrome (FMS) is a widespread, nonarticular, musculo-skeletal pain condition that causes fatigue and multiple tender points. The etiology is unknown, but there is a link between sleep disturbances, lack of exercise, and fibromyalgia, and multiple theories exist. Some include possible CNS involvement with serotonin and substance P, abnormal levels of norepinephrine, hyperfunctioning of the hypothalamic–pituitary–adrenal axis, an increase in cortisol, a decrease in ACTH, a dysfunction in the autonomic nervous system (ANS), viral illness or Lyme disease, a decreased amount of growth hormone, or simply a low pain threshold with increased muscle tenderness.

Clinical Manifestations

Clinical manifestations include widespread burning or gnawing pain that worsens and improves throughout the day. It is difficult to discriminate the origin of the pain.

- Head or facial pain may develop from a stiff neck and shoulder muscles and can accompany temporomandibular joint dysfunction.
- There is joint tenderness at 11 or more of the 18 specific tender point sites.
- The client has difficulty concentrating, has memory lapses, and often feels overwhelmed by multiple tasks.
- Depression, anxiety, numbness or tingling in hands or feet, restless legs syndrome, and irritable bowel syndrome frequently develop.
- The client often has difficulty swallowing, perhaps due to abnormalities in esophageal smooth muscle function.
- The client experiences urinary frequency and urgency and may experience dysmenorrhea with worsening of symptoms.

Diagnostics

Laboratory tests can rule out other suspected disorders. A muscle biopsy may have a nonspecific moth-eaten appearance or show fibre atrophy. Rheumatology classifies a client as having FMS when the following criteria are met: pain is experienced in 11 of 18 tender points on palpation and there is a history of widespread pain for at least 3 months.

Therapeutics and Nursing Considerations

Treatment focuses on restoring sleep and relieving pain. This consists of the following:

- Balancing rest with activity
- Using analgesics for pain relief
- Administering low-dose tricyclic antidepressants or skeletal muscle relaxants for stress, fatigue, and sleep disturbances. Selective serotonin reuptake inhibitors (SSRIs) may be used for depression and benzodiazepines for anxiety.
- Massage combined with ultrasound or application of alternating heat and cold to sore muscles is often beneficial.
- Practising gentle stretching, yoga, Tai Chi, or low-impact aerobics is encouraged.
- Limiting the intake of sugar, caffeine, and alcohol is recommended.
- Vitamin and mineral supplements are suggested to assist the immune system.
- Relaxation strategies are discussed.

Chronic Fatigue Syndrome
Pathophysiology

Chronic fatigue syndrome (CFS) is characterized by unexplained debilitating fatigue and a variety of associated complaints lasting longer than 6 months. Immune abnormalities are also present. This syndrome is more common in women, with the usual onset between 25 and 44 years.

The precise cause is unknown, but viral infections such as herpes, Epstein–Barr virus, CMV, and retroviruses are suspected to be involved.

CFS often follows a cyclical course, alternating between illness and relatively symptom-free intervals. An abnormal immune function appears to be the central event, which leads to decreased immunoglobulin production, reduced NK cell activity, and altered cytokine production. CFS is sometimes referred to as a mental illness due to the mild to moderate depression that develops in these clients. CFS is often difficult to distinguish from FMS.

Clinical Manifestations

Clinical manifestations include sleep disturbances, low-grade fever, generalized musculo-skeletal pain, fatigue, sore throat, cervical or axillary adenopathy, multijoint pain without swelling, and headaches.

Diagnostics

Ruling out other possible causes assists in the diagnosis. No specific laboratory test is used for diagnosis.

Therapeutics and Nursing Considerations

Treatment is aimed at controlling the symptoms. Education of the client with CFS focuses on managing the fatigue while improving functioning and quality of life. Management consists of informing the client about what is known about the disease and recognizing the fears and concerns of the clients as real. The treatments are as follows:

- NSAIDs for relief of pain and fever
- Treatment for any allergic symptoms
- Tricyclic antidepressants and SSRIs for mood and sleep problems
- Clonazepam (Rivotril) for sleep disturbances or panic disorders
- Exercise to improve conditioning and restore energy, with gradual increases in intensity and duration
- Total rest is not advised as it can potentiate the client's self-image of being an invalid; rather, a carefully graduated exercise program is encouraged.
- Clients are taught to maintain a balanced diet as good nutrition is essential to producing adequate energy stores. Referrals to agencies and CFS groups are very helpful for the client.

Osteoarthritis
Pathophysiology

Osteoarthritis (OA) is a noninflammatory disorder of the diarthrodial (synovial) joints. It is slowly progressive, with the majority of adults being affected by age 40. After menopause, more women than men are affected by OA. OA may occur as an idiopathic (of unknown cause) or secondary disorder due to a previous infection, trauma, or skeletal deformity. Estrogen reduction at menopause, as well as genetic factors, seems to play a significant role. Modifiable risk factors include obesity and sedentary lifestyle.

OA causes deterioration of the joint cartilage and reactive new bone formation at the margins and subchondral areas. The progression of OA causes cartilage to gradually become softer, less elastic, and less able to resist wear with heavy use. Continued changes in the cartilage collagen lead to erosion of the articular surface. Uneven joint surfaces create an unequal distribution of stress across the joint, resulting in limited joint movement. Although inflammation is not characteristic of OA, a secondary synovitis may result when phagocytic cells try to rid the joint of small pieces of cartilage torn from the joint surface. These inflammatory changes contribute to the early pain and stiffness of OA. In later stages of OA, contact can occur between exposed bony joint surfaces after cartilage has completely deteriorated.

Clinical Manifestations

Clinical manifestations do not include systemic symptoms. The symptoms are as follows:

- Joint pain is the most common symptom and occurs particularly after exercise or weight-bearing.
- Joint pain may worsen as barometric pressures fall before inclement weather.
- Sometimes crepitation, a grating sensation caused by loose particles of cartilage, can be felt in the joint cavity.
- The joint pain is asymmetrical, and the client may experience early-morning stiffness, but this stiffness is usually resolved within 30 minutes.
- Joints that are commonly involved include the distal interphalangeal, proximal interphalangeal, and carpometacarpal joint of the thumb. Weight-bearing joints such as

the hips and knees are commonly affected, as well as the metatarsophalangeal and the cervical and lower lumbar vertebrae.

- Heberden's nodes are deformities of the distal interphalangeal joint and indicate osteophyte formation. Bouchard's nodes are deformities found on the proximal interphalangeal joint. These deformities often appear red, swollen, and tender.

Diagnostics

Diagnosis is based on a history and physical examination. Bone scans, CT scans, MRIs, and X-rays are used to look for joint changes. Blood work would include ESR and CBC. Synovial fluid analysis will rule out an inflammatory arthritis.

Therapeutics and Nursing Considerations

There is no cure for OA; therefore, treatment is focused on the following:

- Management of symptoms of pain and inflammation
- Prevention of deformity and maintenance of joint function
- Rest and joint protection
- Heat and cold applications, which may help reduce pain and stiffness
- Nutritional therapy
- Exercise
- Complementary and alternative therapies
- Supportive devices such as braces, which can be used to protect the joint

Drug therapy is based on the severity of the symptoms. Clients with mild to moderate joint pain may receive relief from acetaminophen. Salicylates or NSAIDs may provide greater relief for moderate to severe OA pain. Corticosteroids, disease-modifying antirheumatic drugs (DMARDs), immunosuppressants, biological therapy, and antibiotics may be added, depending on the client. As the pain worsens, opioid medications may be added.

Education is a necessary element for the client. The client needs to know about medications and the treatment plan and be a full participant in his or her own care.

Rheumatoid Arthritis
Pathophysiology

Rheumatoid arthritis (RA) is a chronic, systemic disease characterized by inflammation of the connective tissue in the diarthrodial (synovial) joints and surrounding tissues. Systemic manifestations include pulmonary, cardiac, vascular, ophthalmological, dermatological, and hematological effects. RA typically has periods of remission and exacerbation. It affects all ethnic groups and can occur at any time of life; however, the incidence increases with age. Women are affected two to three times more than men. Smoking appears to play a role in the development of RA.

The cause of RA is unknown, although an autoimmune etiology is currently the most widely accepted theory. The unknown antigen triggers the formation of an abnormal IgG. RA is characterized by the presence of autoantibody,

rheumatoid factor (RF). RF and IgG form immune complexes that initially deposit on synovial membranes or superficial articular cartilages in the joints, which leads to activation of complement and an inflammatory response. Joint changes from inflammation begin when the hypertrophied synovial membrane invades the surround cartilage, ligaments, tendons, and joint capsule. Pannus forms with the joint and eventually covers and erodes the entire surface of the articular cartilage. Inflammatory cytokines further contribute to cartilage destruction. The pannus scars and shortens supporting structures, causing joint laxity, subluxation, and contracture. A genetic predisposition appears to be important in the development of RA.

Anatomical changes of RA follow four stages:

- Stage 1—early: There are no destructive changes on X-ray, although there may be evidence of osteoporosis.
- Stage 2—moderate: X-rays reveal evidence of osteoporosis with or without slight bone or cartilage destruction. There is no joint deformity. Adjacent muscle will atrophy, and extra-articular soft tissue lesions may be present.
- Stage 3—severe: X-rays reveal cartilage and bone destruction in addition to osteoporosis. There will be joint deformity with extensive muscle atrophy, and extra-articular soft tissue lesions may be present.
- Stage 4—terminal: Fibrosis, bony ankylosis, or both are present, as well as all the criteria for stage 3.

Clinical Manifestations

The onset of RA is typically insidious. Nonspecific manifestations may precede the onset of arthritic complaints. These may include the following:

- Fatigue
- Anorexia and weight loss
- Generalized morning stiffness

Specific articular involvement of pain, stiffness, limitation of motion, and signs of inflammation develop. The joint symptoms occur symmetrically and frequently. The joints most frequently affected include the small joints of the hands and feet and the larger peripheral joints of the wrists, elbows, shoulders, knees, hips, ankles, and jaw. The cervical spine may also be involved. The client with RA will often experience joint stiffness after periods of inactivity. Morning stiffness may last from 60 minutes to several hours or more. Joints become tender, painful, and warm to the touch. Joint pain increases with movement, varies in intensity, may not be proportional to the degree of inflammation, and may make it difficult for the client to grasp things (tenosynovitis). The inflammation and fibrosis of the joint capsule and supporting structures may lead to deformity and disability.

RA can affect nearly every system of the body. The three most common complications include rheumatoid nodules, Sjögren's syndrome, and Felty's syndrome. Rheumatoid nodules develop in 25% of all clients with RA who have high titres of RF. Sjögren's syndrome affects 10–15% of clients with RA and can occur as a disease by itself or in conjunction with other arthritic disorders. Felty's syndrome occurs most commonly in clients with severe nodule-forming RA.

Diagnostics

Diagnosis depends on an accurate history and physical examination. RF can be found in 75–80% of clients with RA. ESR and C-reactive protein are indicators of active inflammation. X-rays are not specifically diagnostic in the early stages. A bone scan may detect early changes and confirm the diagnosis. Synovial fluid analysis will show increased volume and turbidity but decreased viscosity. The client might be slightly anemic with slight leukocytosis.

Therapeutics and Nursing Considerations

Treatment focuses on drug therapy, education, physical therapy, and occupational therapy. Drug therapy is the cornerstone of RA treatment and is as follows:

- DMARDs such as methotrexate, sulphasalazine (Salazopyrin), leflunomides (Arava), or combinations of these have the potential to lessen the permanent effects of RA.
- Biological or targeted therapy are also used to slow disease progression in RA.
- NSAIDs, salicylates, and steroids are also used.
- In some situations, antimalarials, gold sodium thiomalate, or antibiotics may be used.

The choice of drug depends on the disease activity, the client's level of function, and lifestyle considerations.

Other important treatments include the following:

- Balanced nutrition can control weight loss, which may result from loss of appetite and inability to shop for and prepare food.
- Corticosteroids or immobility may result in unwanted weight gain.
- Exercise reduces stress on arthritic joints. The client is encouraged to alternate rest and activity.
- Lightweight splints help rest inflamed joints and prevent deformity.
- Occupational therapists are helpful in teaching the client about work simplification techniques and time-saving joint protection devices.

Psychological support is important as clients are constantly threatened by problems of limited function and fatigue, loss of self-esteem, altered body image, fear of disability and deformity, and loss of sexuality.

The major goals of therapy for clients with RA include the following:

- Promoting comfort and satisfactory pain relief
- Promoting independence and self-care with minimal loss of functional ability of affected joints
- Reducing fatigue
- Maintenance of a positive self-image
- Preventing injury and promoting mobility and maintenance of activities of daily living

Systemic Lupus Erythematosus
Pathophysiology

Systemic lupus erythematosus (SLE) is a chronic multisystem inflammatory disorder of the connective tissue. SLE affects multiple organ systems, including the skin, and can be fatal. It mostly affects young women of African, Asian, or Indigenous descent, although it does affect people of European descent as well. The etiology is unknown; however, genetic influences, hormones, environmental factors, and certain medications have been known to precipitate the disease. The onset of SLE usually occurs following menarche. The autoimmune reactions are directed at the body producing antibodies against components of its own cells, resulting in immune complex disease. Clients with SLE may produce antibodies against RBCs, neutrophils, platelets, lymphocytes, or any organ or tissue in the body.

Clinical Manifestations

Since SLE has multisystem involvement and characteristics of remission and exacerbation, the clinical manifestations can be many. These may include the following:

- Characteristic facial butterfly rash
- Photosensitivity
- Oral ulcers
- Arthritis
- Pleuritis
- Pericarditis
- Renal disorders (proteinuria)
- Neurological disorders (seizures, psychosis)
- Hematological disorders (hemolytic anemia, leukopenia, lymphopenia, thrombocytopenia)
- Immunological disorders and development of antinuclear antibodies

Diagnostics

There is no specific diagnostic test for SLE, which is primarily diagnosed on examination of criteria relating to client history, physical findings, and laboratory findings. Antinuclear antibodies are positive for most clients with SLE.

Therapeutics and Nursing Considerations

Management of SLE revolves around drug therapy. The following drugs are utilized:

- NSAIDs
- Antimalarial drugs
- Steroid-sparing drugs
- Corticosteroids
- Immunosuppressive drugs

Since SLE is a chronic condition, the client's physical, psychological, and socio-cultural problems should be assessed and managed. Pain and fatigue need to be monitored daily. The client needs to be educated regarding management of these ongoing issues. The overall goals for managing clients with SLE include satisfactory pain relief and adherence to the therapeutic regimen to achieve maximum symptom management. Other goals are to demonstrate awareness of and avoid activities that cause disease exacerbation and to maintain optimal function and a positive self-image.

With an acute exacerbation, it is important to record the severity of symptoms and the client's response to therapy. The client needs to be observed for the following:

- Fever pattern
- Joint inflammation
- Limitation of motion

- Location and degree of discomfort
- Fatigue
- Signs of bleeding
- Weight, fluid, and electrolyte anomalies need to be monitored if on corticosteroid therapy.
- Neurological disorders

The client will require support with explanations through the exacerbation. Once the exacerbation has ended, further client teaching needs to focus on adherence to the treatment plan and minimizing exposure to precipitating factors.

Low Back Pain
Pathophysiology

Low back pain is a common problem that affects 70–85% of the population at least once and can result in significant economic and social costs. The lumbar region is susceptible to injury as this area bears most of the weight of the body and is the most flexible region of the spinal column. This region has poor biomechanical structure, and the nerve roots in the area are vulnerable to injury. Risk factors for developing low back pain are as follows:

- A lack of muscle tone
- Excess weight
- Poor posture
- Cigarette smoking
- Stress
- Repetitive heavy lifting
- Vibrations
- Prolonged periods of sitting

Low back pain is most often due to musculo-skeletal problems, such as acute lumbosacral strain, instability of the lumbosacral bony mechanism, and OA of the lumbosacral vertebrae. Low back pain can also be due to intervertebral disc degeneration or herniation of the intervertebral disc.

Chronic back pain lasts for more than 3 months or is manifested in repeated incapacitating episodes. The causes of chronic back pain include the following:

- Degenerative disc disease
- Lack of physical exercise or prior injury
- Obesity
- Structural and postural abnormalities
- Systemic disease; OA of the lumbar spine is found in clients over the age of 50 years
- Cold, damp weather, which can aggravate back pain

Clinical Manifestations

Acute low back pain lasts 4 weeks or less and is usually associated with some activity that causes undue stress on the tissues of the lower back. The actual lower back pain with or without spasms will often appear later. Straight-leg raises will increase the pain.

Diagnostics

A thorough history and physical examination are needed to rule out serious conditions that may present as low back pain. MRI and CT scanning are not usually done unless trauma or systemic disease is suspected.

Therapeutics and Nursing Considerations

The client is cared for on an outpatient basis with the following treatments:

- Analgesics
- Muscle relaxants
- Massage
- Possible use of a corset to prevent rotation, flexion, and extension
- Rest may also be beneficial.

The client will be encouraged to avoid lifting, bending, twisting, and prolonged sitting. Most cases improve within 2 weeks.

Once an acute episode has resolved, health promotion is very important. Suggestions such as maintaining an appropriate weight, avoiding sleeping in the prone position, and using a firm mattress are beneficial. The client will be instructed not to lean forward without bending the knees, lift anything above the level of the elbows, stand in one position for a prolonged time, or exercise without consulting a healthcare provider. Treatment of chronic low back pain is similar to that for acute low back pain.

Herniated Intervertebral Disc
Pathophysiology

A herniated intervertebral disc is often referred to as a "slipped disc." It is a protrusion of the nucleus pulposus between adjacent surfaces of vertebral bodies and may occur anywhere along the spine. It can result from trauma, a sharp or sudden movement, or natural degeneration due to age. The gelatinous centre of the disc may rupture, causing acute injury and back pain. Common sites of rupture include L4–L5, L5–S1, C4–C5, C5–C6, and C6–C7. Herniation of thoracic discs is less common.

Clinical Manifestations

Clinical manifestations of a herniated disc are dependent on the location and size of the herniation. Manifestations may include low back pain that radiates down the leg in dermatomal distribution. Lying down often relieves pain. Reflexes may be depressed or absent. Muscle weakness is found in the legs, feet, and toes. There may be incontinence and impotence.

Diagnostics

Diagnostic studies include X-ray, myelography, MRI, CT, epidural venography, discography, and EMG to determine the severity of nerve irritation and to rule out other pathological conditions.

Therapeutics and Nursing Considerations

Treatment involves limitation of extremes of spinal involvement; the local application of heat, ice, or both; ultrasound and massage; and traction and transcutaneous electrical nerve stimulation (TENS).

Drug therapy can include NSAIDs, short-term narcotic opioids, and muscle relaxants. Once symptoms subside, back-strengthening exercises are encouraged. The client should be taught the principles of good body mechanics. Surgical therapy is needed when the client is unresponsive to conservative treatment or experiences consistent pain or there is a persistent neurological deficit. Several surgical procedures can be used to treat a herniated disc, which are as follows:

- Laminectomy, removal of a portion of the lamina, is the most common surgery for a herniated disc.
- A discectomy, removal of all or part of the herniated disc.
- A spinal fusion is done to stabilize two or more vertebrae by the insertion of bone grafts with or without the addition of rods, plates, screws, or other hardware.

After surgery, the client will be on a flat bed for 1–2 days, depending on the extent of the surgery. The client will be turned by log-rolling. Pillows will be placed under the thighs of each leg when the client is supine and between the legs when the client is in the side-lying position. The client is often fearful of any movement; therefore, explanation and reassurance are essential. IV narcotics will manage pain. Muscle relaxants may be prescribed. The client should be monitored for CSF leakage, which would manifest by a severe headache or the appearance of clear or slightly yellow fluid at the surgical site. Neurological assessment is ongoing, comparing the movement of the arms and the legs with preoperative movement. The client should be assessed for paraesthesia in all appropriate dermatomes. Movement and muscle strength of all extremities should be monitored. Wound care is done when needed. The donor site for a bone graft must be regularly assessed. The posterior iliac crest is the most common donor site. The donor site often produces more pain than the fused area. A pressure dressing may be needed to prevent excessive bleeding at the site.

Complications following surgery may include the following:

- Paralytic ileus and interference with bowel function may arise.
- Nausea, abdominal distension, and constipation; stool softeners may be ordered.
- Bladder emptying may be altered due to limited activity, the use of narcotics, or anaesthesia.
- Loss of sphincter tone or bladder tone may indicate nerve damage.

The client will have to adjust to a permanent immobility at the graft or fusion site. The client and family will need education regarding proper body mechanics, avoiding standing or sitting for long periods of time, balancing rest with activity, and that bending, lifting, and stooping could be injurious. Walking should be encouraged. Twisting movements of the spine are contraindicated.

Fractures
Pathophysiology

A fracture is a disruption or a break in the continuity of the structure of a bone, usually due to a blow to the body, a fall, or another accident. Fractures are described and classified according to their type and anatomical location and whether there is communication or noncommunication with the external environment. Other classification categories include appearance, position, alignment of the fragments, classic

- **Complete fracture** is when a bone breaks into two parts that are completely separated.

- An **incomplete fracture** is when a bone breaks into two parts that are not completely separated.

- A **comminuted fracture** is one in which the bone is broken and shattered into more than two fragments.

- A **closed (simple) fracture** is one in which there is no break in the skin.

- An **open (compound) fracture** is one in which there is a break in the skin through which the fragments of broken bone protrude.

- A **greenstick fracture,** common in children, is one in which the bone is partially bent and partially broken.

Fig. 8.7 Types of fractures. (From deWit, S. C., Stromberg, H., & Dallred, C. [2017]. *Medical-surgical nursing: Concepts and Practices* [3rd ed., p. 739, Box 32-1]. St. Louis: Elsevier.)

names, and whether they are stable or unstable. Fig. 8.7 illustrates various types of fractures.

Typical complete fractures include the following:
- Closed (simple) fractures are noncommunicating wounds between bone and skin.
- Open (compound) fractures are communicating wounds between bone and skin.
- Other types include comminuted, linear, oblique, spiral, transverse, impacted, pathological, avulsion, extracapsular, and intracapsular fractures.

Typical incomplete fractures include greenstick, torus, bowing, stress, and transchondral fractures.

Clinical Manifestations

Clinical manifestations of fractures include the client reporting a mechanism of injury resulting in immediate localized pain, loss of function, and obvious deformity. Other symptoms could include excessive motion at the site, crepitus, soft tissue edema in the area of injury, warmth over the injured area, ecchymosis of skin surrounding the injured area, paralysis, impairment or loss of sensation distal to the site of injury, signs of shock, and inability to bear weight on or use the affected part.

Therapeutics and Nursing Considerations

Fracture healing is a reparative process of self-healing (union) that occurs in the following stages:
1. Fracture hematoma
2. Granulation tissue
3. Callus formation
4. Ossification
5. Consolidation
6. Remodelling

Treatment focuses on anatomical realignment of fragments (reduction), immobilization to maintain alignment, and restoration of normal function. A closed reduction involves nonsurgical manual realignment. An open reduction is the correction of bone alignment through a surgical incision. Forms of immobilization include skin traction for short-term immobilization and skeletal traction for long-term immobilization.

Traction is the mechanism by which a steady pull is exerted on a part or parts of the body while countertraction pulls in the opposite direction. Traction is used to prevent or reduce muscle spasm, immobilize the limb, reduce the fracture, stretch adhesions, and correct deformities. Suspension is the use of traction equipment, such as frames, splints, pulleys, and weights, to suspend but not exert pull on a body part. Balanced suspension is often used with traction to allow the client more freedom.

Casts are considered temporary circumferential immobilization devices and are commonly used with closed reductions. There are many different types of casts.

External fixation uses metallic devices composed of pins that are inserted into the bone and attached to external rods. Internal fixation uses pins, plates, rods, and screws that are surgically inserted at the time of realignment.

Drug therapy for the treatment of fractures may include the following:

- Muscle relaxants
- Tetanus–diphtheria toxoid or immunoglobulins
- Bone-penetrating antibiotics, such as cephalosporin and analgesics as needed

The overall goals for treatment of the fracture include physiological healing with no associated complications, pain relief, and achievement of maximal rehabilitation potential. The following considerations are important:

- Neurovascular assessment of colour, temperature, capillary refill, peripheral pulses, edema, sensation, motor function, and pain should be ongoing.
- Fractures pose a risk of peripheral neurovascular dysfunction, pain, and infection.
- A high fluid intake and a diet high in fibre are important due to the immobility of the client.
- Traction equipment should be checked for proper functioning, and pin site care must be done.
- Too tight a cast can result in neurovascular complications; extremities must be checked frequently.
- If a cast is applied, the limb should be elevated above the level of the heart if possible when the client is resting.
- The client should be encouraged to exercise the joints above and below the cast to decrease muscle atrophy.
- Assistive devices such as canes, walkers, or crutches may be needed to help mobilize the client.

Complications of fractures include infections. Open fractures and soft tissue injuries have an increased risk of developing infections. Osteomyelitis may become chronic. If infection is present in an open fracture, surgical debridement may be necessary. Antibiotic therapy will be initiated.

Compartment syndrome is a condition in which elevated intracompartmental pressure within a confined myofascial compartment compromises the neurovascular function of the tissues within the space. This causes capillary perfusion to be reduced below a level necessary for tissue viability and is classified as acute, chronic or exertional, or crush. Two basic etiologies create compartment syndrome. There may be a decreased compartment size due to restrictive dressings, splints, or casts, or there may be increased compartment content due to bleeding or edema. Clinical manifestations of compartment syndrome include the following "six Ps":

- Paraesthesia
- Pain
- Pressure
- Pallor
- Paralysis
- Pulselessness

Clients may present with one or all of the six Ps. Absence of a peripheral pulse is considered an ominous late sign. Treatment requires prompt, accurate diagnosis. Early recognition is key. The bandage or cast should be removed and traction weight reduced, and the limb should not be placed above the heart, nor should it receive hot or cold applications. Surgical decompression (fasciotomy) may be needed.

Venous thrombus is another potential complication of fractures. Precipitating factors include venous stasis, caused by incorrectly applied casts or traction, local pressure on the vein, and immobility.

Fat embolism syndrome (FES) is characterized by the presence of fat globules in tissues and organs after a traumatic skeletal injury. The fractures that most often cause FES include fractures of the long bones, ribs, tibia, and pelvis. Tissues that are most affected are the lungs, brain, heart, kidneys, and skin. Symptoms will occur within 24–48 hours after injury and may manifest as interstitial pneumonitis, which may produce symptoms of ARDS (chest pain, tachypnea, cyanosis, decreased PaO_2, dyspnea, apprehension, and tachycardia). The course of FES is rapid, with an acute onset and feelings of impending doom, and the client may be comatose for a short while. Treatment is directed at prevention; careful immobilization of the bone fracture is the most important preventive factor.

Stroke (Brain Attack or Cerebrovascular Accident)

Pathophysiology

A cerebrovascular accident (CVA) occurs when there is a sudden interruption of circulation in one or more of the cerebral blood vessels, resulting in the death of brain cells. Functions such as movement, sensation, and emotion that were controlled by the affected area of the brain are impaired or lost. The severity of the loss of function varies according to the location and extent of involvement.

Nonmodifiable risk factors for developing a stroke include increasing age, male gender, female gender postmenopause, heredity, and being of African descent. Modifiable risk factors include the following:

- Poorly controlled DM
- Heart disease, arrhythmias, hypertension, hypercoagulability, and dyslipidemia

- Obesity, sedentary lifestyle, smoking, and heavy alcohol use
- Sickle cell disease (if sickling episodes can be prevented)
- Oral contraceptives

Blood is supplied to the brain by two major pairs of arteries, the internal carotid arteries and the vertebral arteries. The brain requires a continuous supply of blood to provide the oxygen and glucose that neurons need to function. If blood flow to the brain is totally interrupted, neurological metabolism is altered in 30 seconds. Metabolism stops within 2 minutes, and cellular death occurs in 5 minutes.

Atherosclerosis is the major cause of stroke. It can lead to thrombus formation and contribute to emboli development. In response to ischemia, a series of metabolic events (ischemic cascade) occur, which include inadequate ATP production, loss of ion homeostasis, release of excitatory amino acids, free radical formation, and cell death. Around the core area of ischemia is a border zone of reduced blood flow where ischemia may be reversed. If adequate blood supply can be restored (in less than 3 hours), the ischemic cascade can be interrupted, with the result that there is less brain damage and less neurological function is lost.

Transient ischemic attack (TIA) is a temporary focal loss of neurological function caused by ischemia. TIAs usually resolve within 3 hours but may last as long as 24 hours. TIAs may be due to microemboli that temporarily block the blood flow and are warning signs of progressive cerebrovascular disease.

Strokes are classified based on the underlying pathophysiological findings and are either ischemic or hemorrhagic in nature. Ischemic strokes result from inadequate blood flow to the brain from partial or complete occlusion of an artery. Ischemic strokes constitute 80% of all strokes and are due to either thrombus or emboli damage. Thrombotic stroke occurs in relation to injury to a blood vessel wall and subsequent formation of a blood clot that narrows the blood vessel, resulting in a decreased amount of blood delivered to the tissue. This is the most common type of stroke and is usually associated with hypertension, DM, or both. Thrombotic stroke is often preceded by a TIA.

Embolic stroke occurs when an embolus lodges in and occludes a cerebral artery. This results in no blood to the distal tissues, leading to infarction and edema. This is the second most common cause of a stroke. The majority of emboli originate in the inside layer of the heart, with plaque breaking off from the endocardium and entering the circulation. Clients with an embolic stroke commonly have a rapid occurrence of severe clinical symptoms that may or may not be related to activity. Clients experiencing an embolic stroke usually remain conscious, although they often have a headache. Recurrence is common unless the underlying cause is aggressively treated.

Hemorrhagic strokes account for about 15% of all strokes. They result from bleeding into the brain tissue itself or into the subarachnoid space or ventricles. Intracerebral hemorrhage is bleeding within the brain caused by a rupture of a vessel, usually during activity. Hypertension is the most common cause. The onset is sudden, with a progression of symptoms over minutes to hours due to ongoing bleeding. Manifestations include neurological deficits, headache, nausea, vomiting, hypertension, and decreased levels of consciousness.

Subarachnoid hemorrhage occurs when there is intracranial bleeding into the CSF-filled space between the arachnoid and pia mater. This bleeding is commonly caused by rupture of a cerebral saccular or berry aneurysm. The majority of aneurysms are in the circle of Willis. Clients often describe the pain as "the worst headache in [their] life."

Clinical Manifestations

Motor impairment is the most obvious effect of stroke and can involve the following:

- Mobility
- Respiratory function
- Swallowing, speech, and gag reflex
- Self-care abilities
- Skilled voluntary movement
- The integration of movements, and alteration in muscle tone
- Alterations in reflexes
- An initial period of flaccidity, which may last from days to several weeks and is related to nerve damage
- Spasticity of the muscles, which follows the flaccid stage and is related to interruption of upper motor neuron influence

Stroke can also have the following neurological effects:

- The client may experience aphasia (total loss of comprehension and language) when a stroke damages the dominant hemisphere of the brain.
- Many clients also experience dysarthria (impairments with pronunciation, articulation, and phonation). Dysarthria does not affect the meaning of communication or the comprehension of language, but it does affect the mechanics of speech.

For various neurological deficits of stroke and their nursing considerations, see Table 8.9.

Clients who suffer a stroke may have difficulty controlling their emotions, with the result that their emotional responses may be exaggerated or unpredictable. Depression and feelings associated with changes in body image and loss of function can make this worse. Clients may also be frustrated with immobility and communication problems.

Both memory and judgement may be impaired as a result of stroke. A left-brain stroke is more likely to result in memory problems related to language. Stroke on the right side of the brain is more likely to cause problems in spatial perceptual orientation, although this can also occur with left-brain stroke. Most problems with urinary and bowel elimination occur initially and are temporary. Manifestations for right-brain and left-brain stroke are summarized in Fig. 8.8.

Diagnostics

A CT scan is the primary diagnostic test used when stroke is suspected. The CT scan diagnoses either hemorrhage or

TABLE 8.9   Neurological Deficits of Stroke

Neurological Deficit	Manifestation	Nursing Considerations and Client Teaching Applications
Visual Field Deficits		
Homonymous hemianopsia (loss of half of the visual field)	• Unaware of persons or objects on side of visual loss • Neglect of one side of the body • Difficulty judging distances	• Place objects within intact field of vision. • Approach the client from side of intact field of vision. • Instruct/remind the client to turn his or her head in the direction of visual loss to compensate for loss of visual field. • Encourage the use of eyeglasses if available. • When teaching the client, do so within the client's intact visual field.
Loss of peripheral vision	• Difficulty seeing at night • Unaware of objects or the borders of objects	• Avoid night driving or other risky activities in the darkness. • Place objects in centre of client's intact visual field. • Encourage the use of a cane or other object to identify objects in the periphery of the visual field.
Diplopia	• Double vision	• Explain to the client the location of an object when placing it near the client. • Consistently place client care items in the same location.
Motor Deficits		
Hemiparesis	• Weakness of the face, arm, and leg on the same side (due to a lesion in the opposite hemisphere)	• Place objects within the client's reach on the non-affected side. • Instruct the client to exercise and increase the strength on the unaffected side.
Hemiplegia	• Paralysis of the face, arm, and leg on the same side (due to a lesion in the opposite hemisphere)	• Encourage the client to perform range-of-motion exercises to the affected side. • Provide immobilization as needed to the affected side. • Maintain body alignment in functional position. • Exercise unaffected limb to increase mobility, strength, and use.
Ataxia	• Staggering, unsteady gait • Unable to keep feet together; needs a broad base to stand	• Support client during the initial ambulation phase. • Provide supportive device for ambulation (walker, cane). • Instruct the client not to walk without assistance or supportive device.
Dysarthria	• Difficulty forming words	• Provide the client with alternative methods of communicating. • Allow the client sufficient time to respond to verbal communication. • Support the client and family to alleviate frustration related to difficulty in communicating.
Dysphagia	• Difficulty swallowing	• Test the client's pharyngeal reflexes before offering food or fluids. • Assist the client with meals. • Place food on the unaffected side of the mouth. • Allow ample time to eat.
Sensory Deficits		
Paraesthesia (occurs on the side opposite the lesion)	• Numbness and tingling of extremity • Difficulty with proprioception	• Instruct the client to avoid using this extremity as the dominant limb due to altered sensation. • Perform range-of-motion exercises on affected areas and apply corrective devices as needed.
Verbal Deficits		
Expressive aphasia	• Unable to form words that are understandable; may be able to speak in single-word responses	• Encourage the client to repeat sounds of the alphabet.
Receptive aphasia	• Unable to comprehend the spoken word; can speak but may not make sense	• Speak slowly and clearly to assist the client by modelling sounds.
Global (mixed) aphasia	• Combination of both receptive and expressive aphasia	• Speak clearly and in simple sentences; use gestures or pictures when possible. • Establish alternative means of communication.

Continued

TABLE 8.9 Neurological Deficits of Stroke—cont'd

Neurological Deficit	Manifestation	Nursing Considerations and Client Teaching Applications
Cognitive Deficits	• Short- and long-term memory loss • Decreased attention span • Impaired ability to concentrate • Poor abstract reasoning • Altered judgement	• Reorient the client to time, place, and situation frequently. • Use verbal and auditory cues to orient the client. • Provide familiar objects (family photographs, favourite objects). • Use non-complicated language. • Match visual tasks with a verbal cue; holding a toothbrush, simulate brushing of teeth while saying, "I would like you to brush your teeth now." • Minimize distracting noises and views when teaching the client. • Repeat and reinforce instructions frequently.
Emotional Deficits	• Loss of self-control • Emotional lability • Decreased tolerance to stressful situations • Depression • Withdrawal • Fear, hostility, and anger • Feelings of isolation	• Support the client during uncontrollable outbursts. • Discuss with the client and the family that the outbursts are due to the disease process. • Encourage the client to participate in group activity. • Provide stimulation for the client. • Control stressful situations, if possible. • Provide a safe environment. • Encourage the client to express feelings and frustrations related to the disease process.

From Day, R. A., Paul, P., Williams, B., et al. (2016). *Brunner & Suddarth's textbook of medical-surgical nursing* (3rd Cdn. ed., p. 2047, Table 63.2). Philadelphia: Lippincott, Williams & Wilkins. Reprinted with permission.

Right-brain damage (stroke on right side of the brain)	**Left-brain damage** (stroke on left side of the brain)
• Paralyzed left side: hemiplegia	• Paralyzed right side: hemiplegia
• Left-sided neglect	• Impaired speech–language (aphasias)
• Spatial–perceptual deficits	• Impaired right–left discrimination
• Tends to deny or minimize problems	• Slow performance, cautious
• Rapid performance, short attention span	• Aware of deficits: depression, anxiety
• Impulsive; safety problems	• Impaired comprehension related to language, math
• Impaired judgement	
• Impaired time concepts	

Fig. 8.8 Manifestations of right-brain and left-brain stroke. (From Lewis, S. M., Bucher, L., Heitkemper, M. M., et al. [2019]. *Medical-surgical nursing in Canada: Assessment and management of clinical problems* [4th Cdn. ed., p. 1513, Figure 60-5]. Milton, ON: Elsevier.)

ischemic stroke and thus assists in appropriate treatment. Brain scans reveal ischemia but may not be positive for up to 2 weeks after a stroke. Carotid ultrasonography may detect a blockage, stenosis, or reduced blood flow of the carotid arteries. Ophthalmoscopy may detect signs of hypertension and atherosclerosis in retinal arteries. Angiography can help pinpoint the site of occlusion or rupture. An electroencephalogram (EEG) may help localize the area of damage. Laboratory tests include CBC, platelets, PT, partial thromboplastin time (PTT), electrolytes, glucose, renal and hepatic studies, and lipid profile.

Therapeutics and Nursing Considerations

Goals for collaborative care during the acute phase of a stroke are to preserve life, prevent further brain damage, and reduce disability. The practical nurse monitors and reports vital signs and neurological assessments, including LOC, motor and sensory function, pupil size and reactivity, oxygen saturation, and cardiac rhythm.

Rehabilitation care begins after the stroke has been stable for 12–24 hours. Collaborative care shifts from preserving life to lessening disability and attaining optimal function. Goals at this time include maintaining a stable or improved LOC, attaining maximum physical functioning, attaining maximum self-care abilities and skills, and maximizing communication abilities. A plan to prevent recurrence of stroke is developed with the client and family.

Management of the following systems is very important. Nursing considerations:

• The respiratory system is a priority as the client may be at risk for aspiration pneumonia and airway obstruction.

- The neurological system requires close monitoring for changes that might suggest an extension of a stroke.
- The cardiac system (vital signs and cardiac rhythm) also requires close monitoring due to the potential for a decreased cardiac reserve.
- Monitoring the lungs for sounds of fluid and the heart for the sound of murmurs is important for early detection of heart failure.
- Fluid and electrolyte balance is important.
- Proper positioning with appropriate supports and ROM exercises are needed to help prevent joint contracture and muscle atrophy.
- The skin of a client with stroke is susceptible to breakdown related to loss of sensation, decreased circulation, and immobility. This can be compounded by the client's age, poor nutrition, dehydration, edema, and incontinence. Pressure relief by proper turning and positioning is needed, along with good skin hygiene.
- Early mobility is helpful.
- Stress of the illness contributes to a catabolic state that can interfere with recovery. Good nutrition is essential, but the client must be checked for an active gag reflex before oral feedings are initiated. Feedings should be followed by thorough oral hygiene.
- Constipation is a common bowel problem for clients with stroke. Physical activity will promote bowel function. Stool softeners and suppositories may be needed. Urinary incontinence is more common in the acute stage of the illness. Efforts should be made to promote normal bladder function and avoid the use of in-dwelling catheters.

It is imperative to meet the psychological needs of the client. The client will be assessed for the ability to speak and understand. Speaking slowly and calmly with simple words and sentences assists the client in speech improvement. Blindness in the same half of each visual field is a common problem after a stroke. Other visual problems may be diplopia, loss of the corneal reflex, and ptosis.

Explanations about what has happened to the client and about diagnostic and therapeutic procedures should be clear and understandable to the client and family.

HEALTH CHALLENGES RELATED TO ALTERED SENSORY INPUT

Otitis Media
Pathophysiology

Inflammation or infection of the middle ear is considered the most common cause of conductive hearing loss. It can be caused by viruses or bacteria, with *Streptococcus* infections being the most common causative factor in bacterial otitis media. An accumulation of fluid can build up behind the tympanic membrane, resulting in loss of movement of the membrane, which can prevent the ossicles from moving and result in temporary hearing loss.

Clinical Manifestations

Symptoms of otitis media vary according to the severity of the infection. They may include tugging at the ears, pain and irritability, poor sleeping, diarrhea, vomiting and fever, inability to hear soft sounds, fluid draining from the ear, and possibly loss of balance. See Chapter 10 for more information on otitis media.

Diagnostics

Diagnosis is made based on otoscopic examination, which reveals that the tympanic membrane is red and bulging (Lewis et al., 2019).

Therapeutics and Nursing Considerations

Treatment for this condition includes acetaminophen for pain and fever control and antibiotics specific to the infectious organism.

The practical nurse should monitor the effectiveness of the antibiotic and acetaminophen. Educating the client regarding adherence to the medication regimen, awareness of complications such as a perforated tympanic membrane, and when to seek medical assistance is important.

Cataracts
Pathophysiology

Cataracts are a common cause of vision loss. Vision is lost gradually due to the developing opacity of the lens or lens capsule of the eye. Cataracts commonly occur bilaterally but progress independently. They can be due to the following:
- Blunt force trauma
- Congenital factors
- Radiation and ultraviolet exposure
- Systemic corticosteroids
- Ocular inflammation

Most cataracts occur due to age-related changes in the lens and are called "senile cataracts." Frequent exposure to ultraviolet light may cause cataracts to occur earlier in life.

Clinical Manifestations

The client presents with a decrease in vision and abnormal colour perception. There may be whitening of the pupil, and the client may complain of halos around lights and a blinding glare from headlights at night. The client also is likely to experience glare and poor vision in bright sunlight.

Diagnostics

Diagnostic testing includes a detailed history and physical examination along with a visual acuity measurement. Ophthalmoscopy, slit lamp microscopy, and glare testing will confirm the diagnosis.

Therapeutics and Nursing Considerations

Nonsurgical treatment includes visual aids to compensate for the decreased ability to see. Surgical treatment consists of removal of the opaque lens and insertion of a prosthetic intraocular lens. The procedure is usually done on an outpatient basis. Postoperatively, the client requires antibiotic and anti-inflammatory eye drops and possibly an eye patch and may be advised against activities that increase intraocular eye pressure.

Glaucoma
Pathophysiology

Glaucoma refers to a group of disorders characterized by abnormally high intraocular pressure (IOP, fluid pressure in the eye), which can damage the optic nerve. Glaucoma occurs in three primary forms: open-angle (primary), acute angle-closure, and secondary to other causes. Risk factors for chronic open-angle glaucoma include genetics, hypertension, diabetes, aging, being of African descent, and severe myopia.

Acute angle-closure glaucoma (also called *narrow-angle glaucoma*) results from obstruction to the outflow of aqueous humour from anatomically narrow angles between the anterior iris and posterior corneal surface. It also results from shallow anterior chambers, a thickened iris that causes angle closure on pupil dilation, or a bulging iris that presses on the trabecular meshwork, closing the angle. Precipitating risk factors for acute angle-closure glaucoma include drug-induced mydriasis (extreme dilation of the pupil) and excitement or stress, which can lead to hypertension.

Secondary glaucoma may result from uveitis, trauma, steroids, diabetes, infections, or surgery.

Diagnostics

Ophthalmoscopic examination will show cupping and atrophy of the optic disc. Diagnostic studies include tonometry measurements of IOP, gonioscopy to examine the angle between the iris and the cornea, and peripheral and central vision tests.

Therapeutics and Nursing Considerations

Chronic open-angle glaucoma can be treated by drug therapy, cyclocryotherapy, argon laser trabeculoplasty, or trabeculectomy. Acute angle-closure glaucoma can be treated with miotics, hyperosmotic solutions, laser peripheral iridotomy, or surgical iridectomy. Secondary glaucoma is managed by treating the underlying problem and with antiglaucoma medications.

It is very important that the client is able to understand and comply with the treatment. The client's ability to react to sight-threatening disorders needs to be assessed. The expected goals of treatment are no progression of vision loss, the client and family understanding the disease process and treatment, the client's adherence to the treatment, and no postoperative complications.

Macular Degeneration
Pathophysiology

Age-related macular degeneration (AMD) is a degeneration of the macula, the central area of the retina, which results in varying degrees of central vision loss. AMD is divided into two classic forms: dry (atrophic), which is the most common, and wet (exudative), which is more severe. AMD is the most common cause of irreversible central vision loss in people over the age of 60.

AMD is related to retinal aging. Risk factors include the following:

- Family history is a major risk factor, and a gene responsible for some cases of AMD has been identified.
- Long-term exposure to ultraviolet light
- Hyperopia (farsightedness)
- Cigarette smoking
- Light-coloured eyes

In dry AMD, the client notices reading and other close vision tasks becoming more difficult. This form starts with the abnormal accumulation of yellowish coloured extracellular deposits called *drusen* in the retinal pigment epithelium. Atrophy and degeneration of macular cells then result, leading to a slowly progressive and painless vision loss.

Wet AMD is characterized by the growth of new blood vessels from their normal location in the choroids to an abnormal location in the retinal epithelium. As the new blood vessels leak, scar tissue gradually forms. Acute vision loss may occur in some cases due to this bleeding.

Clinical Manifestations

Symptoms include blurred and darkened vision, the presence of scotomata (blind spots), or metamorphopsia (distortion of vision).

Diagnostics

Diagnosis is based on the history and physical examination, visual acuity measurements, ophthalmoscopic examinations, an Amsler grid test, fundus photography, and IV fluorescent angiography.

Therapeutics and Nursing Considerations

When visual acuity is compromised, laser photocoagulation of abnormal blood vessels has been the therapy of choice, but it can also destroy the retinal pigment epithelium and photoreceptor cells. Photodynamic therapy is a newer therapy that results in fewer complications.

The permanent loss of central vision associated with AMD has serious psychological implications for nursing care. Uncorrectable vision impairment needs specific care and consideration.

HEALTH CHALLENGES RELATED TO OXYGEN PERFUSION

Hypertension
Pathophysiology

Hypertension refers to an intermittent or sustained elevation in the diastolic or systolic BP. Primary (also known as *essential* or *idiopathic*) hypertension is the most common form. Secondary hypertension results from a number of disorders, such as coarctation of the aorta or renal disease. Malignant hypertension is a severe fulminant form of hypertension.

There is no single cause of hypertension, but there are numerous risk factors, including the following:

- Family history
- Being of African descent
- Males are more at risk than females, but the risk level reverses postmenopause.
- Stress
- Obesity
- High dietary fat and sodium intake
- Cigarette smoking
- Hormonal contraception
- Sedentary lifestyle
- Aging
- DM

Complications of hypertension target the heart, brain, kidneys, and eyes. Individuals with poorly controlled hypertension have an increased risk for developing the following diseases:

- Coronary artery disease, left ventricular hypertrophy, and heart failure
- Cerebrovascular disease and peripheral vascular disease
- Nephrosclerosis
- Retinal damage

Clinical Manifestations

Primary hypertension usually begins insidiously and progresses slowly. If left untreated, even mild cases can lead to major complications. Initially, the client is asymptomatic. As the disease progresses, the client may experience the following symptoms:

- Fatigue and reduced activity tolerance
- Palpitations, angina, and dyspnea
- Epistaxis
- Blurred vision

Diagnostics

Along with the client's history and physical examination, the following tests may identify underlying causes: urinalysis, blood glucose, CBC, lipid profile, BUN and creatinine, electrolyte levels, and ECG.

Therapeutics and Nursing Considerations

Treatment of primary hypertension focuses on lifestyle changes and drug therapy. Secondary hypertension is treated by treating the underlying cause. The goal of therapy is to reduce the overall cardiovascular risk factors and control the BP by the least intrusive means possible. Follow-up monitoring is very important, as is gaining the client's trust to help enhance adherence to therapy. Lifestyle modifications may include the following:

- Dietary changes to low-fat, low-sodium products
- Limitation of alcohol intake and avoidance of tobacco use are important.
- Regular physical exercise and stress management are encouraged.

If lifestyle modifications are not enough or the BP remains high, drug therapy will be initiated. Drug therapy is directed at reduction of systemic vascular resistance (SVR) and a decreased volume of circulating blood. The types of medications used include the following:

- Diuretics
- Adrenergic inhibitors
- Direct vasodilators
- Angiotensin inhibitors
- Calcium channel blockers

See Chapter 7, page 135, for more specific information on antihypertensive drugs. The client will require regular follow-up to monitor BP. Explanation and encouragement are necessary with every visit to encourage adherence to treatment.

In rare situations, a client may go into a hypertensive crisis, in which there is a severe, abrupt elevation in BP. This more commonly affects a client who is not compliant with the treatment. A hypertensive crisis puts the client at risk for developing renal insufficiency, heart failure, pulmonary edema, severe diaphoresis, and, in extreme cases, hypertensive encephalopathy. This is an emergency, and the client requires immediate medical assistance.

Coronary Artery Disease
Pathophysiology

Coronary artery disease (CAD) refers to any narrowing or obstruction of arterial lumina that interferes with cardiac perfusion. Deprived of sufficient blood, the myocardium can develop angina pectoris, infarction, arrhythmias, heart failure, and sudden death. The vessels involved are the right coronary artery, the left coronary artery, and the left anterior descending artery.

The right coronary artery supplies blood to the right atrium, right ventricle, inferior portion of the left ventricle, and posterior walls of the septum. The left coronary artery branches off to form the left circumflex artery, which supplies blood to the left atrium, lateral and posterior walls of the left ventricle, and posterior intraventricular septum. The left anterior descending artery supplies blood to the anterior wall of the left ventricle. The majority of blood passes into the coronary arteries when the heart muscle is at rest (diastole).

Every myocardial cell has four unique properties: automaticity, excitability, conductivity, and contractility. When a blockage occurs in an artery, the cells distal to the blockage will suffer, and these unique properties will be damaged or destroyed. The ejection fraction (EF), the percentage of blood ejected from the ventricle per beat, will be affected when any property is compromised.

Risk factors for the development of CAD include the following:

- Family history
- Obesity
- Smoking
- A high-fat diet
- A sedentary lifestyle
- Stress
- Diabetes
- Hypertension
- Dyslipidemia

Atherosclerosis begins as soft deposits of fat accumulate along the inner wall of an artery. As the atherosclerosis progresses, luminal narrowing is accompanied by vascular changes that impair the diseased vessel's ability to dilate. When oxygen demand exceeds what the diseased vessels can supply, localized myocardial ischemia develops. Transient ischemia can cause angina pectoris, a reversible change that can depress myocardial function. If untreated, actual tissue injury or necrosis (infarction) may result. Oxygen deprivation causes a shift to anaerobic metabolism in the myocardium, resulting in the formation of lactic acid. The accumulation of lactic acid—with a subsequent drop in pH—further impairs cardiac function and results in decreased cardiac output (CO). When occlusion of the coronary arteries occurs over a long period of time, there is a greater chance that collateral circulation will develop. Some clients have an inherited predisposition to developing new vessels.

Angina pectoris has three main forms. Stable angina refers to cardiac pain that is predictable in frequency and duration and can be relieved with rest and nitrates. Unstable angina is unpredictable, with increasing cardiac pain. Prinzmetal's angina is a variant of unpredictable angina that is caused by vasospasm.

MI occurs as a result of sustained ischemia causing irreversible cellular death. The degree of altered function depends on the area of the heart involved and the size of the infarct. Within 24 hours of the infarct, leukocytes infiltrate the area of cell death. Enzymes are released from the dead cells, and proteolytic enzymes of neutrophils and macrophages remove all necrotic tissue by the second or third day. Collateral circulation improves areas of poor perfusion. The necrotic zone can be identified on the ECG and by nuclear scanning. Ten to 14 days following an infarct, scar tissue is developing but is still very weak. By 6 weeks, the scar tissue has replaced the necrotic tissue and the area is said to be healed. Ventricular remodelling is an attempt by the heart to compensate for the infarcted muscle and includes hypertrophy and dilation.

Complications of a MI include the following:
- Arrhythmias
- Heart failure (most common)
- Cardiogenic shock
- Papillary muscle dysfunction
- Ventricular aneurysm
- Pericarditis
- Dressler syndrome, which is pericarditis with effusion and fever that can develop 1–4 weeks post-MI
- Pulmonary embolism

Clinical Manifestations

Clinical manifestations of MI include the following:
- Pain in the chest, neck, jaw, arms, or epigastric region
- Dyspnea
- Nausea and vomiting
- Cool, clammy, pale skin
- Low-grade fever within the first 24 hours
- Initially an increase in BP and heart rate, which may later drop due to decreased CO
- Decreased urine output
- Crackles
- Peripheral edema
- Fear with feelings of impending doom

Recent research has shown that women present differently than men. In women, severe fatigue prior to the MI is the most common complaint. Sleep disturbances, shortness of breath, and anxiety are also symptoms of CAD in women. Women can experience chest discomfort, but they are more likely to express discomfort in the diaphragm, neck, or jaw.

Diagnostics

Diagnosis will be based on the client's history and physical examination. Pain is the chief complaint and can be described as a heavy pressure on the chest, up the neck, along the arms, and in the back or as epigastric discomfort. The cardiac pain usually does not change with respiration or position change. An ECG can show ischemia or an infarct. Laboratory work will show elevation in the following blood work:
- Cardiac enzymes (troponin I and T)
- Creatine kinase (CK)
- Cardiac isoenzyme (CK-MB)

Coronary angiography can reveal coronary stenosis or obstruction. A stress ECG may provoke chest pain and signs of myocardial ischemia.

Therapeutics and Nursing Considerations

Treatment for angina consists of the following considerations:
- Rest to decrease the oxygen demand
- Nitrates
- Acetylsalicylic acid (ASA)
- Possible stent placement
- With some clients with angina, beta blockers or calcium channel blockers may be needed.

Invasive interventions may include percutaneous coronary interventions, atherectomy, laser angioplasty and myocardial revascularization with coronary artery bypass graft (CABG), or minimally invasive direct coronary artery bypass grafting (MIDCABG). The same management may be used for treating a client with an infarct, with the addition of thrombolytics to dissolve the clot and allow blood to pass. The main complications following thrombolytic therapy are bleeding arrhythmias and reocclusion. Medications used in the acute management of an infarct include the following:
- Oxygen
- Nitrates
- Morphine
- Antiarrhythmic drugs
- Beta-adrenergic blockers
- Angiotensin-converting enzyme inhibitors
- Stool softeners may also be used.

Once the acute phase has ended, the client will need cardiac rehabilitation to help him or her return to as normal a lifestyle as possible. This rehabilitation includes physical, emotional, and psychological assistance.

Sudden Cardiac Death

Sudden cardiac death is unexpected death from cardiac causes. There is a disruption in cardiac function causing an abrupt loss of cerebral blood flow. Death usually occurs within an hour of the onset of symptoms and is mostly caused by ventricular arrhythmia.

Dysrhythmias
Pathophysiology

The normal electrical pattern of the heart begins at the sinoatrial (SA) node, which is considered the pacemaker of the heart. It is found in the right atrium and usually sets a rate of 60–100 beats per minute (bpm). The electrical signal spreads through the atria and then travels to the atrioventricular (AV) node, where it is held for a short period of time to allow the atria to contract. If there is interference with the SA electrical impulse, the secondary pacemaker nodes (AV and Purkinje fibres) will automatically activate to keep the heart contracting. The AV node is normally the only avenue of connection with the ventricles. If an impulse starts at the AV node, the rate is usually around 40–60 bpm. The impulse then travels down the bundle of His and spreads to the ventricles via the Purkinje fibres. Once all cells in the ventricle are stimulated, the ventricles contract. If the impulse is formed in the ventricle, the normal rate is around 20–40 bpm.

A dysrhythmia is an abnormal heartbeat. It is very important to assess how this abnormal rhythm is affecting the CO.

The ECG is a display of electrical activity of the heart. The ECG can detect rate, rhythm, and conduction abnormalities; left ventricular hypertrophy; electrolyte imbalance; and digoxin (Lanoxin) toxicity.

The ECG also shows the voltage and duration of waves. The voltage gives information regarding the thickness of the chamber walls, and the duration gives information about the formation and conduction.

The action potential is the impulse generated by the movement of ions across a cell membrane. A cell is resting in a polarized state. A change in the electrical charge across the membrane causes an action potential, or cell depolarization. Once the heart is completely depolarized, it will attempt to return to its resting state via cell repolarization. The cycle of depolarizing and repolarizing includes the following five phases:

- Phase 0—The cell receives the impulse and is depolarized. Sodium moves rapidly into the cell, and calcium moves slowly into the cell.
- Phase 1—Early or rapid repolarization occurs, and the sodium channel closes.
- Phase 2—A plateau phase, slow repolarization occurs. Calcium is still slowly moving into the cell, and now potassium flows out of the cell.
- Phase 3—Rapid repolarization returns as the calcium channels are closed, and potassium flows out of the cell rapidly.
- Phase 4—The resting phase, active transport through the sodium–potassium pump returns potassium to the inside of the cell and sodium to the outside of the cell. The cell is now impermeable to sodium. Potassium can still move out of the cell. This is the end of the cycle, and the cell is ready for a new impulse. Cardiac action potential is shown in Fig. 8.9.

Refractory periods refer to the stage of resistance to stimulation. In the absolute refractory period, no depolarization can occur. In the relative refractory period, a strong stimulus is needed to initiate an impulse. In the supernormal refractory period, only a mild stimulus is needed to initiate an impulse. Many dysrhythmias are triggered in the relative and supernormal refractory periods, with the T wave being the most vulnerable.

Antidysrhythmic drugs are classified according to the phase they affect. The classes of antidysrhythmic drugs are as follows:

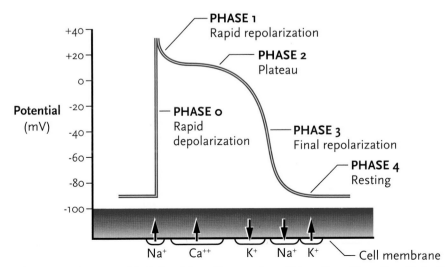

Fig. 8.9 Cardiac action potential. Ca^{++}, calcium; K^{+}, potassium; Na^{+}, sodium. (From Day, R. A., Paul, P., Williams, B., et al. [2016]. *Brunner & Suddarth's textbook of medical-surgical nursing* [3rd Cdn. ed., p. 721, Figure 27-4]. Philadelphia: Lippincott, Williams & Wilkins. Reprinted with permission.)

- Class I drugs block the influx of sodium into the cell in phase 0. These are sodium channel blockers.
- Class II drugs block the beta-receptors; therefore, they block the SNS, depress depolarization, slow the SA node impulses, and increase the AV nodal refractory period. They are considered general myocardial depressants.
- Class III drugs block the potassium movement in phase 3, thereby prolonging the repolarization and refractory periods.
- Class IV drugs block calcium in phase 2 and so are calcium channel blockers or slow channel blockers. They act to prolong conductivity and increase the refractory period and time at the AV node.

Other medications do not fit into these classifications and are as follows:

- Adenosine (Adenocard) decreases conduction at the AV node.
- Atropine sulfate is an anticholinergic that blocks the vagal effect on the SA and AV nodes, thereby increasing the heart rate.
- Digoxin (Lanoxin) is an inotropic medication that strengthens the myocardial contraction and slows conduction at the AV node.
- Epinephrine (Adrenalin) acts on alpha- and beta-adrenergic receptor sites of the SNS, helping to restore normal sinus rhythm in a cardiac arrest.
- Magnesium sulfate decreases excitability and conduction.

Dysrhythmias are triggered by internal forces such as acid–base imbalances, electrolyte imbalances, and hypoxia and by external forces such as illness, medication, and stress. Dysrhythmias are characterized by an alteration in impulse formation affecting the rate, rhythm, and development of entopic beats (those outside the normal pathway) or by alterations in conductivity, where failure or delay of impulse transmission may occur. The rhythms are classified according to the site of impulse formation and the degree of conduction block.

Sinus bradycardia is a slow sinus rhythm with a rate below 60 bpm. This rhythm can be normal in trained athletes. It becomes significant when CO is decreased and hypotension develops. Sinus bradycardia can predispose a client with an acute MI to develop escape arrhythmias and premature ectopic beats. If the bradycardia is compromising the CO, it can be treated with atropine.

Sinus tachycardia is a sinus rhythm with a rate over 100 bpm. It can cause dizziness and hypotension. The increased rate increases the oxygen consumption of the heart. It can create angina and extend the size of an infarct. Treatment depends on determining the underlying cause. Beta-adrenergic blockers are used to decrease heart rate and oxygen consumption.

Atrial flutter is an atrial tachyarrhythmia identified by recurring, regular, sawtooth-shaped flutter waves. It is usually associated with slower ventricular responses and is significant only when the ventricular response is elevated. There is a risk of clot formation with this rhythm. Treatment focuses on slowing the ventricular response by increasing the AV block.

The client may require electrical cardioversion. Diltiazem (Cardizem), digoxin (Lanoxin), and beta blockers may be used. Anticoagulant therapy is needed to prevent the formation of clots.

Atrial fibrillation (AF) is the total disorganization of atrial activity without effective atrial contraction. It may be chronic or intermittent, can result in decreased CO, and carries a risk for stroke. AF is sometimes found in clients experiencing heart failure. Treatment is the same as for atrial flutter.

Premature ventricular contractions (PVCs) are contractions originating in an ectopic focus in the ventricles. Ventricular tachycardia is a run of three or more PVCs. It is considered life-threatening because of decreased CO and the possibility of deterioration to ventricular fibrillation. Ventricular fibrillation is a severe derangement of the heart rhythm. This is an emergency, and the client needs cardiopulmonary resuscitation (CPR) and advanced cardiac life support (ACLS) with drug therapy and defibrillation.

Defibrillation is the most effective method of terminating ventricular fibrillation. Ideally, it is performed 15–20 seconds after the onset of the arrhythmia. It involves the passage of a direct current of electricity through the heart to depolarize all cells with the intent of allowing the SA node to resume its normal role. A pacemaker is a pulse generator that provides electrical stimulus to a heart that cannot conduct its own impulse in order to supply adequate CO. It can be used for transient or permanent conduction defects.

Heart Failure

Pathophysiology

Heart failure (HF) is an abnormal condition involving impaired cardiac pumping. It is not a disease but a syndrome. HF is often associated with long-standing hypertension and CAD. HF occurs when the heart is no longer able to pump an adequate amount of blood to meet the metabolic needs of the client. It is the most common reason for hospitalization in adults over age 65 years.

Risk factors for developing HF include the following:

- CAD
- Advanced age
- Hypertension
- Obesity
- Cigarette smoking
- DM
- High cholesterol
- Being of African descent

Conditions that can precipitate or exacerbate HF include the following:

- Stress
- Dysrhythmias
- Infection
- Anemia
- Thyroid disorders
- Pregnancy
- Paget's disease
- Nutritional deficiency of B vitamins

- Pulmonary disease
- Hypervolemia

HF may be caused by any interference with normal mechanisms regulating cardiac output. CO depends on preload, afterload, myocardial contractility, heart rate, and metabolic rate.

Systolic failure is the most common cause of HF. The left ventricle loses its ability to generate enough pressure to eject blood into the body. The hallmark of systolic failure is a decrease in the left ventricular ejection fraction.

Diastolic failure is the impaired ability of the ventricles to fill during diastole and usually is the result of left ventricular hypertrophy. Pulmonary congestion results from diastolic failure, and there will be a normal ejection fraction until systolic failure develops.

There can also be mixed systolic and diastolic failure, as seen in dilated cardiomyopathy. This is known as *biventricular failure*. The ejection fraction in this case is extremely poor.

The four basic factors that cause HF are as follows:
- An increase in the volume of blood to be pumped
- An increase in the resistance against which the blood must be pumped
- A decrease in contractility
- A decrease in the filling of the cardiac chambers

Cardiac reserve refers to the heart's ability to increase CO in response to stress. A failing heart has limited ability to respond to increased demand.

There are three cardiac compensatory mechanisms: tachycardia, ventricular dilation, and ventricular hypertrophy. Systemic compensatory mechanisms involve the SNS, kidneys, and liver.

Clinical Manifestations

Clinical manifestations of HF depend on the specific ventricle involved, precipitating causes of the failure, the duration of the failure, and any underlying condition the client may have. One-sided failure eventually leads to biventricular failure.

Left-sided (left ventricular) heart failure is the most common classification of HF. With this type of HF, blood backs up through the left atrium into the pulmonary veins, causing congestion and edema. Hypertension is the most common cause of left-sided HF, followed by cardiomyopathies, rheumatic heart disease, and CAD.

Right-sided (right ventricular) heart failure results in the backward flow of blood to the right atrium and venous circulation, which creates venous congestion, peripheral edema, hepatomegaly, splenomegaly, and jugular venous distension. The primary cause of right-sided HF is cor pulmonale.

Complications of HF are pleural effusions, arrhythmias, left ventricular thrombus, and hepatomegaly.

Classifications of HF are based on the person's tolerance to physical activity. Classifications are as follows:
- Class 1 is no limitation of physical ability.
- Class 2 is slight limitation to physical ability.
- Class 3 is a marked limitation.
- Class 4 is the inability to carry on any physical activity without discomfort.

Manifestations of acute HF include the following symptoms:
- Agitation
- Pale and cyanotic skin, and cold and clammy extremities
- Severe dyspnea and tachypnea

If untreated, the client may develop pulmonary edema. Chronic symptoms of HF include the following:
- Fatigue
- Dyspnea, orthopnea, and cough
- Tachycardia, pulse alterans, and AF
- Edema and nocturia
- Restlessness and confusion
- Chest pain
- Weight changes
- Skin with a dusky appearance
- Heart enlargement
- Cheyne-Stokes respirations

Death usually results from asphyxiation, pulmonary acidosis, shock, or dysrhythmias.

Diagnostics

Diagnostic studies are done to determine the underlying cause and extent of present failure, and they include the history and physical examination of the client. Chest X-ray, ECG, electrolytes, liver function tests, CBC, BUN and creatinine, and cardiac enzyme tests are performed. An echocardiogram with measurement of the ejection fraction may be done, along with stress testing and cardiac catheterization.

Therapeutics and Nursing Considerations

Treatment is focused on the following:
- Decreasing intravascular volume
- Decreasing venous return
- Decreasing the afterload
- Improving the gas exchange and oxygenation
- Improving cardiac function
- Reducing anxiety

Drugs that are frequently prescribed for HF include diuretics, beta blockers, nitrates, calcium channel blockers, and angiotensin-converting enzyme inhibitors.

The client will be encouraged to be in a high Fowler's position with the legs down to help decrease blood return to the heart. Oxygen therapy is usually needed as the condition deteriorates. Symptom management is important. Teaching regarding the activity–exercise balance, nutrition with a low-sodium diet, medications, support systems, and possible psychological changes will be helpful for the client with HF.

Abdominal Aortic Aneurysm
Pathophysiology

An abdominal aortic aneurysm is an abnormal dilation in an arterial wall, commonly in the aorta between the renal arteries and iliac branches. Aneurysms commonly result from atherosclerosis, which weakens the aortic wall and gradually distends the lumen. Other causes include fungal infections, congenital disorders, trauma, syphilis, and hypertension.

Degenerative changes in the tunica media create a focal weakness, allowing the tunica intima and tunica adventitia to stretch outward. BP within the aorta progressively weakens the vessel walls and enlarges the aneurysm.

The most serious complication of an aneurysm is rupture. If it is a posterior rupture into the retroperitoneal space, bleeding may tamponade by surrounding structures, preventing exsanguination. If the rupture occurs anteriorly into the abdominal cavity, mortality is very high due to uncontained massive hemorrhage.

Clinical Manifestations

Clients are often asymptomatic. On physical examination, a pulsating mass is found in the periumbilical area. There may be a systolic bruit over the aorta, and the client may experience tenderness on deep palpation. Lumbar pain that radiates to the flank and groin can occur. If the aneurysm ruptures, there is severe, persistent, abdominal and back pain, often mimicking renal colic. Tachycardia, profuse diaphoreses, and hypotension can occur.

Diagnostics

Diagnosis is made by history and physical examination, chest X-ray, echocardiography, ECG, CT scan, and MRI.

Therapeutics and Nursing Considerations

The goal of management is to prevent rupture of the aneurysm. Early detection and prompt treatment are imperative. The aneurysm will be surgically removed and replaced with a Dacron graft. If the aneurysm is small and the client is asymptomatic, surgery may be delayed. Endovascular grafting may be used to repair an abdominal aneurysm. This is a minimally invasive procedure, in which a catheter with an attached graft is inserted through the femoral or iliac artery and advanced over a guide wire into the aorta. The graft is then positioned across the aneurysm. A balloon on the catheter expands, affixing the graft to the vessel wall.

Peripheral Vascular Diseases
Pathophysiology

Peripheral vascular disease (PVD) is an imbalance between the supply and demand of blood and nutrients that results from the degeneration of the peripheral vascular system. PVD includes arterial insufficiency and occlusion and venous insufficiency and occlusion.

Peripheral arterial diseases (PADs) can affect any artery but tend to affect the aorta, iliac, femoral, popliteal, tibial, and peritoneal arteries. Risk factors for developing PAD include the following:

- Increasing age, smoking, diabetes, obesity, sedentary lifestyle, and stress
- Heredity
- Male gender
- Hyperhomocysteinemia
- CVD

There are two forms of PAD: organic and functional. Organic disease is caused by structural damage to the blood vessel with plaque or inflammation blocking blood flow. Functional disease is a reversible disturbance in the SNS. The vasospasm of Raynaud's disease is an example of functional disease.

Clinical Manifestations

The classic symptom of organic PAD is intermittent claudication, in which ischemic muscle ache or pain is precipitated by a constant level of exercise. The pain usually resolves within 10 minutes or less of rest. The pain is reproducible. Other manifestations may be as follows:

- Paraesthesia
- Thin, shiny, and taut skin on lower legs
- Loss of hair on lower legs
- Diminished or absent pedal, popliteal, or femoral pulses
- Pallor
- Reactive hyperemia
  Complications of PAD include the following:
- Atrophy of the skin and underlying muscles
- Delayed wound healing
- Wound infections
- Tissue necrosis
- Arterial ulcers

Diagnostics

Diagnostic studies include Doppler ultrasonography, ankle–brachial index, duplex imaging, angiogram, or magnetic resonance angiography.

Therapeutics and Nursing Considerations

Treatment focuses on preventing further damage to the vessel. The client is encouraged to do the following:

- Stop smoking
- Treat the dyslipidemia, hypertension, and diabetes
- Exercise, as this improves oxygen delivery to the legs
  Pharmacological therapy may include the following:
- ASA (Aspirin)
- Ticlopidine (Ticlid)
- Clopidogrel (Plavix)
- Pentoxifylline (Trental) or cilostazol (Pletal) may be prescribed for intermittent claudication.

If PAD progresses and the intermittent claudication becomes incapacitating, the client has pain at rest, or ulceration and gangrene develop, surgical intervention will be needed.

A percutaneous transluminal balloon angioplasty could be done. The most common surgical procedure is a peripheral arterial bypass operation with autogenous vein or synthetic graft material to bypass the lesion.

An endarterectomy may need a patch graft. A sympathectomy may be done. When gangrene is present, amputation is needed.

Peripheral Venous Disease
Pathophysiology

The most common peripheral disorder of the veins is venous thrombus, which is the formation of a clot in association with inflammation of the vein. Three important factors, known as

Virchow's triad, are involved in the etiology of the clot formation. These factors are venous stasis, damage to the endothelium lining, and hypercoagulability of the blood. Some of the risk factors for developing either superficial or DVT include the following:

- Major abdominal surgery
- Pelvic or orthopaedic surgery
- Oral contraceptives and hormone replacement therapy
- Obesity
- Pregnancy
- Heart disease
- Advanced cancer
- Coagulation disorders

Blood cells, platelets, and fibrin accumulate together to form the thrombus. A common site of clot formation is the cusps of the veins. An enlarged clot may occlude the lumen of the vein. Emboli can break away from the clot and lodge anywhere else in the body. The most serious complications of venous problems include pulmonary emboli and phlegmasia cerulea dolens (swollen, blue, painful legs).

Varicose veins are dilated tortuous subcutaneous veins that usually affect the saphenous system. Risk factors for developing varicosities include the following:

- Congenital defective valves
- Prolonged standing
- Obesity
- Systemic conditions such as pregnancy, ascites, heart disease, and abdominal masses

Clinical Manifestations

Clients with superficial thrombophlebitis may present with the following:

- A palpable, firm, cordlike vein
- Surrounding area may be red and tender and warm to touch
- A slight fever

Many clients with a DVT are asymptomatic. Those clients who are symptomatic experience the following:

- Unilateral leg edema
- Pain
- Warm, red skin

Varicosities present as prominent, superficial, discoloured, tortuous veins. The client usually complains of the following:

- A dull ache or heaviness
- Fatigue
- Leg cramps and edema
- Some varicosities have nodular protrusions.

Diagnostics

Diagnoses can be made from the client's history and physical examination, blood work such as platelet count, bleeding time and international normalized ratio (INR), venous Doppler evaluation, duplex scanning, and venogram.

Therapeutics and Nursing Considerations

Treatment of superficial thrombophlebitis involves elevating the affected limb and applying warm moist heat to the area.

ASA and acetaminophen may be used to relieve discomfort. NSAIDs may be used to treat the inflammation.

To prevent DVT development, early mobilization following surgery is encouraged. If the client is to remain in bed, frequent position changes are encouraged, as well as dorsiflexing the feet and rotating the ankles. Preventive measures such as compression stockings or support hose should be employed.

People with venous disorders should be encouraged not to cross their legs or ankles, not to stand in one place for long periods of time, and not to wear constrictive clothing.

If a DVT does develop, the client is usually started on anticoagulants to prevent the growth of the present clot and the development of any new clots. Unfractionated heparin, low-molecular-weight heparin, and warfarin (Coumadin) derivatives are the most commonly used anticoagulants. Coumadin requires 48–72 hours to have an effect on the PT; therefore, Coumadin is started before the heparin infusion is completed. A venous thrombectomy or insertion of a vena cava interruption device may be done to prevent pulmonary emboli. The client usually remains on prophylactic Coumadin.

Varicose vein management involves education concerning prevention, including lifestyle modifications, exercise, use of support hose, not standing for long periods, and reducing obesity. Surgical therapy for varicose veins may include sclerotherapy, ligation and stripping, or laser therapy for smaller varicosities.

CRITICAL HEALTH CHALLENGES

Burns
Pathophysiology

Burns occur when there is injury to the tissue of the body caused by heat, chemicals, electrical current, or radiation and can lead to many local and systemic problems. Burns are classified according to the depth, extent, and location of the burn, as well as the client's own risk factors. The depth of the burn is now categorized as a partial- or full-thickness burn, as follows:

- A superficial partial-thickness burn involves the epidermis.
- A deep partial-thickness burn involves the dermis.
- A full-thickness burn involves, fat, muscle, and bone.

The location of the burn is related to the severity of the injury. Face, neck, and chest burns can result in respiratory complications. Circumferential burns of the extremities can cause circulatory problems and compartment syndrome. Older clients or clients who have pre-existing cardiovascular conditions, respiratory conditions, renal disease, diabetes, alcoholism, a history of drug use, or malnutrition are slower at healing from a burn.

Clinical Manifestations

Manifestations of burns are as follows:

- Shock
- Blisters
- Dynamic ileus

- Shivering
- Altered mental status
  Many complications can result from burns:
- Cardiovascular complications include arrhythmias, hypovolemic shock, edema, ischemia, necrosis, gangrene, and increased blood viscosity.
- Respiratory complications can be mechanical obstruction and asphyxia, interstitial edema, pneumonia, and pulmonary edema.
- Renal complications because of acute tubular necrosis can result in kidney damage.
- GI changes that can occur from burns include impairment of gastric mucosal integrity and motility. Paralytic ileus may develop. Abdominal distension can occur, and curling ulcer (acute ulcerative gastroduodenal disease) can develop.

Metabolic complications can include hypermetabolism, increasing body temperature, and increasing catabolic rates.

Skin complications occur due to the burn injury's disruption of the protective barrier of the skin, which increases the risk of infection.

Therapeutics and Nursing Considerations

Care begins at the time of the burn. The client must first be removed from the source of the burn. For smaller burns, cover the burn with a clean, cool, tap water–dampened towel. For larger burns, remove burned clothing and wrap the client in a clean sheet, without using any cool water or ice.

Emergent phase. The emergent (resuscitative) phase is from the onset to two to five or more days following the burn. In the first 24–48 hours, the client will lose fluid and form edema until fluid mobilization and diuresis occur. At this time, the client is at risk for the following complications:
- Hypovolemic shock
- Edema, decreased BP, and increased pulse
- Increased insensible water loss
- Thrombosis
- Potassium and sodium shifts
- The immune system is compromised.

Initial management focuses on survival. Goals of management include the following:
- Securing the airway
- Supporting circulation by fluid replacement
- Keeping the client as comfortable as possible with analgesics
- Preventing infection
- Maintaining body temperature
- Providing emotional support
- Airway management
- Fluid management

Wound care is delayed until a patent airway, adequate circulation, and adequate fluid replacement have been established. When time permits, the wound should be cleansed by using a hydrotherapy tub, shower, or bed. Debridement is the removal of loose, necrotic skin and may require sedation. An open wound is covered with a topical antibiotic without a dressing. When dressings are used, they should be in the form of sterile gauze laid over the topical antibiotic. Dressings are changed two to three times per day initially and then less often as the wound heals.

Be aware of the following:
- Allograft or homograft skin grafts are commonly used, but they are often rejected by the client's body.
- Routine blood work is important to monitor for electrolyte imbalance and homeostasis.
- Early ROM exercises help prevent contractures.
- Analgesics and sedatives are given, as well as a tetanus immunization.
- Antimicrobial agents, both topical and systemic, are used.
- Fluid replacement takes priority over nutritional requirements. Oral intake can be started once the bowel sounds return. Due to the increased metabolic state, the client will need high-calorie meals with vitamin and mineral supplements.

Acute phase. The acute phase begins with the mobilization of ECF and subsequent diuresis and ends when the burned area is completely covered by skin grafts or when the wounds are healed. Necrotic tissue will begin to slough off, and granulation tissue will form. A partial-thickness wound will heal from the edges. Full-thickness wounds must be covered by skin grafts. Partial-thickness wounds form eschar initially, and then epithelialization begins once the eschar is removed. Full-thickness wounds require debridement. The interventions required are as follows:
- Wound care in the acute phase includes daily observation, cleansing, and debridement.
- Appropriate coverage of the graft is needed. A fine mesh gauze is placed on the graft, followed by a middle and outer dressing. Sheet skin grafts must be kept free of blebs. Eschar is removed down to the subcutaneous tissue of fascia. Cultured epithelial autographs, grown from biopsies of the client's own skin, or artificial grafts may be used.
- Analgesics and sedation are needed.
- Passive and active ROM exercises should be performed.
- Splints help prevent deformities.
- A high-protein, high-carbohydrate diet helps meet the client's increased metabolic needs.

Rehabilitation phase. The rehabilitation phase begins when the client's burn wounds are covered with skin or healed, and the client is able to resume a level of self-care activity. The burn wound will heal either by primary intention or by grafting. Layers of epithelialization begin rebuilding the tissue structure. Collagen fibres add strength to weakened areas. In about 4–6 weeks, the burn area becomes raised and hyperemic. Mature healing is reached in 6 months to 2 years. The skin will never completely regain its original colour. The following are nursing considerations:
- Skin and joint contractures are the most common complication in the rehabilitation phase.
- Both the client and the family become active learners regarding wound care.
- An emollient water-based cream is recommended.
- Cosmetic surgery may be needed.

- The client will require constant encouragement and reassurances. The family will need to understand the importance of re-establishing the client's independence while participating in client care. It is important to assess for psychoemotional cues and understand that psychiatric intervention may be needed.

Shock
Pathophysiology
Shock is a syndrome characterized by decreased tissue perfusion and impaired cellular metabolism. Cardiogenic shock or low-blood-flow shock involves systolic and diastolic dysfunction and compromised CO. The causes are as follows:
- MI, cardiomyopathies, and blunt cardiac injury
- Severe systemic or pulmonary hypertension
- Severe sepsis can cause cardiogenic shock.

Diastolic dysfunction results from the impaired ability of the ventricle to fill during diastole and a decrease in stroke volume. Early signs of cardiogenic shock include the following:
- Tachycardia
- Hypotension and narrowed pulse pressure
- Increased SVR
- Increased myocardial oxygen consumption, tachypnea, pulmonary congestion, and crackles
- Since the CO is low, renal blood flow and urine output decrease.
- Lack of oxygen to the tissues can result in anxiety.

Hypovolemic shock. Hypovolemic shock is loss of intravascular fluid, either an absolute or relative volume loss. Absolute hypovolemia can be due to the following:
- Hemorrhage
- GI loss
- Fistula drainage
- Diuresis

Relative hypovolemia occurs when fluid moves out of the intravascular space into an extravascular space (third spacing). With hypovolemic shock, the size of the vascular compartment is unchanged, and there is a decreased venous return to the heart, decreased preload, and decreased CO, which results in impaired cellular metabolism. If the loss of blood is more than 30% of total volume, blood replacement is needed.

Neurogenic shock. Neurogenic shock occurs after SCI, at T5 or above. Neurogenic shock results in massive vasodilation, leading to pooling of blood in the vessels. Clinical signs include hypotension and bradycardia. Hypothalamic dysfunction is characteristic, with temperature dysregulation.

Spinal shock. Spinal shock is manifested by decreased reflexes, loss of sensation, and flaccid paralysis below the level of injury. These symptoms may last days to months and may mask postneurological function. Once spinal shock has been resolved in clients with spinal injuries at T6 or higher, return of the reflexes may trigger the development of autonomic dysreflexia, which is a massive uncompensated cardiovascular reaction mediated by the SNS. Autonomic dysreflexia is life-threatening and usually occurs in response to visceral stimulation once the spinal shock is resolved. A distended bladder or rectum is the most common precipitating cause of autonomic dysreflexia. Manifestations of autonomic dysreflexia include extreme hypertension, blurred vision, throbbing headache, marked diaphoresis, piloerection, flushed skin, nasal congestion, nausea, and anxiety (Lewis et al., 2019).

Anaphylactic shock. Anaphylactic shock is an acute life-threatening hypersensitivity reaction that causes massive vasodilation, increased capillary permeability, and release of mediators. This can lead to respiratory distress and circulatory failure. Sudden symptoms are anxiety, confusion, and a sense of impending doom.

Septic shock. Septic shock is a systemic inflammatory response to infection. It is the leading cause of death in noncoronary Critical Care Units (CCUs). The primary causative agents are Gram-negative and Gram-positive bacteria. With septic shock, there is increased coagulation and inflammation. The decreased fibrinolysis results in the formation of microthrombi that can obstruct microvasculature. SVR will decrease, leading to hypotension. The client will be tachypneic and have temperature dysregulation, decreased urinary output, altered neurological status, GI dysfunction, and respiratory failure (Lewis et al., 2019).

Clinical Manifestations
Initial stage of shock. The initial stage of shock may not be clinically apparent. Metabolism changes from aerobic to anaerobic with lactic acid accumulation. Lactic acid must be removed by the blood and broken down in the liver, which requires oxygen that is not available.

Compensatory stage. During the compensatory stage, the body attempts to re-establish homeostasis. Baroreceptors in the carotid and aortic bodies activate SNS in response to the decreased BP. The following actions happen as listed:
- Peripheral vasoconstriction occurs to maintain blood to the visceral organs. The client's extremities will be cool and clammy. However, the septic client will be warm and flushed.
- The decreased renal blood flow activates the renin–angiotensin system in an attempt to increase venous return to the heart and increase CO and BP.
- The impaired GI motility can lead to paralytic ileus.
- The decreased arterial oxygen levels cause increased respirations. SNS stimulation increases myocardial oxygen demand.

Progressive stage. If the perfusion deficit is corrected, the client will recover with no residual sequelae; if the deficit is not corrected, the client enters the progressive stage, which begins when the compensatory mechanisms fail.

Aggressive intervention is needed to prevent multiorgan dysfunction syndrome. Decreased cellular perfusion and altered capillary permeability are hallmarks for the progressive stage of shock.

Refractory stage. The refractory stage involves the exacerbation of anaerobic metabolism, accumulation of lactic acid, and increased capillary permeability. The client may be hypotensive and tachycardic and may experience both cardiac and cerebral ischemia, as well as hypoxia. In the refractory stage, failure of one organ will affect the other organs. Recovery at this stage is unlikely.

Diagnostics

There is no single diagnostic test to determine shock. Integration of the physical examination and medical history is key.

Therapeutics and Nursing Considerations

Treatment focuses on interventions to control or eliminate the cause of decreased perfusion and to protect the organs from dysfunction. Multisystem care is needed, including the following:

- Ensuring a patent airway and optimizing oxygen delivery
- Possible blood transfusions or other fluid replacement therapy
- An in-dwelling catheter allows for frequent checks of output.
- Vital signs and ABGs must be monitored frequently.
- Vasopressor agents may be given for hypotension.
- Vasodilators may be given.
- Cardiac monitoring may be done.
- A pulmonary catheter may be used to monitor venous pressures.
- Chest and bowel sounds should be assessed frequently.

The goals of treatment are to provide adequate tissue perfusion, to restore normal BP, to recover organ function, and to have no complications.

Treatment for life-threatening autonomic dysreflexia includes the following:

- Raising the head of the bed to 45 degrees
- Immediate urinary catheterization if the bladder is distended
- A digital rectal examination with topical anaesthesia may be needed if the client is constipated.
- Constrictive clothing and tight shoes need to be removed to prevent excessive skin stimulation.
- BP must be closely monitored and treated with an alpha-adrenergic blocker or an arteriolar vasodilator (Lewis et al., 2019).

CONCEPTS IN NURSING PRACTICE

Preoperative Care

Surgery can be described as the art and science of treating diseases, injuries, and deformities by operation and instrumentation. Surgery can be performed for purposes of diagnosis, cure, palliation, prevention, exploration, and cosmetic improvement. A surgery may be a planned event (elective surgery) or arise unexpectedly (emergency surgery).

Part of preoperative care includes interviewing the surgical client. The purpose of this interview is to obtain health information, determine client expectations, provide and clarify information about the surgery, and assess the emotional state and readiness of the client. During the interview and any other interactions, the use of a common language is important; therefore, translators may be needed.

Preoperative care also includes nursing assessment of the client undergoing surgery. The goals of the nursing assessment should include the following:

- Determining the client's psychological status in order to reinforce coping strategies
- Determining any psychological factors of the procedure that may contribute to risks
- Establishing baseline data
- Identifying medications and herbs taken that may affect surgical outcomes
- Identifying, documenting, and communicating results of laboratory and diagnostic tests
- Identifying cultural and ethnic factors that may affect the surgical experience
- Determining whether the client has signed the informed consent for surgery

Psychosocial assessment is important as a magnified stress response can affect recovery. During this assessment, the practical nurse can identify any emotional reactions to hospitalization, allay anxieties or fears, assess coping mechanisms, and help restore self-esteem. The nursing assessment includes obtaining information on the following:

- The client's health history
- Medical conditions
- Previous surgeries
- Menstrual and obstetric history
- Familial diseases
- Reaction to anaesthesia
- Current prescribed medications and over-the-counter medications
- Herbs or homeopathic preparations used
- Vitamins
- Recreational drugs
- Alcohol
- Tobacco
- Allergies

There are different methods of performing the physical assessment; however, they should contain a review of the systems of the body: the cardiovascular, respiratory, nervous, urinary, GI, integumentary, musculo-skeletal, endocrine, and immune systems. Other assessments include fluid and electrolyte status and nutritional status.

Preoperative teaching is very important. The client has the right to know what to expect during and after surgery. By having this knowledge, the client will have decreased anxiety and an increased sense of control. Instruction on postoperative deep breathing, coughing, and ambulation, and giving the client the rationale for these actions, increases the client's success and adherence in performing them. Methods of pain control should be discussed. The client and family should be informed about any tubes, drains, monitoring devices, or special equipment that might be present postoperatively. This knowledge will decrease client and family fears and anxiety. Information should be provided to the client and the family about fluid or food restrictions, the need for certain treatments prior to surgery, the need for a shower prior to surgery, and the need to remove jewellery and prosthetics prior to surgery.

Legal preparation is important. Ensure that all forms have been correctly signed and witnessed. These forms could include the informed consent form, a blood refusal form, if needed, an advance directive, a living will, and a power of attorney. With voluntary consent, the client must have a clear understanding and comprehension of what is going to happen prior to signing the consent form. An anaesthesiologist will assess the client for anaesthetic risk and discuss the type of anaesthetic that will be used. The surgeon is responsible for obtaining the client's consent on the agency consent form after the surgical procedure and risks have been clearly explained. The practical nurse may witness the signature if required. The client has the right to withdraw consent at any time. Legally appointed representatives of the family may give consent if the client is a child, unconscious, or mentally incompetent. Medical emergencies may override the need for consent. If no next of kin is available, the surgeon may document the necessity of the surgery.

On the day of surgery, the following nursing interventions are essential for any type of surgery:
- Preoperative teaching should be reinforced.
- Consent should be verified.
- Preoperative charting should be complete.
- Clients cannot wear any cosmetics.
- Dentures should be removed.
- Correct client identification and allergy bands must be in place.
- Valuables are given to the family or locked in a safe.
- The client is encouraged to void prior to surgery.

Intraoperative Care

The surgical suite is a controlled environment designed to minimize the spread of infection and to allow for the smooth flow of clients, personnel, and instruments or equipment. The operating room is geographically, environmentally, and bacteriologically controlled.

The basic surgical team includes the perioperative nurse, the circulating nurse, the scrub nurse, the surgeon, and the anaesthetist. The perioperative nurse ensures that the client is fully prepared for the surgery. The circulating nurse is not scrubbed, gowned, or gloved. The circulating nurse assists the scrub nurse with the surgical count, provides supplies as needed to the scrub team, assists the anaesthesiologist as needed, and documents the procedure. The scrub nurse follows a designated scrub procedure, participates in the surgical count, monitors blood loss and medications used during surgery, requests sterile supplies as needed, passes instruments and implements to the surgeon, and remains within the sterile field. Practical nurses with advanced training perform the scrubbing function in many Canadian institutions. The surgeon is the physician who performs the procedure. The anaesthesiologist administers the anaesthesia, maintains the client's physiological homeostasis, and monitors his or her physical status throughout the surgery.

Proper positioning of the client is important to provide accessibility of the operative site and for the administration of anaesthetic agents, the maintenance of the airway, and the correct skeletal alignment. The client should be protected from pressure on nerves and skin over bony prominences. The eyes should be protected. Adequate thoracic excursion should be provided. Arteries and veins should not be occluded. Modesty in exposure of the body should be respected. Any painful area or deformity should be recognized and respected. Client safety is a priority.

Anaesthetics are classified as general, local, conscious sedation, and regional. General anaesthetics provide loss of sensation with loss of consciousness, skeletal muscle relaxation, and analgesia. General anaesthetics can affect somatic, autonomic, and endocrine responses. General anaesthetics are usually given to clients who require significant skeletal muscle relaxation, must be placed in awkward positions, or require extended surgical time. These anaesthetics are also given to clients who are extremely anxious or refuse or have contraindications for a local or regional anaesthetic. General anaesthetics may be inhaled or administered by IV line. IV administration is rapid, quickly inducing a pleasant sleep. Inhalation agents enter the body through the alveoli and are excreted rapidly by ventilation. Complications of inhalation agents include coughing, laryngospasm, bronchospasm, increased secretions, and respiratory depression. Adjuncts to general anaesthetics include opioids, benzodiazepines, and neuromuscular blocking agents.

Local anaesthesia results in a loss of sensation without loss of consciousness. Local anaesthetics can be administered topically, intracutaneously, and subcutaneously. Local anaesthesia produces ANS blockage and skeletal muscle paralysis in the area of the affected nerve. There is little systemic absorption, and recovery tends to be rapid, with little residual "hangover." Possible complications include discomfort, hypotension, and seizures.

Conscious sedation results in a minimally depressed LOC with maintenance of the client's protective airway reflexes. The goal with conscious sedation is to reduce the client's anxiety and discomfort and facilitate co-operation. A sedative–hypnotic and opioid are frequently used with conscious sedation. The client is able to maintain his or her own airway and to respond to appropriate commands.

Regional anaesthesia results in loss of sensation in a body region without loss of consciousness, when the administration of a local anaesthetic blocks a specific nerve or group of nerves. Spinal anaesthesia and epidural blocks are a form of regional anaesthesia. The client will need to be monitored for ANS blockage, bradycardia, hypotension, nausea, and vomiting.

Other management techniques that may be done during surgery include controlled hypotension, in which the BP is decreased during the administration of the anaesthetic to decrease blood loss during surgery. Hypothermia results from the deliberate lowering of the client's body temperature in order to reduce the demand for oxygen and anaesthesia. Cryoanaesthesia freezes a localized area to block pain impulses. Hypoanaesthesia is hypnosis to alter pain consciousness. Acupuncture decreases sensation to specific areas.

Catastrophic events that may happen in the operating room include anaphylactic reactions, which may be masked by the anaesthesia. Malignant hyperthermia is a rare metabolic disease that can be fatal. Hyperthermia with skeletal muscle rigidity can also occur. This is possibly due to exposure to succinylcholines. Other factors such as trauma, heat, and stress may be triggers of malignant hyperthermia. Some clients have inherited hypermetabolism of the skeletal muscles, resulting in altered control of intracellular calcium.

Manifestations of malignant hyperthermia include the following:
- Tachypnea
- Hypercarbia
- Hyperthermia
- Tachycardia
- Ventricular dysrhythmias, which can result in cardiac arrest and death

Postoperative Care

Care of the client in the postoperative (anaesthesia) care unit (PACU) includes monitoring and managing the following:
- Respiratory and circulatory function
- Pain
- Temperature
- Surgical site
- Airway patency, rate and quality of respiration, and auscultation of breath sounds in all fields will be assessed.
- Oxygen therapy may be established.
- Cardiac monitoring, including the rate and rhythm of the client's heartbeat, will be compared with preoperative findings.
- BP and temperature will also be compared with the previous baseline.
- Neurological assessment will include LOC, orientation, sensory and motor status, and size and equality of pupils.
- Intake and output will be monitored.
- Surgical sites and the condition of dressings will be noted, with the amount and type of drainage.

Fig. 8.10 outlines potential problems in the postoperative period. See Fig. 8.11 for an example of airway obstruction.

In order for the client to be discharged from the PACU, the client must be mobile, alert, and able to provide a degree of self-care. Pain, nausea, and vomiting should be controlled. The PACU nurse will give a report to the receiving nurse on the ward that summarizes the operative and postoperative periods. The client will be transferred to the bed, and then an

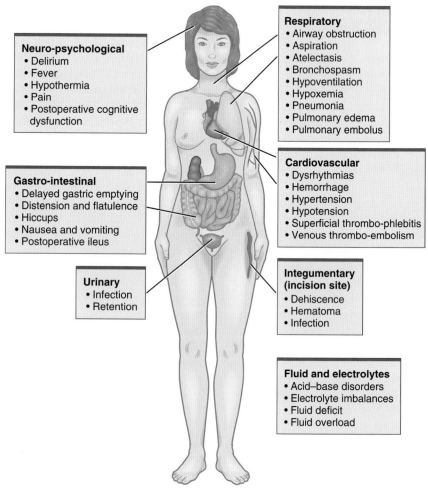

Neuro-psychological
- Delirium
- Fever
- Hypothermia
- Pain
- Postoperative cognitive dysfunction

Respiratory
- Airway obstruction
- Aspiration
- Atelectasis
- Bronchospasm
- Hypoventilation
- Hypoxemia
- Pneumonia
- Pulmonary edema
- Pulmonary embolus

Gastro-intestinal
- Delayed gastric emptying
- Distension and flatulence
- Hiccups
- Nausea and vomiting
- Postoperative ileus

Cardiovascular
- Dysrhythmias
- Hemorrhage
- Hypertension
- Hypotension
- Superficial thrombo-phlebitis
- Venous thrombo-embolism

Urinary
- Infection
- Retention

Integumentary (incision site)
- Dehiscence
- Hematoma
- Infection

Fluid and electrolytes
- Acid–base disorders
- Electrolyte imbalances
- Fluid deficit
- Fluid overload

Fig. 8.10 Potential problems in the postoperative period. (From Lewis, S. M., Bucher, L., Heitkemper, M. M., et al. [2019]. *Medical-surgical nursing in Canada: Assessment and management of clinical problems* [4th Cdn. ed., p. 420, Fig. 22.1]. Milton, ON: Elsevier.)

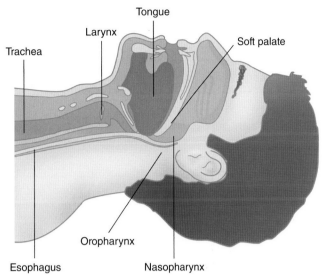

Fig. 8.11 Obstruction of airway by tongue. (From Rothrock, J., & McEwen, D. [2019]. *Alexander's care of the patient in surgery* [16th ed., p. 265, Figure 10.3]. St. Louis: Elsevier.)

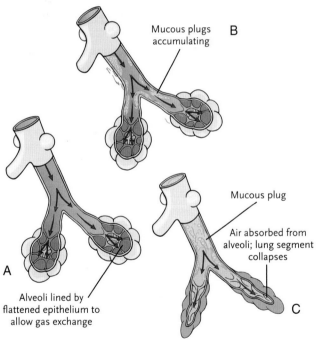

Fig. 8.12 Postoperative atelectasis. **A,** Normal bronchiole and alveoli. **B,** Mucous plug in bronchiole. **C,** Collapse of alveoli due to atelectasis following absorption of air. (From Lewis, S. M., Bucher, L., Heitkemper, M. M., et al. [2019]. *Medical-surgical nursing in Canada: Assessment and management of clinical problems* [4th Cdn. ed., p. 422, Figure 22-3]. Milton, ON: Elsevier.)

in-depth assessment must be done, postoperative orders will be initiated, and ambulation may be encouraged.

Atelectasis and pneumonia are complications that may occur after abdominal and thoracic surgery (see Fig. 8.12). There may be postoperative development of mucous plugs and decreased surfactant related to hypoventilation, a recumbent position, ineffective coughing, or smoking.

To help prevent the development of atelectasis and pneumonia, the practical nurse will encourage the client to breathe deeply and cough. Other techniques to encourage full lung expansion include the use of incentive spirometry, splints, diaphragmatic breathing, and changing position every 2 hours.

Fluid and electrolyte imbalances may contribute to cardiovascular alterations. Fluid retention in the first 2–5 days could occur due to the stress response. Fluid overload may occur when IV fluids are administered too quickly, if chronic disease exists, or if the client is an older adult. Fluid deficits may result from inadequate fluid replacement, causing a decreased CO and tissue perfusion. Hypokalemia can result from urinary or GI losses.

The stress response can contribute to an increase in clotting factors, causing DVT or pulmonary emboli. Symptoms of a pulmonary embolus include the following:

- Tachypnea
- Dyspnea
- Tachycardia
- Chest pain
- Hypotension
- Dysrhythmias
- Heart failure
- Hemoptysis

Syncope can indicate decreased CO, fluid deficits, or deficits in cerebral perfusion.

Vital signs need to be monitored and compared with the preoperative status. Intake and output need to be assessed accurately. Laboratory work, especially electrolytes, needs to be monitored. Mouth care and leg exercises are also part of postoperative care of the client.

A low urinary output can be expected for the first 24 hours due to an increase in aldosterone and ADH levels in the client's body due to the stress response of surgery, fluid losses during surgery, drainage, and diaphoresis. The anaesthesia may depress the nervous system, allowing the bladder to fill to a greater than normal extent before the urge to void is felt. Anticholinergic and narcotic drugs may also interfere with the ability to initiate voiding. Fluid retention is more likely to develop with abdominal or pelvic surgery where pain may alter the perception of a full bladder. The recumbent position may also impair the ability to void. The normal urine output should be at least 0.5 mL/kg body weight per hour. This would mean about 30 mL/hr for an adult. If the client does not have a catheter, he or she should be able to void about 200 mL following surgery. To assist the client to void, place the client in the normal voiding position. Use techniques such as running water, pouring water over the perineum, or ambulation or use the bedside commode.

Nausea and vomiting may be caused by anaesthetic agents or narcotics, delayed gastric emptying, slowed peristalsis, or resumption of oral intake too soon after surgery. Abdominal distension results from a decreased peristalsis caused from the handling of the bowel during surgery or by the client swallowing air. Hiccups occur due to irritation of the phrenic nerve. The client will remain NPO until the gag reflex has returned and the client has bowel sounds. Bowel sounds indicate that peristalsis has resumed. Clear fluids are introduced first and advanced fluids added as tolerated. Regular mouth care is essential when the client is NPO. An NG tube may be inserted if the vomiting persists and to help decompress the abdomen. Early ambulation is helpful to prevent abdominal distension.

The surgical incision disrupts the skin barrier, and healing is a major concern during the postoperative period. Adequate nutrition is important to help fight the catabolic effect of the stress response and assist in wound healing. Wound infections may be caused by oral flora, intestinal flora, or exogenous flora on the skin or in the environment. The incidence of wound sepsis is higher in clients who are malnourished, immunosuppressed, older adults, or experiencing a prolonged hospital stay.

Wound infection usually is not apparent until the third to fifth postoperative day, when the following symptoms may appear:
- Local manifestations of redness
- Edema
- Pain and tenderness around the site
- Purulent drainage leaking from the surgical incision
- Systemic manifestations, including leukocytosis and fever

Accumulation of fluid in the wound may impair healing and may require a drain to be placed in the area. The practical nurse should note the type, amount, colour, and consistency of the drainage. Assessment of position changes on the drainage should also be noted. The physician should be notified of excessive or abnormal drainage.

Postoperative pain may be caused by traumatization of skin and tissues, reflex muscle spasms, and anxiety or fear. Analgesics should be administered on a timely basis to ensure effectiveness during activities and for comfort. The practical nurse should observe for behavioural clues of pain and ask clients about their pain, as well as assess for the location, intensity, and quality of the client's pain. The practical nurse should evaluate the effectiveness of any pain management technique that is utilized and notify the physician if alternative pain management orders are needed.

Anxiety and depression may be more pronounced with clients experiencing a poor prognosis. Attention to a history of neurotic or psychotic disorders is important. The client's response may be part of the grief process. Confusion and delirium may result from psychological or physiological sources, including the following:
- Fluid and electrolyte imbalances
- Hypoxemia
- Drug effects
- Sleep deprivation
- Sensory alteration or overload

Delirium tremors may result from alcohol withdrawal. The practical nurse must provide adequate support for the client. Listen and talk with the client, offer explanations, reassure, and encourage involvement of the significant other.

Planning for discharge begins in the preoperative period. The client is informed and prepared to gradually assume greater responsibility for self-care. The following client teaching topics should be covered:
- Information should be provided regarding care of the wound site and dressing.
- Information should be provided about the action and side effects of medications as well as when and how to take medications.
- Dietary restrictions or modifications should be explained.
- Any symptoms that should be reported should be described.
- Where and when to return for follow-up care should be explained.
- Written instructions to help in reinforcement and remembering should be provided to the client.

The practical nurse should always allow plenty of time for the client to ask questions regarding postoperative care at home.

End-of-Life Care

End-of-life care refers to issues that relate to death and dying, the concluding phase of the normal lifespan. The three main goals of end-of-life care are as follows:
- Providing comfort and supportive care during the dying process
- Improving the quality of the remaining life
- Helping ensure a dignified death

Pathophysiology

Death occurs when all vital organs and systems cease to function. There will be irreversible cessation of circulatory and respiratory function. The body gradually slows down until all functions end. Generally, respirations cease first, with the heart stopping within a few minutes. Hearing and touch are the last senses to disappear. The vision may blur, the eyes may sink and glaze over, the blink reflex is absent, and the eyelids may remain half open. The skin of the hands, arms, feet, and legs becomes mottled and feels cold and clammy. There may be cyanosis on the nose, nail beds, and knees. A waxlike appearance of the skin suggests that death is imminent. Initially, there may be an increase in respiration, followed by Cheyne-Stokes respirations slowing down to terminal gaps of breathing (apneic spells) until respirations cease. Urinary output will gradually decrease. The client may be incontinent of urine or be unable to urinate. The digestive functions slow, with a possible accumulation of gas, resulting in abdominal distension and nausea. The client may experience a loss of sphincter control. A bowel movement may occur before imminent death, at the time of death, or not at all. The client will gradually lose the ability to move, and the jaw will sag as facial muscle tone is lost. Swallowing can become difficult, as can maintaining body alignment. The gag reflex will be lost. The heart rate may increase and then slow with a weakening pulse. The cardiac rhythm often is irregular.

Brain death occurs when the cerebral cortex stops functioning or is irreversibly destroyed. The cerebral cortex is responsible for voluntary movements and actions as well as cognitive functioning.

Psychosocial manifestations include the following:
- Altered decision making
- Anxiety about unfinished business
- Decreased socialization
- Fear of loneliness
- Fear of pain

Often the client and family feel overwhelmed, helpless, powerless, and tired. End-of-life clients need time to ponder their thoughts, review their lives, and express their feelings.

Grief

Grief is the emotional and behavioural response to loss. Grief is an individual experience and can be manifested in many ways. The intensity of grief is driven by the individual's personality, the nature of the relationship with the dying person, concurrent life crises, coping resources, and the availability of support systems. Table 8.10 is a summary of models of grief and bereavement.

Grief is a complex process in which an individual attempts to make sense of the loss. Not everyone experiences all stages of grief, nor do they progress through the stages in a linear fashion. Bereavement is a term used to describe an individual's response to the loss of a significant person. Bereavement may begin prior to the actual death. The normal grief process may take months to years. Goals for the grief process include the following:
- Resolving emotions
- Reflecting on the dying person
- Expressing feelings of loss and sadness
- Valuing what has been shared

Pathological grief refers to grief that has not lessened after the first year. Conflicted grief is when the bereaved person has not resolved ambivalent feelings toward the deceased. Absent grief is seen when the bereaved person appears to be coping by carrying on as if nothing has happened. Maladaptive or dysfunctional grief refers to prolonged, disruptive, or unresolved grief. Adaptive grief is a healthy response, in which the person comes to accept the reality of death. See Chapter 11, page 412, for further information on grief.

TABLE 8.10 Summary of Models of Grief and Bereavement

Kübler-Ross (1969)	Bowlby (1980)	Parkes (1986)
		Shock and alarm
		Searching
		Anger and guilt
		Gaining a new identity
Denial	Numbness	
Anger/bargaining	Yearning and	
Depression	searching	
Acceptance	Disorganization	
	and support	
	Reorganization	

Adapted from Lugton, J. (2005). *Palliative care: The nursing role.* (2nd ed., p. 309, Box 10.1). Philadelphia: Elsevier

Canada is a multicultural society; therefore, healthcare providers need to be aware of the variables that may affect end-of-life care. These variables include attitudes and beliefs, as well as cultural, religious, and family influences, and often the client's beliefs and attitudes are based on his or her culture and religion. However, healthcare providers must be vigilant not to assume that a person from a certain culture will always hold a particular set of cultural, religious, and spiritual beliefs and values. Nursing assessment must be completed on an individual basis to avoid stereotyping.

Advance and Instructional-Living Directives

In Canada, it is recognized that mentally competent people have the right to make decisions regarding their health care, including the right to request or refuse life-sustaining treatment (Lewis et al., 2019). Advance directives give information about future medical care and treatments and include instructional-living wills or treatment directives and proxy directives. Instructional-living directives include living wills and treatment directives. Living wills give instruction about future medical care and treatments and specify whether the client would like to die without heroic or extraordinary measures. Living wills are an important form of communication when the client is unable to communicate verbally. Proxy directives are in the form of a power of attorney for personal care document. The power of attorney for personal care will list the person(s) who may make healthcare decisions on the client's behalf should the client become unable to make informed decisions on his or her own.

If a Do Not Resuscitate (DNR) order is in place, CPR will not be attempted, but the DNR does not preclude the use of other forms of treatment. Another term that is being used to replace DNR or "no code" is "allow natural death" (AND). In this case, the client will still receive pain control and symptom management but no resuscitative treatment.

Ethical issues may arise regarding pain relief, in particular with clients who are terminally ill. According to the principle of nonmaleficence, the practical nurse is expected to prevent or reduce harm to the client and to provide adequate pain control to alleviate suffering in the terminally ill, even if a secondary effect of pain control is an earlier death. Medical assistance in dying (MAID) is now legal in Canada for those who meet eligibility requirements (see Chapter 3, page 20, for further information on MAID).

Palliative Care

Palliative care is intended to improve the quality of life of the client and his or her family as they manage a life-threatening illness through identification and relief of suffering as well as through support (World Health Organization, 2018). Palliative care strives to remain sensitive to personal, cultural, and religious values, beliefs, and practices. The therapies provided during palliative care will change over the course of the illness according to the client's and family's concerns, treatment priorities, and goals of care. See Box 8.3 for further details on the goals of palliative care.

BOX 8.3   Goals of Palliative Care

- Provide relief of symptoms, including pain.
- Regard dying as a normal process.
- Affirm life and neither hasten nor postpone death.
- Support holistic patient care and enhance quality of life.
- Offer support to patients to live as actively as possible until death.
- Offer support to the family during the patient's illness and in their own bereavement.

From Lewis, S. M., Bucher, L., Heitkemper, M. M., et al. (2019). *Medical-surgical nursing in Canada: Assessment and management of clinical problems* (4th Cdn. ed., p. 207, Table 13-1). Milton, ON: Elsevier Canada. Reprinted from *Cancer*, WHO, WHO Definition of Palliative Care, Copyright 2018.

In Canada, the term *hospice palliative care* refers to the convergence of hospice and palliative care. Hospices exist to provide support and care for persons in the last phases of incurable diseases. This care is aimed at relief of suffering and improving the quality of life for these individuals. There are over 600 hospices in Canada, and they are organized under a variety of models. There are free-standing hospices, home hospice care, and hospital-based palliative care units. Hospices are run by a medically supervised interdisciplinary team of professionals and volunteers, the hospice nurse being an integral part of this team. The hospice nurse plays a key role in educating the client and family on pain and symptom management. Grief support is incorporated into the plan of care for the family members and significant others during the illness and after the client's death.

The decision to begin hospice care is sometimes difficult due to a lack of information about hospice palliative care, difficulty in accessing palliative care services, the attitudes of healthcare providers, who sometimes regard palliation as a personal failure, and the fact that clients and families may regard palliative care as "giving up." Coordination of palliative care focuses on the needs of the client and his or her family and significant others, as well as on education, counselling, advocacy, and support. The goals of palliative care focus on ensuring that the client is able to express and share his or her feelings with others and that comfort measures and physical maintenance care are provided during the last stages of life.

Education of the palliative client and family involves providing ongoing information about the disease, the dying process, the care needed and offered, coping strategies, and barriers to grief.

Nursing Considerations

Nursing considerations for the dying client focus on comfort and improving the quality of life. Psychosocial care and physical care are interrelated for both the dying client and the family (Lewis et al., 2019). Anxiety is a feeling of uneasiness caused by a source that is not easily identified. Anxiety in end-of-life clients is frequently related to fear. Anxiety and depression may be exhibited during the end-of-life period and can be caused by pain that is not well controlled, psychosocial

factors related to the disease process or impending death, altered physiological states, or the effects of drugs. Encouragement, support, and education can help decrease some of the anxiety. Pharmacological and nonpharmacological measures may also be used.

Fear is a typical feeling for palliative clients. Fear of pain, loneliness and abandonment, and meaninglessness are common fears. Clients and families fear pain as they often associate death with pain. There is no physiological evidence that death is always painful. Psychologically, pain may occur based on anxieties. Terminally ill clients should receive enough analgesic so that they are comfortable. They should not be in physical pain, nor should they be deprived of the ability to interact with others.

There can be a real fear of loneliness and abandonment if the clients fear their loved ones cannot cope and will abandon them. Palliative clients appreciate loved ones comforting and supporting them at this stage. Holding hands, touching, and listening are greatly valued. Simply providing companionship allows the dying person a sense of security.

Fear of meaninglessness often leads palliative clients to review their lives, often examining their intentions and actions. Some clients may express regret, but many clients are able to recognize the value of their lives. Practical nurses should encourage clients and families to identify the positive qualities of the client's life. Practical nurses should also respect and accept practices and rituals associated with the client's life review without being judgemental.

Physical care centres around physiological and safety needs. Symptom management is key. The palliative client deserves the same care as people who are expected to recover from their illnesses. See Table 8.11 for the nursing management of physical care at the end of life.

Therapeutic Communication

Therapeutic communication is an important nursing intervention that includes the essential components of empathy and active listening. Clients and their families should be allowed time to express their thoughts and feelings. Sometimes unusual communication by the client may take place at the end of life. The client's speech may be confused, disoriented, or garbled. The client may even speak with family or friends who have predeceased them. At other times, the client may leave instructions for family members or speak of projects that have to be completed. Active careful listening allows identification of specific patterns in the client's communication and decreases the risk for inappropriate labelling of behaviours.

The resolution of grief is the primary focus of interventions for anticipatory and dysfunctional grief. Specific interventions for both types of grief are similar and include providing an environment that allows the client to express his or her feelings. Clients should be free to express feelings of anger, fear, or guilt without others' judgement. Both the client and the family need to understand that the grief reaction is normal. The client's privacy should be respected. Honesty in answering questions and giving information is essential.

TABLE 8.11   Nursing Management: Physical Care at the End of Life

Characteristic	Nursing Management
Pain • Pain may be a major symptom associated with terminal illness and is the most feared. • Pain can be acute or chronic. • Physical and emotional irritations can aggravate pain.	• Assess pain thoroughly and regularly to determine the quality, intensity, location, and pattern, as well as the contributing and relieving factors. • Minimize possible irritants such as skin irritations from moisture, heat or cold, or pressure. • Administer medications around the clock in a timely manner and on a regular basis. • Provide complementary and alternative therapies, such as guided imagery, massage, acupressure, heat and cold, therapeutic touch, distraction, and relaxation techniques, as needed. • Evaluate the effectiveness of pain relief measures frequently to ensure that the client is on an adequate drug regimen. • Do not delay or deny pain relief measures to a terminally ill client.
Delirium • Delirium is characterized by confusion, disorientation, restlessness, clouding of consciousness, incoherence, fear, anxiety, excitement, and often hallucinations. • It may be misidentified as depression, psychosis, anger, or anxiety. • The use of opioids, corticosteroids, or both (as well as many other medications) in end-of-life care may cause delirium. • The underlying disease process may contribute to delirium. • It is generally considered a reversible process.	• Perform a thorough assessment for reversible causes of delirium, including pain, constipation, and urinary retention. • Provide a room that is quiet, well lit, and familiar to reduce the effects of delirium. • Reorient the dying person to person, place, and time with each encounter. • Administer ordered benzodiazepines, sedatives, and antipsychotics as needed. • Stay physically close to a frightened client. Reassure in a calm, soft voice with touch and slow stroking of the skin.
Restlessness • This may occur as death approaches and cerebral metabolism slows.	• Assess for spiritual distress as a cause for restlessness and agitation. • Do not restrain. • Use soothing music and slow, soft touch and voice. • Limit the number of persons at the bedside. • Limit other stimuli and activity.
Dysphagia • This may occur because of extreme weakness and changes in level of consciousness.	• Identify the least invasive alternative routes of administration for drugs needed for symptom management. • Suction orally as needed. • Administer frequent oral care.
Dehydration • Dehydration may occur during the last days of life, but hunger and thirst are rare. • As the end of life approaches, clients tend to take in less food and fluid.	• Assess the condition of mucous membranes frequently to prevent excessive dryness, which can lead to discomfort. • Maintain complete, regular oral care to provide for comfort and hydration of mucous membranes. • Do not force the client to eat or drink. • Encourage the consumption of ice chips and sips of fluids or use moist cloths to provide moisture to the mouth. • Use moist cloths and swabs for unconscious clients to avoid aspiration. • Apply lubricant to the lips and oral mucous membranes as needed. • Reassure the family that reduced food and fluid intake is a natural part of the process of dying.
Dyspnea • This is a subjective symptom, often accompanied by anxiety and the fear of suffocation. • An underlying disease process can exacerbate dyspnea.	• Assess respiratory status regularly. • Elevate the head or position the client on his or her side, or both, to improve chest expansion. • Use a fan or air conditioner to facilitate the movement of cool air. • Administer supplemental oxygen as ordered.

Continued

TABLE 8.11   Nursing Management: Physical Care at the End of Life—cont'd

Characteristic	Nursing Management
	• Administer drugs (depending on the underlying cause of the dyspnea) such as opioids, sedatives, diuretics, antibiotics, corticosteroids, and bronchodilators as ordered to relieve congestion and coughing and to decrease apprehension.
Pooling of Secretions • Coughing and expelling secretions become difficult.	• Perform gentle oropharyngeal suctioning as needed to remove accumulated secretions. • Position the client on his or her side supported with pillows with head down, or in a semiprone position if there are excessive secretions. • Use anticholinergic medications (scopolamine or glycopyrrolate [Robinul]) as ordered.
Weakness and Fatigue	• Assess the client's tolerance for activities. • Time nursing interventions to conserve the client's energy. • Assess the client to identify and complete valued or desired activities. • Provide support as needed to maintain positions in a bed or chair. • Provide frequent rest periods.
Myoclonus • This is mild to severe jerking or twitching, which is sometimes associated with the use of large doses of opioids. • Clients may complain of involuntary twitching of the upper and lower extremities.	• Assess for the initial onset and duration of this effect and any discomfort or distress experienced by the client. • If myoclonus is distressing or becoming more severe, discuss possible drug therapy modifications with the physician. • Changes in opioid medication may alleviate or decrease myoclonus.
Skin Breakdown • Skin integrity is difficult to maintain at the end of life. • Immobility, urinary and bowel incontinence, dry skin, nutritional deficits, anemia, friction, and shearing forces lead to a high risk for skin breakdown. • Disease and other processes may impair skin integrity. • As death approaches, circulation to the extremities decreases, and they become cool, mottled, and cyanotic.	• Assess the skin for signs of breakdown. • Implement protocols to prevent skin breakdown by controlling drainage and odour and keeping the skin and any wound areas clean and dry. • Perform wound assessments as needed. • Follow appropriate nursing management protocol for dressing wounds. • Consider the use of special pressure-relieving air mattresses. • Follow appropriate nursing management to prevent skin irritations and breakdown from urinary and bowel incontinence. • Use blankets to provide warmth; never apply heat. • Prevent the effects of shearing forces.
Bowel Patterns • Constipation can be caused by immobility, the use of opioid medications, a lack of fibre in the diet, and dehydration. • Diarrhea may occur as muscles relax or from a fecal impaction related to immobility, the use of opioids, or both.	• Assess bowel function. • Assess for and remove fecal impactions. • Encourage movement and physical activities as tolerated. • Encourage fibre in the diet if appropriate. • Encourage fluids if appropriate. • Use suppositories, laxatives, or enemas if ordered.
Anorexia, Nausea, and Vomiting • They may be caused by complications of the disease process. • Drugs may contribute to nausea. • Constipation, impaction, and bowel obstruction can cause anorexia, nausea, and vomiting.	• Assess the client for complaints of nausea, vomiting, or both. • Assess possible contributing causes for nausea or vomiting. • Have family members provide the client's favourite foods. • Discuss modifications to the drug regimen with the healthcare team. • Provide frequent mouth care, especially if the client has vomited.

Adapted from Lewis, S. M., Bucher, L., Heitkemper, M. M., et al. (2019). *Medical-surgical nursing in Canada: Assessment and management of clinical problems* (4th Cdn. ed., pp. 217–218, Table 13.11). Milton, ON: Elsevier Canada.

Families and clients need encouragement to continue their usual activities as much as possible. Planning for the future or for the funeral may be needed based on the client's or family's coping abilities. Anger must be recognized as a normal response to dying. When a client or family member acts out in anger, the practical nurse must not react on a personal level. Practical nurses need to encourage realistic hope within the limits of the situation. A sense of power can be restored for the client by encouraging him or her to identify goals and make decisions pertaining to his or her own care.

Care of the Body

After the client is pronounced dead, the practical nurse prepares or delegates preparation of the body for immediate viewing by the family. Considerations when preparing the body include cultural customs, provincial and territorial laws, and agency policies and procedures.

PRACTICE QUESTIONS

Case 1

Fred Kingsley, a 52-year-old country and western singer, has been diagnosed with vocal cord polyps, requiring surgical laser removal.

Questions 1–3 refer to this case.

1. What is the practical nurse's priority assessment in Mr. Kingsley's immediate postoperative period?
   1. Hemorrhage
   2. Pain
   3. Difficulty swallowing
   4. Oral pharyngeal edema
2. What is the recommended postoperative position for Mr. Kingsley?
   1. Prone with his head on a pillow
   2. Reverse Trendelenburg with the neck extended
   3. Semi-Fowler's with the neck flexed
   4. Supine with his neck hyperextended and supported with a pillow
3. What nursing action can best alleviate Mr. Kingsley's throat discomfort?
   1. Having him drink warm fluids
   2. Giving him ASA (Aspirin)
   3. Giving him acetaminophen (Tylenol) elixir or pills
   4. Placing a heating pad around his throat

Case 2

Consuela Gomez, age 58, moved to Canada from Mexico 10 years ago. For the past few months, she has been experiencing fatigue, cough, and occasional blood-tinged sputum. The practical nurse administers a Mantoux tuberculin skin test, and Mrs. Gomez returns to the clinic for the test to be read.

Questions 4–7 refer to this case.

4. Mrs. Gomez's Mantoux test yields an induration area of 10 mm. What is the most accurate interpretation of a 10-mm result?
   1. Active disease is present.
   2. She has been exposed to *M. tuberculosis* or has been vaccinated with bacille Calmette-Guérin.
   3. The disease is not active, but preventive treatment should be initiated.
   4. The reaction is questionable and should be repeated.
5. Which of the following tests is most reliable to confirm a diagnosis of tuberculosis (TB) for Mrs. Gomez?
   1. A chest X-ray
   2. Acid-fast bacilli in a sputum smear
   3. A nucleic acid amplification test
   4. Second-step Mantoux test with induration of 10 mm or greater
6. Mrs. Gomez is started on a multiple-drug regimen. The practical nurse teaches Mrs. Gomez about the medications. Which of the following drugs have side effects of ototoxicity and nephrotoxicity?
   1. Ethambutol (Myambutol)
   2. Isoniazid (INH)
   3. Rifampin (Rifadin)
   4. Streptomycin (Streptomycin)
7. The practical nurse discusses with Mrs. Gomez the importance of adherence to her medication regimen. How long will Mrs. Gomez be required to take the pharmacological treatment for TB?
   1. 1–2 months
   2. 3–4 months
   3. 5–6 months
   4. 6–9 months

Case 3

Ms. Juliet Mathias, age 34, has been overweight most of her life. Because she began feeling light-headed and dizzy, she came to the health clinic for a checkup. She was diagnosed with primary hypertension following serial blood pressures of 150/100 mm Hg. The community practical nurse visits her in her home.

Questions 8–10 refer to this case.

8. Which of the following statements about primary hypertension is true?
   1. It requires management by drug therapy.
   2. It has no identifiable cause.
   3. It is related to another underlying condition.
   4. Obesity is not a factor.
9. Ms. Mathias is started on hydrochlorothiazide (HydroDIURIL) by the physician for her hypertension. Which dietary modification, related to the HydroDIURIL, would the practical nurse teach Ms. Mathias in order to prevent an electrolyte imbalance?
   1. Increase potassium-containing foods.
   2. Decrease sodium-containing foods.

3. Increase sodium-containing foods.

4. Decrease potassium-containing foods.

10. The practical nurse determines that Ms. Mathias's hypertension is not well controlled on the diuretic. She is referred back to the physician, who prescribes a calcium channel blocker. What would be priority teaching for her regarding this medication?

1. She should watch for decreased urine output.

2. She may develop hair loss.

3. She may develop high blood pressure.

4. She may feel dizzy when she stands quickly.

Case 4

Linda Hynes, age 52, is admitted to the hospital in preparation for surgery for an adrenal tumour that has caused Cushing's syndrome. A health assessment reveals Ms. Hynes to be manifesting truncal obesity, thin arms and legs, a round face, and a "buffalo hump" on her upper back. She is irritable during the assessment and says she just wants to be left alone.

Questions 11–12 refer to this case.

11. In addition to the manifestations noted in the initial health assessment, which of the following, observed by the practical nurse, may be additional manifestations of Cushing's syndrome?

1. Petechiae and abdominal purplish red striae on the abdomen

2. Decreased axilla and pubic hair

3. Tachycardia and bulging eyes

4. Hypotension and hypoglycemia

12. Later in the day, Ms. Hynes apologizes for her irritability and tells the practical nurse she just does not like anyone examining her because she looks so bad. Which response by the practical nurse is most appropriate?

1. "You really shouldn't worry about how you look. It's what you are on the inside that counts."

2. "There are some really good ways to dress so that the changes wouldn't seem so noticeable."

3. "You are going to look much better right after your surgery."

4. "Most of the physical and mental changes caused by the disease will gradually improve after your surgery."

Case 5

Brian Wilson, a 17-year-old student, sustains a mandibular fracture while playing rugby. There was no loss of teeth. His treatment includes intermaxillary fixation surgery.

Questions 13–15 refer to this case.

13. Postoperatively, how should the practical nurse position Brian?

1. Prone to facilitate lung expansion

2. On his side with his head slightly elevated to prevent aspiration

3. Supine with his head to the side to promote the drainage of secretions

4. Slight Trendelenburg to prevent aspiration of fluids

14. What is the most important postoperative goal for Brian?

1. Adequate nutrition

2. Jaw immobilization

3. Oral hygiene

4. Patent airway

15. Which of the following is the most important to be available at Brian's bedside?

1. Nasogastric suction tube

2. Nasopharyngeal suction catheter

3. Wire cutter

4. Oxygen cannula

Case 6

Mrs. Cheng, age 78 years, fell on the ice and injured her hip. She was transported to the nearest emergency department, where a fractured hip was diagnosed.

Questions 16–17 refer to this case.

16. Mrs. Cheng is on bed rest with immobilization of her hip while she is waiting for an operating room to be available for surgery later in the day. What assistive device will the practical nurse provide for Mrs. Cheng?

1. A urinary catheter, as a bedpan may not be used

2. A trapeze to facilitate lifting movement

3. Side rails in the "up" position for Mrs. Cheng to use for moving herself

4. A "geri-chair" so Mrs. Cheng may sit up for meals

17. It is determined that Mrs. Cheng has osteoporosis. Prior to discharge from rehabilitation, the practical nurse discusses measures to prevent further fractures. Which of the following would be important to discuss with Mrs. Cheng?

1. Calcium supplements and prescribed bisphosphonate medication

2. Incorporating non–weight-bearing exercise into her daily routine when allowed by the physician

3. Vitamin D, 200 international units (IU)

4. Planning for a move from her residential home to an assisted living facility

Case 7

The practical nurse in a walk-in, ambulatory clinic assesses Sandra Procinski, 33 years old. She states she experienced a sore throat about a week ago but has not had any problems until today. This morning she awoke to find her face swollen, particularly around her eyes. She also has noted that her urine appears foamy.

Questions 18–19 refer to this case.

18. The practical nurse suspects that Ms. Procinski is manifesting symptoms of which of the following?

1. Urinary tract infection

2. Pyelonephritis

3. Nephrotic syndrome

4. Acute glomerulonephritis

19. What is the likely initial treatment for Ms. Procinski?

1. A diet low in potassium

2. Rest

3. Antihypertensives

4. Antibiotics

Case 8

Bernard Cowler, 36, was admitted to hospital with a diagnosis of pulmonary embolism.

Questions 20–21 refer to this case.

20. Mr. Cowler is started on heparin (Hepalean) therapy. What blood test result does the nurse need to monitor closely?
    1. International normalized ratio (INR)
    2. Partial thromboplastin time (PTT)
    3. Platelet function assay (PFA)
    4. Prothrombin time (PT)
21. Several days later, the nurse transcribes a physician order for Mr. Cowler: "Discontinue heparin, start warfarin (Coumadin) at 5 mg OD each morning." What action should the nurse take?
    1. Stop the heparin and notify the pharmacy to prepare Coumadin for Mr. Cowler.
    2. Stop the heparin and give Mr. Cowler his first dose of Coumadin.
    3. Question the doctor regarding the dose of Coumadin.
    4. Question the doctor about discontinuing heparin before therapeutic levels of Coumadin are reached.

Case 9

The practical nurse interviews Arnold Hampton, age 69 years, at the clinic. He states he has been experiencing muscle cramps in his legs that are getting worse, and he is not able to walk as much as he once did. He tells the practical nurse the pain gets better when he sits but starts again shortly after he gets up and begins walking.

Questions 22–24 refer to this case.

22. When performing the physical assessment on Mr. Hampton, the practical nurse instructs him to abduct his leg. What does *abduction* mean?
    1. Movement of part toward midline of body
    2. Movement of part away from midline of body
    3. Rotating the joint outward
    4. Rotating the joint inward
23. The practical nurse and physician suspect Mr. Hampton may have peripheral arterial disease (PAD). What assessment would the practical nurse perform with a client with presumed PAD?
    1. Assess for diminished or absent pulses in the extremities.
    2. Assess for pallor or blanching of the foot when in a dependent position.
    3. Assess for lower leg edema.
    4. Assess blood pressure in both thighs.
24. What self-care activities would the practical nurse suggest to Mr. Hampton?
    1. Use a heating pad to help him become comfortable while resting.
    2. Purchase support stockings to wear daily.
    3. Walk at least 30 minutes a day.
    4. Inspect his feet for redness once a week.

Case 10

Sarah Sawchuk is an 18-year-old female who is admitted to the hospital with severe diarrhea, anorexia, weight loss, and abdominal cramps. She is diagnosed with ulcerative colitis.

Questions 25–27 refer to this case.

25. What symptoms of fluid and electrolyte imbalance caused by ulcerative colitis should the practical nurse report immediately?
    1. Thirst and dry, sticky mucous membranes
    2. Extreme muscle weakness and tachycardia
    3. Development of tetany and muscle spasms
    4. Numbness and tingling of fingers, mouth, and toes
26. Ms. Sawchuk's condition deteriorates, and she requires an ileostomy. What would her postoperative care include?
    1. Removing rectal packing 4 hours after surgery
    2. Continuous, slow feedings via nasogastric tube
    3. Monitoring intake and output accurately
    4. Removing the nasogastric tube on arrival at the unit
27. The practical nurse teaches Ms. Sawchuk about nutrition related to her ileostomy. Which of the following foods may cause an obstruction and should be avoided by Ms. Sawchuk?
    1. Raw fruits and vegetables
    2. Beans and legumes
    3. Eggs
    4. Cheese

Case 11

Mrs. Edna O'Brien, age 90 years, lives in a retirement home. Although she is generally healthy, she has bilateral cataracts that she has been reluctant to have treated. Mrs. O'Brien is presently almost totally blind.

Questions 28–29 refer to this case.

28. The practical nurse instructs the dietary aide in assisting Mrs. O'Brien with her meals. What direction might the practical nurse give to the aide?
    1. Do not give Mrs. O'Brien sharp utensils.
    2. Provide Mrs. O'Brien with finger foods that she can feel and pick up easily.
    3. Help Mrs. O'Brien locate the food on her plate by comparing it to a clock; for example, say, "The toast is at nine o'clock."
    4. Stay with Mrs. O'Brien throughout the meal and feed her when necessary.
29. Mrs. O'Brien consents to have her cataracts treated. At a local clinic, she has an initial right cataract extraction with intraocular lens implant and is discharged the same day. What discharge instructions would the practical nurse provide to Mrs. O'Brien?
    1. "I will give you a stool softener to prevent constipation."
    2. "You need to drink at least six glasses of water or fluids this evening."
    3. "You will not be allowed to bathe until you return to see the doctor in 2 days."
    4. "You are allowed to watch TV, but you should not read for the next 48 hours."

Case 12

Mrs. Gardner, age 84, was diagnosed with heart failure 2 years ago. She has been a pack-a-day cigarette smoker for over 50 years. She has never had a myocardial infarction. Mrs. Gardner has been admitted to her local hospital with severe shortness of breath and only able to speak in one-word sentences. She is pale, diaphoretic, and cool to the touch. Her pulse is rapid and irregular.

Questions 30–33 refer to this case.

30. What position should the practical nurse encourage Mrs. Gardner to assume while being treated for the shortness of breath?
    1. Prone, to allow her to rest more effectively
    2. Semi-Fowler's, to allow her to breathe more easily
    3. Trendelenburg, to encourage drainage of fluids from the upper respiratory airway
    4. High Fowler's with legs down, to decrease preload

31. Mrs. Gardner is given furosemide (Lasix) to initiate urinary output. When she starts to void, what is the priority assessment?
    1. Electrolyte levels
    2. Blood pressure
    3. Hourly output
    4. Respiratory rate

32. It is determined that Mrs. Gardner has left-sided heart failure. Which of the following would the practical nurse assess for in Mrs. Gardner?
    1. Pitting edema
    2. Jugular venous distension
    3. Hepatomegaly
    4. Lung crackles

33. During Mrs. Gardner's hospitalization, blood work showed elevated BUN and creatinine levels, with reduced creatinine clearance. Chronic renal failure was diagnosed, and she was placed on a renal diet. The practical nurse should teach Mrs. Gardner to avoid which of the following foods?
    1. Red meat and shellfish
    2. Potatoes and citrus fruit
    3. Cookies and cake
    4. Lean meat and chicken

Independent Questions

Questions 34–60 do not refer to a particular case.

34. Mr. Sharapov, aged 74, was admitted with an exacerbation of chronic obstructive pulmonary disease (COPD). His condition has stabilized, and he is to be discharged on home oxygen therapy. What action by the nurse would best assist Mr. Sharapov in managing home oxygen therapy?
    1. Provide a teaching session on the use of a portable oxygen compressor.
    2. Give Mr. Sharapov a pamphlet on oxygen therapy that he could refer to when he is at home.
    3. Arrange for a home consultation with a respiratory therapist or technologist.
    4. Make an appointment for Mr. Sharapov to have pulse oximetry 1 week after discharge.

35. Harold Hart, an 82-year-old man, has a history of hypertension. He was admitted to hospital with a myocardial infarction (MI). What laboratory tests will confirm the diagnosis of MI?
    1. PT, PTT, INR
    2. Troponin, CK-MB, LDH
    3. Na^+, K^+, CK-BB
    4. BUN, Cr, CK-MM

36. A practical nurse attends a summer pool party. One of the male guests dives into the shallow end of the pool and sustains a high neck fracture and spinal cord injury. The practical nurse suspects a C2-level injury. What priority first aid measure will the practical nurse likely need to provide until paramedics arrive?
    1. Immobilize him on a firm board, such as a Styrofoam "flutter board."
    2. Fashion a roll out of clothes to stabilize the neck.
    3. Maintain him in the pool without attempting to lift him out.
    4. Provide rescue breathing.

37. Minh Tam Tran is a 16-year-old who has been diagnosed with asthma. She has been prescribed salbutamol (Ventolin) and beclomethasone (Beclovent) metered-dose inhalers. Minh asks the school practical nurse why she needs to take these medications. What is the practical nurse's most appropriate response?
    1. "The Beclovent is a steroid, and the Ventolin is a bronchodilator."
    2. "You take both of these so that you don't have another asthma attack."
    3. "The Ventolin opens your airways, and the Beclovent decreases the swelling, so together they stabilize your asthma."
    4. "You must be careful to take both of these inhalers exactly as they are prescribed to prevent another attack."

38. Mr. Sanders visits the neurology clinic, where he receives a diagnosis of Parkinson's disease from the physician. The practical nurse sees Mr. Sanders following his meeting with the physician. What would be the most helpful approach by the practical nurse?
    1. "I am really sorry about your diagnosis, but the drugs can keep you stable for a long time."
    2. "What did the physician explain to you about your diagnosis of Parkinson's disease?"
    3. "There is a lot of research about Parkinson's disease these days, so many new treatments may be available."
    4. "I understand that you are upset by this very bad diagnosis. I will sit here with you for a while."

39. Ms. Singh has a hemoglobin of 100 mmol/L. What will be the most likely manifestation of her condition?
    1. Headache
    2. Bradycardia
    3. Yellow sclera
    4. Fatigue

40. Mrs. Angelina has experienced several weeks of diarrhea as a result of a viral gastroenteritis. Mrs. Angelina is at

risk of being deficient in which of the following due to the diarrhea?
1. Magnesium
2. Calcium
3. Potassium
4. Sodium

41. Mr. Wheeler has symptoms of gastroesophageal reflux disease (GERD). What would the community practical nurse recommend while he is waiting for his appointment with the physician?
    1. "I will refer you to a therapist who will evaluate and treat your swallowing difficulties."
    2. "I recommend you place a heating pad on your stomach area to ease the pain."
    3. "You might try an antacid preparation to soothe the heartburn."
    4. "Eating small, frequent meals will prevent nausea and vomiting."

42. Mr. Tibor, age 64 years, is unable to be discharged from the surgical unit after a hip replacement because of a sudden onset of frank gastric bleeding. He has a history of peptic ulcer disease. What priority intervention should the practical nurse anticipate?
    1. Sengesten-Blakemore tube insertion
    2. An intravenous bolus of normal saline
    3. Insertion of a nasogastric tube and saline lavage
    4. Administration of oxygen

43. Which of the following is a manifestation of diverticulitis?
    1. High fever
    2. Chronic diarrhea
    3. Epigastric discomfort
    4. Left lower quadrant pain

44. Mr. Wilmox, age 45, has been admitted to the surgical unit because appendicitis is suspected. The practical nurse assesses Mr. Wilmox. Which of the following is a possible manifestation of appendicitis?
    1. Increased abdominal pain with coughing
    2. Esophageal reflux
    3. High-grade fever
    4. A negative Rovsing's sign

45. In a client with viral hepatitis, the practical nurse should closely monitor for indications of which of the following abnormal laboratory values?
    1. Decreased vitamins C and E
    2. Elevated serum potassium
    3. Prolonged prothrombin time
    4. Decreased calcium

46. During recovery from hepatic coma, a high-fibre diet is recommended. What is the primary rationale for recommending this diet?
    1. To prevent dyslipidemia
    2. To prevent diarrhea
    3. To decrease hypokalemia
    4. To decrease serum ammonia

47. Mr. Hawkins has radical neck surgery for cancer of the larynx. Which of the following is the most important assessment postsurgery?

1. Pain
2. Temperature of 38°C
3. Stridor
4. Serosanguinous oozing from the operative site

48. Mrs. Cohen has primary adrenal insufficiency (Addison's disease). The practical nurse assessing Mrs. Cohen should anticipate which of the following manifestations?
    1. Exophthalmos and goitre
    2. Polydipsia and polyuria
    3. Moon face and buffalo hump
    4. Bronze pigmentation and hypotension

49. Which of the following is descriptive of cluster headaches?
    1. Constant, squeezing tightness at the base of the skull
    2. A throbbing, synchronous, pulsing pain that is commonly unilateral and anterior
    3. Palpable neck and shoulder muscles, stiff neck, and tenderness
    4. Severe "bone-crushing" pain radiating up and down from one eye

50. Mr. Gianopoulos, 35 years old, had just recovered from an upper respiratory infection when he suddenly experienced muscle weakness in his feet and lower legs. He sought medical assistance and was diagnosed with Guillain-Barré syndrome. Which of the following would be the priority of nursing care?
    1. Treating the infection that triggered onset of the syndrome
    2. Managing respiratory muscle dysfunction
    3. Strengthening and stretching targeted muscles
    4. Preventing major complications due to immobility

51. Mr. Andersson, age 32, experienced a cerebrovascular accident (CVA) resulting from a ruptured aneurysm with a subarachnoid hemorrhage. He is gradually improving; however, his family has been informed that he has apraxia as a result of the CVA. The family asks the practical nurse to tell them what apraxia means. What should the practical nurse respond?
    1. "Apraxia is loss of comprehension of verbal or written language."
    2. "Apraxia is the inability to use objects properly."
    3. "Apraxia is an inability to recognize objects, sights, sounds, or other sensory stimuli."
    4. "Apraxia is the loss of production of verbal or written language."

52. Mrs. Tetrault, an 83-year-old widow, has a history of type 2 diabetes and chronic arterial occlusive disease. She is hospitalized due to gangrene of all her right toes. The doctor has informed her that she will need a below-the-knee amputation. The practical nurse goes into Mrs. Tetrault's room and finds her crying about this upcoming procedure. How should the practical nurse respond to Mrs. Tetrault?
    1. "Don't cry; this really isn't such a bad thing. They do wonderful things with prostheses now."
    2. "I know you will be just fine. You are so strong, and you can get through this."

3. "I can see that you are upset. Would you like to talk about your concerns?"
4. "It's okay to be upset. This is devastating news. I'd be upset too."

53. The clinic practical nurse performs a physical examination on Mr. Fredericks, age 60. What assessment data would support the diagnosis of abdominal aortic aneurysm (AAA)?
    1. Epigastric discomfort
    2. Pyrosis
    3. Abdominal bruit
    4. Tearing abdominal pain

54. Mrs. Olsen, age 84, is admitted to hospital from a nursing home due to extreme lethargy. Her hematocrit is 54% and sodium is 120 mmol/L. Which intervention should the practical nurse anticipate will be implemented?
    1. Pushing oral fluids
    2. Establishing an intravenous (IV) line of 10% dextrose solution
    3. Starting an IV line of normal saline (0.9% NaCl)
    4. Inserting a nasogastric tube for enteral feeding

55. Mr. Frank Ulrinski is a farmer who lives in the Prairies. He is bald and spends most of his working day in the sun. The practical nurse performs a skin assessment. What type of skin cancer is Mr. Ulrinski most at risk for?
    1. Adenocarcinoma
    2. Basal cell carcinoma
    3. Malignant melanoma
    4. Spongioblastoma

56. Which of the following is presumed to be the most effective prevention for cancer of the cervix?
    1. Routine Papanicolaou (Pap) tests
    2. Colposcopy
    3. Human papilloma virus (HPV) vaccine
    4. Laser treatment for genital herpes

57. Catherine Blinker, age 92, has osteoporosis. She is generally well but uses a walker frame to assist with mobility. What activity would the practical nurse recommend to improve her osteoporosis?
    1. Swimming
    2. Walking
    3. Aerobics
    4. Range-of-motion exercises

58. Brenda Chaisson is pregnant with her second child when she is diagnosed with multiple sclerosis. What manifestations is she likely to have initially experienced?
    1. Sensory disturbances that include blurred vision and tinnitus
    2. Bradykinesia, rigid muscle tone, tremors, and impaired postural reflexes
    3. Fluctuating weakness of certain skeletal muscle groups
    4. Unpleasant motor and sensory abnormalities (paraesthesias)

59. Six hours following a transurethral resection of the prostate (TURP), Mr. Douglas experiences abdominal pain and bladder distension. What action will the practical nurse implement?
    1. Pain assessment
    2. Flushing of the continuous bladder irrigation catheter
    3. Decreasing the flow rate in the bladder irrigation
    4. Notifying the physician

60. A practical nurse on the palliative care team is supporting the family of Mrs. Millar, who has chosen to die at home. The family asks the practical nurse how they will know death is imminent. What would the practical nurse respond?
    1. "Her skin may become mottled."
    2. "Her respirations will be slow and deep."
    3. "Her pulse will increase."
    4. "Her temperature will decrease."

REFERENCES

Black, J. M., & Hawks, J. H. (2009). *Medical-surgical nursing: Clinical management for positive outcomes* (8th ed.). St. Louis: Saunders.

Day, R. A., Paul, P., Williams, B., et al. (2016). *Brunner & Suddarth's textbook of medical-surgical nursing* (3rd Cdn. ed.). Philadelphia: Lippincott, Williams & Wilkins.

deWit, S. C., Stromberg, H., & Dallred, C. (2017). *Medical-surgical nursing: Concepts and practices* (3rd ed.). St. Louis: Elsevier.

Huether, S., Power-Kean, K., El-Hussein, M. T., et al. (2018). *Understanding pathophysiology* (Cdn. ed.). Milton, ON: Elsevier.

Ignatavicius, D. D., Workman, M. L., & Rebar, C. (2018). *Medical-surgical nursing: Concepts for interprofessional collaborative care* (9th ed.). St. Louis: Elsevier.

Lewis, S. M., Bucher, L., Heitkemper, M. M., et al. (2019). *Medical-surgical nursing in Canada: Assessment and management of clinical problems* (4th Cdn. ed.). Milton, ON: Elsevier.

Lewis, S. M., Heitkemper, M. M., Dirksen, S. R., et al. (2014). *Medical-surgical nursing in Canada: Assessment and management of clinical problems* (3rd Cdn. ed.). Toronto: Elsevier.

Lugton, J. (2005). *Palliative care: The nursing role*. Philadelphia: Elsevier.

Rothrock, J., & McEwen, D. (2019). *Alexander's care of the patient in surgery* (16th ed.). St. Louis: Elsevier.

World Health Organization. (2007). *WHO case definitions of HIV for surveillance and revised clinical staging and immunological classification of HIV-related disease in adults and children*. Geneva, Switzerland: Author. Retrieved from http://www.who.int/hiv/pub/guidelines/HIVstaging150307.pdf.

World Health Organization. (2018). WHO definition of palliative care. Retrieved from http://www.who.int/cancer/palliative/definition/en/.

BIBLIOGRAPHY

Hockenberry, M., Rodgers, C., & Wilson, D. (2017). *Wong's essentials of pediatric nursing* (10th ed.). St. Louis: Elsevier.

Skidmore-Roth, L. (2016). *Mosby's 2016 nursing drug reference.* St. Louis: Elsevier.

WEB SITES

- **Health Finder.gov** (https://www.healthfinder.gov/): This U.S. Department of Health and Human Services site includes a health library that has information on a wide variety of topics and a search engine on health topics. It also provides access to DrugDigest, a medication database that provides a wealth of information (including interactions) on medications, vitamins, and herbs.

- **National Center for Complementary and Integrative Medicine** (https://nccih.nih.gov/health/integrative-health): This U.S. National Institutes of Health site offers comprehensive health information on a variety of herbs and other dietary supplements. It also includes information on alternative treatment modalities, such as acupuncture and relaxation techniques.

- **Public Health Agency of Canada** (https://www.canada.ca/en/public-health.html): This federal government site provides many resources on health promotion and health prevention. It includes information on diseases and conditions, immunization and vaccines, and drug and health products.

Maternal–Newborn Nursing

In a woman's life, and within her family experiences, pregnancy and giving birth are profound, life-changing events influenced by many factors. These factors include the woman's health and well-being; her life experiences, beliefs, and culture; and the diverse Canadian society in which she lives. Family-centred maternal–newborn nursing reflects an evidence-informed practice that respects pregnancy and childbirth as a normal physiological event unique to each woman and her family.

This approach also acknowledges the complexity of the childbirth experience and the potential for health and social complications. Practical nurses respond by providing care through a collaborative relationship that is founded on respect and adaptation to the varied and changing needs of the family.

WELL-WOMAN CARE: HEALTH IN THE CHILD-BEARING YEARS

Although the child-bearing years begin with the onset of puberty and sexual maturation, a woman's lifetime supply of immature eggs is present in the ovaries at the time of her own birth. Puberty and menarche represent not only a time of rapid and multiple physical changes but also psychological and social development. Throughout a woman's child-bearing years, many health, societal, and personal issues will influence her decisions regarding sexual and reproductive choices and the lifestyle she chooses to live. Practical nurses need to consider the determinants of health in Canadian society, which also have an important influence on women's reproductive health and well-being.

Puberty

Physical sexual maturity and reproductive potential begin when the primary and secondary sexual characteristics develop during puberty in response to neuroendocrine hormonal changes. The timing of puberty varies widely, beginning about 2 years earlier for girls than for boys. For both, puberty is usually completed by the mid- to late teens. The psychological and cognitive developmental stages of adolescence also greatly affect an individual's identity and relationships with peers and family.

Female Manifestations

Between the ages of 8 and 14, the maturing brain begins to produce and secrete hormones that stimulate the ovaries and uterus of the young girl to mature in preparation for potential pregnancy. Growth hormones are also produced, which, over 3 to 4 years, bring about the characteristic physical changes in appearance and size that announce the transition from childhood into adolescence and early adulthood. These changes include the following:

- Reproductive changes—The uterus, ovaries, and vagina increase in size and blood supply, and hormones stimulate maturation of an ovum each month at the time of menarche. Menstruation may be irregular for the first year or two, and the first few menstrual cycles may be anovulatory (infertile). Ovulation marks the onset of fertility.
- The development of secondary sexual characteristics—Growth of pubic, leg, and axillae hair; breast development and growth; subcutaneous fat stores with characteristic curves and softness to body shape; sweat gland activity increases; and facial acne may develop.
- Skeletal changes—The pelvis widens, and there is sudden skeletal growth, with adult height typically reached at 2–2½ years after menarche.

Male Manifestations

Between the ages of 13 and 15, the maturing brain stimulates a marked increase in the production of androgens, the male sex hormones, especially testosterone. In boys, this stimulates the following changes:

- Reproductive changes—Testosterone stimulates sexual interest, the production of sperm, and the growth and maturation of the penis, scrotum, testes, prostate gland, and seminal vesicles. Onset of fertility begins with ejaculation of mature sperm and continues throughout life, with new sperm formed about every 10 weeks.
- The development of secondary sex characteristics—Increased body hair on the face, chest, axillae, and pubic area; thickening of the vocal cords and deepening of the voice; enlargement and thickening of the muscles; and increased sebaceous gland activity and acne formation take place.
- Skeletal and other physical changes—Rapid growth takes place in skeletal bones, including length and density, that continues until almost 18 or 20 years of age; widening of the shoulders, increased cellular metabolism, and increased red blood cell (RBC) production also takes place.

Nursing Considerations

There are many important nursing considerations in regard to these developmental stages. These considerations include the following:

- Provide factual, nonjudgemental information.
- Be aware that teenagers may obtain inaccurate information from peers and be reluctant to discuss their concerns with adults.
- Recognize that both girls and boys may have body-image conflicts as they naturally gain weight and experience body changes.
- Offer reassurance and clarification of normal variations in puberty changes.

Chapter 10 has more detailed information on adolescent growth and development.

The Menstrual Cycle

The female reproductive cycle begins at puberty and ends at menopause. It is composed of the ovarian and endometrial cycles or phases, which are influenced by hormones released by the brain. All work in unison in preparation for a potential pregnancy. If pregnancy does not occur, hormone levels decrease, menstruation occurs, and the cycle repeats. A cycle typically lasts 28 days, plus or minus 5 days, but may vary and last as long as 38 days. See Fig. 9.1 for an illustration of the menstrual cycle.

The Ovarian Cycle

Follicular phase. The follicular phase of the cycle occurs in the following sequence:

- The follicular phase occurs in the first half of the cycle, approximately 14 days prior to ovulation. In women who experience irregular menstrual cycles, the follicular phase varies in length.
- The anterior pituitary in the brain releases follicle-stimulating hormone (FSH) and luteinizing hormone (LH). FSH stimulates the ovarian follicle, and the immature oocyte grows. As the follicle matures, it releases estrogen. LH stimulates the final maturation of the follicle just prior to ovulation. A mature graafian follicle develops by the midpoint of the cycle under the influence of both FSH and LH.
- Under the influence of progesterone, body temperature increases 0.3°C to 0.6°C for 24–48 hours after the time of ovulation and remains elevated until menstruation begins.
- Ovulation usually occurs on the 14th day, or midpoint, of the cycle; the follicle ruptures, and the mature ovum is released.

Luteal phase. The luteal phase of the cycle occurs in the following sequence:

- The luteal phase begins when the ovum leaves the follicle, which occurs between day 15 and day 28 of a 28-day cycle.
- LH influences the development of the corpus luteum from the ruptured follicle. As it reaches a peak, estrogen levels drop, and progesterone secretion begins.
- When fertilization occurs, the corpus luteum is maintained until weeks 10–12 of the pregnancy; it secretes human chorionic gonadotropin (HCG), estrogen, and progesterone to maintain the pregnancy until the placenta is mature.
- If fertilization does not occur, the corpus luteum degenerates, causing a decrease in estrogen and progesterone hormone levels, and menstruation follows by day 28 of the cycle.

The Endometrial Cycle

The menstrual phase. The menstrual phase of the cycle occurs in the following sequence:

- The menstrual phase occurs during days 1–5, when estrogen and progesterone levels are low.
- Menstrual discharge or uterine blood loss is dark red and may contain small clots.

The proliferative phase. The proliferative phase of the cycle occurs in the following sequence:

- On days 7–14, the proliferative phase of the endometrium corresponds to the follicular phase of the ovary.
- Estrogen causes the endometrial lining of the uterus to thicken in anticipation of the implantation of a fertilized ovum, and the cervical mucus becomes more hospitable to sperm: clear, thin, elastic, and alkaline.
- Mittelschmerz (midcycle abdominal pain), midcycle spotting, or both may occur as the ovum is released from the follicle at the time of ovulation.

The secretory phase. The secretory phase of the cycle occurs in the following sequence:

- The secretory phase occurs on days 15–26, corresponding to the luteal phase of the ovary.
- Estrogen decreases as progesterone levels remain high and the vascularity of the endometrium and uterus increases. If fertilization and implantation occur, the endometrium remains thickened and continues to develop.

The ischemic phase. The ischemic phase of the cycle occurs in the following sequence:

- On days 27–28, if fertilization does not occur, the corpus luteum degenerates, and estrogen and progesterone levels fall. The endometrium becomes ischemic and pale as the vasculature constricts.

Nursing Considerations

It is important to be aware of and sensitive to religious and cultural beliefs that may affect practices and behaviours at the time of menstruation.

Client teaching points with regard to the menstrual cycle include the following:

- Basal body temperature and cervical mucus changes may be used to predict ovulation.
- Super-absorbent tampons should be used with caution; they are associated with the rare but serious condition of toxic shock syndrome.
- The best time for performing (and teaching) breast self-examination is following the menstrual phase, when hormonal levels are lowest.

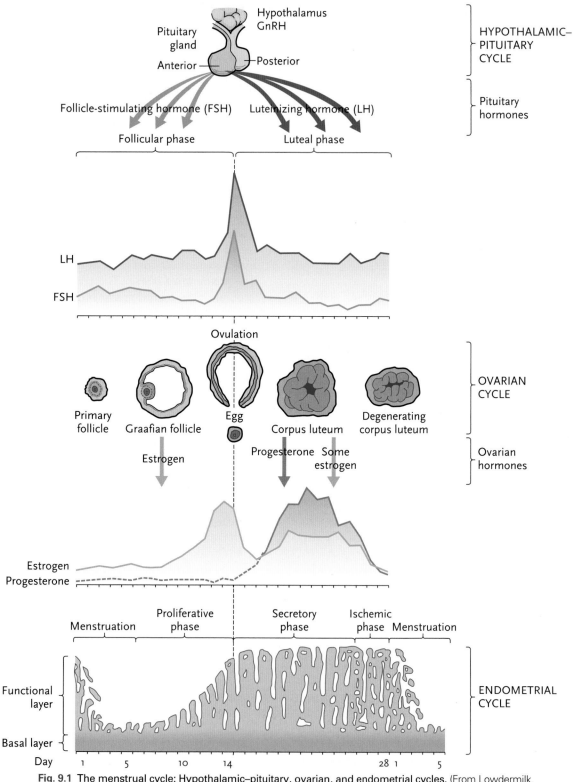

Fig. 9.1 The menstrual cycle: Hypothalamic–pituitary, ovarian, and endometrial cycles. (From Lowdermilk, D. L., Perry, S. E., Cashion, K., et al. [2016]. *Maternity & women's health care* [11th ed., p. 67, Figure 4-7]. St. Louis: Mosby.)

CANADIAN FAMILIES

No one definition or example can accurately describe a typical Canadian family. The concept of "family" encompasses many meanings and values, some of which are influenced by social circumstances, ethnicity, culture, and the belief systems of each family unit. Maternal–newborn nursing focuses on a family-centred approach. It is important for practical nurses to recognize and respect the diversity of family structures found within their communities and professional practices.

In addition to the traditional biological and legal definitions of family, in maternal–newborn nursing practice, the concept of family is identified by the social relationships that are personally significant and important to the woman. Understanding family within a framework that is broad and inclusive reflects an attitude of respect and responsiveness to the unique needs and structure of each family.

Family Diversity

In Canadian society, the diversity of maternal–newborn families is influenced by many factors, including culture, ethnicity, race, language, socio-economic status, maternal age, delayed child-bearing trends, employment of women outside the family home, social supports, community resources, and isolation from extended families and support (Health Canada, 2000c). Refer to the definitions in Box 9.1, which capture the diversity of family forms in Canada.

Principles of Providing Family-Centred Care

Health Canada's principles of family-centred care (Health Canada, 2000c) include the following:

- The process of pregnancy and birth is usually a normal, healthy, and unique experience for each woman and her family.
- Care is based on research evidence and directed at maximizing the probability of a healthy woman giving birth to a healthy baby.
- Relationships between healthcare providers, women, and their families are based on mutual respect and trust. Women are cared for within the context of their families; and within the childbirth experience, a woman defines her family and support system.
- To make informed choices, women and their families need knowledge about their care.
- Women have autonomy in decision making and are empowered to take responsibility.
- Healthcare providers have a powerful effect on women who are giving birth and their families. A woman's subjective experience is included in assessing the quality of care.
- Family-centred care includes many disciplines of practice, including nurses, midwives, physicians, doulas, and childbirth educators.
- Technology is used judiciously and appropriately and does not replace direct supportive care and observation.
- Language is important and should ease communication by conveying openness and appreciation for the importance of families (Health Canada, 2000c).

FAMILY COMPOSITION AND CHILDBIRTH TRENDS

National and regional trends in family composition and childbirth practices are relevant to maternal–newborn nursing as they influence the required resources, choices, needs, and even expectations of women and their families. The healthcare system and practical nurses who provide

---

BOX 9.1   Family Forms

Blended Family

Formed when both parents bring children from previous relationships into a new, joint living situation or when children from the current union and children from previous unions are living together

Extended Family

Includes the nuclear family and other relatives (perhaps grandparents, aunts, uncles, cousins)

Lone-Parent Family

Consists of one parent and one or more children. The lone-parent family is formed when one parent leaves the nuclear family because of death, divorce, or desertion or when a single person decides to have or adopt a child.

Step-Family

Formed when at least one child in a household is from a previous relationship of one of the parents

Traditional Nuclear Family

Consists of a mother and father (married or common-law) and their children

Family Forms—Increasing Diversity

Family forms and family relationships within Canada have become increasingly diverse. They include married and common-law couples without children, families in which grandparents provide care for their grandchildren, adults living alone, and same-sex couples (with or without children). The rates of traditional families (two married parents and children living together) in Canada is declining, while the proportion of common-law and lone-parent families is increasing. Today, the average Canadian household consists of 2.5 people, and for the first time in 2011, there were more one-person households (27.6%) (a number now totaling 28.2%, based on the 2016 Census*) than couple households with children (26.5%).[†] These changes hold significant societal implications. For instance, smaller families and more people living alone have led to an increasing need for affordable child care in Canada. Further, the care and support of young children or older Canadians is now spread among a decreasing number of family members.

*Statistics Canada. (2017). The shift to smaller households over the past century. Retrieved from http://www.statcan.gc.ca/pub/11-630-x/11-630-x2015008-eng.htm.
[†]Statistics Canada. (2017). 2016 Census topic: Families, households and marital status. Retrieved from http://www12.statcan.gc.ca/census-recensement/2016/rt-td/fam-eng.cfm.
From Potter, P. A., Perry, A. G., Stockert, P., et al. (2019). *Canadian fundamentals of nursing* (6th ed., Box 19-1). Milton, ON: Elsevier.

---

direct care must recognize and respond to the many significant changes taking place in Canadian families.

Changes in Canadian Families
Factors Influencing Canadian Families

- A lower birthrate across the country: The annual number of births continues to decline (Statistics Canada, 2018a).

- Delayed motherhood: In 2016, 45.9% of first-time mothers were aged 30 or older. Moreover, the number of women giving birth after the age of 40 has increased by 53% (Statistics Canada, 2016). An exception to this trend is Indigenous women: based on the 2006 census, a higher proportion of young Indigenous women tended to become teen mothers as compared with non-Indigenous women (Arriagada, 2016).
- Smaller families: Large families are now rare; the number of families with three or more children has decreased. In addition, families have, on average, 1.8 children (Battams, 2018).
- A decrease in married couples: Married couples remain the predominant family structure, although their number has declined over time (Statistics Canada, 2018b).
- A rise in common-law families: The number of common-law families has increased (Battams, 2018).
- A rise in same-sex families: The number of same-sex married and common-law families has risen significantly (Statistics Canada, 2017b). Many same-sex families have children through adoption, through donor insemination, or from previous heterosexual relationships.
- A rise in LGBTQ family building using assisted reproductive technologies (ART): There has been a significant increase within the lesbian, gay, bisexual, transgender, and queer (LGBTQ) community of those seeking out ART at infertility clinics to have children.
- A rise in step and blended families: Step and blended families have also increased over the past decade (Battams, 2018).
- A rise in the number of lone parents raising children: In 2016, 16% of all Canadian families were lone-parent families, compared with 11% in 1961. Women head 87% of these families. Male lone-parent families are also increasing (Battams, 2018).
- Changes in the Indigenous population and Indigenous families: In 2011, close to half of the Indigenous population in Canada was under the age of 25, compared with 30% of the non-Indigenous population (Kelly-Scott & Smith, 2015). The Indigenous population is experiencing rapid growth: from 2006 to 2016, the First Nations population grew by 39.3%, the Métis population grew by 51.2%, and the Inuit population grew by 29.1% (Statistics Canada, 2017a). The size of the Indigenous youth population living in urban areas, especially in Western Canada, has more than doubled in the last 20 years.

Childbirth Choices and Trends

Within the philosophy of family-centred care, families have many options and decisions to make when planning for prenatal care, the birth of the baby, and the family's postpartum transition. These plans include the following:

- Prenatal education and birth preferences—Community or private classes and programs, specialized programs such as Lamaze, breathing techniques, hypnosis, therapeutic touch, acupuncture, medication and pain control options and preferences

- Family participation—Identifying participants and their roles at each stage of the birth experience, attendance of the father or other support persons at childbirth classes and during labour and birth, the involvement of siblings and extended family members
- Healthcare setting—Deciding upon home birth, a birthing centre, a community hospital, or a high-risk pregnancy hospital
- Healthcare providers and support—Doula, registered or nonregistered midwife, family general practitioner, obstetrician, nurses, lactation consultant
- Postpartum—Breast- or formula feeding, circumcision, early discharge programs, in-home support and community follow-up, newborn and maternal assessment, family involvement

Nursing Considerations

Nursing considerations are many and include the following:
- Provide information on available pregnancy and birth choices in the community.
- Refer as appropriate to community and hospital resources.
- Consider and respect cultural beliefs and preferences when discussing choices with families.
- Recognize that when families are provided with current, accurate information regarding choices, they are the experts at understanding which options will best fit their beliefs, preferences, and needs.
- Provide support to families whose personal birth plans may require adaptation due to the need for specialized care or medical intervention.

Midwifery

Historically, midwifery has a long and respected role as a childbirth option for families. Midwives, often working in teams of two, provide holistic care for the woman and family throughout the pregnancy and birth process. Birth options may include hospital, clinic, or home-birth settings. Postpartum care and support is an integral part of midwifery practice.

Access to regulated midwifery care varies across Canada. Most provinces now offer publicly funded, legislated midwifery services. Midwives must be registered with the regulatory body/college in the province in order to legally work as midwives (Canadian Midwifery Regulators Council, 2017). The Canadian Association of Midwives (CAM) and various provincial groups continue to be active in raising public awareness and lobbying governments to provide this option to all Canadian families.

- Midwives collaborate with other healthcare providers, including nurses, as appropriate and as indicated by the needs of the mothers and families they care for.
- In 1994, Ontario became the first province to regulate and publicly fund midwives. Midwives are legislated under the *Regulated Health Professions Act* (RHPA).
- Midwifery as a legislated and regulated profession is currently available to families in British Columbia, Alberta, Saskatchewan, Manitoba, Ontario, Quebec, Nova Scotia,

Newfoundland, and the Northwest Territories (Canadian Association of Midwives, 2017).

- The National Aboriginal Health Organization (NAHO) continues to lobby for Indigenous midwifery to be recognized and supported as a safe and culturally sensitive birth option with a long and respected history within the Indigenous community (NAHO, 2012).
- In some parts of Canada, Indigenous midwives, trained in community-based programs, are exempt from midwifery regulations (NAHO, 2012).

ACCESS TO CARE: REGIONALIZATION

Regionalization of care refers to the coordination of the many facilities and professional services needed to provide optimal maternal–newborn care to families. Regions are catchment areas within defined geographical boundaries that are structured to provide all the necessary maternal–newborn services required for both uncomplicated and high-risk births. The provision of comprehensive services may be affected by challenges such as geography, funding constraints, and the availability of healthcare providers. Despite these challenges, advantages to regionalization include lower maternal and newborn morbidity and mortality rates, improved reproductive outcomes, and more efficient, economical utilization of facilities and personnel. Regionalization uses the principles of risk assessment and referral to provide access to the care that is appropriate to the needs of the mother, baby, and family at a location that is as close to their home as possible.

The Goals of Regionalization

The goals of regionalization are as follows:
- The provision of quality care for all women, newborns, and their families (preconception, pregnancy, birth, postpartum, newborn) and the provision of referral mechanisms
- The coordination of services, the appropriate use of personnel and facilities, the provision of professional education, and the incorporation of research and evaluation (Health Canada, 2000c)

Regional Care Levels

Three levels of care are directed at ambulatory prenatal care, labour and birth, and postpartum and newborn care.

Primary Level: Level 1

- It covers about 85% of pregnancies, identified as uncomplicated normal, including healthy mothers and newborns, of a pregnancy or gestational age of 36 weeks or older, and newborns weighing more than 2.5 kg.
- The facility and personnel are able to provide assessment, education, and monitoring of normal pregnancies, as well as identification of at-risk pregnancies with appropriate referrals.
- Personnel provide and manage immediate care for emergency maternal and newborn complications, including stabilization until support from and transportation to a level 2 or 3 facility are possible (Health Canada, 2000c).

Secondary Level: Level 2

- It covers about 12% of pregnancies, identified as having a low to moderate obstetrical or neonatal risk. It includes mothers with pregnancy greater than 32 weeks and newborns with gestational age greater than 32 weeks and weighing more than 1.5 kg.
- Intensive care services are available for mothers with obstetrical risks and complications. The facility is able to provide short-term (48 hours) assisted ventilation to newborns.
- It is able to provide immediate and ongoing care of newborns with problems expected to resolve quickly, as well as care of stabilized newborns transferred from level 3 facilities.
- Neonatology expertise and follow-up are available in the form of neonatologists and advanced practice clinical nurse specialists (Health Canada, 2000c).

Tertiary Level: Level 3

- It covers about 3% of pregnancies.
- It provides level 1 and 2 services and also manages and provides all services required for very high-risk, complicated pregnancies, births, and newborns.
- It includes intensive care services under the direction of neonatologists and advanced practice clinical nurse specialists, as well as specialized services and resources, including advanced diagnostics, specialty consultations, surgery, and follow-up care (Health Canada, 2000c).

FERTILITY CONTROL AND INFERTILITY HEALTH CHALLENGES

Fertility Control

More than any other time in history, women today have many options by which they can exercise control over the planning and prevention of pregnancies. Men, too, share in the responsibility for fertility control. Despite this, Canadian statistics show that even in stable relationships, 45–50% of pregnancies are unplanned.

In Canada, under the *Health Information Act*, minors can refuse to consent to the disclosure of information to their parent, including information on their use of birth control, as long as they have the mental capacity to make this decision (Office of the Information and Privacy Commissioner, 2001).

Each contraceptive method has associated advantages and disadvantages, and its success at preventing pregnancy varies. Birth control methods are most effective when used consistently and correctly all the time. Only total sexual abstinence is 100% effective in preventing pregnancy and the transmission of sexually transmitted infections (STIs). In educating women in making a choice of the best contraceptive method, several considerations must be taken into account:

- The woman's overall health status, sexual patterns and frequency, the number of sexual partners, if children are desired in the future, effectiveness, potential side effects and risks, and financial costs and availability

- Ease of use and comfort level with using the method
- Cultural beliefs and religious practices that may limit acceptable birth control options

Client teaching points on contraception:

- Most birth control methods *do not* offer protection from STIs such as human immunodeficiency virus (HIV), Chlamydia, herpes, or gonorrhea. The use of a male condom, known as *dual protection*, is recommended in addition to the primary method of birth control.
- Emergency hormonal contraceptive is available in Canada from a pharmacist without a medical prescription. It should be taken within 72 hours of unprotected sexual intercourse (MyHealth.Alberta.ca, 2018).
- Breastfeeding is *not* a reliable method of birth control unless the woman accurately uses the lactational amenorrhea method (LAM). LAM is not recommended in North America because most breastfeeding mothers do not maintain the required feeding patterns.

Common Methods of Contraception and Nursing Considerations

Fertility Awareness Methods

- Sexual intercourse is avoided on the seventh day or later, when a woman with regular menstrual cycles is fertile.
- Awareness, knowledge, and careful monitoring of menstrual patterns, cervical mucus changes, and basal body temperature changes are required. Effectiveness can be 80% when used with considerable knowledge, motivation, and consistency.

Male Condoms

- Male condoms can be purchased without a prescription; this is a barrier method that blocks the sperm from reaching the ovum and protects against HIV and STIs.
- Effectiveness is 85–98%, depending on correct use and early application during sexual activity. Condoms are most effective when used with a vaginal spermicide.
- Oil- and petroleum-based lubricants can cause latex to break down, resulting in the condom tearing or breaking. Only water-soluble lubricants should be used if needed. Condoms should be made from latex or polyurethane; animal- or natural-product condoms have micro-openings that can allow HIV to be transmitted.

Female Condoms

- Effectiveness is 80–90% with this barrier method.
- Female condoms can be inserted up to 24 hours in advance of sexual intercourse; they offer protection against HIV and STIs.

Oral Contraceptives

- Oral contraceptives are commonly known as "the pill" and are taken daily. The pill contains the hormones estrogen and progestin, which suppress the release of the ovum.

Effectiveness is 95–99%. The pill does not protect against HIV and STIs.

- Extended-cycle pills containing levonorgestrel/ethinylestradiol were approved in July 2007 by Health Canada and are taken for 12 consecutive weeks followed by 1 week of nonhormonal pills. This limits menstruation to four cycles per year, which can help manage endometriosis.
- Some antibiotics may interfere with effectiveness. Women who are prescribed antibiotics should be advised to use an additional method of birth control.
- In the province of Quebec, registered nurses may prescribe oral contraceptives to teenagers without a medical prescription or parental consent (Jelowicki, 2015).
- Women over 35 years of age or who smoke may be advised to choose an alternative method of birth control to minimize the known risks of high blood pressure, blood clots, and arterial blockage. The pill may be contraindicated in women with a history of blood clots or breast, liver, or endometrial cancers.

The "Mini" Oral Contraceptive

- The "mini-pill" contains only the hormone progestin and acts by thickening the cervical mucus so that sperm cannot reach the egg. In addition, if the egg does become fertilized, it is prevented from implanting in the uterine wall.
- The mini-pill may be an option for those women who cannot take estrogen-based contraceptives.
- Effectiveness is 92–99%, but only if taken at the same time each day.

Intrauterine Devices (IUDs)

- The device is placed inside the uterus, preventing sperm from reaching the egg, the implantation of the fertilized egg, or both. The device may use copper or the hormone progesterone as an active ingredient to prevent pregnancy.
- Effectiveness is 98–99%. The device can offer up to 5 years of protection.

Depo-Provera

- This is an injection of the hormone progestin given every 3 months. Its effectiveness is 97%.
- Use of medroxyprogesterone (Depo-Provera) has been associated with loss of bone mineral density that may not be completely reversible. It is to be used for the shortest time period possible (Pfizer, 2018).

Diaphragm, Cervical Cap

- These are barrier methods, used with spermicidal gel or foam prior to sexual intercourse. Both must be properly fitted to cover the cervix; if used correctly, they can be 85–91% effective.
- They must be left in place 6–8 hours after intercourse to prevent pregnancy and be removed no later than 24 hours after intercourse.

Surgical Sterilization

- Tubal ligation prevents the egg from reaching the fallopian tube and uterus and is a permanent method of birth control with 99.9% effectiveness.
- Vasectomy, with 99% permanent effectiveness, involves ligation, the removal of a piece of the vas deferens, or both, thereby eliminating sperm from the semen.

Emergency Contraception

- Emergency contraception is also referred to as the "morning-after pill." Hormones interfere with ovulation, and possibly implantation, preventing pregnancy from occurring. This pill can be used up to 72 hours after unprotected intercourse or contraceptive failure such as a broken condom, providing 75% effectiveness.
- This contraception is sold in Canada under the name "Plan B" and is available from pharmacists without a medical prescription.
- This pill does not prevent the transmission of HIV or STIs.
- Side effects may include nausea, vomiting, irregular vaginal bleeding, fatigue, headache, breast tenderness, and dizziness (MyHealth.Alberta.ca, 2018).

Pregnancy Termination Through Induced Abortion

While induced abortions are legal in Canada and many countries in the world, they continue to be a source of controversy among those with strongly opposing views based on moral, religious, and ethical beliefs. Pregnancies may be ended by medical or surgical means depending on the gestational age, with the majority occurring in the first trimester of pregnancy. Factors influencing a woman's decision to choose to have an abortion may include the following:

- Contraceptive failure
- Diseases or a life-threatening medical condition affecting the mother or fetus
- Psychosocial factors, including distress due to the timing and circumstances of the pregnancy

Medical Abortion

Medical abortions are available up to 9 weeks' gestation using methotrexate and misoprostol (Cytotec).

Surgical Abortion

- First trimester surgical methods include dilatation and curettage (D & C), vacuum suction or aspiration, and vacuum curettage.
- Second trimester surgical methods include dilatation and extraction, systemic or intrauterine prostaglandins, and intrauterine hypertonic saline administration.
  Risks and side effects of surgical abortion include cramping, bleeding, perforation of the uterus, and laceration to the cervix.

Nursing Considerations

- Be aware of your own beliefs regarding elective induced abortion.
- Know the applicable and relevant rules and guidelines of the nursing regulatory body for your province or territory regarding providing nursing care for clients seeking or undergoing elective abortions.
- Provide accurate information regarding side effects to be expected following the abortion, including cramping, bleeding, and pain.
- Provide emotional support throughout and possibly request a referral by a physician or nurse practitioner for follow-up psychological support and possible contraceptive planning.

Infertility

Infertility, which affects 10–20% of couples trying to conceive, is diagnosed when pregnancy does not occur following a year without contraception. Primary infertility refers to a couple who has never conceived. Secondary infertility describes a couple who experiences fertility problems after having at least one previous conception. Sterility is an absolute inability to conceive. Many infertility issues may respond to interventions. The psychological impact on the couple dealing with infertility must not be underestimated and can be extremely challenging.

Female Infertility Factors

Female infertility factors include the following:

- Age—Delaying child-bearing until age 30 and beyond may lead to corresponding lowered fertility.
- Weight—Excessive weight gain or loss can decrease fertility levels.
- Reproductive organs—Tubal obstructions, cervical stenosis, infections, especially with pelvic inflammatory disease, scarring of the uterus, congenital anomalies, uterine fibroids, inhospitable cervical mucus, in utero exposure to diethylstilbestrol (DES), polycystic ovarian syndrome, antibodies to partner's sperm, and endometriosis can contribute to infertility.
- Endocrine disorders—Abnormal hormone production in the hypothalamus, anterior pituitary, ovary, thyroid, or adrenal glands can contribute to infertility.
- Unknown causes—Ten to 15 percent of female infertility is due to unknown causes.

Male Infertility Factors

Male factors account for 35–40% of infertility causes. Male infertility factors include the following:

- Social factors—Prolonged bicycling, hot tubs, malnutrition, or trauma can decrease fertility levels.
- Environmental factors—Testicular radiation, heavy marijuana, cocaine, or alcohol use can contribute to infertility.
- Reproductive organs—Congenital anomalies, hypospadias, varicocele, cryptorchidism, infections, STIs, retrograde ejaculation, ejaculatory failure, impaired circulation, diabetes, obstructions, and faulty spermatogenesis can contribute to infertility.
- Endocrine disorders—Cushing's syndrome, pituitary tumour, or acromegaly can contribute to infertility.

- Unknown causes—Ten percent of male infertility is due to unknown causes.

Diagnostic Assessment

Diagnostic assessments include the following:

- Complete health and reproductive history, respecting individual confidentiality issues
- Physical examination, which may also include tests for anatomical abnormalities, tubal patency, endometrial biopsy, transvaginal ultrasonography, laparoscopy to evaluate peritoneal factors, a postcoital examination of cervical mucus and the quantity and quality of sperm present, and basal body temperature monitoring
- Analysis of semen: Volume, sperm count, motility
- Laboratory assessment for STIs and infections, hormonal analysis of endocrine and ovarian function, ovulation predictor kits or LH surge kits to detect ovulation

Therapeutics

Therapeutic interventions for infertility are directed at the underlying cause or causes.

Male factors.

- Sperm washing and assisted intrauterine insemination, use of donor sperm, antibiotic treatment for infections, androgen (testosterone) hormone therapy
- Referral to a urologist for treatment of reparable structural disorders

Female factors.

- Surgery for tubal occlusions, pelvic adhesions, fibroids, or reparable structural abnormalities
- Pharmacological therapy is often directed toward treating ovulatory dysfunction

Assisted reproductive technologies (ARTs).

These technologies include any therapeutic intervention in which the sperm, eggs, or both are managed outside the body. There are several techniques, and the use of donor sperm and eggs may be part of the intervention. National guidelines have been established to regulate the process. There has been an increase in the use of assisted reproduction services by the LGBTQ community (Best Start Resource Centre, 2012).

Often multiple steps are required to prepare the woman's body for ART interventions. The medications used may have several adverse effects.

Nursing Considerations

- Psychological support and counselling are essential when managing fertility problems as infertility issues are often accompanied by feelings of helplessness, frustration, and grief.
- Women need to be informed of and closely monitored for side effects and risks when undergoing hormonal therapies and ART interventions. Maternal and fetal morbidity and mortality rates in pregnancy, birth, and postpartum are higher for ART interventions.
- It is important to be sensitive to the language used during the ART process when working with LGBTQ clients.

NORMAL PREGNANCY

A woman's body undergoes tremendous physiological changes as it adapts to the demands of supporting a pregnancy. This major life event inevitably also brings many developmental and psychosocial adjustments as roles and relationships change within a family. Whether in antenatal community health settings or labour birthing rooms, nurses play a significant role in educating and supporting a woman and her family during this profoundly important event.

Conception, Fertilization, and Implantation

The sequencing of these stages includes the following:

- At the time of ovulation, the ovum is released and swept up by cilia in the ampulla of the fallopian tube. The ovum is fertile and viable for about 24 hours after ovulation.
- Spermatozoa are viable and optimally fertile for 24 hours postejaculation, although they may survive and remain mobile in the cervical mucus for 2–3 days. Although 200–500 million sperm may be contained in the ejaculate, only one will penetrate and fertilize the ovum. Prostaglandins in the semen stimulate uterine smooth muscle contractions and help propel the sperm to the fallopian tube, where fertilization commonly takes place.
- Capacitation—Enzymes in the sperms' heads are released, changing the outer coating of the ovum to allow one sperm to penetrate the ovum.
- Zonal reaction—Once a sperm has penetrated the ovum, cellular changes occur on the ovum's surface membrane, preventing other sperm from entering.
- At the time of fertilization, the nuclei of the sperm and ovum fuse, and the 23 chromosomes from each combine to restore the diploid number of 46. Sex is determined by the 23rd pair of chromosomes, the male contributing either an X chromosome for an XX (female) or a Y chromosome for an XY (male) chromosome pair.

Chromosomal disorders may or may not be linked to hereditary causes. Hazards such as radiation or chemical exposure may also cause chromosomal defects.

Multiple Pregnancy

A multiple pregnancy occurs naturally in about one in 80 pregnancies. It arises from two different processes:

- Monozygotic or identical twins occur due to the spontaneous division of one fertilized ovum early in development.
- Dizygotic or fraternal twins occur when two or more separate ova are fertilized by two or more different spermatozoa. Fetuses have separate placentas and individual chromosomal genotypes.

ART fertility treatments may produce multiple fertilized ova. The Society of Obstetricians and Gynaecologists of Canada (SOGC) currently recommends implantation of no more than two or three zygotes, depending on maternal age and reproductive status, due to the increased maternal–fetal morbidity and mortality risks (Min, Claman, & Hughes, 2006).

Embryonic and Fetal Development

Development is divided into three stages: the ovum, embryonic, and fetal stages. The amniotic cavity provides a climate-controlled environment for the developing fetus. The placenta is a key structure with multiple functions. As the uterus receives 10% of the maternal cardiac output, anything that impairs uteroplacental circulation will adversely affect the fetus. Knowledge of this relationship is crucial for nurses when assessing risk factors for maternal–fetal well-being.

Ovum Stage

The ovum stage lasts from conception to day 14. It is characterized by cellular division, formation of the blastocyst and beginnings of the embryonic membranes, and differentiation of the primary germ layers.

- The two-celled zygote continues to undergo mitotic cellular division (also known as *cleavage*) while travelling through the fallopian tube toward the uterine cavity.
- With each mitotic division, two-, four-, and eight-celled groups called *blastomeres* form until a solid ball of 16 cells called a *morula* reaches the uterus and prepares to implant into the uterine wall.
- Inside the morula, development continues as a solid inner mass of cells called the *blastocyst* forms. This marks the first important differentiation from which specific structures will develop, including the embryo, which will develop into a fetus.
- Implantation occurs 7–10 days after fertilization, as chorionic villi on the blastocyst implant into the top one-third of the fundus of the uterine wall.
- Following implantation, the endometrium is now called the *decidua*.
- The chorionic villi then secrete the hormone HCG, maintaining the corpus luteum until the placenta develops enough to take over hormone production. HCG is the hormone detected in pregnancy testing.
- The primary germ layers form (ectoderm, mesoderm, and endoderm), from which all tissues and organs will develop.
- The ectoderm is the source of the central and peripheral nervous systems, sensory epithelium, tooth enamel, nails and hair, and lens of the eye.
- The mesoderm produces the skeletal bones and cartilage, muscles, connective tissue, cardiovascular and reproductive systems, kidneys, and spleen.
- The endoderm's lower layer forms the pancreas, liver, bladder, epithelial lining of the respiratory tract, and vagina.

Embryonic Stage

The embryonic stage lasts from gestational day 15 until the embryo reaches a crown-to-rump length of 3 cm, or approximately to the end of the eighth week. This is a critical time of development of all organ systems and external body features and a high-risk time for teratogenic substances to interfere with and harm organ and tissue development.

- From the blastocyst, the amnion (innermost layer) and chorion (outermost layer) membranes form to protect the developing embryo.
- The amnion continues to grow, enclosing the developing embryo in a protective, fluid-filled cavity.
- The chorion becomes the fetal side of the placenta and contains the umbilical blood vessels—two arteries and one vein—surrounded by Wharton's jelly connective tissue.

Fetal Stage

This stage begins at week 9 and lasts until birth or the end of the pregnancy. Major developmental milestones are outlined in Table 9.1, and high-risk critical times of development are depicted in Fig. 9.2.

Amniotic Fluid

- Amniotic fluid is derived initially from maternal blood filtrates and eventually consists mostly of fetal urine. Normal volume is 500 mL to a maximum of 1 000 mL.
- Oligohydramnios is a volume of less than 300 mL, which impairs fetal movement and symmetrical growth and may be associated with fetal abnormalities, and if prolonged, does not allow for normal alveoli development.
- Polyhydramnios is a volume greater than 1.5–2 L and is also associated with fetal abnormalities.
- The amniotic fluid functions to control temperature, protect the fetus from trauma, and allow symmetrical growth, fetal breathing, and motor movements.

The Placenta

- The placenta is structurally complete by week 12 gestation; it continues to grow and expand until 20 weeks.
- Fetal and maternal blood are independent, although separated only by a thin layer of cells.
- Functions include gas exchange, heat transfer, antibody transfer, transportation of nutrients, excretion of metabolic wastes, and hormone production essential for maintaining the pregnancy.
- Most substances are of a molecular size that allows for transfer across the maternal circulation and into the fetal circulation. This can include protective maternal immunoglobulins but also harmful antibodies, viruses, most drugs, and other external teratogenic substances, including alcohol, nicotine, caffeine, and cocaine.
  Hormone production.
- Estrogen is a steroid that stimulates growth of the uterus and breast tissue, increases in amount as the pregnancy reaches term, and helps stimulate uterine muscle contractility, thereby helping to stimulate the onset of labour.
- Progesterone is a protective hormone that may help maintain the pregnancy by decreasing uterine contractility. It also decreases smooth muscle contractions in maternal circulation and helps maintain the endometrium.
- HCG is detected by pregnancy tests, found in maternal serum and urine 8–10 days postconception, and maintains the function of the corpus luteum until the placenta is fully developed.

TABLE 9.1   Essentials of Fetal Development by Pregnancy Trimester

FIRST TRIMESTER	SECOND TRIMESTER	THIRD TRIMESTER
Up to 12 Weeks' Gestation	**13–24 Weeks' Gestation**	**25–40 Weeks' Gestation**
Weight: 45 g Heart beats at 28 days; fetal circulation complete; fetal heartbeat (FHB) heard by Doppler; all body organs are formed; differentiation of sex glands; sex determination possible; fingers and toes are distinct; face appears human; eyelids closed; tooth buds appear; skin pink and smooth; palate has developed and closed; outlines of bones visible on ultrasonogram; lungs acquire shape; kidneys produce urine, contribute to amniotic fluid; able to move limbs.	Weight: 60–780 g By 16 weeks, there is rapid growth; transparent skin; blood vessels visible; active movements present; sucking motions; meconium produced; sweat glands developing; skeletal system obvious. At 20 weeks, mother feels fetal movement ("quickening"); lung alveoli appear; surfactant begins production; respiratory movements occur, called *fetal breathing movements* (FBM); eyes are closed; there is rapid growth. By 24 weeks, eyebrows and lashes are formed; skin is red, wrinkled; there is little subcutaneous fat; fingerprints, footprints are present; vernix covers the body; lanugo is abundant; myelination of the spinal cord begins; fetal suck and swallow reflexes are present; peristalsis begins; teeth form; grasp reflex is present.	Weight: 900–3 500 g By 28 weeks, weight 1200 g; eyes open and close; gas exchange possible; two-thirds of final size; testes descend; nervous system begins some regulation; germinal matrix of brain rich in blood, increasing risk of bleeding if born now. By 32 weeks, weight 2000 g; central nervous system regulation rapidly developing, bones fully developed; iron stores begin; subcutaneous fat stores develop; skin less wrinkled and red; pupils react to light. By 35 weeks, lung surfactant peaks, signalling lung maturity; lanugo and vernix decrease. By 38 to 40 weeks, the pregnancy is considered full term.

Fig. 9.2 Critical periods in human prenatal development. (From Moore, K., & Persaud, T. [2008]. *Before we were born: Essentials of embryology and birth defects* [7th ed. p. 313, Figure 19-11]. Philadelphia: Saunders.)

- Human placental lactogen (HPL) is a growth-type hormone that supports fetal growth by stimulating maternal metabolism and increasing the transport of glucose to the fetus. It also prepares the breasts for milk production and lactation.

Uteroplacental Circulation

- The uterus receives 10% of maternal cardiac output by the end of the pregnancy.
- Anything that adversely affects maternal circulation will impair placental function and put the fetus at risk.

Uterine blood flow.

- Uterine blood flow is decreased by maternal hypotension, supine hypotensive disorder, prolonged labour contractions, and vigorous or prolonged cardio exercises.
- Uterine blood flow is increased by maternal positioning to a left or right lateral position.

Nursing Considerations

- Key considerations:
  - Normal placental function depends almost entirely on normal maternal circulation. Any health conditions that decrease maternal circulation may adversely affect placental function.
  - Blood flow is decreased by maternal vasoconstriction related to diabetes, hypertension, either chronic or pregnancy induced (PIH), vasopressor medications, nicotine, and cocaine.
- Assess the learning needs of families and provide resources for understanding fetal growth and development. Assess the need for genetic counselling based on family history or teratogenic exposure and refer as appropriate.
- Teach the mother measures by which to maximize uteroplacental circulation throughout her pregnancy: avoiding unsupported supine position, following treatment plans for medical and circulatory problems, utilizing a left or right lateral sleeping and resting position, and avoiding excessive or prolonged cardio exercise practices.
- Be aware that maternal elevated core body temperature or a fever of 38.5°C or higher may increase the risk of harm in embryological development. Teach the mother the balance between benefits and risks regarding avoiding excessive body temperature overheating. For example, hot tubs and saunas should be avoided, especially during the sensitive embryonic development stage, to protect the embryo. Reducing fever with medications such as acetaminophen (Tylenol) is a safely used fever reduction practice, even in pregnancy.

Calculating Length of Pregnancy

- The length of a pregnancy is calculated from the first day of the last menstrual period (or cycle) (LMP). It can be described as approximately 280 days, 40 weeks, 9 calendar months, or 10 lunar months. Nine calendar months are divided into three trimesters of 3 months each.
- Term refers to the normal length of a pregnancy, with labour and birth occurring between 38 and 42 weeks' gestation. Preterm refers to labour and birth between 20 and 37 weeks' gestation. Post-term is labour and birth after 42 weeks' gestation.
- Naegle's rule—The estimated date of confinement (EDC, that is, labour and birth) is calculated as follows: EDC = LMP + 7 days − 3 months + 1 year.

Key Terms Related to Pregnancy

- *Gravida* is a woman who is pregnant.
- *Nulligravida* is a woman who has never been pregnant.
- *Primigravida* is a woman who is pregnant for the first time.
- *Multigravida* is a woman who has been pregnant more than once.
- *Viability* refers to an infant sufficiently developed enough to live outside the womb, technically after 20 weeks' gestation or weighing more than 500 g. True viability is more realistic after 23–24 weeks' gestation and would still require neonatal intensive care support.
- *Para* is a woman who has given birth after 20 weeks' gestation. The outcome or number of infants born is not taken into account.
- *Nullipara* is a woman who has not given birth to an infant of viable age. Note that the woman may have been pregnant but may have had a spontaneous abortion (miscarriage) or induced abortion.
- *Primipara* is a woman who has given birth at more than 20 weeks' gestation, regardless of outcome and regardless of how many infants were born (e.g., twins count as one para event).
- *Multipara* is a woman who has had two or more viable births.
- *TPAL* (*t*erm, *p*reterm, *a*bortions, *l*iving) is a more accurate way of describing parity and outcome.

  See the section "Labour and Birth Processes" for additional key terms.

PRECONCEPTION

Ideally, women of child-bearing age should have preconception access to information and health practices that will increase the likelihood of a healthy pregnancy. To improve healthy outcomes and lower risk factors, pregnancy health promotion should take place in the classroom, the public media, and any healthcare setting before a pregnancy is planned or occurs. Practical nurses, by virtue of their wide range of professional practice settings, are ideally situated to assess and support women in all stages of pregnancy planning and care.

Antenatal Health Assessment

This assessment includes nursing assessment, teaching, support, and referral in the following areas identified by Health Canada as variables that influence pregnancy outcomes (Health Canada, 2000b):

- Social support—Factors include life stressors, economic status, stability of housing and accommodations, employment, community resources, quality and nature of relationships and available support, and family support.
- Abuse and violence—There is an increased incidence of violence in intimate relationships during pregnancy.
- Female genital mutilation (FGM)—The diversity of the Canadian population and the worldwide prevalence of this cultural practice mean that nurses may provide counselling and care to women who have undergone FGM, despite the practice being banned in Canada.
- Lifestyle practices—The type and amount of exercise and activity, as well as tobacco, alcohol, and medicinal and nonmedicinal drug use, are identified as potentially

adverse lifestyle practices; support, education, and resources are provided.

- Exposure to environmental chemicals and toxic hazards—Previous and current exposure is identified, including exposure in home, recreational settings, and the workplace. Hazardous substances include anaesthetic gases, radiation, lead, and pesticides.
- Health history—Factors include past medical and family history, especially cardiovascular disease, diabetes, congenital disorders, genetic family history, STIs, past illnesses and hospitalizations, chronic conditions, mental health, bleeding disorders, surgeries, partner's health history, and family mortality and causes.
- Current health status—Factors include weight, age, occupation, current medications and herbal supplements, allergies, teratogenic exposure or risks, chronic conditions, nutrition and dietary patterns, and immunizations, especially rubella and varicella.
- Socio-cultural factors—They include cultural, spiritual or religious, and ethnic considerations and practices and language barriers.
- Pregnancy plans—Factors include pregnancy and birth plan preferences, education, and family involvement and roles.
- Psychological factors—They include psychological readiness for pregnancy, attitudes toward this pregnancy (e.g., excitement, ambivalence, anxiety, emotionally labile).
- Gynecological and reproductive history—Factors include age at menarche, STIs or other infections, menstrual cycle, last Pap smear, contraceptive history, infertility, past pregnancies, postpartum depression, TPAL, breastfeeding history, complications of past pregnancies or births, prenatal education, blood type, and Rh factor.
- Current pregnancy—This includes calculating the first day of LMP; pregnancy test results, if known; weight gain; discomforts of pregnancy or complications such as spotting, cramping, or bleeding; any medications, vitamins, or supplements; attitude regarding this pregnancy; and family and support system.

High-Risk Pregnancy Screening

High-risk pregnancy screening identifies health and social issues that may adversely affect the mother or fetus during the pregnancy, labour, and birth. Early identification of these factors provides an opportunity to monitor, intervene, or make referrals promptly, thereby providing the best chance for a healthy pregnancy outcome.

Many provincial and territorial health systems utilize standardized antenatal risk screening assessment profiles to identify those at risk and needing referral for specialized monitoring or care. The assessment tool is completed at the first prenatal visit and updated at each visit. For example, pregnancy risk levels may be differentiated and defined as a healthy pregnancy with no predictable risk, a pregnancy at risk, or a pregnancy at high risk.

Social risk factors. There are many social risk factors, including the following:

- Low socio-economic status and education level, housing problems, and social isolation
- Living in a high-altitude geographical location
- Extremes in weight—Obesity (greater than 90 kg) or extreme underweight (less than 46 kg)
- Extremes in age—Adolescent (younger than 16 years) or mature (older than 35 years)
- Lifestyle—Alcohol, tobacco, or recreational drug use
- Exposure to occupational or environmental hazards or toxin exposure, past or present (Health Canada, 2000a)

Reproductive health risk factors.

- Past or pre-existing conditions: Cardiovascular disease, diabetes, thyroid disorders, blood or bleeding disorders, blood incompatibility or Rh sensitization, renal disease, mental health disorders, and congenital or genetic disorders
- Past and current obstetrical complications with pregnancy or birth: DES exposure; ectopic pregnancy; cervical insufficiency (premature dilation of cervix); surgeries; stillbirths; Caesarean births; premature or prolonged rupture of membranes; multiple gestation; STIs or other infections, especially rubella, cytomegalovirus (CMV), herpes, and syphilis; abruption or placenta previa; PIH; or gestational diabetes
- Fetal or past neonatal complications of morbidity or mortality: Prematurity or postmaturity, teratogen exposure, small for gestational age (SGA) or large for gestational age (LGA), or fetal compromise

Initial Prenatal Physical Examination

In addition to a detailed history, the physical examination will include vital signs, height, weight, weight gain, pelvic examination, including assessment of pelvic type and adequacy, and breast examination.

Initial Laboratory Assessment

- Blood work entails a complete blood count (CBC); ABO and Rh typing; screening for syphilis, HIV, gonorrhea, and CMV; rubella titre; hepatitis B screening; glucose; screening for sickle cell disease if parent is of African descent; and screening for thalassemia trait if parent is of Mediterranean descent
- Urinalysis
- Pap smear

Danger Signs of Pregnancy

At any time during the pregnancy, the following signs and symptoms should be reported at once:

- Cramping and uterine contractions, vaginal spotting or bleeding
- Persistent vomiting
- Painful, frequent urination or oliguria
- Temperature above 38°C
- Persistent or severe headache, edema of hands or face, dizziness, muscle irritability, epigastric pain related to PIH
- Unusual pain, especially abdominal or uterine pain, absence of fetal movement

- Signs of preterm or impending labour—Rupture of membranes, bloody show, uterine contractions that are regular and increasing in intensity and duration, expulsion of mucous plug

Nursing Considerations

- Key client teaching point:
  - Teach the mother the danger signs and symptoms of pregnancy that should be reported immediately. Provide health teaching for immediate interventions.
- Create an interview atmosphere that ensures privacy, safety, and sensitivity to encourage honest, open communication and responses. Ask direct questions, especially regarding abuse and risk factors for abuse.
- Provide information and refer to community and professional services for any identified preconception and antenatal risks, including information about antenatal screening procedures and rationales for testing.
- Advise that moderate exercise appears advantageous if already part of a women's prepregnancy lifestyle. Emphasize the avoidance of hot tubs, saunas, or strenuous, prolonged activity, which may cause overheating.

PERINATAL ASSESSMENT AND CARE

Health Assessment in Normal Pregnancy

Routine health assessment for a normal pregnancy is performed according to the following schedule:

- Every 4 weeks until 28 weeks' gestation
- Every 2 weeks until 36 weeks' gestation
- Thereafter, every week until birth of the infant

Routine assessment includes physical assessment, maternal weight and weight gain patterns, adjustment to pregnancy, discomforts of pregnancy, presence of edema, nutritional assessment, family life and psychosocial status, vital signs, urine testing, fundal height and uterine growth, fetal heart rate (FHR), and a pelvic examination at 36 weeks' gestation to assess for signs of impending labour. For biophysical profile scoring, see Table 9.2.

Laboratory and Maternal Screening

- Urinalysis for protein, glucose, ketones; trace glucose may reflect normal alterations to renal function in pregnancy
- Glucose tolerance testing at 24–28 weeks' gestation if there is excessive glucose in urine or a history of diabetes or gestational diabetes
- Indirect Coombs test on Rh-negative women at 28 weeks to assess for Rh sensitization
- Fetal ultrasonogram at 16–18 weeks
- Group B *Streptococcus* (GBS) at 35–37 weeks' gestation
- Maternal CBC at 28 weeks' gestation to assess for anemia

Expected Physical Assessment Findings in Normal Pregnancy

Vital Signs

- Temperature: 36.5–37.5°C
- Heart rate: 60 to 90 bpm; heart rate may increase by 10 bpm due to cardiovascular adaptations
- Blood pressure: 90–120/60–80 mm Hg, with a decrease in the second trimester due to smooth muscle relaxation of blood vessels

Fetal Heart Rate and Movement

- 110–160 bpm
- Detected at 10–12 weeks by Doppler ultrasonography, 16–20 weeks by stethoscope

Fundal Height

After 20–22 weeks' gestation, fundal height in centimetres for a woman of average weight corresponds approximately to the gestational age in weeks. Individual differences in growth make this inaccurate after 36 weeks' gestation.

Weight Gain

Women of normal prepregnancy weight (body mass index [BMI] 18.5–24.9) can expect to gain an average of 11.5–16 kg (25–35 lb.) during a 40-week pregnancy. According to Health Canada's *Prenatal Nutrition Guidelines for Health*

TABLE 9.2   Biophysical Profile

Biophysical Variable	Adequate Score (Score = 2)	Inadequate Score (Score = 0)
Nonstress test	2 accelerations in 20 minutes, 15 beats above baseline lasting 15 seconds	<2 accelerations in 20 minutes
Fetal breathing movements	≥1 episodes of rhythmic fetal breathing of ≥20 seconds within 30 minutes	<30 seconds of sustained fetal breathing movements
Fetal movements	≥2 discrete body/limb movements in 20 minutes of observation*	<2 episodes of fetal movement
Fetal tone	≥1 Episode of active extension with rapid return to flexion of fetal limb(s), trunk, or hand	Either slow extension with return to partial flexion or movement of limb in full extension or absent fetal movement
Amniotic fluid volume	Single pocket of fluid present measuring ≥2 cm in a vertical axis†	Evidence of decreased amniotic fluid or oligohydramnios†

*Simultaneous limb and trunk movements are considered one movement.
†Some protocols use a single-pocket measurement, and some use the amniotic fluid index: ≤5.0 = oligohydramnios; 5.1–8 = low normal; 8.1–24 = normal; >24 = polyhydramnios.
From Blackburn, S. T. (2018). *Maternal, fetal, and neonatal physiology: A clinical perspective* (5th ed.). St. Louis: Saunders.

Professionals, gestational weight gain is based on preconception BMI (Health Canada, 2010a). In addition to the fetal weight, expected increases in weight are due to increased blood volume, reproductive tissue growth (especially uterine growth), as well as the placenta, amniotic fluid, and products of conception.

The weight gain for the average BMI weight is as follows:
- First trimester—Approximately 1–2 kg (2–4 lb.), almost all of which is due to maternal physiological changes and growth
- Second and third trimester—On average, 0.4 kg (1.0 lb.) per week

Nursing Considerations

- Key consideration:
  - Weight gain of more than 1 kg (2 lb.) in 1 week may be a sign of excess fluid retention or hypertension and should be assessed further.
- Quickening or maternal awareness of fetal movement occurs at around 20 weeks' gestation, earlier in multiparas.
- Higher than expected fundal height may be related to polyhydramnios, or multiple gestation.
- Lower than expected fundal height may be due to oligohydramnios, a fetus that is SGA, and/or intrauterine growth restriction.
- Women may need to be reassured regarding body image and weight gain fears and be made aware of the risks of excessive weight gain or being underweight.
- Women should be aware that the varied and changing emotional responses to pregnancy are normal and expected. Encourage discussion between partners regarding feelings of ambivalence, uncertainty, and insecurities regarding changing roles and body image. These feelings are an expected part of adapting to a major life change. If feelings continue beyond the first trimester to be a source of distress or conflict, encourage and offer resources and referral to appropriate counselling services. Also promote childbirth preparation classes in a group setting for health information and peer support.

Physical and Physiological Adaptations to Pregnancy

In order for the woman's body to accommodate the demands of a pregnancy, all body systems undergo normal changes. While the reproductive system undergoes the most significant and noticeable changes, all body systems adapt as necessary.

Reproductive System Changes

Reproductive body system changes are as follows:
- Uterus—There is increased growth, elasticity, and enlargement of pre-existing muscles; and increased vascularity and blood supply (10% of cardiac output by term). Irregular Braxton Hicks contractions provide regulatory blood flow to placenta and are felt after the second trimester.
- Cervix—It becomes softer (Goodell's sign), shorter (especially as term approaches), and closed by a protective mucous plug; increased vascularity makes it appear cyanotic on a prenatal examination (Chadwick's sign).
- Ovaries—They may be enlarged on palpation in the first trimester due to hormone-producing corpus luteum.
- Vagina—There is an increase in vascularity, elasticity, and secretions, and the pH changes to alkaline with added risk of infections.
- Perineum—There is increased vascularity (Chadwick's sign) and hypertrophy of tissues.
- Breasts—There is greater sensitivity, increased vascularity with more prominent veins, increased size of periareolar glands and areola, and increased pigmentation in response to increased melanin production.

Cardiovascular System Changes

Significant changes occur in the cardiovascular system as the body supports the added blood volume, flow, and transportation demands:
- Blood volume and flow—Blood volume increases 30–45% as plasma volume peaks at 22 weeks, with a marked increase in flow to the uterus and kidneys.
- Blood constituents—RBCs increase by 10–15%, but not in proportion to the increase in plasma volume, creating the condition known as *physiological anemia*. Hemoglobin should remain at or above 120 mmol/L, or the client should be assessed for true anemia. Fibrinogen increases by 50% (to help prevent excess bleeding at birth and postpartum), and the erythrocyte sedimentation rate (ESR) increases.
- Cardiac output—It increases by 30–50%, peaking at 20–24 weeks' gestation.
- Heart rate—It increases by 10–15 bpm. A systolic murmur may be heard.
- Blood pressure—It decreases slightly in the second trimester due to progesterone; low blood pressure may lead to postural hypotension or fainting.

Respiratory System Changes

Respiratory system changes during pregnancy include the following:
- Respiratory rate and tidal volume increase due to progesterone and slight respiratory alkalosis, 30–40% increased volume. Oxygen requirements increase 15–20%.
- The diaphragm is displaced upward, leading to shortness of breath as the pregnancy progresses; there is lateral expansion of the ribs and chest wall with increased elasticity and dilation of airways.
- Increased vascularity is secondary to estrogen; resulting nasal congestion and nosebleeds are common.

Gastro-Intestinal System Changes

Gastro-intestinal system changes during pregnancy include the following:
- Carbohydrate metabolism with insulin secretion increases, although its effectiveness is impaired by the action of hormones, and demand may exceed the pancreas's ability, resulting in symptoms of gestational diabetes. Fasting

blood sugar decreases secondary to the accelerated utilization of glucose to meet fetal demands, and hypoglycemia may lead to fainting and dizziness.

- Gastric motility decreases with prolonged gastric emptying, slower peristalsis secondary to progesterone, and increased risk of constipation and hemorrhoids.
- Esophageal smooth muscle relaxation is secondary to progesterone and regurgitation.
- The gallbladder has decreased tone, distension, and slower emptying, and there is increased risk for gallstone formation.
- The liver has increased alkaline phosphatase and cholesterol and decreased albumin.
- Gingivitis is secondary to increased estrogen.

Renal System Changes

Renal system changes during pregnancy include the following:

- Bladder has decreased tone, increased capacity, and urinary stasis with increased risk of urinary tract infections.
- Renal blood volume and flow changes the glomerular filtration rate, which increases by 50%; kidneys receive one-fifth of cardiac output.
- There is impaired reabsorption of glucose and nitrogen with excretion into urine.

Integumentary System Changes

Skin system changes during pregnancy include the following:

- Increased melanin from the anterior pituitary leads to linea nigra darkening down the mid-abdomen, facial chloasma (mask of pregnancy) with brown patchy pigmentation over cheeks and forehead, darkening of areola, and development of secondary areola.
- Pruritis (itching) is due to increased estrogen and liver changes.
- Increased sweat and sebaceous gland stimulation can lead to acne, perspiration, and night sweats.
- Striae gravidarum, or stretch marks, are due to underlying connective tissue weakening and breakage; they are dark red or bluish during pregnancy and fade to silver.
- Spider nevi, which are fine red dilated arterioles over the face, neck, and thorax, are secondary to increased estrogen.

Musculo-skeletal System Changes

Musculo-skeletal system changes during pregnancy including the following:

- Joints become hypermobile secondary to the hormones relaxin and progesterone with increased risk for injury.
- Postural changes consist of an accentuated lumbar spinal curvature and a waddling gait.

Metabolic System Changes

Metabolic system changes during pregnancy are as follows:

- Basal metabolic rate increases by 15–20%.
- In carbohydrate metabolism, insulin production increases and fasting blood sugar decreases.

Endocrine System Changes

The endocrine system is affected by pregnancy as follows:

- Increased hormone production by the hypothalamus–pituitary–ovarian axis—Menstruation ceases, and estrogen and progesterone increase.
- Adrenal cortex—There is increased antidiuretic hormone (ADH), aldosterone, and cortisol.
- Pancreas—There is increased insulin demand and production but increased maternal resistance to insulin.
- Thyroid—The thyroid experiences a slight enlargement, and thyroxine (T_4) increases.

Light-headedness and fainting in early pregnancy is secondary to hypoglycemia or postural changes.

Common Discomforts of Pregnancy

Some of these changes will lead to what are commonly referred to as minor or normal discomforts of pregnancy. Although minor from a health viewpoint, many pregnant women view these discomforts as a source of concern and distress. Practical nurses can use prenatal visits to educate their clients concerning what to expect and to help plan interventions for relieving these discomforts.

First Trimester Discomforts and Nursing Considerations

Discomforts of early pregnancy can include the following:

- Nausea and vomiting—50–80% of women complain of nausea, with 50% of them also reporting episodes of vomiting
- Urinary frequency—Related to uterine pressure on the bladder until the uterus expands out of the pelvis
- Fatigue
- Breast tenderness—Secondary to progesterone and estrogen hormone changes
- Vaginal discharge—Leukorrhea
- Nasal congestion and nosebleeds—Secondary to increased estrogen

Recommend that pregnant clients do the following:

- Eat small, frequent meals, eat dry foods separate from liquids, and eat dry crackers early in the morning to help relieve nausea.
- Avoid large fluid intakes prior to sleep and void frequently during the day.
- Try to plan times for increased rest and naps.
- Wear a supportive bra, adjust it for increased breast size, and even wear a bra to bed if helpful.
- Shower daily and avoid douching.

Second and Third Trimester Discomforts and Nursing Considerations

Common discomforts of the second and third trimesters include the following:

- Heartburn and regurgitation of gastric contents
- Leg cramping due to imbalance in the phosphorus–calcium ratio and postural changes
- Varicose veins
- Hemorrhoids and constipation

- Backache
- Ankle edema—Related to poor venous return and increased sodium levels
- Carpal tunnel syndrome related to medial nerve compression, especially in the dominant hand
- Shortness of breath
- Sleep disturbances

Recommend the following to clients:

- Continue to eat small, frequent meals, avoid spicy, high-fat meals, and use extra pillows to elevate the head.
- Evaluate dietary intake and increase calcium intake, eat fewer phosphorus-rich foods, and increase fluids and fibre for constipation and hemorrhoids.
- Elevate legs; take frequent breaks when driving long distances or sitting for prolonged periods; wear supportive stockings and dorsiflex ankle to relieve cramping.
- When lightening occurs as the uterus moves lower in the pelvis in the primigravida, shortness of breath will be relieved; in bed, elevate the head with pillows.

Psychological Tasks of Pregnancy

Pregnancy involves a myriad of emotional responses and psychological adjustments as a new developmental role is undertaken and family members adjust to accepting a new member into their lives. In addition to the pregnant woman, all family members, including involved extended family such as grandparents, must adjust to the changes in their roles and responsibilities. This can be a time of both happiness and anticipation but also of ambivalence and stress. Practical nurses can help families in understanding the feelings and role changes and can provide support and reassurance.

A number of steps are important to attachment between mother and baby:

1. Planning the pregnancy
2. Confirming the pregnancy through testing and medical confirmation
3. Accepting the pregnancy; even planned pregnancies are associated with feelings of ambivalence and conflict
4. Perception of fetal movements
5. Accepting the fetus as an individual, role-playing, and fantasizing
6. After birth, reconciling the imagined infant with reality
7. Sensory interactions, such as seeing, touching, and giving care to the baby (Gardner, Carter, Enzman-Hines, et al., 2016)

All family members, especially the woman and her partner, need the opportunity to discuss their emotions and adaptations to the pregnancy. Pregnancy, even when carefully planned for, represents a major developmental change for the woman and her partner. The challenges of integrating all the practical, physical, financial, and role changes into a relationship and family can threaten the stability a family may or may not have. The adaptations, conflicts, and changing roles need to be acknowledged. Community childbirth classes, prenatal programs, and prenatal visits provide an opportunity for open discussion, support, and, when needed, referral to counselling services. Many community programs also offer classes

to prepare siblings for the changes that happen when a new family member arrives.

Sexuality in Pregnancy

Body image, sensuality, and sexuality are all affected by the demands and changes pregnancy brings—on both an individual and a relationship level. Concerns may include fear of harming the developing fetus, fear of miscarriage, and cultural beliefs and practices. Physical changes may also influence desire and comfort with sexual practices.

Contraindications

There are few absolute contraindications to sexual activity or intercourse during pregnancy. They include vaginal spotting or bleeding, premature rupture of membranes, active vaginal infection, uterine cramping, and a history of spontaneous abortions.

Nursing Considerations

- Assess for beliefs, fears, and concerns and offer reassurance and factual information.
- Assess for contraindications and offer support and alternative suggestions.
- First trimester: Sexual desire may be decreased due to nausea, fatigue, breast tenderness, psychological ambivalence, and fear of harming the fetus. Suggest alternatives to sexual intercourse if desire is decreased; reassure that unless risk factors are present, there is no risk of harming the fetus during sexual intercourse.
- Second trimester: Increased interest and satisfaction takes place due to increased vaginal and perineal vascularity; the discomforts of the first trimester decrease.
- Third trimester: Increased size and discomfort may affect comfort level. Suggest changes in positions or alternatives to sexual intercourse that will offer closeness and intimacy.

PERINATAL NUTRITION

The anatomical and physiological changes of pregnancy result in increased daily requirements for energy, nutrients, and vitamins. Ideally, optimal nutrition is part of preconception planning for pregnancy. Meeting nutritional needs during pregnancy is an important factor in promoting healthy outcomes for both mother and infant. For many women, due to inadequate preconception dietary intake, special attention should be paid to ensuring that there is an adequate intake of calcium, vitamin D, folate, iron, and essential fatty acids. *Eating Well with Canada's Food Guide* suggests adding two or three food-guide servings each day to meet the needs of pregnancy (Health Canada, 2011).

Nutritional Supplements

- Prenatal multivitamin: A prenatal daily multivitamin is recommended because it contains the additional minerals, vitamins, and folic acid necessary to support the woman and fetus during pregnancy. A multivitamin with folic acid is recommended for women who could become pregnant or are planning a pregnancy.

- Calcium and vitamin D: Calcium is essential for the development and maintenance of bone mass, both prior to and during pregnancy. Adequate intake is also needed for fetal skeletal development. The body needs vitamin D to enhance the intestinal absorption of calcium. The recommended daily intake for calcium during pregnancy is between 1 200 and 1 500 mg, depending on age. Vitamin D daily requirement is under review to increase the daily recommended intake (Health Canada, 2010b). During the summer months in Canada, daily sun exposure of 15 minutes meets recommended requirements. From November to April, vitamin D production from sun exposure ceases due to low sunlight levels; therefore, additional vitamin D supplements are required (Health Canada, 2010b).
- Iron: Additional iron is needed to support the increase in maternal RBC production. Iron supplementation is recommended during the second and third trimesters based on the assumption that prepregnancy iron stores are inadequate in most women. Recommended iron intake increases from 13 to 18 mg in the second trimester and to 23 mg by the third trimester (Health Canada, 2018b).
- Folate: Folate (folic acid) supplementation significantly reduces the risk of neural tube defects, which affect about one in 1 000 babies born in Canada (live births and stillbirths). A supplement of 400 mcg daily in addition to dietary intake is recommended. A dose of 4 000–5 000 mcg starting 1 month before pregnancy and through the first trimester is recommended for women who have compromised health; are at increased risk for diabetes or obesity; or previously gave birth to a baby with a neural defect.
- Essential fatty acids: They are important during pregnancy for proper fetal neural and visual development. The fetus is dependent on maternal sources, especially during the rapid growth period of the last trimester of pregnancy. Women are encouraged to increase dietary intake of foods rich in essential fatty acids, including nonhydrogenated vegetable oils, nuts, eggs, meat, and fatty fish such as wild salmon.

Nursing Considerations

- Assess and work to develop a plan toward optimal preconception and perinatal nutrition practices, including adequate caloric intake of nutrient-dense foods that meet the requirements of pregnancy and follow *Eating Well with Canada's Food Guide.*
- Be aware of and sensitive to the reality that dietary habits and practices are influenced by socio-economic status, cultural diversity, and religious dietary practices and beliefs.
- When taking into account individual differences for caloric energy increases, suggest that women use appetite as a guide to satisfying hunger. Review strategies for managing nausea in the first trimester.

- Refer clients to dietary supplement programs sponsored by Health Canada and administered by local community agencies, such as the Canada Prenatal Nutrition Program (CPNP).
- Provide suggestions for dietary sources of foods rich in folate, calcium, and iron.
- Increase awareness and understanding of potential adverse effects of excessive use of some vitamins, especially vitamin A, and over-the-counter herbal supplements.
- Ensure that vegetarians understand sources for increased protein and iron dietary intake.
- Assess for risk factors for inadequate iron stores and probable need for supplementation, including a diet deficient in meat, fish, poultry, or vitamin C, as well as frequent consumption of tea or coffee close to meal time, multiple gestations, and parity of three or more (Health Canada, 2018b).
- Include in teaching that there is increased absorption of iron from heme sources such as meat, poultry, and fish. Particularly for vegetarians, nonheme iron is found in vegetables, fruit, grains, nuts, eggs, iron-enriched cereals, and pastas. Vitamin C and meat, poultry, and fish enhance the absorption of nonheme iron. Iron absorption is inhibited when consumed with tea, coffee, whole grains, and calcium.
- Assess for risk factors of low calcium intake, including low socio-economic status, pregnant adolescents, and vegetarians who do not consume milk products.
- Assess for risk factors for inadequate vitamin D production, including dark-pigmented skin, inadequate exposure to sunlight due to northern geographical location during the winter months (most of Canada) (Whiting, Langlois, Vatanparast, et al., 2011).
- Promote the consumption of healthy essential fatty acids through increased dietary intake. Reassure women who may have misconceptions that all dietary fats are harmful.

MATERNAL HEALTH PROBLEMS AND PREGNANCY

With advances in technology, research, high-risk referral, and professional expertise, women with health concerns and their infants are experiencing better outcomes. It is essential, however, to recognize the very real risks and complications that are associated with many maternal health issues. Women need to be informed of the potential risks for increased maternal and fetal morbidity and mortality and educated on the early monitoring and intervention provided.

Cardiac and Blood Disorders

As previously discussed, the cardiovascular system is challenged during pregnancy to accommodate a 50% increase in circulating volume and an increase in cardiac output. For women with a pre-existing heart condition, the needed cardiac reserve to accommodate those changes may not be sufficient. Heart disease is a significant cause of maternal morbidity and mortality, and puts a woman into a high-risk pregnancy classification.

- If the condition is associated with cyanosis and decreased systemic circulation, regardless of treatment, pregnancy should be avoided.
- If maternal oxygenation and systemic circulation are impaired, the fetus will suffer the effects of decreased uterine blood flow and hypoxia. This can result in fetal compromise, fetal death, SGA, or spontaneous abortion.
- Antibiotic prophylaxis may be recommended during labour and birth because of an increased risk of bacterial endocarditis.

Nursing Considerations

- Emphasize a preventive approach to minimizing complications of known conditions.
- Provide realistic information about the risks and a plan of care will enable the mother to participate in her care and reduce anxiety.
- Be aware that throughout pregnancy, labour, and birth, care is directed at minimizing cardiac workload for those clients at high risk for hypoxemia. Bed rest or restricted activity may be recommended. Cardiology referral and high-risk care will be required.
- Know that the first hours following birth present a high-risk time as the body begins to remobilize the extra circulating blood volume acquired during pregnancy. This adds to the workload of the heart. Assess the client for signs of respiratory distress and pulmonary edema.

Infections

During pregnancy, the woman's immune system is suppressed, leading to an increased risk of acquiring infections. TORCH infections (toxoplasmosis, other [syphilis, varicella zoster, parvovirus B19], rubella, CMV, and herpes) are those caused by a group of organisms that can cross the placenta. In the mother, symptoms may be flulike but may cause significant developmental problems in the fetus that increase the risk of illness and death.

Toxoplasmosis

- Detected in maternal serum antibodies, this infection can be acquired by handling cat feces or garden soil or through raw meat consumption. Abortion is common; surviving newborns may present with severe neurological problems, seizures, hepatic splenomegaly, jaundice, and developmental delay.
- Pregnant women should be advised to wear gloves while gardening and to avoid handling cat litter and eating raw meat products.

Rubella

- Exposure in the first trimester has a high incidence of spontaneous abortion and congenital anomalies, including heart, eye, ear, and brain defects.

- Preconception titre testing is recommended and vaccination with 3 months of contraception. Vaccination is often offered during the postpartum period.

Cytomegalovirus (CMV)

Pregnant women may be asymptomatic, but the fetal effects of CMV can be severe. CMV is easily transmitted in all body fluids and crosses the placenta to infect the fetus. Fetal effects include microcephaly and severe intellectual and developmental problems, seizures, hydrocephaly, SGA, cerebral calcifications, and deafness.

Herpes Simplex Virus (HSV)

Type 1 infections cause cold sores; type 2 infections are sexually transmitted. Transmission is via the birth canal; however, Caesarean birth is recommended only when active lesions are present.

Fetal and newborn effects include microcephaly, severe intellectual and developmental impairment, patent ductus arteriosus, and eye defects.

Human Papilloma Virus (HPV)

- HPV is the most common sexually transmitted virus, and certain strains are correlated with precancerous lesions, which can lead to cervical cancer. Transmission to the fetus is unknown, but infection can result in respiratory tract papillomatosis.
- An HPV vaccine is available and recommended for all young women prior to becoming sexually active (Public Health Agency of Canada, 2018).

HIV and AIDS

- All pregnant women should be offered voluntary HIV screening and counselling at their first prenatal visit.
- Advances in the past 25 years now give pregnant women the opportunity to be treated with antiretroviral prophylaxis to effectively help prevent HIV transmission to the fetus, and treating the pregnant women decreases risk from 25 to 2%.
- Birth by Caesarean section is preferred.

Group B Streptococcus (GBS)

- GBS is a bacterial infection vertically transmitted from mother to infant.
- Maternal problems include preterm labour and preterm rupture of membranes.
- Fetal neonatal problems, including blindness, deafness, developmental delay, neonatal sepsis, and meningitis, may appear within 72 hours of birth with significant morbidity and mortality.
- Prenatal assessment and treatment intrapartum with penicillin is recommended.

Varicella (Chicken Pox)

- Maternal varicella infections can cause serious complications to the fetus or neonate.

- In first trimester exposure, fetal defects include microcephaly, skin, eye, and limb anomalies, and low birth weight.
- Third trimester infection may rarely result in neonatal complications. A varicella zoster immune globulin (VZIG) is available to exposed pregnant women.

Varicella vaccine is recommended to all susceptible women (those lacking immunity) of reproductive age. It cannot be given during pregnancy. Pregnant women who are not immune should have the vaccination offered postpartum (Health Canada, 2018a).

Chlamydia

- This epidemic infection is the result of a parasitic transmission that occurs by direct sexual contact or exposure at birth. Infection, often asymptomatic in the mother, is associated with increasing infertility rates in Canada.
- Fetal and newborn effects are common and include prematurity, low birth weight, and stillbirth.
- Prophylaxis erythromycin eye treatment is given to all newborns at birth to prevent conjunctivitis and potential eye sequelae.

Gonorrhea

- This bacterial infection is spread by direct contact in the lower genital tract, causing only minor maternal symptoms but potentially serious infections.
- Fetal effects include preterm birth and the premature rupture of membranes. Newborns are at risk for pneumonia and eye infections. Prophylaxis erythromycin eye treatment is given to all newborns at birth to prevent conjunctivitis and potential eye sequelae.

Nursing Considerations

- Know that routine screening for STIs should be part of all initial prenatal assessments. Practical nurses need to know reportable STIs.
- Know that thorough history-taking in a private setting with a nonjudgemental approach is important for honest disclosure of high-risk behaviours.
- Stress the importance of consistency and adherence to treatment protocols for infections.
- Refer to appropriate community resources for information and follow-up care.
- Administer prophylactic treatment to all newborns as indicated.

Respiratory Disorders
Asthma

For unknown reasons, the incidence and severity of asthma during pregnancy may improve (30%), remain unchanged (50%), or worsen (22%) (Gardner & Doyle, 2004).

Infections

- Most upper respiratory tract infections are self-limiting and pose no added risk to the fetus.

- Bacterial pneumonia should be treated with antibiotics that are considered safe in pregnancy, including those in the penicillin family.

Nursing Considerations

- For all respiratory conditions, the approach to care centres around the prevention of hypoxemia in the mother. This includes promoting effective control of asthma attacks.
- Systemic steroid when used in the treatment of maternal asthma in the first trimester may be teratogenic.
- Over-the-counter cold and cough remedies cause vasoconstriction of blood vessels, which may elevate blood pressure and therefore should be avoided. Herbal treatments may have unknown side effects, including potential harm to the fetus, and should be avoided.
- Hypoxemia associated with acute respiratory distress or pneumonia may cause fetal compromise, and chronic hypoxia may increase the risk for SGA.

Connective Tissue Disorders

These disorders are characterized by an autoimmune-mediated abnormality and include rheumatoid arthritis, multiple sclerosis, scleroderma, myasthenia gravis, and systemic lupus erythematosus (SLE). SLE has the most significant and serious consequences for the mother, fetus, and infant.

Nursing Considerations

- When health teaching, emphasize the importance of adequate rest, especially with the increased metabolic demands of pregnancy. Teach the mother to recognize the signs of preterm labour.
- Educate the woman as to the antenatal fetal well-being monitoring techniques.

Cancers

The occurrence of pregnancy and cancer together during the child-bearing years is relatively rare but represents a devastating time of fear and crisis for the woman and her family. Pregnancy is a growth event as the hormones of pregnancy work to prepare and sustain the woman's body to support the pregnancy and developing fetus. Hormone-responsive cancers may also experience accelerated growth as a result.

Nursing Considerations

- A multidisciplinary approach in collaboration with the family is essential in all stages of treatment and care.
- Decisions regarding treatment options and continuing with the pregnancy are deeply personal and need to be supported and informed by the best available research.

Hypertension

Hypertension in pregnancy can be a pre-existing chronic condition or can be associated with the pregnancy itself. PIH, also known as *pre-eclampsia* and *eclampsia*, poses a more significant risk for the mother and the fetus.

Primary Hypertension

- Includes pre-existing chronic hypertension and chronic renal diseases
- Increases the risk for uteroplacental insufficiency and placental abruption
- May lead to intrauterine growth delay

Hypertensive Disorders of Pregnancy

Predisposing Factors

- Primigravida
- Adolescent or advanced maternal age: Younger than 18 years or older than 35 years
- Diabetes mellitus
- Chronic hypertension or chronic renal disease
- Multiple pregnancy
- Previous or family history of hypertensive disorders of pregnancy (HDP)

Pathophysiology

Placental arteries do not widen as needed to increase placental perfusion, and the resulting ischemia leads to damage of all blood vessel walls. This damage results in generalized vasoconstriction, which leads to poor tissue perfusion, elevated blood pressure and damage to cell wall permeability, and fluid leakage and loss. Other consequential changes include the following:

- A decrease in placental perfusion (placental vascular insufficiency), renal blood flow, glomerular filtration rate, and oliguria
- Central nervous system (CNS) effects such as edema, cerebral hemorrhage, hyper-reflexia, and severe headache with progression to seizure activity

Clinical Manifestations

- Cardinal signs are hypertension, proteinuria, and obvious generalized edema after 20 weeks' gestation.
- Subjective signs are complaints of headache, photophobia, blurred or double vision, oliguria, nausea and vomiting, epigastric or right upper quadrant pain, hematuria, and severe headache.
- Pulmonary edema

Manifestations quickly resolve following the birth of the infant within 48 hours.

Maternal and Fetal Risks

- Maternal risks: Placental abruption leading to hemorrhage or disseminated intravascular coagulation (DIC), maternal seizures, pulmonary edema, stroke, renal failure, and ruptured liver
- Fetal risks: SGA, prematurity, fetal hypoxia or demise, neonatal hypocalcemia

Diagnostics and Therapeutics

Diagnostics.

- Mild pre-eclampsia: Hypertension and proteinuria—If diastolic blood pressure is greater than 90 mm Hg and systolic blood pressure is greater than 140 mm Hg, monitor closely for diastolic hypertension; monitor for generalized edema of the face or hands, 1+ proteinuria, 1–2+ deep tendon reflexes, and adequate urine output.
- Severe pre-eclampsia: Monitor for blood pressure greater than 160–180/110 mm Hg, oliguria (less than 400 mL/24 hr), 2+ proteinuria, 3+ to 4+ deep tendon reflexes, visual disturbances, retinal detachment, severe headache, epigastric pain, pulmonary edema, generalized edema, and weight gain of more than 1 kg in 1 week.
- Eclampsia—Seizures or coma are preceded by severe headache, visual disturbances, epigastric pain, or right upper quadrant abdominal pain (London, Ladewig, Davidson, et al., 2017).

Therapeutics for mild pre-eclampsia.

- Therapeutics include rest; fetal antenatal monitoring, including ultrasonography, non-stress testing (NST), and intrapartum monitoring; laboratory work-up for liver, blood, clotting factors, and renal function. Magnesium sulphate may be administered.

Therapeutics for severe pre-eclampsia.

- Hospitalization includes advanced hemodynamic monitoring; an early birth is planned if symptoms worsen or the fetus is compromise; the fetus should be monitored.
- Antihypertensive therapy and magnesium sulphate ($MgSO_4$) are recommended.

Therapeutics for eclampsia.

- A patent airway is maintained, and oxygen support is provided.
- A bolus amount of $MgSO_4$ is given, as well as diazepam (Valium), if needed.
- Vaginal birth is preferred when the mother has been stabilized.

Nursing Considerations

- Assess for worsening cardinal and other manifestations through careful monitoring and teach the mother, if still at home, to assess blood pressure and urine protein.
- Diet should be high in protein and moderate in salt.
- Assess weight daily and carefully monitor fluid intake and output.
- Promote and teach methods to maximize uteroplacental circulation, including lying in the left or right lateral position.
- Monitor fetal well-being with FHR monitoring and NST.
- Promote rest and a quiet environment to minimize distress from cerebral manifestations.
- Observe for signs of placental abruption and be prepared for an emergency birth.
- Provide psychological support to all family members.

Diabetes Mellitus and Gestational Diabetes

Pregnancy is a diabetogenic event. The normal carbohydrate and hormonal changes that occur in the body during pregnancy create a situation that challenges the pancreas to produce more insulin while some of the hormones of pregnancy make the cells more resistant to the effects of insulin. For a woman with pre-existing diabetes mellitus, pregnancy is a high-risk event requiring careful ongoing management. For other women, the manifestations of diabetes will become apparent only during the pregnancy. In this situation, a diagnosis of gestational diabetes is made. For the woman with gestational diabetes, the disease process stops after the birth of the infant, although she will carry a higher risk of developing type 2 diabetes later in life. In both types of diabetes, maternal risks are present, and the fetus and newborn are also at risk for complications and must be carefully monitored.

Pathophysiology

- Placental hormones cause an anti-insulin effect, allowing the fetus, in the first half of the pregnancy, to receive the increased amounts of glucose that it needs for growth and development. Maternal glucose crosses the placenta; maternal insulin does not.
- At around 20 weeks' gestation, the maternal pancreas is challenged to produce increasing amounts of insulin, which it normally does. A woman with pre-existing diabetes cannot meet this challenge, and her symptoms of diabetes will worsen. In other women, if the pancreas fails to match the increased demand for insulin, signs and symptoms of diabetes will appear.
- If the resulting hyperglycemia is not diagnosed or well controlled, the fetus will continue to receive high amounts of glucose, resulting in excessive growth. This creates added risk during labour and at the time of birth.
- The fetal pancreas produces increased amounts of insulin to match the high levels of glucose it is receiving. Following birth, the infant no longer receives high amounts of glucose, but the pancreas needs time to adjust and continues to produce large amounts of insulin. This can quickly lead to moderate to severe hypoglycemia in the newborn.

Clinical Manifestations

Maternal:
- In the first trimester, hypoglycemia is present.
- At around 20 weeks' gestation, the development of hyperglycemia and glucosuria, ketonuria, increased risk for urinary tract infections due to glucosuria, increased risk of PIH and spontaneous abortion if there is pre-existing diabetes, risk of polyhydramnios, risk of postpartum hemorrhage due to increased macrosomia.
 Fetal:
 Risks include increased growth, LGA (over 4 kg), risk of congenital anomalies, preterm birth, birth trauma, and hypoglycemia.

Diagnostics and Therapeutics

- Monitor for glucosuria and ketonuria at all prenatal visits. Normal values are a fasting glucose level of 5.8 mmol/L or less. If the result is abnormally high, a three-hour oral glucose tolerance test is done with an oral load of glucose. Blood glucose levels are taken hourly for 3 hours, which

exceeds normal limits; a diagnosis of impaired glucose tolerance (IGT) is made.
- Management includes consultation between the pregnant woman, dietitian, endocrinologist, obstetrician, pediatrician, and nurse.
- Frequent monitoring of blood glucose levels, up to four times daily, and administration of insulin injections to maintain a normal glucose level. A dietary plan is developed with the dietitian.
- Additional, frequent prenatal visits and possible planned earlier delivery at 37–38 weeks' gestation, depending on NST results and maternal well-being. Morbidity and mortality are lowest if the birth takes place as close to term as possible.
- Fetal monitoring may include additional ultrasonograms, NST, biophysical profile, amniocentesis, an alphafetoprotein test, and electronic fetal monitoring during labour.
- During labour and birth, the woman is kept nothing by mouth (NPO), and an intravenous (IV) with 5% glucose is used to maintain normal serum glucose levels. Insulin is given as needed. Postpartum, insulin requirements decrease, especially for the first 48 hours.
- Breastfeeding is encouraged as it lowers the amount of insulin required.
- The newborn is monitored closely for respiratory distress and hypoglycemia. Care in a level 2 or 3 nursery may be required.

Nursing Considerations

- Know that because oral hypoglycemics cross the placenta, they are considered teratogenic and are not used in the first trimester. Glyburides are used in later trimesters.
- Teach the pregnant woman the manifestations of hyperglycemia and insulin reaction and measures to take for each.
- Support and encourage adherence to and diligence in glucose testing, insulin self-administration, dietary control, balancing rest and activity levels, accurate record-keeping, and follow-up visits to specialists.
- Provide information and support for additional tests monitoring fetal well-being.
- Prepare the woman and family for a possible earlier planned birth and the potential need for a Caesarean birth.
- Observe for signs of hypoglycemia in the newborn, including lethargy, jitteriness, poor sucking reflex, and a blood glucose level of less than 2–2.5 mmol/L.
- Observe the newborn for signs of respiratory distress, birth trauma, hypothermia, and possible congenital anomalies.
- Promote and support breastfeeding as the ideal feeding option for mothers with diabetes.

PREGNANCY COMPLICATIONS

Adolescent Pregnancy

The teen pregnancy rate continues to decline in Canada (Statistics Canada, 2017c). Pregnancy during the teen years presents many life challenges and interrupts the normal developmental tasks of adolescence. Pregnant adolescents and their newborns are at an increased risk for complications; the younger the teen, the higher the risk. All of the determinants of health need to be addressed during and after the pregnancy, and if the young mother chooses to raise her child, community support is essential.

Risk Factors

- Obstetrical: Premature birth; high risk of PIH, anemia, and poor nutrition; lack of knowledge about the harm of using tobacco and alcohol; poor prenatal care if the pregnancy is hidden; cephalopelvic disproportion; SGA infants; postpartum hemorrhage
- Psychosocial: Lack of partner and family support, interruption to education, feelings of isolation and fear, lack of knowledge and life experience to manage changes and transitions, risk of poor coping strategies, lack of community support in isolated areas with minimal resources, negative attitudes and judgement from others
- Socio-economic: Unless community support through services directed at adolescent parents is available and accessible, teen parents are at risk for not completing high school or progressing to postsecondary education, low earning potential, lack of affordable housing, continued social isolation, chronic stress and poor self-esteem, and increased risk of inadequate nutrition for themselves and their child.

Nursing Considerations

- Provide collaborative, early intervention and prenatal care that focuses on the young woman's strengths in a trusting and supportive environment of care. Assess the adolescent's maturity, coping strategies, health history, and support systems, both available and needed. Use a collaborative approach to decision making and planning for the birth of the baby and understanding the demands of the pregnancy.
- Identify the needs of the adolescent and her obstetrical risk factors.
- Arrange referral to community resources and programs for teen mothers, including those sponsored by Health Canada. Needs may include programs for prenatal nutrition; healthy-baby programs; parenting programs; social services for housing, child care, and employment; and educational opportunities to finish high school.
- Provide counselling and nonjudgemental support to assist the new mother with postpartum decisions regarding appropriate birth control options.

Spontaneous Abortion (Miscarriage)

A spontaneous abortion is the natural termination of the pregnancy before viability is established, which is usually at 20 weeks' gestation. Early miscarriage occurs in the first 12 weeks of pregnancy.

Pathophysiology

- Maternal factors: Infection, cervical insufficiency, failure of the placenta to develop or implant normally, trauma, teratogenic exposure
- Fetal factors: Genetic or developmental abnormality, faulty implantation into endometrium

Clinical Manifestations

- Threatened: No cervical dilatation, cramping, vaginal spotting or bleeding; the pregnancy may or may not terminate
- Imminent or inevitable: Bleeding, cramping, with cervical dilatation
- Incomplete: Bleeding, expulsion of only some of the products of conception
- Complete: All products of conception expelled
- Missed abortion: Embryo or fetal death without cervical dilatation, cramping, or bleeding; no FHR detected; a negative pregnancy test
- Habitual: Three or more consecutive miscarriages

Diagnostics and Therapeutics

- Threatened: Rest, avoidance of sexual intercourse, restricted activities
- Incomplete: Outpatient day surgery for D & C
- Missed abortion: Vaginal or abdominal ultrasound, HCG hormone test, D & C to remove products of conception; if the missed abortion is between 16 and 20 weeks, induction of labour may be required with prostaglandins
- Complete: No medical treatment necessary; emotional support and follow-up provided
- Habitual: Referral for infertility investigation, possible surgical intervention for incompetent cervix

Grief reaction to the loss of the pregnancy includes shock, disbelief, sadness, anger, depression, and fear for fertility and the future ability to carry a pregnancy.

Nursing Considerations

- Provide an injection of Rh-immune globulin (WinRho) to any woman who is Rh-negative to prevent a maternal immune antibody response.
- Know that for each woman, a pregnancy has very individual meaning and significance. Support the woman's emotional reaction and response; dispel any feelings of blame or guilt.
- Teach what to expect with either natural completion of the miscarriage process or operative D & C procedure.
- Assess vital signs and vaginal bleeding; provide pain relief and emotional support.
- Refer as appropriate to community resources for follow-up counselling, including local grief support and infertility groups.

Placenta Previa
Pathophysiology

- The placenta implants in the lower uterus, at or near the internal os at the cervix, instead of the top one-third of the uterine fundus. The cause is unknown, but this condition affects about 1 in 300 pregnancies, and the following risk factors have been identified: multiparity, previous Caesarean birth or uterine surgery, previous placenta previa, tobacco use, and maternal age greater than 35 years.

- Close to term, around 30 weeks' gestation or later, placental villi become separated from the uterine wall as the uterus contracts and the cervix thins and dilates.
- Placenta previa is classified by the position of the placenta:
  - Total or complete—The placenta completely covers the internal os.
  - Partial or incomplete—The placenta covers some of the internal os.
  - Low-lying or marginal—The placenta reaches but does not cover the internal os.

Clinical Manifestations

Placenta previa manifests as painless, bright red vaginal bleeding with a uterus that is soft and relaxed or relaxes between contractions.

Diagnostics and Therapeutics

- Many low-lying placenta previas are commonly detected on early antenatal ultrasonograms and resolve by term as the uterus elongates. Repeat ultrasonography in the third trimester is needed for confirmation of true placenta previa. The need for Caesarean birth is determined by the classification of the previa, the amount of vaginal bleeding, and fetal well-being.
- In unconfirmed placenta previa, vaginal examination may be deferred until emergency operative interventions are in place.
- The decision to allow a vaginal birth is based on ultrasound findings, which locate the placenta.
- Outpatient management may be used if the woman is stable, home support is available, bed rest is an option, and there is close proximity to the hospital with readily available transportation and telephone access (Oppenheimer, 2007).
- If blood loss is significant or worsens, interventions must include maternal resuscitation for blood loss and shock. Immediate delivery must be done to treat fetal distress due to hypoxia.
- Blood typing, cross-match, and available blood products for maternal resuscitation are needed.

Nursing Considerations

- Reinforce the need for bed rest and accurate pad counts to monitor bleeding. Teach the client to report immediately any changes in condition.
- Ensure that women who are discharged home prior to labour and birth understand and are able to comply with outpatient management. Sexual intercourse is contraindicated.
- Observe for signs of shock and be prepared to insert a large-bore IV catheter to administer blood products and proceed to emergency operative birth.

- Provide emotional support and an opportunity to discuss fears and anticipatory grieving response.
- Monitor for fetal well-being and FHR and conduct an NST; birth will be delayed if possible to allow for fetal lung maturity. Steroids may be given to advance lung maturity.

Placental Abruption

Placental abruption occurs when a normally implanted placenta prematurely separates or partially separates in the second half of pregnancy or during labour. Abruption is an emergency situation with a high risk of maternal and fetal morbidity and mortality.

Pathophysiology

- The exact cause or causes are unknown, but theories include the degeneration, necrosis, and separation of the placental arterioles at the site of implantation.
- The bleeding can be concealed (no vaginal bleeding) due to formation of retroplacental clot.
- Risk factors include primary hypertension or PIH, multiparity, abdominal trauma short umbilical cord, previous Caesarean birth, large placenta, smoking, vasoconstrictive drugs, decompression of overdistended uterus, delivery of first twin, and older mothers.
- Complete abruption with massive hemorrhage can lead to complications including fetal demise, maternal shock, DIC, and death.

Clinical Manifestations

- Sudden, intense pain with or without bright red vaginal bleeding
- Concealed bleeding
- A hard uterus hard that does not relax between contractions
- Sudden onset of acute, severe fetal compromise
- Signs of maternal shock with tachycardia, hypotension, cold clammy skin, pallor, loss of consciousness

Diagnostics and Therapeutics

- Often this is an obstetrical emergency, and interventions may be initiated based on clinical findings without confirmation by ultrasound, especially if maternal and fetal compromise is present. If maternal and fetal vital signs are stable, an ultrasound may be used to confirm bleeding but not to diagnose concealed abruption.
- Immediate birth is planned for, vaginal or Caesarean, depending on the stage and progression of labour.
- Nursing staff need to be prepared for the possible resuscitation of the mother and infant.

Nursing Considerations

- Key consideration:
  - Note the distinguishing difference between placenta previa (painless) and placental abruption (painful) bleeding in your immediate assessment.
- Initiate emergency measures to assist in prompt resuscitation efforts and emergency birth: establish an IV and

administer volume expansion fluids, administer oxygen 6–8 L/min at 100%, monitor FHR continuously, perform ultrasonography if time and condition allow, cross-match and administer blood when necessary (prn).

- Provide information and support to the mother and family members.

Ectopic Pregnancy

An ectopic pregnancy occurs when the fertilized ovum implants itself in a location outside the uterine endometrium.

Pathophysiology

- Implantation can occur anywhere, including the abdominal cavity, but, overwhelmingly, implantation occurs in the fallopian tube, mainly on the right side, for reasons that are unknown.
- Risk factors include fallopian tube damage secondary to pelvic inflammatory disease, STIs, structural abnormalities, tumours, scarring and partial obstruction, IUD contraceptive, endometriosis, history of ectopic pregnancy, tobacco use, maternal age greater than 35 years.

Clinical Manifestations

- Early rupture: The woman experiences a missed menstrual period or abnormal period, signs and symptoms of early pregnancy and positive pregnancy test, abdominal tenderness over lower abdomen.
- Rupture: If the fallopian tube ruptures, acute lower quadrant abdominal pain occurs, often on the right side, along with referred shoulder pain, low-grade fever, and possible shock due to blood loss.

Diagnostics and Therapeutics

- Careful history-taking is important, as manifestations mimic other conditions, including appendicitis, ovarian cyst, and urinary tract infection.
- Pelvic examination and ultrasonography confirm the ectopic pregnancy; laparoscopic surgery is used to remove the products of conception, possibly repair or remove the fallopian tube, and control bleeding.
- Systemic methotrexate may be considered for unruptured or chronic ectopic pregnancies as it destroys the pregnancy over several weeks while preserving the fallopian tube.

Nursing Considerations

- Be sure to take menstrual history carefully; in particular, take note of missed or unusual menstrual periods, use of IUD, or past history of STIs or infections.
- Observe for signs of shock and prepare for surgery.
- Offer support and counselling, as often the woman may not have been aware a pregnancy had occurred.
- Be aware that women with an Rh-negative blood type must have Rh-immune globulin administered to prevent blood incompatibility antibody formation.

Hyperemesis Gravidarum

This condition of severe, unrelenting nausea and vomiting occurs in about 1% of pregnancies and greatly impacts the quality of life of the women affected.

Pathophysiology

This condition is poorly understood and likely related to many factors. Theories have included high levels of circulating HCG. It is also associated with multiple gestation and hydatidiform molar pregnancy.

Clinical Manifestations

- Physiological aspects: Symptoms include persistent vomiting that leads to a 5% prepregnancy weight loss with associated electrolyte balance and ketonuria (Arsenault & Lane, 2002).
- Psychosocial aspects: Anxiety, worry, exhaustion, and depression related to quality-of-life issues, including absence from employment and relationship and family stress. The severity of the personal impact has led some women to consider or undertake elective termination of the pregnancy.

Diagnostics and Therapeutics

- Diagnosis is made on the basis of history-taking and presenting manifestations, including confirmation by blood electrolytes and urinalysis and weight loss confirmation.
- Oral pharmacological interventions considered safe for use in pregnancy include doxylamine–pyridoxine combination as the standard of care. Other medications may be used for breakthrough episodes or as adjunct therapy.
- Corticosteroids are avoided in the first trimester due to their teratogenic effect.

Nursing Considerations

- Provide information and reassurance regarding current pharmacological interventions.
- Know that supportive therapies may include ginger, acupuncture, acupressure, and meditation.
- Encourage dietary and lifestyle changes that support the woman's choices in choosing foods that are appealing.
- Know that early recognition and prompt treatment can restore metabolic balance and quality of life.
- Provide accurate intake and output; monitor weight, assess for fetal well-being.
- Offer reassurance and counselling to address psychosocial distress, fears, and concerns.
- Refer to social services as appropriate if hospitalization is prolonged.

Teratogens and Substance Abuse

A teratogen is any agent, drug, toxin, chemical, or infection that can harm the developing embryo or fetus. Depending on molecular size and fat solubility, many, if not most, substances cross the placenta. During the embryonic stage of development in the first trimester, exposure to teratogens can have devastating consequences for the developing embryo, resulting in spontaneous abortion, congenital defects, or death (see Fig. 9.2). Even with over-the-counter and prescription medications, teratogenic effects are still poorly understood, and decisions to use medications must be made balancing the risks and benefits to maternal and fetal well-being. A few commonly used teratogenic substances and their effects are described next.

Alcohol

- The severity of fetal effects is influenced by development at the time of exposure, genetic sensitivity, and quantity of alcohol exposure. No safe amount of alcohol consumption is known.
- Adverse effects of fetal alcohol spectrum disorder (FASD) and fetal alcohol syndrome (FAS) include congenital defects, including craniofacial deformities, skeletal abnormalities, cardiac anomalies, moderate to severe intellectual and development delays, recurrent ear infections, behavioural problems including impulsivity, attention-deficit/hyperactivity disorder (ADHD), and short-term memory impairment. These abnormalities persist into adulthood with ongoing negative outcomes and adverse effects on quality of life.
- The newborn may exhibit irritability, a high-pitched cry, inconsolability, jitteriness, and poor sucking and feeding.
- Nursing considerations include careful antenatal assessment and teaching that no amount of alcohol is safe. Screen for alcohol use. Referral to community agencies and ongoing support to stop drinking should be provided. Referral should be made to FAS follow-up programs and provision made for long-term support for newborn effects.

Tobacco

- Nicotine in tobacco products, inhaled via smoking or exposure to second-hand smoke, is a powerful alkaloid vasoconstrictor that can affect uteroplacental blood flow.
- Fetal effects include prematurity, SGA, increased incidence of childhood asthma, and increased risk of sudden unexpected infant death (SUID).

Cocaine

- Cocaine is a powerful vasoconstrictor that leads to decreased cardiac output, uteroplacental insufficiency, and an increased level of fetal neurotransmitters.
- Maternal effects include onset of premature labour, risk of spontaneous abortion, cardiovascular failure, hypertensive crisis, seizures, and placental abruption.
- Fetal complications include prematurity, SGA, brain damage, cardiac anomalies, CNS abnormalities including cerebral infarcts, and fetal compromise.
- Neonatal complications include neurobehavioural abnormalities at birth, including hyper-reflexia, high-pitched cry, extreme sensitivity to environmental stimuli, poor feeding, diarrhea, and an increased risk for SUID.

Prescription Medications

The Society of Obstetricians and Gynaecologists of Canada (2018) recommends that women should not take medications during pregnancy, ideally. If medication is prescribed for a diagnosed medical condition, the decision to continue needs to be made on an individual basis.

FETAL EVALUATION AND MONITORING

Essentials of Fetal Evaluation

Some of the most frequently used tests to assess for fetal well-being in the antenatal and intrapartum periods are described next. Daily monitoring of fetal movements starting at 26–32 weeks should be done in clients at risk for adverse outcomes. The contraction stress test is used when biophysical profile is not accessible.

Non-Stress Test (NST)

The fetal brain is extremely sensitive to the amount of oxygen it receives. Any maternal condition that adversely affects blood and oxygen supply to the placenta can lead to fetal hypoxia and distress. A sign that the fetus is receiving enough oxygen for the CNS to respond normally is seen when the FHR increases in response to fetal activity. This is considered a reassuring sign of fetal well-being. This ability to respond is assessed during an NST. When the fetus does not respond as expected, it may be an indication of acute or chronic conditions of hypoxia.

An NST is indicated for any high-risk maternal condition that may cause uteroplacental insufficiency, including hypertension, HDP, renal disease, diabetes, cardiac disease, or multiple gestation. Also, if the mother reports decreased fetal activity, an NST may be used along with ultrasound to assess well-being. This test is also part of the biophysical profile test.

Nursing considerations.

- Educate the woman about the purpose and procedure; the test is completed in 30–45 minutes and is noninvasive and not painful.
- Be aware that occasionally, the fetus will be sleeping and nonactive. In that case, the test may have to be repeated. The mother should be reassured that this is not uncommon.

Ultrasonography

High-frequency sound waves are painlessly transmitted via a vaginal or abdominal transducer. Sound waves reflect different body tissue densities and are displayed on a monitor. This diagnostic tool is widely used to assess the status of the pregnancy and fetal growth and well-being.

- First trimester indications: If used before 20 weeks' gestation, fetal gestational age can be calculated within 3 days' accuracy by measuring crown–rump length and biparietal skull diameters. Ultrasound at 8–12 weeks is most accurate.
- Second and third trimester indications: Ultrasound is used to assess placental location, source of vaginal bleeding,

polyhydramnios, congenital anomalies, fetal presentation and position.

- Procedure: Before 20 weeks' gestation, the woman drinks enough fluids to have a full bladder to lift the uterus up out of the pelvis for better visualization. Gel is applied to the abdomen with the woman lying on her back. It takes about 20 minutes to complete the test.

Ultrasonography is widely used because to date no harmful effects have been found. It is considered inappropriate to use ultrasound to view the fetus to only determine the gender (College of Physicians and Surgeons of Ontario, 2010).

Amniocentesis

This is a test used to obtain a sample of amniotic fluid for biochemical and genetic analysis. It is performed at 15–17 weeks' gestation when enough amniotic fluid is available to sample. Clinical trials using early amniocentesis before 12 weeks' gestation showed increased risk of complications and spontaneous abortion. In Canada, the test is not performed before 15 weeks' gestation.

- Indications: Amniocentesis is indicated for pregnant women over 35, karyotyping assessment for chromosomal abnormalities, assessing bilirubin levels, assessing alpha-fetoprotein levels, and assessing fetal lung maturity.
- Procedure: The woman is prepped and empties her bladder, and abdominal ultrasonography is used to locate a pocket of amniotic fluid and avoid fetal and placental structures. By needle aspiration, 15–20 mL of amniotic fluid is removed. The mother and fetus are monitored throughout the procedure.
- Complications: They are less than 1% but may include spontaneous abortion, hemorrhage, Rh isoimmunization, infection, fetal injury, leaking of amniotic fluid, and premature rupture of membranes. The woman may experience mild cramping postprocedure.
  - Rh-immune globulin is administered to Rh-negative women to prevent antibody formation.

LABOUR AND BIRTH PROCESSES

The intrapartum period, composed of four stages, begins with the onset of regular, true contractions that result in cervical dilatation and end with the recovery and stabilization of mother and infant following the birth.

Factors That Affect the Labour Process

The four factors, also known as the *four Ps*, are the passage, the passenger, the powers, and the psyche of the mother.

The Passage

The passage is made up of the maternal structures of the pelvis and soft tissues that the fetus must navigate through in the process of being born.

- Bony pelvis: Of the four types of pelvis (android, anthropoid, platypelloid, and gynecoid), the gynecoid pelvis is the most common (50%) and is ideally suited in its shape and dimensions to accommodate the movements of the fetus toward birth.
- Soft tissues: The lower uterus, cervix, vaginal canal, and introitus (opening) must all thin, stretch, and open to allow the fetus to pass through.

The Passenger

The fetus, or passenger, travels through the passage with an ease or degree of difficulty that is influenced by several factors:

- Fetal head size—The skull of the fetus is made up of bony plates connected by unfused suture lines and two fontanelles. The anterior and posterior fontanelles can be palpated vaginally to help determine the position and presentation of the fetus. The fetal skull can fit through the bony pelvis with the help of a slight overlapping of the bones, called *moulding*, during labour. Following birth, the head resumes its normal shape within a few days.
- Fetal lie—This describes the relationship between the long axis of the mother and the long axis of the fetus. Normal lie for a vaginal birth is longitudinal.
- Fetal presentation—The bony part of the fetus that presents or enters the pelvic inlet first. A cephalic, or head, presentation occurs in 97% of births. A breech presentation occurs in about 3%.
- Fetal attitude—The relationship of fetal body parts to each other. A normal attitude is one of moderate flexion, with the fetal chin tucked in toward the chest. A flexed attitude ideally allows for the smallest diameter of the head, the suboccipitobregmatic diameter, to enter the true pelvis. The biparietal diameter of the fetal head is the widest diameter.
- Fetal position—The relationship of the bony presenting part of the fetus to the four quadrants of the maternal pelvis. Using three letters, the position indicates if the presenting part (occiput, sacrum) is to the right or left of and anterior or posterior to the pelvis. ROA (right occipitoanterior) means that the occiput is facing toward the front and right of the pelvis. Posterior positions may result in persistent back pain during labour and a more prolonged labour.
- Engagement—This occurs when the largest transverse diameter (usually the biparietal) of the presenting part has passed through the pelvic inlet and into the true pelvis. Engagement can be determined by vaginal examination. For the primipara, engagement may occur a few weeks before the onset of labour.
- Station—Station is the relationship of the presenting part to the ischial spines of the maternal pelvis. The ischial spines are designated as station zero; above the spines is noted as a negative number from 1–5 cm and below is plus 1–5 cm. Station is assessed during a vaginal examination. Birth is imminent at +4 or +5 cm.

The Powers

Primary powers. These are the involuntary uterine contractions, measured by their frequency, duration, and intensity as they thin and dilate the cervix. Contractions are initiated by pacemaker points at the top of the fundus and radiate down over the uterus in rhythmic waves.

- The relaxation phase (minimum 60 seconds) between contractions is essential for restoring blood flow to the uterus and placenta.
- Frequency is measured as the time from the beginning of one contraction to the beginning of the next contraction. For example, contractions can be 3 minutes apart in frequency.
- Duration is the length a contraction lasts in seconds. Normal contractions last a maximum of 90 seconds in duration. After 90 seconds, there is a risk of fetal compromise and hypoxia.
- Intensity indicates the strength of the contraction, assessed by palpating the firmness of the uterus, and is recorded as mild, moderate, or strong.
- Effacement is measured as a percentage from 0–100%. During a contraction, the upper half of the uterus shortens and pulls up the lower uterine segment, stretching and thinning the cervix until only a thin edge can be palpated. In primiparas, effacement is quite advanced by the time contractions begin. In multiparas, effacement and dilatation occur together.
- Dilatation is the opening of the cervix and cervical canal from less than 1 cm to full dilatation, about 10 cm. Full dilatation marks the end of stage 1 of labour.

Secondary powers. When the cervix is completely dilated, the secondary powers are an important aid in assisting with the descent of the fetus through the birth canal. When the presenting part of the fetus descends to the pelvic floor, the contractions become expulsive. The mother experiences the urge to "bear down," which is the secondary power and is additional help in expelling the fetus.

- Uterine contractions continue.
- The mother feels an overwhelming urge to bear down and push, contracting her abdominal muscles and diaphragm with each contraction.
- Maternal position can aid the secondary powers. Being in an upright or squatting position improves uterine blood flow and uses gravity to help with the descent and birth of the fetus.

The Psyche

This important factor encompasses all of the psychosocial influences, past experiences, preparation, hopes, and beliefs the woman brings to the labour and birth experience. This event and the support she receives will impact the memories and beliefs she will integrate into her life after the experience. Supporting, educating, and collaborating with the mother and family during all stages of the labour and birth process are essential parts of the nursing role.

Pain Management During Labour and Birth

Intrapartum pain is complex and has both physiological and psychological components. Uterine contractions cause visceral hypoxic pain, while traction, pressure, and stretching can also cause various pain sensations to be felt. The woman's previous experience with pain and her coping strategies, fears, support systems, and beliefs about her control over the pain will also influence her perception of pain. The goal of pain management is to collaborate with the mother in finding measures that provide comfort and superior pain relief that is safe and appropriate to the stage of labour. The need for pharmacological agents is often reduced when timely information is provided about the progress of labour and supportive comfort measures are used.

Alternatives to pharmacological pain relief can include breathing techniques, walking or rocking motions, warm showers, hypnosis, meditation, effleurage, transcutaneous electrical nerve stimulation (TENS), therapeutic touch, and acupuncture.

Pharmacological Interventions

- Systemic opioids such as morphine sulphate provide pain relief and mild sedation; however, they cross the placenta, causing fetal CNS depression. They are avoided if birth is anticipated within 2–3 hours.
- Barbiturates and tranquilizers are not recommended for use in labour as they cross the placenta, cannot be reversed, and have a long half-life that may lead to respiratory and CNS depression in the mother and newborn.
- General anaesthesia is used less often for emergency Caesarean births. Maternal aspiration is a risk. Fetal CNS depression (including bradycardia, respiratory depression) may result from the drugs used and can be reversed with a narcotic antagonist.
- Regional anaesthesia usually provides very effective pain relief without affecting the woman's level of consciousness. Narcotic and anaesthetic agents are injected into a localized area and block the transmission of sensory nerve impulses to the brain. Limitations include only achieving partial pain relief, nerve damage (rare), and the need for skilled administration and careful monitoring for potential side effects.
- Regional anaesthesia methods include local infiltration of perineal tissues, pudendal block of perineal pain via local injection near the nerve plexus beside the ischial spines of the pelvis, and epidural block. In 2016–17 in Canada, the percentage of births using epidural anaesthesia ranged from 13.5% in the North West Territories to 72.1% in Quebec (Canadian Institute for Health Information, 2018).

Epidural Regional Anaesthesia

The anaesthetic agent is usually administered when the mother is in active labour. Injection is performed by a skilled anaesthetist into the lumbar epidural space between L2 and L3 or L3 and L4. Dermatome testing is done to assess for pain and respiratory distress. Epidural anaesthesia can be used for vaginal or Caesarean births.

- Preparation: Consent is obtained, an IV is established, and vital signs are recorded. A bolus of fluid is often given to increase maternal circulating volume and prevent hypotension. The mother is positioned in a curled side-lying or upright position leaning over to open the epidural spaces for maximum exposure. The nurse supports the mother in holding still during the needle insertion and alerts the physician to the onset of any contractions. If the catheter is left in place, it is securely taped to the woman's back.

- Monitoring: Pain relief is often obtained within 5–10 minutes, and the woman will experience a heaviness and numbness of the abdomen and legs. Turning the mother from one side to the other may help with even distribution of pain relief. Maternal vital signs and FHR are monitored frequently (q2–5 minutes initially) for hypotension and adverse effects.
- Complications: Although very rare, they may include inadvertent puncture of the dura with leakage of cerebrospinal fluid and respiratory distress. Injection into a vein rarely occurs but may result in seizures, loss of consciousness, cardiovascular collapse, and even death.

Nursing Considerations

- Discuss and plan for comfort and pain management strategies early in the labour process based on assessment findings and the wishes of the mother.
- Be aware that effective support includes promoting open communication, providing anticipatory teaching, offering praise and encouragement, and providing information about the progress of labour.
- Prepare the mother for the administration of any pharmacological agents and continuously monitor the mother and fetus for any potential adverse effects. Document all findings.
- Assist with epidural block by positioning the client during the procedure, securing a continuous epidural line, establishing IV access, administering fluids, monitoring volumetric solution changes, especially hypotension, monitoring contractions and FHR, assessing the effectiveness of pain relief, assessing for bladder distension, and monitoring the progress of labour.
- Have emergency equipment and narcotic antagonists such as naloxone (Narcan) available to reduce the effects of CNS depression if narcotic analgesics have been used.
- Evaluate the effectiveness of the pain management plan and modify strategies as needed.

Intrapartum Fetal Monitoring

Assessment of the FHR is the accepted standard of care to assess for fetal well-being and detect fetal compromise during active labour (London et al., 2017, p. 348). FHR can be assessed using noninvasive periodic auscultation with a stethoscope or electronic transducer or via continuous electronic FHR monitoring devices. All have their advantages and disadvantages. The most appropriate and least invasive means is used to provide the information needed for optimal care of the mother and the fetus during labour.

Intermittent Auscultation of FHR

This is the preferred method of FHR monitoring for women in active labour with no identified fetal or maternal risks (London et al., 2017, p. 348).

- The FHR is heard best over the fetal back via Leopold's manoeuvre. Take the maternal pulse at the same time to ensure the fetal pulse is not the mother's.
- Fetoscope or Doppler transducer: Listen for 1 full minute; apply gel to the woman's abdomen when using a transducer to improve sound wave transmission.

Continuous Electronic FHR Monitoring

This method monitors the response of and relationship between the FHR and the uterine contractions.

- Indications: It is used in high-risk pregnancies with a risk of uteroplacental insufficiency, apparent signs of fetal compromise, or oxytocin induction in labour.
- External monitoring: A flexible disc attached to an elastic belt, called a *tocotransducer*, is strapped over the fundus to detect and monitor contractions, but does not accurately measure uterine intensity or resting tone. An intrauterine pressure catheter measures uterine pressure. A second transducer is placed over the fetal back to assess FHR.
- Internal monitoring (scalp clip): This method is used when electronic fetal monitoring patterns are non-reassuring. The scalp clip can only be applied to the fetal scalp if the amniotic membranes are ruptured, the cervix is at least 2 cm dilated, and the fetal position and presentation are known.
  - Advantages: Allows ongoing assessment and early intervention for signs of fetal distress during active labour; potential decrease in fetal morbidity and mortality
  - Disadvantages: Potential interference with the labour process due to restriction on the mother's activity, inaccurate interpretation and increased risk for medical and surgical interventions, including Caesarean birth, increased risk of infection with scalp clip monitoring, false reassurance, or increased fears and anxiety regarding fetal well-being

Baseline FHR Patterns

- Baseline FHR is 110–160 bpm over 10 minutes.
- Fetal tachycardia is considered to be a rate greater than 160 bpm over a 10-minute period. The tachycardia may be related to maternal anxiety, infection, or prematurity or may indicate distress if accompanied by other changes in FHR patterns, such as poor variability.
- Fetal bradycardia is an FHR of less than 110 bpm for 10 minutes. The bradycardia may be related to maternal hypotension, fetal hypoxia, placental separation, or cord compression. Bradycardia associated with poor variability and late deceleration patterns requires clinical assessment. It may be necessary to prepare for an early delivery.

Variability

FHR variability is the term used to describe the normal small fluctuations in heartbeat rate observed over 1 minute. The average FHR variability is 6–25 bpm. Count maternal and fetus pulse. Variability that is absent or minimal (≤5 bpm) for 40 minutes is atypical and requires ongoing close monitoring.

If this pattern continues for greater than 80 minutes, immediate intervention is needed.

Periodic Changes in FHR

The following periodic changes in FHR last less than 2 minutes and are in response to uterine contractions. They occur early, late, or variably during the course of the contractions.

- Accelerations: FHR normally increases with fetal activity 15 bpm for 15 seconds for the term infant, and is a sign of normal sympathetic nervous system response.
- Early decelerations: They occur early in the contraction with a return to normal baseline by the time the contraction is over. They are repetitious. They are associated with head compression as labour progresses. They do not require intervention.
- Variable decelerations: They vary in duration, degree of severity, length of time, and timing during the contractions. They are associated with umbilical cord compression, and as the cord becomes compressed during or between contractions, the FHR drops and then recovers. These decelerations are considered ominous, with an immediate need for intervention if variability is also depressed and the decelerations are 60 bpm below normal baseline and last longer than 60 seconds in duration. Reduce maternal anxiety and coach to change breathing or pushing.
- Late decelerations: They occur late in the contraction, with recovery during the resting phase between contractions. They are associated with uteroplacental insufficiency as seen with maternal hypertension disorders, diabetes, or obstetrical emergencies such as placental abruption. Persistent, late decelerations are ominous, even if the FHR does not decrease dramatically, since they represent fetal compromise and hypoxia. If there is also poor variability, intrauterine resuscitation measures should be initiated promptly.

Nursing Considerations for FHR Monitoring

- Assess the most appropriate means of monitoring FHR. Provide explanations and answer questions regarding the use of electronic monitoring.
- Document electronic fetal monitoring patterns with uterine contractions; they are every 15 minutes in the active phase of labour and every 5 minutes in the second stage of labour once pushing.
- Respond to changing situations in FHR patterns by providing the mother with information and ongoing rationales for actions.
- Initiate intrauterine resuscitation measures to correct early distress by increasing uterine blood flow and perfusion, decreasing umbilical cord compression, improving fetal oxygen supply, and allowing time for preparing for an emergency Caesarean birth if needed.

Premonitory Signs of Labour

There are many theories concerning what triggers labour, including decreasing progesterone levels, increasing oxytocin and prostaglandins that stimulate contractions, and placental aging and uterine distension that irritate the uterus and stimulate contractions. The following list includes some of the most significant indicators that labour is imminent:

- "Lightening" is the perceived sensation that the fetus is lower in the pelvis. It occurs anytime in the last 4 weeks of pregnancy for the primipara and closer to or at the time of labour for the multipara.
- Braxton Hicks contractions (involuntary uterine tightening) become stronger and more frequent.
- A nesting instinct or a burst of energy may result from lowered progesterone levels.
- Diarrhea or loose stools occur.
- Weight loss of 1–2 kg occurs a few days before onset of labour.
- Increased vaginal secretions or bloody show may indicate that the mucous plug has been expelled.
- Spontaneous rupture of membranes is confirmed with nitrazine paper; amniotic fluid is alkaline and will fern on a glass slide; it should be clear and odourless.

Stages and Mechanisms of Labour and Birth
First Stage of Labour

The first stage of labour is from the onset of regular uterine contractions to the full effacement and dilatation of the cervix. It is divided into three phases: latent, active, and transitional. Primiparas tend to labour longer than multiparas (20 hours versus 14 hours, on average).
- Latent phase: Up to 3 cm dilatation, regular contractions, mostly progress in effacement
- Active phase: 4–7 cm dilatation, contractions every 2–5 minutes, descent of the fetus begins
- Transitional phase: 7 cm to full dilatation; contractions every 2 minutes are very intensely felt by the mother

Second Stage of Labour

- From complete cervical dilatation and effacement to the birth of the infant, up to 2 hours for a primipara, often much less time for a multipara
- The term *crowning* means that the widest diameter of the head is encircled by the introitus. Pushing is stopped to allow for controlled delivery of the head and to prevent perineal trauma.

Third Stage of Labour

- From the birth of the infant to the expulsion of the placenta, lasting up to 30 minutes
- The uterus maintains a contracted state, constricting the blood vessels and controlling bleeding.

Fourth Stage of Labour

The fourth stage is the immediate recovery and stabilization time, from the delivery of the placenta to 2–4 hours after the birth.

Mechanisms of Labour

Also known as the *cardinal movements*, these are the various positions the fetus assumes in a cephalic presentation as it

Fig. 9.3 Cardinal movements of the mechanism of labour. **A,** Engagement and descent. **B,** Flexion. **C,** Internal rotation to occipitoanterior (OA) position. **D,** Extension. **E,** External rotation beginning (restitution). **F,** External rotation. (From Lowdermilk, D. L., Perry, S. E., Cashion, K., et al. [2016]. *Maternity & women's health care* [11th ed., p. 377, Fig. 16.12]. St. Louis: Mosby.)

moves through the confines of the pelvis and birth canal. See Fig. 9.3.

1. Engagement and descent: The fetus moves downward into the pelvic passageway.
2. Flexion: The head flexes downward, chin to chest.
3. Internal rotation: The head rotates 45 degrees.
4. Extension: The head passes under the symphysis pubis and reaches the perineum.
5. External rotation: The head rotates back to its original position (restitution), followed by shoulder rotation.
6. Expulsion: The shoulders pass under the pubic arch and perineum; the body is delivered.

Nursing Considerations During Labour and Birth

In a hospital birth, the nurse spends more time with the woman and her family during the labour and birth process than any other healthcare provider. This presents a significant responsibility to provide safe, effective care while enjoying a place of privilege in welcoming a new family member and person into the world.

Labour Nursing Considerations for the First Stage of Labour

- Undertake initial maternal and fetal assessment: This includes past history, length of pregnancy, onset of labour and progression, spontaneous rupture of membranes, contractions, bloody show, preparation and plans for pain management and childbirth, family support, vital signs, FHR, gestational age, risk factors or complications, plans for infant feeding, vaginal examination for cervical dilatation, effacement, station, and fetal presentation and position.
- Provide ongoing support: It is recommended that women in active labour receive ongoing support with 1:1 nursing care (Liston, Sawchuck, & Young, 2007).
- Monitor labour: Observe and check the progress of labour and the maternal and fetal responses to labour according to unit protocols or more frequently as indicated by assessment findings. The minimum should be vital signs, vaginal show q1h, contractions and FHR q15–30 minutes during

active labour and more frequent assessment of bloody show, contractions, FHR monitoring (q5–10 minutes) during transition.

- Monitor for bladder fullness: Do so especially if an epidural block is used.
- Monitor for spontaneous or artificial rupture of membranes (AROM): Assess FHR for distress due to possible cord prolapse or compression; fluid should be clear and odourless, with no meconium.
- Assess for complications of labour: They include duration of contractions longer than 90 seconds, resting phase shorter than 60 seconds, FHR outside normal limits or periodic changes, maternal temperature above 38°C, rupture of membranes more than 24 hours before, foul-smelling amniotic fluid or maternal show, persistent dark or bright red vaginal bleeding, sustained abdominal pain with rigid abdomen.
- Keep vaginal examinations to a minimum to reduce the risk of infection: After the initial examination, a repeat examination may be done prior to giving additional pain medication or when the mother feels increased perineal pressure and the urge to bear down.
- Prepare for the birth: Birth is imminent when the multiparous woman reaches transition and when the nulliparous woman is fully dilated.

Nursing Considerations for the Second and Third Stages of Labour

- Prepare the mother: Ensure that her bladder is empty prior to pushing, assist her into a birthing position, give support for relaxing between contractions and pushing effectively during contractions, and monitor contractions and FHR.
- Prepare for the infant: Have warm and dry blankets, a preheated radiant overhead warmer, and resuscitation equipment available.
- Provide immediate newborn care: Assess and maintain a patent infant airway, use maternal–fetal skin-to-skin contact and immediately dry the infant to minimize hypothermia, note the time of birth, assess Apgar scores at 1 and 5 minutes, document first voiding or passing of meconium, assess for gestational age and obvious defects, provide resuscitation as needed, administer vitamin K (1.0 mg intramuscular [IM] if birth weight is greater than 1 500 g) and eye prophylaxis, verify and apply identification, weigh and measure the infant, and promote attachment with the mother and family through early breastfeeding, holding the infant, and interacting.
  - Apgar scores are used to assess adaptation to extrauterine transitions. Parameters are heart rate, respiratory effort, muscle tone, reflex irritability, and colour. A score of 8–10 is normal.
- Provide maternal care: Assist with placental delivery; obtain cord blood samples if required; monitor vital signs, perineal trauma, vaginal bleeding, lochia, and uterine contractility; administer oxytocin for uterine contractility;

assess the bladder; and provide pain medication and a perineal ice pack.

Nursing Considerations for the Fourth Stage of Labour

- Assess for uterine contractility. Check fundal height (midway between the umbilicus and symphysis). The uterus rises to just below the umbilical height after several hours. Assess the position (midline) and tone (firm).
- Assess the perineum and lochia. Check the amount of lochia, its character, and whether there are clots or hemorrhage. Hemorrhage (blood loss greater than 500 mL) is suspected if uterine tone is soft and a perineal pad is saturated within 15 minutes. Assess the perineum for hematomas, swelling, and hemorrhoids; offer ice packs.
- Assess maternal vital signs, bladder tone, and ability to void.
- Promote early parental attachment and provide support for breastfeeding choice.
- Assess fetus for ongoing ease of transition to extrauterine life, monitor vital signs and responsiveness, and prevent heat loss.

Essentials of Labour and Birth Complications
Dystocia

Dystocia is a prolonged, abnormal labour related to maternal factors (uterus or pelvis) or fetal factors (size, presentation, position, number of fetuses):

- Abnormal uterine contractions—Hypertonic contractions in the latent phase are abnormally painful and irregular but ineffective in effacing or dilating the cervix. Narcotic analgesia may allow the mother to rest and uterine patterns to revert to normal. Hypotonic contractions become ineffective or stop at the active phase. Oxytocin may be used to augment labour once fetal pelvic relationship problems have been ruled out.
- Precipitous labour—It lasts less than 3 hours, with increased risk of uterine rupture, amniotic fluid embolism, and postpartum hemorrhage. Fetal complications include distress and hypoxia.
- Pelvic dystocia—This relates to a pelvic shape that does not allow for descent of the fetus, leading to prolonged labour, increased risk of assisted birth with forceps or vacuum, risk of birth trauma, or Caesarean birth.
- Cephalopelvic disproportion—Excessive fetal size causes problems with descent through the pelvis or under the pubic arch. Assisted birth with forceps, vacuum suction, or Caesarean birth may be needed.
- Breech position—The breech position occurs in 3% of presentations, with the sacrum (buttocks) most commonly presenting to the pelvis. There is an increased risk of birth trauma, prolonged labour, asphyxia, cord prolapse, and the need for Caesarean birth.
- Multiple fetuses—More than one fetus increases the risk of preterm labour, breech or shoulder presentation of one or more fetuses, cord prolapse, fetal compromise, and operative birth.

Induction or Augmentation of Labour

Methods, including AROM or medications, are used to initiate labour prior to the onset of spontaneous contractions.

- AROM usually stimulates contractions within 12 hours. Amniotic fluid is slowly released. The fetal head should be engaged to prevent cord prolapse. Nursing considerations include noting the time of rupture and the colour, amount, and presence of meconium and monitoring maternal temperature q2h as the risk of infection increases 24 hours after rupture of membranes.
- Cervical ripening methods include Foley catheter insertion into the cervix, cervical prostaglandin gel, and augmentation 24 hours later with oxytocin infusion.
- Oxytocin (Pictosin) infusion requires following a careful protocol for administering IV oxytocin with an infusion pump. The dosage should be increased no more frequently than q30 minutes followed by frequent maternal and fetal monitoring. Fetal monitoring is used and contractions are closely monitored for excessive uterine activity or tetanic contractions (greater than 90 seconds). At any sign of maternal or fetal compromise, the oxytocin infusion is stopped until further assessment can be made (London et al., 2017, p. 455).

Caesarean Birth

- Indications for a Caesarean section are often related to preventing or intervening in situations of fetal compromise or maternal medical emergencies that require an immediate response or operative birth.
- Surgical incision is most commonly low segment transverse (bikini line) with improved healing and lower risk of hemorrhage or subsequent rupture. The classic and longitudinal incision increases the risks of hemorrhage, pain, healing time, and future uterine rupture is related to location of incision.
- Regional anaesthesia is the preferred method for pain management as the mother is awake and there are fewer complications than with general anaesthesia. General anaesthesia is primarily used when rapid birth is necessary in emergency situations.
- Maternal risks and complications include aspiration, infection, hemorrhage, anaesthesia complications, prolonged postpartum recovery, thrombophlebitis, pain, and immobility.
- Fetal risks include transient tachypnea with "wetter lungs" as fetal lung fluid was not removed during passage through the birth canal, as well as CNS depression from the general anaesthetic.
- Additional nursing considerations include postoperative vital sign monitoring, assessment of incision, pain management, extra assistance with infant care and feeding, monitoring for complications, and encouraging early ambulation.

Vaginal Birth After Caesarean (VBAC)

Following a Caesarean birth, it may be possible for a woman to attempt to give birth vaginally in subsequent pregnancies. Recommended parameters for VBAC are the desire to have a vaginal birth, the absence of previous indications for Caesarean section, uncomplicated pregnancy, fetal vertex presentation, normal labour, and a previous incision that was low segment transverse (Martel & MacKinnon, 2005).

Preterm Labour and Birth

- Labour between 20 and 37 weeks' gestation with uterine contractions and cervical dilatation is considered preterm and presents the risk of premature birth of an immature fetus.
- Maternal risk factors include underweight (less than 45 kg), smoker, strenuous physical activity, physical abuse, no antenatal care, chronic illness, premature rupture of membranes, infection, multiple pregnancy (50% of twin gestations are premature), past history of preterm labour, maternal age less than 18 years, polyhydramnios, cervical insufficiency, cardiovascular disease, placental disorders, and unknown causes (London et al., 2017, p. 407).
- Therapeutic interventions include early risk screening, early detection of onset, stopping uterine contractions, and preparing for care of the premature infant. High-risk mothers should be knowledgeable and know how to immediately report all signs of preterm labour; activities may be restricted or admission to hospital indicated.
- If birth is inevitable, an episiotomy may be used to reduce the risk of intraventricular hemorrhage from pressure on the fragile premature skull. A pediatrician or neonatologist should be present to assist in the resuscitation and transportation of the newborn. Nursing considerations in addition to assisting with the birth include supporting the parents with factual information, avoiding false hope, acknowledging their concerns, taking photos if the infant is to be admitted to a neonatal intensive care unit, and providing ongoing psychological support and information.

Perinatal Loss and Bereavement

When perinatal loss occurs during the course of a pregnancy, it is a tragedy and crisis for the parents and family. For many young families, it may be their first encounter with the death of a family member. Maternal newborn nurses and staff are also affected by the death of a fetus or newborn. Perinatal loss is unique in that it often occurs suddenly, with little warning, and interrupts the normal developmental processes of pregnancy and parenthood. Practical nurses need to understand the grief process as it applies to perinatal loss and provide skilful, sensitive care during this highly vulnerable time.

Losses include stillbirths, prematurity, newborns with anomalies, and neonatal deaths.

Grief is a personal experience of deeply felt sorrow at the loss of something highly valued. Grief occurs in stages, slowly over a period of time, allowing the individuals to work their way through the various defences the psyche uses to protect itself from the full impact of the loss. Grief does not follow a linear path—it is a dynamic process.

Stages of Grief

- Parents experience disbelief and shock as they cannot take in the reality of the news. In being overwhelmed, parents may appear not able to hear or understand what is being said to them; they may be immobile or emotionally numb in their initial reactions.
- Anger may be expressed as the reality of the situation is absorbed. Women often have more difficulty than men in expressing anger; this may result in depression and feelings of guilt. Anger may be directed at staff.
- Bargaining occurs when there is an understanding of the reality of the situation but hope that something can change it.
- Depression, overwhelming sadness, and withdrawal represent a greater level of acceptance of the impact of the loss.
- Acceptance is the process of integrating the experience and its meaning into one's life. Normal activities slowly resume, and memories of both sorrow and joy can be recounted.
- Acute grief reactions are intensely felt for 6–10 weeks, but the full process of grieving usually takes time, frequently over 1–2 years.

Behavioural and Physical Symptoms of Grief

- Somatic manifestations include weight gain or loss, nausea, hyperventilating, sighing respirations, tightening of the throat, heavy feeling in the chest, palpitations, headaches, loss of muscle strength, and extreme fatigue.
- Behavioural manifestations include preoccupation; nightmares; feelings of guilt, shame, apathy, loneliness, isolation, anger, sorrow, and irritability; decreased sexual interest; social withdrawal; crying; exhaustion; loss of concentration and motivation; and restlessness.

Nursing Considerations

- Promote an empathetic environment that openly acknowledges the death of the newborn and supports the reactions of the mother and family. Provide time for the parents to see, touch, and be with the infant. Take photos and collect as many mementos as possible: locks of hair (requires parental permission), footprints, ID band, and weight and length information.
- Provide information about community resources on grief counselling and bereavement, and follow-up in the postpartum period.
- Be sensitive to and accommodate cultural and religious practices.
- Grieving parents are vulnerable to well-meaning but harmful comments and clichés that minimize their loss. Educate others as to why these comments are harmful. Offer suggestions for helping the family acknowledge and cope with the loss.
- Understand that immediate and extended family members are all affected by the loss. Sibling responses will be dependent on their age and stage of development. Simple language that is honest and clear in its meaning and uses words such as "death" lessens confusion and fears.

- Practical nurses need to take the time to understand their own beliefs and reactions to loss and death in order to be emotionally available to others who are grieving. Finding ways to nurture oneself following these painful experiences is beneficial and important.

THE POSTPARTUM STAGE

Sometimes referred to as the *fourth trimester*, this 6-week puerperium is when the mother's body returns to its prepregnant state, the newborn adapts to an extrauterine life, and family members begin to adjust to the many changes a newborn brings into their lives.

Maternal Adaptations
Physiological Changes

- Reproductive changes: The uterus remains firmly contracted and undergoes involution, descending from the height of the umbilicus about one fingerbreadth per day until it can no longer be palpated by days 10–14. By 6 weeks postpartum, the uterus has returned to its nonpregnant state. The cervix becomes thicker and firmer and contracts over several weeks to an elongated rather than a circular opening. The perineum remains swollen, perhaps bruised for a few days, and the vaginal rugae and tone return within 6–10 weeks.
- Sexual intercourse: Assuming that there is no infection or complications, intercourse may resume when the woman feels physically and emotionally comfortable and ready. Appropriate methods of birth control should be discussed and planned for as part of postpartum teaching prior to discharge home.
- Lochia, or uterine discharge: It changes over the course of about 3 weeks from lochia rubra (dark red, with small clots) for 3–4 days to lochia serosa (pinkish, serosanguinous) from days 3–10, to lochia alba (whitish to clear, no odour) from day 10 to week 3.
- Breast changes: Colostrum is present at the time of birth, and breast milk is produced by the third or fourth day postpartum. Engorgement is common when milk production starts and lasts 24 hours. Newborn suckling and feeding stimulates prolactin, which stimulates more milk production. (See the section "Newborn Nutrition").
- Cardiovascular changes: They are significant as the circulating blood volume decreases rapidly and is lost through diuresis and diaphoresis (perspiration). Blood pressure remains stable; transient bradycardia (as low as 50 bpm) lasts up to 3 months.
- Renal changes: The glomerular filtration rate is elevated to help mobilize excess vascular volume; overdistension of the bladder and difficulty voiding in the first 24 hours are fairly common. A full bladder may displace the uterus in the early postpartum stages.
- Endocrine changes: Estrogen and progesterone drop rapidly following birth, and prolactin rises, reaching a peak at day 3, when breast milk production begins. Menstruation is often delayed with breastfeeding until 12–24 weeks

postpartum. Menstruation returns for nonbreastfeeding mothers by 6–12 weeks postpartum.

Psychological Adaptations and Attachment

- The disruption to normal sleep patterns, the increased need for rest and recovery, the needs of a newborn, and changing roles and relationships all add to the stress of adapting to parenting in the postpartum period.
- The transition to parenting is aided by family and community support, positive past experiences, cultural beliefs and practices that promote attachment, and learned adaptive behaviours for coping with change.
- The term *attachment* is preferred to the older term *bonding* when describing the process by which the parents interact and form a relationship with their newborn. The newborn is more awake and sensitive to its surroundings in the first hour of life than it will be for the next 2 weeks, so it is an ideal time for interaction. While this time is ideal, parents should not feel guilty if circumstances do not allow for this first intimate contact to happen. Attachment is the reciprocal relationship that develops over time as parents and newborn interact with each other, using cues and responses to learn to understand each other and to connect on an emotional level.
- Most women experience postpartum blues, often on days 3–5, when milk production begins and prolactin levels surge. This condition is characterized by feelings of inexplicable sadness, letdown, and increased crying and usually resolves within 10 days.

Maternal Complications

Postpartum Hemorrhage

- Risk factors include polyhydramnios, multiple gestation, rapid labour, prolonged rupture of membrane, placenta previa, high parity, a history of coagulation disorder, uterine atony, retained placenta, and trauma.
- Early postpartum hemorrhage is a blood loss of 500 mL or more that occurs in the first 24 hours after giving birth. It is usually related to the uterus not contracting or staying contracted following delivery of the placenta, lacerations of the cervix or vagina, parts of the placenta being retained, or clotting disorders. It presents a greater risk of morbidity and mortality to the mother than does a late hemorrhage.
- Late postpartum hemorrhage occurs after 24 hours following birth and is most often related to retained placental fragments.

Nursing considerations.

- Assess uterine involution and teach the mother what to expect with vaginal discharge and what signs of complications to report, including fever greater than 38°C, lochia that changes back to rubra or bright red bleeding, a pad that soaks through in 15 minutes, foul-smelling lochia or urine, or feelings of inability to cope and sadness that last more than 1 or 2 weeks.
- Know that an inability to void and a full bladder may displace the uterus from its midline position, impairing the normal contractility and increasing the risk of

hemorrhage. Assess the bladder frequently early in the postpartum period and encourage frequent voiding.

- Monitor the uterus and vaginal blood loss q15 minutes following birth for the first hour and as per unit protocol for the next 24 hours. Gentle massage of the uterus may stimulate uterine contractility, as will breastfeeding. Know the policy and procedure for responding to a postpartum hemorrhage.
- Following birth, it is recommended to administer oxytocin to promote uterine contractility and prevent postpartum hemorrhage.

Infection

Infection is a significant cause of maternal morbidity and may include the uterus, post–Caesarean section incision, urinary tract, or breasts (mastitis).

Nursing considerations.

- Assess the mother for signs of infection, including a temperature of 38°C or higher, tachycardia, pain and tenderness, redness or swelling, nausea and feeling unwell, foul-smelling discharge, and excessive fatigue.
- Teach the mother how to recognize and report any signs of fever and infection. Teach the importance of taking all doses of antibiotics as prescribed. In the case of mastitis, continued breastfeeding or manual expressing of breast milk is recommended.

Postpartum Depression

Unlike those of the postpartum blues, the manifestations of depression continue and worsen over time. They include feelings of despair, hopelessness, inadequacy, ambivalence or apathy toward the newborn, inability to feel joy, and somatic symptoms of headache, appetite changes, sighing, excessive fatigue, or hyperactivity. This disorder is more common than thought or reported in the past and must be part of health teaching and follow-up care.

Nursing considerations. It is essential that practical nurses teach the parents to be aware of the manifestations of depression and to seek support and medical help promptly. Depression is a disease process of neurochemical imbalance; it is not a personal failure or weakness. It is crucial to seek help, follow the treatment plan, and involve others who may provide support, including extended family and community programs.

Newborn Adaptations

Beginning with the process of labour, the fetus undergoes many changes on a physiological and developmental level. These transitional changes allow the newborn to adapt to life outside the uterine environment. While remaining dependent on others for nutrition, warmth, and a nurturing environment, the newborn is remarkably well equipped to interpret, respond to, and make known his or her needs.

Transition to Extrauterine Life

Transition is a critical time period in the first 6–24 hours of life, when many newborn anatomical and physiological changes occur, especially in the cardiovascular and respiratory systems. The fetus has three unique cardiac features that change during transition, beginning with the stimulation of labour and the newborn's first breath. External and internal stimuli initiate these changes. Nurses assess the newborn's ability to adapt during the different transitional periods of reactivity.

Respiratory adaptations.

- By 35–37 weeks, the fetal lungs are structurally developed enough to do the work of breathing. Surfactant, a phospholipid that lubricates the lungs and helps keep them partially inflated after each breath, peaks, with an L:S ratio of 2:1.
- Fetal anatomical structures that change during transition as the newborn initiates breathing are the ductus venosus, ductus arteriosus, and foramen ovale.
- Stimuli that initiate respirations include chemical, mechanical, and sensory factors:
  - Chemical stimuli—Uterine contractions temporarily decrease fetal oxygen supply, causing a mild acidosis that stimulates the respiratory centre of the brain to initiate breathing.
  - Mechanical stimuli—Most of the lung fluid is squeezed out as the fetal chest is compressed in the birth canal. There is a passive intake of breath once the chest is past the birth canal.
  - Sensory stimuli—The abrupt change in environmental temperature at birth is a major stimulus to breathe, in addition to touch, light, sound, noise, and pain.
- After the first breath, pressure changes occur in the lungs and circulation. The lungs open and pulmonary vessels dilate, changing from a closed high-pressure system to an open low-pressure system.

Circulatory adaptations.

- The fetal circulatory system changes from a low-pressure to a higher-pressure system, causing the fetal circulatory structures to close.
- The foramen ovale, located between the right and left atrium, closes as blood flow and pressure on the left side of the heart become greater than on the right side of the heart.
- The ductus venosus, located between the inferior vena cava and the umbilical vein, closes when the umbilical cord is clamped.
- The ductus arteriosus, located between the pulmonary artery and the aorta, closes when pulmonary blood flow and pressures increase. Rising oxygen levels are detected by chemoreceptor sites on the ductus, which also helps stimulate the ductus arteriosus to close.
- **Note:** These anatomical structures functionally close within 15–20 minutes of birth, but a murmur may be heard for 6–12 hours in the newborn. If the infant is hypoxic or asphyxiated, the ductus arteriosus may open again. Refer to Fig. 9.4, which illustrates fetal circulation.

Temperature adaptation.

- All newborns are at increased risk for heat loss (via convection, radiation, evaporation, and conduction) due to their large body surface compared with body mass, blood vessels close to the skin surface, an inability to shiver, and immature CNS temperature-control mechanisms. Newborns can also easily overheat if wrapped in too many layers of clothes.
- Maintaining a neutral thermal environment means that the newborn must use only minimum amounts of oxygen, glucose, and metabolic energy to keep warm.
- Newborns use nonshivering thermogenesis to metabolize their unique brown fat stores to generate body heat.

Renal adaptations.

- Full-term infants normally void in the first 24 hours of life. They have a limited ability to concentrate urine and may lose 10% of their body weight in the first 3 days of life due to fluid shifts and losses. They will regain the weight within 1 week with normal feeding.
- **Note:** In the first week, a newborn that is receiving adequate hydration through feeding should have one heavy wet diaper for each day of life.

Gastro-intestinal adaptations.

- The gut is sterile at birth, bowel sounds begin within the first few hours, the first meconium stool passes within 24 hours, and the newborn requires frequent feedings of 30–90 mL—or until satisfied at the breast—every few hours.
- There is an increased risk of bleeding in the first week of life, and vitamin K IM is routinely administered.
- The cardiac sphincter between the esophagus and stomach is immature, and regurgitation of feeding is common. Burping following feeding will help.
- Stool characteristics change from meconium (thick, sticky, black, passed in the first 24 hours) to transitional stools (thin, brownish-green). Breastfed stools are bright mustard yellow, loose, and frequent. Formula-fed stools are pasty, pale yellow, and less frequent. Elimination patterns may vary, from once to five or six per day in the first few weeks.
- The fetal liver is immature and unable to conjugate bilirubin well at term. Most preterm and 50% of full-term infants will experience physiological jaundice in the first week of life.
- **Note:** Physiological jaundice or hyperbilirubinemia (indicated by yellowed skin, mucous membranes, and eye sclera) appears after 24 hours of life in infants who are otherwise well, peaks at 3 days, and resolves itself by 10 days. Phototherapy may be used as ultraviolet light aids in conjugating bilirubin into a water-soluble form that can be excreted in urine and stools. Frequent feedings help resolve physiological jaundice.

Nursing Considerations

- Be aware that adequately hydrated newborns should wet 6–8 diapers each day.
- Monitor for physiological jaundice, encourage early and frequent feedings, and implement phototherapy as needed, covering eyes while exposing skin to ultraviolet lights. Phototherapy side effects include a sleepy newborn, loose stools, and an increased need for fluids of 10%.

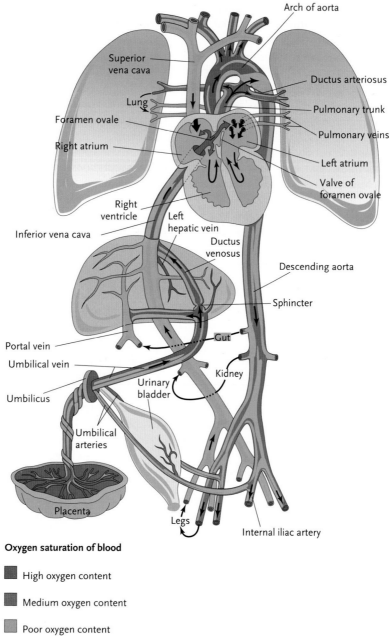

Fig. 9.4 Fetal circulation. (Moore, K & Persaud, T.V.N. [2008] *Before we are born: essentials of embryology and birth defects* [7th ed., p. 221, Fig 14.32] Philadelphia, PA. Saunders/Elsevier.)

- As newborns are obligate nose breathers from birth up until 3 months of age, ensure that nasal passages are clear.
- Closely monitor for expected vital signs and physical and behavioural adaptations.
- First period of reactivity:
  - Immediately after birth, tachypnea up to 80 breaths per minute with nasal flaring
  - Tachycardia up to 180 bpm
  - Murmur may be heard; hands and feet may appear blue (acrocyanosis) as peripheral circulation is sluggish
  - Neurologically awake and alert

- Period of relative inactivity:
  - Heart and respiratory rate and effort decrease to normal range of heart rate 120–160 bpm
  - Respiratory rate of 30–50
  - Newborn falls asleep
- Second period of reactivity:
  - Very responsive and awake
  - Increased oral mucus may lead to gagging and cyanosis
  - May have tachycardia
  - Bowel sounds present; may pass meconium and void for the first time
- Monitor temperature frequently; prevent heat loss by drying newborn immediately, protecting from drafts

Essential Newborn Assessment

A systematic assessment of the full-term newborn reveals findings in appearance, reflexes, and responses to the environment that are normal, a variation on normal, or abnormal (Fig. 9.5). These findings also vary depending on the gestational age of the newborn. Assessment should include the following:

- Vital signs—Temperature is labile, prone to hypothermia due to large body surface area, not a reliable indicator of infection, and 36.5–37°C; blood pressure is 60/40 to 80/50 mm Hg; respiratory rate is 30–60; listen for heart rate at apex for 1 full minute (120–170 bpm when awake, 80–90 bpm when sleeping).
- Weight and length—Average weight is 3 500 g; average length is 50 cm.
- Skin—Skin is pink or ruddy; body fat is present; acrocyanosis resolves after 12 hours; waxy vernix is present in creases; lanugo (fine downy hair) is present; erythema toxicum or newborn rash and milia on nose are common and resolve spontaneously. Birthmarks may be permanent, such as port wine stain, or they may resolve, as in strawberry hemangioma (or "stork bite marks").
- Head—The head appears large compared with the flexed body. Measure the head circumference at the widest diameter of the occiput and over the eyebrows; average is 33–35 cm. Moulding resolves in the first week, anterior fontanelle is soft and pulsating and may be tense with crying. Assess for symmetrical facial features. Outer edge of eye should be in line with the top of the ear; eyes are slate blue and tearless and can focus 45 cm; ear cartilage springs back when folded. Palate in mouth is intact; Epstein's pearls (small white gum cysts) that look like teeth may be visible, but they disappear spontaneously.
- Chest—The chest moves in unison with the abdomen when breathing; it typically has a 32-cm circumference over nipple line. Engorged breasts are common due to maternal estrogen effect.
- Back and extremities—The back is smooth and straight; no dermal sinus or defect appear at base of spine. The extremities are symmetrical and flexible; full-term nails extend beyond fingertips; skin creases on soles of feet.
- Abdomen—The abdomen is cylindrical, protrudes, and bowel sounds are audible after 30 minutes of birth. The umbilical cord has two arteries and one vein, and dries and falls off within 7 days. A patent anus passes meconium within 24 hours and voids within 24 hours. Reddish-brick dust spots in urine are harmless urate crystals.
- Genitals—In girls, the labia majora covers the minora, and pseudomenstruation is common due to the effect of maternal hormones. In boys, assess that both testes are in scrotum and full-term scrotum has rugae; inspect penis for central position of the urethra.
- Reflexes in full-term newborn include Moro (startle), rooting (turns head toward stroked cheek), grasp/palmar (grasps fingers around object), tonic neck (head turned to one side, same side arm and leg extend, opposite arm and leg flex), stepping (held upright, legs move as if stepping), and positive Babinski (when the sole of the foot is stroked upward, the toes extend outward).
- Behaviour states—These include crying, quiet, and alert (ideal time to interact, assess, feed), deep sleep (tunes out environment, very still, regular respiratory rate), and active alert (irregular breathing, easily startled, eyes wide, may cry, turns from eye contact).

Nursing Care, Parent Teaching, and Follow-Up Considerations

- Safety: Teach the parents to never leave the newborn unattended in a bath, on a change table, or with a family pet. Also, Canadian law requires that all newborns be transported in an approved car seat. The safest position is rear-facing with the car seat in the back seat of the vehicle.
- *Candida albicans*: A pinpoint bright red diaper rash that does not resolve within 24 hours may be caused by *C. albicans* and should be assessed for antifungal skin treatment. Oral thrush (coated or red tongue and throat) will also require treatment.
- Sudden unexpected infant death (SUID): Newborns should sleep on their backs, in their own crib, on a firm mattress with no pillows or thick blankets in the crib.
- Ongoing assessment: Following stabilization in the transitional stage, ongoing assessment at each shift and as needed includes monitoring of vital signs and skin colour and integrity; nutrition and elimination patterns; behavioural responses; and interactions with the mother and family.
- Vitamin K injection/eye prophylaxis: If not part of labour and birth procedures, administer vitamin K 1.0 mg IM within 6 hours of birth to prevent hemorrhagic disease of the newborn (into the middle one-third of the side of the thigh muscle—the vastus lateralis—using a 25-gauge needle) and eye prophylaxis (erythromycin [E-Mycin] ointment onto the lower lid of the eye).
- Hygiene: A sponge or tub bath daily or twice per week using mild soap is recommended. Prevent excess heat loss and assess water temperature (24°C) using a thermometer or dorsal part of the hand, not the fingers; do not use baby powder as particles may be aspirated. Bathing prior to feeding will avoid the risk of regurgitation and promote alertness for better feeding success.
- Client teaching on newborn problems: Provide phone numbers and resources and teach parents to seek help if the newborn is experiencing difficulty breathing, not successfully feeding, not voiding 6–8 wet diapers per day, crying inconsolably, lethargic, or jaundiced or appears unwell.
- Infection avoidance: Everyone having contact with the newborn should first wash their hands and avoid contact if they are infectious as the newborn immune system is immature.
- Diaper rash: Diaper rash may be treated with exposure to air (avoid cold stress), petroleum jelly or zinc oxide barrier products, and frequent diaper changes with each feeding.

MOULDING
A. Significant moulding, soon after birth.
B. Schematic of bones of skull when moulding is present.

CAPUT SUCCEDANEUM
Caput succedaneum (left) and
cephalhematoma (right) are common birth injuries.

CEPHALHEMATOMA

NEVUS FLAMMEUS
(Port-wine stain)

**SUBCONJUNCTIVAL
HEMORRHAGE**

MILIA
(Vernix-filled sebaceous glands)

FORCEPS MARKS

CUTIS MARMORATA
(Mottling)

MONGOLIAN SPOT
Mongolian spots are common in dark-skinned
children. These bluish skin discolorations
should not be confused with bruises.

Fig. 9.5 Common variations in the newborn. (From **[top left]** Lowdermilk, D. L., Perry, S.E., Cashion, K., et al. [2016]. *Maternity & women's health care* [11th ed., p. 537, Figure 23-9]. St. Louis: Mosby. **A,** Courtesy Kim Molloy, Knoxville, IA; **[top right]** Bowden, V., Dickey, S., & Greenberg, C. [1998]. *Children and their families: The continuum of care.* Philadelphia: Saunders; **[middle left]** Zitelli, B. J., & Davis, H. W. [2002]. *Atlas of pediatric physical diagnosis* [4th ed.]. St. Louis: Mosby; **[middle centre]** Beischer, N. A., Mackey, E. V., & Colditz, P. B. [1997]. *Obstetrics and the newborn* [3rd ed.]. Oxford: Baillière Tindall; **[middle right]** Beischer, N. A., Mackey, E. V., & Colditz, P. B. [1997]. *Obstetrics and the newborn* [3rd ed., p. 599]. Oxford: Baillière Tindall; **[bottom left]** Leifer, G. [2007]. *Maternity nursing: An introductory text* [10th ed., p. 169, Table 10-1]. St. Louis: Saunders; **[bottom centre]** Eichenfield, L. F., Frieden, I. J., & Esterly, N. B. [2001]. *Textbook of neonatal dermatology.* Philadelphia: Saunders; **[bottom right]** Hockenberry, M. J., Wilson, D., Winkelstein, M., et al. [2003]. *Wong's nursing care of infants and children* [7th ed.]. St. Louis: Mosby.)

- Umbilical cord care: The cord normally dries within 24 hours and falls off within 7 days. Teach the mother to dry around the cord carefully and report any signs of bleeding, foul odour, or discharge.
- Holding and positioning: Newborns require interaction and nurturing, ideally during quiet alert states. They are consoled by being contained in a moderately flexed body posture with a receiving blanket and with skin-to-skin contact covered with a blanket. Newborn necks have weak muscles, and the heavy head must be supported at all times when holding the infant.
- Male circumcision: Male circumcision is most often practised to comply with religious or cultural beliefs. Routine circumcision is not recommended (Canadian Paediatric Society [CPS], 2015). If circumcision is performed, teach the parents to observe for first voiding and complications including bleeding (apply direct pressure and seek medical help) and infection. Pain medication should be used during the procedure.
- Follow-up appointment and information on additional support: Upon discharge, ensure that the mother and family have a follow-up appointment usually at week 1 or 2 and then monthly. Provide information for breastfeeding or nutrition support, public health nursing, telephone help lines, and emergency contact numbers.

Newborn Nutrition

Newborns require adequate fluids and calories to promote hydration and growth. Breastfeeding is widely recognized and recommended as the ideal feeding method to meet the newborn's nutritional requirements. There are few contraindications to breastfeeding, and there are numerous health advantages. Practical nurses support the mother in meeting the newborn's nutritional needs by providing evidence-informed information, teaching, and practical support. Some mothers, for a variety of reasons, will instead use formula feedings, and their decision also needs to be respected and appropriate teaching and information provided.

Requirements

- A healthy full-term newborn requires about 100–120 kcal/kg/day. Expected rates of growth include a weight gain of 15 g/kg/day or an average of 1 kg per month for the first 3 months of life. Growth charts are used to monitor acceptable growth patterns.
- Newborns go through growth spurts at 2 weeks, 4–6 weeks, 3 months, and 6 months, and demands to be fed will increase accordingly.
- Fluoride supplementation is not recommended in the first 6 months of life.
- Breastfed infants need vitamin D supplementation of 400 IU/day, available in infant drops. In areas of Canada north of 55° latitude (such as Edmonton) or for dark-skinned infants, 800 IU/day is needed between October and April, when sunlight levels are low (CPS, 2007; First Nations, Inuit and Métis Health Committee, 2007).

Breastfeeding

- Exclusive breastfeeding is recommended for the first 6 months of life and can be continued for 2 years and beyond (CPS, 2013; Government of Canada, 2015).
- Contraindications include mothers who are HIV positive, have undergone long-term chemotherapy, or have galactosemia, untreated infectious tuberculosis, or herpes simplex lesions on or near the nipple (Government of Canada, 2015).
- Breastfeeding is ideally suited to newborn metabolic needs and digestion and is associated with decreased infections, lower risk of SUID, prevention of allergies, enhanced brain development, and lower costs for newborn feeding.
- Colostrum is available at the time of birth. It is rich in proteins, vitamins, minerals, and immunoglobulins. Breast milk is produced by day 3 or 4 postpartum under the influence of the hormone prolactin. Oxytocin hormone causes the letdown reflex that releases the milk when the baby begins to feed. The amount of milk produced is dependent on the breast being stimulated and emptied with frequent feedings. Mothers are encouraged to feed on demand. Newborns may initially feed 8–12 times in 24 hours.

Formula Feeding

- Commercial formulas that are cow's milk based and iron enriched are the most acceptable alternative to breast milk until 9–12 months of age.

- Soy-based formulas are recommended only if dairy-based milk is not used for health, religious, or cultural reasons, as in the case of a vegan lifestyle or infants with galactosemia.
- Water for formula should be boiled and then cooled for infants in order to remove pathogens (Government of Canada, 2015).

Nursing Considerations

- Practical nurses have an important role in promoting and supporting breastfeeding as the optimal choice for infant nutrition; educate and support parents, create a supportive environment to learn breastfeeding techniques, and provide follow-up resources.
- Breast milk can be expressed and stored in glass bottles (or bisphenol A–free plastic) in the fridge for 24 hours or the freezer for 14 days. It is important not to microwave breast milk because it destroys the antimicrobial agents and vitamin C.
- The newborn will feed best if correctly attached to or "latched on" to the breast. The mother should be comfortable and supported. Signs a baby is feeding well include a wide open mouth encircling the breast; movement of the baby's jaw, not just lips; the baby swallowing at regular intervals; the baby being content after feeding; the mother not being in pain; and the baby wetting 6–8 diapers in a 24-hour period. Most newborns, properly latched, will empty the breast within 30 minutes. The mother should break the seal by placing a clean finger between the breast and the baby's mouth. Upright burping will help release any swallowed air. Small amounts of regurgitation are normal.
- Nutrient-rich solid foods can be introduced at 6 months of age in addition to breast milk or formula feedings, including iron-fortified cereals, meat, or other protein sources. To prevent newborn botulism, no honey or honey products should be given in the first year of life. Herbal teas are not recommended.
- Criteria for postpartum discharge should include demonstration of a clear understanding of feeding needs and techniques, written instructions, community resources and referrals, and at least two successful infant feedings independently performed by the mother. Professional follow-up within 48 hours of discharge is recommended to assess infant hydration, feeding, and the presence of jaundice (Provincial Council for Maternal and Child Health, 2018).

Newborn Complications
Maturity and Size

Preterm or post-term newborns may be SGA (10th percentile), LGA (90th percentile), or average for gestational age (AGA; 50th percentile), depending on their percentile score against weight and age categories on a growth assessment chart. SGA newborns score below the 10th percentile, meaning that 10% of other newborns weigh less than them and 90% weigh more. LGA babies should be investigated as infants of diabetic mothers. SGA newborns may be associated with conditions that impaired uteroplacental circulation during the pregnancy.

Preterm Newborn
Pathophysiology.

- A preterm baby is one born after 20 weeks and before the end of 37 weeks' gestation, regardless of weight. Assessment tools to determine age include the Dubowitz and Ballard scoring systems.
- Cause is often unknown; leading cause of morbidity and mortality; for maternal risk factors, see the section "Preterm Labour and Birth."
- Preterm complications are numerous depending on age and include an inability to establish and maintain independent respirations (respiratory distress syndrome [RDS]), heart murmurs, cold stress, electrolyte and calcium imbalances, increased risk of infection, poor skin integrity, hypoglycemia, risk of neurological impairment and bleeding, anemia, poor digestive ability and malnourishment, and retinopathy of prematurity.

Clinical manifestations. Physical characteristics are dependent on gestational age but may include extended body position, fine downy hair on the head, soft pliable ear without cartilage, lack of body fat, tissuelike or gelatinous skin with visible veins, lack of rugae on the scrotum, labia minor and clitoris visible on female, no sole creases, fine downy lanugo hair widely distributed, and vernix covering the body.

Nursing considerations.

- Observe for signs of respiratory distress, including grunting, chest indrawing, nasal flaring, oxygen saturation of less than 85%, tachypnea, or apnea.
- Maintain a neutral thermal environment; monitor temperature, preventing cold stress using a hat and booties; and maintain skin integrity.
- Establish early frequent feedings to counter hypoglycemia. If the respiratory rate is greater than 60, nasogastric feedings will be required. Carefully monitor intake and output and weight gains or losses.
- Support parents in understanding the needs of the preterm infant, especially if intensive care is required; allay feelings of guilt; and anticipate grieving and the need for open discussion.

Post-Term Newborn
Pathophysiology.

- A post-term newborn is one born after 42 weeks' gestation, a condition associated with primiparas, past history of postmaturity, and congenital anomalies, including anencephaly (lack of brain development).
- Morbidity and mortality risks are associated with increasingly poor uteroplacental circulation and hypoxia and include meconium aspiration, pneumothorax, hypoglycemia, hypothermia, asphyxia, and birth trauma.

Clinical manifestations. Physical characteristics include a long thin body with wasted appearance, little body fat, long nails, dry and cracked skin, meconium staining, and no vernix or lanugo.

Nursing considerations.

- Monitor for uteroplacental insufficiency with regular NST beginning at pregnancy term.
- Be prepared for complications at the time of birth and the need for respiratory support.
- Closely monitor respiratory rate and effort, observe for complications, prevent cold stress, monitor for hypoglycemia and establish frequent regular feedings, and provide information for follow-up care in the community and referral to a pediatrician if needed.

Birth Trauma

Most instances of birth trauma are temporary and self-resolve over time. Trauma may result from medical interventions, including forceps, or be related to pelvic or fetal dystocia factors. Examples include the following:

- Cephalohematoma—It is a well-defined, soft, localized swelling, an accumulation of blood between the skull and periosteum that does *not* cross the cranial suture lines. It emerges on day 2 or 3 following birth and then slowly disappears over weeks or months. There is a risk of jaundice secondary to the blood loss and reabsorption.
- Caput succedaneum—It is a poorly defined, localized soft tissue edema caused by cervical pressure on the fetal head, present at birth, crosses the suture lines, and disappears within hours or days.
- Forceps injury—Facial bruising may be apparent over the cheeks from forceps application. Compression may cause one-sided facial nerve palsy, with one side of the newborn's face appearing asymmetrical, especially when crying. The bruising resolves within a few days. The facial paralysis is rarely permanent and usually resolves within a few hours or days.
- Brachial plexus injury—It is the most common nerve injury and is caused by traction on the nerves in the neck and head during birth. The affected arm is extended and limp, with absent reflexes. Recovery is within weeks with immobilization and physiotherapy. Some infants require surgical intervention. LGA infants with shoulder dystocia and breech infants are especially at risk.
- Fractured clavicle—Redness, swelling, or crepitus is noted over the collar bone, and the infant may be irritable and crying. The fracture is confirmed by X-ray and immobilized.
- Bruises and edema—The infant may have bruising and edema on the other parts of the body due to birth trauma, particularly in difficult deliveries, which disappears in a few days. These bruises can be mistaken for Mongolian spots. Mongolian spots are bluish-black areas of pigmented skin that can occur in babies of Mediterranean, Latin American, Asian, or African descent. They disappear eventually in months or years.

Hemolytic Disease

ABO and Rh blood incompatibilities in the fetus and newborn are caused by maternal immune reactions against blood group factors on the fetal RBCs. While fetal and maternal blood supplies are separate, minute amounts of fetal blood cross into maternal circulation with placental breaks and at the time of birth.

Pathophysiology.

- ABO incompatibility affects about 20% of pregnancies of group A or B infants with group O mothers. Group O mothers have natural anti-A or anti-B antibodies, or both, which initiate a hemolytic response against the fetal RBCs.
- Rh incompatibility affects about 2% of pregnancies. The mother is Rh-negative, while the fetus is Rh-positive. During the first pregnancy, the hemolytic response is initiated when the mother's blood is sensitized and antibodies are produced. The first pregnancy may be unaffected, but unless treated, each subsequent pregnancy will result in a stronger immune hemolytic response with resulting destruction of fetal RBCs and stimulation of the fetal liver and spleen to produce more RBCs.
- Immunization and antibody formation can also occur with a spontaneous or induced abortion, amniocentesis, or ectopic pregnancy.

Clinical manifestations.

- ABO incompatibility: Neonatal jaundice occurs in the first 24 hours, with mild anemia but rarely with an enlarged liver or spleen.
- Rh incompatibility: In affected pregnancies, jaundice occurs in the first 24 hours, with moderate to severe anemia, hepatosplenomegaly, cardiac or pulmonary failure, ascites, edema, or even stillbirth in severe cases.

Diagnostics and therapeutics.

- ABO incompatibility: Diagnosis is via direct and indirect Coombs test (detecting maternal antibodies), bilirubin, and CBC. It usually resolves without complications using phototherapy.
- Rh incompatibility: Blood tests are the same as for ABO. Diagnosis may also require testing amniotic fluid for bilirubin levels or performing cordocentesis for fetal blood analysis.
  - Provide Rh-immune prophylaxis (WinRho) for all at-risk women to prevent and suppress the maternal antibody response.
- Exchange blood transfusion: The newborn's blood is replaced with type O blood, which will not react to the maternal antibodies. The newborn will revert back to his or her natural blood type over time without a subsequent hemolytic reaction.

Nursing considerations.

- Monitor antibody, bilirubin, and CBC levels in the mother and newborn.
- Provide information and teaching to the Rh-negative woman about the importance of receiving prophylaxis in all high-risk situations. It is given at 28 weeks' gestation, within 72 hours postpartum, or following the at-risk episodes noted earlier.
- Provide antenatal fetal monitoring for Rh incompatibility, including ultrasonography and amniocentesis.
- Assess the newborn for early-onset jaundice and implement appropriate treatment.

PRACTICE QUESTIONS

Case 1

Ms. Viraj gave birth to her first child 18 hours ago in an uncomplicated vaginal birth. She is preparing to be discharged home later today with her newborn son and her common-law partner. The baby has successfully breastfed several times since birth. The practical nurse is performing a postpartum assessment and preparing the family for discharge.

Questions 1–6 refer to this case.

1. The practical nurse notes that the lochia is a moderate amount of rubra on the perineal pad. She palpates Ms. Viraj's uterus and assesses that it is firm, 2 cm above the height of the umbilicus, and located toward the left side of the abdomen. What is the most likely cause for this assessment finding?
   1. Postpartum hemorrhage
   2. A uterine infection
   3. A full bladder
   4. Normal uterine involution

2. Ms. Viraj is concerned that she will not know if the baby is getting enough breast milk. Which of the following provides the best information for Ms. Viraj to assess if the baby is receiving enough nourishment?
   1. The baby sleeps for 5 or 6 hours between feedings.
   2. The baby wets 6–8 diapers in a 24-hour period.
   3. The baby's weight increases after each feeding.
   4. The baby passes a stool each day.

3. The practical nurse explains to Ms. Viraj that while breast milk provides the ideal nutrition, she will need to give the baby supplemental drops. What nutrients, not found in adequate amounts in breast milk, will need to be supplemented?
   1. Vitamin D
   2. Iron
   3. Vitamin A
   4. Essential fatty acids

4. Ms. Viraj's partner tells the practical nurse that he can't understand why she keeps talking about what happened during the labour and birth, telling the story over and over again. Which of the following is the best response by the practical nurse to Ms. Viraj's partner?
   1. "You seem tired. Perhaps you should try to get some extra rest."
   2. "I can provide referral information for counselling services."
   3. "It's an essential part of the bonding experience for her."
   4. "Reliving the experience helps her with the reality of the experience and is a normal part of adjusting to parenthood."

5. The baby's physical assessment reveals a poorly defined, soft mass across the top of the head. The practical nurse explains to the parents that this is a temporary condition that will resolve over the next few days. What is this assessment finding called?

   1. Moulding
   2. Caput succedaneum
   3. Cephalohematoma
   4. Mongolian spot

6. Ms. Viraj and her partner have been discussing whether they are going to have their son circumcised. Ms. Viraj tells the practical nurse that she has heard it is healthier for the baby. The practical nurse's best response would include which of the following information?
   1. That circumcision should be performed only for religious reasons.
   2. The practical nurse's personal beliefs regarding the need for circumcision should be shared.
   3. Circumcision is not recommended as a routine practice.
   4. There is clear evidence that circumcision is beneficial and should be performed in infancy.

Case 2

Ms. Smitherman, age 42, gravida 1, para 0, is admitted to the labour unit at 33 weeks' gestation after she experienced painless vaginal bleeding that soaked through several sanitary pads. An ultrasonogram is ordered. Preparations are made for a possible early birth. Six hours later, Ms. Smitherman goes into premature labour and her vaginal bleeding worsens.

Questions 7–10 refer to this case.

7. What is the primary purpose for the ultrasonogram in this situation?
   1. To assess fetal well-being
   2. To detect fetal abnormalities
   3. To determine the location of the placenta
   4. To calculate fetal growth and gestational age

8. What is the most likely cause of Ms. Smitherman's painless vaginal bleeding in the third trimester?
   1. Placenta previa
   2. Placental abruption
   3. Spontaneous abortion
   4. Hemolytic Rh incompatibility

9. The practical nurse prepares Ms. Smitherman for a Caesarean birth. Ms. Smitherman is anxious about this unplanned Caesarean surgery. She wants to know whether this will be the only way she can deliver future children. The practical nurse indicates that
   1. her future deliveries will be by a Caesarean section.
   2. she should have a vaginal birth with the next pregnancy.
   3. caesarean births are easier to recover from than vaginal births.
   4. she will need to discuss the possibility of a future vaginal delivery with the obstetrician.

10. In the operating room, a neonatal team of physician, nurse, and respiratory therapist attends the premature infant when it is born. What is the most important assessment by the team after delivery?

1. Respirations
2. Apical heart rate
3. Colour
4. Identification of any congenital defects

Case 3

Mr. and Ms. Cane's full-term newborn son is 3 days old. Ms. Cane is recovering from a difficult birth. The baby has forceps bruising on his face and a cephalohematoma on the right side of his head. The morning assessment of the baby reveals that the sclera of the eyes, oral mucous membranes, and skin are yellowed. Blood work shows an elevated bilirubin. Phototherapy is prescribed for the baby.

Questions 11 and 12 refer to this case.

11. Mr. Cane asks the practical nurse whether the baby has a liver disease that caused the jaundice. In explaining physiological jaundice to the parents, which explanation would best describe this condition?
    1. It occurs after 24 hours in many babies who are in good health and will resolve in a few days.
    2. Physiological jaundice was caused by the bruising and cephalohematoma.
    3. Physiological jaundice occurs on the first day of life, and more tests will be needed.
    4. A blood exchange transfusion will be required to prevent brain damage.

12. What side effect of phototherapy should the practical nurse teach the parents to expect?
    1. Fluid requirements for the baby decrease by 10% while undergoing phototherapy treatment.
    2. The baby may experience constipation with fewer, firmer stools.
    3. The baby may be more awake, irritable, and difficult to settle.
    4. The baby's eyes will be covered for protection, but the majority of skin will be exposed and may darken temporarily.

Independent Questions

Questions 13–25 do not refer to a particular case.

13. Ms. Cooke is 39 weeks' gestation with her first pregnancy. She calls the obstetrician's office and tells the practical nurse she is having regular contractions 7 minutes apart, but her membranes have not ruptured. What advice would the practical nurse provide?
    1. Wait until her membranes have ruptured before going to the hospital.
    2. Have her partner drive her to the hospital.
    3. Walk around the house to see if the contractions become less regular.
    4. Come to the hospital when the contractions are 4 minutes apart.

14. By what physiological mechanism do newborns stay warm?
    1. Shivering
    2. Metabolizing brown fat stores
    3. Decreasing oxygen consumption
    4. Keeping an extended body posture

15. Which of the following is an indicator used in assessing gestational age?
    1. Weight
    2. Head circumference
    3. Ear cartilage
    4. Body length

16. During the transitional changes at birth when the newborn breathes independently, what causes the foramen ovale to close?
    1. Oxygen levels increase.
    2. The umbilical cord is clamped.
    3. Pressure in the left atria of the heart becomes greater than that in the right atria of the heart.
    4. Pulmonary blood vessels constrict, and pulmonary blood pressure increases.

17. Ms. Morrissey, age 34, is in active labour and is 6 cm dilated. She has a history of chronic hypertension. Continuous electronic fetal heart rate monitoring reveals a baseline heart rate of 110 bpm with a variability of 16–18 bpm. What are these findings most indicative of?
    1. Fetal well-being
    2. Head compression
    3. Umbilical cord compression
    4. Uteroplacental insufficiency

18. Rh-immune prophylaxis treatment with WinRho should be administered in certain situations to prevent maternal antibody formation. In which one of the following situations would WinRho be administered to the mother?
    1. Following the birth of an Rh-negative newborn
    2. Following a spontaneous or induced abortion
    3. Following all births, regardless of blood type and Rh factor
    4. Following an ABO-incompatible birth

19. Teaching parents ways to reduce the risk of sudden unexpected infant death (SUID) is an important part of discharge planning. Which one of the following statements best reflects current recommendations?
    1. Newborns should sleep in a bed with their mothers so they can be closely monitored.
    2. Newborns should sleep on their backs in their own crib on a firm mattress without a pillow.
    3. Newborns should sleep on their sides or stomachs after feeding to avoid aspiration.
    4. Newborns should be dressed in several layers and well covered to avoid cold stress.

20. Which of the following scenarios represents the greatest risk for female infertility?
    1. Ms. Cartwright, who has delayed child-bearing until after age 35 to improve her socio-economic stability
    2. Ms. Allbright, who is in a same-sex relationship
    3. Ms. Abruzzon, who has had more than five sexual partners
    4. Ms. Gusen, who experienced early onset of puberty and menarche, before the age of 13 years

21. Which of the following is a risk factor for the infant of a mother with gestational diabetes?

1. Hypoglycemia
2. Small for gestational age (SGA)
3. Hyperglycemia
4. Insulin resistance

22. The practical nurse is assessing a client whose membranes have just ruptured and notices that the amniotic fluid is greenish in colour. What is the cause of this greenish discoloration?
    1. Blood from placenta previa
    2. Uric acid from the fetus urine
    3. Meconium from fetal distress
    4. Presence of Chlamydia

23. The practical nurse at the community health centre is conducting a prenatal class on maternal nutrition in pregnancy. He tells the class that during pregnancy, the need for most nutrients increases. But he cautions that one nutrient taken in excessive amounts has been associated with teratogenic effects on the newborn. Which nutrient should not be taken in increased or supplemented amounts in pregnancy?
    1. Calcium
    2. Folic acid
    3. Iron
    4. Vitamin A

24. Systemic opioid analgesics, such as morphine sulphate, may be used for maternal pain management. Which statement best describes the nursing considerations for administering systemic opiate analgesics?

    1. Systemic opioids are often administered up to the second stage of labour.
    2. An opioid antagonist such as naloxone (Narcan) should be administered to the mother to reverse the effects if birth is imminent.
    3. An opioid antagonist such as naloxone (Narcan) should be administered to the newborn if signs of central nervous system (CNS) depression are present.
    4. Systemic opioids should not be used for postpartum pain management, as these drugs cross into breast milk and may cause CNS depression in the newborn.

25. A 2-day-old 36-week gestation infant is receiving oxygen in the neonatal intensive care unit. He is not able to tolerate oral feeds as yet. His mother is upset as she had planned to breastfeed. What would be appropriate for the practical nurse to say to her?
    1. "I will bring you the electric breast pump so that you may start pumping your breasts for when your baby can start feedings."
    2. "Your baby will probably need feeds through an intravenous infusion for several weeks and perhaps after that you may be able to provide him with breast milk."
    3. "It is best to give premature infants formula when they start feedings as the exact amounts of milk can be determined."
    4. "As soon as the baby is out of oxygen, you will be able to put him to breast."

REFERENCES

Arriagada, P. (2016). *First nations, métis and inuit women.* Ottawa: Statistics Canada. Retrieved from https://www150.statcan.gc.ca/n1/en/pub/89-503-x/2015001/article/14313-eng.pdf?st=GMzvdUyt.

Arsenault, M., & Lane, C. (2002). The management of nausea and vomiting of pregnancy. *Journal of Obstetrics and Gynaecology Canada,* 24(10), 817–823.

Battams, N. (2018). *A snapshot of family diversity in Canada.* Ottawa: The Vanier Institute of the family. Retrieved from http://vanierinstitute.ca/snapshot-family-diversity-canada-february-2018/.

Beischer, N. A., Mackey, E. V., & Colditz, P. B. (1997). *Obstetrics and the newborn* (3rd ed.). Oxford: Baillière Tindall.

Best Start Resource Centre. (2012). *Welcoming and celebrating sexual orientation and gender diversity in families, from preconception to preschool.* Toronto: Author. Retrieved from http://lgbtqpn.ca/wp-content/uploads/woocommerce_uploads/2014/11/Best-Start-Manual-Welcoming-and-Celebrating-Sexual-Orientation-and-Gender-Diversity-in-Families-from-preconception-to-preschool.pdf.

Blackburn, S. (2013). *Maternal, fetal & neonatal physiology: a clinical perspective.* Maryland, MO: Saunders.

Bowden, V., Dickey, S., & Greenberg, C. (1998). *Children and their families: the continuum of care.* Philadelphia: Saunders.

Canadian Association of Midwives. (2017). Midwifery in Canada. Retrieved from http://www.canadianmidwives.org/.

Canadian Institute for Health Information. (2018). *Inpatient hospitalizations, surgeries, newborns, and childbirth indicators, 2016–2017.* Ottawa: Author. Retrieved from https://secure.cihi.ca/free_products/hospch-hosp-2016-2017-snapshot_en.pdf.

Canadian Midwifery Regulators Council. (2017). *Midwifery in Canada: Legal status and employment.* Winnipeg: Author. Retrieved from http://cmrc-ccosf.ca/.

Canadian Paediatric Society. (2007). Vitamin D supplementation: Recommendations for Canadian mothers and infants [Reaffirmed 2017]. Retrieved from https://www.cps.ca/en/documents/position/vitamin-d.

Canadian Paediatric Society. (2013). Nutrition for healthy term infants: Recommendations from Birth to six months [Reaffirmed 2018]. Retrieved from http://www.cps.ca/en/documents/position/nutrition-healthy-term-infants-overview.

Canadian Paediatric Society. (2015). Position statement: Newborn male circumcision. Retrieved from http://www.cps.ca/en/documents/position/circumcision.

College of Physicians and Surgeons of Ontario. (2010). Fetal ultrasound for Non-medical reasons. Retrieved from https://www.cpso.on.ca/cpso/media/uploadedfiles/policies/policies/policyitems/ultrasound.pdf.

Eichenfield, L. F., Frieden, I. J., & Esterly, N. B. (2001). *Textbook of neonatal dermatology.* Philadelphia: Saunders.

First Nations, Inuit and Métis Health Committee. (2007). Vitamin D supplementation: Recommendations for Canadian mothers and infants. *Paediatrics & Child Health,* 12(7), 583–589.

Gardner, M., & Doyle, N. (2004). Asthma in pregnancy. *Obstetrics and Gynecology Clinics of North America,* 28(3), 385–413.

Gardner, S. L., Carter, B. S., Enzman-Hines, M. I., et al. (2016). *Merenstein & Gardner's handbook of neonatal intensive care* (8th ed.). St. Louis: Elsevier.

Government of Canada. (2015). Nutrition for healthy term infants: Recommendations for birth to six months. Retrieved from https://www.canada.ca/en/health-canada/services/food-nutrition/healthy-eating/infant-feeding/nutrition-healthy-term-infants-recommendations-birth-six-months.html.

Health Canada. (2000a). Chapter 2: Organization of services. In *Family-centred maternity and newborn care: National guidelines* (4th ed.). Ottawa: Health Promotions and Programs Branch. Retrieved from http://www.lhsc.on.ca/About_Us/SPL/projects/completed/SWOPP/guidelin.pdf.

Health Canada. (2000b). Chapter 3: Preconception care. In *Family-centred maternity and newborn care: National guidelines* (4th ed.). Ottawa: Health Promotions and Programs Branch. Retrieved from http://www.publications.gc.ca/site/eng/9.647663/publication.html.

Health Canada. (2000c). The guiding principles of family-centred maternity and newborn care. In *Family-centred maternity and newborn care: National guidelines* (4th ed.). Ottawa: Health Promotion and Programs Branch. Retrieved from http://www.publications.gc.ca/site/eng/9.647663/publication.html.

Health Canada. (2010a). *Prenatal nutrition guidelines for health professionals: Gestational weight gain*. Ottawa: Services Canada. Retrieved from https://www.canada.ca/content/dam/hc-sc/migration/hc-sc/fn-an/alt_formats/pdf/nutrition/prenatal/ewba-mbsa-eng.pdf.

Health Canada. (2010b). Vitamin D and calcium: Updated dietary reference intakes. Retrieved from https://www.canada.ca/en/health-canada/services/food-nutrition/healthy-eating/vitamins-minerals/vitamin-calcium-updated-dietary-reference-intakes-nutrition.html.

Health Canada. (2011). *Eating well with Canada's food guide*. Ottawa: Author. Retrieved from http://www.hc-sc.gc.ca/fn-an/food-guide-aliment/index_e.html.

Health Canada. (2018a). Canadian immunization guide part 4: Active vaccines: Varicella (chicken pox) vaccine. Retrieved from https://www.canada.ca/en/public-health/services/publications/healthy-living/canadian-immunization-guide-part-4-active-vaccines/page-24-varicella-chickenpox-vaccine.html#p4c23a5c.

Health Canada. (2018b). Pregnancy and breastfeeding: Folic acid and iron. Retrieved from https://www.canada.ca/en/health-canada/services/food-nutrition/canada-food-guide/choosing-foods/advice-different-ages-stages/pregnancy-breastfeeding.html.

Hockenberry, M. J., Wilson, D., Winkelstein, M., et al. (2015). *Wong's nursing care of infants and children* (10th ed.). St. Louis: Mosby.

Jelowicki, A. (2015). Quebec nurses granted new powers to prescribe pills. *The Globe and Mail*. Retrieved from http://globalnews.ca/news/2266760/quebec-nurses-granted-new-powers-to-prescribe-pills/.

Kelly-Scott, K., & Smith, K. (2015). *Aboriginal peoples: Fact sheet for Canada*. Ottawa: Statistics Canada. Retrieved from https://www150.statcan.gc.ca/n1/en/pub/89-656-x/89-656-x2015001-eng.pdf?st=7Dw9s8xL.

Leifer, G. (2007). *Maternity nursing: An introductory text* (10th ed.). St. Louis: Saunders.

Liston, R., Sawchuck, D., & Young, D. (2007). Fetal health surveillance: Antepartum and intrapartum consensus guideline. *Journal of Obstetrics and Gynaecology Canada, 29*(9, Suppl. 4). Retrieved from http://www.sogc.org/guidelines/documents/gui197CPG0709.pdf.

London, M., Ladewig, P., Davidson, M., et al. (2017). *Maternal and child nursing care* (5th ed.). Upper Saddle River, NJ: Pearson.

Lowdermilk, D. L., Perry, S. E., Cashion, K., et al. (2016). *Maternity & women's health care* (11th ed.). St. Louis: Mosby.

Martel, M.-J., & MacKinnon, C. (2005). Guidelines for vaginal birth after a previous caesarian birth. *Journal of Obstetrics and Gynaecology Canada, 27*(2), 164–174.

Min, J. K., Claman, P., & Hughes, E. (2006). Guidelines for the number of embryos to transfer following in vitro fertilization. *Journal of Obstetrics and Gynaecology Canada, 28*(9), 799–813. Retrieved from https://doi.org/10.1016/S1701-2163(16)32246-0.

Moore, K. L., & Persaud, T. V. N. (2003). *The developing human: Clinically oriented embryology* (7th ed.). Philadelphia: Saunders.

Moore, K., & Persaud, T. (2008). *Before we were born: Essentials of embryology and birth defects* (7th ed.). Philadelphia: Saunders.

Murray, S., & McKinney, E. (2014). *Foundations of Maternal-Newborn and women's health nursing* (6th ed.). St. Louis, Missouri: Saunders.

MyHealth.Alberta.ca. (2018). Emergency contraception. Retrieved from https://myhealth.alberta.ca/health/Pages/conditions.aspx?hwid=tb1838.

National Aboriginal Health Organization. (2012). *Midwifery*. Ottawa: Author.

Office of the Information and Privacy Commissioner. (2001). Health information a personal matter: A practical guide to the Health Information Act. Retrieved from https://ia800806.us.archive.org/8/items/healthinformatio2001albe/healthinformatio2001albe.pdf.

Oppenheimer, L. (2007). Diagnosis and management of placenta previa. *Journal of Obstetrics and Gynaecology Canada, 29*(3), 261–266.

Pfizer. (2018). Depo-Proveria (medroxyprogesterone acetate injectable suspension, USP). Retrieved from https://www.pfizermedicalinformation.ca/en-ca/depo-provera#.

Potter, P. A., Perry, A. G., Stockert, P., et al. (2019). *Canadian fundamentals of nursing* (6th ed.). Milton, ON: Elsevier.

Provincial Council for Maternal and Child Health. (2018). Standards of postnatal care for mothers and newborns in Ontario: Birth to one week postnatal period. Retrieved from http://www.pcmch.on.ca/wp-content/uploads/2018/05/Standards-of-Postnatal-Care-for-Mothers-and-Newborns-in-Ontario-Final-Report-Part-I-2018May16.pdf.

Public Health Agency of Canada. (2018). Section 5-5: Canadian guidelines on sexually transmitted infections—Management and treatment of specific infections—Human papillomavirus (HPV) infections. Retrieved from https://www.canada.ca/en/public-health/services/infectious-diseases/sexual-health-sexually-transmitted-infections/canadian-guidelines/sexually-transmitted-infections/canadian-guidelines-sexually-transmitted-infections-33.html#t_03a.

Society of Obstetricians and Gynaecologist of Canada. (2018). Medications and drugs during pregnancy. Retrieved from https://www.pregnancyinfo.ca/your-pregnancy/healthy-pregnancy/medications-and-drugs-during-pregnancy/.

Statistics Canada. (2016). The average age of Canadian mothers is increasing. Retrieved from https://www150.statcan.gc.ca/n1/daily-quotidien/180430/dq180430f-eng.htm.

Statistics Canada. (2017a). Aboriginal people in Canada: Key results from the 2016 census. Retrieved from https://www150.statcan.gc.ca/n1/daily-quotidien/171025/dq171025a-eng.htm.

Statistics Canada. (2017b). Census in brief: Same-sex couples in Canada in 2016. Retrieved from https://www12.statcan.gc.ca/census-recensement/2016/as-sa/98-200-x/2016007/98-200-x2016007-eng.cfm.

Statistics Canada. (2017c). Teenage pregnancy. Retrieved from http://www.statcan.gc.ca/eng/help/bb/info/teen.

Statistics Canada. (2018a). Births, 2015 and 2016. Retrieved from https://www150.statcan.gc.ca/n1/daily-quotidien/180430/dq180430f-eng.htm.

Statistics Canada. (2018b). Portrait of families and living arrangements in Canada. Retrieved from https://www12.statcan.gc.ca/census-recensement/2011/as-sa/98-312-x/98-312-x2011001-eng.cfm.

Whiting, S., Langlois, K., Vatanparast, H., et al. (2011). The vitamin D status of canadians relative to the 2011 dietary reference intakes: An examination in children and adults with and without supplement use. *The American Journal of Clinical Nutrition*, 94(1), 128–135. Retrieved from https://doi.org/10.3945/ajcn.111.013268.

Zitelli, B. J., & Davis, H. W. (2002). *Atlas of pediatric physical diagnosis* (4th ed.). St. Louis: Mosby.

BIBLIOGRAPHY

Anderson, C. (2007). Pre-eclampsia: Exposing future cardiovascular risk in mothers and their children. *Journal of Obstetric, Gynecologic, & Neonatal Nursing*, 36(1), 3–8.

Beck, C. (2003). Recognizing and screening for post-partum depression in mothers of NICU infants. *Advances in Neonatal Care*, 3(1), 37–46.

Benjamin, K. (2005). Distinguishing physical characteristics and management of brachial plexus injuries. *Advances in Neonatal Care*, 5(5), 240–251.

Boland, M. (2005). Exclusive breastfeeding should continue to six months. *Paediatrics & Child Health*, 10(3), 148.

Callister, L. (2005). What has the literature taught us about culturally competent care of women and children? *American Journal of Maternal/Child Nursing*, 30(6), 380–396.

Campbell, S. (2003). Prenatal cocaine exposure and neonatal/infant outcomes. *Neonatal Network*, 22(1), 19–21.

Canadian Institute for Health Information. (2018). Giving birth in Canada. Retrieved from https://secure.cihi.ca/estore/productSeries.htm?pc=PCC226.

Canadian Nurses Association. (2005). Nursing and genetics: Are you ready? *Nursing Now*. Retrieved from https://www.cna-aiic.ca.

Canadian Paediatric Society. (2007). Breastfeeding; Vitamin D [Reaffirmed 2017]. Retrieved from http://www.cps.ca/en/search-recherche?q=breastfeeding%20and%20vitamin%20D.

Cherniak, D., Grant, L., Mason, R., et al. (2005). Intimate partner violence consensus statement. *Journal of Obstetrics and Gynaecology Canada*, 27(4), 365–388.

Clemmens, D. (2004). Post-partum depression as profiled through the depression screening scale. *The American Journal of Maternal/Child Nursing*, 29(3), 180–185.

College of Midwives of Ontario. (2017). *About midwifery*. Toronto: Author. Retrieved from http://www.cmo.on.ca/wp-content/uploads/2015/11/5.-Brochure_About-Midwifery_RESOURCES_2012.pdf.

College of Nurses of Ontario. (2017). Professional conduct: Professional misconduct. Retrieved from http://www.cno.org/globalassets/docs/ih/42007_misconduct.pdf.

Fetus and Newborn Committee. (2004). Routine administration of vitamin K to newborns. *Paediatrics & Child Health*, 2(6), 429–431.

Fraser Askin, D. (2004). Intrauterine infections. *Neonatal Network*, 23(5), 23–31.

Gilliland, F. D., Berhane, K., McConnell, R., et al. (2000). Maternal smoking during pregnancy, environmental tobacco smoke exposure and childhood lung function. *Thorax*, 55, 271–276.

Government of Canada. (2006). *Chapter 3: The well-being of Canada's young children: Government of Canada report 2006*. Ottawa: Minister of Public Works and Government Services Canada. Retrieved from http://publications.gc.ca/site/eng/245490/publication.html.

Greene, C. M., & Goodman, M. H. (2003). Neonatal abstinence syndrome: Strategies for care of the drug-exposed infant. *Neonatal Network*, 22(4), 15–25.

Gregory, K. (2005). Update on nutrition for preterm and full term infants. *Journal of Obstetric, Gynecologic, & Neonatal Nursing*, 34(1), 98–108.

Hackman, P. (2001). Recognizing and understanding the cold-stressed term infant. *Neonatal Network*, 20(8), 35–41.

Hamelin, K., Saydak, M. I., & Bramadat, I. A. (1997). Interviewing mothers of high risk infants. What are their support needs? *Canadian Nurse*, 93(6), 35–38.

Health Canada. (2001). Fetal alcohol syndrome/fetal alcohol effects and the effects of other substance use during pregnancy. Retrieved from http://publications.gc.ca/collections/Collection/H49-156-1-2001E.pdf.

Health Canada. (2016). *Smoking cessation during pregnancy and relapse after childbirth in Canada*. Ottawa: Author. Retrieved from https://www.canada.ca/en/public-health/services/publications/healthy-living/smoking-cessation-during-pregnancy-relapse-after-childbirth-canada.html.

Higgins, L. (2005). Screen for abuse during pregnancy. *The American Journal of Maternal/Child Nursing*, 30(2), 109–114.

Hockenberry, M., & Wilson, D. (2015). *Wong's nursing care of infants and children* (10th ed.). St. Louis: Elsevier/Mosby.

Jarvis, C., Browne, A. J., MacDonald-Jenkins, et al. (2019). *Physical examination and health assessment* (3rd Cdn. ed.). Philadelphia: Saunders.

Keenan-Lindsay, L., & Yudin, M. (2006). HIV screening in pregnancy. *Journal of Obstetrics and Gynaecology Canada*, 28(12), 1103–1107.

Kidner, M., & Flanders-Stepans, M. (2004). A model for the HELLP syndrome: The maternal experience. *Journal of Obstetric, Gynecologic, & Neonatal Nursing*, 33(1), 44–55.

Kim-Godwin, Y. (2003). Post-partum beliefs & practices among non-western cultures. *The American Journal of Maternal/Child Nursing*, 28(2), 74–77.

Lachat, M., Scott, C. A., & Relf, M. V. (2006). HIV and pregnancy: Considerations for nursing practice. *The American Journal of Maternal/Child Nursing*, 31(4), 233–242.

MacMullen, N., Tymkow, C., & Shen, J. (2006). Adverse maternal outcomes in women with asthma: Differences by race. *The American Journal of Maternal/Child Nursing*, 31(4), 253–268.

Magee, L., Helewa, L. A., Moutquin, J., et al. (2008). Diagnosis, evaluation, and management of the hypertensive disorders of pregnancy. *Journal of Obstetric, Gynecologic, & Neonatal Nursing*, 30(3), 9–24.

McManus, A., Hunter, L., & Renn, H. (2006). Lesbian experiences and needs during childbirth: Guidance for health care providers. *Journal of Obstetric, Gynecologic, & Neonatal Nursing*, 35(1), 11–23.

Midwives Association of British Columbia. (2018). Frequently asked questions: What is a midwife? Retrieved from http://www.bcmidwives.com/node/1.

Money, D., & Dobson, S. (2004). The prevention of early-onset neonatal group B streptococcal disease. *Journal of Obstetrics and Gynaecology Canada, 26*(9), 826–832.

Murphy, P., & Chez, R. (2000). Management of nausea and vomiting in pregnancy: Alternative therapies. *Contemporary OB/GYN, 45*(4), 55–64.

Olds, S., London, M., Ladewig, P., et al. (2014). *Maternal-newborn nursing & women's health care* (10th ed.). Upper Saddle River, NJ: Pearson Prentice Hall.

Ontario Maternity Care Expert Panel. (2006). *Executive report of the Ontario maternity care expert panel: Emerging crisis, emerging solutions.* Toronto: Ontario Women's Health Council. Retrieved from http://www.cmo.on.ca/downloads/Executive_Report _FINAL.pdf.

Parker, L. (2005). Early recognition and treatment of birth trauma: Injuries to the head and face. *Advances in Neonatal Care, 5*(6), 228–297.

Parker, L. (2006). Birth trauma: Injuries to the intra-abdominal organs, peripheral nerves, and skeletal system. *Advances in Neonatal Care, 6*(1), 7–14.

Perinatal HIV Guidelines Working Group. (2018). *Recommendations for use of antiretroviral drugs in pregnant HIV-infected women for maternal health and interventions to reduce perinatal HIV transmission in the United States.* Rockville, MD: AIDSinfo. Retrieved from https://aidsinfo.nih.gov/ contentfiles/lvguidelines/PerinatalGL.pdf.

Picard, A., & Cullen, C. (2005). School nurses can now prescribe the pill to quebec teens. *The Globe and Mail*, A19. Retrieved from http://www.sogc.org/media/pdf/news/schoolnursescan nowprescribethepillforquebecteens_april272005.pdf.

Poole, J. (2003). Analgesia and anesthesia during labor and birth: Implications for mother and fetus. *Journal of Obstetric, Gynecologic, & Neonatal Nursing, 32*(6), 780–786.

Public Health Agency of Canada. (2017). Human papillomavirus (HPV) prevention and HOV vaccines: Questions and answers. Retrieved from https://www.canada.ca/en/public-health/ services/infectious-diseases/sexual-health-sexually -transmitted-infections/hpv-prevention-vaccines -questions-answers.html.

Public Health Agency of Canada. (2017). *Perinatal health indicators for Canada 2017.* Ottawa: Her Majesty the Queen in Right of Canada. Retrieved from http://publications.gc.ca/collections/ collection_2018/aspc-phac/HP7-1-2017-eng.pdf.

Roberts, S. (2006). Health care recommendations for lesbian women. *Journal of Obstetric, Gynecologic, & Neonatal Nursing, 35*(5), 583–591.

Secco, M., Profit, S., Kennedy, E., et al. (2007). Factors affecting post-partum depressive symptoms of adolescent mothers. *Journal of Obstetrics and Gynaecology Canada, 36*(1), 47–54.

Sherman, T., Greenspan, S., St. Clair, N., et al. (2006). Optimizing the neonatal thermal environment. *Neonatal Network, 25*(4), 251–260.

Simpson, K. (2004). Monitoring the preterm fetus during labour. *The American Journal of Maternal/Child Nursing, 29*(9), 380–388.

Simpson, K. (2005). The context and clinical evidence for common nursing practices during labour. *The American Journal of Maternal/Child Nursing, 30*(6), 356–363.

Society of Obstetricians and Gynaecologists of Canada. (2004). SOGC clinical practice guidelines: Canadian contraception consensus. *Journal of Obstetricians and Gynaecologists of Canada, 26*(2), 143–156. Retrieved from http://www.sogc.org/ guidelines/public/143E-CPG1-February2004.pdf.

Society of Obstetricians and Gynaecologists of Canada. (2008). Diagnosis, evaluation, and management of hypertensive disorders. *Journal of Obstetrics and Gynaecology Canada, 30*(3, Suppl. 1), S1–S56.

Society of Obstetricians and Gynaecologists of Canada. (2015). SOGC clinical practice guidelines: Adolescent pregnancy. *Journal of Obstetricians and Gynaecologists of Canada, 37*(8), 740–756. Retrieved from http://comingsoon.jogc.com/article/ S1701-2163(15)30180-8/pdf.

Society of Obstetricians and Gynaecologists of Canada. (2018). Spread the word, not the disease: The facts on the human papillomavirus from Canada's experts. Retrieved from http://hpvinfo.ca.

Statistics Canada. (2017). Census in brief: Diverse family characteristics of Aboriginal children aged 0 to 4. Retrieved from http://www12.statcan.gc.ca/census-recensement/2016/as -sa/98-200-x/2016020/98-200-x2016020-eng.cfm.

Stringer, M. (2004). Nursing care of the patient with preterm premature rupture of membranes. *The American Journal of Maternal/Child Nursing, 29*(3), 144–150.

Vieira, T. (2003). When joy becomes grief: Screening tools for post-partum depression. *AWHONN Lifelines, 6*(6), 506–513.

Wiseman, C., & Kiehl, E. (2007). Picture perfect: Benefits and risk of fetal 3d ultrasound. *The American Journal of Maternal/Child Nursing, 32*(2), 102–109.

Wyatt, S., & Rhoads, S. (2006). A primer on antenatal testing for neonatal nurses: Part 2: Tests of fetal well-being. *Advances in Neonatal Care, 6*(5), 228–241.

WEB SITES

- **First Nations and Inuit Health—Health Pregnancy** (https:// www.canada.ca/en/indigenous-services-canada/services/ first-nations-inuit-health/family-health/healthy-pregnancy -babies.html): This government of Canada site provides information specifically for First Nations and Inuit people on a variety of topics, including becoming a mother, eating well, and being active. It also includes links to additional resources.

- **Health Canada, Guide to Healthy Pregnancy** (https:// www.canada.ca/en/health-canada/services/healthy-living/ healthy-pregnancy.html): This site has extensive information on healthy living during pregnancy.

- **Motherisk** (http://www.motherisk.org/women): This site is hosted by the Hospital for Sick Children. It is designed to provide information and guidance about the risk and safety of maternal exposure to medications, chemicals, diseases, radiation, and environmental agents.

- **Society of Obstetricians and Gynaecologists of Canada** (http:// www.sogc.org): This site includes information on women's health, including pregnancy. As well, the site includes many resources for health professionals.

- **Women's Health Matters** (http://www.womenshealthmatters .ca): This site was created by Women's College Hospital experts on women's health and has an English and a French version. It has a section on pregnancy and newborn care on such topics as prepregnancy planning, childbirth, multiple births, and life with a newborn.

10

Pediatric Nursing

This chapter on pediatric nursing encompasses the care of children of all ages, from newborns to adolescents, focusing on injury prevention and the promotion of optimal health in a variety of health conditions. An awareness of growth and development patterns in children, as well as the unique physical changes that occur at each stage of development, is essential to the delivery of quality pediatric nursing care.

Pediatric care is provided within the context of the family. Effective care is respectful of social and cultural differences and beliefs and involves the development of trusting and collaborative relationships between family members and the practical nurse.

FAMILY INFLUENCES ON CHILD HEALTH

Family is defined in many ways by scholars and individuals. As a matter of policy and practice, the Vanier Institute of the Family defines family as follows:

Any combination of two or more persons who are bound together over time by ties of mutual consent, birth and/or adoption or placement and who, together, assume responsibilities for variant combinations of some of the following:
• Physical maintenance and care of group members
• Addition of new members through procreation or adoption
• Socialization of children
• Social control of members
• Production, consumption, distribution of goods and services
• Affective nurturance—love (Vanier Institute of the Family, 2015)

This definition is purposely broad and promotes respect and support for all types of families.

It is important to keep in mind that numerous social, cultural, religious, and economic factors influence the family as well as the health and well-being of the child. A family-centred care model is recognized to promote child health and well-being.

In pediatric nursing, a thorough family assessment is essential and should include the collection of data concerning both family structure and family function.

Family Structure

"The family structure, or family composition, consists of individuals, each with a socially recognized status and position, who interact with one another on a regular, recurring basis in socially sanctioned ways" (Hockenberry, Rodgers, & Wilson, 2017, p. 17). With the transition from the nuclear family to non-traditional family structures, the pediatric practical nurse is challenged to understand the influences each family structure has on the health and well-being of a given child.

Common Types of Family Structures

Nuclear family. A nuclear family (referred to as a *census family* by Statistics Canada) comprises two parents cohabiting with their children; the parents may be married or common-law and of the opposite sex or same sex (Statistics Canada, 2016).

A nuclear family has the following characteristics:
• Parent relationships and sibling relationships can be biological, step, adoptive, or foster.
• No other relatives or persons live in the household.

Nursing considerations for a dual-income nuclear family include developing strategies for the family to meet the conflicting demands of career and child-rearing while promoting optimal health.

Blended family. A blended family has at least one step-parent, stepsibling, or half-sibling. In 2016, 6.1% of Canadian children were living with one biological or adoptive patent and one step-parent (Statistics Canada, 2016).

Nursing considerations include providing resources for families on parenting styles and strategies to reduce conflicts that can arise between the stepchild and the step-parent.

Extended family. In an extended family, household expenses and child-rearing responsibilities are shared with a couple and a grandparent or other relative. This type of family structure is common for recently immigrated families as well as working-class families.

Nursing considerations include ensuring that resources are in place for aging family members (e.g., an older grandparent) participating in child-rearing, who may have financial difficulties and increasing health problems.

Lone-parent family. A lone-parent family is a household led by one parent (the mother or the father) following death, divorce, separation, or illegitimacy. In 2016, 19.2% of Canadian children were being raised in a lone-parent family. In all, 15.6% of lone-parent families were led by the mother, and 3.6% were led by the father (Statistics Canada, 2016).

Nursing considerations include focusing on resources for social, emotional, and financial support.

Binuclear family. In a binuclear family, parents continue their parenting roles with their biological children in two independent households (in a joint custody or co-parenting arrangement).

Nursing considerations include ensuring consistency in health promotion teaching and guidance with each parent in the event of an acute or chronic illness in the child.

Family Function

"*Family function* refers to the interactions of family members, especially the quality of those relationships and interactions" (Hockenberry et al., 2017, p. 19). Assessment of family strengths and unique functioning styles is important for a pediatric practical nurse, as these factors can promote a stronger family unit and will influence how a family copes with illness in their child.

Parenting

Parents assume a leadership role in the family to guide children to learn acceptable behaviours. Ideally, parents instill beliefs, morals, and cultural values in their children in an effort to develop socially responsible and contributing members of society. The parenting style, along with the child's personality traits, will influence that child's developmental outcomes.

Parenting Styles

There are three main parenting styles. Families will generally display one style but may assume a different style in certain situations.

Authoritarian parents
- Rules and standards of conduct are set by the parent and followed rigidly.
- Children do not participate in family decision making.
- Children develop with poor communication and negotiation skills.
- Children are generally shy and self-conscious.

Authoritative parents
- Firm controls and limits are set by the parent.
- Children participate in open discussions on family issues and decisions.
- Children develop a sense of high self-esteem and self-reliance.

Permissive parents
- Parents exercise little or no control over their children.
- Children are permitted to regulate their own activity as much as possible.
- Children often control the parents and are disobedient, rebellious, and aggressive.

Parenting in Special Circumstances

Even in the most ideal circumstances, parents encounter many challenges when raising their children. When the family unit deviates from the norm, parents and children can face challenges that can potentially lead to family disruption.

Adoption. Adoption is not merely a simple matter of the legal transfer of parental rights from one party to another but includes the social and emotional health of the adopted child, the birth parents, and the adoptive families. Practical nursing can support families by helping to identify sources of adoptive agencies, by assisting families in preparing other siblings for the arrival of the adoptive child, and by helping to integrate the adoptive child into the family system.

Divorce. An estimated 35% of Canadian children are affected by divorce (Ambert, 2009). Potential effects of divorce on children are as follows (Hockenberry & Wilson, 2015):
- Children may experience more emotional and behavioural problems.
- Factors that influence the impact include the age and sex of the child, the outcome of the divorce, the quality of the parent–child relationship, and parental care following the divorce.
- Children may experience two major phases post-divorce: (a) a crisis phase lasting for a year or longer and characterized by emotional upheaval and (b) an adjustment phase involving adaptation to the new family structure.
- Children may feel more loyal to one parent and may become the "message carrier" between the divorced parents.

Family-centred care. It is common practice in most pediatric centres to approach care using a family-centred philosophy. Families and health care providers work together to plan, provide, and evaluate care.

Family-centred care comprises the following:
- "Recognizing that the family is the constant in a child's life, while the service systems and personnel within those systems fluctuate.
- Facilitating child/family/professional collaboration at all levels of service.
- Sharing with the family, on a continuing basis and in a supportive manner, the best information regarding their child's health care.
- Understanding and incorporating the developmental needs of infants, children, adolescents, and their families in health care delivery.
- Recognizing family strengths and individuality and respecting different methods of coping.
- Recognizing and honouring diversity, strengths and individuality within and across all families, including racial, spiritual, social, economic, educational and geographical diversity.
- Encouraging and facilitating family-to-family support and networking.
- Implementing comprehensive policies and programs that provide support to meet the diverse health care needs of families.
- Designing accessible service systems that are flexible, sensitive, and responsive to family-identified health care needs." (Johnson, Jeppson, & Redburn as cited in SickKids, 2017)

GROWTH AND DEVELOPMENT

It is essential to understand the stages of growth and development when caring for children. As children progress through infancy to adolescence, their nutritional, cultural, and social

TABLE 10.1   Developmental Theories of Freud, Erickson, and Piaget

Age Group	Freud	Erickson	Piaget
Infancy (birth to 1 year)	Oral stage	Trust versus mistrust	Sensorimotor
Toddler (1–3 years)	Anal stage	Autonomy versus shame and doubt	Sensorimotor (ends at 2 years) Preoperational (begins at 2 years)
Preschool (3–6 years)	Phallic stage	Initiative versus guilt	Preoperational
School age (6–12 years)	Latency stage	Industry versus inferiority	Concrete operational
Adolescence (12–18 years)	Genital stage	Identity versus role confusion	Formal operational

situations will impact their development. Pediatric practical nurses integrate their knowledge of growth and development in each encounter with a child, and care is delivered in an age-appropriate manner.

Key Terms Related to Growth and Development

- *Growth* refers to increases in physical parameters, for example, height, weight, vital signs.
- *Development* refers to increases in capability or function, including motor, psychosocial, and cognitive function.
- *Cephalocaudal* means developmental progression from head to toe. For example, a child gains control of the head and neck before the trunk and limbs.
- *Proximodistal* means developmental progress that proceeds from the centre of the body outward to the extremities. For example, a child gains control of the hands before the fingers.

Major Theories of Development

Many theorists have organized their observations of childhood development into stages based on these approximate age groups:

- Infancy: Birth to 1 year
- Toddler: 1–3 years
- Preschool: 3–6 years
- School age: 6–12 years
- Adolescence: 12–18 years

A few of the major theories of childhood development follow.

Freud's Theory of Psychosexual Development

Freud's theory suggests that sexual energy is centred in specific parts of the body at certain ages. Unresolved conflict and unmet needs at a certain stage lead to a fixation of development at that stage (Lerner, 2002).

Erickson's Theory of Psychosocial Development

Erickson's theory suggests that individuals progress through life experiencing developmental crises at certain stages in life. Critical developmental needs must be met at each stage in order to move on to future stages and prevent future maladaptive social relationships (Erickson, 1963).

Piaget's Theory of Cognitive Development

Piaget's theory suggests that children are greatly influenced by age, experience, and maturational ability. Children learn from

TABLE 10.2   Kohlberg's Theory of Moral Development

Preconventional (4–7 years)	Decisions are based on the desire to please others and to avoid punishment.
Conventional (7–11 years)	A conscience or internal set of standards is based on beliefs and teaching of others, such as parents. Rules are important and to be followed to please others and "be good."
Postconventional (12 years and older)	The individual has internalized ethical standards on which to base decisions, and uses awareness of the common good and ethical principles rather than relying on the standards of others. Social responsibility is recognized. The value in each of two offering moral approaches can be considered and a decision made.

From Ball, J. W., Bindler, R. C., & Cowen, J. (2014). *Child health nursing: Partnering with children & families* (3rd ed. p. 116). Upper Saddle River, NJ: Pearson/Prentice Hall.

new experiences by integrating these experiences into their learning base. The child will then manage new experiences through accommodation (Piaget, 1972). The three theories are summarized in Table 10.1.

Kohlberg's Theory of Moral Development

Kohlberg's theory explains the development of moral decision making and judgement. Older children and adolescents start to develop a value system that is autonomous from that of their parents and other authority figures. The theory has been controversial because of sexual bias and the lack of cultural sensitivity (Ball, Bindler, & Cowen, 2014). Kohlberg's theory of moral development is summarized in Table 10.2.

Spiritual Development (Fowler)

Spiritual beliefs are closely related to the moral and ethical portion of the child's self-concept and, as such, must be considered as part of the child's basic needs assessment. Children need to have meaning, purpose, and hope in their lives. Also, the need for confession and forgiveness is present, even in very young children. Extending beyond religion (an organized set of beliefs and practices), spirituality affects the whole person, including the mind, body, and spirit.

Fowler (1981) identified seven stages in the development of faith, five of which are closely associated with and parallel cognitive and psychosocial development in childhood.

Stage 0: Undifferentiated—This stage encompasses the period of infancy, in which there is no concept of right or wrong, no beliefs, and no convictions to guide behaviour. The beginning of faith is established with the development of basic trust through the relationship with the primary caregiver.

Stage 1: Intuitive-projective—Toddlers imitate the religious gestures and behaviours of others without comprehending any meaning or significance to the activities. In preschool years, children assimilate some of the values and beliefs of their parents. Parental attitudes toward moral codes and religious beliefs convey to children what they consider to be good and bad. Children still imitate behaviour at this age and follow parental beliefs as part of their daily lives rather than through an understanding of the basic concepts underlying those beliefs.

Stage 2: Mythical-literal—During the school-age years, spiritual development parallels cognitive development and is closely related to children's experiences and social interaction. Many children have a strong interest in religion. They may accept the existence of a deity, and petitions to an omnipotent being are important and expected to be answered; good behaviour is rewarded, and bad behaviour is punished. Their developing conscience bothers them when they disobey. They have reverence for thoughts and matters and are able to articulate their faith. They may question the validity of their faith.

Stage 3: Synthetic-convention—As children approach adolescence, they become increasingly aware of spiritual disappointments. They realize that prayers are not always answered (at least on their own terms) and may begin to abandon or modify some religious practices. They begin to reason, to question some of the established parental religious standards, and to drop or modify some religious practices.

Stage 4: Individuating-reflexive—Adolescents are more skeptical. They compare the religious standards of their parents with those of others and attempt to determine which standards to adopt and incorporate into their own set of values. They begin to compare religious standards with the scientific viewpoint. They are uncertain about many religious ideas but will not achieve profound insights until late adolescence or early adulthood.

INFANCY: BIRTH TO 1 YEAR OF AGE

Biological Changes

Infancy is the most rapid period of growth, with increases in length, weight, and head and chest circumference and changes in fontanelles. Growth should be charted on standardized growth charts for boys and girls to observe for comparable gains in length, weight, and head circumference.

Length
- Increases in length occur in spurts rather than through slow and steady growth.
- Elongation of the trunk dominates, with height increasing by 2.5 cm per month during the first 6 months and then by 1.25 cm per month during the second 6 months.
- Length should increase by 50% by the end of the first year.

Weight
- Weight increases 680 g per month for the first 5 months, at which point, the birth weight is doubled.
- Weight increases at half this rate for the next 6 months, with an average of 340 g per month; by 12 months, the birth weight should have tripled.
- Breastfed infants tend to weigh slightly less than formula-fed infants during the second 6 months of life.

Head and Chest Circumference
- Head growth is rapid and is a major indicator of brain development.
- Head circumference increases on average 1.5 cm per month for the first 6 months, then 0.5 cm per month for the next 6 months.
- By the end of the first year, head size has increased on average 33%.
- Chest circumference is normally 2 cm less than head circumference.

Fontanelles
- The anterior (diamond-shaped) fontanelle typically measures 5 cm at birth and closes at between 12–18 months.
- The posterior (triangular-shaped) fontanelle typically measures 1 cm and closes at 1 to 2 months.

Vital Signs
Temperature. Body temperature measurements differ in children based on the method used.
- The rectal route gives the closest temperature to the core temperature.
  - Rectal temperatures may lag behind a core temperature during rapid temperature changes.
  - Rectal thermometers should not be used in newborns under 1 month due to the risk of anal perforation.
- The axillary route is recommended unless a core temperature is necessary.
- For safety reasons, use of an oral thermometer is not recommended for children under 4 years old.

For further information on temperature-taking, refer to Chapter 6, page 85.
Heart rate
- Heart rate decreases as age increases.
- The apical impulse (heard through a stethoscope held to the chest at the apex of the heart) is most reliable.
- It is important to count the apical rate for 1 full minute, as young children may have irregularities in rhythm.

TABLE 10.3   Comparison of Pediatric Differences in Vital Signs

	Temperature (°C)	Pulse (Bpm)	Respirations (Number Per Minute)	Blood Pressure (mm Hg)
Newborn	37.5	100–180	35	65–80/40–50
1–12 months	37.7	80–150	30	95–110/60–70
1–3 years	37.2	70–110	23–25	100–115/74–85
3–6 years	37.0	70–110	21–23	105–115/63–75
6–12 years	36.7	70–110	19–21	115–125/75–82
12–18 years	36.8	55–90	16–19	125–132/82–86

bpm, beats per minute.
From Hockenberry, M. J., & Wilson, D. (2015). *Wong's nursing care of infants and children* (10th ed., inside back cover). St. Louis: Elsevier/Mosby.

Respirations
- The rate decreases as age increases.
- It is important to count for 1 full minute due to irregular movements.
- Abdominal movements should be monitored since respirations are primarily diaphragmatic.

Blood pressure
- The most important factor in accurate assessment is use of an appropriately sized cuff that covers three-quarters of the upper arm.

  See Table 10.3 for normal-range vital signs for newborns and infants.

Gross and Fine Motor Development

Gross motor development includes maturation in posture, head balance, sitting, creeping, standing, and walking. Fine motor development includes the use of hands and fingers to grasp objects. See Table 10.4 for a summary of growth and development during infancy.

Nutrition

Both the rate and the pattern of growth can be modified by nutrition.
- Breast milk is the most desirable, complete diet for infants during the first 12 months.
- Breastfed infants will feed on demand.
- Breastfed infants require a daily supplement of 10 mcg (400 IU) of vitamin D from birth until the equivalent amount is obtained from other dietary sources or until they reach 1 year of age. If the infant lives north of the 55th parallel, this level should increase to 20 mcg (800 IU) from all sources between October and April (Canadian Paediatric Society [CPS], 2007; Health Canada, 2012b). Formula-fed infants receive vitamin D in formula but still require supplements of an additional 10 mcg (400 IU) if they live north of the 55th parallel. The CPS has recommended further research in response to studies that have shown that supplemental vitamin D levels may still be inadequate, particularly in at-risk populations such as First Nations, Inuit, and Métis populations in northern climates. The CPS also recommends that pregnant and lactating women consult their physicians about taking up to 2000 IU of vitamin D daily to ensure adequate amounts (CPS, 2007).

- An acceptable alternative to breastfeeding is a commercial iron-fortified formula.
- Formula-fed infants will take about 5–8 feedings every 24 hours.
- All drinking water and water used for formula must be boiled.
- Infant fluid requirements average 125–150 mL/kg/day from birth to 6 months of age and 120–135 mL/kg/day from 6–12 months.
- Use of a cup at 6–9 months will help reduce nursing bottle caries when diluted apple juice is introduced.
- Solids can be introduced at 6 months, starting first with rice cereal, which is easy to digest, contains iron, and rarely causes an allergic reaction.
  - Other cereals, fruits, vegetables, and finally meats should be introduced one at a time and usually 3 days apart to test for possible food allergies.
  - Finger foods such as toast, teething crackers, soft fruits, and cooked vegetables should be introduced at 6–7 months. Parents should be advised to monitor for choking.
  - Chopped table food or commercially prepared junior food can be introduced around 9–12 months.
- Weaning from the breast or bottle to a cup may occur after 6 months and should be based on the readiness of the mother and infant.

Sleep
- Sleep patterns vary greatly among infants.
- By 3–4 months, most infants will sleep 15 hours a day, of which 9–11 hours will be overnight.
- By 12 months, morning and afternoon naps are common.
- Breastfed infants will usually sleep for shorter periods than bottle-fed infants.

Dental
- Fluoride is an essential mineral to promote healthy teeth.
- Most Canadian municipalities add fluoride to drinking water.
- Primary teeth erupt around 6 months of age, beginning first with the upper central incisors.
- Parents should begin a routine of good dental hygiene before teeth are present by using a soft-bristled toothbrush or a damp cloth with water rather than toothpaste.

TABLE 10.4 Growth and Development During Infancy

Age	Physical	Gross Motor Development	Fine Motor Development	Vocalization
1 month		Can turn head side to side when prone Marked head lag when pulled from lying to sitting position	Hands predominantly closed Grasp reflex is strong	Cries to express displeasure Small throat sounds Comfort sounds during feeding
2 months	Posterior fontanelle closed	Less head lag	Hands often open Grasp reflex fading	Vocalizes, distinct from crying Coos Vocalizes to familiar voices
3 months	Primitive reflexes fading	Able to hold head more erect when sitting but still bobs forward	Holds rattle but will not reach for it Grasp reflex gone Pulls at blankets and own hands	Squeals aloud to show pleasure Coos, babbles, chuckles
4 months	Drooling begins	Balances head well in sitting position Able to sit erect if propped up Rolls from back to side	Inspects and plays with hands Tries to reach for objects but overshoots Cannot carry objects to mouth	Laughs aloud Makes consonant sounds n, k, g, p, b Vocalization changes according to mood
5 months	Beginning signs of tooth eruption Birth weight has doubled	Able to sit for longer periods of time with back supported Can turn from abdomen to back	Able to grasp objects voluntarily Takes objects directly to mouth Plays with toes	Squeals Makes cooing vowel sounds with interspersed consonants (i.e., ah-goo)
6 months	Growth rate may decrease Teething may begin with two lower central incisors	When supine, puts feet in mouth When prone, can lift chest and bear weight on hands Rolls from back to abdomen	Grasps and manipulates small objects Drops one cube when given another Holds bottle	Begins to imitate sound Vocalizes to toys and mirror images Enjoys hearing own sounds
7 months	Eruptions of upper central incisors	Bears full weight on feet Bounces when held in standing position Sits erect momentarily	Transfers objects from one hand to the other Holds two cubes more than momentarily Bangs cubes on table	Produces vowel sounds and chained syllables (i.e., "baba," "dada," "kaka")
8 months	Begins to show regular bladder and bowel patterns	Sits steadily unsupported Readily bears weight on legs when supported and stands holding onto furniture	Has beginning pincer grasp Reaches for and pulls toys Rings bell purposely	Listens selectively for familiar words Utterances signal emphasis and emotion
9 months	Eruption of upper lateral incisor may begin	Creeps on hands and knees Pulls self to standing position by holding onto furniture	Uses thumb and index finger in crude pincer grasp Shows preference for use of dominant hand	Responds to simple commands Comprehends "no-no"
10 months	Labyrinth righting reflex is strongest (when in prone or supine position, infant is able to raise head)	Cruises by holding onto furniture Can change from prone to supine position Recovers balance easily while sitting	Release of object from crude pincer grasp begins Grasps bell by handle	Says "dada" or "mama" with meaning May say one word (i.e., "hi," "bye," "no")
11 months	Eruption of lower lateral incisors may begin	When sitting, will pivot to reach objects behind Cruises or walks while holding onto furniture	Examines objects more closely Has neat pincer grasp Drops object deliberately to be picked up	Imitates definite speech sounds
12 months	Birth weight has tripled	Walks with one hand held and cruises well Can sit down from standing position without any help	Can turn pages in a book, many at a time Attempts to build two-block tower but fails	Recognizes objects by name Imitates animal sounds Understands simple verbal commands (i.e., "give it to me")

Adapted from Hockenberry, M. J., & Wilson, D. (2015). *Wong's nursing care of infants and children* (10th ed., pp. 481–485, Table 12.3). St. Louis: Elsevier/Mosby.

Swallowing too much toothpaste containing fluoride can lead to fluorosis (Canadian Dental Association, 2017a).

- To prevent dental caries, parents should avoid breast- and bottle-feeding while the infant sleeps and avoid fruit juices in a bottle, particularly before 6 months of age.
- Foods with concentrated sugar should be used in limited quantity.
- The practice of coating a pacifier with honey should be discouraged; this can cause infant botulism.
- The use of hard-candy pacifiers should be discouraged, not only due to the sugar content but also as parts of the candy can break off and be aspirated.

Immunizations

See Table 10.5A–B for the recommended Canadian routine immunization schedule (Public Health Agency of Canada, 2018a).

Nursing Considerations

When administering immunizations, do the following:
- Ensure proper storage of the vaccine.
- Rotate sites and administer the injections as painlessly as possible.
- Consider use of topical anaesthetics such as EMLA cream to prevent a painful injection
- Give acetaminophen (Tylenol) prior to the injection; this medication will provide pain relief and make the child more comfortable after the immunization.
- Monitor for signs of allergic reaction.
- Ensure adequate penetration of the muscle when administering intramuscularly.
- Provide adequate information to parents on the risks and benefits of immunizations. See Chapter 5, page 75, for more information on vaccinations and risk communication.
- Maintain accurate documentation in an immunization record for parents to keep.

Safety

- Almost half of all deaths among children aged 1 to 4 years are due to injury (Health Canada, 2011).
- Some of the leading causes of injury include suffocation, choking, strangulation, drowning, falls, poisonings, burns, and motor vehicle accidents.
- As the infant develops fine and gross motor skills and begins to explore the environment, the risk of injury should be addressed with parents with appropriate injury prevention teaching. See Table 10.6 for a list of preventable hazards for infants.
- The Government of Canada Toy Safety Web site provides consumer information on potentially hazardous products, particularly toys that present choking hazards and toxic compositions. This site also includes product recalls, for example, toys that are manufactured with unacceptable levels of lead paint. See the end of this chapter for this and other Web sites focused on child safety.

Play

- In infancy, play is mostly used for physical development and for gaining awareness of the environment.
- Play is basically solitary and will become more interactive during the first year.
- Toys should be simple to match the child's attention span.
- Toy safety is of primary concern, to prevent aspiration and injury.
  See Table 10.7 for a list of suggested toys for infants.

Reactions to Illness and Hospitalization

The impact of hospitalization on an infant under 3 months is minimized if it is a short time period and there is a nurturing person who can meet the child's physical needs. At 4–6 months, the infant starts to recognize the parents as separate from itself and develops a fear of strangers, which can lead to separation anxiety if the child is hospitalized.

Nursing Considerations During Hospitalization

- Be present with the parents within sight of the infant to build a sense of safety in the child.
- Encourage parents to participate in the child's care as much as possible.
- Follow home routines as much as possible.
- Give the infant a sense of security by holding the child and moving gently, cuddling, talking, and responding to the child's reactions.
- Ensure that sensorimotor stimulation is provided.
- Provide physical care, comfort, and safety.
- Keep the infant warm and dry and plan treatments and tests around the home feeding schedule to prevent hunger and discomfort.
- Encourage breastfeeding or the use of the same type of formula used at home.
- Make sure crib rails are up and provide safe crib toys and an area to play in.
- Encourage cognitive stimulation through the use of various stimulating toys, such as rattles, mobiles, and music boxes with different textures.
- Encourage vocal stimulation and language development by talking to the infant and making sounds.
- Develop and maintain a relationship with the parents and encourage parent participation throughout the hospitalization whenever possible.
- Encourage the parents to voice their concerns and address them as much as possible.
- Try to keep the same core nurses as much as possible.

TODDLER: 1 TO 3 YEARS OF AGE

Biological Changes

Growth slows considerably during childhood, as compared with the first year. The toddler will experience steplike growth with spurts and lags versus the more linear growth of infancy.

Toddlers have the traditional pot-belly abdomen as a result of underdeveloped abdominal muscles. Legs will remain

TABLE 10.5A Routine Childhood Immunization Schedule, Infants and Children (birth to 17 years of age)

Vaccine	Birth	2 mos	4 mos	6 mos	12 mos	15 mos	18 mos	23 mos	2 years	4 years	5 years	6 years	9 years	12 years	14 years	15 years	16 years	17 years
DTaP-IPV-Hib		A	A	A			A											
Or		Or	Or	Or			Or 4th dose											
DTaP-HB-IPV-Hib		B	B	B			Generally at 18 months of age											
DTaP-IPV		1st dose	2nd dose	3rd dose														
Or																		
Tdap-IVP										C								
Tdap															D			
Rot		E																
		2 or 3 doses	Complete series before 8 months															
Pneu-C-13		F	G		F													
Men-C-C			According to P/T schedule															
Men-C-C			G		G													
Or					Generally at 12 months													
Men-C-ACYW														H				
MMRV					K					OR	K							
											Generally at 4-6 years							
HB			L															
			3 doses															
HB										OR						M		
																2 or 3 doses		
HPV															N			
															2 or 3 doses			

Continued

TABLE 10.5A   Routine Childhood Immunization Schedule, Infants and Children (birth to 17 years of age)—cont'd

Vaccine	Birth	2 mos	4 mos	6 mos	12 mos	15 mos	18 mos	23 mos	2 years	4 years	5 years	6 years	9 years	12 years	14 years	15 years	16 years	17 years
HPV									OR							O 3 doses		
Inf									P 1 0 or 2 doses Recommended annually							P 1 dose Recommended annually		

Obtained information from Government of Canada Healthy living Vaccines and immunization, Canadian Immunization Guide (2018) https://www.canada.ca/en/public-health/services/publications/healthy-living/canadian-immunization-guide-part-1-key-immunization-information/page-13-recommended-immunization-schedules.html#p1c12a2. *Canadian immunization guide.* Adapted and reproduced with permission from the Minister of Health, 2013.

A = Diphtheria toxoid-tetanus toxoid-acellular pertussis-inactivated polio-*haemophilus influenza type b* (DTaP-IPV-Hib). For infants and children beginning primary immunization at 7 months of age and older, the number of doses of Hib vaccine required varies by age.

B = Diphtheria toxoid-tetanus toxoid-acellular pertussis-hepatitis B-inactivated polio-*haemophilus influenza type b* (DTaP-HB-IPV-Hib). Alternative schedules may be used: DTaP-HB-IPV-Hib at 2, 4 and 12-23 months of age with DTaP-IPV-Hib vaccine at 6 months of age; or DTaP-HB-IPV-Hib at 2, 4 and 6 months of age with DTaP-IPV-Hib vaccine at 12-23 months of age.

C = Diphtheria toxoid-tetanus toxoid-acellular pertussis-inactivated polio OR tetanus toxoid – reduced diphtheria toxoid-reduced acellular pertussis-inactivated polio

D = Tetanus toxoid-reduced diphtheria toxoid-reduced acellular pertussis (Tdap): 10 years after last dose of DTaP or Tdap containing vaccine

E = Rotavirus: rotavirus pentavalent vaccine – 3 doses, 4 to 10 weeks apart; rotavirus monovalent vaccine-2 doses at least 4 weeks apart. Give the first dose starting at 6 weeks and before 15 weeks of age. Administer all doses before 8 months of age.

F = Pneumococcal conjugate 13-valent (Pneu-C-13) Healthy infants beginning primary immunization at 2-6 months of age; 3 or 4 dose schedule. For a 3 dose schedule: 2, 4 months of age, followed by a booster does at 12 months of age. For a 4 doses schedule: minimum of 8 weeks interval between doses beginning at 2 months of age, followed by a booster dose at 12–15 months of age. Healthy infants beginning primary immunization at 7–11 months of age: 2 doses, at least 8 weeks apart followed by a booster dose at 12–15 months of age, at least 8 weeks after the second dose. Children who have received age-appropriate pneumococcal vaccination with a pneumococcal conjugate vaccine but not Pneu-C-13 vaccine: 12–35 months of age-1 dose: 36–59 months of age and of aboriginal origin or attended group care – 1 dose: other heathy children 36–59 months of age – consider 1 dose.

G = Meningococcal conjugate monovalent: children 12–48 months of age: 1 doses routinely provided at 12 months of age, regardless of any doses given during the first year of life. Immunization may be considered for unimmunized children 5–11 years

I = Measles-mumps-rubella: first dose at 12–15 months of age; second dose at 18 months of age or anytime thereafter, but should be given no later than around school entry.

J = Varicella (chickenpox): first dose at 12 month of age; second dose at 18 months of age or anytime thereafter, but should be given no later than around school entry.

K = Measles-mumps-rubella-varicella: first dose at 12–15 months of age; second dose at 18 months of age or anytime thereafter, but should be given no later than around school entry.

L = Hepatitis B: months 0, 1, and 6 (first dose = month 0) with at least 4 weeks between the first and second dose, at least 2 months between the second and third dose, and a least 4 months between the first and third dose. Alternatively, can be administered as DTsP-HB-IPV-Hib vaccine with first dose at 2 months of age

M = Hepatitis B: 9-17 years of age – months 0, 1 and 6 (first dose = month 0) with at least 4 weeks between the first and second dose, at least 2 months between the second and third dose, and at least 4 months between the first and third dose. 11-15 years of age – 2 doses; schedule depends on the product used.

N = Human Papillomavirus (HPV): Girls, 9-14 years of age: HPV bivalent (HPV2) or HPV quadrivalent (HPV4) vaccine or HPV nonavalent (HPV9) vaccine – months 0 and 6-12 (first dose = month 0). Alternatively, a 3 dose schedule may be used for HPV2 vaccine – months 0, 1 and 6 (first dose = month 0), for HPV4 vaccine – months 0, 2 and 6 (first dose = month 0), and HPV nonavalent (HPV9) vaccine – months 0, 2 and 6 (first dose = month 0). Boys, 9-14 years of age: HPV4 or HPV9 vaccine – months 0 and 6-12 (first dose = month 0). Alternatively, a 3 dose schedule may be used for HPV4 vaccine – months 0, 2 and 6 (first dose = month 0), and HPV9 vaccine – months 0, 2 and 6 (first dose = month 0). For a 2 or 3 dose schedule, the minimum interval between first and last doses is 6 month

O = Human Papillomavirus: Girls, 15-17 years of age: HPV2 vaccine – months 0, 1 and 6 (first dose = month 0), HPV4 vaccine – months 0, 2 and 6 (first dose = month 0) or HPV9 vaccine – months 0, 2 and 6 (first dose = month 0). Boys, 15-17 years of age: HPV4 vaccine – months 0, 2 and 6 (first dose = month 0) or HPV9 vaccine – months 0, 2 and 6 (first dose = month 0). In individuals who received the first dose of HPV2 or HPV4 or HPV9 vaccine between 9-14 years of age, a 2 dose schedule can be used with the second dose administered at least 6 months after the first dose.

P = Influenza: recommended annually for anyone 6 months of age and older without contraindications. Children 6 months-less than 9 years of age, receiving influenza vaccine for the first time – 2 doses, at least 4 weeks apart. Children 6 months-8 years of age, previously immunized with influenza vaccine and children 9 years of age and older – 1 dose.

TABLE 10.5B Recommended Immunizations Schedule, Children (less than 7 years of age), NOT Previously Immunized as Infants

| Vaccine | 1st visit | Time after 1st visit | | | | | 6–12 mos after last dose |
		4 weeks	8 weeks	3 mos	4 mos	6 mos	
DTaP-IPV-Hib Or DTap-HB-IPV-Hib	A		A		A		A B
Pneu-C-13	C		C				
Men-C-C	D						
MMR	E	E					
VAR	F				F		
				OR			
MMRV	G			G			
HB	H	H				H	
Inf	I	I					

slightly bowed in appearance due to the weight of a comparatively large trunk.

Height

- The rate of increase in height slows, with an average increase of 7.5 cm per year.
- Increase occurs mainly in elongation of the legs rather than the trunk.
- Adult height is about twice the height of the child at age 2.

Weight

- Average weight gain is 1.8–2.7 kg per year.
- Birth weight is quadrupled by age $2\frac{1}{2}$.

Head and Chest Circumference

Chest circumference surpasses head and abdominal circumferences, giving the toddler a taller, leaner appearance.

Vital Signs

See Table 10.3 for normal-range vital signs for toddlers.

Temperature
- Recommended routes include axillary, tympanic, and rectal (if a core temperature is required).
- Use of an oral thermometer is not recommended in children under 4 years old.

Heart rate. A satisfactory radial pulse can be obtained in children over 2.

Gross and Fine Motor Development

- The major gross motor development of the toddler is locomotion.
- Fine motor development is demonstrated by increasingly skilful manual dexterity.
  See Table 10.8 for a summary of growth and development during the toddler years.

Nutrition

- As growth slows, so will the toddler's requirements for calories, protein, and fluids.

- By 12 months, most children will eat the same food prepared for the rest of the family.
- Parents should be encouraged to follow *Eating Well with Canada's Food Guide* for children 2 years of age and older (Health Canada, 2011). (For more on *Eating Well with Canada's Food Guide*, see Chapter 5, page 69.)
- Toddlers will fully transition from the bottle to a cup by age 18 months, with some spilling.
- Proper control of a spoon is seen after 18 months of age.
- Emphasis should be placed on the introduction of a variety of foods and in developing healthy eating habits.
- Food should be presented in an appealing manner and served in small sizes; toddlers enjoy finger foods.
- By 18 months, most toddlers will display a phenomenon called *physiological anorexia*, evidenced by a decrease in nutritional needs and appetite.
- Toddlers become picky eaters and may eat voraciously 1 day and almost nothing the next; however, most toddlers will continue to consume enough nutrients for growth.
- Toddlers may experience "food fads" or "jags," eating one particular type of food for several days in a row and then suddenly refusing to eat it again.
- Toddlers need to feel a sense of control over food choices.

Sleep

- Total sleep decreases slightly during the second year, with an average of 12 hours per day.
- Most toddlers will require one nap per day and most often will give up napping by age 3.
- Toddlers will commonly experience difficulty going to bed and falling asleep as a result of separation anxiety.
- Parents should establish bedtime rituals with a consistent bedtime and the use of a transitional object such as a stuffed animal or a blanket for comfort and security.

Dental

- The Canadian Dental Association encourages the assessment of infants by a dentist within 6 months of the

TABLE 10.6   Preventable Hazards for Infants

Hazard	Nursing Considerations When Educating Caregivers
Falls	Keep car seat or baby carrier on the floor rather than on a table or counter.
	Always use safety straps in strollers and high chairs.
	Always raise crib rails.
	Never leave a child alone on a change table. Keep all supplies at hand.
	Be aware that wheeled baby walkers, which have been banned in Canada since 2004, should not be used as they can cause serious injuries to children, including falls, head injuries, and burns.
	Use a baby gate at the top of stairs; the baby gate must be fastened to the wall with screws, not suction.
Burns	Check the temperature of bath water and foods and liquids.
	Keep hot items out of reach.
	Place guards in front of fireplaces or heating devices.
	Avoid hanging tablecloths as children may pull down hot items.
	Avoid overexposure to the sun and use sunscreen if the infant is over 6 months of age.
Motor Vehicle Accidents	Motor vehicle crashes are the leading cause of preventable injury and death to children between one and nine years.
	Every year about 10 000 children 12 years or under are injured, some fatally, in traffic collisions in Canada.*
	The Transport Canada Web site provides information on child car seat requirements for individual provinces and territories. The site includes installation instructions, airbag safety tips, and recall alerts.
	For children up to 10 kg, use rear-facing car seats.
	For children over 10 kg, use forward-facing seats until they outgrow the seats.
	For children who have outgrown forward-facing seats, use booster seats until the child is able to use the seat belt safely (each province has a minimum age, weight and height requirement)
	For children 36 kg or 145 cm tall and 9 years of age, use seat belts.
	The safest location for children 12 years or younger is in the back seat, away from airbags.*
Drowning	Drowning is the second leading cause of death for Canadian children.†
	Children can drown in as little as 5 cm (2 in) of water in just seconds.
	Never leave an infant alone in a bath, even for a few seconds.
	Avoid the use of a baby bath seat as it is not a safety device.
Poisoning	Do not store toxic substances in food containers.
	Keep medications locked up.
	Do not administer medications as candy.
	Keep the phone number of a poison control centre readily available.
	Refer to Table 10.9 for additional poisoning risks.
Suffocation and Strangulation	Position infants to sleep on their backs.
	Do not place pillows, bumper pads, or stuffed toys in a crib.
	Do not use plastic in a crib.
	Avoid latex balloons.
	In Canada, cribs made before 1986 are dangerous and should not be used as the part supporting the mattress can fall, entrapping an infant.
	Crib bars should be no more than 6 cm (2⅜ in.) apart to prevent the infant's head from getting caught in the bars.
	Keep the infant's crib away from windows as children have died when their heads got caught in the cords of blinds.
	Do not use pacifiers with cords attached.
	Do not use baby gates made before 1990 as children have died when their heads were trapped in the gates (these are usually gates with large diamond- or V-shaped openings).
Choking	Hold infant for feeding and do not prop a bottle.
	Use pacifiers with one-piece contraction and a loop handle.
	Keep small objects such a buttons, beads, and small toys away from the infant.
	Avoid the use of baby powder.
	Use caution with toys and ensure that no small parts can come off and choke the infant.

*Public Health Agency of Canada 2008; †Parachute Preventing injuries, saving lives (2018), Government of Canada: Consumer product safety, child car seat safety (2018).

TABLE 10.7 Suggested Toys for Infants

Age	Visual Stimulation	Auditory Stimulation	Tactile Stimulation	Kinetic Stimulation
Birth to 1 year	Nursery mobiles Unbreakable mirrors Contrasting coloured sheets	Music boxes Music mobiles Crib dangle bells Small-handled clear rattle	Stuffed animals Soft clothes* Soft or furry quilt* Soft mobiles	Rocking crib or cradle Weighted or suction toy Infant swing
6–12 months	Coloured blocks Nested boxes or cups Books with rhymes and bright pictures Strings of big beads Simple take-apart toys Large ball Cup and spoon Large puzzles Jack-in-the-box	Squeaky toys and animals Rattles of different sizes, shapes, tones, and bright colours Recordings with light, rhythmic music	Soft, different-texture animals and dolls Sponge toys Floating toys Squeeze toys Teething toys Books with textures, such as fur and zippers	Activity box for cribs Push–pull toys Wind-up swing

*Toys must be removed from the crib when the infant is sleeping to avoid suffocation. Adapted from Hockenberry, M. J., & Wilson, D. (2015). *Wong's nursing care of infants and children* (10th ed., p. 428, Table 10.2). St. Louis: Elsevier/Mosby.

TABLE 10.8 Toddler Growth and Development

Age	Physical	Gross Motor Development	Fine Motor Development	Language
12–15 months	Steady growth in height and weight	Walks alone without help Creeps up stairs Assumes standing position without support	Can grasp a very small object Can drop a small object into a narrow opening Repeatedly throws objects and retrieves them Scribbles spontaneously with a crayon Cannot insert a particular shaped object into a matching hole Drinks from cup Uses spoon but will rotate it	Says 4–6 words Asks for objects by pointing Shakes head to denote "no" Understands simple commands
18 months	Physiological anorexia from decreased growth needs Anterior fontanelles closed Physiologically able to control sphincters	Tries to run but falls easily Walks up stairs with one hand held Jumps in place on both feet Can throw a ball over head without losing balance	Can build a tower of 3–4 blocks Can insert a particular shaped object into the matching hole Manages spoon without rotation	Says 10 words or more Forms word combinations Points while naming the object
24 months	Chest circumference exceeds head circumference May be ready to toilet train Primary dentition of 16 teeth	Walks up and down stairs on own	Can build a tower of 6–7 blocks Imitates a circular and a vertical line with a crayon Turns door knobs and unscrews lids Turns pages in a book one at a time	Has a vocabulary of about 300 words Uses pronouns *I*, *me*, and *you* Refers to self by name Talks continuously
2½ years	Quadruples birth weight May have bladder and bowel control during the day Primary dentition is complete at 20 teeth	Can jump using both feet Stands on one foot for a second or two Can take a few steps on tiptoe	Can build a tower of eight or more blocks Holds a crayon with fingers rather than in fist	

Adapted from Hockenberry, M. J., & Wilson, D. (2015). *Wong's nursing care of infants and children* (9th ed., p. 499, Table 12.2). St. Louis: Elsevier/Mosby.

eruption of the first tooth or by 1 year of age (Canadian Dental Association, 2017b).
- All 20 baby (or primary) teeth should erupt by 2 to 3 years.
- Dental hygiene includes brushing with a soft-bristled toothbrush and flossing.
- As with infants, toothpaste should be avoided.
- Foods high in sugar should be limited.

Immunizations

See Table 10.5A–B for the recommended Canadian routine immunization schedule.

Safety

- Injuries are one of the major causes of death and morbidity for children and youth after the age of 1 (Health Canada, 2011).
- Leading causes of injury include suffocation, choking, strangulation, drowning, falls, poisonings, burns, and motor vehicle accidents.
- As the infant develops fine and gross motor skills and begins to explore the environment, injury prevention should be addressed with parents.

See Table 10.9 for a list of preventable hazards for toddlers.

Play

- Toddlers engage in parallel play by playing alongside, but not with, other children.
- Toddlers will play freely and spontaneously without following rules.
- This is an active stage of development that involves intense exploration of the environment.
- Due to their short attentions spans, toddlers will change activities often.
- Appropriate toys will help develop locomotion (push–pull toys), imagination, language, and gross and fine motor skills. See Box 10.1 for a list of appropriate toddler toys.

BOX 10.1 Appropriate Toys for the Toddler

- Dolls
- Play telephones, furniture, and dishes
- Puzzles with few, large pieces
- Pedal toys such as a riding truck or tricycle
- Push–pull toys
- Clay, sand box, crayons, finger paints
- Large blocks and pounding toys

TABLE 10.9 Preventable Hazards for Toddlers	
Hazard	**Nursing Considerations/Parent Education**
Falls	Due to a developing sense of balance, toddlers will quite often fall while climbing, jumping, or running.
	Parents should continue to keep crib rails up, monitor the toddler around stairs, and secure windows and screens.
Burns	Keep hot items well back from the edge of a countertop as with increased height, the toddler can easily reach for items on top of counters.
	Turn pot handles in on stoves.
	Avoid hanging tablecloths as children may pull down hot items.
	Teach the toddler what "hot" means.
	Check bath water and do not allow the toddler to play with the faucets.
	Avoid overexposure to the sun and use sunscreen.
Motor Vehicle Accidents	Rear-facing child seats are required for children up to 10 kg (22 lb), then front-facing seats are necessary until seats are outgrown.
	Supervise the toddler at all times during outdoor play and teach the safety rules around roads and parked cars.
	Head injuries are the number one cause of serious injury and death to children riding wheeled vehicles, including bicycles, in-line skates, scooters, etc. Parachute: Preventing injuries, saving lives *Toddler safety* (2018).
	Fit the toddler properly with a bike helmet that meets safety standards of the Canadian Safety Association (CSA).
Drowning	Never leave a toddler alone in a bath, even for a few seconds.
	Supervise the toddler around all sources of water at all times, including buckets.
	Keep bathroom doors closed and toilet seats down.
Poisoning	Poisonings by household chemical products, such as bleaches, paint thinners, ammonia, and abrasive cleaners, are among the top causes of injuries and deaths in children under the age of 5.
	A small amount of a chemical product can be harmful to a child, and bad tastes and odours do not keep children away from chemical products.
	Keep other harmful products, such as cosmetics, drugs, vitamins, and first-aid treatment products, out of the sight and reach of children.
Suffocation	Remove draw strings from clothing.
	Dispose of old appliances properly by removing doors.
	Select safe toy boxes without heavy hinged lids.
	Keep window covering cords out of the toddler's reach.
Choking	Avoid foods that are choking hazards, such as whole hot dogs, large chunks of meat, fruit with pits, fish with bones, dried beans, chewing gum, nuts, popcorn, grapes, round candies, and marshmallows.

Toilet Training

One of the major tasks for the toddler to master is toilet training. See Box 10.2 for a summary of the factors involved in determining readiness to toilet train.

Reactions to Illness and Hospitalization

The toddler age group has a poorly defined body image and body boundaries. Painful and invasive procedures can cause extreme anxiety. Toddlers react to pain in a similar way to infants but also can recall previous painful experiences. Most toddlers have separation anxiety and look at hospitalization as being abandoned.

Toddlers respond to stressful situations by using regression as a coping mechanism. They can have a feeling of loss of control when they are physically restricted, if there is a disruption of routines and rituals, or when there is a fear of injury, pain, or dependency. The peak age for separation anxiety is 18 months (Ball et al., 2014). The following are the three stages of separation anxiety:

- Protest—This is the usual reaction to hospitalization. The child cries for the parents, verbally or physically attacks others, tries to find parents, clings to them, and is inconsolable.

BOX 10.2 Assessing Toilet Training Readiness

Physical Readiness
- Voluntary control of anal and urethral sphincters, usually by 22–30 months of age
- Ability to stay dry for 2 hours, decreased number of wet diapers, waking dry from naps
- Regular bowel movements
- Gross motor skills of sitting, walking, and squatting
- Fine motor skills to remove clothing

Mental Readiness
- Recognition of urge to defecate and urinate
- Verbal or non-verbal communication skills to indicate when child is wet or has the urge to defecate or urinate
- Cognitive skills to imitate appropriate behaviour and follow directions

Psychological Readiness
- Expressing willingness to please parent
- Ability to sit on toilet for 5–8 minutes without fussing or getting off
- Curiosity about adults' or older siblings' toilet habits
- Impatience when in soiled or wet diapers, desire to be changed immediately

Parental Readiness
- Recognition of child's level of readiness
- Willingness to invest the time required for toilet training
- Absence of family stress, such as a divorce, moving, new sibling, or imminent vacation

From Hockenberry, M. J., & Wilson, D. (2015). *Wong's nursing care of infants and children* (10th ed., p. 501). St. Louis: Elsevier/Mosby.

- Despair—The child shows disinterest in surroundings and play, passive reactions, depression, loss of appetite.
- Detachment or denial—The child appears to adapt to surroundings, but the adaptation is superficial, and the child remains detached. This adaptation usually happens after a long period of separation.

Nursing Considerations for Separation Anxiety
- Encourage the toddler to protest.
- Encourage parents to stay if possible.
- Encourage the use of transitional or parent objects associated with the parents that can be left with the child.
- Request that parents leave the room only when the child is awake and truthfully tell the child their return time.
- Try to keep to home routines, such as bedtime rituals, and use the words that the child is familiar with, such as "bye bye," to promote security.
- Provide activities and a play area to enhance muscle development.
- Encourage self-care with assistance in feeding, toileting, dressing, and hygiene.
- Encourage sensorimotor learning by imitation.
- Promote language skills by reinforcing mastered vocabulary and using activities that require language.
- Provide simple explanations to prepare for treatments.
- Enhance the toddler's sense of autonomy by offering choices.
- Use parents' photographs and encourage parental visiting.

PRESCHOOL: 3 TO 6 YEARS OF AGE

The preschooler has a slow and uniform rate of growth. Preschool children tend to be slight, sturdy, and nimble and have improved posture.

The major milestone for a preschooler is to prepare to enter school. Achievements that prepare them for school include gaining control of bodily systems, experiencing brief and prolonged periods of separation, ability to interact cooperatively with other children and adults, use of language, increased attention span, and memory preparation (Hockenberry & Wilson, 2015).

Biological Changes

The rate of physical growth slows down and stabilizes:
- Increases in height remain steady at an increase of about 6.5–9 cm per year.
- Increases in weight continue to be steady as well at a rate of 2–3 kg per year.
- A typical 4-year-old will be 103 cm tall and will weigh an average of 16.5 kg.
- Boys and girls will have a similar body shape and size and may at times be distinguishable only by dress and hairstyle.
- Muscles and bones continue to mature as the preschooler gains strength by walking, running, and jumping.
- A balance of good nutrition, exercise, and rest is essential for growth and development.

TABLE 10.10 Growth and Development During Preschool Years

Age	Physical	Gross Motor	Fine Motor	Language
3 years	May have night-time control of bowel and bladder	Rides tricycle, jumps off bottom step, goes up and down stairs using alternate feet, may dance, stands on one foot for a few seconds	Builds tower of nine to 10 cubes, builds bridge of three cubes, copies a circle, imitates a cross, names what has been drawn, cannot draw stick figure	Says 900 words, uses three- to four-word sentences, talks incessantly, asks many questions
4 years	Length at birth is doubled	Skips, jumps, goes downstairs using alternate feet, catches a ball reliably, throws a ball overhead	Uses scissors successfully to cut out picture following outline, laces shoes, copies a square, adds three parts to stick figure	Says 1 500 words, uses four- to five-word sentences, tells exaggerated stories, sings simple songs; questioning is at its peak
5 years	Permanent teeth may begin to erupt Handedness is determined (90% are right-handed)	Skips and hops on alternate feet, throws and catches a ball well, balances on alternate feet well with eyes closed	Ties shoe laces; uses scissors, simple tools, and pencil well; copies a diamond and a triangle; prints a few numbers, letters, or words such as first name	Says 2 100 words, uses six- to eight-word sentences, names four or more colours, knows days of the week and the months

Adapted from Hockenberry, M. J., & Wilson, D. (2015). *Wong's nursing care of infants and children* (10th ed., p. 858, Table 15.1). St. Louis: Elsevier/Mosby.

- Blood pressure should be measured annually in children over 3 years of age.

Gross and Fine Motor Development

Gross motor skills improve and become more refined:

- An average preschooler can hop, skip, and run, which can lead to the introduction of a sport such as soccer, skating, or swimming.
- Encouraging physical activity in children of this age will help create a pattern that may benefit them for the rest of their lives.

Fine motor skill advancement is most evident in improvements in the preschooler's ability to draw:

- The preschooler will begin to hold a pencil or crayon with the fingers rather than the fist.
- Drawings demonstrate advancements in perception of shape as well as developing fine motor skills.

See Table 10.10 for a summary of growth and development in the preschooler years.

Nutrition

As they do in the toddler, the nutritional and fluid requirements in the preschooler continue to decrease slightly, with the exception of protein requirements, which will increase.

- Parents should be encouraged to follow *Eating Well with Canada's Food Guide* to determine the correct amount and portions of each food group for toddlers (Health Canada, 2011).
- Preschool children will change their eating patterns daily, and parents may find that the quantity consumed varies day to day.
- Parents should be concerned with the quality versus the quantity of food as children have the ability to self-regulate their caloric needs and intake. What they do not eat at one meal they will make up at the next.
- An average preschool child will consume slightly more food than a toddler, or about half an adult portion.
- Food habits such as fad foods and strong food preferences will continue in the preschool years.
- At age 4, the child may become more rebellious and refuse to try new foods.
- By age 5, the child will become more open to trying new foods and will enjoy being included in food preparation with a family member.
- Parents should introduce table manners but should be cautioned not to be too strict. The preschooler may find it difficult to sit still for long periods of time.

Sleep

The preschooler will sleep an average of about 12 hours a night and very rarely naps during the day. It is common to see most sleep disturbances during the preschool years.

- Mastery of autonomy, separation, and object permanence can lead to sleep disturbances (Hockenberry & Wilson, 2015; Thiedke, 2001).
- Nightmares can occur and are typically defined as a scary dream followed by full waking. They typically occur in the second half of the night, when dreams are more intense. Once fully awake, the child will be aware of the parent's presence and can be comforted and reassured.
- Sleep terrors can also occur and are typically defined as a partial arousal from a deep sleep. They typically occur 1–4 hours after falling asleep. The child will not be aware of the parent's presence and hence is not easily consoled. The child should simply be observed during the sleep terror until it subsides and the child returns

to a calm state. He or she should be guided back to bed if needed.

- Establishing good bedtime routines is essential to promote good sleep patterns.
- Behaviour that delays bedtime and is determined to be attention-seeking should be ignored by the parent.
- Preschoolers can be very active during the day, and slowing down before bedtime can lead to less resistance in going to bed.

Dental

The focus for preschoolers is on dental hygiene and prevention of decay:

- They should be encouraged to brush their own teeth, but they will require adult supervision of how well they manipulate the toothbrush.
- Professional care and routine follow-ups are encouraged every 6 months (Canadian Dental Association, 2017b).
- Dental injuries are not uncommon at this age and should be examined by a professional.

Immunization

See Table 10.5A–B for the recommended Canadian routine immunization schedule.

Safety

Preschoolers are less accident-prone than toddlers; however, injuries among children in this age group are common. The most common causes of injury in the home to children less than 5 years of age are falls from heights, burns and scalds, and poisonings (Health Canada, 2012a).

- To reduce the risk of injury caused by falls from heights in this age group, ensure that there is a mechanism to prevent the child from falling down stairs or from opening windows more than 15 cm (LeBlanc, Pless, King, et al., 2006).
- To reduce the risk of injury caused by burns and scalds, ensure that the maximum temperature of tap water is less than 54°C; cords do not dangle from the kettle or other appliances in the kitchen; there is a stove guard to prevent a child from grabbing pots; and matches and lighters are well out of reach.
- To reduce the risk of injury by fire, ensure that the home has functioning smoke detectors and fire extinguishers (LeBlanc et al., 2006).
- To reduce the risk of injury caused by poisonings, ensure that all choking hazards in the home are out of reach of the child; all bathroom supplies, cleaning supplies, and medications are out of reach; all bathroom bottles and medications have child-resistant lids (especially grandparents' and visitors'); and a functioning carbon monoxide detector is in the home (LeBlanc et al., 2006).

Play

Preschoolers engage in associative play. This age group enjoys group play in similar activities but without rigid organization or rules.

- Activities should promote physical growth and motor skills and include running, jumping, and climbing.
- Toys that help develop muscles and coordination include tricycles, wagons, gym and sports equipment, sandboxes, and wading pools.
- Activities to help promote muscle strength and coordination include swimming, skating, and skiing.
- Large blocks, puzzles, crayons, paints, and simple crafts can help develop fine motor skills.

Reactions to Illness and Hospitalization

Preschoolers still have poor differentiation between themselves and their environment. They still have a limited understanding of language and can see only one part of an object or situation at a time.

Preschoolers believe that unrelated events cause illness. They also have magical thinking that cause them to perceive illness as a punishment. There is also a fear of mutilation.

Reactions to hospitalization at this stage are primarily regression and a lack of co-operation as coping mechanisms for separation. Preschoolers can experience a loss of control because they feel a loss of their own power. Fear of injury and pain leads to a fear of mutilation and invasive treatments. They lack knowledge about the body. This creates, for example, a fear of castration from enemas or rectal thermometers or a fear that the insides of their body may leak out during the insertion of an intravenous (IV) line. They perceive hospitalization as a punishment and separation from parents as a lack of love.

Nursing Considerations for Separation Anxiety

- Use puppets and dolls to demonstrate treatments with an appropriate level of vocabulary.
- Use adhesive bandages to "stop the insides from coming out."
- Stay with the preschooler during treatments.
- Give rewards such as stars or stickers.
- Use hospital therapeutic play kits to work through anxieties.
- Help prevent a sense of guilt by reassuring the preschooler that he or she is not responsible for the illness.
- Provide motor stimulation and praise achievements.
- Promote autonomy by encouraging choices and self-care, such as a choice of clothing.
- Promote language skills by telling stories and teaching new words.
- Encourage parental involvement, rooming in with the child and visiting as well as contact with siblings and peers to decrease separation anxiety.

SCHOOL AGE: 6 TO 12 YEARS OF AGE

At this age, the child has a slow and uniform rate of growth. This is a generally healthy age group with fewer visits to the pediatrician and fewer immunizations.

- It is important to focus on establishing good health habits, proper nutrition, and physical activity.
- There may be an increased risk of obesity at this stage.

Biological Changes

This is generally a period of gradual growth and development with a growth spurt at prepuberty.

- Height changes are slow and steady, adding 5 cm per year to gain about 30–60 cm.
- Weight will almost double, with increases of 2–3 kg per year.
- Boys and girls vary little during this phase, although girls will begin to surpass boys in both height and weight toward the end of the stage.
- At prepubescence (2 years preceding adolescence), the difference in girls and boys in biological terms can be as much as 2 years, with girls starting prepubescence first.
- In girls, prepubescence is a period of rapid growth, with puberty beginning at approximately age 12. This may cause anxiety in girls who develop earlier or later than their peers.
- In boys, prepubescence is a period of steady growth, with puberty beginning at approximately age 14.
- Changes in height and weight will differ greatly among children; therefore, some may appear older physically than their behavioural, emotional, or mental development would indicate.
- Heart rate and respirations tend to decrease, whereas blood pressure will increase in this stage.

Gross and Fine Motor Development

Generally, school-aged children are steadier on their feet and more graceful than those at the previous stage. Bodies will take on a more slender look, and certain activities, such as biking and climbing, will be easier.

Muscle mass will increase, but it is important not to overwork muscles to the point of fatigue. See Table 10.11 for a summary of growth and development in the school-age years.

Nutrition

The focus for this age group is independence and forming good habits for the years to come. Children become more independent in their food choices at home and school, have strong likes and dislikes for foods, are exposed to choices of foods and are very influenced by friends and the media.

- Good choices and habits will lead to good nutrition and healthy weight gain, whereas poor choices and habits will lead to excessive weight gain and poor nutrition.
- Caloric needs tend to decrease.
- There are fewer stomach upsets, blood sugar levels balance out and are better maintained, and there is an increase in stomach capacity, meaning that food is retained for longer periods of time.

Sleep

It is very important for school-aged children to have enough energy for school and other activities.

- They begin to take charge of bedtime routines; however, they will need reminders to go to bed.
- They no longer take naps and will sleep through the night with typically 8–12 hours of sleep.

TABLE 10.11	**Growth and Development During the School-Age Years**			
Age	**Physical**	**Gross Motor**	**Fine Motor**	**Language**
6 years	Continues to grow slowly, loses first tooth, vision reaches maturity	A very active age with constant activity Demonstrates gradual increase in dexterity	Likes to draw, print, and colour	Develops concept of numbers, knows morning from the afternoon, defines objects in terms of use (i.e., fork, chair), knows left from right hand
7 years	Begins to grow at least 5 cm per year Jaw begins to expand to accommodate permanent teeth	More cautious approach to new performances Repeats performances to master them	Can copy a diamond	Notices certain items missing from a picture, repeats three numbers backward, develops concept of time
8–9 years	Continues to grow at least 5 cm per year	Dresses self completely More limber, bones grow faster than ligaments Always on the go and hard to quiet down	Produces simple paintings and drawings	Gives similarities and differences Can count backward from 20 Describes common objects in detail, not just by use
10–12 years	Slow growth in height and rapid weight gain, possibly leading to obesity Posture more similar to that of an adult	Reaches adult levels	Continues to refine	Writes brief stories Writes occasional short letters to friends Reads for practical information or own enjoyment

Adapted from Hockenberry, M. J., & Wilson, D. (2015). *Wong's nursing care of infants and children* (10th ed., p. 584, Table 15.1). St. Louis: Elsevier/Mosby.

Dental

Many changes to the mouth at this stage require regular visits to the dentist.

- Most children lose their first tooth by age 6 (usually the front).
- Eventually, they will lose all 20 deciduous teeth, and permanent teeth will begin to erupt.
- Permanent teeth appear large in proportion to the rest of the face, a stage that is sometimes known as the ugly duckling phase.
- The jawline elongates, and the new teeth move into their new positions.
- Regular flossing, brushing, and dental visits will promote good oral hygiene.
- Sweets and sugary snacks should be limited.

Immunization

See Table 10.5A–B for the recommended Canadian routine immunization schedule.

Safety

School-aged children tend to have frequent minor injuries, such as falls from bikes, skin rashes from environmental exposures, and bruises from ball sports.

- Due to the increasing need for independence, this age group tends to engage in activities without an adult. Therefore, it is important to teach about safety, risks, and consequences.
- Parents should ensure that children use protective gear, such as bike helmets (which are mandatory in most provinces).
- Parents should ensure that children use a booster seat until the vehicle seat belts fit correctly (Transport Canada, 2018).
- Safety strategies should be put into place for "latch key" children.
- Streetproofing and learning how to avoid abduction allow children to achieve independence and autonomy, safely.
- Parents may participate in community programs in which fingerprints and other identification systems are organized in case the child is missing.
- After-school programs keep children occupied during times when parents are unavailable to supervise.
- Emergency numbers and contact people need to be readily available to the child.

Play

Learning good physical activity habits will influence future involvement in an activity or sport. A proper amount of physical activity will help with weight control, encourage good socialization, help develop gross and fine motor skills, and give the child a sense of accomplishment.

- Play involves increased physical skill, intellect, and fantasy.
- Groups and cliques foster a sense of belonging to a team or club, which leads to a sense of importance.
- Games now have well-established rules, and knowing the rules means belonging (conformity and ritual will guide play).
- Children have increased interest in complex games and electronic games.
- Children have increased interest in reading.
- Quiet and solitary play is valued at this stage as school-aged children enjoy collecting objects and toys, which they tend to keep in disorganized piles.

Mental Health

This is an age at which one's self-concept and self-esteem are developed (Ball et al., 2014).

- Self-concept is the mental idea one has of oneself.
- Self-esteem reflects a positive self-concept.
- The family has a great influence on the child's development of self-esteem and self-concept.
- Children at this age are beginning to form a concept of sexuality and need to have good information and openness to discuss ideas, questions, misconceptions, and fears.
- They are beginning to develop ways to problem-solve situations and develop solutions, for example, around doing homework, making choices, or setting limits.
- This is the concrete stage of cognitive development; therefore, when teaching, provide opportunities to touch, feel, and become engaged in learning.
- Three types of temperament categories in this stage are as follows (Ball et al., 2014):
  - Easy: adapts readily to new situations
  - Slow to warm up: is uncomfortable with new situations and takes time to adapt
  - Difficult: is easily distracted and needs to be prepared for a situation

Reactions to Illness and Hospitalization

The school-aged child can be stressed by immobilization, fear of mutilation and death, and modesty. This child can also be stressed by necessary dependency, which gives a sense of loss of control. It may still be difficult for these children to be able to express themselves verbally, and they may be self-conscious with their care. However, they are curious about their body and are eager to learn about it.

Children at this stage think of illness as being caused by external forces. School-agers are aware of the implications of the different illnesses. They react to separation by exhibiting loneliness, boredom, isolation, and depression. They may show aggression, irritability, and inability to relate to siblings and peers.

Nursing Considerations for Illness and Hospitalization

- Encourage verbalization and reassure the child that it is acceptable to cry.
- Promote autonomy, self-care, and choices with participation in care.
- Celebrate successes when the child succeeds at tasks in order to enhance feelings of accomplishment.

- Encourage peer interaction and use group teaching.
- Provide diversions that help with the development of fine motor skills, such as computer skills, as well as with stress control.
- Increase understanding of bodily functions and the illness and prepare for procedures using pictures to teach the child about the body.
- Work through emotions and stress through various expressive means such as art, music and drama therapy

ADOLESCENCE: 12 TO 18 YEARS OF AGE

Adolescence is the second most rapid growth period. It is defined as the transition period between childhood and adulthood and is a time of development in which one makes educational and occupational choices for the future. It is common for adolescents to take chances and engage in risk-taking behaviour, which may lead to health concerns and injury.

Biological Changes

The period of development referred to as *puberty* involves complex biological, cognitive, psychological, and social changes—more so than any other time in life.

- Puberty involves a predictable series of hormonal and physical changes in both sexual maturation and physical growth.
- Puberty is triggered by a series of hormonal changes in the body controlled by the anterior pituitary gland in response to stimulus from the hypothalamus (Hockenberry & Wilson, 2015).

The Tanner stages of development, which comprise five stages, depict the typical sequence of changes in external secondary sexual characteristics in females and males (Hockenberry & Wilson, 2015). The Tanner stages are used to describe changes in females and males in the text that follows.

Changes in the Female

The primary sexual change in girls is the buildup of enough estrogen to force the release of an egg, or ovum, from the ovaries every 28 days.

   Female breast development
- Stage 1 is the prepubertal stage.
- Stage 2 is characterized by the development of breast buds.
- Stage 3 is characterized by the further enlargement of the breasts and areolae, with no separation of contours.
- Stage 4 is characterized by projection of areolae and papillae to form secondary mounds.
- Stage 5 is characterized by adult configuration.
   Pubic hair development (male and female)
- Stage 1 is the prepubertal stage.
- Stage 2 is characterized by sparse, long, straight, downy hair.
- Stage 3 is characterized by darker, coarser, curly hair that is sparse over the entire pubis.
- Stage 4 is characterized by dark, curly, and abundant hair in the pubic area only.
- Stage 5 is characterized by an adult pattern.

Changes in the Male

The primary male sexual characteristic is the development of viable sperm.

- Follicle-stimulating hormone (FSH) and luteinizing hormone (LH) act on testicular cells to stimulate the production of testosterone and viable sperm.
- The production of viable sperms tends to follow the boy's first ejaculation.
   Male genitalia development
- Stage 1 is the prepubertal stage.
- Stage 2 is characterized by enlargement of the scrotum and testes and rugation and reddening of the scrotum.
- Stage 3 is characterized by lengthening of the penis and further enlargement of the scrotum and testes.
- Stage 4 is characterized by an increase in the length and width of the penis, development of the glans, and darkening of the scrotum.
- Stage 5 is characterized by an adult configuration.

Gross and Fine Motor Development

In the adolescent, gross motor development reaches adult levels. Fine motor development continues to be refined.

Nutrition

Puberty marks the beginning of accelerated physical growth, which can result in as much as double the adolescent nutritional requirements for iron, protein, zinc, and calcium.

Many factors influence an adolescent's nutrition, including growing independence, the need for peer acceptability, concerns over physical appearance, and an active lifestyle.

- It is common for the adolescent to choose snacks of "empty calories," those devoid of any appropriate vitamins and minerals.
- Adolescents are at increased risk for obesity, as well as for eating disorders such as anorexia and bulimia.

Sleep

Adolescents commonly feel fatigued. Factors contributing to fatigue include rapid growth, overexertion, a tendency to stay up late, insufficient sleep, and poor nutrition. In an effort to catch up on missed sleep, many adolescents like to sleep in.

Dental

Continued dental hygiene must be encouraged, including proper brushing, flossing, and regular dental visits.

- Orthodontics are common and may lead to teasing and embarrassment.
- Good snack choices and reduce exposure to empty calories should be encouraged.

Immunization

See Table 10.5A–B for the recommended Canadian routine immunization schedule.

Safety

Adolescents rarely consider the risk or consequence of their actions and often feel invulnerable.

- The use of safety devices decreases in this age group, resulting in increased injury, such as the failure to use helmets or seat belts.
- Health teaching should focus on managing peer pressure to engage in risky activities.

Reactions to Illness and Hospitalization

For adolescents, hospitalization can have a significant impact, causing stresses due to issues around body image, separation from peers, and reduced independence due to necessary restrictions. In children up to 14 years, illness may still be viewed as a punishment.

Reactions to illnesses include the adolescent coping mechanisms of denial and displacement. A sense of a loss of control occurs because of dependency and loss of identity, causing the adolescent to react with rejection, uncooperativeness, self-assertion, anger, frustration, or possibly withdrawal, even from peers. Adolescents also fear mutilation and sexual changes, fears demonstrated by a lot of questioning, rejecting others, questioning adequacy of care, psychosomatic complaints, and sexual reactions. Separation, particularly from the peer group, may result in further withdrawal, loneliness, and boredom.

Nursing Considerations for Illness and Hospitalization

- Relate to adolescents at their level and be authentic.
- Allow them to wear their own clothes, keep their belongings, and decorate their rooms.
- Understand that staying connected through social media is important for family and peer interaction.
- Respect their privacy.
- Set limits.
- Teach about puberty-related issues such as personal hygiene, breast self-examination, testicular self-examination, sexuality and safer sexual practices, contraception, human immunodeficiency virus (HIV), and other relevant topics.
- Provide clear explanations based on science.
- Encourage as much mobility and exercise as possible.
- Encourage the adolescent to participate and be an active decision maker in his or her own health care.
- Promote independence.
- Explore body image and self-esteem.
- Encourage family participation and support.
- Encourage the teen to keep up with schoolwork and in contact with teachers and encourage career goals.

THERAPEUTIC RELATIONSHIP

A therapeutic relationship with the child and the family is the foundation of pediatric practical nursing. See Chapter 3, page 14, for more information on this topic. The hallmarks of effective communication are as follows:

- Establish trust.
- Respect and maintain confidentiality.
- Be truthful.
- Convey respect.
- Implement appropriate communication strategies.

Inherent in every group of nursing considerations in this chapter is the importance of the practical nursing role in developing therapeutic relationships, encouraging clients and families to participate in their care and verbalize their concerns, being a client and family advocate, teaching disease prevention and health promotion, providing support and counselling, and making ethical decisions. The impact of hospitalization according to the age and stage of development is outlined in the previous sections. These principles should be referred to in relation to each of the following health challenges.

PAIN MANAGEMENT

Pain management is an important aspect of pediatric practical nursing care. Nurses perform pain assessments and provide non-pharmacological and pharmacological pain-relieving interventions that bring relief and comfort to children and their families.

Physiological Measures of Pediatric Pain

Physiological reactions to pain, particularly in the non-verbal younger age groups and children with communication and cognitive impairments, can help practical nurses assess the child's level of pain.

Developmental Characteristics of Children's Responses to Pain

The response to pain depends on the child's developmental stage. Characteristics of pain response based on development are summarized in Box 10.3.

Pain Tools

Practical nurses can use a variety of pain tools to help assess children's level of pain. These tools are adapted to the different developmental stages and include behavioural, physiological, or self-report measurements.

Pain scale for preterm infants. A unique pain scale was developed for preterm infants, called the *PIPP* (Premature Infant Pain Profile). There is a higher pain score for infants with a lower gestational age. Sleeping infants also receive additional points for reduced reactions. See Table 10.12 for a summary of the PIPP scale.

Pain scale for 1- to 5-year-olds. CHEOPS, or Children's Hospital of Eastern Ontario Pain Scale, was developed for 1- to 5-year-olds by McGrath, Johnson, Goodman, and others in 1985 in collaboration with recovery room nurses. Six categories of behaviours are identified: cry, facial, verbal, torso, touch, and legs. See Table 10.13 for a summary of this scale.

BOX 10.3 Developmental Characteristics of Children's Responses to Pain

Young Infant
- Generalized body response of rigidity or thrashing, possibly with local reflex withdrawal of stimulated area
- Loud crying
- Facial expression of pain (brows lowered and drawn together, eyes tightly closed, and mouth open and square-shaped)
- No association demonstrated between approaching stimulus and subsequent pain

Older Infant
- Localized body response with deliberate withdrawal of stimulated area
- Loud crying
- Facial expression of pain or anger
- Physical resistance, especially pushing the stimulus away after it is applied

Young Child
- Loud crying, screaming
- Verbal expressions such as "Ow," "Ouch," "It hurts"
- Thrashing of arms and legs
- Attempts to push stimulus away before it is applied
- Lack of co-operation, need for physical restraint
- Requests termination of procedure
- Clings to parent, nurse, or other significant person
- Requests emotional support, such as hugs or other forms of physical comfort
- May become restless and irritable with continuing pain
- Behaviours occur in anticipation of actual painful procedure

School-Aged Child
- May exhibit all behaviours of young child, especially during actual painful procedure, but fewer in anticipatory period
- Stalling behaviour, such as "Wait a minute" or "I'm not ready"
- Muscular rigidity, such as clenched fists, white knuckles, gritted teeth, contracted limbs, body stiffness, closed eyes, wrinkled forehead

Adolescent
- Less vocal protest
- Less motor activity
- More verbal expressions, such as "It hurts" or "You're hurting me"
- Increased muscle tension and body control

From Hockenberry, M. J., & Wilson, D. (2015). *Wong's nursing care of infants and children* (10th ed., p. 153, Box 5–1). St. Louis: Elsevier/Mosby.

Pain scale for 3- to 12-year-olds. The Wong-Baker FACES Pain Rating Scale is a self-reporting tool for children 3–12 years old. See Fig. 10.1 for the FACES tool.

Pain assessment in the child with communication and cognitive difficulties. Children with communication and cognitive difficulties present a significant challenge

to practical nurses in accurately assessing their pain level. These children may not react in the usual way to pain. Parents are very important in helping practical nurses interpret the child's pain reactions. The most reported pain reactions in this type of child are as follows (Hockenberry & Wilson, 2015):
- Moaning, crying, or being irritable
- Being less active
- Seeking comfort
- Not cooperating
- Being stiff, spastic, tense, or rigid
- Sleeping less
- Being difficult to satisfy or pacify
- Flinching or moving body part away and being agitated or fidgety.

Non-Pharmacological Strategies for Pain Management
Many non-pharmacological strategies can be used to help children cope with pain. A number of these strategies are listed in Box 10.4.

Pharmacological Strategies for Pain Management
The following are routes used to deliver pain analgesics:
- Oral, sublingual, buccal, or transmucosal
- IV
- Subcutaneous, continuous
- Patient-controlled analgesia (PCA), family-controlled analgesia, or nurse-activated analgesia
- Intramuscular (this route is discouraged)
- Intranasal
- Intradermal
- Topical or transdermal

Groups of Drugs
Many types of drugs can be used in pediatric pain control. See Chapter 7 for more specific information on the drugs listed here. For the pediatric population, the types of drugs that can be used are as follows (Hockenberry & Wilson, 2015):
- Nonsteroidal anti-inflammatory drugs (NSAIDs) approved for children
  - Indomethacin, ibuprofen, naproxen
- Acetaminophen
- Opioids formulated for children
  - Morphine, fentanyl, codeine, hydromorphone, hydrocodone and acetaminophen, levorphanol, methadone, oxycodone
- Antidepressants
  - Amitriptyline, nortriptyline
- Anticonvulsants
  - Gabapentin, carbamazepine
- Anxiolytics
  - Lorazepam
- Corticosteroids
  - Dexamethasone
- Others
  - Clonidine, mexiletine

TABLE 10.12 Premature Infant Pain Profile (PIPP)

Ages of Use	Reliability and Validity	Variables	Scoring Range
28–40 weeks' gestational age	Internal consistency using Cronbach alpha = 0.75–0.59; standardized item alpha for 6 items = 0.71 Construct validity using handling versus painful situations: statistically significant differences (paired t = 12.24, two-tailed p <0.0001, and Mann-Whitney U = 765.5, p <0.0001) and using real versus sham heelstick procedures with infants aged 28–30 weeks' gestational age (t = 2.4, two-tailed p <0.02, and Mann-Whitney U = 132, p <0.016) and with full-term males undergoing circumcision with topical anaesthetic versus placebo (t = 2.6, two-tailed p <0.02, or non-parametric equivalent Mann-Whitney U test, U = 145.7, two-tailed p <0.02)	Gestational age (0–3) Eye squeeze (0–3) Behavioural state (0–3) Nasolabial furrow (0–3) Heart rate (0–3) Oxygen saturation (0–3) Brow bulge (0–3)	0 = no pain; 21 = worst pain

From Stevens, B., Johnston, C., Petryshen, P., et al. (1996). Premature Infant Pain Profile: Development and Initial validation. *The Clinical Journal of Pain, 12*(1), 13–22. Reprinted with permission.

TABLE 10.13 Children's Hospital of Eastern Ontario Pain Scale (CHEOPS)

Ages of Use	Reliability and Validity	Variables	Scoring Range
1–5 years	Interrater reliability = 90–99.5% Internal correlation = significant correlations between pairs of items Concurrent validity between CHEOPS and visual analogue scale (VAS) = .91; between individual and total scores of CHEOPS and VAS = 0.50–0.86 Construct validity with preanalgesia and postanalgesia scores = 9.9–6.3	Cry (1–3) Facial (0–2) Child verbal (0–2) Torso (1–2) Touch (1–2) Legs (1–2)	4 = no pain; 13 = worst pain

From McGrath, P. J., Johnson, G., Goodman, J. T., et al. (1985). The CHEOPS: A behavioural scale for rating post-operative pain in children. In H. L. Fields, R. Dubner, & F. Cervero (Eds.), *Advances in pain research and therapy* (p. 207). New York: Raven Press. Reprinted with permission.

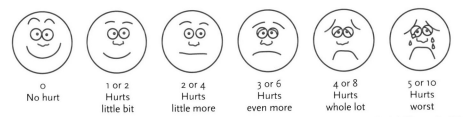

Fig. 10.1 Wong-Baker FACES Pain Rating Scale. (From Hockenberry, M., Rodgers, C., & Wilson, D. [2017]. *Wong's essentials of pediatric nursing* [10th ed., p. 117, Table 5-2]. St. Louis: Elsevier.)

SKIN AND HAIR CARE

Pediculosis Capitis

Pediculosis capitis, or head lice, is an infestation in the hair and is a common condition that can be difficult to eliminate. It can also spread to other family members. It occurs in all socio-economic groups. Outbreaks can occur, particularly in elementary schools and daycare facilities.

Pathophysiology

Head lice live only on humans and are transmitted by direct hair-to-hair contact or by sharing brushes, combs, towels, and so on. They can move quickly but do not jump. The female louse will lay her eggs along the hair shaft. The eggs, which stick to the hair and look like teardrops, hatch in 8–10 days.

Clinical Manifestations

The child will complain of severe itching of the scalp, and the scalp has the appearance of dandruff. Secondary infections can develop because of scratching lesions.

Therapeutics and Nursing Considerations

The CPS recommends a topical insecticide shampoo treatment, which contains pyrethrins or permethrin (Cummings, Finlay, MacDonald, et al., 2018). These pediculicides affect

---

BOX 10.4 Non-Pharmacological Strategies for Pain Management

General Strategies

- Use non-pharmacological interventions to supplement, not replace, pharmacological interventions and use for mild pain and pain that is reasonably well controlled with analgesics.
- Form a trusting relationship with the child and the family.
- Express concern regarding their reports of pain and intervene appropriately.
- Take an active role in seeking effective pain management strategies.
- Prepare the child before potentially painful procedures but avoid "planting" the idea of pain.
- Use "non-pain" descriptors when possible, such as "It feels like heat" rather than "It is a burning pain." This avoids suggesting pain and gives the child control in describing reactions. Avoid evaluative statements or descriptions such as "It will hurt a lot."
- Stay with the child during a painful procedure.
- Allow parents to stay with the child if so desired by both child and parent and encourage the parent to talk softly to the child and to remain near the child's head.
- Involve the parent in learning specific non-pharmacological strategies and in assisting the child with their use.
- Educate the child about the pain, especially when explanation may lessen anxiety, and ensure that the child understands he or she is not responsible for the pain.

Specific Strategies

Distraction

- Employ play, music, computer games, singing, and rhythmic breathing.
- Have the child use deep breathing and blowing it out.
- Encourage the child to concentrate on yelling or saying "ouch."
- Have the child look through a kaleidoscope and concentrate on designs.

- Use humour by watching cartoons, telling jokes or funny stories, or acting silly with the child.
- Help the child read, play games, or visit with friends.

Relaxation

- Hold infant in a comfortable position and rock or sway back and forth.
- Repeat one or two reassuring words softly.
- Use relaxation techniques, such as going limp as a rag doll while exhaling or asking the child to yawn.

Guided Imagery

- During a painful episode, have the child identify and describe some pleasurable or imaginary experiences, including as many senses as possible.
- Write down or record a script.
- Combine the script with relaxation and rhythmic breathing.

Positive Self-Talk

- Teach the child positive statements to say when in pain.

Thought Stopping

- Identify positive facts about the painful event.
- Identify reassuring information.
- Condense positive and reassuring facts into a set of brief statements and have the child memorize them and repeat whenever he or she thinks about or is experiencing a painful event.

Behavioural Contracting

- May be used with children as young as 4 or 5, with stars, tokens, or stickers as rewards.
- Identify rewards or consequences that are reinforcing and goals that can be evaluated.
- Reinforce identified rewards or consequences.
- Use a formal written contract, dated and signed by all persons involved in any of the agreements.

Adapted from Hockenberry, M. J., & Wilson, D. (2015). *Wong's nursing care of infants and children* (10th ed., p. 165). St. Louis: Elsevier/Mosby.

---

the lice but do not affect the nits (eggs); therefore, the treatment must be repeated to kill the hatched lice. Lindane shampoo may be used as a secondary treatment, but only with caution and not with children under 2 because of potential toxicity and resistance. A new non-insecticidal product has been recently approved that contains isopropyl myristate and cyclomethicone for use in children who are over 4 years old.

Dermatitis

Dermatitis is a skin inflammation that develops in response to various stimuli. The types of dermatitis that are the most common in children and adolescents are contact, diaper, seborrheic, and atopic, or eczema. A child's skin is sensitive, and it is important to keep the skin clean, moisturized, and protected from skin breakdown to prevent infections.

Contact Dermatitis

Contact dermatitis is an inflammatory reaction of the skin to an allergen or irritating substance. It commonly affects infants of 9–12 months.

Pathophysiology and Clinical Manifestations

The clinical manifestations are erythema, edema, pruritis, vesicles, or bullae that rupture, ooze, and crust over. Contact dermatitis is usually present only in the contact area, where fissures, dryness, scaling, and necrosis can also appear. Sometimes there is a rash that is distal to the originating area after about 1 week that can last about 3–4 weeks without treatment.

Irritants can cause an inflammatory response, and allergens can be absorbed into the skin, creating an initial sensitization. The allergen is carried to the T lymphocytes to create an immune memory. It takes repeated exposures to the allergen to create an allergic inflammatory reaction. The exception is poison ivy or poison oak, which requires only one or two exposures to elicit the immune reaction.

Therapeutics and Nursing Considerations

The treatment is to remove the irritant or allergen and wash the skin, decrease itching, and promote healing. The child may need patch testing for the allergen. Antihistamines, calamine lotion, wet dressings, or colloidal oatmeal–based bath products will help decrease the itching. Burow's solution soaks (aluminum acetate) will encourage drying. Topical corticosteroids after dressing soaks followed by an emollient will increase the absorption and decrease the itching. If the rash covers more than 10% of the body, oral corticosteroids may be required to decrease the inflammation and start the healing (Ball et al., 2014).

Diaper Dermatitis

Diaper dermatitis is caused by a skin reaction to urine, feces, moisture, or friction that causes abrasion.

Pathophysiology and Clinical Manifestations

The skin reacts to the irritants and becomes increasingly permeable to the irritants and microbes. Irritants such as urine and stool can lead to a rash and subsequent skin breakdown. Common diaper rash, or diaper dermatitis, occurs frequently and affects approximately one-third of infants. Breastfed babies have a lower pH, which helps decrease the occurrence of dermatitis (Ball et al., 2014).

The clinical manifestations are as follows:
- Red glazed plaques appear in the diaper area.
- In most cases, the rash is not in the skin folds of the groin area but affects the rest of the diaper region.
- If the rash becomes severe, it is characterized by a raised, red, and confluent rash, and pustules may also occur.
- *Candida albicans* infection can occur as a primary or secondary infection and is indicated by red, scaly plaques with sharp margins. Small papules and pustules can be present, including in the groin area.

Diagnostics

A skin scraping for microscopic testing with potassium hydroxide can diagnose *Candida* (Ball et al., 2014).

Therapeutics and Nursing Considerations

A barrier cream with zinc oxide paste can treat a mild dermatitis. Moderate or severe dermatitis can by treated with a mild hydrocortisone cream (0.25–1%) with each diaper change for 5–7 days. For candidiasis, an antifungal cream such as clotrimazole can be added. Sometimes an oral antifungal drug may be used to decrease the candidiasis in the bowels (Ball et al., 2014).

It is important to teach the family how to prevent dermatitis. The following interventions can help (Ball et al., 2014):
- Using superabsorbent disposable diapers, change the child every 2 hours during the day and once at night.
- Cleanse skin with mild soap and use diaper barrier creams frequently.
- Do not use tight diapers or waterproof pants.

Seborrheic Dermatitis

Seborrheic dermatitis is an inflammatory skin condition that recurs.

Pathophysiology and Clinical Manifestations

This form of dermatitis is probably caused by an overgrowth of *Pityrosporum* yeast, which is generally found near sebaceous glands in the scalp (cradle cap), forehead, postauricular and periorbital regions, eyelids, inguinal area, skin neck folds, or nasolabial folds. It often occurs in infants and adolescent age groups. It presents with the following manifestations (Ball et al., 2014):
- A waxy, scaly rash with yellow-red patches
- Skin flakes (dandruff)

Therapeutics and Nursing Considerations

The treatment is as follows:
- In young babies, daily shampooing with a baby shampoo
- In the adolescent age group, antidandruff shampoo on the scalp with selenium sulphide or salicylic acid and baby shampoo on the eyes and eyebrows
- It often occurs on the scalp in the infant age group because parents may be reluctant to shampoo over the soft fontanelle. In this case, the scalp needs to be soaked with oil, and then the scales are gently combed out and the area is shampooed (Ball et al., 2014).

Eczema or Atopic Dermatitis

Eczema is a chronic, superficial inflammatory condition that is very itchy.

Pathophysiology and Clinical Manifestations

Eczema is due to a genetic predisposition and external triggers that cause T cells to activate and produce an excess amount of immunoglobulin E (IgE). A child with eczema tends to have allergies and has an increased risk of developing asthma. Frequent triggers are dust mites, animal dander, pollens, food allergies, soaps, chemicals, hormonal changes, and emotional stress. Flare-ups tend to be related to high or low temperatures, perspiration, scratching, and irritant fabrics, such as wool. Severe atopic dermatitis in the infant age group tends to be related to food allergies (Ball et al., 2014, p. 1315).

The symptoms are as follows:
- Pruritis
- Erythematous patches with vesicles, exudate, and crusts
- Chronic symptoms, which include pruritis, dryness, scaling, and lichenification (thickening of the skin)

It occurs most often in dry or cold weather and usually on the face, upper arms, back, upper thighs, and back of the hands and feet. Skin folds are frequently affected.

Diagnostics

Eczema is diagnosed by family history and through the presence of a generalized rash without any known exposure to an allergen. Culture of the skin may be done if there is a secondary infection. A food elimination test can be done to see if food allergies are a factor. Most often, cow's milk, wheat, eggs, soy, citrus, and peanuts are the food allergens (Ball et al., 2014).

Therapeutics and Nursing Considerations

- Wet dressings or colloidal oatmeal cleansing will help decrease the itching; lubricate with emollients while the skin is still moist to enhance moisture trapping.
- If there is oozing, Burow's solution soaks (aluminum acetate) will encourage drying.
- Topical corticosteroids after dressing soaks followed by an emollient will increase the absorption and decrease the itching.
- In the case of a severe flare-up, oral corticosteroids may be required to decrease the inflammation and start the healing.
- Immunomodulators that inhibit T-lymphocyte action are a second line of topical drug that is more often used on the face.

Burns

Burns can range from a minor scald to a major, life-threatening deep tissue injury. In children under 5 years, burns comprised 54.3% of the injury cases reported to the Canadian Hospital Injury Reporting and Prevention Program (Crain, McFaull, Rao, et al., 2017). Thermal burns are the most frequent injuries, from scalding, flames, or contact with a heated object such as a hot cooking pot. Some of these burns are caused by child abuse. Because of the sensitivity of children's skin, they burn more quickly than adults.

Special age groups are at greater risk for certain types of burns, and they are as follows (Ball et al., 2014):

- Infants—They are mostly injured by thermal burns as a result of scalding and house fires.
- Toddlers—They are mostly injured by thermal burns as a result of pulling hot liquids and grease onto themselves.
- Preschoolers—They are mostly injured by thermal burns as a result of scalding or hot objects such as irons or ovens.
- School-agers and adolescents—They are mostly injured by thermal burns (from matches or fireworks). Other risks are electrical burns (due to climbing high-voltage towers and contact with electrical wires), and chemical burns (from combustion experiments).

Children are at more risk from fluid balance shifts and electrolyte imbalances that result with a burn because their bodies have a greater surface area. Refer to Chapter 8, pages 236–237, for burn treatment and nursing considerations for the practical nurse. Burns can be devastating to a child, causing pain, scarring, decreased range of motion (ROM), and damage to self-image and self-esteem.

FLUID AND ELECTROLYTE IMBALANCES

The percentage of body water varies with the age of the child:

- In the infant age group, total body water constitutes 80% of body weight.
- At age 3, total body water constitutes about 65% of body weight.
- At age 15, total body water constitutes about 60% of body weight.

TABLE 10.14   Daily Maintenance Fluid Requirements

Body Weight	Amount of Fluid Per Day
1–10 kg	100 mL/kg
11–20 kg	1 000 mL plus 50 mL/kg for each kg >10 kg
>20 kg	1 500 mL plus 20 mL/kg for each kg >20 kg

From Hockenberry, M. J., & Wilson, D. (2015). *Wong's nursing care of infants and children* (10th ed., p. 947, Table 24.1). St. Louis: Elsevier/Mosby.

The daily maintenance fluid requirements by body weight are shown in Table 10.14.

Fluid and electrolyte imbalances occur more often and more quickly in infants and young children. They are more at risk for these imbalances because of the following:

- A greater body surface area permits a higher proportion of water to be lost through the skin.
- A higher metabolic rate increases the water turnover, and the body fluid needs to be replaced.
- The immature kidney function and buffer system in young children make it harder for them to regulate homeostasis.
- There is a higher proportion of fluid in the extracellular spaces.
- There are higher insensible water losses through the skin and respiratory system.
- Young children lack the ability to control body temperature by sweating or shivering.

Dehydration

Dehydration is an excessive loss of water from the body tissues. It occurs in infants and children whenever total fluid intake is less than fluid output. It is caused by problems that result in an increase in water loss from the kidneys and gastro-intestinal (GI) system and insensible water loss from the skin and respiratory tract. Possible causes include the following:

- Excessive vomiting and diarrhea
- Insufficient oral fluid intake
- Prolonged high fever
- Diabetic ketoacidosis (DKA)
- Extensive burns

Pathophysiology

A child can become dehydrated and can lose both fluid and electrolytes, depending on the cause of the loss. Dehydration is categorized as isotonic, hypotonic, or hypertonic. For further information on fluid and electrolytes, see Chapter 8, pages 159–163.

The degrees of dehydration can be estimated by comparing the child's current weight with his or her weight before the illness. As with diarrhea, dehydration can be classified by severity as follows (Hockenberry & Wilson, 2015):

- Mild dehydration is a loss up to about 5% of pre-illness weight.
- Moderate dehydration is a loss of 5–10% of pre-illness weight.
- Severe dehydration is a loss of more than 10% of pre-illness weight.

TABLE 10.15	**Clinical Manifestations of Dehydration**		
Manifestation	**Isotonic (Loss of Water and Salt)**	**Hypotonic (Loss of Salt in Excess of Water)**	**Hypertonic (Loss of Water in Excess of Salt)**
Skin			
Colour	Grey	Grey	Grey
Temperature	Cold	Cold	Cold or hot
Turgor	Poor	Very poor	Fair
Feel	Dry	Clammy	Thickened, doughy
Mucous Membranes	Dry	Slightly moist	Parched
Tearing and Salivation	Absent	Absent	Absent
Eyeball	Sunken	Sunken	Sunken
Fontanelle	Sunken	Sunken	Sunken
Body Temperature	Subnormal or elevated	Subnormal or elevated	Subnormal or elevated
Pulse	Rapid	Very rapid	Moderately rapid
Respirations	Rapid	Rapid	Rapid
Behaviour	Irritable to lethargic	Lethargic or comatose; convulsions	Marked lethargy with extreme hyperirritability on stimulation

From Hockenberry, M. J., & Wilson, D. (2015). *Wong's nursing care of infants and children* (10th ed., p. 952, Table 24-4). St. Louis: Mosby.

Clinical Manifestations

Clinical manifestations of dehydration are summarized in Table 10.15.

Diagnostics

The following diagnostic tests are used to assess the level of dehydration:

- Abnormal values of serum electrolyte (sodium [Na^+], potassium [K^+], chloride [Cl^-])
- Decreased serum pH value if there is acidosis
- Increased hematocrit
- Increased blood urea nitrogen (BUN) level
- Urine is concentrated with a high specific gravity (>1.030) and high osmolarity
- Decreased urine sodium concentration

Therapeutics and Nursing Considerations

Nursing consideration goals are to correct fluid and electrolyte imbalances and to treat the underlying cause.

- Assess the child's health history, health assessment findings, and laboratory tests to help find the cause of the dehydration.
- Weigh the child to get an accurate initial weight and monitor weight changes indicating fluid balance increases and decreases.
- Administer oral rehydration solution (ORS) or other oral fluids in small quantities—about 30–60 mL (1–2 oz) every hour—and do not give a full diet to the child until the child's hydration has improved, the reason for the dehydration has been corrected, and the fluid balance is normal.
- If the child cannot drink enough fluid to rehydrate or has significant dehydration, start an IV line and administer an appropriate replacement solution, as prescribed. The ordered solution is usually a saline solution containing 5% dextrose. The selection of solution depends on the type and cause of dehydration. Sodium bicarbonate and K^+ may be additives to balance the pH and electrolytes if needed.

- Observe the IV site frequently for signs of infiltration.
- Do not add K^+ to the IV solution until the child voids.
- Assess the child's level of hydration by watching the fluid balance and watching for signs of dehydration.
- Observe and record accurate intake and output and urine specific gravity values.
- Prevent infection by using aseptic technique to insert the IV line and keeping the skin clean at the site.
- Maintain good handwashing and isolation techniques, if required, to prevent spreading infection.
- Slowly increase the child's diet until a full diet is tolerated and chart the response.
- Provide family teaching and support for the following:
  - Oral fluid rehydration and diet increases
  - Care of a child with an IV line
  - Cause and signs and symptoms of dehydration
  - Education regarding handwashing and other hygiene techniques
  - Follow-up medical appointments as necessary after discharge

Fever

Fever or hyperpyrexia occurs when there is an increase in the hypothalamic set point, the body's thermostat-like mechanism, and when the body's heat loss mechanism cannot dissipate excess heat production, leading to an abnormally elevated body temperature.

- Hyperthermia occurs when the body's set point is normal, but other internal or external conditions exceed the ability of the body to eliminate excess heat. These conditions could include heat stroke, Aspirin toxicity, and hyperthyroidism (Hockenberry & Wilson, 2015).
- Frequent causes of pyrexia in pediatrics include otitis media, respiratory tract infections, general viruses, and enteric viral infections.
- More serious causes of fever include urinary tract infections (UTIs), bacteremia, meningitis, pneumonia,

osteomyelitis, cancer, immunological disorders, septic arthritis, poisoning or drug overdose, and dehydration.

Pathophysiology

Fever most commonly results from interference with the hypothalamic set point as a result of allergy, infection, endotoxins, or tumour and leads to increased heat production and decreased heat loss. Clinical assessment of associated symptoms will help the practical nurse decide how serious the fever is. For example, infants, with their larger body surface, are at higher risk for fluid imbalances due to a fever.

Clinical Manifestations

- Temperature of 38.9–40.6°C by axilla (refer to Table 10.3 for normal-range pediatric vital signs)
- Reddened skin with diaphoresis and chills
- Sluggishness or restlessness

Diagnostics

Laboratory tests and results will vary depending on the etiology of the fever.

Nursing Considerations

- Check the temperature as indicated. It is important for the nurse to remember that the degree of fever does not necessarily indicate the severity of the illness.
- Be aware that fever can be a serious concern, and the child needs immediate medical assessment in the following circumstances (Hockenberry & Wilson, 2015):
  - Infant is under 3 months of age
  - Fever is over 40.5°C
  - Child is appearing or acting very ill
- Administer antipyretics as prescribed if the child has pyrexia.
- As prescribed, administer acetaminophen instead of Aspirin because of the association with Reye's syndrome. Acetaminophen is given as an antipyretic and to alleviate discomfort and can be given every 4 hours but not more often than five times per 24 hours.
- Administer NSAIDs or ibuprofen, if prescribed. Ibuprofen also is approved for reducing fever in children as young as 6 months.
- Know that loosening clothing, decreasing room temperature, applying a cool washcloth to the forehead, and increasing the amount of circulating air are effective measures if provided about 1 hour after an antipyretic drug, but only if the child is not shivering. Shivering increases the metabolic rate and can increase the core temperature.
- Teach parents how to take the child's temperature accurately and control fever.

Febrile Seizures

A febrile seizure is a seizure that is associated with an illness that has caused a fever. It is the most common seizure in children.

- Febrile seizure affects approximately 3–5% of children. It usually occurs after 6 months and before 3 years and is unusual after 5 years; the usual onset is between 18 and 22 months (Hockenberry & Wilson, 2015).
- Most children have only one seizure, but some will have recurrences, particularly if febrile seizure runs in families.
- The etiology is unknown, but it is usually associated with common childhood illnesses such as upper respiratory tract infections and UTIs.

Pathophysiology

Febrile seizure usually is a tonic–clonic seizure, associated with an acute febrile illness.

- Febrile seizure usually results when the child hits a peak temperature threshold over 38.8°C, and not from the rapid rise in temperature (Hockenberry & Wilson, 2015).
- It is considered benign if the electroencephalogram (EEG) is normal and other neurological and physical abnormalities are not found.

Clinical Manifestations

Seizure activity generally ceases by the time the child is brought in for medical attention. Most seizures are tonic–clonic and last less than 1 minute.

Diagnostics

Diagnostic tests to check for other underlying problems that contributed to the seizure include lumbar puncture to rule out meningitis and an EEG to rule out a seizure disorder. Computed tomography (CT) and magnetic resonance imaging (MRI) are other tests that may be performed.

Therapeutics and Nursing Considerations

- Observe for signs and symptoms of illness.
- Provide a safe environment in case of a seizure, have suction and oxygen ready, and roll the child on the side to maintain a patent airway.
- Prepare the client and family for procedures and provide emotional support.
- Use temperature-reducing interventions, as noted earlier.
- Educate parents on how to lower a fever and how to protect the child during a seizure.
- Administer anticonvulsant therapy as prescribed if the child is still seizing when he or she arrives at hospital.

Diarrhea

Diarrhea is defined as frequent, abnormally watery stools. Diarrhea can be mild, moderate, or severe. There is also acute or chronic diarrhea, which can be inflammatory or non-inflammatory. Diarrhea is a very common childhood illness that can be life-threatening if the child becomes dehydrated and has an electrolyte imbalance with hypovolemia. The children who are most at risk are young, attend daycare centres, and have poor sanitation at home.

Pathophysiology

- Acute diarrhea is caused by a rotavirus, which is the most common non-bacterial gastroenteritis. Bacterial causes include *Escherichia coli*, *Salmonella*, *Campylobacter*, and

Shigella. Clostridium difficile may occur after antibiotic treatment.

- Chronic diarrhea is commonly related to malabsorption syndromes, immune deficiencies, allergies, and inflammatory bowel disease.

In cases of infectious diarrhea, the pathogens produce enterotoxins that attack the intestinal walls and cause an increase in fluid and electrolyte secretions.

Clinical Manifestations

The severity of the diarrhea needs to be determined:

- Mild diarrhea is a slight increase in frequency with a liquid consistency.
- Moderate diarrhea is several loose or watery stools, possibly accompanied by nausea, vomiting, or irritability, which resolves in 1–2 days.
- Severe diarrhea is frequent or continuous stools with moderate to severe fluid and electrolyte imbalances, cramping, and irritability. The child may appear lethargic, with inappropriate responses, and may become comatose (Ball et al., 2014).

Diagnostics

A stool specimen can be sent for culture and sensitivity to confirm the presence of an infectious or parasitic agent. A stool pH of less than 6 and the presence of reducing substances suggest carbohydrate malabsorption or a lactase deficiency. In stools with a fatty or oily appearance, a three-day stool collection can determine fat malabsorption.

- Stool positive for occult blood can be an indicator of irritation or inflammation.
- It is important to also test for serum complete blood count (CBC), electrolytes, creatinine, and BUN.

Therapeutics

The fluid and electrolyte imbalances need to be corrected and the cause of the diarrhea treated. Premixed ORS is the initial treatment for mild or moderate dehydration. If there is significant dehydration and electrolyte imbalance, IV treatment is started. Reintroduction of a normal diet is done gradually as tolerated by the dehydrated child (Leung, Prince, Canadian Paediatric Society, et al., 2006). A child who is not dehydrated should be fed a normal diet.

Nursing Considerations

- Obtain an accurate history in order to identify the causative factor, such as travelling or eating contaminated foods.
- Assess the type of diarrhea.
- Assess for signs of dehydration, which are outlined in Table 10.15.
- Give ORS frequently to the child with dehydration, and increase the volume as tolerated.
- Check for specific gravity of urine and daily weights and maintain strict intake and output to monitor fluid balance.
- Administer prescribed parenteral fluid and antimicrobials if needed.

- Cleanse the skin area around the perineum and apply protective cream such as zinc oxide to prevent skin breakdown and reduce the potential for infection.
- Provide education to help the family assess the child's diarrhea and level of hydration and to know when to seek medical attention.
- Teach parents oral rehydration treatment with commercial products such as Pedialyte, Rehydralyte, Gastrolyte, Enfalyte, or Cera. It is important to instruct the family not to give the child water, fruit juices, carbonated beverages, gelatin, or any caffeine-containing products when rehydrating the child.
- Restart the child's normal nutrition, in particular breastfeeding and solids, unless the child has developed a lactose intolerance from the diarrhea. A lactose-free formula or half-strength lactose-containing product can be used briefly if there is intolerance until the bowel returns to normal.
- Teach proper handling of stools and hand hygiene to prevent the spread of infection.

Sepsis

Sepsis is a generalized bacterial infection with a systemic inflammatory response. Infants within the first year of life, particularly if they are low birth weight, have a high risk of developing sepsis. All neonatal infections are potentially opportunistic, and any bacteria are capable of causing sepsis. Group B *Streptococcus* is the most common bacteria, and *E. coli* and streptococcus viridans are also common causes of sepsis (Jefferies & Canadian Paediatric Society, 2017). The neonatal inflammatory and immune defence mechanisms are immature, which allows rapid invasion, spread, and multiplication of infecting micro-organisms. The young infant is unable to localize infections.

Clinical Manifestations

The initial signs and symptoms may be subtle and may include temperature instability (the child may be hypo- or hyperthermic), tachycardia, poor peripheral perfusion with pallor, cyanosis or mottling, and respiratory distress. The manifestations may also include poor sucking and feeding, weak cry, lethargy, irritability, decreased pain response, hypotension, jaundice, dehydration, GI disturbances, seizures, hypotonia, tremors, full fontanelle, and cardiac arrest.

Late-onset sepsis (up to age 4 months) usually appears with meningitis.

Diagnostics

- Blood culture, urine culture, and lumbar puncture for cerebrospinal fluid (CSF) analysis are done to try to determine the focal site of the infection.
- CBC with an elevated white blood cell (WBC) count with increased immature neutrophils indicates infection, and C-reactive protein (CRP) levels may or may not be elevated.
- A chest X-ray is done when the infant has respiratory symptoms.

Therapeutics

The infant is treated immediately with antimicrobials after the cultures have been collected. Ampicillin and gentamicin are usually prescribed and are based on drug sensitivities to the common organisms cultured from the infant with sepsis. If the cultures are negative in 48 hours, then the drug therapy can be discontinued (Jefferies & Canadian Paediatric Society, 2017).

Nursing Considerations

Nursing management is focused on the following goals and is similar to that given to a high-risk newborn:

- Assess the newborn for signs and symptoms of onset infection and sepsis, particularly in infants having invasive procedures done that can elevate the risk of infection.
- Provide a neutral thermal environment due to the infant's immature abilities to regulate temperature.
- As prescribed, administer antibiotic therapy for 7–10 days if culture results are positive and discontinue therapy if culture results are negative (usually in 2 days).
- Monitor hydration and intake and output.
- Monitor the infant for signs of a worsening condition or shock (Ball et al., 2014).

Meningitis

Meningitis is an inflammation of the meninges caused by a bacterial or viral infection. Neonates and infants are at increased risk of developing bacterial meningitis, and it can be fatal if not treated immediately. Viral meningitis is less virulent. The outcome of the meningitis depends on the organism, as well as the child's age and response to treatment.

- Most cases occur between 1 month and 5 years, with infants under 12 months being the most susceptible to bacterial meningitis. The risk of mortality is higher in adolescents and young adults.
- Meningitis in Canada has decreased significantly with the introduction of universal immunization programs delivering conjugate vaccines for *Haemophilus influenzae* type b (Hib), *Neisseria meningitidis*, and *Streptococcus pneumoniae*. Pneumococcal meningitis has also decreased significantly in all age groups following the introduction of the vaccine PCV7 (Le Saux, Canadian Paediatric Society, & Infectious Diseases and Immunization Committee, 2014).
- Viral meningitis or aseptic meningitis is caused mainly by enteroviruses and less commonly by arboviruses, herpes simplex, and varicella zoster. It is a self-limiting disease that lasts 7–10 days.
- In bacterial meningitis, the bacteria from a focal infection site, such as otitis media, enter the meninges through the bloodstream and spread through the CSF. The infection can also be introduced as the result of an invasive procedure or through a surgical or trauma site. The bacteria toxin creates a meningeal inflammatory response and causes a release of purulent exudates that spreads the infection rapidly. The brain surface becomes covered in exudate and

is edematous. The ventricles can then become obstructed by pus, fibrin, or adhesions, blocking the CSF flow and potentially producing increased intracranial pressure (ICP). Serious damage to the brain cells, some of which can be permanent, is caused by necrosis (Ball et al., 2014).

Clinical Manifestations

The manifestations vary depending on the child's age, the type of bacterial infection, and the onset of the infection. Newborns have non-specific symptoms that are different from those of older children. Symptoms in this age group may include poor sucking ability, vomiting, or diarrhea. Neonates with meningitis tend to have poor muscle tone with little movement and a weak cry. The fontanelle may be bulging, but this is a late sign. The newborn may be irritable, lethargic, jaundiced, and drowsy and have seizures, apnea or irregular respirations, cyanosis, fever (varies with level of maturity), and weight loss. If the infant is not treated, there is deterioration leading to cardiovascular collapse, seizures, and apnea (Hockenberry & Wilson, 2015).

Infants who are between 3 months and 2 years of age show signs of fever, poor feeding, vomiting and a bulging or tense fontanelle and often have a high-pitched cry. Nuchal rigidity (resistance to neck flexion) and Brudzinski's and Kernig's signs are not usually present in children under 12–28 months of age. Older children may initially have respiratory or GI problems and then develop nuchal rigidity (stiff neck), headache, and tripod posturing. Kernig's sign is present with meningitis when the supine or sitting child's knee is flexed, and there is pain and resistance upon extension of the knee. Brudzinski's sign is present with meningitis when the supine child's head is flexed, and the hips and knees flex involuntarily. A petechial rash may also appear.

Diagnostics

- A lumbar puncture is done in order to diagnose meningitis. CSF may be cloudy, with an elevated WBC count, elevated protein level, and decreased glucose level. The CSF is cultured, and a Gram stain is done to determine the causative agent. A CT scan may be done before this test if increased ICP is present to prevent brain herniation.
- CBC reveals increased WBC count.
- Blood culture may pinpoint the causative agent as well.

Therapeutics

The prognosis of meningitis depends on treating the infection before clinically severe disease ensues. Therefore, the timely administration of empirical antimicrobial therapy, specifically third-generation cephalosporin, is crucial (Le Saux et al., 2014).

Nursing Considerations

Perform careful assessments to monitor the child for changes in illness and signs of complications.

- Monitor temperature, vital signs, and level of consciousness frequently, particularly for shock or respiratory distress.

- Accurately monitor intake and output and fluid and electrolyte balance; children with decreased levels of consciousness should receive nothing by mouth; others are allowed fluids and diet as tolerated.
- Assess neurological signs and level of consciousness, including signs of increased ICP. Measure head circumference to monitor for the development of subdural effusions and obstructive hydrocephalus.
- Administer antibiotics as prescribed (the type depends on the organism), and maintain IV line.
- Provide fever-reducing measures.
- Monitor for signs of a secondary infection.
- Know that steroids may be prescribed to relieve cerebral edema.
- Set up respiratory isolation for 24–48 hours after antibiotic administration begins.
- Be aware that the child will be sensitive to sound and bright lights; keep the room as quiet as possible to decrease environmental stimuli.
- Assess the level of pain and give prescribed acetaminophen Tylenol with codeine as needed.
- Position the child in a side-lying position without a pillow with the head of the bed slightly raised to increase comfort from neck stiffness (Hockenberry & Wilson, 2015).

PSYCHOSOCIAL AND MENTAL HEALTH CHALLENGES

Child Maltreatment

Child maltreatment refers to the harm, or risk of harm, that a child or youth may experience while in the care of a person whom he or she trusts or depends on, including a parent, sibling, other relative, teacher, caregiver, or guardian. Harm may occur through the direct actions by the person (acts of commission) or through the person's neglect to provide a component of care necessary for healthy child growth and development (acts of omission).

The five types of child maltreatment are as follows:
- Physical abuse (assault)—The application of unreasonable force by an adult or youth to any part of a child's body
- Sexual abuse—Abuse involving a child, by an adult or youth, in an act of sexual gratification, or exposure of a child to sexual contact, activity, or behaviour
- Neglect—Failure by a partner or caregiver to provide the physical or psychological necessities of life to a child
- Emotional harm—Adult behaviour that harms a child psychologically, emotionally, or spiritually
- Exposure to family violence—Circumstances that allow a child to be aware of violence occurring between a caregiver and his or her partner or between other family members

Child abuse is a very serious situation that has long-term implications for the child and the family. A full 32% of adults in Canada have reported having experienced some form of maltreatment as a child. Based on 2015 police-reported data, of the children and youth who were victims of violence, 30% were victims of family violence; that is, acts perpetrated by parents, siblings, extended family members, or spouses (Public Health Agency of Canada, 2018b).

Three types of factors put a child at increased risk of being abused: parental factors, child factors, and environmental factors.

Parental factors
- Severe punishment as children
- Poor impulse control
- Free expression of violence
- Social isolation
- Poor social–emotional support system
- Low self-esteem
- Substance abuse

Child factors
- Temperament: doesn't "fit" as well into the family
- Illness, disability, or developmental delay
- Illegitimacy
- Hyperactivity
- Resemblance to someone the parent does not like
- Failure to bond
- Problem pregnancy, delivery, or prematurity
- Other siblings who are not attached

Environmental factors. These factors apply to all socioeconomic groups.
- Chronic stress, such as divorce or poverty
- Frequent relocation
- Substitute caregivers who can be abusive (Hockenberry & Wilson, 2015)

Clinical Manifestations

Physical abuse. Physical indicators:
- Skin injuries, such as bruising, with different stages of healing in unusual locations and often shaped like the object that was used
- Burns, such as cigarette burns
- Fractures, such as spiral fracture
- Head injuries, particularly in a young child
- Fatal intracranial trauma without signs of external injuries caused by violent shaking, especially in infants under 6 months (CPS, 2008).
- Subdural or retinal hemorrhages in the absence of external signs
- Traumatic eye injuries such as conjunctival hemorrhages
- Mouth injuries
- Poisonings
- Drowning
- Repeated accidents

Behavioural indicators:
- The child may be wary of adults and fearful of parents as well as afraid of going home.
- The child suffers pain without crying.
- The child has superficial relationships or is overly friendly.
- The child reports injury by parents.
- The child exhibits attention-seeking behaviour (Hockenberry & Wilson, 2015).

Nursing Considerations

Practical nurses often identify potential or actual abuse situations. Any suspected child maltreatment must be immediately reported to the appropriate authorities, such as a hospital child abuse team or a children's aid society. The following interventions are critical to ensuring a child's safety, as well as helping the child and the child's family cope with the situation:

- Carefully perform a physical examination and history-taking for signs of abuse. This is essential.
- Know that accurate documentation is very important to preserve the facts.
- Encourage the child to verbalize concerns without any undue questioning.
- Encourage positive self-concept in the child.
- Use play to help the child work out stress.
- Collaborate with the interdisciplinary team and refer the family to social services.
- If the child has been apprehended, help the child cope with the loss of the family and ease his or her transition into foster care.

Emotional abuse. Emotional abuse is a deliberate attempt to destroy a child's self-esteem or confidence.

Indicators:
- Failure to thrive, developmental delays
- Feeding problems
- Sleep problems
- Enuresis
- Habit disorders such as rocking, biting, or hair-pulling
- Withdrawn
- Unusual fearfulness
- Behavioural problems of extremes, either withdrawal or aggression
- Age-inappropriate behaviours
- Attempted suicide (Hockenberry & Wilson, 2015)

Neglect. The definition of the term *neglect* is to deprive a child of necessities.

Physical indicators:
- Failure to thrive, malnutrition, constant hunger
- Poor hygiene and inappropriate clothing
- Bald patches on an infant's head
- Lack of adequate supervision, abandonment
- Poor health

Behavioural indicators:
- Dull, inattentive infant
- Begging or stealing food
- School attendance issues
- Use of drugs and alcohol
- Delinquency
- Child reports having no caretaker (Hockenberry & Wilson, 2015)

Sexual abuse. Sexual abuse includes incest, molestation, exhibitionism, child pornography, child prostitution, and pedophilia (Hockenberry & Wilson, 2015).

The following are characteristics of the abuser and the child:

- Anyone can be an abuser, but usually it is a male whom the child knows.
- Child maltreatment involves all socio-economic groups.
- The abuser may be a prominent community member or someone who works with children, such as a teacher or coach.
- Pornography or prostitution can involve the parents or strangers.
- Stepfathers may put a child more at risk.
- The child is often a runaway.
- The child is often afraid to expose the abuser because of a fear of retaliation or that he or she will not be believed.
- Boys are less likely to report abuse (Hockenberry & Wilson, 2015).

Physical indicators of sexual abuse include the following:
- In many children, no obvious signs
- Difficulty walking or sitting
- Torn, stained, bloody underwear
- Gross evidence of trauma (genital, oral, anal), pain, itching, sexually transmitted infections, discharge
- Pregnancy
- Weight loss, eating disorder
- Vague somatic complaints

Behavioural indicators:
- Under age 5—Regression, feeding or toileting disruptions, temper tantrums, requests for frequent underwear changes, seductive behaviour
- Ages 5–10—School problems, night terrors, sleep problems, anxieties, withdrawal, refusal of physical activity, and inappropriate behaviours
- Adolescents—School problems, running away, delinquency, promiscuity, drug and alcohol abuse, eating disorders, depression, and other significant psychological problems, such as suicide attempts (Hockenberry & Wilson, 2015).

Munchausen syndrome by proxy. This syndrome occurs when a parent, usually the mother, induces the symptoms of an illness, such as poisoning, in a child. It is very hard to verify. Indicators:

- The history does not match the clinical findings.
- Unexplained, prolonged, or extremely rare illness that does not respond to treatment and occurs only when the parent is present.
- The parent shows unusual interest in the health care team members and pays special attention to the child.
- Family members display similar symptoms (Hockenberry & Wilson, 2015).
- The child and family need to be referred to the child abuse team. There can be significant physical effects that can potentially cause serious physical illness and death. As well, significant emotional trauma can be caused to the child.

Suicide

Suicide is taking action to intentionally end one's life. Suicide is the second most common cause of death among Canadian adolescents, representing one-quarter of all deaths among youth 15 to 19 years of age in 2016 (Statistics Canada, 2018). The First Nations and Inuit populations are at a significantly higher risk. The risk factors for suicide in this age group are as follows:

- Previous suicide attempts
- A friend who has tried to or has committed suicide
- School issues and grade changes
- Substance abuse
- Problems with a love relationship
- Depression, loneliness, and isolation
- Chronic family issues
- Chronic condition
- Change in behaviour or weight
- Family history of suicide
- Abuse—physical, emotional, sexual
- Low self-esteem
- Giving away possessions
- Access to guns and ammunition
- Minority sexual practice (Ball et al., 2014)

Clinical Manifestations

- Depression usually precedes suicide. Symptoms of depression may be obvious or subtle.
- Danger signs include lethargy, feeling unwell, insomnia or early-morning awakening, poor appetite or overeating, excessive crying, giving away important possessions, a preoccupation with death or death themes, and statement of intent.

Nursing Considerations

- Provide education for groups such as teachers, families, and youth about risk factors.
- Provide youth counselling, stress management, and problem-solving techniques.
- Assess if the child has a suicide plan.
- Arrange for counselling, crisis intervention, and hospitalization if necessary and refer the youth and family to a professional therapist.
- Provide counselling after a suicidal death for the adolescent's family and friends to help them understand and work through their bereavement.

Attention-Deficit/Hyperactivity Disorder
Pathophysiology

Attention-deficit/hyperactivity disorder (ADHD) is a neurodevelopmental condition with an unknown cause. Scientists believe that genes and environmental factors cause subtle brain alterations. In turn, these brain alterations cause problems with behaviour and learning. It causes inattention, hyperactivity/impulsivity, or both. ADHD is very common; it is estimated that between 5 and 12% of children have ADHD (AboutKidsHealth, 2017).

Clinical Manifestations

There are three subtypes of ADHD. Depending on their symptoms, a child may be diagnosed with one of the following:

- Predominantly Hyperactive/Impulsive subtype—Mainly hyperactive or impulsive symptoms, few or no inattentive symptoms; this subtype is rare compared with the others
- Predominantly Inattentive subtype—Mainly inattentive symptoms, few or no hyperactive symptoms
- Combined subtype—Both inattentive and hyperactive symptoms

Subtypes can change as children grow older. As children grow older, they may show fewer hyperactive and impulsive symptoms. Therefore, people who were diagnosed with the Combined subtype of ADHD as children may become Predominantly Inattentive as teens or adults.

About one-third of children with ADHD continue to have ADHD in adulthood. Another third of children with ADHD continue into adulthood with some attention problems but not enough to qualify for a clinical diagnosis of ADHD. The remaining third of children with ADHD outgrow their symptoms by the time they reach adulthood.

Therapeutics

Medication is an important component of the treatment ADHD. Medication is very effective for treating the symptoms which improves behaviour in the classroom and in social situations. In turn, this improves children's relationships with their peers, teachers and parents.

Behavioural treatment can help the child become responsible for their own behaviour and to provide support in the process. It is important to address all areas of the child's life. This means making the child's whole environment supportive, including home and school.

A combination of both medication and behavioural treatment is recommended (AboutKidsHealth, 2017).

Nursing Considerations

The practical nurse is an active member of the health care team in managing a child with ADHD and acts as a link between other health care providers and educators. In this role, he or she should do the following:

- Encourage parents to express their concerns and express their emotions.
- Participate in child and family teaching, arranges referrals to support groups, and discusses school settings and classroom placement for special assistance.
- Provide information on the medication and treatment plan

Environment manipulation education is needed to help the family and the child. The use of organizational charts, decreasing distractions, and modelling positive behaviours in a consistent approach may help (Hockenberry & Wilson, 2015).

Autistic Spectrum Disorders

Autism Spectrum Disorder (ASD) is a complex developmental brain disorder caused by a combination of genetic and environmental influences. Autism appears to have its roots in very early brain development. The etiology is still uncertain. However, the most obvious signs and symptoms of autism tend to emerge between 2 and 3 years of age.

It is considered to be a lifespan disorder. An estimated 1 in 68 children is identified with ASD (Autism Speaks Canada, 2017).

Clinical Manifestations

ASD is characterized by social-interaction difficulties, communication challenges, and a tendency to engage in repetitive behaviours. However, symptoms and their severity vary widely across these three core areas. Taken together, they may result in relatively mild challenges for someone on the high functioning end of the autism spectrum. For others, symptoms may be more severe, as when repetitive behaviours and lack of spoken language interfere with everyday life.

Some children with autism have an identifiable genetic condition that affects brain development. These genetic disorders include fragile X syndrome, Angelman syndrome, tuberous sclerosis, and chromosome 15 duplication syndrome and other single-gene and chromosomal disorders.

It is estimated that between 40–70% of people with ASD have at least one co-occurring mental health problem. Common problems include anxiety, depression, and anger (Autism Speaks Canada, 2017).

Diagnostics

Diagnosis is based on the presenting deficits as well as the severity. When the child exhibits persistent deficits in social communication and social interaction across multiple contexts:

- Deficits in social-emotional reciprocity
- Deficits in non-verbal communicative behaviours used for social interaction
- Deficits in developing, maintaining, and understanding relationships

Severity is based on social communication impairments and restricted repetitive patterns of behaviour (Autism Speaks Canada, 2017).

Therapeutics

Early diagnosis, referral, and concentrated intervention are critical for the child to progress and increase the level of social development. Some children can improve when language and communication skills can be acquired. Intervention can include intensive behaviour treatments and medication. Early intensive behavioural intervention involves the entire family working closely with a team of professionals.

Nursing Considerations

Children with autism do not adapt easily to new situations and require directed activities, minimal stimulation, established routines, and close supervision. It is important to encourage the family to stay with the child when hospitalization is required because of the difficulties surrounding new people and situations.

The child and the family require highly specialized care and treatment. They need to be referred to community treatment centres and support networks. Families need support and education on how to manage the child at home. The treatments can be very expensive and can be a significant drain on the family's finances.

Anorexia Nervosa and Bulimia Nervosa

Anorexia nervosa is a potentially life-threatening eating disorder that affects mainly females. The peak incidence is at 12–13 years; there is another peak again at 17–18 years. Bulimia nervosa also occurs mainly in females and with a teenage onset. See Chapter 11, pages 436–439.

End of Life
Developmental Stages and Reactions to End of Life

Refer to the earlier sections on reactions to hospitalization in this chapter, pages 308, 315, 317, 319 and 321, for the different developmental stages.

Infants and toddlers. There is currently no consensus as to whether this age group grieves or mourns. Children in this age group will perceive that the family is very upset and sad even though they do not understand why. Encourage the family members to stay with the dying child and provide physical comfort, such as cuddling and rocking. Establishing routines and rituals with familiar objects will give a sense of security.

Preschoolers. Children at this stage are familiar with the term *death*, but they see it as a going away or possibly as sleep. Preschoolers take statements literally; when family members tell a preschooler that they have put their dog to sleep, the child may fear sleeping. Death is equated with sleep and separation and is reversible.

- In the magical thinking of preschoolers, the dead can be alive and do things such as breathing, eating, and sleeping.
- Preschoolers who have a seriously ill sibling may feel that their own actions have caused the death and that the anger and sadness of the family are being directed at them; as a result, they may view the illness as a punishment for their actions and thoughts.
- Separation from parents is the biggest fear for this group, and the preschooler may feel that the parents will go away and not come back.
- Encourage the family to minimize separations, use concrete language, and be alert for a sense of punishment and guilt.

School-aged children. For these children, death is only temporary and is personified by figures such as the "bogeyman" or the devil. The child may think that death can be avoided by being good. There are degrees of being dead; therefore, people are not really dead; life and death are transposable. By 7–9 years, there is a deeper understanding that death is universal and irreversible, and the child will defy death and joke about it.

When the school-aged child or a sibling has a terminal illness, the child fears the unknown and loss of control, which leads to a decreased sense of security and self-confidence. Clear explanations of what is going to happen will give the child a sense of control and maintain his or her self-esteem. The child at this stage can appear to be uncooperative or rude but is trying verbally to gain some sense of control and power.

- Encourage the child to express his or her feelings and provide physical activities to relieve stress.
- Provide as much choice and control as possible.

Adolescence. Adolescents normally respond with appropriate grief and react to death with an almost adult understanding. This age group is starting to look for the meaning in death and religious meaning, such as life after death.

- Adolescents are unable to prioritize their losses; therefore, the loss of a friend may be just as upsetting as the loss of a parent.
- A loss due to death can interfere with the search for identity, and physical changes in the body of a terminally ill adolescent can be more devastating than the actual illness.
- The ill adolescent is often isolated from his or her peer group; encourage contact and communication with friends because the child may be unable to communicate with his or her parents and get support. Peer support groups can be helpful.
- The practical nurse can facilitate communication between these groups and provide as much independence and control as possible.

Clinical Manifestations

When evaluating a child's psychological state in relation to death and dying, assessment findings usually take into consideration the following:

- The developmental stage of the child
- Cultural and spiritual concerns
- Socio-economic factors
- Support network and family connections
- Grief manifestations
- Unfinished business between parents and child
- Anticipatory grieving
- Dysfunctional grieving (Hockenberry & Wilson, 2015)

Nursing Considerations

The end of life is a very sensitive topic. The child and the family need guidance in understanding the process of death and dying and to maintain as healthy a grieving process as possible.

Nursing considerations for end of life are as follows:

- Encourage discussion of the child's past experiences with death and dying.
- Determine and develop strategies to help decrease anxiety.
- Determine comfort measures and objects and promote a sense of security.
- Encourage the use of the child's and family's rituals, routines, and customs.
- Provide a member of the clergy if the child and the family would like the referral.
- Encourage the child and the family to verbalize feelings and concerns.
- Refer the family to social services or community resources if the family needs financial assistance.
- Organize and help activate support systems.
- Refer the family to a grief counsellor if needed (Hockenberry & Wilson, 2015).

Sudden Unexpected Infant Death

Sudden unexpected infant death (SUID) (also called *sudden infant death syndrome* [SIDS]) is the sudden, unexplained death of any infant for whom a post-mortem examination fails to determine the cause of death. The death usually occurs during sleep. In 2004, SUID accounted for 5% of all infant deaths. From 1999 to 2004, Canada observed a 50% decrease in the rate is SUID (Public Health Agency of Canada, 2018c). The drop in rates may be due to how infants' deaths are classified, but likely it is mainly due to the changes in recommendations for safe sleeping positions for young infants.

The risk factors for infants are as follows:

- Sleeping position other than on the back
- Sleeping alone in a room
- Bed sharing with mothers who are cigarette smokers
- Bed sharing with an adult who is extremely fatigued or impaired by drugs or alcohol
- Use of soft bedding, a pillow, and covers that can cover the head
- Sleeping with an infant on a sofa, which is of particular high risk
- Bed sharing with other than parents or usual caregiver (Cyr, Canadian Paediatric Society, & Injury Prevention Committee, 2012)

Infants who are at higher risk of SUID include the following groups:

- Infants requiring cardiopulmonary resuscitation or vigorous stimulation with a combination of apnea, colour change, marked change in muscle tone to limpness, and choking or gagging (ALTE, apparent life-threatening events)
- Preterm infants with apnea spells when discharged home
- Siblings of two or more SUID occurrences
- Infants with certain types of diseases or conditions, particularly with central hypoventilation (Hockenberry & Wilson, 2015)

The peak age for SUID ranges from 2–4 months, with most cases occurring before 6 months. SUID affects male infants more than females and usually occurs in winter.

Pathophysiology

The cause of SUID is unknown, but the most accepted theory is an abnormality of the brainstem, the area that regulates the neurological system of cardiopulmonary control, which can cause sleep apnea, dysrhythmic breathing, and impaired arousal to increased carbon dioxide and decreased oxygen. However, sleep apnea does not cause SUID. There may be a genetic predisposition. Maternal smoking may be an important factor in SUID. Prone sleeping is also a major factor, one that can impair arousal, cause oropharyngeal obstruction and carbon dioxide rebreathing, and affect thermal balance. Soft bedding may prevent infants from turning their heads to the side, creating the same dangers as prone sleeping (Hockenberry & Wilson, 2015).

Clinical Manifestations

There are no characteristic findings before death. Usually, parents discover that the infant has died in the crib. The infant is often found with blankets over the head, face down, with frothy, blood-tinged secretions in the nose and mouth. The diaper usually has both urine and stool in it. The child's appearance causes acute distress to the family (Hockenberry & Wilson, 2015).

Diagnostics

No laboratory tests are diagnostic of SUID.

Nursing Considerations

- To decrease the risk of SUID, teach families to place their infant on their backs to sleep and decrease exposure to smoking before and after the birth (Public Health Agency of Canada, 2018c).
- Encourage the family to verbalize concerns and validate feelings.
- Assess the family's grieving patterns and ability to cope.
- Refer the family for counselling if needed. Bereavement counsellors and support groups are often very helpful.
- Provide a supportive environment and time for the family to say goodbye to the child.
- Offer a memory package with a lock of hair, foot and hand prints, and other important mementos.

EAR DYSFUNCTION

Acute Otitis Media

Acute otitis media (OM) is the inflammation of the middle ear, with the signs and symptoms of acute infection, fever, and ear pain. It is the most common reason that antibiotics are prescribed. It is usually caused by *H. influenzae*, *Moraxella catarrhalis*, or *S. pneumoniae*. The viral cause is usually respiratory syncytial virus (RSV) and influenza. It occurs more commonly in boys. Seventy percent of all children will develop OM (Hockenberry & Wilson, 2015).

Pathophysiology

Children more predisposed to OM are as follows:

- Children who have short, horizontally positioned eustachian tubes, which allow secretions to easily migrate into the middle ear
- Children with immaturely developed cartilage that lines the eustachian tube opening; this makes the tubes more likely to open up, allowing secretions to migrate into the middle ear
- Children who have immature immune systems, which increases the risk of infection
- Children with enlarged lymph tissue, which can block the eustachian tube openings
- Children who are in environments with smokers; passive smoking increases inflammation and decreases secretion drainage

Breastfed infants have a lower incidence because of their semi-upright feeding position and immunity acquired from the mother, whereas bottle-fed infants who are fed in the supine position have a higher incidence of infection

due to the possibility that formula may reflux into the eustachian tubes.

Treatment of OM with antibiotics remains controversial because of the risk of bacteria such as *S. pneumoniae* developing antibiotic resistance. Although controversial, antibiotic therapy is the main treatment, with amoxicillin being most frequently used, unless the child has been on antibiotics in the last month. Other antibiotics include amoxicillin–clavulanates (Clavulin), azithromycin (Zithromax), and cephalosporins (Cefazolin). It is generally agreed that waiting up to 72 hours for the infection to clear in healthy children is acceptable, but for children under 2 years, caution is needed because of the risk of sepsis (Hockenberry & Wilson, 2015).

Possible complications include hearing loss, scarring of the tympanic membrane, tympanic perforation, chronic suppurative otitis media, mastoiditis, meningitis, and cholesteatoma, in which the epithelial lining forms scales and can destroy bone and middle ear structures.

Myringotomy tubes are tiny drainage tubes that may be inserted into the tympanic membrane to drain excess secretions in the middle ear and equalize pressure.

Follow-up is important to ensure that the antibiotic therapy has cleared the infection and that there are no complications, such as hearing loss.

Clinical Manifestations

Health history and physical assessment data may reveal the following:

- Irritability, pulling at the affected ear, and complaints of ear pain
- Fever
- Decrease in appetite
- Nasal congestion, rhinorrhea, cough, and vomiting and diarrhea, showing a concurrent infection
- Otoscopic findings, including erythematous tympanic membrane; bulging tympanic membrane, membrane with no visible landmarks, including no light reflex; or diminished tympanic membrane mobility and discoloured effusion
- Purulent discharge

Diagnostics

Culture and sensitivity tests may identify organisms in ear discharge. An audiology referral for hearing tests can be done if hearing impairment is suspected.

Nursing Considerations

- Reduce fever by administering antipyretics as prescribed and dressing the child lightly.
- Relieve pain with prescribed analgesics by offering soft foods to reduce chewing and through the application of local heat or warm compresses to the affected ear. Note that heat may aggravate the pain in some children. Ice packs on the affected ear may relieve pain by reducing edema.
- Facilitate drainage by having the child lie on the affected ear.
- Prevent skin breakdown by keeping the external ear clean and dry and by using a moisture barrier.

- Assess for hearing loss and recommend referral for audiological testing if indicated.
- Administer prescribed antibiotics; prophylactic antibiotic treatment may be prescribed for children with recurrent infections.

RESPIRATORY DYSFUNCTION

Upper Respiratory Infection

Upper respiratory tract infections include nasopharyngitis, pharyngitis, and tonsillitis.

Nasopharyngitis and Pharyngitis

Also called the *common cold*, nasopharyngitis is a viral infection of the nose and throat. It is usually caused by viruses such as rhinoviruses, RSV, adenoviruses, influenza, and parainfluenza viruses. Pharyngitis is an inflammation of the pharynx. Nasopharyngitis is the most common illness in infancy and childhood.

Pathophysiology

The disease course of upper respiratory tract infections is usually self-limiting and lasts from about 4 days and up to 10 days if there are complications. If the infection is caused by group A beta-hemolytic *Streptococcus*, there is the potential for complications such as acute glomerulonephritis or rheumatic fever (Hockenberry & Wilson, 2015). Young children are more susceptible to catching these infections because of their immature immune systems.

Clinical Manifestations

The symptoms often include fever, irritability, restlessness, decreased appetite and fluid intake, and decreased activity. Rhinorrhea and nasal congestion can occur because of inflammation and can lead to skin irritation from wiping away secretions.

Therapeutics

- Antipyretics and other fever-reducing measures are given.
- The Canadian Paediatric Society (2017) recommends saline drops to help clear nasal congestion. Over-the-counter decongestants and cough medicines may not be very effective and are not recommended for children under 3 years unless recommended by a physician or nurse practitioner.

Nursing Considerations

Teaching family members to care for their children at home is important; considerations are as follows:
- Elevate the head of the bed to help the secretions drain.
- Provide suction with a nasal bulb to clear congestion and use vaporization.
- Ensure fluid intake, which is necessary to prevent dehydration.
- Be aware that preventing infection is difficult but necessary. When possible, keep children away from other infected people and encourage family members to wash their hands frequently.

Tonsillitis

Tonsillitis is inflammation of the tonsils and often occurs with pharyngitis. In young children, the tonsils commonly are enlarged and become smaller as the child ages. The infection can be caused by bacteria or viruses.

Clinical Manifestations

The symptoms are caused by inflammation and include the following:
- The child may have difficulty eating and swallowing because of swelling and pain. If the tonsils are very large, there can be breathing issues due to airway obstruction.
- The child's breath can have an odour, and he or she may have decreased ability to smell and taste.
- Frequent sore throats and ear infections can occur.
- There may be a muffled and nasal tone of speech if the adenoids are enlarged.
- Throat cultures may show streptococcal organisms; if so, the child needs to be treated with an antibiotic.
- Non-bacterial tonsillitis is mild and self-limiting. It is characterized by a gradual onset, low-grade fever, mild headache, sore throat, hoarseness, and a cough.
- Bacterial tonsillitis is marked by the rapid onset of high fever, headache, generalized muscle aches, and vomiting.

Nursing Considerations

- Tonsillectomy is not recommended unless there are recurrent, frequent streptococcal infections or a history of peritonsillar abscess (Hockenberry & Wilson, 2015).
- Treatment is focused on symptom relief: Antibiotics are used if it is a bacterial infection, analgesics–antipyretics such as acetaminophen (Tylenol) or an opioid combination (Tylenol with codeine), salt–water throat gargles for older children, lozenges or hard candy, fluids or soft foods, and rest.

  If surgery is required:
- Preoperatively—Prepare the child and family for hospitalization and surgery as with any procedure, with the teaching adapted to the child's developmental level. Explain that the child will have a sore throat after surgery but will be able to talk and swallow normally.
- Postoperatively—Observe for unusual bleeding; monitor vital signs; assess child's colour; be alert for restlessness, which can indicate hemorrhaging; help prevent bleeding by discouraging the child from coughing, clearing the throat, and blowing the nose; until the child is fully alert after the anaesthetic, position him or her on the side or the abdomen to facilitate drainage from the throat.

  Clear fluids that are not red in colour, which could disguise bleeding, and that are cool or iced should be given first; milk products should not be used because they tend to coat the throat and cause throat-clearing; analgesics should be given on a regular basis (Hockenberry & Wilson, 2015).

  Postoperative teaching:
- Avoid gargling and vigorous tooth-brushing.
- Avoid persons with infections.
- Provide a soft diet that does not include acidic, spicy, or other irritating foods.
- Avoid coughing and clearing the throat and do not use straws.

- Monitor for bleeding, especially immediately postoperatively and 5–10 days postoperatively, when tissue sloughing occurs. Return to hospital immediately if bleeding occurs.
- Limit activity to decrease the risk of bleeding, including when the child returns to school.

Pneumonia

Pneumonia's main feature is an acute inflammation of the bronchioles, alveolar ducts and sacs, and alveoli that impairs gas exchange.

Pneumonia is classified according to the etiological agent and the location and extent of pulmonary involvement:

- Lobar pneumonia involves a large segment of one or more lobes; when both lungs are affected, it is called *bilateral pneumonia.*
- Bronchopneumonia begins in the terminal bronchioles, which become clogged with mucopurulent exudates, and then consolidates in patches in the nearby lobules.
- Interstitial pneumonia is an inflammation confined to the alveolar walls and peribronchial and interlobular tissues (Hockenberry & Wilson, 2015).

Pathophysiology

Pneumonia most commonly results from infection from viruses, bacteria, mycoplasma, or fungi.

- In children less than 5 years old, viral pneumonia is the most common type, including RSV, adenovirus, rhinovirus, influenza, parainfluenza, and enterovirus.
- Bacterial pneumonia in the newborn is commonly caused by group B *Streptococcus* and *Chlamydia trachomatis.*
- In children over 5, bacterial pneumonia is most common and is most often caused by *Staphylococcus aureus* and *S. pneumoniae.*
- In school-aged children, *Mycoplasma pneumoniae* is a common cause of pneumonia.
- *H. influenza* type b and *S. pneumoniae* decreased as causative agents as a result of current immunizations against these agents (Ball et al., 2014).
- Pneumonia typically begins with a mild upper respiratory tract infection. As the disorder progresses, lung inflammation occurs.
- Bacterial pneumonia flows through the bloodstream to the lungs, usually causing inflammation and edema with cellular debris and mucus, in turn leading to airway obstruction and consolidation within one lung.
- Viral pneumonia agents enter the lung through the upper respiratory system into the alveoli near the bronchi and spread to nearby lung tissue in a patch pattern. Infants' small airways make them vulnerable to atelectasis and edema.
- Aspiration pneumonia can be caused by a child aspirating formula or vomitus or experiencing gastric reflux and can cause chemical injury and an inflammatory response that leads to pneumonia as a secondary infection.

Clinical Manifestations

Manifestations vary, depending on the causative agent. Common signs and symptoms in viral pneumonia include the following:

- Variations ranging from mild fever, slight cough, and malaise to high fever, severe cough, and prostration
- Non-productive or productive cough with whitish sputum
- Wheezing or fine rales

Common signs and symptoms in bacterial pneumonia include the following:

- High fever
- Unproductive to productive cough with whitish sputum, tachypnea, wheezing, rales, dullness on percussion, chest pain, retractions, nasal flaring, pallor or cyanosis (depending on severity)
- Irritability, restlessness, lethargy
- Nausea, vomiting, anorexia, diarrhea, and abdominal pain (Hockenberry & Wilson, 2015)

Diagnostics

- Chest X-ray studies may show diffuse or patchy infiltrates, consolidation, disseminated infiltration, or patchy clouding, depending on the type of pneumonia.
- Blood tests may reveal an elevated WBC count.
- A causative agent may be grown in blood culture or Gram stain and culture of sputum.

Nursing Considerations

Administer medication as prescribed.

- Viral pneumonia: Treatment is usually supportive, with fever and pain control, although antibiotic therapy may be recommended to reduce the risk of a secondary bacterial infection.
- Bacterial pneumonia: Antibiotic therapy is indicated; oral amoxicillin (Amoxil) or a second-generation cephalosporin such as cefuroxime (Kefurox) should be given if the child is not completely immunized for *H. influenzae.* Erythromycin (Novo-Rythro) is given to older children and adolescents until *M. pneumoniae* has been diagnosed. If the child is hospitalized:
- Be aware that humidified oxygen, chest physiotherapy, and deep breathing, as well as incentive spirometry may be helpful.
- Assess for respiratory distress by monitoring respiratory status and vital signs.
- Change the child's position frequently and elevate the head of the bed.
- Monitor fluid balance and encourage oral fluid intake to ensure hydration.
- Promote rest by maintaining bed rest and organizing nursing care to minimize disturbances.
- Provide client and family teaching.
- Discuss home care and follow-up measures.

Atypical Pneumonia

Some children have an atypical type of pneumonia that is caused by *M. pneumoniae.* It occurs commonly in the school-aged child who is living in crowded conditions.

A serious new form of atypical pneumonia appeared in Asia in 2003, called *severe acute respiratory syndrome* (SARS). SARS is caused by a previously unrecognized coronavirus called *SARS-CoV.* Although rare in Canada, persons who are

in contact with clients with SARS, or who have travelled in areas where SARS is present, are at risk of being infected. Strict isolation with a fitted respiratory mask is required. The clinical manifestations include the following:
- Fever higher than 38°C
- Headache
- Cough, shortness of breath, difficulty breathing
- A dry, non-productive cough after 2–7 days
- In the young child, milder symptoms and a runny nose and cough
- In the adolescent group, malaise, myalgia, chills, and rigour (Denison, 2005)

Some individuals may require ventilation. Treatment is mostly supportive, with no clear improvement from using steroids, antibiotics, or antivirals (Hockenberry & Wilson, 2015).

Asthma

Asthma is a chronic inflammatory respiratory disease that causes difficulty breathing following exposure to certain triggers. A trigger is anything that causes inflammation in the airways and is specific to the individual. Inflammatory triggers include dust mites, animals, cockroaches, moulds, pollens, viral infections, and certain air pollutants. Symptom triggers, which do not cause inflammation but instead provoke "twitchy" airways, include smoke, exercise, cold air, strong smells such as perfumes, food additives such as sulphites, air pollutants, moulds and mildew, dust, and intense emotions. Because it is a chronic condition, asthma must be monitored and controlled over a lifetime. Asthma is one of the leading causes of pediatric admissions to hospital in Canada (Canadian Institute for Health Information, 2018).

Pathophysiology

In response to triggers, the following changes occur in the airways:
- Bronchoconstriction, which is tightening and narrowing of the circular muscles in the airway
- Edema of the airways as an inflammatory response
- Mucus production, which is also part of the inflammatory response to triggers

The result is a narrowing of the airways primarily on expiration, causing restricted airflow and subsequent respiratory distress.

Clinical Manifestations

Children typically present with signs of asthma between the ages of 3 and 8. In younger children, an attack usually follows a respiratory infection. Symptoms typically occur at night or in the early morning. Asthma can vary in symptoms from mild or moderate to severe and can vary from person to person. The clinical manifestations are as follows:
- Wheezing on expiration is a classic sign.
- Suprasternal and substernal retractions
- Shortness of breath, dyspnea, increased respiratory rate
- Tightness in the chest
- Coughing that may be dry, non-productive, or productive and that commonly occurs at night

- Diaphoresis, worried look, anxiety, pale skin
- Hunched shoulders, tripod position, refusal to lie down
- In more severe attacks, difficulty speaking, behavioural signs of hypoxia
- "Silent chest," an ominous sign of impending respiratory arrest

Diagnosis is typically determined on the basis of clinical manifestations, history, and physical examination. Generally, chronic cough in the absence of infection or diffuse wheezing during expiration is sufficient enough for a diagnosis.

Diagnostics

Peak flow measurements and spirometry test lung volumes and expiratory capacities. Pulmonary function tests are more comprehensive tests to determine airway parameters.

Therapeutics

- Controller medicines (usually inhaled steroids) stabilize the airways and decrease the inflammatory response. They are maintenance therapy and are of no use during an acute attack.
- Reliever medicines (usually inhaled bronchodilators) open the airways during attacks and are used prior to steroid inhalations to provide maximum airway dilation.
- Allergy desensitization has proven to be of little value.

Nursing Considerations

- Be aware that asthma can best be managed if an asthma plan is in effect. This plan is best formulated with the input of the health care team and family. The focus is on avoidance of triggers, appropriate and timely medication therapy, proper use of inhalers, avoidance of upper respiratory infections, symptom monitoring, involvement of the child and the family, and maintenance of a normal lifestyle.
- Ensure the proper use of inhalers as this is a frequent cause of poorly managed asthma. Use appropriate devices, such as a spacer, to improve medication delivery. Allow several minutes between bronchodilator inhalations.
- Know that the child may benefit from using the bronchodilator prior to exercise or in cold weather.
- Advise the child to rinse the mouth following steroid inhalation.
- Teach parents when to bring the child to hospital for emergency care.
  In hospital:
- Observe the chest, including size, shape, symmetry, and movement.
- Perform lung auscultation to assess for adventitious breath sounds.
- Take vital signs.
- Administer inhaled bronchodilator via a mask with compressed air or oxygen. Monitor the response to the inhalation.
- Maintain the child on clear and increased fluids.
- Know that extreme shortness of breath or the absence of breath sounds accompanied by a sudden rise in respiratory

rate is an ominous sign indicating respiratory failure and imminent asphyxia.

- Provide support and reassurance: An asthma attack is very frightening for both the child and the parent.

Respiratory Syncytial Virus (RSV) and Bronchiolitis

RSV is the most common respiratory pathogen for bronchiolitis and pneumonia among infants and children under 2 years of age. Approximately 80% of infants are infected with RSV during their first year of life, and virtually all children will have been infected by the age of 2 years (Hockenberry & Wilson, 2015). In many cases, RSV will cause symptoms similar to a cold; however, serious infection in the lungs can occur in premature infants, babies with chronic lung disease or congenital heart disease, or those infants who are immuno-compromised. The infection rate rises in the late fall, peaks midwinter, and decreases in frequency in the spring in countries with temperate climates, such as Canada. This highly contagious pathogen is typically spread from hand to eye, nose, or other mucous membranes. The virus will live on surfaces such as clothing, toys, countertops, and facial tissues for hours.

Pathophysiology

RSV affects the epithelial cells of the respiratory tract, causing obstruction due to accumulated debris from infected cells, mucus, and exudate. This leads to small airway obstruction, air trapping, poor gas exchange, increased work of breathing, and a characteristic expiratory wheeze.

Clinical Manifestations

The signs and symptoms of RSV vary, depending on the age and condition of the child and the severity of the infection. Peak incidence of RSV bronchiolitis is 2–5 months. The infection progresses as follows:

- Early—Runny nose, sneezing, pharyngitis, coughing, wheezing, and crackles; there may be intermittent fever
- As illness progresses—Increased coughing and sneezing, shortness of breath, tachypnea and accessory muscle use, and cyanosis
- In severe illness—Tachypnea at more than 70 breaths per minute, listlessness, poor air exchange, significantly decreased breath sounds, and apneic spells, which may rapidly progress to respiratory failure
  Symptoms will appear 3–5 days after exposure and will last approximately 12 days.

Diagnostics

Positive diagnosis of RSV is based on the initial upper respiratory infection symptoms, the time of year (late fall to early spring), history of exposure, chest X-ray to rule out other respiratory conditions, and a nasal swab culture.

Therapeutics

RSV infections are treated symptomatically with high humidity, adequate fluids, and caloric intake and rest. Most children can be managed at home. Hospitalization is required for those with advanced symptoms of the illness or an underlying respiratory or cardiac disease. RSV immune globulin, or, less frequently, RSV monoclonal antibody, may be administered prophylactically for high-risk infants. Bronchodilators and steroids can be used but are controversial in terms of effectiveness (Hockenberry & Wilson, 2015).

Nursing Considerations

- Monitor for respiratory distress, noting respiratory rate and rhythm, breath sounds, and adventitious sounds, especially wheezing.
- Assess skin colour and hydration status.
- Take appropriate isolation precautions.
- Administer prescribed medications.
- Ensure high humidity with oxygen as prescribed; increase fluids to maintain adequate hydration, offering small amounts frequently to prevent aspiration.
- Know that the child may need IV fluids if tachypnea creates a potential for aspiration.
- Maintain proper positioning to promote increased air exchange, usually high Fowler's.
- Provide support for parents.
  Treatment with ribavirin:
- Note that use of this medication is controversial as it may cause toxic effects in health care workers who inhale the aerosol, and the effectiveness in children has not been definitely proved.
- Ribavarin (Virazole) may be used for high-risk children, such as premature or very young infants, and infants at increased risk for progressing from mild to severe disease.

Laryngotracheobronchitis

Laryngotracheobronchitis (LTB), or croup, is an inflammation and narrowing of the laryngeal and tracheal areas. The cause is usually viral, and the common infectious agents are RSV, influenza viruses, parainfluenza viruses, adenoviruses, and measles virus. As a result of effective immunization campaigns, the number of *H. influenzae* LTB infections has decreased. LTB also may be of bacterial origin (as in diphtheria or pertussis).

LTB affects boys more than girls, usually between the ages of 3 months and 8 years, and peaks in the winter months (Hockenberry & Wilson, 2015).

Pathophysiology

LTB usually follows an upper respiratory infection, which may spread to the larynx, trachea, and sometimes the bronchi. The elastic larynx of a young child can go into spasm and can cause a significant airway obstruction. Severe airway edema can cause airway obstruction and seriously affect air exchange.

Clinical Manifestations

In spasmodic croup with rapid onset, the child wakes at night with a barklike or seal-like cough.

- Acute LTB: gradual onset from upper respiratory tract infection, progressing to signs of respiratory distress with pallor or cyanosis

- Hoarseness, inspiratory stridor, indrawing, and possibly severe respiratory distress
- Possibly low-grade fever
- Restlessness and irritability
- Wheezing, crackles, and localized areas of diminished breath sounds

Therapeutics

Treatment is commonly humidity with cool mist via a croupette, despite the fact that it has not been shown to decrease subglottal edema.

- Racemic epinephrine, which causes vasoconstriction and decreases subglottal edema, is administered by nebulizer for children who are not improving.
- Steroids may be effective when administered orally or intramuscularly if oral steroid cannot be tolerated.

Nursing Considerations

- Assess for airway obstruction by evaluating respiratory status by colour, respiratory effort, evidence of fatigue, and vital signs.
- Know that in severe cases of LTB, intubation to manage the airway may be necessary.
- Administer oxygen and increase humidity to decrease hypoxia if oxygen saturation is below 92%.
- Administer IV or oral fluids as prescribed to ensure good fluid balance.
- Reduce the child's anxiety by maintaining a quiet environment and promoting rest and relaxation.
- Provide parental support and teaching.
- Teach home management with cool, moist air: For example, to decrease subglottal edema, measures include having the child breathe in the cool night air, taking the child to a cool basement, or having the child breathe in air from an open freezer.

Epiglottitis

Epiglottitis is an acute and severe inflammation of the epiglottis that causes a supraglottic airway obstruction. It is mainly caused by parainfluenza A and B, adenovirus, and RSV. *H. influenzae* immunizations have decreased the occurrence of that type of infection. Now it usually affects older children and is caused by viruses.

Pathophysiology

Swelling and inflammation of the soft tissue of the epiglottis cause life-threatening obstruction of the airway. Progressive obstruction results in hypoxia, hypercapnia, and acidosis, closely followed by decreased muscle tone, altered level of consciousness, and, if obstruction becomes complete, sudden death. Endotracheal intubation or tracheostomy usually is considered. IV antibiotics are initiated, and steroids may be used for edema.

Clinical Manifestations

- Sudden onset of fever, sore throat, dyspnea, and lethargy
- Restlessness and anxiety due to respiratory obstruction

- Hyperextension of the neck, drooling, severe sore throat with refusal to drink
- Stridor, hoarseness
- Rapid, thready pulse
- Adoption of a characteristic "tripod" position by the child: sitting upright, leaning forward with chin thrust out, mouth open, and tongue protruding
- Late signs of hypoxia: listlessness, cyanosis, bradycardia, decreased respiratory rate with decreased aeration
- A red and inflamed throat with a large, red, edematous epiglottis (Hockenberry & Wilson, 2015).

Diagnostics

- Lateral neck X-ray shows epiglottal enlargement.
- Elevated WBC count and increased bands and neutrophils may be seen on the differential count.
- Causative bacteria may be identified by blood cultures (Hockenberry & Wilson, 2015).

Nursing Considerations

If epiglottitis is suspected, throat examination should be by a specially trained person. Ensure that intubation and tracheostomy equipment is nearby, as the throat examination may cause laryngospasm and precipitate a complete airway obstruction. Provide care as for other respiratory conditions.

Cystic Fibrosis

Cystic fibrosis (CF) is a chronic autosomal recessive hereditary disorder that affects the pancreas, respiratory system, GI tract, salivary glands, and reproductive tract. The majority of clients with CF (95%) are people of European descent.

The gene responsible for CF was identified in 1989 on chromosome 7. Advancements in treatments with gene and protein therapy, in addition to aggressive chest physiotherapy, inhalation therapy with antibiotics, and nutritional support, have improved the prognosis. In Canada, people with CF live until they are about 50 years old, which is 20 years longer than they did in 1990 (Canadian Institutes of Health Research, 2016).

Pathophysiology

The underlying defect is in the *CFTR* gene, causing impaired chloride movement and abnormally viscous and thick mucus that obstructs bronchioles and ducts in the pancreas and other exocrine glands, creating multisystem problems. The child with CF has an increase in sodium and chloride in the saliva and sweat.

In the lungs, ciliary movement is slower and the thickened secretions accumulate, creating obstruction, air trapping, and infection. Respiratory infections recur and cause bronchiectasis and fibrotic scarring. The pancreas becomes obstructed and significantly decreases production of the digestive enzymes, leading to major malabsorption of proteins and fats. The small intestine can become obstructed.

Clinical Manifestations

Manifestations vary with severity and time of emergence; they may appear at birth or take years to develop. Children with CF often taste salty because of the high salt content of their sweat.

Respiratory signs and symptoms:

- Wheezing, dyspnea, cough, cyanosis
- Respiratory infections that are usually caused by staphylococci, *Pseudomonas aeruginosa,* and, eventually, as the disease progresses, *Burkholderia cepacia*; the child can develop resistance to antibiotics
- Chronic sinusitis, bronchitis, bronchopneumonia, or ear, nose, and throat problems

As CF progresses, atelectasis and generalized obstructive emphysema result from mucus blockage in the small airways, producing a barrel-shaped chest and finger clubbing.

Gastro-intestinal signs:

- Meconium ileus at birth; rectal prolapse (common); loose, bulky, frothy, fatty stools; large appetite; weight loss; marked tissue wasting; failure to thrive; distended abdomen; thin extremities; evidence of vitamin A, D, E, and K deficiencies

Reproductive signs:

- Females—Decreased fertility apparently from increased viscosity of cervical mucus, which blocks the entry of sperm
- Males—Sterility in 95%, which may be caused by blockage of the vas deferens with abnormal secretions or failure of the vas deferens tubes to develop

Cardiovascular signs:

- Cor pulmonale, right-sided heart enlargement, and heart failure resulting from obstruction of pulmonary blood flow (Hockenberry & Wilson, 2015)

Diagnostics

- Elevated chloride levels on the sweat test (iontophoresis with pilocarpine); chloride level is >60 mmol/L
- Absence of pancreatic enzyme activity
- Steatorrhea detected in stool analysis
- Generalized obstructive emphysema on chest X-ray
- Fetal diagnosis in utero (Ball et al., 2014)

Therapeutics

The child with CF receives aggressive treatments for respiratory infections from oral, inhaled, and IV antibiotics. Aminoglycosides, such as tobramycin and gentamicin, and cephalosporins are often used. Sputum cultures are required because clients with CF become colonized with *P. aeruginosa* and then the more antibiotic-resistant strain of *B. cepacia*, and antibiotics must match the sensitivity of the organisms. Clients with CF who are colonized with *B. cepacia* have a poorer prognosis. Inhaled bronchodilators, which may include inhaled tobramycin, are used before daily chest physiotherapy sessions with postural drainage. Huff breathing techniques, positive expiratory pressure, use of a spirometer flutter valve, and high-frequency chest wall oscillation all help clear mucus and prevent infection. DNAse can also be given by nebulizer to help thin respiratory secretions. Exercise also helps clear the mucus.

Replacement pancreatic enzymes in the form of one to five capsules are given with meals to help improve digestion of food. Fat-soluble vitamins are needed because of the difficulty of digesting fat. Esophageal reflux is common and is treated as usual.

Breast milk or hydrolysate formula can be given. Lactulose may prevent early distal intestinal obstructions and prevent recurrence; abdominal obstructions are treated with propylene glycol electrolyte solution (Golytely). Constipation, which can contribute to obstruction, is treated as usual. A high-calorie, high-protein, and high-fat diet is important to prevent malnutrition (Ball et al., 2014).

Nursing Considerations

- Perform pulmonary mucus clearance to help increase sputum clearance, such as chest physiotherapy, postural drainage, inhalation treatments with bronchodilators, and breathing exercises.
- Monitor respiratory status.
- Encourage good nutrition with meals high in fat and protein. Increasing salt intake is important when the child experiences increased salt losses through the skin, as when he or she is in a hot environment or has a fever.
- Assess nutritional status by doing calorie counts, monitoring intake and output, and recording daily weights.
- Administer medications as prescribed, pancreatic enzymes with food, fat-soluble vitamins (A, D, E, and K), bronchodilators, and antibiotics when prescribed for infections.
- Promote growth and development by providing activities that enhance developmental stages.
- Monitor for signs of infection; prevent infection by promoting good health and hygiene practices, as well as by avoiding exposure to people with infections.
- Encourage adequate rest by organizing nursing activities around rest periods.
- Help the child maintain a positive self-concept by active listening, encouraging verbalization, and identifying strengths and coping strategies.
- Foster communication and allow the family and child to express their feelings about the chronic nature of the disorder and its long-term implications, the potential need for a lung transplant, and death and dying.
- Provide client and family teaching regarding pulmonary care, dietary instructions, medication dosage, administration and side effects, infection prevention, and the need for routine follow-up (Hockenberry & Wilson, 2015).

GASTRO-INTESTINAL SYSTEM DISORDERS

The GI system has numerous important functions. The major purposes are to break down and digest foods so that the nutrients may be absorbed through the digestive tract and waste products may be eliminated.

During fetal development, the GI system begins to form during the fourth week of the embryonic stage, starting with the mouth and anal tube. The GI tract becomes more mature in the last few weeks of development. If there is any interruption in normal fetal growth, then malformations can occur anywhere along the GI tract. Congenital anomalies of the GI tract can be present at birth or shortly after birth.

Obesity
Pathophysiology

Increasingly, obesity is becoming a health concern in Canada and around the world. As childhood obesity rates rise, so do unusual childhood complications such as type 2 diabetes. There is widespread concern that children with obesity will have significant health issues as adults as a direct result of their condition. Childhood obesity is a predictor of adult obesity; therefore, prevention is the best intervention.

There are many reasons for increasing obesity rates, including the following:
- Parental overweight
- Overweight at birth
- Physical inactivity
- Irregular snacking
- Poor food choices
- Lack of availability of a variety of nutritious foods (Health Canada, 2012a)
  Complications of obesity include the following:
- Decreased levels of growth hormone prolactin in girls and testosterone in boys
- Increased rates of amenorrhea and dysfunctional uterine bleeding in girls
- Dyslipidemia and hypertension
- Choledocholithiasis
- Slipped capital femoral epiphyses, Legg–Calvé–Perthes disease
- Obstructive sleep apnea and Pickwickian syndrome (increased daytime sleepiness and hypoventilation)
- Increased respiratory illness in toddlers under 2
- Psychosocial disturbances, such as low self-esteem, abnormal body image, difficulty developing peer relationships, social withdrawal, and isolation
- Adult obesity

Diagnostics

Tests include random blood glucose, thyroid-stimulating hormone (TSH) and thyroxine (T_4) levels (if short in stature), and urinalysis for glucose and lipid profile. In addition, in adolescent girls with amenorrhea or dysfunctional uterine bleeding, pelvic ultrasonography should be performed to rule out polycystic ovaries.

Therapeutics and Nursing Considerations

Goals of the treatment are family centred and are designed to modify behaviour so that more energy is used by the child for growth, activity, and metabolic processes than is consumed. Practical nurses play an important role in planning, teaching, and monitoring the child's progress.

Considerations include the following:
- Decreased caloric intake and making healthier choices using *Eating Well with Canada's Food Guide* (Health Canada, 2011).
- Increased exercise over time
- Decreased sedentary activities, such as watching television and playing video games
- Employing a population-based approach to prevent childhood obesity (Health Canada, 2012a)

Follow-up visits are necessary to monitor height and weight.

Cleft Lip and Palate Conditions

The most common craniofacial malformation is cleft lip (CL), with or without a cleft palate (CP). It occurs in approximately one in 700 live births (Hockenberry & Wilson, 2015). CL with or without CP occurs more commonly in males, and CP alone occurs more in females. There is an increased occurrence in relatives and in monozygotic twins.

Pathophysiology

CL occurs in the upper lip when the tissue does not completely close during the sixth week of fetal development. CL can occur unilaterally or bilaterally, with varying degrees of depth. CP occurs when the embryonic palate plates do not completely close at about the seventh and twelfth weeks of gestation. CL and CP conditions can occur separately, or both malformations may be present in a newborn.

See Fig. 10.2 for variations in clefts of the lip and palate at birth.

Clinical Manifestations

The defects are present at birth. Other investigations need to be done to rule out other midline birth malformations.

Diagnostics

There are no specific tests to be performed.

Therapeutics

The treatment for CP and CL is surgical intervention.
- Early surgical correction of CL within 1 month permits a more normal sucking pattern and increases parental bonding. It also promotes a more normal speech pattern.
- For larger clefts, surgery for scar revision may be needed in the future.
- An extensive treatment plan developed by a multidisciplinary palate team is required for CP.
- The timing of surgical repair of the palate is controversial; it can be done in the neonate but is usually done at 12–15 months, before the incompletely fused palate can cause a speech impediment. A posterior pharyngeal flap is performed, and a bone graft may be done later to build up the palate density.
- The child with CP will have corrections performed in stages and usually requires speech therapy as well as orthodontics and prosthodontics to correct misaligned, missing, or malformed teeth.
- An obturator is a temporary appliance that blocks the defect in the palate until surgery is done, but it is controversial and may not be used.

Fig. 10.2 Variations in clefts of lip and palate at birth. **A,** Notch in vermillion border. **B,** Unilateral cleft lip and cleft palate. **C,** Bilateral cleft lip and cleft palate. **D,** Cleft palate. (From Hockenberry, M. J., & Wilson, D. [2015]. *Wong's nursing care of infants and children* [10th ed., p. 429, Figure 11-16]. St. Louis: Elsevier/ Mosby.)

- Ineffective eustachian tube function creates impaired drainage of the middle ear, with the result that recurrent bouts of OM can occur. Bilateral myringotomies may be required.
- There is the potential for damage to the child's self-image, particularly related to a speech impairment.
- Delayed development has also been observed.

Nursing Considerations

Nursing care involves facilitating feeding, providing emotional support, preoperative and postoperative care, and assisting parents through the health care system.

Feeding implications
- Know that openings in the palate make it difficult for the infant to suck. It is challenging for the child with CP to get enough pressure to adequately squeeze the nipple in the bottle or the areola of the breast.
- Be aware that CL and CP babies may be more successful at breastfeeding than at using adaptive enlarged nipples, soft bottles, or syringes.
- During feeding, there is a risk of aspiration, so hold infants more upright and direct the milk away from the cleft, toward the side of the mouth.
- Ensure adequate nutritional intake by monitoring height and weight gain.
- Feed slowly and burp frequently to prevent excessive air swallowing and regurgitation.

Psychosocial implications
- Encourage the family to express feelings and concerns to facilitate acceptance and bonding.
- Model acceptance of the child and the condition to the family members.
- Reassure parents that surgery usually is successful.
- Show the parents pictures of successful surgical repairs and refer them to a support group.

Postoperative care
- Assess airway clearance and vital signs to monitor for edema and respiratory distress.
- Place an infant with CL in a baby seat or on one side to avoid contact with the surgical site. Position a child with CP prone to facilitate drainage.
- Clean the suture line and apply prescribed antibacterial ointment for CL to prevent infection and help prevent scarring.
- Apply elbow restraints to prevent rubbing of the suture line. Remove restraints every 2 hours to provide ROM exercises and give skin care.
- Feed the infant with adaptive devices such as droppers with a rubber tip, bulb syringes, Breck feeders, or soft bottle nipples, to help decrease pressure on the suture line.
- For older children, do not provide straws or sharp objects and try to keep them from rubbing the suture line with their tongue.

- Administer analgesics as prescribed to provide pain control.
- Check temperatures of warm liquids to prevent burns; the child with a new palate may lack nerve endings and sensation in the area.
- Provide mouth care to prevent the mucous membranes from drying out due to the child tending to mouth-breathe.

Family teaching requirements include care of the surgical wound; feeding strategies and positioning; prosthetic care if utilized; long-term follow-up with the multidisciplinary team services; referral to community services; and a genetic counselling referral, if requested.

Gastroesophageal Reflux and Gastroesophageal Reflux Disease

Gastroesophageal reflux (GER) occurs when stomach contents flow back up the esophagus due to an incompetent or relaxed cardiac sphincter. Gastroesophageal reflux disease (GERD) is reflux into the esophagus or oropharynx, causing symptoms. Approximately 1 in 300 to 1 in 1 000 children has GERD (Hockenberry & Wilson, 2015). It usually does not require surgery unless it causes significant complications and continues into late infancy. This is the most common esophageal disorder in the infant age group. GER is often associated with other pediatric disorders, such as tracheoesophageal fistulas or esophageal atresia, neurological disorders, scoliosis, asthma, or cystic fibrosis.

Pathophysiology

The cause of GER is not known but may be related to immature lower esophageal neuromuscular function or hormonal control system.

- Cardiac sphincter incompetence allows reflux of stomach contents into the esophagus.
- Delayed gastric emptying may also be a cause of the reflux.
- Repeated episodes of reflux may harm the mucosal lining of the esophagus.
- Small amounts of reflux are considered normal in all age groups.
- Long-term problems with GER can cause esophageal strictures from a scarred esophagus and recurrent respiratory problems due to aspiration.
- Usually, infants improve by 12–28 months of age and respond to conservative treatment.

Clinical Manifestations

The most common sign in infants is passive regurgitation or vomiting; occasionally, hematemesis is seen. Other manifestations include the following:

- Weight loss and poor growth
- Aspiration and frequent respiratory infections
- "Blue spells" or apnea
- Esophagitis and bleeding due to gastric acid irritating the esophageal lining
- Melena stools
- Heartburn and abdominal pain

Diagnostics

- A history of vomiting and a health assessment examination can confirm the presence of GER.
- Barium swallow and upper GI radiology demonstrate reflux.
- An esophageal pH probe can measure the level of acidity, the timing of acid clearance, and the reflux amount. It can determine the impact of feedings and positioning.
- Intraesophageal pH monitoring measures reflux gastric acid from the stomach.
- Scintigraphy can detect delayed gastric emptying (Hockenberry & Wilson, 2015).

Therapeutics

Most infants are treated conservatively until the reflux disappears. Small, frequent feedings of thickened rice cereal using enlarged bottle nipples and frequent burping decrease the number and volume of emesis. Placing the infant in the prone position decreases reflux but is controversial due to an increased risk of SUID in infants placed in this position (Hockenberry & Wilson, 2015).

- Pharmaceutical treatments include H_2 antagonists to treat the esophagitis and proton pump inhibitors to suppress gastric acid; as well, prokinetics are often prescribed to promote esophageal peristalsis and increase gastric emptying, but they are of limited value. Antacids are not generally recommended for children due to the aluminum content of the formulations, possible neurotoxicity, and lack of research.
- Surgery is performed on children who have not responded to conservative measures or when there are contributing anatomical anomalies.
- The most common surgical procedure is called a *Nissen fundoplication*, which creates an antireflux valve by bringing a portion of the fundus of the stomach around the esophagus. Children with delayed gastric emptying may have a pyloroplasty.
- Fundoplications can result in complications including small bowel obstruction, no relief from GER, wrap hernia, retching, gas-bloat syndrome, and dumping syndrome (Hockenberry & Wilson, 2015).
- For children who require long-term tube feeding, an alternative to a plication is the insertion of a percutaneous gastrojejunostomy.

Nursing Considerations

- Manage acute and chronic pain.
- Assess hydration and the frequency, amount, and characteristics of the vomitus.
- Assess whether positioning, postfeed handling, or the type of activity affects the vomiting.
- Provide small, frequent feedings of thickened formula and burp often.
- Be aware that although positioning the infant upright after meals has not necessarily proven to be effective, it is generally used as a method to help prevent postfeeding reflux.

Minimize handling of infants postfeeds and place children over 1 year in a left-sided position with the head of the bed elevated.

- Assess for signs of aspiration pre- and postfeeding.
- Monitor with a cardiac or apnea monitor if appropriate.
- Administer prescribed medications.
- Know that fundoplication requires routine abdominal postoperative care, including surveillance for wound infections, return of bowel motility, gagging, distension from gas, or intolerance of some foods, such as spicy meals. See Chapter 6, pages 111–113.
- Provide client and family teaching related to medications, hydration, nutrition, and feeding techniques.
- Be aware that treatment may involve temporary gastric decompression by nasogastric (NG) tube and gradual clamping of the tube until the infant tolerates the feeds.

Hypertrophic Pyloric Stenosis

Hypertrophic pyloric stenosis (HPS) occurs when a narrowed circular pyloric sphincter obstructs the flow of gastric contents into the intestine. It requires a surgical pyloromyotomy to correct the constricted valve and the obstruction. HPS is shown in Fig. 10.3.

Pathophysiology

The narrowed pyloric sphincter leads to increasing hypertrophy of the valve. The pyloric canal narrows, leading to blockage of the pyloric sphincter, obstruction, gastric distension, and forceful vomiting. The cause is unknown but may be related to local innervation problems and can be associated with other conditions, such as intestinal malrotation and esophageal and duodenal atresia. HPS occurs more commonly in first-borns, boys, and full-term infants and has a tendency to run in families.

Clinical Manifestations

- Non-bilious vomiting usually begins at about 3 weeks of age, but the timing can vary.
- Vomiting increases in frequency and strength until it is projectile.
- Vomitus may be brown tinged from blood if gastritis develops.
- The infant is hungry and irritable.
- The condition progresses to dehydration, weight loss, and failure to thrive, with upper abdominal distension.
- Gastric peristalsis and the pylorus olive-shaped mass can be visible and palpable in the epigastrium to the right of the umbilicus.

Diagnostics

- Ultrasonograms and upper GI series show slowed gastric emptying with an abnormally stretched and thinned pylorus.
- The child has metabolic acidosis with increased serum pH and bicarbonate levels.
- There are decreased levels of serum chloride, sodium, and potassium due to vomiting.

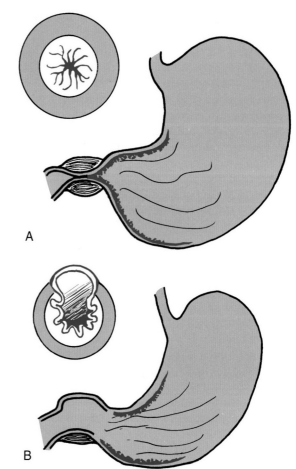

Fig. 10.3 Hypertrophic pyloric stenosis. A, Enlarged muscular tumour nearly obliterates pyloric canal. **B,** Longitudinal surgical division of muscle down to submucosa establishes adequate passageway. (From Hockenberry, M. J., & Wilson, D. [2015]. *Wong's nursing care of infants and children* [10th ed., p. 1322, Figure 33-6]. St. Louis: Elsevier/Mosby.)

- Dehydration leads to increased hemocrit, hemoglobin, and BUN levels.

Therapeutics

Rehydration and correction of electrolyte imbalance occur before surgery. A laparoscopic pyloromyotomy splits the pyloric muscle longitudinally. An NG tube may be inserted to decompress the stomach.

Nursing Considerations

- Maintain hydration and electrolyte balance by assessing for dehydration, monitoring intake and output and daily weights, evaluating urine specific gravity, and administering prescribed IV fluids of glucose and electrolytes (potassium is added to the IV fluid after voiding has occurred).
- Provide NG tube care if in situ. See Chapter 6, pages 107–108.
- Provide mouth care and a pacifier when a child is on a nothing by mouth (NPO) order.
- Start small amounts of clear fluids within 24 hours postsurgery; increase diet progressively, as tolerated, up to 48 hours postsurgery.

- Be aware that infants may be bottle- or breastfed for shorter-than-usual intervals.
- Feed slowly and burp frequently; place the child in a high Fowler's position on the right side after feeding.
- Administer analgesics as prescribed.
- Assess for wound infection as infants are more prone to wound healing problems.
- Encourage parent and family involvement in care; demonstrate feeding, positioning, and wound care.

Intussusception

Intussusception occurs when a portion of intestine invaginates, or folds into, an adjacent portion. This folding causes an obstruction that does not resolve and needs emergency medical intervention if the child is to survive.

Pathophysiology

Invagination usually begins close to or at the ileocecal valve. It can also occur in the ileum or the colon. Peristalsis pulls the invaginated section and causes edema and resulting obstruction that shuts off the flow of blood and lymph to the area. If intussusception is untreated for more than 24 hours, bowel strangulation can occur and cause ischemia, perforation, peritonitis, hemorrhage from venous engorgement, mucus buildup, and shock.

The cause of intussusception is usually not known but may be connected to viruses, intestinal polyps, lymphoma, CF, and Meckel's diverticulum. It is one of the most common causes of bowel obstruction in children under 5 years, more common in males and peak age is 3–9 months (Ball et al., 2014).

Fig. 10.4 shows the invagination of the bowel in a child with intussusception.

Clinical Manifestations

- Sudden, severe, spasmodic abdominal pain causes the child to cry and draw the legs up to the abdomen.
- As intussusception progresses, the child will vomit gastric contents and blood will appear in the stools.
- The classical presentation of a tender, distended abdomen, with a possibly palpable sausage-shaped abdominal mass and "currant jelly" stools, occurs in 20% of children.
- The child may present with a more chronic picture of diarrhea, anorexia, weight loss, occasional vomiting, and periodic pain. The older child may have only pain.
- If the obstruction is not relieved, symptoms are lethargy, "currant jelly" stool (containing blood and mucus), bile-stained or fecal emesis, and shocklike syndrome, which can progress to death (Hockenberry & Wilson, 2015).

Diagnostics

- Initially, an abdominal X-ray is done to detect intraperitoneal air, which contraindicates a barium enema.
- A barium enema detects the obstruction to the flow of barium, confirming the diagnosis.
- A rectal examination produces mucus and blood and can detect a low intussusception.

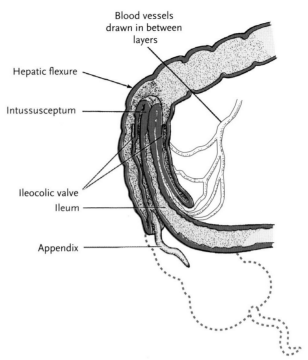

Fig. 10.4 Ileocecal valve (ileocolic) intussusception. (From Hockenberry, M. J., & Wilson, D. [2015]. *Wong's nursing care of infants and children* [10th ed., p. 1093, Figure 26-7]. St. Louis: Elsevier/Mosby.)

Therapeutics

- IV fluids, NG decompression, and antibiotic therapy may be given before the enema.
- If there are no signs of shock or perforation, the initial barium enema is frequently replaced by air pressure and water-soluble contrast to prevent barium peritonitis and to reduce the intussusception by using hydrostatic forces.
- If the enema is unsuccessful in resolving the invagination, a surgical bowel resection is required.

Nursing Considerations

- Monitor vital signs, NG drainage, and signs of bowel bleeding.
- Postsurgery, encourage clear fluid intake and increase diet as tolerated.
- Monitor for signs of infection; assess wound healing for redness, swelling, and drainage; and monitor temperature.
- Perform pain assessment and management.
- Provide parental support and discharge teaching for diet and wound care.

Appendicitis

Appendicitis is the most common condition that requires surgery in the pediatric population. The vermiform appendix becomes obstructed, leading to increased lumen pressure and bacterial infiltration with subsequent necrosis, perforation, and peritonitis.

Surgical removal of the appendix is required. Appendicitis occurs slightly more often in males and in older children, age 10–12 years. It is unusual in children under 4 years and is rare in infants less than a year. Perforation occurs more often in the younger child, possibly related to later detection.

Pathophysiology

The appendiceal lumen may become obstructed from a peritoneal skin fold, submucosal lymphoid tissue, fecaliths (hardened stool), foreign body, and parasites.

Clinical Manifestations

- The most common symptom is a spasmodic pain in the periumbilical area, which moves to the right lower quadrant near McBurney's point (located midway between the right anterior superior iliac crest and the umbilicus) with rebound tenderness.
- The pain causes difficulty with walking or when moving abdominal muscles over the inflamed area.
- Anorexia, nausea, and vomiting (common early sign but is less common in older children)
- Low-grade fever in the early stages; sharp rise with peritonitis
- Decreased or absent bowel sounds
- Constipation or small watery stools
- Irritability
- Complications, which can include perforation or peritonitis if appendicitis remains undiagnosed
  - Peritonitis leads to a sudden increase in fever, the release of and increase in pain, abdominal distension and guarding, tachycardia, and pallor, can be difficult to diagnose and can mimic other common conditions.

Diagnostics

- There is no definitive test; diagnosis is based mainly on history and physical examination.
- Blood tests mirror other common conditions.
- WBC count is elevated but is similar to counts for other types of infections.
- Urinalysis is done to rule out UTI.
- Ultrasonography and CT of the abdomen will visualize the appendix and show fluid around it.

Therapeutics

- Treatment for dehydration and electrolyte imbalance with IV therapy
- NG tube decompression if vomiting
- Preoperative antibiotics
- Appendectomy through an incision in the right lower quadrant removes the appendix.
- If perforated, abdominal lavage is done; the suture line may be left open for a drain, and a catheter may be inserted to instill antibiotics.
- Ampicillin, clindamycin (Dalacin C), metronidazole (Flagyl), or gentamicin (Garamycin) for 7–10 days if perforated, with an elective appendectomy at a later date

Nursing Considerations

- Preoperatively: Monitor hydration levels, administer prescribed IV fluid and electrolytes, assess the level of abdominal pain, perform light palpation only, and observe for signs of shock.
- Postoperatively: Maintain NPO, administer IV fluids and electrolytes, assess for abdominal distension and signs of peritonitis, listen for bowel sounds and observe for normal bowel movements, and provide pain management.
  - If a drain has been left in to prevent infection, monitor drainage, assess for wound healing and signs of infection and fever, and apply saline-soaked wet dressings.

Constipation and Encopresis

Constipation is a common condition in pediatrics. Functional constipation occurs with disruption of the normal pattern of bowel movements, a change in regularity or consistency, or in how easy it is to pass stool. This type of constipation has no underlying problem and occurs because of a brief illness, holding stool in due to a negative experience, or as a result of a diet lacking in fluid and fibre. Diet changes, enemas, and mild stool softeners usually solve the problem.

Pathophysiology and Clinical Manifestations

Constipation is diagnosed when a child has not passed a stool for more than 3 days, stool is hard and can be blood streaked, bowel movements may be painful, and stool is retained with or without soiling. All children have their own pattern of bowel movements.

Infants:
- Meconium should be passed within 24–48 hours of birth.
- Meconium plugs that have less fluid can be removed digitally or with irrigation and may be caused by lack of innervation in the bowel, hypothyroidism, meconium ileus, or obstruction resulting from CF.
  - Other causes include low-fibre intake, mild cow's milk allergy, hard stools, infection of the perianal area, some antiseizure and diuretic medications, dehydration, CF, and anal or rectal anomalies.

Toddlers and school-aged children:
- Passing painful, hard stools may cause the child to withhold stool for fear of pain. This causes further dilation of the colon and decreases the urge to defecate. Subsequently, the child avoids passing stool, creating even more constipation.
- Encopresis can occur when stool is withheld and stool leaks around the stool plug, causing incontinence and embarrassment.
- When the child enters school, there is a change in toileting patterns, such as new daily schedules and a lack of privacy in the school toilets, and children can be teased if they are incontinent.
- Constipation can be caused by physical problems such as disorders of the GI tract, neurological disorders, and decreased activity.

Diagnostics

The child needs to be assessed for any physical abnormalities or underlying psychological factors that are contributing to the constipation.

Therapeutics

- Mild constipation does not need treatment.
- Breastfed babies have fewer problems with constipation.
- Constipation usually improves when solids are introduced or fluids and fibre in the diet are increased.
- Stool softeners such as lactulose work well.
- Hard, impacted stool can be removed with suppositories, enema flushing, and occasionally propylene glycol electrolyte solution (Golytely) orally or by NG tube.
- Rectal stimulation is discouraged because it can be a negative experience and result in more constipation due to retention.
- Institute regular toileting routines for bowel retraining.

Nursing Considerations

Client and family teaching should cover diet changes to increase fibre, instituting a toileting routine, and the administration of medications, bowel irrigations, or other stool evacuation procedures.

Psychological factors need to be explored and a plan devised by the client and family.

Hirschsprung's Disease

Hirschsprung's disease, or congenital aganglionic megacolon, is a lack of colon innervation that causes poor GI motility in the region of the colon or rectum and results in obstruction and dilatation. In rare cases, a child can be treated conservatively with stool softeners and enemas, but, generally, surgery is required to remove the aganglionic portion of the intestine. A temporary colostomy is created with a later pull-through procedure to close the colostomy.

Pathophysiology

Hirschsprung's disease is the absence of autonomic parasympathetic ganglia in one or many sections of the intestine. It may involve the entire intestine. As a result, intestinal contents collect in the abnormal part of the colon. The intestine then becomes distended because of the lack of GI motility and peristalsis.

Hirschsprung's disease is a congenital condition occurring in 1 in 5 000 births and about four times as often in males than in females. It is found in children with the genetic trait and less commonly in children with trisomy, Down syndrome, GI malformations, and craniofacial defects. There may be an accompanying tight anal sphincter, which interferes with the evacuation of stool. Fig. 10.5 illustrates the dilated colon in Hirschsprung's disease.

Clinical Manifestations

Clinical manifestations vary, depending on the age of the child when diagnosed.

In neonates, symptoms are commonly as follows:
- Failure to pass meconium stools and abdominal distension in the first 48 hours
- Poor feeding and vomiting that is bile-stained
- Irritability

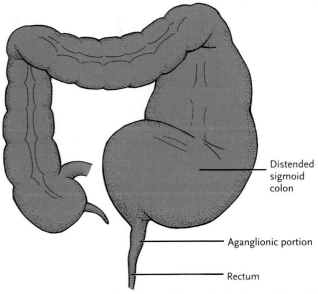

Fig. 10.5 Hirschsprung's disease. (From Hockenberry, M. J., & Wilson, D. [2011]. *Wong's nursing care of infants and children* [9th ed., p. 1305, Figure 33-5]. St. Louis: Elsevier/Mosby.)

In infants, symptoms are commonly as follows:
- Poor weight gain
- Vomiting and bowel obstruction
- Abdominal distension, ribbonlike stools, constipation, and bouts of diarrhea

In older children, symptoms are commonly as follows:
- Chronic constipation, ribbonlike, foul-smelling bowel movements, abdominal distension, palpable fecal mass, observable peristalsis, malnourishment, and anemia and hypoproteinemia

A complication of Hirschsprung's disease is enterocolitis. The symptoms include explosive, watery stools, fever, and severe prostration. This complication can be life-threatening.

Diagnostics

- Rectal examinations show a lack of stool in the rectal area with stool overflow and a tight anal sphincter.
- Barium enema shows a dilated megacolon and a narrow distal portion in children over 2 months.
- Rectal biopsy demonstrates aganglionic cells.
- Anorectal manometry measures a lack of reflex relaxation.

Therapeutics

The majority of children affected with Hirschsprung's disease need to have surgical intervention. Very few can be managed with regular enemas and a low-fibre diet.

The surgery is usually very successful and is done in two stages. The bowel is resected, the aganglionic section is removed, and an ostomy is created. When the child has gained weight, a second-stage pull-through surgery eliminates the colostomy. If the bowel is not too distended, the ostomy may not be required. Some children who have a large part of the intestine involved may need a permanent ileostomy.

Following pull-through surgery, the child may have some incontinence or require bowel retraining or anal dilatation.

Nursing Considerations

- Neonate: Observe bowel movements and prepare parents for the surgery and colostomy.
- Child: Assess bowel history and patterns and observe for clinical manifestations of Hirschsprung's disease.
- If required, provide parental teaching regarding either pharmacy-prepared or correct homemade saline enemas.
- If the child is malnourished, the surgery may be delayed and managed with small, frequent, low-fibre, high-protein, and high-calorie meals; periodic enemas; and, if severely malnourished, total parenteral nutrition.
- Observe the bowel movement patterns and stool characteristics.
- Administer stool softeners and enemas as prescribed.
- Elevate the head of the bed to decrease discomfort, change the child's position frequently, and assess for respiratory distress due to abdominal distension.
- Preoperatively, prepare the child and the family for the surgery and resulting colostomy.
  - If enterocolitis develops, emergency care is required.
  - Monitor the child's vital signs for signs of shock, check fluid balance and IV fluid and electrolyte therapy, administer blood derivatives if prescribed, and measure abdominal circumference and mark with a pen for accuracy.
  - Assess for signs of bowel perforation, such as fever, increasing pain, irritability, dyspnea, and cyanosis.
- Postoperatively:
  - Perform NG tube decompression with suction and monitor fluid balance, including NG tube losses and stool from the ostomy.
  - Keep diapers below the suture line to prevent urine contamination.
  - Assess bowel sounds and bowel movements before oral fluids and solids are given.
  - Provide pain control.
  - Monitor wound healing and provide ostomy care.
  - Provide client and family teaching on ostomy care, signs of infection, wound care, monitoring bowel patterns and stool characteristics, signs of bleeding, and referral to home care for follow-up.

Celiac Disease

Celiac disease (CD) is a gluten-sensitive enteropathy in which the child has a permanent intolerance to grain gluten and associated proteins. Exposure to gluten causes villous atrophy in the small bowel. The most serious complication can be an increased risk of developing a lymphoma, particularly in the region of the small intestine. Management of diet with restricted intake of gluten will decrease the symptoms and the lymphoma risk. In Canada, CD occurs in approximately 1:100 people (Canadian Celiac Association, 2016).

Pathophysiology

CD is a genetic immune condition that causes an inability to digest the gliadin part of gluten found in wheat, barley, rye, and oats. As a result, the amino acid glutamine accumulates and is toxic to the intestinal mucosal cells. The resulting villous atrophy leads to malabsorption of nutrients due to decreased absorptive surface area.

Clinical Manifestations

- Symptoms usually appear at the age of 1–5 years, a few months after pasta and beans become part of the solid diet.
- Poor fat absorption causes steatorrhea and very foul-smelling stools.
- Poor absorption of nutrients can cause failure to thrive, weight loss, anemia, and muscle-wasting.
- Chronic diarrhea with abdominal distension, anorexia, vomiting, irritability, and abdominal pain is common.
- A lack of vitamin K due to malabsorption can cause epistaxis, bruising, or melena.
- Celiac crisis can occur episodically with acute, severe, watery diarrhea and vomiting.

Diagnostics

- Duodenal biopsy showing villous atrophy and hyperplasia of the crypts
- Three-day fecal fat stool collection test
- Clinical improvement with removal of gluten from the diet
- Blood tests show positive for immunoglobulin A tissue transglutaminase antibody (IgA-TTG) and need to be combined with serology tests to confirm the diagnosis (Canadian Celiac Association, 2016).

Therapeutics

A gluten-free diet is necessary for life. In addition, supplemental vitamins, iron, and folate are needed until malnutrition is corrected.

Nursing Considerations

- Provide child and family teaching regarding a gluten-free diet.
- Avoid fibre until the bowel symptoms have improved.
- Be aware that when the bowel is inflamed, the child may develop lactose intolerance.
- Provide a referral to a dietitian for nutritional counselling.
- Be aware that for a celiac crisis, an NG tube is inserted for decompression, and IV fluid and electrolyte imbalances are corrected.
- Teach the family that recognition of early symptoms of celiac crisis is important.

Hernias and Hydroceles

A hernia occurs when part of the bowel protrudes through an abnormal hole in the abdominal wall. In the pediatric population, it occurs most often at the umbilicus and in the inguinal canal. Hernias can occur in association with other congenital anomalies. Inquinal hernias occur most often in males in a 5:1 ratio to girls and account for the majority of all hernias. A hydrocele occurs when abdominal fluid is trapped in the scrotal sac.

Pathophysiology

In an umbilical hernia, the umbilical ring is not completely closed and results in parts of the omentum and intestine protruding through the opening. The opening closes spontaneously by 3–5 years. Surgical intervention is needed if the opening does not close or if the herniated bowel becomes incarcerated.

Inguinal hernias occur because the processus vaginalis does not close between the abdomen and the scrotum (or uterus in females), and a section of the intestine pushes downward. Incarceration results when the lower section becomes trapped in the hernia sac and the blood supply is reduced.

Emergency surgical intervention is required when a hernia is incarcerated. A hernia that is not incarcerated may still require elective surgical intervention.

There are two types of hydrocele. At birth, a non-communicating hydrocele occurs when some peritoneal fluid is caught in the lower section of the processus vaginalis (the tunica vaginalis) with no communication with the peritoneal space. Normally, the fluid is reabsorbed and disappears in the first few months without any intervention.

A communicating hydrocele is often present with an inquinal hernia due to lack of closure of the opening in the processus vaginalis from the scrotum to the abdominal space. Surgical intervention is undertaken if the fluid is not absorbed by 1 year of age.

Clinical Manifestations

Hernias
- An umbilical hernia manifests as a soft protrusion around the umbilical region and usually can be reduced or decreased by pushing gently with a finger.
- An inguinal hernia is a painless, soft protrusion in the inguinal region that can be reduced and increases with crying, straining, coughing, or standing for long periods.
- An incarcerated hernia manifests with irritability, tenderness, anorexia, abdominal distension, and difficulty having a bowel movement. It can lead to a complete abdominal blockage, and a lack of blood flow can cause gangrene.

Hydroceles
- A non-communicating hydrocele is a soft protrusion that does not increase with activity and is easily transilluminated.
- A communicating hydrocele is an inguinal protrusion that changes in size depending on the child's position and is not reducible.

Nursing Considerations
- Teach the family to avoid ineffective and potentially harmful home remedies such as taping a hernia.
- Teach early recognition of an incarceration.

- Inform the family that hernia repair is usually done as day surgery.
- Postsurgery family teaching: Change diapers as soon as they are damp, use an occlusive dressing to protect the incision and decrease the risk of irritation and infection, assess for signs of a wound infection, and administer analgesics as needed.
- Older children should avoid strenuous activity for about 3 weeks.

CARDIAC SYSTEM DISORDERS

Review of Circulation Changes at Birth
See Fig. 10.6 for differences between prenatal and postnatal circulation.

Congenital Heart Defects
In Canada about 1 in 80 to 100 individuals are born with a congenital heart defect (CHD) (Government of Canada, 2013). In the majority of cases, the cause of the CHD is unknown. Factors associated with the increased incidence of CHD include the following:
- Fetal and maternal infections in the first 3 months of gestation, especially rubella
- Chronic maternal illnesses, such as type 1 diabetes
- Exposure to toxins such as maternal use of alcohol or drugs with teratogenic effects
- Having a sibling or parent with CHD
- Chromosomal abnormality such as Down syndrome
  CHDs are classified as *acyanotic* and *cyanotic*. These terms can be misleading because acyanotic cardiac conditions can also have cyanosis associated with the condition.

Acyanotic Cardiac Conditions
In acyanotic cardiac disorders, there is little or no reduction of blood flow to the lungs; therefore, deoxygenated venous blood does not enter the systemic arterial circulation. Defects that involve the left to right shunting of blood through an abnormal opening include patent ductus arteriosus (PDA), atrial septal defect (ASD), and ventricular septal defect (VSD). Malformations or lesions that obstruct or restrict ventricular outflow, such as aortic valvular stenosis, pulmonary stenosis, and coarctation of the aorta, are also acyanotic defects.

Pathophysiology and Clinical Manifestations

Patent ductus arteriosus defect. PDA occurs when the ductus arteriosus remains open, instead of closing, at about 3–4 days after birth. As a result, blood flows from the aorta through the PDA and back to the pulmonary artery and lungs. It usually affects premature infants but is seen in 5–10% of all cardiac anomalies and is more frequent in females.

Clinical manifestations
- Children with a small defect may be asymptomatic.
- A loud, machinelike murmur is common.
- The child may have frequent respiratory infections. The child may develop heart failure (HF) with tachypnea,

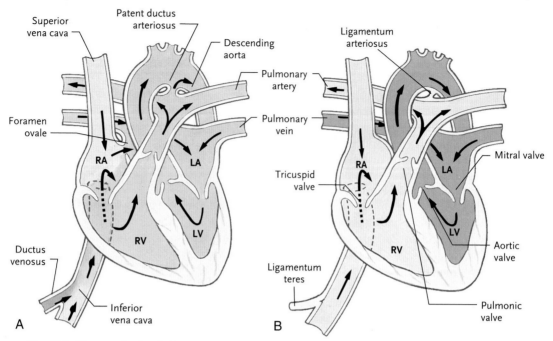

Fig. 10.6 Changes in circulation at birth. **A,** Prenatal circulation. **B,** Postnatal circulation. Arrows indicate direction of blood flow. Four pulmonary veins enter the LA; for simplicity, only two are shown here. *LA,* left atrium; *LV,* left ventricle; *RA,* right atrium; *RV,* right ventricle. (From Hockenberry, M. J., & Wilson, D. [2015]. Wong's nursing care of infants and children [10th ed., p. 1253, Figure 29-2]. St. Louis: Elsevier/Mosby.)

failure to thrive, poor feeding, hepatosplenomegaly, and irritability.

Atrial septal defect. ASD occurs when atrial septal tissue does not fuse properly during fetal development, creating an abnormal opening. The pressure of blood within the heart is normally higher in the left atrium than in the right; therefore, blood shunts from the left to the right side of the heart through the abnormal opening. The right ventricle and pulmonary artery dilate because of the increased workload of more blood.

Clinical manifestations

- Many infants are asymptomatic until early childhood; about half of ASDs close on their own through time, with 20% closing within the first year (UCSF Pediatric Cardiothoracic Surgery, 2018).
- Symptoms vary depending on the size of the ASD.
- The usual symptoms are dyspnea and fatigue on exertion.
- Slow weight gain is also a common symptom.
- The child may have frequent respiratory infections.
- A characteristic systolic murmur is usually heard at the second intercostal space.

Ventricular septal defect. VSD is an abnormal opening in the ventricular septum that can vary from very tiny to a large defect, such as a missing septum. The higher pressure in the left ventricle causes the blood to flow through the abnormal opening to the right ventricle, leading to an increase in pulmonary vascular resistance and right heart enlargement.

In all, 20–25% of total cardiac anomalies are VSDs, making it the most common defect (Cincinnati Children's Hospital, 2016).

Clinical manifestations. Manifestations vary, depending on the size of the VSD, the child's age, and the amount of resistance.

- The child is usually asymptomatic.
- The child fails to thrive.
- The child experiences excessive diaphoresis and fatigue.
- The child may have increased respiratory infections.
- The child may have signs and symptoms of HF.

Aortic valvular stenosis defect. A narrowing of the aortic valve causes an obstruction to the flow of blood from the left ventricle into the aorta. The long-term result is a left ventricular hypertrophy. Restricted and poor blood flow to the myocardium can develop because the oxygen need of the hypertrophied left ventricle is not met.

Clinical manifestations

- In infants with a severe defect, practitioners would expect to see decreased cardiac output, faint pulse, hypotension, tachycardia, and poor feeding.
- Older children may present with exercise intolerance, chest pain, and dizziness when standing for a long time.
- A characteristic systolic ejection murmur is heard at the second intercostal space.

Pulmonary stenosis. Pulmonary stenosis is a narrowing at the entrance of the pulmonary artery from the right ventricle. The obstruction to blood flow increases right ventricular pressure. Over a period of time, right ventricular hypertrophy failure may result. Pulmonary stenosis occurs in 5–8% of all cardiac lesions, and many children have other associated cardiac anomalies (UCSF Pediatric Cardiothoracic Surgery, 2018).

Clinical manifestations

- The child may be asymptomatic or have a mild cyanosis and signs of HF.
- Characteristic systolic murmur may be heard over the pulmonic area, and a thrill may be felt if stenosis is severe.
- In a child with a severe defect, there is decreased exercise tolerance, dyspnea, pain in the precordial region, and generalized cyanosis.

Coarctation of the aorta. Coarctation of the aorta (COA) is a narrowing of the aorta. The three types of COA depend on the location of the narrowing:

- Preductal—Located proximal to the insertion of the ductus arteriosus
- Postductal—Located distal to the ductus arteriosus
- Juxtaductal—Located at the insertion of the ductus arteriosus

There is an increase in pressure proximal to the defect and a decrease in pressure distal to it. The narrowed aorta restricts the blood flow, causing an increase in left ventricular pressure, dilation of the proximal aorta, left ventricular hypertrophy, and possibly failure. Over a period of time, collateral blood vessels bypass the coarcted area and supply improved blood flow to the lower part of the body.

Clinical manifestations

- The child may be asymptomatic.
- The child may have a marked difference in blood pressure and pulse quality between the upper and lower extremities. The upper extremity pulses are bounding with high blood pressure, and femoral pulses are weak or absent.
- The child may experience epistaxis, headaches, fainting, and lower leg muscle cramps.
- There is a risk of stroke, aneurysm, and ruptured aorta.
- A characteristic systolic murmur may be heard over the left anterior precordium and between the scapula posteriorly.

Diagnostics for Acyanotic Heart Defects

- Chest X-rays may show cardiac enlargement.
- Electrocardiograms (ECGs) may show an enlargement of the atria and ventricles, unclosed ductus arteriosus, size of shunts, and degrees of obstruction.
- Echocardiography can accurately detect specific cardiac conditions and may help the child avoid having to have a cardiac catheterization.
- Cardiac catheterization identifies defects and measures pressure variations.

Therapeutics

Patent ductus arteriosus defect:

- This condition is managed either conservatively or surgically and has a risk of less than a 1% mortality rate (Hockenberry & Wilson, 2015, p. 1275).
- Medical management includes administration of prostaglandin–synthetase inhibitors, such as indomethacin, to stimulate closure of the open ductus.
- In clients with uncomplicated PDAs, non-surgical management involves placing coils via cardiac catheterization to block the PDA.

- Surgical management involves ligating or dividing the PDA via a thoracotomy or clipping the PDA via video-assisted thoracoscopic surgery.
- Surgery is performed at 1–2 years old, or in infancy if HF is present.

Atrial septal defect

- This condition is managed either surgically or non-surgically, with a mortality rate of less than 1% (Hockenberry & Wilson, 2015, p. 1275).
- Non-surgical treatment includes the placement via cardiac catheterization of a septal occluder for more centred and smaller defects.
- Surgical treatment includes the placement of a pericardial or Dacron patch, which requires a cardiopulmonary bypass and is usually done before school age.

Ventricular septal defect

- This condition is managed surgically or non-surgically, with a mortality rate of less than 2% in uncomplicated VSDs (Hockenberry & Wilson, 2015, p. 1276).
- Non-surgical treatment is currently being investigated, using closure devices via cardiac catheterizations.
- Surgical treatment includes suturing small defects or placing a Dacron patch via cardiopulmonary bypass if the defect is larger.
- Palliative care, used only in children with complex cardiac anomalies, involves banding the pulmonary artery to decrease pulmonary blood flow.

Pulmonary stenosis

- This condition is managed surgically or non-surgically and has a mortality rate of less than 1%—slightly higher rate in neonates (Hockenberry & Wilson, 2015, p. 1276).
- The most common non-surgical treatment is balloon angioplasty via cardiac catheterization. The balloon catheter is inserted into the narrowed valve, and the balloon is blown up and pulled back through the valve. The procedure dilates the pulmonary valve and improves blood flow.
- Surgical treatment consists of a pulmonary valvotomy, in which the valve is reconstructed via cardiopulmonary bypass.

Coarctation of the aorta

- This condition is managed surgically or non-surgically, with a mortality rate of less than 5% (Hockenberry & Wilson, 2015, p. 1276)
- Non-surgical treatment, usually used in older children, is the balloon procedure to dilate the narrowed portion of the aorta.
- Surgical treatment is used in infants of less than 6 months and in older children with a complex cardiac defect. The narrowed part of the aorta is removed, and the ends are reconnected. The alternative is to dilate the aorta using a prosthetic graft or a graft from a subclavian artery.

Nursing Considerations

Management of hypoxia

- Assess for signs of tachypnea, cyanosis, bradycardia, tachycardia, restlessness, cyanosis, grunting, nasal flaring, cough, and syncope:

- Place the child in a knee–chest position.
- Administer oxygen as prescribed.
- Administer medication as prescribed.
- Decrease the child's oxygen needs by organizing care around periods of rest, preventing crying, and providing quiet activities for the older child.

Management of nutrition

- Be aware that good nutrition, especially an iron-rich diet, is needed in these clients for normal growth patterns and electrolyte balance and to prevent anemia and infections.
- Provide a balanced diet rich in iron (to prevent anemia) and potassium and low in sodium.
- If the child is on potassium-losing diuretics, provide a high-potassium diet and administer potassium supplements when prescribed.
- Give small, frequent meals if the child tires easily.
- Know that the duration of breast- or bottle-feedings may need to be limited, or it may be necessary to feed the child more often for shorter periods to avoid fatigue.
- Evaluate weight gain daily.

Assessing for signs of HF

- Observe for signs of bacterial endocarditis: fever, pallor, petechiae, anorexia, and fatigue.
- Antibiotics may be prescribed prior to dental work or before surgery or suturing repair.
- Observe for manifestations of thrombosis, including irritability, restlessness, seizure activity, coma, paralysis, edema, hematuria, oliguria, and anuria.
  Other nursing considerations:
- To decrease the risk of thrombosis, keep the child well hydrated.
- Institute infection control measures.
- Encourage the child's self-esteem through self-care activities.
- Encourage activities within the child's exercise tolerance.
- Provide client and family education regarding hypoxic episodes, weight gain, exercise tolerance, avoiding infections, and medication management.
- Provide referrals to home care agencies, support groups, and follow-up care.

Cyanotic Cardiac Conditions

Cyanotic cardiac conditions are heart defects in which deoxygenated blood enters the systemic arterial circulation. Cyanotic heart defects include tetralogy of Fallot, transposition of the great vessels, truncus arteriosus, and hypoplastic left heart syndrome. In each of these defects, cyanosis is caused by the right to left shunting of blood through abnormal cardiac openings, resulting in a mixing of oxygenated and deoxygenated blood. Most cyanotic conditions require complex surgery.

Pathophysiology, Clinical Manifestations, and Therapeutics

Tetralogy of Fallot. Tetralogy of Fallot is the most common cyanotic heart defect, consisting of four major abnormalities: VSD, right ventricular hypertrophy, pulmonary stenosis, and aorta overriding VSD. The combination of these defects results in the aorta receiving blood from both the right and left ventricles.

Clinical manifestations and therapeutics. Manifestations vary, depending on the size of the VSD and the degree of pulmonary stenosis.

- Some infants are cyanotic at birth; others gradually develop cyanosis over the first year, with an increase in the degree of pulmonary stenosis.
- It is common for infants to have cyanotic spells or "Tet spells," in which there is an acute cyanotic episode, especially during feeding or crying. These episodes can lead to a transient cerebral ischemia.
- After a cyanotic spell, there is a risk of emboli, seizures, and loss of consciousness.
- In older children, squatting is an adaptation that decreases the return of venous blood from the lower parts of the body, increases systemic vascular resistance, and increases pulmonary blood flow.
- The child fails to thrive.
- The child has clubbing of the fingers, exertional dyspnea, fainting, or slowness due to hypoxia.
- Characteristic pansystolic murmur is heard at the mid–lower left sternal border.
- The only treatment is surgery, either complete or palliative, if complete surgery cannot be done.
- A Blalock–Taussig shunt is inserted, which provides blood flow to the pulmonary arteries from the left or right subclavian artery via a tube graft. The shunt has the potential to distort the pulmonary artery.
- Complete repair is usually done during the first year, when there is an increasing level of cyanosis and Tet spells. A cardiopulmonary bypass and sternal entry are used. Improved techniques have reduced the surgical mortality rate to less than 3% (Hockenberry & Wilson, 2015, p. 1280).

Transposition of the great vessels. The pulmonary artery and aorta exit abnormally from the opposite ventricle. This abnormality leads to two separate circulatory patterns, in which the right heart manages systemic circulation and the left heart manages pulmonary circulation. To survive, the child must have an associated defect that allows oxygenated and deoxygenated blood to mix in the heart chambers. These infants are often referred to as "blue babies." There are many serious potential complications, including HF, endocarditis, brain abscess, and cerebrovascular accident resulting from hypoxia or thrombosis.

Clinical manifestations and therapeutics

- Varying degrees of cyanosis are seen, depending on the size of the associated defect.
- Cardiomegaly occurs within the first few weeks of birth.
- Severe cyanosis at birth
- In a child with associated defects, there is less cyanosis, but the child has HF symptoms.
- Failure to thrive
- No murmur is evident, or there is a murmur characteristic of an associated defect.

- This condition requires surgical intervention.
- Initial treatment is to provide mixing of oxygenated and deoxygenated blood.
- The administration of prostaglandin E keeps the ductus arteriosus open.
- A balloon atrial-septostomy may be performed to enlarge the ASD in order to increase the mixing of oxygenated and deoxygenated blood.
- Surgical intervention in the first few weeks of life involves performing an arterial switch, which re-establishes normal circulation, with the left ventricle acting as the systemic pump.
- The mortality rate varies, depending on the anatomy and the procedure; for neonates with intact ventricular septum, the operative mortality rate is 6% (Hockenberry et al., 2017, p. 750).
- Long-term problems include suprapulmonic stenosis and aortic dilation and regurgitation.

Truncus arteriosus. This is a defect of a single blood vessel instead of a separate pulmonary artery and aorta. Newborns with this abnormality may initially appear normal, but as pulmonary vascular resistance decreases after birth, severe pulmonary edema and HF usually develop.

Clinical manifestations and therapeutics
- Significant cyanosis, particularly when active
- Clinical manifestations of HF
- Left ventricular hypertrophy, dyspnea, significant exercise intolerance, and failure to thrive
- Characteristic loud systolic murmur best heard at lower left sternal border and radiating throughout the chest
- Treatment is performed in the first month of life.
- The condition requires a complex surgery that involves closing the VSD and forming conduits to establish continuity between the right ventricle and pulmonary artery.
- Postoperative complications include persistent HF, bleeding, pulmonary artery hypertension, dysrhythmias, and residual VSD.
- The mortality rate is higher than 10% (Hockenberry & Wilson, 2015, p. 1280).
- Conduits do not grow with the child and may require one or more replacements.

Hypoplastic left heart syndrome. Hypoplastic left heart syndrome involves a variety of abnormalities, including an underdeveloped or hypoplastic left ventricle, aortic valve, mitral valve, and ascending aorta. In order for the child to survive, the ductus arteriosus must remain open. When the ductus closes, low cardiac output leads to hypoxia and inevitable death.

Clinical manifestations and therapeutics
- This condition is usually evident by 2 weeks of age.
- Mild cyanosis and HF become more severe with closure of the ductus.
- Signs and symptoms of HF
- Single S_2 heart sound
- Characteristic soft ejection murmur is present.
- Neonates require inotropes and stabilization with mechanical ventilation.

- Prostaglandin E is administered to maintain ductal patency and ensure adequate systemic blood flow.
- Complex two-stage surgical interventions are needed for the infant to survive.
- Prognosis for the first-stage operation varies widely, but survival rates have improved over the past 10 years.
- If surgeries are unsuccessful, or if the defect is profound, heart transplantation may be the only option.

Heart Failure

HF results from an inability of the heart to produce enough cardiac output to meet the body's oxygen and metabolic needs. There is a decrease in myocardial contractility, or the cardiac output is not sufficient to meet the needs of pathological conditions that require a higher cardiac output.

Pathophysiology

HF is caused by volume or pressure overload, decreased contractility, or a need for high cardiac output. There are two types of HF, right- and left-sided. Right ventricular failure occurs when the right ventricle is unable to pump effectively, causing pooling of systemic venous circulation and edema of the extremities. Cor pulmonale is the term for HF resulting from obstructive lung diseases such as CF or bronchopulmonary dysplasia. Left ventricular failure occurs because the left ventricle is unable to pump blood effectively into the systemic circulation. This leads to lung congestion, increased pulmonary pressure, and pulmonary edema.

Causes of HF. The primary cause in the first 3 years of age is CHD. Other causes include the following:
- Cardiomyopathies, arrhythmias, and hypertension
- Pulmonary embolism or chronic lung disease
- Severe hemorrhage or anemia
- Adverse effects of an anaesthetic or surgery, transfusions or infusions, or drugs such as doxorubicin
- Increased body demands resulting from conditions such as fever or infection
- Severe physical or emotional stress
- Excessive sodium intake

Clinical Manifestations

It may be difficult to distinguish right- from left-sided ventricular failure because when one side of the heart is failing, it causes an impact on the other side.

The clinical manifestations are as follows:
- Weakness, fatigue
- Poor feeding, ascites, weight loss or weight gain from edema, and pleural effusions
- Irritability
- Pallor, cyanosis, and diaphoresis
- Dyspnea, tachypnea, orthopnea, wheezing, cough, weak cry, and grunting
- Tachycardia, cardiomegaly, and gallop rhythm
- Hepatomegaly and abdominal pain or distension
- Distended jugular, neck, and peripheral veins and edema

Diagnostics

- Chest radiology shows an enlarged heart and increased pulmonary vascular markings due to increased pulmonary blood flow.
- Blood values display dilution hyponatremia, hypochloremia, and hyperkalemia.
- Ventricular hypertrophy appears on an ECG.
- Echocardiology detects the cause of HF, such as a specific CHD.

Therapeutics

The aim of the therapeutic management program for a child with HF is to manage the HF and stabilize the condition until the underlying cause can be treated.

- Angiotensin-converting enzyme (ACE) inhibitors (such as Vasotec) reduce the afterload on the heart, making it easier for the heart to pump.
- Digoxin (Lanoxin) administered in an elixir or parenterally is the primary drug to improve myocardial contractility.
- Doses of digoxin must be exact and must be individually regulated for each client.

Nursing Considerations

- Monitor for signs of respiratory distress, suction as needed, administer oxygen as prescribed, keep the head of the bed elevated, and monitor arterial or capillary blood gas values.
- Monitor for signs of altered cardiac output, pulmonary edema, arrhythmias, including extreme tachycardia and bradycardia, and characteristic ECG and heart sound changes.
- Evaluate fluid balance by intake and output measurements, monitoring daily weights, assessing for edema and severe diaphoresis, and monitoring electrolyte and hematocrit levels, as well as maintaining fluid restrictions as prescribed.
- Prevent infections by using hand hygiene and keeping the child away from individuals with infections.
- Reduce cardiac demands by keeping the child warm, scheduling nursing interventions around rest periods, restricting infant feeding to less than 45 minutes at a time, and providing gavage feeding if the infant is fatigued or needs supplemental feeding.
- Help ensure adequate nutrition by feeding the child small, frequent, high-calorie, low-sodium meals as prescribed.
- Help decrease anxiety by providing developmentally appropriate explanations and encouraging parental involvement in the child's care as appropriate.
- Administer medications as prescribed: Digoxin is used to increase cardiac performance; diuretics such as furosemide, hydrochlorothiazide, and spironolactone to reduce venous and systemic congestion; and iron and folic acid supplements to improve nutritional status.
- Monitor for digitalis toxicity: Extreme bradycardia and increased serum levels are cardinal signs of toxicity; withhold digoxin if the child's heart rate falls below the normal range for his or her age.
- Provide referrals to follow-up community services as needed.
- Offer client and family teaching for signs and symptoms of HF, nutrition and fluid restrictions, and the dosage, administration, and side effects of prescribed medications.

HEMATOLOGICAL AND IMMUNOLOGICAL SYSTEM DISORDERS

Iron Deficiency Anemia

Iron deficiency anemia (IDA) is one of the most common nutritional disorders. IDA is most often caused by an insufficient quantity of iron in the diet, poor absorption of iron, or a significant loss of blood. Premature infants, children between the ages of 6 months and 3 years, and adolescents are most at risk. Infants fed cow's milk can develop intestinal irritation and lose blood through the stools.

Pathophysiology

- IDA is caused by an insufficient supply of iron that is required for normal red blood cell (RBC) formation.
- Lack of iron leads to smaller cells, a reduced RBC mass (microcytic), a decreased hemoglobin concentration, and decreased oxygen-carrying capacity of the blood.
- Over time, the depleted RBC mass leads to a decreased hemoglobin concentration and reduces blood capacity.

Clinical Manifestations

- The child may be asymptomatic.
- Pallor, irritability, fatigue
- Pica or eating non-food items
- Tachycardia and systolic heart murmur
- Headaches and dizziness
- Muscle weakness and delayed growth
- Developmental delay may occur.
- Nail deformities

Diagnostics

Diagnostic blood tests include the following:
- CBC: RBC is normal or slightly decreased; hemoglobin and hematocrit are low; mean corpuscular volume (MCV) is decreased (microcytic); and mean corpuscular hemoglobin (MCH) is decreased (hypochromic).
- Erythrocyte protoporphyrin (EP) is greater than 0.75 mcml/L.
- Low serum iron capacity
- Elevated total iron binding capacity

Therapeutics

- The underlying etiology should be treated, if it can be corrected.
- Adequate nutritional intake of iron is essential; boost iron intake via breast milk, iron-fortified formula, and cereal.
- Oral supplements of elemental iron should be provided to create iron stores. Ferrous iron is usually used because it is absorbed easily. Iron has side effects of nausea, GI irritation, anorexia, diarrhea, and constipation.

- Parenteral iron, administered intravenously or intramuscularly, is reserved only for children who do not respond to oral supplements and iron-rich diets as it is painful and expensive.
- Reticulocyte count is done after about 10 days to evaluate the effectiveness of the therapy.
- Blood transfusions are administered only to children with severe anemia.
- Supplemental oxygen is administered if the tissue hypoxia is severe.
- Some children have vitamin B_{12} deficiency and require intramuscular B_{12} injections.

Nursing Considerations

- Encourage sufficient intake of iron-rich foods, including iron-fortified formula and cereals, lean meat, fish, leafy dark green vegetables, beans, and whole-grain breads.
- Discourage milk as the predominant food source when the child is on solid food.
- Administer intramuscular injections of iron, using the Z-track method.
  Child and family teaching points regarding iron:
- Administer an oral iron supplement by giving it in two to three divided doses in a small amount of vitamin C–containing liquid (such as orange juice) before meals to enhance absorption and minimize side effects.
- Administer iron with a dropper to an infant or through a straw to an older child to minimize staining of the teeth.
- Brush the child's teeth after administration to minimize teeth staining.
- Be aware of the side effects of nausea and vomiting, diarrhea or constipation, and dark green or black stools.
- Ensure safety precautions, as iron is very toxic.

Sickle Cell Anemia

Sickle cell anemia (SCA) is an inherited autosomal recessive disorder and a chronic, serious, hemolytic disorder found predominantly in people of African descent. With each pregnancy, there is a 25% chance of the child having sickle cell disease when both parents carry the trait. The sickle cell trait is not usually symptomatic, unless there is an extreme or prolonged lower level of oxygen. SCA may lead to significant long-term complications. The major cause of death in children under 5 with SCA is bacterial sepsis.

Pathophysiology

Low oxygen and pH in the blood trigger hemoglobin S (HgbS) to transform RBCs into a sickle (crescent) shape. Because of the sickle shape, the cells tend to clump, creating thrombosis, blockage of arteries, thickening of the blood, early breakdown of the cell, tissue anoxia, and necrosis. Acute and eventually chronic changes occur as the sickling progresses. Sickle cell crisis may be precipitated by infection, dehydration, fever, cold exposure, hypoxia, strenuous exercise, extreme fatigue, or extreme changes in altitude.

Clinical Manifestations

- Enlarged spleen because of clogging from sickled cells
- Enlarged liver, which causes pain due to poor blood flow
- Hematuria, inability to concentrate urine, enuresis, and occasionally nephritic syndrome, bone weakness, and dactylitis (symmetrical swelling of the hands and feet)
- Pain, often severe, especially during a vaso-occlusive crisis
  Complications include the following:
- Stroke
- Myocardial infarction (MI)
- Poor growth, delayed sexual maturation, decreased fertility, priapism
- Recurrent severe infections
- Splenic sequestration: A life-threatening condition in which the spleen collects a large amount of blood, causing a severe drop in blood volume and resultant shock. Symptoms include paleness, abdominal distension, pain and irritability, low blood pressure, and increased heart rate. Treatments are transfusions and splenectomy (Hockenberry & Wilson, 2015).
  See Fig. 10.7 for the effects of sickled RBCs on circulation and potential complications.

Diagnostics

Blood tests:

- The Sickledex screening blood test can identify if HgbS is present; however, hemoglobin electrophoresis is needed to differentiate between sickle cell trait and SCA.

Therapeutics

- Treatment varies depending on the specific complications for individual children.
- Standard immunizations for pneumococcal *H. influenzae* type b and meningococcal vaccine should be given.
- Prophylactic penicillin may be prescribed for the first 5 years to prevent life-threatening sepsis.
- Hydroxyurea decreases recurrent severe painful episodes. This may reduce long-term complications and prolong survival (Sickle Cell Disease Association of Canada, n.d.).
  During vaso-occlusive crises:
- Ensuring good hydration levels by administering IV and oral fluid to increase the blood fluid volume will help prevent sickling and, potentially, blood clots.
- Electrolyte replacement is used to offset the acidosis caused by hypoxia, which can increase sickling.
- Oxygen therapy is used to offset hypoxia.
- Blood transfusions decrease the viscosity of the blood and treat anemia.
- Morphine is administered for pain control, often via PCA, which may be used in children as young as 5 years.
- Acetaminophen and codeine-containing compounds are administered for mild pain.

Nursing Considerations

- Monitor vital signs when the child is at rest and when active, particularly when there is reduced tissue perfusion.

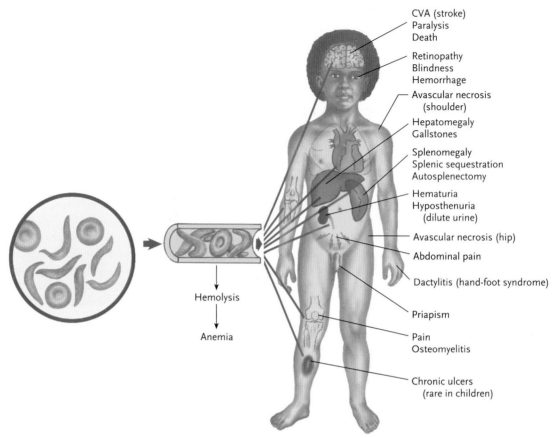

Fig. 10.7 Effects of sickled red blood cells on circulation and potential complications. *CVA,* cerebrovascular accident. (From Hockenberry, M. J., & Wilson, D. [2015]. *Wong's nursing care of infants and children* [10th ed., p. 1340, Figure 30-4]. St. Louis: Elsevier/Mosby.)

- Assess for signs of HF.
- Monitor height, weight, and developmental status; growth can be delayed in children with SCA due to profound anemia.
- Carefully assess skin colour and mucous membranes, particularly in children with darker skin tones.
- Encourage bed rest or reduced activities as necessary to conserve energy and avoid overexertion to promote tissue oxygenation. Passive exercises promote circulation and ROM.
- Help the child develop coping strategies when under emotional stress and to increase oxygen perfusion.
- Perform pain assessment and management, with a PCA pump, if possible.
- Use pain control techniques such as heat to affected areas, relaxation, and meditation, as well as placing the child in the most comfortable position.
- Administer prescribed analgesics around the clock.
- Monitor for signs of dehydration and electrolyte imbalance and ensure adequate hydration by encouraging oral fluid intake or administering IV fluids; maintain strict intake and output and daily weight records.
- Provide a nutritionally balanced diet.
- Help the child avoid known sources of infection.
- Monitor for signs of infection and administer antibiotics as prescribed.

- Provide emotional support to the child and family, particularly in relation to issues around anger, self-esteem, positive body image, and the effects of chronic pain.
- Child and family teaching: Explain the disease process, genetic aspects, and early signs and symptoms of sickling crises and discuss home management measures for a mild crisis; how to avoid factors known to precipitate crises; the recognition of early signs of infection; the importance of regular health, dental, and eye examinations; and maintaining as normal a lifestyle as possible.
  - Provide referrals for possible genetic counselling.

Thalassemia

Thalassemia is the term used to describe genetic blood disorders characterized by insufficient synthesis of specific globulin chains of the hemoglobin molecule. The most common thalassemia is beta-thalassemia. The most serious form is thalassemia major (beta-thalassemia, or Cooley's anemia) and usually is seen in children of Mediterranean descent (particularly those of Italian and Greek heritage) or Asian descent.

Pathophysiology

- In thalassemia, a problem in the production of specific globin chains (beta) in hemoglobin ultimately results in the destruction of RBCs.

- The body tries to increase the production of RBCs to cope with the RBC destruction, but these cells are immature and break down quickly. The excess iron that is released when the RBCs disintegrate is stored in different organs, causing a condition called *hemosiderosis*.

Clinical Manifestations
- Thalassemia minor usually creates mild to moderate anemia that may be asymptomatic and often goes undetected.
- Thalassemia major produces clinical manifestations around the age of 6 months, when the protective effect of the fetal hemoglobin diminishes.

The following are signs of thalassemia (Hockenberry & Wilson, 2015):
- Early signs include pallor, anemia, unexplained fever, poor feeding, poor weight gain, and an enlarged spleen or liver.
- Later signs include chronic hypoxia; headache; bone and precordium pain; decreased exercise tolerance; damage to the liver, spleen, heart, pancreas, and lymph glands from hemochromatosis, the excess storage of iron, which results in cellular damage in these organs; slight jaundice or a bronze skin colour; thick cranial bones with prominent cheeks and a flat nose; and growth delay and delayed sexual development.
- Long-term complications result from hemochromatosis, including splenomegaly, usually requiring splenectomy; skeletal complications, such as thickened cranial bones and an enlarged head; prominent facial bones, malocclusion of the teeth, and susceptibility to spontaneous fractures; cardiac complications, such as arrhythmias, pericarditis, HF, and fibrosis of cardiac muscle fibres; gallbladder disease; cirrhosis; jaundice and brown pigmentation due to iron deposits; growth delay; and endocrine complications, such as delayed sexual maturation and diabetes.

Diagnostics
- CBC shows abnormalities in hemoglobin and RBCs: decreased hemoglobin, hematocrit, and reticulocyte counts.
- Hemoglobin electrophoresis shows that HgbA and HgbF values are increased, confirming the type and severity of the hemoglobin variants.
- Increase in RBC precursors appear in bone marrow.
- Results show folic acid insufficiency.
- Prenatal screening is done through chorionic villus sampling or fetal blood cell analysis.

Therapeutics
- Supportive therapy with transfusions to maintain sufficient hemoglobin levels has the goal of preventing tissue hypoxia and promoting normal growth and development, more physical activity, decreased cardiomegaly and hepatosplenomegaly, and fewer bony changes and infections (Hockenberry & Wilson, 2015).
- Desferoxamine (Desferal), an iron chelator, is administered with transfusions to minimize hemosiderosis (excess iron in tissues).

- Home chelation therapy with desferoxamine is done 5–7 days a week via an IV infusion pump, usually during the night.
- Splenectomy may be necessary to decrease abdominal pressure from the enlarged spleen and increase the lifespan of RBCs.
- Amniocentesis sampling of fetal blood cells can diagnose thalassemia.
- Bone marrow transplantation (BMT) has been used with some success.

Nursing Considerations
- Administer blood transfusions and observe for complications of transfusions, which can lead to an overload of iron.
- Monitor for signs of iron toxicity related to blood transfusions: abdominal pain, vomiting, bloody diarrhea, decreased level of consciousness, shock, and metabolic acidosis.
- Administer chelation therapy and monitor vital signs, observing for hypotension or allergic reaction; visual acuity (ocular toxic) and hearing (ototoxic); intake and output; and colour of urine (may turn red).
- Provide information regarding splenectomy, if applicable.
- Administer folic acid as prescribed.
- Monitor for signs of infection and avoid sources of infection.
- Encourage the child to be careful with physical activities and to avoid situations of risk in order to prevent fractures.
- Promote adequate rest and good nutrition.
- Help minimize dietary iron ingestion as much as possible.
- Assess for signs and symptoms of hepatitis and iron surplus.
- Support and educate the child and family as to coping strategies and how to deal with a chronic illness and treatment protocols.
- Refer to family support groups as appropriate.
- Provide instructions for home chelation therapy (Hockenberry & Wilson, 2015).

Hemophilia

Hemophilia is a group of hereditary bleeding disorders in which there is a deficiency in a blood clotting factor. The most common types of hemophilia are factor VIII deficiency (classic hemophilia, hemophilia A) and factor IX deficiency (Christmas disease, hemophilia B). Eighty percent of hemophiliacs have factor VIII deficiency. Hemophilia is mainly an X-linked recessive disorder transmitted by females or caused by a gene mutation. The occurrence is about 1 in 5 000 males.

Pathophysiology

Hemophilia is classified as mild, moderate, or severe, depending on the degree of coagulation involved.
- In hemophilia A, there is a defect in the clotting function, although the factor VIII molecule is present.
- In hemophilia B, there is an impaired ability to form a fibrin clot caused by a defect or deficiency of factor IX (Hockenberry & Wilson, 2015).

Clinical Manifestations

Hemophilia is initially suspected in the case of a newborn with excessive bleeding from the umbilical cord or after circumcision.

The manifestations of hemophilia include the following:
- Bruising easily and prolonged bleeding from wounds
- Nosebleeds
- Spontaneous hematuria
- Hemarthrosis (hemorrhages in the joints causing pain, swelling, and decreased ROM), which can be crippling

Complications of hemophilia include the following:
- Airway obstruction, which can occur due to bleeding into the neck, mouth, or thorax
- Bone changes, osteoporosis, and muscle atrophy from hemarthrosis
- Intracranial bleeding, which is a very serious potential complication that can lead to death
- GI hemorrhage, which can lead to intestinal obstruction
- Bleeding into the spinal cord, which can result in paralysis (Hockenberry & Wilson, 2015)

Diagnostics

- The platelet count and bleeding time may be normal.
- Tests that evaluate clotting factor function, such as prothrombin time (PT), partial thromboplastin time (PTT), and whole blood clotting time, may be normal.
- Factor VII or IX level may be low.
- Prenatal diagnosis is done through amniocentesis and carrier identification.

Therapeutics

- Factor VIII concentrates acquired through genetic engineering or pooled plasma are used to replace the missing clotting factors. Home factor VIII treatments are taught to families and clients when children are old enough to perform self-administration.
- Corticosteroids are used to reduce joint inflammation and control hematuria.
- Anti-inflammatory drugs such as ibuprofen can be used for chronic synovitis but must be administered carefully because they inhibit platelets.
- Acetaminophen—with or without codeine—can be given for pain.
- Early intervention with home factor treatments is helping to prevent the severe joint damage from hemarthrosis that has occurred in the past. Exercise programs and physical therapy have also contributed to joint health.

Nursing Considerations

- Be vigilant for acute or chronic bleeding, particularly for signs of internal bleeding, such as hypovolemia and black, tarry stools, and signs of cranial hemorrhage, such as headache, slurred speech, vomiting, blurred vision, and decreased level of consciousness. This is very important.
- Assess for changes in neurological status: vision, hearing, and neurological development. This is very important.
- If there is bleeding into a joint from an injury, initiate factor treatment and the RICE protocol (rest, ice, compression, and elevation) immediately, followed by ROM exercises after the acute phase is over in order to prevent stressing and overstretching of the joint.
- Monitor for side effects of therapy.
- Implement a physical therapy program to help prevent joint dysfunction and injury.
- Encourage normal activities and non-contact sports.
- Support the child's self-esteem and positive self-image.
- Child and family teaching: Include home factor administration and information on support groups such as the Canadian Hemophilia Society.
  - Maintain good oral hygiene and avoid vigorous tooth-brushing, which might cause gums to bleed. Recommend that clients clean their teeth by wetting a very soft toothbrush or using a sponge-tipped swab or water irrigation device.

Idiopathic Thrombocytopenic Purpura

Idiopathic thrombocytopenic purpura (ITP) is an acquired hemorrhagic disorder in which the number of circulating platelets is reduced through the destruction of platelets (thrombocytopenia), there is purpura or bruising from petechiae, and the bone marrow, though normal, features an unusual number of large, young platelet cells. ITP occurs most frequently between the ages of 2 and 10 but may occur at any age. The etiology is unknown, but it is likely an autoimmune reaction and often occurs after an upper respiratory infection, measles, or chicken pox. The child usually recovers completely within 6 months. ITP can be either an acute illness, lasting 6 months or less (80%), or it can become a chronic illness that lasts longer than 6 months (20%) (Hockenberry & Wilson, 2015).

Pathophysiology

The number of circulating platelets is reduced as a result of the action of an antiplatelet antibody that is produced in the spleen. This results in bleeding into the tissues (purpura). It is self-limiting.

Clinical Manifestations

- The child bruises easily, with petechiae, hematomas, and blood in the mucous membranes, stool, or urine.
- The child does not look sick.

Diagnostics

- Platelet count drops below $10 \times 10(9)$/L.
- Blood tests that depend on platelet function, such as bleeding time, as well as clot retraction and tourniquet tests, are not normal.
- Bone marrow aspiration needs to be done to rule out other conditions that cause low platelets, such as leukemia and lupus.

Therapeutics

- Treatment is supportive, as ITP is usually self-limiting.
- Steroids can be prescribed for children at high risk for serious bleeding.
- Intravenous immunoglobulin (IVIG) may be used to increase platelet production.
- The anti-D antibody protects the platelets from destruction but can be used only if the child is not bleeding and meets specific criteria, such as having an Rh+ blood type.
- A splenectomy may be required if the child is unresponsive to treatment or if bleeding is severe (Hockenberry & Wilson, 2015).

Nursing Considerations

- Observe for bleeding and new areas of petechiae and bruises.
- Focus on safety and injury prevention until the platelet count returns to normal.
- Avoid acetylsalicytic acid (Aspirin) or Aspirin-containing products, rectal temperatures, and intramuscular injections.
- Teach the importance of follow-up care to monitor the child's platelet level, usually every 1–2 weeks.

HIV and AIDS

HIV leads to a wide range of diseases and a variety of clinical courses. Acquired immune deficiency syndrome (AIDS) is the most serious condition of these diseases. Advances in treatments have been able to turn AIDS from a non-survivable disease into a chronic disease.

Pathophysiology

AIDS is caused by HIV, a retrovirus that infects a subset of T lymphocytes (CD4$^+$ T cells) and suppresses the immune system, reducing the number of CD4$^+$ T cells. Abnormal B-cell function can be detected early in pediatric HIV infection. The child with HIV cannot fight bacterial infections because helper T cells that control B-cell function have been reduced, decreasing cell-mediated and humoral immunity.

Modes of HIV transmission in children are as follows:

- Perinatally, mother-to-infant transmission occurs before or at birth and also through breastfeeding. Most infected children are born to families in which one or both parents are infected. The risk of infection for an infant whose mother is HIV-positive is 13–30% without medical intervention (Hockenberry & Wilson, 2015).
- Sexual contact from HIV-positive individuals can transmit HIV.
- Percutaneous exposure to contaminated needles can also transmit HIV.
- Transfusion of blood, blood components, or clotting factor concentrates is now a rare mode of transmission.

There is dissemination of the virus throughout the lymphoid organ. At the same time, the virus suppresses the function of the T lymphocytes, which no longer function effectively in the peripheral bloodstream. The suppression of the CD4$^+$ function creates an immune response that maintains the HIV plasma level. During the latency period, the virus does not increase in number, and in the adult population, this period can last at least 10 years.

The incubation period of a symptomatic HIV infection ranges from months to years. Over this time period, the CD4$^+$ cells gradually continue to decrease in number, and, eventually, the child will develop opportunistic infections that can lead to death. In infants infected perinatally, the median age for onset of symptoms is 3 years, with the disease progressing more quickly because of the immaturity of the immune system.

Clinical Manifestations

The typical manifestations of HIV are as follows:

- Lymphadenopathy, hepatosplenomegaly, oral candidiasis, chronic or recurrent diarrhea, failure to thrive, developmental delay, and parotitis

  The typical manifestations of AIDS are as follows:
- *Pneumocystis carinii* pneumonia (PCP), lymphocytic interstitial pneumonitis (LIP), recurrent bacterial infections, wasting syndrome, candidal esophagitis, HIV encephalopathy, cytomegalovirus disease, *Mycobacterium avium intracellulare* complex infection, pulmonary candidiasis, herpes simplex disease, and cryptosporidiosis (Hockenberry & Wilson, 2015)
- Developmental disabilities: Many children with AIDS have developmental disabilities, including problems with motor skills, communication, use of language, memory loss, and behaviour changes (Hockenberry & Wilson, 2015).

Diagnostics

- For children over 18 months, traditional enzyme-linked immunosorbent assay (ELISA) and Western blot assay tests are used.
- Accurate testing in infants is complicated due to the presence of maternal antibodies for up to 18 months; the result may be a false-positive ELISA. HIV cultures, detection of HIV–DNA sequences using the polymerase chain reaction (PCR), and identifying specific HIV antigens can be used for these infants. Most infants are diagnosed within 1–3 months of age.

Therapeutics

- There is currently no cure; management is primarily supportive, with treatment for opportunistic infections.
- Goals of therapy include slowing the growth of HIV, preventing and treating opportunistic infections, ensuring good nutritional support, and relieving symptoms.
- Medication regimens include combinations of the antiretroviral drugs that help prevent the production of new viral particles. New antiretroviral drugs are being developed, and the use of these in combination, as well as strict adherence to the medication regimen, prevents the development of drug resistance (Anabwani, Woldetsadik, & Kline, 2005).
- Trimethoprim-sulfamethoxazole (Septra) is prescribed as well as a prophylaxis drug of choice to prevent and treat

PCP, the most opportunistic infection in this population, particularly in clients between 3 and 6 months of age.

- Children exposed to or infected with HIV should be immunized with pneumococcal and influenza vaccines as scheduled (Hockenberry & Wilson, 2015).

Nursing Considerations

- Observe blood and excretion precautions (use gloves to change dressings; clean up spilled body fluids with a 1:10 bleach solution; keep garbage in a closed container; flush feces, urine, and other body fluids down the toilet; use proper containers for needles).
- Protect the child from infection, for example, by maintaining distance from people with infections, using hand hygiene, or through reverse isolation.
- Promote optimum nutrition.
- Administer antibiotics and other medications as prescribed.
- Assist the child in maintaining self-esteem, appropriate developmental tasks, and normalization of lifestyle.
- Assist with pain management.
- Provide health teaching concerning the disease and its transmission (particularly for sexually active adolescents); protection from infections; adherence to drug regimens, blood tests, and follow-up care; and referral to appropriate community agencies.
- Teach at-home body fluid precautions: Avoid mixing the ill child's secretions with those of the family; have separate linens, a separate toothbrush, a separate razor, and separate eating utensils.

Cancer

Childhood cancer is a rare occurrence in Canada, and most children diagnosed with cancer will survive. However, it is the leading cause of death from disease in children over 1 month of age. In Canada, between 2009 and 2013, an average of 943 children were diagnosed with cancer each year. The annual mortality rate between 2008 and 2012 was 12%. The incidence rate of childhood cancer is not increasing, the mortality rate is decreasing, and today the 5-year survival rate is on average 91%. Improved diagnostic methods and better treatment plans have improved this rate (Canadian Cancer Society, 2018a).

Cure criteria include cessation of therapy, continuous freedom from clinical and laboratory evidence of cancer, and minimal or no risk of relapse, as determined by previous experience with the disease. Time that must elapse ranges from 2–5 years (Hockenberry & Wilson, 2015).

Pathophysiology

Categories of malignant cells include the following:

- Embryonal—Cells that arise from embryonic tissue, such as blastomas
- Lymphomas—Cells arising from the lymphatic system
- Leukemias—Cells that arise from blood-forming organs
- Sarcomas—Cells derived from connective and supportive tissue, such as bone

- Carcinomas—Those derived from epithelial cells
- Adenocarcinomas—Carcinoma of glandular tissue, such as breast tissue (Hockenberry & Wilson, 2011)

Properties of tumour cells include the following:

- The growth rate usually is rapid.
- Anaplasia is the loss of differentiation and organization of cells for a specific function.
- Invasion—Cancer cells invade adjacent tissue and replace normal cells.
- Metastasis—Cancer cells spread to distant sites (via the blood or lymphatic system, or by iatrogenic methods, such as biopsy) to form colonies of malignant growth.
- Competition—Cancer cells compete with normal cells for essential nutrients.
- Expansion—Unrestricted growth of cancer cells compresses adjacent tissue and causes organ damage.
- Staging criteria and terminology are used.
- Criteria to describe and classify the extent of malignant neoplasms and their metastases depend on the specific tumour or treatment centre.
- Staging systems are used to guide therapy and evaluate progress (Hockenberry & Wilson, 2011).

Clinical Manifestations

Specific clinical findings vary, depending on the particular body system involved.

The cardinal signs and symptoms of cancer in children are as follows:

- Fever, night sweats
- Persistent, localized pain or limping
- Tendency to bruise easily
- Palpable mass
- Sudden changes in behaviour, gait, balance, or vision
- Sudden, unexplained weight loss and anorexia
- Unexplained paleness and fatigue

Diagnostics

- CBC, such as increased production of immature cells, chemistry, and urinalysis
- Bone marrow aspiration or biopsy and other tissue biopsies for definitive diagnosis of cancer
- Lumbar puncture to analyze CSF for leukemic cells, as well as brain tumours and other cancers
- Imaging techniques (CT, ultrasonography, MRI) to detect solid tumours and areas of metastases

Therapeutics

- Protocols may include the following therapies: surgery, chemotherapy, radiotherapy, immunotherapy, and BMT.
- Supportive therapy, such as nutritional supplements, is needed when serious damage occurs to normal cells as the result of cancer treatment.
- Complications that may occur from therapy include oncological emergencies, such as acute tumour lysis syndrome, obstruction, superior vena cava syndrome, and infections (Hockenberry & Wilson, 2015).

Nursing Considerations

- Childhood cancer has a significant impact on the family and profound psychosocial implications.
- The child and family need to adapt to living with the various phases of a life-threatening illness.
- The child's reaction largely depends on his or her age, the information the child is given, and the physical impact of the disease on his or her energy level and coping skills.

Leukemia

Leukemia is the most common cancer found in children, affecting about one-third of all children with cancer. Leukemia may be diagnosed at any age but has a peak onset between 2 and 6 years. The etiology is unknown. Several genetic diseases have been associated with increased incidences of leukemia, including Down syndrome and Fanconi's hypoplastic anemia.

Leukemia is a proliferation of abnormal WBCs. There are different types of leukemia, based on the morphology of the cells and the course of the disease. Each type has a different prognosis and different characteristics.

Most leukemia in children is acute lymphoblastic leukemia (ALL), involving a proliferation of very immature WBCs, or blasts. Acute leukemia has a short history of symptoms and, without treatment, a rapidly declining course leading to death in 3–6 months. Acute myelogenous leukemia (AML) is less common (Canadian Cancer Society, 2018b).

Pathophysiology

- Malignant leukemia cells arise from precursor cells in blood-forming elements.
- Cells accumulate and crowd out normal bone marrow elements, spill into peripheral blood, and eventually invade all body organs and tissues, depriving all body cells of nutrients necessary for survival.
- Replacement of normal hematopoietic elements by leukemic cells results in bone marrow suppression, marked by decreased production of RBCs, normal WBCs, and platelets.
- Bone marrow suppression results in anemia, decreased RBC production, the predisposition to infection due to neutropenia, and bleeding tendencies due to thrombocytopenia.
- Infiltration of reticuloendothelial organs (spleen, liver, and lymph glands) causes marked enlargement and, eventually, fibrosis.
- Leukemic infiltration of the central nervous system (CNS) results in increased ICP.
- Other possible sites of long-term infiltration include the kidneys, testes, prostate, ovaries, GI tract, and lungs (Hockenberry & Wilson, 2015).

Clinical Manifestations

- Anemia from RBC suppression causes fatigue, tachycardia, and pallor.
- Bleeding from platelet suppression causes petechiae, purpura, hematuria, epistaxis, and melena stools.
- Immunosuppression from WBC suppression causes fever, infection, and poor wound healing.
- Reticuloendothelial involvement causes hepatosplenomegaly, bone pain, and lymphadenopathy.
- If CNS metastasis occurs, manifestations include headache, meningeal irritation, and signs of increased ICP.
- General symptoms include weight loss, anorexia, vomiting, and fever (Hockenberry & Wilson, 2015).

Diagnostics

- CBC findings show a normal, decreased, or increased WBC count with immature cells (blasts), decreased RBCs, and decreased platelets.
- Diagnosis is confirmed with bone marrow aspiration showing extensive replacement of normal bone marrow elements by leukemic cells.
- Lumbar puncture is performed to assess the migration of abnormal cells to the CNS.

Therapeutics

Therapy involves a combination of chemotherapy and possibly cranial irradiation therapy, provided at four levels:

1. Remission induction treatment is chemotherapy designed to eradicate the cancer cells.
2. Intensification or consolidation therapy involves the use of a combination of medications designed to eradicate any cancer cells that may remain after remission induction.
3. CNS prophylactic therapy prevents leukemic cells from invading the CNS and usually consists of intrathecal administration of chemotherapy.
   - Radiation to the brain, spinal cord, or testis is rarely done unless it is a high-risk client or there is existing infiltration of the CNS.
   - Prepubertal male clients may require androgen replacement therapy; sterility may also occur.
4. In the remission phase, maintenance chemotherapy is given to decrease the risk of recurrence.
   - If relapse occurs and leukemic cells appear in the bone marrow, reinduction therapy includes a combination of other medications not previously used. The prognosis worsens with each relapse.
   - BMT, when successful, destroys leukemic cells and replenishes bone marrow with healthy cells. BMT is usually done following a second relapse with ALL and is considered in the first phase for AML, which has a poorer prognosis (Hockenberry & Wilson, 2015).
   - There are three categories of BMTs:
     - Allogenic refers to tissue from a histocompatible donor, usually a sibling, but may also involve an unmatched donor.
     - Autologous refers to tissue that is collected from the child's own tissue, frozen, and sometimes processed to remove undesired cells.
     - Syngeneic refers to tissue that is identical to the child's tissue, which comes from an identical twin.

Nursing Considerations

Set realistic goals depending on the type of therapy prescribed:

- Prepare the child and family for diagnostic tests and treatments by assessing the child's level of understanding, addressing specific fears, providing information appropriate to the child's age and developmental level, and specifying what the child will see, smell, hear, and feel.
- Help prevent complications related to bone marrow suppression, such as infection, bleeding, and anemia.
- Promote optimal nutrition to maintain and rebuild healthy tissue.
- Promote adequate rest.
- Minimize the risk of infection secondary to diagnosis and chemotherapy: Avoid contact with others who have infections, monitor the child's temperature every 4 hours, practise handwashing, and avoid live plants and uncooked fruits and vegetables, which may contain pathogens.
- Prevent injury secondary to thrombocytopenia and chemotherapy.
- Minimize injections; when necessary, apply pressure to sites for 3–5 minutes to stop bleeding.
- Avoid rectal temperatures.
- Monitor hemoglobin and hematocrit.
- Monitor and report hemorrhagic bleeding.
- Minimize nausea and vomiting secondary to chemotherapy by administering an antiemetic 30 minutes before chemotherapy begins, continuing antiemetics as prescribed, and employing non-pharmacological measures such as visualization and music.
- Minimize discomfort from stomatitis secondary to chemotherapy by assessing the mouth frequently and providing mouth care every 2 hours using a soft toothbrush. Avoid potential irritants such as firm toothbrushes, commercial mouthwashes, and lemon–glycerine swabs, any of which can irritate the gums and mucous membranes; instead, offer cool, soothing, bland foods and liquids and administer anaesthetic mouthwashes.
- Minimize body image disturbances related to alopecia by reassuring the child that hair loss is temporary; educating him or her that the new hair may have different texture; using hats, scarves, and wigs; and avoiding the use of hair chemicals when hair grows back.
- Support the child and family by encouraging verbalization of concerns, fostering family support systems, and using appropriate resources.
  - Provide palliative care counselling as appropriate and use appropriate resources.
  - Encourage normal growth and development by fostering activities appropriate for the child's age and condition.
  - Provide child and family teaching.
  - Refer to appropriate home care and follow-up services (Hockenberry & Wilson, 2015).

Wilms' Tumour (Nephroblastoma)

Wilms' tumour is a malignant neoplasm of the kidney, which is the most common intra-abdominal tumour in children and the most curable solid tumour. Wilms' tumour occurs most often in young children but may occur in adolescents. The median age at diagnosis is between 3 and 4 years, with 80% of cases under the age of 5. Siblings of children with Wilms' tumour have an increased risk of developing this cancer than do children in the general population (Hockenberry & Wilson, 2015).

Pathophysiology

- The tumour originates in the renal parenchyma.
- It is well encapsulated in the early stages but may later extend into the lymph nodes and the renal vein or vena cava and metastasize to the lungs and other sites. Wilms' tumours are classified into five stages, from stage 1 (confined to one kidney) to stage 5 (involving both kidneys).
- Usually, the tumour is unilateral and occurs with other abnormalities, such as an absent iris or genitourinary problems.
- This type of tumour has one of the highest survival rates of all childhood cancers (Hockenberry & Wilson, 2015).

Clinical Manifestations

- There may be no symptoms.
- Characteristics may include a firm, non-tender upper quadrant mass, fever, abdominal pain, hematuria, anemia (due to hemorrhage within the tumour), hypertension (due to secretion of excess renin from the tumour), anorexia, weight loss, and lethargy.
- If the tumour has metastasized to the lungs, shortness of breath, cough, and chest pain may be present.

Diagnostics

- Blood studies may show anemia secondary to bleeding from the tumour.
- Abdominal ultrasonography, CT, and MRI may disclose a mass or evidence of metastasis.

Therapeutics

- Nephrectomy, with removal of regional nodes and any resectable regional tumour, as well as the adjacent adrenal gland may be used.
- Chemotherapy may be used.
- Radiation may be used, but not for stages 1 and 2 (Hockenberry & Wilson, 2015).

Nursing Considerations

- Prepare the child for diagnostic tests and treatments.
- Help prevent rupture of an encapsulated tumour by avoiding abdominal palpation and by careful bathing and handling.
- Monitor bowel sounds and perform an assessment for signs and symptoms of intestinal obstruction resulting

from abdominal surgery, vincristine-induced adynamic ileus, and radiation-induced edema.
- Help prevent infection by practising hand hygiene and limiting the child's exposure to persons with infections; observe for signs of infection.
- Monitor blood pressure.
- Help prevent postoperative pulmonary complications by providing frequent position changes and by encouraging coughing and deep-breathing exercises as well as ambulation.
- Provide child and family teaching as for a child with leukemia.

Brain Tumours

Brain tumours include astrocytoma, medulloblastoma, brainstem glioma, and ependymoma. CNS tumours account for about 25% of all childhood cancers (Hockenberry & Wilson, 2015).

Pathophysiology
- Tumours arise from anywhere in the cranium: glial cells (astrocytomas), nerve cells, neuroepithelium, cranial nerves, blood vessels, pineal gland, or hypophysis.
- About half are infratentorial, occurring primarily in the cerebellum or brainstem, and cause symptoms of increased ICP. The others are supratentorial and occur mainly in the cerebrum (Hockenberry & Wilson, 2015).

Clinical Manifestations
- Recurrent and progressive headache, especially on waking
- Loss of balance and coordination
- Increase in head circumference and tense fontanelles
- Behavioural changes such as irritability or lethargy
- Severe morning vomiting and failure to thrive
- Cranial nerve neuropathy
- Signs of increased ICP
- Seizures

Diagnostics
- MRI is used to diagnose brain tumours and assess the growth of the tumour before and after treatment.
- CT permits direct visualization of the brain parenchyma, ventricles, and surrounding subarachnoid space.
- Angiography provides information about the tumour's blood supply.
- A definitive diagnosis is made by biopsy during surgery.

Nursing Considerations
- Assess for signs and symptoms when a diagnosis of brain tumour is suspected.
- Prepare the child and family for diagnostic tests and protocols.
- Prevent postoperative complications by monitoring vital signs, positioning, regulating fluids, and administering medication.
- Monitor for signs of increased ICP and seizures.

- For chemotherapy, follow the planning and interventions used for leukemia.
- Provide child and family teaching as for a child with leukemia.

ENDOCRINE SYSTEM DISORDERS

The endocrine system regulates energy production, growth, fluid and electrolyte balance, response to stress, and sexual reproduction. Most endocrine disorders are chronic in nature and require ongoing care related to health maintenance, education, development, and psychosocial needs.

Diagnostics
- Blood chemistry, including thyroid function tests and hormone, calcium, phosphorus, alkaline phosphatase, and electrolyte levels
- Urine studies, to evaluate sodium, calcium, phosphorus, and glucose levels and specific gravity
- Radiographic studies, to evaluate bone age and density and soft tissue calcification
- Genetic studies, to detect enzyme deficiencies, such as congenital adrenal hypoplasia (Hockenberry & Wilson, 2015)

Nursing Considerations

There are important psychosocial implications for a child and family with an endocrine disorder:
- Young children may interpret treatments, such as hormonal injections, as punishment for wrongdoing.
- Injections may be a source of fear and may enhance a child's body mutilation anxieties.

Hypopituitarism

Hypopituitarism results from a diminished or deficient secretion of pituitary hormones, usually growth hormone (GH).

Pathophysiology
- Hypopituitarism may be caused by several conditions, including developmental disorders, lesions such as tumours, trauma, or certain hereditary or functional disorders, such as anorexia nervosa or dwarfism.
- The most frequent organic cause of undersecretion of GH is a tumour in the pituitary or hypothalamic region, especially a craniopharyngioma.
- More than half of the cases are idiopathic and related to GH deficiency.

Clinical Manifestations
- GH deficiency produces varied effects, depending on the degree of dysfunction, which include decreased linear growth, decreased muscle mass, thin hair, poor skin quality, delayed growth, excessive subcutaneous fat, hypoglycemia, and deficiencies of adrenocorticotropic hormone (ACTH), TSH, LH, and FSH, which produce effects related to the functions of these hormones.
- The chief presenting complaint is short stature.

- Children generally grow during the first year; then growth slows, remaining below the third percentile.
- Children with hypopituitarism appear younger than their chronological age.
- Premature aging is common later in life.
- Primary teeth usually appear when expected, but secondary tooth eruption is delayed.
- Sexual development is usually normal but delayed.
- Most children have normal intelligence.
- Emotional and academic problems are common.

Diagnostics

- Family history, including parental height, is an important predictor of the child's ultimate height.
- A history of the child's growth patterns and previous health status is required to rule out prenatal maternal disorders that affect growth, such as malnutrition, and to check for evidence of chronic illness in the child.
- Bone age is younger than chronological age.
- Definitive diagnosis is possible with a subnormal GH level.

Therapeutics

- Early diagnosis and treatment are crucial for children to achieve their genetic growth potential.
- The treatment of GH deficiency resulting from organic etiology is directed at correcting the underlying cause.
- Treatment for children with functional GH deficiency is replacement therapy Other hormone deficiencies also require replacement therapy.

Nursing Considerations

- Monitor children for growth curves below the third percentile on growth charts.
- Prepare the child for diagnostic tests and procedures; explain that endocrine studies may require multiple blood draws.
- Monitor for early signs and symptoms of hypoglycemia, particularly during provocative tests for GH. If hypoglycemia occurs, increase the child's blood glucose level rapidly by giving orange juice.
- Administer GH replacement therapy at the same time of day.
- Assess for GH overdose, indicated by initial hypoglycemia followed by hyperglycemia.
- Promote the child's self-esteem and a positive self-image related to short stature.
- Provide realistic expectations for the child's growth and the effectiveness of GH replacement therapy and encourage the family to provide normal growth and development activities.

Diabetes Mellitus

Diabetes mellitus (DM) is a deficiency of pancreatic insulin that results in chronic high blood glucose levels and problems with fat and carbohydrate metabolism. The differential diagnosis of DM has become more complex and now includes type 1 DM (T1DM), type 2 DM (T2DM), and monogenic and secondary forms of diabetes. DM is either a complete deficiency (T1DM) or a partial deficiency (T2DM) of the hormone. Type 2 diabetes in children has previously been rare, but the incidence is increasing due to the rise in childhood obesity.

T1DM is the most common endocrine disease of childhood. When pancreatic beta cells (which produce insulin) are destroyed, a lack of insulin is the result. T1DM has two forms. The first form of T1DM results from an autoimmune reaction, causing the destruction of pancreatic beta cells. This occurs when a child with a genetic predisposition is exposed to a trigger, most often a virus. The second form of T1DM is rarer and idiopathic, with no known etiology. In children with T2DM, obesity and genetic predisposition are factors. Children of Indigenous, African or Caribbean, Hispanic, or Asian descent are at particular risk for this form of DM (Saylor, 2010). See Chapter 8, pages 196–200.

Secondary forms of DM can be due to an underlying medical condition such as CF or Cushing's syndrome. Other secondary forms are caused by treatments such as steroid and L-asparaginase. The latter form can resolve itself when the underlying conditions are treated or the medication treatments are finished. The early recognition and treatment of secondary diabetes can help improve the outcome and avoid longer term complications (Ho, Seller, Dean, et al., 2010).

Pathophysiology

Insulin, produced by the beta cells of the pancreas, is needed to support carbohydrate, protein, and fat metabolism and to facilitate the entry of these substances into cells. The destruction of 90% or more of the pancreatic beta cells leads to a cascade of metabolic events, including hyperglycemia (increased glucagon, epinephrine, GH, and cortisol levels), lipolysis, fatty acid release, and ketone production.

- Excessive ketone production can cause DKA, a life-threatening condition characterized by marked hyperglycemia, metabolic acidosis, dehydration, and altered level of consciousness ranging from lethargy to coma.
- See the section in Chapter 8, pages 196–200, on T1DM.

Clinical Manifestations

The classic symptoms of T1DM are the three Ps: polydipsia, polyuria, and polyphagia, along with fatigue. Other symptoms include weight loss, dry skin, and blurred vision. Some children present with an abrupt onset of DKA.

Diagnostics

- A fasting blood glucose level >6.5–7 mmol/L
- A level 2 hours postprandial of >7.8 mmol/L
- Glycosuria
- In DKA, there is hyperglycemia, acidosis, glycosuria, and ketonuria.

Therapeutics

Treatment for T1DM in the child involves an interprofessional approach to manage the complexity of the disease and to foster self-care.

- Insulin therapy: The dose is calculated individually for each child based on carbohydrates to be consumed and blood glucose levels and is administered via subcutaneous injection or an insulin pump. Doses will be adjusted during stress, illness, exercise, growth, and puberty. Future therapies may include nasal administration of insulin and islet cell or pancreas transplantation.
- Glucose monitoring: Blood sugar must be monitored multiple times daily. There are many easy-to-use glucometers for home use.
- Glycosylated hemoglobin monitoring: Measuring glycosylated hemoglobin every 3 months is the best method for assessing glucose control.
- Nutrition: Food intake should be planned according to, exercise, insulin injection times, and food preferences. Although concentrated sweets are not advised, there are no longer any absolute rules about foods that are not permitted.
- Exercise: Physical activity is encouraged; children will need to learn about food and insulin adjustments during exercise.

Nursing Considerations

- Nursing considerations are similar to those in the section "Diabetes Mellitus" in Chapter 8, pages 196–200.
- Know that children are able to learn at a young age about self-care: glucose testing, injection of insulin, and diet.
- Teach according to the developmental age of the child and include the child in health teaching.
- Teach the child and family about the signs and treatment of hypoglycemia.
- Know that children may have periods of fluctuating blood sugars with difficulty achieving stabilization. Glucose needs to be monitored frequently, along with increased follow-up with the diabetes team.
- Know that adolescents may rebel at the need for injections, glucose monitoring, and lifestyle changes. Parents and the health care team must be aware of the risk of non-adherence in these clients.

RENAL SYSTEM DYSFUNCTION

Kidney development is complete at the end of the first year. Glomerular filtration and absorption do not reach adult capabilities until between 1 and 2 years.

Kidney functions include maintaining body fluid volume, secreting erythropoietic stimulating factor (ESF), which stimulates the production of RBCs, and producing renin, which stimulates the production of angiotensin. Urine is formed in the nephron and then passes into the renal pelvis, through the ureter, into the bladder, and out of the body through the urethra.

Urinary Tract Infections

UTIs lead to inflammation, usually caused by bacterial infections, of the urethra (urethritis), bladder (cystitis), ureters (ureteritis), or kidneys (pyelonephritis). Peak incidence occurs between 2 and 6 years, with increased incidence also noted in adolescents who are sexually active. Females have a 10–30 times greater risk of developing UTIs than do males (except in neonates) (Couture, Labbe, & Cyre, 2003).

Pathophysiology

- In uncomplicated UTI, inflammation usually is confined to the lower urinary tract.
- Recurrent cystitis may produce anatomical changes in the ureter that lead to vesicoureteral valve incompetence and resultant urine reflux, conditions that provide organisms with access to the upper urinary tract.
- Pyelonephritis usually results from an ascending infection from the lower urinary tract and can lead to acute and chronic inflammatory changes in the pelvis and medulla, with scarring and loss of renal tissue. Recurrent or chronic infection results in increased fibrotic tissue and kidney contraction.
- *E. coli* and other gram-negative organisms account for most UTIs.
- In the neonate, the urinary tract may be infected via the bloodstream; in older children, bacteria ascend the urethra.
- There is an increased incidence of UTI in females due to the shorter urethra and proximity to the anus.
- The incidence of UTI in male infants is often due to congenital malformations of the urinary tract and should be investigated.
- Contributing factors include urinary stasis, urinary reflux, poor perineal hygiene, pregnancy, non-circumcision, in-dwelling catheters, tight clothes or diapers, bubble baths, antimicrobial agents that alter normal urinary tract flora, local inflammation, such as vaginitis, and sexual intercourse.

Clinical Manifestations

Manifestations vary, depending on age and the location of the infection. Approximately 40% of UTIs are asymptomatic.
- Infants: Fever, weight loss, failure to thrive, vomiting, and diarrhea
- Older children: Dysuria, frequency, urgency, incontinence, foul-smelling urine, abdominal pain, and possibly hematuria
- Pylenonephritis: Fever, chills, flank pain, and costovertebral abdominal tenderness

Diagnostics

- Urinalysis: Urine is tested for hematuria, proteinuria, and pyuria.
- Urine characteristically has a foul odour, cloudiness, and strands of mucus.
- Diagnosis is confirmed by bacteria in urine culture.

Therapeutics

- Antibiotics such as penicillins, sulphonamides (including trimethoprim-sulfamethoxazole [Septra]), cephalosporins, nitrofurantoin (Teva-Nitrofurantoin), and tetracyclines are prescribed to treat a current disease or to provide prophylaxis, depending on the sensitivity identified through urine culture.

- All antibiotics can eventually cause resistant strains.

Nursing Considerations

- Evaluate urinary status by observing the appearance and odour of urine and by noting signs and symptoms such as frequency, burning, enuresis, urinary retention, or flank pain. Follow-up urine cultures may be required.
- Maintain sterile technique when performing urinary catheterization.
- Provide comfort measures: analgesics, antipyretics, and urinary anaesthetics.
- Encourage increased fluid intake to reduce fever and dilute urine.
- Employ and teach preventive measures, including good perineal hygiene, cleaning a girl from the urethra back toward the anus, avoiding irritants such as bubble bath and tight clothing, wearing cotton underwear instead of synthetics such as nylon, maintaining adequate fluid intake, voiding regularly and completely emptying the bladder with each urination, and maintaining acidic urine by drinking beverages such as cranberry juice and blueberry juice.
- Drinking cranberry juice or blueberry juice helps prevent bacteria from sticking to the bladder and urethra walls, in turn minimizing the incidences of UTIs. Research now shows that acidic urine is not the reason for UTIs but rather the sticking of bacteria. This non-sticking effect works to prevent UTIs.
- For the sexually active adolescent, teach the importance of voiding both before and after sexual intercourse.

Vesicoureteral Reflux

Vesicoureteral reflux (VUR) occurs when there is a backward flow of urine in the urinary tract when voiding. The prevalence of VUR in healthy children is estimated at less than 1%. However, it is found in 29–50% of children following UTIs and is the most common radiographic abnormality associated with UTIs in children. Development of VUR may in part be genetic; siblings are 10 times more likely to develop it than other children (Hockenberry & Wilson, 2015).

Pathophysiology

- VUR usually occurs a result of an incompetent valvular mechanism at the ureterovesicular junction.
- VUR is graded according to the degree of reflux from the lower ureter to the kidney.
- VUR is a major cause of renal damage; refluxed urine ascending into the collecting tubules of nephrons initiates renal scarring from infective organisms.
- If the amount of refluxed urine is large, the child feels an urge to void shortly after having urinated.
- If the amount is small, it may remain in the bladder, causing urinary stasis and increasing the risk of infection. VUR causes:

- Primary reflux results from congenital abnormalities at the point of insertion of the ureters into the bladder.
- Secondary reflux results from infection and ureterovesicular junction incompetency; it may also result from neurogenic bladder or progressive dilation of ureters following surgical urinary diversion (Hockenberry & Wilson, 2015).

Clinical Manifestations

- Dysuria
- Urinary frequency, urgency, and hesitancy
- Urine retention
- Cloudy, dark, or blood-tinged urine

Diagnostics

- Urinalysis may reveal RBCs or pyuria.
- Structural abnormalities may be detected by intravenous pyelogram (IVP), voiding cystourethrography, and cystoscopy.

Therapeutics

- Antibiotics and urinary antiseptics
- Possible antireflux surgery, involving the reimplantation of ureters

Nursing Considerations

- Administer or teach parents to administer prescribed medications, such as continuous low-dose antibiotics, usually given as nitrofurantoin (Teva-Nitrofurantoin) or trimethoprim-sulfamethoxazole (Septra).
- Encourage increased fluids to dilute urine and develop a regular (3-hour) voiding plan.
- Encourage a high-fibre diet to prevent constipation in order to facilitate muscular relaxation, thereby helping to reduce residual urine.
- Some children with a lower grade reflux can have endoscopic correction instead of a surgical procedure.
- As appropriate, explain antireflux surgery, involving reimplantation of ureters.
- Provide preoperative and postoperative care after antireflux surgery:
  - Observe and protect urinary drainage tubes, in-dwelling catheters, suprapubic catheters, and ureteral stents.
  - Considerations are as in a child with UTI (Hockenberry & Wilson, 2015).

Nephrotic Syndrome

Nephrotic syndrome is characterized by massive proteinuria, hypoalbuminemia, dyslipidemia, altered immunity, and edema. The condition is of idiopathic origin 95% of the time. The prognosis is usually good for the most common type, called *minimal change nephrotic syndrome* (MCNS), which is self-limiting and usually responds to steroidal therapy.

Pathophysiology

- Pathogenesis in MCNS is not understood, but a disturbance in the membrane of the glomeruli causes an increased permeability to protein.

- Proteins, especially albumin, leak through the glomerular membrane and are excreted in the urine.
- Once the albumin is excreted, colloidal osmotic pressure decreases, allowing fluid to escape from the intravascular spaces to the interstitial spaces, resulting in ascites in the abdomen.
- The plasma volume decrease stimulates the antidiuretic hormone (ADH) and aldosterone to reabsorb water and increase the intravascular volume.
- Secondary nephrotic syndrome usually occurs after glomerular damage of known or presumed cause (e.g., due to systemic lupus erythematosus, DM, or sickle cell disease).

Clinical Manifestations

- Manifestations may include periorbital, pedal, and pretibial edema initially, progressing to generalized edema (anasarca), weight increase, ascites, pleural effusion, decreased urine output, pallor, anorexia, fatigue, abdominal pain, and diarrhea.
- With significant edema, the child may appear pale and have respiratory distress.
- Blood pressure may be normal or slightly decreased.
- Children are more prone to infection from decreased immunity.

Diagnostics

- Urinalysis shows marked proteinuria, hyaline casts, few RBCs, and high urine specific gravity.
- The serum protein level is markedly decreased, especially the albumin level.
- A renal biopsy may be performed.

Therapeutics

- Diuretics such as loop diuretics, usually furosemide (Lasix) in combination with metolazone (Zaroxolyn), are sometimes effective, and restrictions are placed on high-sodium foods and salt to manage edema.
- Prednisone (Apo-Prednisone) is usually prescribed for 3 months to reduce proteinuria.
- Immunosuppressant therapy (usually cyclophosphamide [Procytox]) is recommended for the child who fails to respond to steroids. Immunosuppressants decrease the rate of relapse but can have long-term implications, particularly in terms of causing male sterility if used for more than 2–3 months.
- A broad-spectrum antimicrobial agent may be given if infection is present.
- Plasma expanders, such as salt-poor albumin, may be needed to manage severe edema (Hockenberry & Wilson, 2015).

Nursing Considerations

- Assess for a decrease in blood volume by monitoring for increased edema and by measuring abdominal girth, weight, intake and output, blood pressure, and pulse rate. Test urine for protein and specific gravity.
- Monitor for signs of infection and take precautions to prevent infection (the child is susceptible to secondary infection because immunoglobulin is lost in the urine).
- Promote skin integrity by checking areas of edema for skin breakdown, ensuring frequent position changes, using scrotal supports for boys, and providing good skin care.
- Provide a high-protein, high-calorie diet without added salt. Fluids may be restricted if severe edema is present.
- Conserve the child's energy by encouraging bed rest and quiet activities.
- Perform urine testing for albumin.
- Provide parent and child teaching such as monitoring for relapses and signs of infection, medication administration, urine testing, and signs of skin breakdown.

Acute Glomerulonephritis

Acute glomerulonephritis (AGN) is an immune complex disease that may be a primary condition or can be symptomatic of a systemic disorder. It is likely caused by an immune injury secondary to *Streptococcus,* pneumococci, and viruses. Recovery occurs in most cases.

Acute poststreptococcal glomerulonephritis (APSGN) is the most common form. APSGN can occur at any age but is usually seen in school-aged children, peaking at 6 to 7 years. It is uncommon in children under the age of 2.

The majority of infections do not cause AGN. A latent period of 10–14 days occurs between the infection—usually of the throat or skin—and the onset of clinical symptoms.

Pathophysiology

It is speculated that the original infectious organism releases material into the circulation that is antigenic, and antibodies are formed in response. Antibodies interact with antigens that remain in the glomeruli, leading to immune complex formation and tissue injury, a decrease in filtration, and reduced excretion of sodium and water (Hockenberry & Wilson, 2015).

Clinical Manifestations

Manifestations appear approximately 10–14 days after an infection, although some children do not appear to have been ill. These include mild to moderate or high blood pressure, pallor, irritability, fatigue, lethargy, periorbital and generalized edema, weight gain, oliguria and hematuria (urine is brown—cola- or tea-coloured—and cloudy), costovertebral tenderness, and anorexia.

Diagnostics

- Urinalysis: Urine contains RBCs, epithelial cells, granular casts, WBCs, and protein.
- Serum chemistry: Results show elevated BUN and creatinine levels, elevated erythrocyte sedimentation rate (ESR), and elevated antistreptolysin O (ASO) titre and complement level (C3).
- Cultures of the pharynx are done on the child and family members, and if there is a positive culture of group A streptococci, all family members should be treated with an antistreptococcal agent.

- A renal biopsy is not usually performed unless an atypical nephritis is suspected.

Therapeutics

- Treatment usually includes medications to control hypertension, decrease fluid overload, and treat infection.
- Treatment for severe hypertension includes calcium channel blockers, beta blockers, or ACE inhibitors.
- Treatment for mild or moderate hypertension involves loop diuretics.
- Diuretics, usually furosemide (Lasix), are given for edema and fluid overload if no renal failure is present.
- The diet is usually no added salt; if edema is present or the client is hypertensive, there may be moderate sodium restrictions. During periods of oliguria, potassium is also restricted. Protein is restricted only if severe azotemia has developed due to prolonged oliguria.
- Antibiotics are used to treat an existing streptococcal infection.
- Rarely, dialysis may be required to manage severe AGN or heart failure.
- Caloric intake may be increased to balance protein breakdown.
- Diuresis indicates the beginning of recovery.

Nursing Considerations

- Assess fluid status by monitoring intake and output, recording daily weights, and monitoring for edema.
- Closely monitor blood pressure and respiratory rate to identify early signs of complications.
- Administer medications and observe for side and therapeutic effects.
- Maintain adequate caloric intake and nutrition with any dietary restrictions.
- Provide child and family teaching on the need for medical follow-up for urine testing and blood pressure monitoring, as well as on home care measures, including activity and diet instructions, infection prevention measures, and the signs and symptoms of potential complications.

Enuresis

Enuresis is repeated involuntary urination, usually at night, in a child who should have bladder control (usually by age 4 or 5). Enuresis is primary when the child has never achieved continence and secondary if the child starts bedwetting after continence is achieved. Boys are affected more than girls, and night-time bedwetting usually stops between the ages of 6 and 8. Enuresis may have a familial component; 75% of children with enuresis have a first-degree relative with the problem (Hockenberry & Wilson, 2015).

Pathophysiology

Enuresis is primarily a problem of delayed or incomplete neuromuscular maturation of the bladder. Most children with enuresis sleep long periods as infants, have a family history of enuresis, and exhibit slower development up to 3 years of age. The condition is benign and self-limiting.

Therapeutics

- Bladder retention training, motivational therapy, or behaviour modification
- Drug therapy, such as imipramine, which has an anticholinergic effect on the bladder, or desmopressin (DDAVP) nasal spray, which decreases night-time output
- Urine-alarm mattresses, which sound an alarm when wet and can be very effective

Nursing Considerations

- Help the family accept the child's problem and avoid placing blame or adopting attitudes that may foster feelings of low self-esteem in the child.
- Discuss strategies to manage night-time incontinence, such as rubber sheets on beds. Suggest the use of incontinence "pull-ups," which do not look like diapers.

Hypospadias

Hypospadias occurs when the urethral opening is located below the glans penis or anywhere along the ventral surface (underside) of the penile shaft. The rate of occurrence is approximately one in 500 newborns. Testes are undescended in approximately 10% of boys with hypospadias, and inguinal hernias are a common associated finding.

Pathophysiology

- The urethral folds fail to fuse completely over the urethral groove.
- Ventral foreskin is lacking, and the distal segment looks like a hood.

Clinical Manifestations

- Abnormal placement of the meatus should be evident at birth.
- In mild cases, the meatus is just below the tip of the penis.
- In severe cases, the meatus is located on the perineum between the halves of the scrotum.
- Chordee (a ventral curve of the penis) results from the replacement of normal skin with fibrotic tissue and usually accompanies severe hypospadias.
- Severe hypospadias with undescended testes must be differentiated from ambiguous genitalia.

Therapeutics

Surgical repair improves the child's ability to stand when urinating and to urinate in a straight stream and improves the appearance of the penis, as well as preserving sexual adequacy. It is usually performed at 6–12 months of age to avoid issues with body image.

Nursing Considerations

- Inform the parents to avoid circumcision as the foreskin is usually used for surgical repair.

- Allow the parents to verbalize their feelings about the child's condition.
- Prepare the parents and child for the surgical procedures and the possibility of urinary diversion while the new meatus is being constructed.
- Prepare the parents for the expected cosmetic result and show them pictures of successful repairs.
- Monitor intake and output and urinary patterns, encourage fluids, maintain patency, and prevent and observe for infection if the child is catheterized postoperatively.

MUSCULOSKELETAL AND NEUROMUSCULAR DYSFUNCTION

Bone growth occurs in diameter and length. Growth in bone length occurs at the epiphyseal plate, a vascular area of active cell division. These cells are highly sensitive to the impact of GH, estrogen, and testosterone. In adolescence, the epiphyseal plate turns to bone and growth stops.

In children, the epiphyseal plate represents an area of bone weakness that is prone to injury through fracture, crushing, or slippage. Injury to the epiphyseal plate can disturb bone growth. Because a child is still growing, some bony deformities due to injury can be remodelled or straightened over time. Conversely, this can also cause some deformities to worsen with growth.

Because a child's bones are more plastic than an adult's, more force is required to fracture a bone, and specific forces may produce different types of fractures. A child's bones generally heal much faster than those of an adult, often greatly reducing the time required for immobilization.

Pathophysiology

Physical activity is essential for the growth and development of bones and muscles. Conditions that may limit mobility include congenital defects, degenerative neurological disorders, integumentary disorders, musculoskeletal trauma, imposed bed rest to assist healing and restoration, and mechanical restraint as part of therapy.

Clinical Manifestations

General signs and symptoms of musculoskeletal disorders in children are as follows:
- Joint contracture and pain
- Muscular atrophy and weakness
- Fatigue
- Diminished reflexes
- Delayed healing
- Orthostatic hypotension
- Thrombus formation
- Shallow respirations
- Anorexia and constipation
- Renal calculi
- Urinary incontinence or signs of urinary infection
- Skin breakdown and pressure ulcers
- Sensory changes

Diagnostics

- Radiographs (the most common study to assess injury and healing)
- CT scan
- Bone scan
- Arthrography and arthroscopy
- Joint aspiration
- Electromyography (EMG)

Therapeutics

- Therapy is specific to the disorder.
- Immobilization may be required to stabilize disrupted muscle or protect bone integrity.

Nursing Considerations Related to Immobilization

- Know that treatment for musculoskeletal problems often requires immobilization (casts, traction, or body frames), which can be frightening and painful.
- Know that play, social interaction, and self-care help the immobilized child gain self-esteem and independence and promote normal growth and development.
- Protect skin integrity by turning the child frequently and inspecting the skin for early signs of breakdown.
- Promote adequate hydration and nutrition by offering high-protein, high-calorie foods in small, frequent amounts.
- Promote bowel elimination by encouraging fluids and a high-fibre diet. Administer stool softeners as prescribed.
- Promote urinary elimination by encouraging fluids, monitoring intake and output, and assessing for bladder distension.
- Prevent respiratory complications by keeping the child well hydrated, changing the child's position frequently, and encouraging deep-breathing exercises.
- Protect the child from injury by moving and positioning the child carefully and by monitoring physical activities closely; postural hypotension and falling may result if the child resumes usual activities too quickly.
- Help prevent UTIs by keeping the child well hydrated, promoting frequent voiding, providing foods such as blueberry juice and cranberry juice, which prevents bacteria from sticking to the epithelium in the bladder area, and limiting high-calcium foods.
- Prevent contractures by maintaining proper body alignment and providing ROM exercises.
- Administer medications, which may include antibiotics to treat infection; diuretics to remove high levels of calcium; calcium-mobilizing drugs; anticoagulants to prevent clot formation; and stool softeners to prevent constipation. Be alert for the side effects of these medications.
- Be aware that preschoolers may view immobilization as punishment.
- Provide child and family teaching as appropriate, such as cast care, positioning, skin care, nutrition and hydration to repair bone and muscle damage and prevent constipation and UTIs, as well as how to observe for thrombus and

circulatory problems and what medical follow-up is required.

Developmental Dysplasia of the Hip

Developmental dysplasia of the hip (DDH) is a spectrum of hip abnormalities that may arise in the fetus, infant, or child. Hip instability may involve subluxations and dislocations, which, if uncorrected, will lead to permanent disability. The etiology of DDH is unknown, but predisposing factors may be categorized as physiological (lax joints due to maternal hormones), genetic (family history), and mechanical (breech birth). DDH occurs most often in females and most frequently in the right hip.

Pathophysiology

- Subluxation, the most common form of DDH, is defined as an incomplete dislocation, in which the femoral head remains in contact with the acetabulum, but a stretched capsule and ligament tears cause the head of the femur to be partially displaced.
- Dislocation describes the situation in which the femoral head loses contact with the acetabulum and is displaced posteriorly and superiorly over the fibro-cartilaginous rim.

Clinical Manifestations

- In the newborn: Ortolani's sign, Barlow's sign, asymmetrical gluteal folds, limited abduction of affected hip
- In older children: limp, Trendelenburg's sign

Diagnostics

- Radiographic examination is not reliable until between 3 and 6 months of age.
- Ultrasonography may be helpful in diagnosing dysplasia in the newborn.

Therapeutics

Newborn to 6 months. The infant is usually placed in a Pavlik harness, which centres the femoral head into the acetabulum in flexion and deepens the acetabulum by pressure.

- The harness is worn continuously until the hip joint is clinically and radiographically stable.
- By 3–6 months, the child usually is transferred to a protective abduction brace, which is worn for less than a year.

Six to 18 months. The child is placed in traction for gradual reduction, followed by cast immobilization until the joint is stable. If soft tissue blocks reduction, an open reduction is performed, followed by a spica cast for 4–6 months. Then an abduction splint is worn.

Older children. Correction is difficult because secondary changes create complications.

- Surgical reduction is required.
- Successful reduction after 4 years of age is difficult and may require preoperative traction, tenotomy of contracted muscles, and an innominate osteotomy procedure and casting. Reduction is inadvisable after 6 years of age.

Nursing Considerations

- Provide care as indicated in the section "Nursing Considerations Related to Immobilization."
- Be aware that children may be prone to putting toys, food, etc. inside the cast.
- Petal cast edges with waterproof tape, particularly in the diaper area.
- Place a disposable diaper beneath the entire perineal opening in the cast.
- Provide child and family teaching regarding holding techniques, moving, feeding, care of restrictive devices, and signs and symptoms of complications such as increased temperature, pain or blood on voiding, and difficulty breathing.

Cerebral Palsy

Cerebral palsy (CP) is a group of neurological disorders caused by injury or insult to the brain either before or during birth or in early infancy. CP has an early onset, and there is abnormal muscle tone and coordination. CP is the most common permanent disability in childhood. Risk factors include prematurity, asphyxia, ischemia, perinatal trauma, congenital and perinatal infections, and perinatal metabolic problems, such as hyperbilirubinemia and hypoglycemia. Infection, trauma, and tumours can cause CP in early infancy. For most babies born with CP, the cause is unknown (Cerebral Palsy Alliance Research Foundation, 2018). The estimated occurrence in the United States is 1.2–3 of every 1 000 births. CP can range from mildly hypertonic muscles to severe physical and neurological impairment (Hockenberry & Wilson, 2015).

Pathophysiology

- Disabilities usually result from injury to the cerebellum, the basal ganglia, or the motor cortex.
- CP is non-progressive but may become more apparent as the child grows older.
- It can be difficult to establish the precise location of neurological lesions because with a few exceptions, there is no typical pattern of pathology. In some children with CP, there is gross brain malformation, and in others, there is vascular occlusion, neuron loss, and laminar degeneration.
- Anoxia appears to be an important factor in neurological damage.
- CP is often secondary to a wide range of causative factors (Hockenberry & Wilson, 2015).

Classification of CP

- Spastic: This type is the most common and may involve one or both sides. It involves upper motor neuron muscular weakness with intact reflex arc, increased stretch reflexes, increased muscle tone, and often weak muscles. Hallmarks include hypertonicity with poor control of posture, balance, and coordinated movement; impairment of fine and gross motor skills; and active attempts at motion increase abnormal postures and the overflow of movement to other parts of the body. In the infant up to 1 year, hypotonia is present; then spasticity begins to develop.

- Dyskinetic: This type is defined by abnormal involuntary movements that disappear in sleep and increase when the child is stressed; the major manifestation is athetosis (wormlike movement), in addition to dyskinetic movement of the mouth, drooling, dysarthria, and choreiform (jerky) movements.
- Ataxic: This type is characterized by a wide-based gait, rapid, repetitive movements performed poorly, and disintegration of movements of the upper extremities when the child reaches for objects.
- Mixed type: This type features a combination of spasticity and athetosis (Hockenberry & Wilson, 2015).

Clinical Manifestations

- The most common clinical manifestation is universal delayed gross motor development.
- Additional typical manifestations include abnormal motor performance (early dominant hand preference, abnormal and asymmetrical crawl, poor sucking, feeding problems, and persistent tongue thrust), poor head control after 3 months, alterations of muscle tone (such as increased or decreased resistance to passive movements, the child feels stiff when he or she is being handled or dressed, difficulty in diapering, and opisthotonos), the child exhibits abnormal postures (such as scissoring the legs or persistent infantile posturing), and reflex abnormalities (persistent primitive reflexes, such as tonic neck or hyper-reflexia).
- Behavioural manifestations include extreme irritability, little interest in the environment, and sleeping for unusually long periods.
- Associated disabilities include intellectual delays, seizures, attention deficit disorder, and sensory impairment (Hockenberry & Wilson, 2015).

Diagnostics

- Perinatal history
- Persistence of primitive reflexes
- Neurological examination
- Related diagnostic tests, such as an MRI, to rule out other pathologies

Therapeutics

Although there is no cure, the child can be assisted to reach his or her optimum developmental potential.

- Therapeutic goals are as follows:
  - To establish locomotion, communication, and self-help
  - To gain optimal appearance and integration of motor functions
  - To correct associated deficiencies as effectively as possible
  - To provide educational opportunities based on the child's needs and abilities
- Successful therapy relies on a multidisciplinary approach and collaboration among health care team members to manage various aspects of treatment.

- The child may require orthotic devices, such as braces, splints, or casting.
- The child may use assistive and adaptive devices, such as walkers, scooters, motorized wheelchairs, communication boards, and computers.
- Medications for spasticity, pain, seizures, and constipation may be required.
- Adaptive education and learning programs and educational support services should be investigated.
- Speech and language therapy may be employed.
- Physical and occupational therapy may be recommended.
- Some children may require surgery, such as tendon transfers, to correct deformities and decrease spasticity (Hockenberry & Wilson, 2015).

Nursing Considerations

- Prevent injury by providing the child with a safe environment, appropriate toys, and protective gear (helmet, knee pads), if needed.
- Minimize physical deformity by ensuring the correct use of braces and other assistive devices and by providing ROM exercises.
- Promote mobility by encouraging the child to be involved with age- and condition-appropriate motor activities.
- Ensure good nutrition by providing a high-protein, high-calorie diet.
- Administer prescribed medications, which may include sedatives, muscle relaxants, anticonvulsants, and analgesics.
- Encourage self-care by urging the child to participate in activities of daily living (ADLs) that are appropriate for the child's age and condition; normalize as much as possible.
- Facilitate communication by talking to the child directly and slowly, using pictures to reinforce speech, and using communication devices.
- Encourage early speech therapy to prevent poor or maladaptive communication habits and to provide a means of articulate speech; technology, such as computer use, may help children with severe articulation problems.
- Seek referrals as necessary for corrective lenses and hearing devices to decrease sensory deprivation related to vision and hearing deficits.
- Help promote a positive self-image in the child by praising his or her achievements and appearance, setting realistic goals, and encouraging his or her involvement with age- and condition-appropriate peer group activities.
- Refer the family to support organizations, such as the Cerebral Palsy Association of British Columbia
- Discuss with the parents that achievement of new tasks will require patience and help from caregivers.
- Encourage the family to seek appropriate functional, adaptive, and vocational education for the child.
- Encourage family members to achieve balance in their lives between caring for the disabled child and pursuing other family and personal interests.
- Facilitate respite care as appropriate (Hockenberry & Wilson, 2015).

Duchenne Muscular Dystrophy

Duchenne muscular dystrophy (DMD) is the most common and severe form of a group of disorders that cause progressive degeneration and weakness of skeletal muscles. Half of all cases are X-linked, and males are almost exclusively affected. Muscle weakness is progressive, and the disorder is eventually fatal, usually in adolescence, due to infection or cardiopulmonary failure. The incidence is 1 in 3 500 births (Theadom, Rodrigues, Roxburgh, et al. 2014).

Pathophysiology

DMD occurs when a gene mutation occurs in the gene that encodes dystrophin. Dystrophin, a protein product in skeletal muscle, is absent in the muscles of children with DMD. This lack of dystrophin leads to a gradual degeneration of muscle fibres and is characterized by progressive weakness and muscle-wasting.

Clinical Manifestations

- Symptoms begin between the ages of 3 and 5, starting with weakness in the pelvic girdle.
- Key manifestations are delays in motor development; delayed walking and difficulties in running, riding a bicycle, and climbing stairs are among the first symptoms reported.
- Later, a waddling gait, lordosis, and problems with sitting and standing up appear as muscles degenerate.
- Gowers' sign may appear: From a supine position, the child rolls over, kneels, and presses his or her hands against the ankles, shins, knees, and thighs in a "climbing" action to rise to a standing position.
- Profound muscular dystrophy appears in later stages, commonly with deformities and contracture in the large and small joints; by age 12, children with the disorder are usually unable to walk.
- Eventually, the diaphragm and accessory muscles are affected and cardiomegaly usually appears. Respiratory or cardiac failure is often the cause of death.

Diagnostics

- Blood test shows increased serum creatinine phosphokinase.
- Muscle biopsy discloses degeneration of muscle fibres and a lack of dystrophin through DNA analysis. The DNA can also be tested for genetic problems by a serum sample.
- An ECG and pulmonary function tests may help diagnose compromise of heart and lungs.
- EMG results may show a decrease in amplitude and duration of motor unit potentials.

Therapeutics

Therapy is supportive to minimize deformity, prolong ambulation, and assist with ADLs.

Nursing Considerations

- Be aware that therapy is provided by an interprofessional team.
- Maintain optimal physical mobility by facilitating the maximum level of activity that the child can manage, including muscle strengthening and ROM exercises.
- Provide care as indicated in the section "Nursing Considerations Related to Immobilization."
- Monitor temperature when children with DMD receive an anaesthetic because they are at risk for malignant hyperthermia.
- Support the child and family in coping with this degenerative and fatal disorder.
- Refer the family to support agencies, such as Muscular Dystrophy Canada.
- Facilitate respite care for the family as required.
- Assist the family in obtaining genetic counselling.

Scoliosis

Idiopathic scoliosis is a lateral curvature of the spine. It may result from leg length discrepancy, hip or knee contractures, pain, neuromuscular disorders, or congenital malformations but usually is idiopathic. Scoliosis is often of unknown cause and usually is seen in females. Evidence points to a probable genetic autosomal dominant trait or to multifactorial causes. The most common spinal deformity, scoliosis affects 3–5% of all children (Hockenberry & Wilson, 2015, p. 1528). The curvature can be minor, causing no disability, or severe.

Pathophysiology

- The deformity progresses during periods of growth, particularly during adolescent growth spurts, and stabilizes when vertebral growth is completed.
- As the spine grows and the lateral curve develops, the vertebrae rotate, causing rib asymmetry and thoracic hypokyphosis.
- The child attempts to maintain an erect posture, resulting in a compensatory curve.
- Vertebrae become wedge-shaped, and vertebral discs undergo degenerative changes.
- Muscles and ligaments either shorten and thicken or lengthen and atrophy, depending on the concavity or convexity of the curve.
- A hump may form as a result of the ribs rotating backward on the convex side of the curve.
- If the deformity is severe, the thoracic cavity becomes asymmetrical, leading to compromised respiratory function, decreased vital capacity, and potential pulmonary hypertension, cor pulmonale, and respiratory acidosis.

Clinical Manifestations

- If slight, scoliosis can be asymptomatic and can remain undetected until age 10.
- In more moderate to severe degrees of the condition, there may be a curve, asymmetry of the scapula and extremities, unequal distance between arms and waist, a pronounced hump, or twisting of the body.

Diagnostics

- Physical examination may detect scoliosis; when the child bends forward and dangles the arms, the curvature is apparent.
- Radiographic examination reveals the degree and location of the curvature.

Therapeutics

- Early detection is important to prevent a more severe curvature.
- Exercise and bracing are used in milder idiopathic scoliosis to slow the progression of the curvature until growth is completed. Devices such as the Boston and Wilmington braces are plastic shells that mould to the body, and the thoracolumbosacral orthotic brace is a plastic mould that fits under the arms.
- In more severe cases, surgery may be attempted for spinal realignment and straightening by external or internal fixation and instrumentation combined with bony fusion of the realigned spine. Several surgical techniques are used in the surgery, and different instrument systems are available, such as the Harrington, Dwyer, Zielke, Luque, Cotrel-Dubousset, Isola, Texas Scottish Rite Hospital, and Miami–Moss systems.

Nursing Considerations

- Be aware that practical nurses are often the first to diagnose scoliosis during health assessments of adolescents (scoliosis is more common in females).
- Evaluate the child's acceptance of any prescribed brace and exercise to determine his or her compliance level and the need for further teaching.
- Emphasize the positive aspects of wearing the brace, including improved posture and symptom relief. Encourage the child to verbalize any concerns about wearing the brace in relation to body image, which is very important to adolescent females.
- Teach skin care to children wearing a brace: ensuring its proper fit, wearing a cotton shirt under the brace, and early treatment of skin breakdown.
- Provide the child and family with information about scoliosis and its treatment, including equipment.
- See Chapter 6, pages 111–113, for postoperative care.

Fracture

Fractures are breaks in the continuity of a bone when more stress is placed on the bone than it can resist. The bone is realigned or reduced by closed or open reduction followed by immobilization with a splint, traction, or a cast.

Pathophysiology

The fracture types that are most commonly seen in children are as follows:

- Bend—The bone bends to the breaking point and will not straighten without intervention. These are most commonly in the ulna and fibula.
- Buckle—This fracture results from a compression of porous bone, with the bone telescoping on itself.
- Greenstick—The bone does not fracture completely through.
- Complete fracture—The bone divides into bone fragments that are subclassified as transverse, spiral, oblique, comminuted, or butterfly.

Common sites include the following:

- The clavicle
- The humerus (in supracondylar fractures, which occur when a child falls backward onto the hands with the elbows straight, there is a high incidence of neurovascular compromise due to the closeness of the brachial artery and nerves to the fracture site)
- Radius, ulna, and femur (often associated with child abuse)
- Epiphyseal plates (with the potential for growth deformity)

Precautions must be taken to prevent complications, such as cast syndrome, infections, and compartment syndrome. Fractures in children may be the result of falls, sports injuries, motor vehicle accidents, or child abuse.

Clinical Manifestations

Fracture manifestations vary, depending on the location, cause, and type of fracture. Usual symptoms are the five Ps: pain, pulse, pallor, paraesthesia, and paralysis.

Other symptoms include deformity, swelling, bruising, muscle spasms, tenderness, pain, impaired sensation, loss of function, abnormal mobility, crepitus, shock, and refusal to walk or crawl (in small children).

Diagnostics

X-ray examination reveals the initial injury and subsequent healing progress. Ultrasonography, bone scan, and MRI might be required to further differentiate the injury.

Nursing Considerations

Emergency management includes the following:
- Assess the five Ps.
- Determine the mechanism of injury.
- Immobilize the part, moving the injured parts as little as possible.
- Apply traction if circulatory compromise is present.
- Elevate the injured limb if possible.
- Apply cold to the injured area.

Later treatment includes the following:
- Monitor the child for neurovascular status (circulation, sensation, and movement) and signs of compartment syndrome, edema and swelling, skin integrity, and signs of infection.
- Provide cast care, including cast petalling, keeping the cast dry, and checking for foul odour and soft spots. It is very important to check for tightness of the cast when edema is present as it can decrease circulation and cause nerve damage.
- Assist with pain management.

- Provide care as indicated in the section "Nursing Considerations Related to Immobilization."

Osteomyelitis

Osteomyelitis is an infection of the bone, most commonly caused by *S. aureus*. It may occur acutely as a result of a bloodborne organism or infection through a break in the skin or as a chronic condition that may lead to dead bone tissue and orthopedic disability. Typically, the joints and long bones of the leg are involved.

Pathophysiology

- In acute hematogenous osteomyelitis, organisms from sites such as infected tonsils and abscessed teeth travel through the bloodstream and infect the bone.
- In exogenous osteomyelitis, there is a direct inoculation of the organism through trauma close to the bone, for example, a fracture or puncture wound.
- Chronic osteomyelitis occurs when the infection is resistant to treatment, which may lead to dead bone or bone loss.

Clinical Manifestations

- Fever, pain, and tenderness manifests at the site of infection.
- There may or may not be signs of inflammation.

Diagnostics

- Cultures are ordered to identify the organism.
- Bone scans, CT scans, and MRIs are helpful in determining areas of infected bone.
- A bone biopsy may be done if necessary.

Therapeutics

- IV antibiotics are administered, usually for at least 4 weeks.
- Surgery may be required if there is a poor response to the antibiotics.

Nursing Considerations

- Assist with positioning and support of the painful limb.
- Know that weight-bearing activities should not be permitted until healing is established, to prevent stress fractures.
- Consider venous access devices for long-term IV antibiotic administration.
- Administer analgesics as required.
- Provide physical therapy and ROM exercises as indicated.
- Monitor for signs of improvement in the area of infection.

NEUROLOGICAL COGNITIVE DYSFUNCTION

Increased Intracranial Pressure

Increased ICP is excessive pressure from tissue or fluid volume within the rigid cranial vault that disrupts neurological function. While an infant's fontanelles are still open, the sutures can widen and expand slightly pend compensate for some of the increased pressure.

Pathophysiology

- Normally, ICP remains relatively constant within a fluctuating range as a result of a system of compensatory mechanisms among the cranium's contents: the brain tissue, meninges, CSF, and blood.
- Any increase in the proportional volume of one component must be accompanied by an equivalent reduction in one or more of the others.
- After cranial sutures are fused, only two alterations can compensate for increasing intracranial volume: the displacement of CSF to the spinal subarachnoid space and increased CSF absorption.
- An increase in intracranial volume that exceeds the ability of these mechanisms to compensate produces clinical manifestations of increased ICP.
- Conditions that produce increased ICP include craniocerebral trauma, hydrocephalus, brain tumour, meningitis, encephalitis, and intracerebral hemorrhage.

Clinical Manifestations

Early signs and symptoms of increased ICP usually are subtle. Manifestations in infants include the following:

- A tense, bulging anterior fontanelle and separated cranial sutures
- Increased occipital frontal circumference
- "Setting sun" sign
- Macewen's sign ("cracked pot sound")
- Irritability and restlessness with a high-pitched cry
- Changes in feeding habits
- Crying when picked up or disturbed
  Manifestations in older children include the following:
- Headache upon awakening that improves with emesis
- Anorexia, nausea, and vomiting, usually projectile
- Cognitive, personality, and behavioural changes, including irritability, restlessness, indifference, lethargy, decreased school performance, decreased physical activity and motor performance, drowsiness, increased sleeping, and inability to follow commands
- Diplopia, blurred vision
- Seizures
  Late manifestations of extremely high ICP include the following:
- Confusion or decreased loss of consciousness (LOC), ranging from drowsiness to coma
- Decreased motor response to commands
- Decreased sensation to painful stimuli
- Decreased pupil size and reactivity
- Extension or flexion posturing
- Papilledema and strabismus
- Cheyne–Stokes respirations
- Bradycardia

Diagnostics

- ICP is measured by various devices, from a non-invasive transducer to the more commonly used invasive devices, such as a subarachnoid bolt, an epidural transducer, an

intraventricular catheter transducer, and an anterior fontanelle pressure monitor.
- Normal pressure ranges are 0–15 mm Hg.

Nursing Considerations
- Assist in reducing intra-abdominal and intrathoracic pressures, which contribute to ICP, by elevating the head of the bed by 15–30 degrees.
- Monitor for early changes in ICP by assessing vital signs (increased systolic blood pressure, wide pulse pressure, and bradycardia indicate increased ICP), LOC, respiratory status, motor activity, behaviour, and pupil size and reactivity.
- If appropriate, use a transducer to monitor ICP.
- Assist with treatments and supportive measures, such as hyperventilation, mechanical ventilation, and hypothermia.
- Prevent overhydration, which can lead to cerebral edema and can be fatal, and underhydration for adequate cerebral perfusion pressure; monitor intake and output, and impose fluid restrictions if prescribed.
- Avoid positions or activities that may increase the child's ICP, such as neck vein compression, flexion or extension of the neck, turning the head from side to side, painful or stressful stimuli, and respiratory suctioning or percussion. Use a pressure mattress to avoid skin breakdown and use sand bags to keep the head midline.
- Avoid a noisy environment that can raise ICP and use touch to help decrease ICP.
- Promote normal bowel elimination to prevent an intra-abdominal pressure increase from straining.
- As appropriate, prepare the child for surgical intervention to relieve the increased ICP, such as a subdural tap, ventriculotomy, epidural evacuation, placement of ventricular shunt, decompressive craniectomy, or tumour resection.
- Administer medications as prescribed, including corticosteroids to decrease cerebral edema, osmotic diuretics such as mannitol or urea, sedatives for combative children, and antiseizure agents if seizuring.
- Control hyperthermia from fever with antipyretics and cooling devices to decrease oxygen needs.

Seizure Disorders

Seizures are interruptions in normal brain function resulting from excessive and disorderly abnormal electrical discharges in the brain, which can cause LOC, involuntary body movements, and changes in behaviours, sensation, and the autonomic system. Seizures are more common before 2 years than at any other time. Up to 4% of all children experience at least one seizure by adolescence (Friedman & Ghazala, 2006).

Pathophysiology
- Many conditions can cause seizures. They result from overly active and hypersensitive neurons in the brain that trigger excessive electrical discharges. Seizures are normally contained in a focal area, but if a specific trigger, such as hypoglycemia, is present, they can become generalized.
- The location of the hypersensitive cells and the pattern of discharges determine the clinical manifestations.

- There are three categories of seizures:
  - Generalized seizures involve both hemispheres of the brain, are bilateral and symmetrical, and do not have a local onset.
  - Partial, or focal, seizures involve a small area of the cerebral cortex and have a local onset; these seizures may be simple or complex.
  - Unclassified epileptic seizures, such as neonatal seizures, do not provide enough evidence to allow categorization, so they are put in this classification.
- Underlying possible causes include prenatal or perinatal hypoxia, infections, hemorrhages, allergies, syncope, congenital malformations, metabolic disturbances, lead poisoning, head injuries, drug abuse, alcohol misuse, or tumours.
- Most seizures are idiopathic.
- There is some evidence of a genetic etiological factor in which the seizure threshold is lower in affected individuals.

Clinical Manifestations
For generalized seizures:
- Tonic–clonic (formerly called *grand mal*)—Tonic rigidity, extension of extremities, LOC, eyes roll up, fixed jaw and increased salivation, respiratory cessation, dilated pupils; clonic–rhythmic jerking of extremities, autonomic symptoms, possible incontinence
- Myoclonic—Sudden brief contractions of muscle groups, similar in appearance to an exaggerated startle reflex
- Atonic and akinetic—Sudden, brief loss of muscle tone and postural control, and child falls
- Infantile spasm—Brief flexion of the neck, trunk, or legs or, less frequently, extension
- Absence seizure (formerly called *petit mal*)—Brief periods of unconsciousness, may have tonic or atonic phase or automatisms (such as lip-smacking); often mistaken for daydreaming

For partial seizures:
- Simple partial—Motor or sensory signs—consciousness is usually maintained; may include focal motor component (abnormal movement of leg); sensory component (tingling); autonomic (sweating) or psychic manifestations (déjà vu, anger)
- Complex (psychomotor)—Begins as a simple seizure but progresses to unconsciousness
- Status epilepticus involves recurrent, continuous, generalized seizure activity with the danger of cardiac arrest and brain damage.
- Some children experience an aura prior to the seizures, which is actually a partial seizure that reflects the area of abnormal activity. The aura occurs prior to the seizures and may take the form of odd smells, hallucinations, or a feeling of déjà vu.

Diagnostics
- EEG is done to document abnormal activity.
- Long-term video-EEG is performed to correlate observed seizures with brain electrical activity.

- Blood tests are done to screen for infections and metabolic imbalances.
- MRI may be performed to rule out a brain tumour.
- A lumbar puncture can rule out meningitis.
- A full physical examination and history are necessary.

Therapeutics

- Anticonvulsant medications may be prescribed to raise the threshold of neuronal excitability in predisposed persons. A few of the commonly used agents are phenobarbital, phenytoin, carbamazepine, valproic acid, clonazepam, and gabapentin, with the dosage adjusted as the child grows. Drug levels must be measured.
- Surgery may be indicated to remove the area of involvement if the seizures are caused by a cerebral lesion. For children with incapacitating refractory seizures that cannot be controlled by medication, surgery may be performed.
- A therapeutic diet, such as a ketogenic diet (high-fat, low-carbohydrate, low-protein diet, to induce ketosis), may be recommended in children with absence or other kinds of seizures; this diet is very difficult to maintain.
- Vagus nerve stimulation may be recommended as an additional treatment in clients 12 years of age and older. A subcutaneous signal stimulates the left vagal nerve at the onset of a seizure.

Nursing Considerations

- Obtain a thorough clinical history (birth trauma, medications, injuries, illnesses, family history, seizure descriptions).
- Maintain safety; provide a helmet, pad the bed's side rails, and have oxygen and suction equipment at the bedside.
- During a seizure, do not restrain the child, do not place anything in his or her mouth, remove harmful objects from the area, extend the neck to maintain the airway, position the child on one side to allow secretions to flow from the mouth, loosen clothing, and screen the child for privacy if possible.
- Document all seizure activity and encourage the family to keep a seizure journal, including the following:
  - The apparent trigger, if known or suspected
  - The child's behaviour before the seizure and whether or not there was an aura
  - The time the seizure began and ended
  - The clinical manifestations of the seizure
  - The child's postictal seizure behaviour and symptoms
- Help prevent seizures by preventing the child's exposure to known triggers, such as emotional stress or blinking lights.
- Use precautions with anticonvulsant medications and observe for side effects.
- Provide child and family teaching concerning the nature of the disorder and its possible triggers, seizure precaution measures, diagnostic tests and procedures, potential medication side effects, the importance of not discontinuing medication and of not switching to a different brand of the same medication, the need for periodic re-evaluation of medication effectiveness as well as follow-up and close monitoring of blood work, urinalysis, and vital signs; the importance of encouraging a normal lifestyle, activity limitations, the need to share information about the child's special needs with others, such as teachers and school nurses; adolescent needs, such as information about drugs and alcohol, peer pressure, dating, and getting a driver's licence.

Neural Tube Defects

Neural tube defects (NTDs) are a group of related defects of the CNS involving the cranium or spinal cord, which vary from mildly to severely disabling. NTDs include anencephaly, encephalocele, and spina bifida. Heredity and environmental factors have been implicated; NTDs have also been associated with the interaction of genetic predisposition and folic acid deficiency.

Pathophysiology

- During the third to fourth week of gestation, the embryonic neural plate closes to form the neural tube, which eventually forms the spinal cord and brain.
- The vertebral column develops, along with the spinal cord.
- Normally, the spinal cord and cauda equina are enclosed in a protective sheath of bone and meninges. If the sheath fails to close, leaving either a small opening or an opening the entire length of the spinal cord, this creates various degrees of defects.

Clinical Manifestations

Manifestations vary with the degree of the defect.
- The degree of neurological dysfunction is directly related to the anatomical location of the defect and thus to the nerves involved; sensory disturbances usually parallel motor dysfunction.

Diagnostics

- Diagnosis is made on the basis of a clinical examination; if the sac transilluminates, it usually is a meningocele.
- Other tests include ultrasonography, CT, MRI, and myelography.
- Prenatal detection involves ultrasonography and identifying elevated levels of alpha-fetoprotein in the amniotic fluid between 16 and 18 weeks.

Therapeutics

- No treatment is indicated for spina bifida occulta unless there is neurological damage; if a dermal sinus is present, it may need to be closed surgically.
- Meningocele requires closure as soon after birth as possible; the child should be monitored for postoperative complications that could include hydrocephalus, meningitis, and spinal cord disruption.
- Myelomeningocele requires management by a coordinated interdisciplinary team, including neurology, neurosurgery, pediatrics, urology, orthopedics, rehabilitation, and nursing.
- Skin grafting may be required, and shunting is performed for hydrocephalus.
- Antibiotics are initiated to prevent infection.

- The child will need correction of musculoskeletal deformities and management of urological deficits and bowel control.

Nursing Considerations

For myelomeningocele:

- Before surgery, prevent infection by applying sterile, moist saline soaks to the sac or open lesion and keep them moist.
- Avoid placing a diaper or other covering directly over the lesion, to prevent infection from fecal contamination.
- Prevent trauma and tears to the sac by gently placing the infant prone in an isolette or warmer.
- Know that the infant may require clean intermittent catheterizations if neurogenic bladder is present.
- Help prevent hip subluxation by positioning the legs in abduction with a pad between the knees and the feet in a neutral position with a roll under the ankles.
- Monitor vital signs, measure head circumference, and monitor neurological status, including signs of ICP.
- After surgery, place the child in a prone position if a side-lying position, which is permitted by many neurosurgeons, aggravates the hips.
- Refer parents to the Spina Bifida and Hydrocephalus Association of Canada for resources.
- Provide family teaching for associated problems in the growing child, such as neurogenic bladder and bowel, impaired mobility, skin breakdown, ICP, and possible neurological impairment related to hydrocephalus.
- Carefully assess the family's ability to care for the child and refer them for further assistance if needed.

Hydrocephalus

Hydrocephalus is a condition caused by a blockage to the flow of CSF, or an imbalance in the production and absorption of CSF in the ventricular system. When production exceeds absorption, CSF accumulates, usually under pressure, creating ventricular dilatation. The condition occurs in 1 to 2 births in 1 000 (National Institute of Neurological Disorders and Stroke, 2014). Hydrocephalus is caused by congenital defects, such as myelomeningocele, or acquired conditions, such as intraventricular hemorrhage or CSF infection.

Pathophysiology

- CSF flows from the lateral ventricles through the foramen of Monro to the third ventricle, then through the aqueduct of Sylvius into the fourth ventricle through the foramen of Luschka, and the midline foramen of Magendie into the cisterna magna. From there, it flows to the cerebral and cerebellar subarachnoid spaces, where it is absorbed.
- Causes of hydrocephalus are varied but result in either impaired absorption of CSF within the arachnoid space or obstruction to the flow of CSF through the ventricular system

Therapeutics

- Surgery is the preferred intervention to remove the obstruction.

- A shunt provides primary drainage of the CSF to an extracranial compartment, usually the peritoneum.
- Ventriculoperitoneal shunts consist of a ventricular catheter, a flush pump, a unidirectional flow valve, and a distal catheter.
- Major complications of shunts are infections and malfunction; others include subdural hematoma caused by a too rapid reduction of CSF, peritonitis, abdominal abscess, perforation of organs, fistulas, hernias, and ileus.

Clinical Manifestations

- In infants: The child's head grows at an abnormal rate; signs and symptoms include a bulging fontanelle, a tense anterior fontanelle, often bulging and non-pulsatile; dilated scalp veins; Macewen's sign ("cracked pot sound"); frontal bossing; setting sun sign; sluggish and unequal pupils; irritability and lethargy with varying LOC; abnormal infantile reflexes; and possible cranial nerve damage.
- In children: Signs of ICP include headache on awakening with improvement following emesis; papilledema; strabismus; ataxia, irritability, lethargy, apathy, and confusion.

Diagnostics

- Ultrasonograms can diagnose hydrocephalus at 14 weeks' gestation.
- Cranial transillumination shows varying degrees of localized fluid accumulation.
- CT and MRI scans confirm fluid accumulation and enlarged ventricles.

Nursing Considerations

Preoperative considerations:

- Assess head circumference, fontanelles, cranial sutures, and LOC; also assess for signs of ICP: irritability, altered feeding habits, and high-pitched cry.
- Irritability, seizures, poor feeding, lethargy, and altered vital signs point to an advanced condition.
- Prepare the child and family for diagnostic procedures.
- Carefully support the head and neck when holding or repositioning the child.
- Provide skin care, particularly for the back of the head.
- Offer small, frequent feedings to decrease the risk of vomiting.
- Encourage parental participation in the child's care and promote bonding.
  Postoperative considerations:
- Assess for signs of increased ICP.
- Measure head circumference daily; check the anterior fontanelle for size, tenseness, and fullness.
- Position the child on the side opposite the shunt to prevent pressure on the valve.
- Keep the child flat for the first 24 hours so as not to drain the CSF too quickly.
- Monitor dressings for bloody and clear drainage (the presence of glucose in drainage indicates CSF).
- Monitor the fluid balance.

- Promote natural bowel elimination in children with ventriculoperitoneal shunts, who may have constipation.
- Administer antibiotics as prescribed, IV or intraventricular.
- Monitor for infection, particularly CSF or peritonitis; watch for abdominal distension, which can mean peritonitis from the shunt insertion, or postoperative ileus because of shunt catheter placement.
- Administer osmotic diuretics as prescribed to reduce increased ICP.
- Provide child and family teaching concerning ICP, possible neurological impairment, skin care, and the need for frequent follow-up care.

Head Injury

A head injury is a pathological process that can involve the scalp, skull, or meninges. It can range from a mild injury to severe damage to the head.

Pathophysiology

- Pathophysiology and management are directly related to the force of the impact. Intracranial contents are damaged when the force is too great to be absorbed by the skull and the musculoskeletal support of the head.
- Types of head traumas include skull fractures, contusions, diffuse injuries, and hematomas.
- Head injury is one of the most common causes of disability and death in children.
- Head injury is most frequently caused by motor vehicle accidents, abuse, falls, and birth trauma, with the etiology related to the child's age.

Clinical Manifestations

Skull fractures. The type, extent, and accompanying symptoms of skull fractures depend on the velocity, force, and mass of the object that struck the skull; the area of the skull involved; and the age of the child.

Skull fracture types include the following:

- Linear: This is the most common type of fracture. It resembles a thin line and is from a low-velocity blow. Linear fractures are not often seen in children under 2 or 3 years. There are usually no signs other than those found on X-ray; the child is observed for neurological changes; the fracture heals on its own.
- Comminuted: This type has a "cracked eggshell" appearance and may also be categorized as depressed.
- Depressed: The skull is indented at the point of impact, which may cause compression on the brain, shifting of brain tissue, and intracranial damage; symptoms depend on the area damaged. This fracture may require surgery to lift the bone off the cerebrum. Bone fragments could also tear the dura and cause bleeding.
- Basilar: A linear fracture involving the basilar portion of the frontal, ethmoid, temporal, or occipital bones of the skull, often resulting in a dura tear; classic signs are "raccoon eyes," "Battle's sign" (bruising behind the ear from bleeding into the mastoid sinus), and a possible blood or CSF leak into the ears, nasopharynx, or nose.

Brain injury. Signs and symptoms depend on location and severity; post-traumatic syndromes (seizures, hydrocephalus, focal neurological deficits), and metabolic complications (diabetes insipidus, hyponatremia or hypernatremia, hyperglycemic hyperosmolar states) may occur; all of these may occur up to 2 years after the injury.

Hematomas. Epidural (between the skull and the dura) and subdural (between the dura and arachnoid layer) are the most common types.

- Epidural: life-threatening, with rapid onset, characterized by rapid deterioration, headache, seizures, coma, and brain herniation with compression of the brainstem
- Subdural: occurs within 48 hours of injury, characterized by headache, agitation, confusion, drowsiness, decrease in LOC, and increased ICP; chronic subdural hematomas may also occur

General manifestations of minor head trauma

- May or may not involve LOC
- Transient confusion
- Listlessness and irritability
- Pallor and vomiting
  Signs of deterioration are as follows:
- Altered mental status
- Increasing agitation
- Significant changes in vital signs
- Reflexes hyporesponsive, hyper-responsive, or non-existent

Diagnostics

Fractures may be visualized by X-ray; brain injuries and hematomas are viewed by CT or MRI.

Therapeutics

- Therapeutic interventions depend on symptoms, which must be closely observed and monitored.
- Surgical evacuation of hematomas may be needed and may be facilitated by burr holes for evacuation and relief of increased ICP; depressed skull fractures need to be elevated surgically.
- Scalp and dural lacerations may require sutures.

Nursing Considerations

- Promote prevention of injury, especially of falls.
- Promote safety practices, including the use of bike helmets, seat belts, and protective sports equipment; encourage safe driving.
- Perform neurological assessments of cerebral functioning (alertness, orientation, memory, speech), vital signs (check for increased blood pressure, decreased pulse), pupils, and motor and sensory function.
- Assess for cervical and other injuries.
- To help decrease cerebral edema, and if there is no cervical injury, raise the head of the bed to 30 degrees.
- Monitor for complications, which can develop rapidly; monitor vital signs and neurological status frequently; and check for increased ICP and for drainage (of CSF or blood) from the nose and ears.

- Be aware that seizures may occur for up to 2 years after injury.
- Be aware that the child may also require rehabilitation following an extensive brain injury.
- Provide child and family teaching:
  - Discuss complications and what to observe for in post-traumatic syndrome.
  - Refer family members to the Brain Injury Canada.

Intellectual Disability

Intellectual disability (ID), or cognitive impairment (formerly known as "mental retardation"), is part of a broad category of developmental disability. The condition is now defined by the American Association on Intellectual and Developmental Disabilities as "a disability characterized by significant limitations both in intellectual functioning and in adaptive behaviour as expressed in conceptual, social, and practical adaptive skills. This disability originates before the age of 18" (American Association on Intellectual and Developmental Disabilities, 2008).

Pathophysiology

- Pathophysiology depends on cause.
- Early diagnosis and prompt treatment may be particularly important in cases involving an identifiable and possibly correctable cause, such as hypothyroidism phenylketonuria, malnutrition, or child abuse.
- A diagnosis of ID cannot be made on the basis of intellectual ability alone; there must be both adaptive (personal independence and social responsibility) and intellectual impairment.
- Causes include infection and intoxication, trauma or physical agents, metabolic or nutritional abnormalities, gross postnatal brain disease, unknown prenatal conditions, chromosomal abnormalities, gestational disorders, psychiatric disorders with onset during the child's developmental period, such as autism, and environmental influences (Hockenberry & Wilson, 2015).

Diagnostics

- Diagnosis usually is made after a period of suspicion, although it may be made at birth from recognition of a specific syndrome, such as Down syndrome.
- Diagnosis and classification are based on a variety of standardized IQ test scores.

Clinical Manifestations

Manifestations vary, depending on the classification or degree of disability.

Mild ID (50–70 IQ):
- Preschool—Often the child is not noted as having a disability but is slow to walk, talk, and feed himself or herself.
- School age—The child can acquire practical skills and learn to read and do arithmetic to a sixth grade level; with special education, the child achieves a mental age of 8–12 years.

- Adult—Adults can usually achieve social and vocational skills, may need occasional guidance, and may handle marriage but have difficulty with parenting.

Moderate ID (35–55 IQ):
- Preschool—The child has noticeable delays, especially in speech.
- School age—The child can learn simple communication, health and safety habits, and simple manual skills; he or she has a mental age of 3–7 years.
- Adult—Adults can perform simple tasks under sheltered conditions and can travel alone to familiar places but usually need help with self-maintenance.

Severe ID (20–40 IQ):
- Preschool—The child exhibits marked motor delays and few communication skills; he or she may respond to training in elementary self-help, such as feeding.
- School age—The child usually walks with difficulty, has some understanding of and may respond to speech, can respond to habit training, and has the mental age of a toddler.
- Adult—Adults can conform to daily routines and repetitive activities but need constant direction and supervision in a protective environment.

Profound ID (<20 IQ):
- Preschool—The child exhibits gross intellectual disability, has some capacity for function in sensorimotor areas, and needs total care.
- School age—The child displays obvious delays in all areas; shows a basic emotional response; may respond to skilful training in the use of the legs, hands, and jaws; needs close supervision; and has the mental age of a young infant.
- Adult—A profoundly delayed adult may walk but has primitive speech and needs complete custodial care; he or she usually benefits from regular physical activity.

Therapeutics

- The treatment goal is to promote optimal development.
- Preventive measures include regular prenatal care, support for high-risk infants, rubella immunization, genetic counselling, education, and injury reduction.

Nursing Considerations

- Support the family at the time of the initial diagnosis.
- Facilitate the child's self-care abilities through an early stimulation program, self-feeding, independent toileting, and independent grooming.
- Promote optimal development by encouraging self-care goals and emphasizing the universal needs of children, such as play, social interaction, and parental limit-setting.
- Assist the family in planning for the child's future needs.
- Refer parents to appropriate community agencies.
- Discuss the need for patience with the child's slow attainment of developmental milestones.
- Discuss stimulation and safety.
- Demonstrate communication strategies; accentuate non-verbal cues, such as facial expressions and body language, to help cue speech development.

- Explain the need for discipline that is simple, consistent, and appropriate to the child's development.
- Review an adolescent's need for simple, practical sexual information.
- Discuss the importance of positive self-esteem, built by accomplishing small successes, in motivating the child to accomplish other tasks.

Down Syndrome

Down syndrome is the most common chromosomal abnormality. This condition occurs more in individuals of European descent than in other groups.

Pathophysiology

- Approximately 95% of cases may be attributed to an extra chromosome on chromosome 21—hence the name *non-familial trisomy 21* (Canadian Down Syndrome Society, 2018a).
- Two out of three cases may be caused by translocation of chromosomes 15 and 21 or 22; this usually is hereditary and is not related to maternal age (Canadian Down Syndrome Society, 2018a).
- Children with Down syndrome are born to parents of all ages.
- There is a higher statistical risk for mothers over age 35, but most are born to mothers under this age, likely due to prenatal screening for women in older age groups as well as the option of abortion.
- The level of cognitive and physical impairment is related to the percentage of cells with the abnormal chromosome makeup.

Clinical Manifestations

- The most common findings include separated sagittal suture, oblique palpebral fissures, small nose, depressed nasal bridge, high-arched palate, skin excess and laxity, wide space between the big and second toes, plantar crease between the big and second toes, hyperextensible and lax joints, and muscle weakness.
- Other common findings include a small penis, short, broad hands (with a transverse [simian] palmar crease), protruding tongue, small ears, Brushfield spots, and dry skin.
- Associated problems and features include the following:
  - Intelligence varies from severely disabled to low-normal but is generally within the mild to moderate range.
  - Social development may be 2–3 years beyond mental age; temperament range is similar to that of normal children, with a trend toward the "easy" child.
  - Forty to 45% have congenital heart disease, especially septal defects (Canadian Down Syndrome Society, 2018b).
  - Other defects include renal agenesis, duodenal atresia, Hirschsprung's disease, tracheoesophageal fistula, and skeletal deformities.
  - Sensory problems include strabismus, nystagmus, myopia, hyperopia, cataracts and excessive tearing, and conductive hearing loss.

- Other physical disorders may include altered immune function, respiratory infections, leukemia, thyroid dysfunction, and early aging.
- Individuals have a shortened stature with a tendency for rapid weight gain.
- Sexual development may be delayed, incomplete, or both.
- Male genitalia and secondary characteristics are underdeveloped; men are infertile.
- Female breast development is mild to moderate with menarche at an appropriate age; women may be fertile.

Diagnostics

Diagnosis is made by physical examination and chromosomal analysis.

Therapeutics

- Surgery may be used to correct some accompanying defects.
- Behaviour modification may be recommended for dealing with negative behaviours.
- Developmental, social, and educational supports will likely be required.

Nursing Considerations

- Implement nursing care as with ID.
- Support parental genetic counselling.
- Explain hypertonicity and joint hyperextensibility to parents.
- Know that feeding can take longer in the infant due to the large tongue and weak suck.
- For the older child, use a small, straight-handled spoon to push food to the side and back of the mouth.
- Monitor for common associated congenital anomalies, especially cardiac.

COMMUNICABLE DISEASES OF CHILDHOOD

Measles (Rubeola)

Rubeola, or "red measles," is a communicable disease that has been largely eradicated in Canada. Occasional outbreaks are primarily related to people who have been inadequately immunized.

Pathophysiology

- Rubeola, or measles, is a communicable virus that is usually transmitted by direct contact with droplets.
- Incubation time is 10–20 days, and infected individuals are contagious from 4 days before to 5 days after the rash appears.

Clinical Manifestations

- Stage 1: The prodromal stage includes fever and malaise; 24 hours later, acute rhinitis, cough, conjunctivitis with photophobia, and Kolick spots (white spots in the mouth) develop.

- Stage 2: Three to 4 days after the prodromal stage, a rash appears, causing red maculopapular lesions on the face and spreading down toward the trunk and extremities. The rash changes to a browner colour in 3–4 days; fine peeling of the skin begins in the more severely affected regions.
- Potential complications include otitis media, pneumonia, laryngotracheitis, and encephalitis.

Diagnostics

- Assessment of rash
- Antibody titres

Nursing Considerations

- Provide comfort measures, including antipyretics, skin care with oatmeal, cleansing the eyes if conjunctivitis develops, and sunglasses and dim lights for the photophobia.
- Promote childhood immunization. Rubeola is preventable with a vaccine.

Rubella

Rubella, or "German measles," is a communicable disease that, like rubeola, is now largely eradicated in Canada. However, outbreaks are of concern to the public as this disease may cause severe birth defects if contracted by pregnant women.

Pathophysiology

- The rubella virus is transmitted by direct and indirect contact.
- The incubation period is 14–21 days.
- The child is communicable for 7 days before to approximately 5 days after the rash appears.

Clinical Manifestations

- A reddish-pink maculopapular rash begins on the face and spreads downward to the trunk and extremities.
- The rash disappears first in the initial lesions.
- Symptoms also include a low-grade fever, malaise, and lymphadenopathy.
- Complications include possible damage to the fetus in a pregnant woman and, rarely, encephalitis, arthritis, or purpura.

Diagnostics

Diagnosis is generally based on observation of rash and antibody titres.

Nursing Considerations

- Provide comfort measures for the child.
- Advise the parents of the danger to pregnant women of exposure to a communicable child.
- Promote childhood immunization. Rubella is preventable with a vaccine.

Chicken Pox (Varicella)

Chicken pox is an uncomfortable, communicable disease of children and adults. It may leave scars and create a significant health risk for the immuno-compromised child.

Pathophysiology

- Varicella zoster is the communicable agent.
- Infection is transmitted by direct contact and via contaminated objects.
- The child is communicable for 1–2 days before the rash appears and remains infectious until all of the lesions are crusted over.

Diagnostics

Diagnosis is based on assessment of rash and antibody titres.

Clinical Manifestations

- The prodromal stage involves low-grade fever, malaise, and loss of appetite.
- Rash starts on the face with macules that turn to papules, then vesicles, then pustules, and finally crusts. The rash then spreads to the proximal extremities, with fewer lesions in distal areas.
- Lesions can also appear on the mucous membranes.
- The lesions cause severe itching.
- Other symptoms include fever, lymphadenopathy, and irritability from itching.
- Complications are secondary infections, such as encephalitis, pneumonia, and hemorrhagic varicella in immuno-compromised children.

Nursing Considerations

- Know that strict isolation until vesicles are dry is necessary to prevent spread.
- Provide comfort measures: a cool environment, cool oatmeal baths to soothe itchy and irritated skin and decrease the risk of secondary infection and scarring from scratching, loose clothing, antihistamines, and antipyretics.
- Know that zoster immune globulin (ZIG) and acyclovir are given to children who are immuno-compromised.
- Promote childhood immunization. Varicella is preventable with a vaccine.

Pertussis (Whooping Cough)

Pertussis is a potentially serious disease in the infant. Occasional outbreaks of pertussis occur in Canada despite adequate immunization.

Pathophysiology

- The infectious bacterium is *Bordetella pertussis*.
- The incubation period is 6–20 days, with an average of 7 days.
- Stage 1: The catarrhal stage, when the child has signs of an upper respiratory infection; 1 or 2 weeks later, the hacking cough increases in severity.
- Stage 2: The paroxysmal stage, which usually lasts 4–6 weeks. The child has the classic paroxysmal "whoop" cough, which usually occurs at night; the child is flushed or has a cyanotic face, bulging eyes, and a protruding tongue and coughs until he or she coughs up a mucous plug, often vomiting afterward.
- Stage 3: The convalescent stage, in which the cough slowly decreases, vomiting stops, and strength returns.

- Complications include atelectasis, otitis media, seizures, hemorrhage, weight loss, and dehydration.
- In infants, apnea and respiratory arrest from a mucous plug can occur.

Diagnostics

Diagnosis is based on the characteristic cough and a throat swab for culture.

Nursing Considerations

- Maintain isolation.
- Use respiratory precautions.
- Provide a quiet environment, encourage fluids, and monitor for respiratory distress.
- Promote childhood immunization. Pertussis is preventable with a vaccine.

Mumps

Mumps is an infectious disease of the parotid glands. Occasional outbreaks occur in Canada despite adequate immunization.

Pathophysiology

- The infectious agent is paramyxovirus.
- Transmission is by direct contact or droplet.

- The incubation period is 14–21 days.
- The child is communicable immediately before the swelling occurs until immediately after.
- Symptoms of the prodromal stage are pyrexia, headache, and loss of appetite followed by earache, which worsens with chewing.
- The second acute stage occurs by the second day with parotid gland swelling, which is painful and peaks in 1–3 days.
- Complications include meningoencephalitis, orchitis, epididymitis, arthritis, and, rarely, sterility in males.

Diagnostics

Mumps is generally diagnosed by the characteristic facial swelling produced.

Nursing Considerations

- Ensure isolation and bed rest with respiratory precautions.
- Administer analgesics and fluids and provide warmth and support for orchitis.
- Promote childhood immunization. Mumps is preventable with a vaccine.

PRACTICE QUESTIONS

Case 1

Simon is a 6-year-old boy who is brought by his parents to the emergency department of a local hospital. The triage practical nurse assesses that Simon has tachypnea, wheezing, and diminished air entry. The physician diagnoses asthma.

Questions 1–5 refer to this case.

1. In addition to wheezing and tachypnea, Simon manifests other clinical signs of an acute asthma attack. Which of the following are signs of respiratory distress seen in childhood asthma?
   1. Tripod position with refusal to lie down
   2. Harsh, barking cough on inspiration
   3. Shallow breathing with periods of apnea
   4. Continuous respiratory stridor
2. Simon's initial treatment is salbutamol (Ventolin) by inhalation. During the inhalation, Simon begins to shake. What should the practical nurse do?
   1. Stop the inhalation immediately.
   2. Reassure Simon that this is a side effect of the Ventolin.
   3. Provide Simon with a warm blanket.
   4. Reduce the flow of air or oxygen in the inhalation.
3. Which of the following is an appropriate and appealing diet for Simon while he is experiencing respiratory distress?
   1. Ice cream
   2. Macaroni and cheese
   3. Clear beef soup
   4. Ice pops (Popsicles)

4. Simon's parents ask the practical nurse how they can prevent further episodes of asthma. What would be the most appropriate response by the practical nurse?
   1. "We can discuss developing a plan to manage the asthma."
   2. "It is difficult to prevent asthma attacks in children Simon's age, so you need to know how to treat each attack."
   3. "You need to find out what particular triggers cause Simon's attacks."
   4. "Simon needs to take his asthma medications all the time, even when he is not wheezing."
5. The practical nurse assesses that Simon's environment has many potential allergens, for example, pet dander, dust, and second-hand smoke. Prior to discharge, the practical nurse reviews strategies for Simon's parents to modify the environment in order to reduce these allergens. Before discharge home, which of the following is the most important action that can be immediately implemented by the parents?
   1. Remove Simon's dog from the home.
   2. Stop smoking cigarettes in the car.
   3. Have a high-energy particulate air (HEPA) filter installed.
   4. Wet dust all floors and surfaces, particularly in Simon's bedroom.

Case 2

Leah is a healthy 9-month-old infant brought to the community health clinic by her parents. The nurse performs an assessment and health teaching.

Questions 6–10 refer to this case.

6. Leah's parents ask the practical nurse what to do when their daughter has a "cold" with a low-grade temperature. What would the practical nurse respond?
   1. Take Leah to the doctor if the symptoms continue for 2 days.
   2. Give her infant acetylsalicylic acid (Aspirin) as directed on the bottle.
   3. If she is uncomfortable, give her pediatric acetaminophen (Tylenol) or ibuprofen.
   4. Administer an over-the-counter cold remedy formulated for infants.

7. Leah's parents ask for advice on toys that are best for developing her motor abilities. Which of the following are most appropriate for motor development?
   1. Putting her in an infant walker with rollers
   2. Giving her several types of baby rattles
   3. Reading a book to her at bedtime every night
   4. Letting her play with kitchen utensils, such as bowls and spoons

8. The practical nurse discusses infant safety with Leah's parents. Which of the following safety precautions would the practical nurse advise?
   1. Do not give Leah finger foods until she is 18 months of age.
   2. Place pillows around Leah when she is in her crib.
   3. Dress Leah in clothes with Velcro fasteners.
   4. Check all toys for small movable parts.

9. As part of Leah's assessment, the nurse reaches out to Leah to take her vital signs. Leah begins to scream and cling to her father. What should the practical nurse do?
   1. Remove Leah gently from her father.
   2. Postpone the taking of vital signs for another visit.
   3. Talk softly at eye level with Leah.
   4. Hold her arms out and smile at Leah.

10. The practical nurse discusses developmental milestones with Leah's parents. She asks them about Leah's ability to vocalize and understand language. What vocalization milestone is appropriate for a 9-month-old infant?
    1. Responds to simple verbal commands and understands "no-no"
    2. Produces repetitive vowel sounds such as "baba" and "kaka"
    3. Begins to imitate sounds
    4. Says three to five words in addition to "mama" and "dada"

Case 3

A daycare that provides care for children with health problems asks a community practical nurse for a consultation about safe health practices.

Questions 11–15 refer to this case.

11. One of the children who attends the daycare centre has a severe peanut allergy. What would the practical nurse recommend to best prevent potential sources of peanuts from coming in contact with the children?
    1. Do not allow parents to bring homemade food to share with the other children.
    2. Send home a letter to the parents informing them of a ban on foods containing peanuts.
    3. Identify all children at the daycare centre who have a documented allergy to peanuts.
    4. Examine all food given to the children for sources of peanuts.

12. Many of the children develop communicable diseases, particularly upper respiratory infections and diarrhea during the fall and winter seasons. The practical nurse is asked about best practices for caregivers to reduce the incidence of infectious diseases with the children. Which of the following would the practical nurse recommend?
    1. All workers should wash their hands with alcohol-based cleaner after changing diapers.
    2. Child care staff should wash their hands several times throughout the day.
    3. All equipment and toys should be washed with an antibacterial solution between uses by children.
    4. Any child who develops signs of a communicable disease during the day should be immediately separated from the other children.

13. Jayden is a 4-month-old infant with heart failure secondary to a congenital heart defect. The practical nurse discusses optimal feeding strategies for Jayden with the daycare workers. Which of the following should the practical nurse advise?
    1. Feed Jayden on an every-2-hour schedule.
    2. Provide frequent rest breaks when feeding Jayden by bottle.
    3. Dilute formula feeds so that excess energy is not required for sucking.
    4. Gavage feed Jayden to conserve his energy.

14. The practical nurse has heard that there is a community outbreak of chicken pox. She is concerned about the children in the daycare centre as many are immunocompromised. What immunization should the practical nurse ensure that each child has received?
    1. Varicella
    2. MMR
    3. Hib
    4. DTaP

15. Shobana, one of the children attending the daycare centre, has been discovered to have head lice. What would the practical nurse recommend to the staff of the centre to control the spread of the head lice?
    1. Notify all families that Shobana has head lice and if their children have been playing with her, they should examine their children's hair.
    2. Send a letter to all parents about the outbreak with instructions for examining their child's hair and recommended treatment.
    3. Examine the hair of all children as they arrive at the daycare centre and prohibit attendance if lice are found.
    4. Treat all of the children with the recommended pediculicide shampoo.

Independent Questions

Questions 16–25 do not refer to a particular case.

16. James, age 2 months, has diaper dermatitis (diaper rash). What would the practical nurse recommend to the parents to treat this problem?
    1. Expose the diaper area to air whenever possible.
    2. Use a hair dryer or heat lamp to dry the area.
    3. Wash the area completely with commercial wipes after every diaper change.
    4. Use talc on the diaper area to absorb moisture.

17. A 6-year-old has been admitted to the pediatric unit with a new diagnosis of type 1 diabetes mellitus. The practical nurse is to health teach about monitoring blood glucose levels. This health teaching needs to include:
    1. Taking the blood glucose level is completed only once in the morning before breakfast.
    2. The ideal blood glucose level is between 4 to 7 mmol/L.
    3. Dietary restrictions need to be followed to keep the blood glucose levels low.
    4. The child will need to monitor his or her own blood glucose levels at school.

18. Mr. and Mrs. Kaplan are the parents of a newborn who has Down syndrome. They ask the practical nurse what to expect when they take their infant home. What potential problems might the practical nurse discuss with the parents?
    1. Possible difficulty with feedings
    2. An increase in infections due to a decreased immune system
    3. An inability to respond to affection
    4. A gradual deterioration in developmental milestones

19. Candace, age 16 years, is hospitalized during a vaso-occlusive sickle cell crisis. Which of the following is an appropriate nursing intervention?
    1. Administer analgesics prn.
    2. Monitor intake and output.
    3. Promote exercise.
    4. Apply cold compresses to painful joints.

20. A mother brings her 2-month-old infant to the health clinic, stating that the child has long episodes of crying with apparent abdominal pain and cannot be comforted. The infant is formula-fed. What would be an appropriate initial nursing intervention?
    1. Obtain a detailed history of the infant's diet, daily routine, and description of the crying episodes/
    2. Suggest a change to another formula as the symptoms are likely colic caused by an allergy to cow's milk/
    3. Discuss the advisability of initiating breastfeeding using techniques to re-establish the production of breast milk.
    4. Tell the mother that her infant is displaying classic manifestations of colic, and burping the infant more often along with comfort measures will correct the problem.

21. What are the most common forms of childhood malignancy in Canada?
    1. Leukemias
    2. Lymphomas
    3. Central nervous system tumours
    4. Renal tumours

22. Jamal, age 17 years, is a refugee who has recently arrived in Canada. He speaks with a male practical nurse in the clinic concerning an "embarrassing problem" he would like to have fixed. The practical nurse examines Jamal and finds he has hypospadias. What would the practical nurse explain to Jamal?
    1. "A doctor can bring your testicles down into your scrotum, but you may be infertile."
    2. "Your urethra opens on the top side of the penis and can probably be fixed by a surgeon."
    3. "Your penis is small as a result of an inherited condition, but it can be enlarged."
    4. "I will refer you to a urologist who will surgically repair the abnormal opening on the underside of your penis."

23. A practical nurse works on a pediatric surgical unit with children experiencing postoperative pain. Which of the following is correct concerning pain in children?
    1. It is not possible to accurately assess pain in children.
    2. Use of narcotics in children is not recommended for pain control.
    3. Children are often undertreated for pain.
    4. Children always tell the truth about pain.

24. The practical nurse must administer a suspension of oral prednisone to a toddler. The prednisone solution is known to have a bitter taste. The child spat out the previous dose and is refusing to take the medicine. What is the most effective action to administer the prednisone?
    1. Have the parent assist the practical nurse in administering the prednisone.
    2. Ask the physician to change the liquid form to a suppository.
    3. Restrain the child and administer the prednisone via oral syringe.
    4. Mix the prednisone in applesauce.

25. A practical nurse is being orientated to the pediatric unit at the hospital. The unit's philosophy is to provide family-centred care. Which of the following is an example of this approach to care?
    1. The family is included in the morning discussions with the health care team.
    2. The family receives lab values through a Web site at the hospital.
    3. The children are given free access to the Internet to complete school work.
    4. The children will need to follow a bedtime schedule based on their age.

REFERENCES

AboutKidsHealth. (2017). Attention-deficit/hyperactivity disorder (ADHD) resource centre Retrieved from http://www.aboutkidshealth.ca/En/ResourceCentres/ADHD/Pages/default.aspx.

Ambert, A. (2009). *Divorce: facts, causes and consequences* (3rd ed.). Toronto: York University Sociology Department. Retrieved from http://canadianbudgetbinder.com/wp-content/uploads/2016/10/FELDSTEIN-FAMILY-LAW-Divorce-Fact-Sheet-2016.pdf.

American Association on Intellectual and Developmental Disability. (2008). Definition of intellectual disability. Retrieved from http://aaidd.org/education/education-archive#.WYob9LpFy71.

Anabwani, M. G., Woldetsadik, E. A., & Kline, M. W. (2005). Treatment of human immunodeficiency virus (HIV) in children using antiretroviral drugs. *Seminars in Pediatric Infectious Disease*, 16, 116–124.

Autism Speaks Canada. (2017). About autism, diagnosis, screening and treatments. Retrieved from http://www.autismspeaks.ca/about-autism/diagnosis/screen-your-child/.

Ball, J. W., Bindler, R. C., & Cowen, J. (2014). *Child health nursing: Partnering with children & families* (3rd ed.). Upper Saddle River, NJ: Pearson/Prentice Hall.

Canadian Cancer Society. (2018a). Childhood cancer statistics. Retrieved from http://www.cancer.ca/en/cancer-information/cancer-101/childhood-cancer-statistics/?region=on.

Canadian Cancer Society. (2018b). What is childhood leukemia? Retrieved from http://www.cancer.ca/en/cancer-information/cancer-type/leukemia-childhood/childhood-leukemia/?region=on.

Canadian Celiac Association. (2016). Screening and diagnosis of celiac disease. Retrieved from https://www.celiac.ca/healthcare-professionals/diagnosis/.

Canadian Dental Association. (2017a). Cleaning teeth. Retrieved from http://www.cda-adc.ca/en/oral_health/cfyt/dental_care_children.

Canadian Dental Association. (2017b). First visit first tooth. Retrieved from http://www.cda-adc.ca/en/oral_health/cfyt/dental_care_children.

Canadian Down Syndrome Society. (2018a). About Down Syndrome: Types of Down syndrome. Retrieved from http://cdss.ca/resources/about-down-syndrome/.

Canadian Down Syndrome Society. (2018b). Down syndrome health and medical information. Retrieved from http://cdss.ca/resources/health/.

Canadian Institute for Health Information. (2018). Asthma hospital stays by children and youth 2015–2016. Retrieved from https://www.cihi.ca/en/asthma-hospital-stays-by-children-and-youth.

Canadian Institutes of Health Research. (2016). The future of cystic fibrosis treatment. Retrieved from http://www.cihr-irsc.gc.ca/e/49665.html.

Canadian Paediatric Society. (2007). Vitamin D supplementation: Recommendations for Canadian mothers and infants [Reaffirmed 2017]. Retrieved from https://www.cps.ca/en/documents/position/vitamin-d.

Canadian Paediatric Society. (2008). Multidisciplinary guidelines on the identification, investigation and management of suspected abusive head trauma. Retrieved from https://www.cps.ca/en/documents/position/multidisciplinary-guidelines-abusive-head-trauma.

Canadian Paediatric Society. (2017). Caring for kids: Using over-the-counter drugs to treat cold symptoms. Retrieved from https://www.caringforkids.cps.ca/handouts/over_the_counter_drugs.

Cerebral Palsy Alliance Research Foundation. (2018). Causes of Cerebral palsy. Retrieved from https://research.cerebralpalsy.org.au/what-is-cerebral-palsy/causes.

Cincinnati Children's Hospital. (2016). Ventricular septal defects. Retrieved from https://www.cincinnatichildrens.org/health/v/vsd.

Couture, E., Labbe, V., & Cyre, C. (2003). Clinical predictors of positive urine cultures in young children at risk for urinary tract infection. *Paediatrics & Child Health*, 8(3), 145–149.

Crain, J., McFaull, S., Rao, D. P., et al. (2017). Emergency department surveillance of burns and scalds, electronic Canadian hospitals injury reporting and prevention program, 2013. *Health Promotion and Chronic Disease Prevention in Canada: Research, Policy and Practice*, 37(1), Retrieved from https://www.canada.ca/content/dam/phac-aspc/migration/phac-aspc/publicat/hpcdp-pspmc/37-1/assets/pdf/ar-03-eng.pdf.

Cummings, C., Finlay, J. C., MacDonald, N. E., et al. (2018). Practice point: Head lice infestations: A clinical update. Retrieved from https://www.cps.ca/en/documents/position/head-lice.

Cyr, C., & Canadian Paediatric Society, & Injury Prevention Committee. (2012). Preventing choking and suffocation in children. *Paediatrics & Child Health*, 17(2), 91–92.

Denison, M. R. (2005). Severe acute respiratory syndrome: coronavirus pathogenesis, disease and vaccines: an update. *The Pediatric Infectious Disease Journal*, 23(11, Suppl.), S207–S214.

Erickson, E. (1963). *Childhood and society*. New York: W.W. Norton.

Fowler, J. (1981). *Stages of faith: the psychology of human development and the quest for meaning*. New York: HarperCollins.

Friedman, M. J., & Ghazala, S. Q. (2006). Seizures in children. *Pediatric Clinics of North America*, 53(4), 257–277.

Government of Canada. (2018). Child car seat safety. Retrieved from http://www.tc.gc.ca/en/services/road/child-car-seat-safety/choosing-child-car-seat-booster-seat.html.

Government of Canada. (2013). Congenital anomalies in Canada 2013. Retrieved from http://publications.gc.ca/collections/collection_2014/aspc-phac/HP35-40-2013-eng.pdf.

Government of Canada. (2018). Consumer Product Safety. Retrieved from https://www.canada.ca/en/health-canada/services/consumer-product-safety/reports-publications/industry-professionals/industry-guide-second-hand-products-including-children-products/guidance-document.html#a8.9.

Health Canada (2011). *Eating well with Canada's food guide*. Ottawa: Author. Retrieved from http://www.hc-sc.gc.ca/fn-an/food-guide-aliment/index_e.html.

Health Canada. (2012a). Clinical practice guidelines for nurses in primary care—Pediatric and adolescent care. Retrieved from https://www.canada.ca/en/public-health/services/health-promotion/stop-family-violence/snapshot-family-violence-canada-infographic.html.

Health Canada. (2012b). Nutrition for healthy term infants: Recommendations from birth to six months. Retrieved from https://www.canada.ca/en/health-canada/services/food-nutrition/healthy-eating/infant-feeding/nutrition-healthy-term-infants-recommendations-birth-six-months.html.

Ho, J., Seller, E., Dean, H., et al. (2010). Prevalence and associated risk factors for secondary diabetes in Canadian children followed in pediatric tertiary care centre. *Canadian Journal of Diabetes*, 34(2), 107–112. Retrieved from https://www.canadianjournalofdiabetes.com/article/S1499-2671(10)42006-7/pdf.

Hockenberry, M., Rodgers, C., & Wilson, D. (2017). *Wong's essentials of pediatric nursing* (10th ed.). St. Louis: Elsevier.

Hockenberry, M., & Wilson, D. (2011). *Wong's nursing care of infants and children* (9th ed.). St. Louis: Elsevier/Mosby.

Hockenberry, M., & Wilson, D. (2015). *Wong's nursing care of infants and children* (10th ed.). St. Louis: Elsevier/Mosby.

Jefferies, A., & Canadian Paediatric Society. (2017). Position statement: management of term infants at increased risk for early onset bacterial sepsis. *Paediatrics & Child Health*, 22(4), 223–228. doi:10.1093/pch/pxx023.

Le Saux, N., & Canadian Paediatric Society, & Infectious Diseases and Immunization Committee. (2014). Position statement: Guidelines for the management of suspected and confirmed bacterial meningitis in Canadian children older than one month of age [Reaffirmed 2017]. https://www.cps.ca/en/documents/position/management-of-bacterial-meningitis.

LeBlanc, J. C., Pless, I. B., King, W. J., et al. (2006). Home safety measures and the risk of unintentional injury in young children: a multi-centre case-control study. *Canadian Medical Association Journal*, 175, 883–887.

Lerner, R. M. (2002). *Adolescence*. Upper Saddle River, NJ: Pearson Education.

Leung, A., Prince, T., Canadian Paediatric Society, et al. (2006). Oral rehydration therapy and early refeeding in the management of childhood gastroenteritis. *Paediatrics & Child Health*, 11(8), 527–531.

McGrath, P. J., Johnson, G., Goodman, J. T., et al. (1985). The CHEOPS: A behavioural scale for rating post-operative pain in children. In H. L. Fields, R. Dubner, & F. Cervero (Eds.), *Advances in pain research and therapy*. New York: Raven Press.

National Institute of Neurological Disorders and Stroke. (2014). Hydrocephalus fact sheet. Retrieved from http://www.ninds.nih.gov/disorders/hydrocepha-lus/detail_hydrocephalus.htm.

Parachute: Preventing Injuries, Saving Lives. (2018). About child injury prevention. Retrieved from http://www.parachutecanada.org/child-injury-prevention.

Piaget, J. (1972). *The child's conception of the world*. Totowa, NJ: Littlefield, Adams.

Public Health Agency of Canada. (2018a). Canadian immunization guide. Retrieved from https://www.canada.ca/en/public-health/services/publications/healthy-living/canadian-immunization-guide-part-1-key-immunization-information/page-13-recommended-immunization-schedules.html.

Public Health Agency of Canada. (2018b). Family violence: How big is the problem in Canada? Retrieved from https://www.canada.ca/en/public-health/services/health-promotion/stop-family-violence/problem-canada.html.

Public Health Agency of Canada. (2018c). Safe sleep. Retrieved from https://www.canada.ca/en/public-health/services/health-promotion/childhood-adolescence/stages-childhood/infancy-birth-two-years/safe-sleep.html.

Saylor, K. (2010). Risk reduction for type 2 diabetes in Aboriginal children in Canada. Retrieved from https://www.cps.ca/en/documents/position/risk-reduction-type-two-diabetes-aboriginal-children.

SickKids. (2017). Family-centred care. Retrieved from http://www.sickkids.ca/Nursing/Education-and-learning/Nursing-Student-Orientation/Family-Centered-Care/index.html.

Sickle Cell Disease Association of Canada. (n.d.). Novel drugs. Retrieved from http://sicklecelldisease.ca/care_treatment.php.

Statistics Canada. (2016). Census in brief: Portrait of children's family life in Canada in 2016. Retrieved from http://www12.statcan.gc.ca/census-recensement/2016/as-sa/98-200-x/2016006/98-200-x2016006-eng.cfm.

Statistics Canada. (2018). Deaths and age-specific mortality rates, by selected grouped causes. Retrieved from https://www150.statcan.gc.ca/t1/tbl1/en/tv.action?pid=1310039201&pickMembers%5B0%5D=2.6&pickMembers%5B1%5D=3.1.

Stevens, B., Johnston, C., Petryshen, P., et al. (1996). Premature infant pain profile: development and initial validation. *The Clinical Journal of Pain*, 12(1), 13–22.

Theadom, A., Rodrigues, M., Roxburgh, R., et al. (2014). Prevalence of muscular dystrophies: a systematic literature review. *Neuroepidemiology*, 43, 259–268. Retrieved from https://www.karger.com/Article/FullText/369343.

Thiedke, C. C. (2001). Sleep disorders and sleep problems in childhood. *American Family Physician*, 63(2), 277–284.

Transport Canada. (2018). Stage 3: booster seats. Retrieved from https://www.tc.gc.ca/en/services/road/child-car-seat-safety/installing-using-child-car-seat-booster-seat-seat-belt/stage-3-booster-seats.html#move.

UCSF Pediatric Cardiothoracic Surgery. (2018). Congenital heart disease. Retrieved from https://pediatricct.surgery.ucsf.edu/conditions--procedures/congenital-heart-disease.aspx.

Vanier Institute of the Family. (2015). Definition of the family. Retrieved from https://vanierinstitute.ca/family-definition-diversity/.

BIBLIOGRAPHY

Jarvis, C., Browne, A. J., MacDonald-Jenkins, J., et al. (2018). *Physical examination & health assessment* (3rd Cdn. ed.). Toronto: Saunders.

Muscari, M. E. (2005). *Pediatric nursing* (4th ed.). Lippincott's Review Series. Ambler, PA: Lippincott Williams & Wilkins.

Potter, P., Perry, A., Stockert, P., et al. (2019). *Canadian fundamentals of nursing* (6th ed.). Milton, ON: Elsevier.

WEB SITES

- **AboutKidsHealth** (http://www.aboutkidshealth.ca): This site is hosted by the Hospital for Sick Children. It has information for families and children on a variety of pediatric conditions including prematurity, cardiac defects, and seizure disorders. This site also includes fun and interactive games and contests that teach children how their bodies work.

- **Canadian Paediatric Society** (http://www.cps.ca): This site was created by Canadian pediatricians to provide child health care information for physicians and other interdisciplinary health care providers.

- **Canadian Toys Regulations** (http://laws-lois.justice.gc.ca/eng/regulations/SOR-2011-17/FullText.html): This federal government site lists regulation requirements for toys sold in Canada.

- **Caring for Kids** (http://www.caringforkids.cps.ca): Caring for Kids is a CPS site that provides child health and wellness information to families and children. It covers a variety of topics, such as pregnancy and babies, immunizations, care for sick children, and the use of natural products.
- **Clinical Practice Guidelines for Nurses in Primary Care—Pediatric and Adolescent Care** (https://www.canada.ca/en/health-canada/services/first-nations-inuit-health/health-care-services/nursing/clinical-practice-guidelines-nurses-primary-care/pediatric-adolescent-care.html): This federal government site includes pediatric clinical practice guidelines for nurses on different subjects, such as health assessment, prevention, fluid management, and child abuse.
- **Government of Canada: Toy Safety** (https://www.canada.ca/en/health-canada/services/toy-safety.html): This federal government site provides general toy safety tips and information on playing smart and playing safe.
- **Parachute** (http://www.parachutecanada.org/corporate): This Canadian charitable organization is dedicated to preventing injuries and saving lives.

Mental Health Nursing

Mental health, like physical health, affects a person's well-being. Often the two go hand in hand due to the complex relationships among biological, genetic, psychological, and social or environmental factors. People with a mental illness often develop physical symptoms, and vice versa. Mental illness does not discriminate among ages, cultures, or income or education levels. Each year, approximately 1 in 5 Canadians experiences a mental illness (Canadian Institute for Health Information, 2017).

Mental health and mental illness occur along a continuum, just as physical health and illness do. Consequently, just as we speak of health within illness, a person can have a mental illness but manage that illness in healthy ways. People, in general, may have varying qualities and experiences that could be designated as healthy or unhealthy, but only when the unhealthy outweighs the healthy will help be sought or required from a mental health professional. Practical nurses care for clients with a mental health condition in every type of setting and play an essential role in helping these clients and their families on the road to achieving their optimal level of health.

LEGAL, ETHICAL, AND INTERPERSONAL CONSIDERATIONS FOR MENTAL HEALTH NURSING

As professionals, practical nurses are bound by legal, moral, and ethical principles that govern their practice. Because laws, morals, and ethics are grounded in providing for the good of society, they offer guidelines that help practical nurses provide exemplary care for their clients. Sometimes, however, these guidelines are not completely clear, and often they can contradict one another. Ethical dilemmas occur when a practice decision must be made between two competing but imperfect and not completely desirable choices. Mental health practice challenges practical nurses to use their judgement to interpret the guidelines and make ethical decisions, often when the circumstances are ambiguous.

Canadian practical nurses uphold and promote the code of ethics of the Canadian Council for Practical Nurse Regulators (CCPNR, 2013), in which a practical nurse's responsibilities are defined under the following five ethical principles:

1. Responsibility to the public
2. Responsibility to clients
3. Responsibility to the profession
4. Responsibility to colleagues
5. Responsibility to oneself

Registered/licensed practical nurses follow this code of ethics in conjunction with their provincial and jurisdiction standards and competencies, workplace policies, and the legal requirements that govern their practice and behaviour. The CCPNR code of ethics is discussed in more detail in Chapter 3. Refer to the CCPNR Web site, listed at the end of the chapter in the "Web Sites" section, for more information.

In Canada, health care is the responsibility of the provincial and territorial governments. Consequently, each province and territory has its own *Mental Health Act* outlining the regulations for voluntary and involuntary admission to hospital, consent for treatment, and the rights of (and safeguards for) mental health clients. Similarly, legislation defining guardianship and substitute decision makers varies across the country. Federal laws that impact mental health clients include the *Canadian Charter of Rights and Freedoms* and the *Criminal Code of Canada* (Gray, Shone, & Liddle, 2008).

Psychological, neurobiological, and genetic pathology cause mental health disorders that result in disorganization and impairment of thinking, memory, mood, behaviour, or all of these. Consequently, people with a mental illness suffer significant distress and difficulties in everyday functioning.

Impairments of cognition and emotion can interfere with an individual's ability to make appropriate decisions in his or her own best interest, or they may cause the client to make decisions or exhibit behaviours that interfere with the rights of others. Thus, the client's condition may require practical nurses to make ethical and legal choices between competing values. For example, in the case of a client with a psychotic disorder, denying a client's right to autonomy may preserve his or her health or the rights and safety of others.

Mental illness does not discriminate; anyone can suffer from a mental illness. The characteristics of different population groups may pose particular legal and ethical issues for mental health nurses. Here, issues related to different cultures and the homeless population are discussed.

Cultural Differences

Mental health care in Canada is decidedly influenced by Western ideology and practices, yet we are a multicultural society, and people of different cultures may define normal and abnormal behaviour differently. Often healthcare providers require a translator to understand the client's history and healthcare needs. There is a difference between an interpreter and a translator. An *interpreter* is more likely to unconsciously try to make sense of (interpret) what the client is saying and therefore inserts his or her own understanding of the situation into the database. A *professional translator*, on the other hand, tries to avoid interpreting. DeAngelis (2010) strongly advises against the use of untrained interpreters such as family members, friends, and neighbours. These individuals might censor or omit certain content (e.g., profanity, psychotic thoughts, and sexual topics) due to fear or a desire to protect the client. They can also make subjective interpretations based on their own feelings, share confidential details with outsiders, or leave out traumatic topics because they hit too close to home for them (Halter, Pollard, & Jakubec, 2019).

To be culturally sensitive and competent, mental health nurses need to do the following:

- Critically examine their personal cultural beliefs, values, and any ethnocentric tendencies.
- Become familiar with a variety of different cultures and ethnic groups.
- Plan culturally congruent care after conducting a thorough cultural assessment (Shen, 2015).
- Assess how cultural groups define mental illness and what methods of healing are acceptable.
- Learn about cultural and religious rituals, protective symbols, and standards of modesty in various belief systems.
- Respect a person's dietary restrictions and customs.
- Exhibit sensitivity, openness, and flexibility in approach and interactions.
- Understand that "cultural difference is not limited to a difference based on membership in an ethnic or racial group, but rather encompasses differences in experience, meaning, and what is significant to particular individuals and families" (Hartrick Doane & Varcoe, 2015, pp. 139–140).

Homelessness

The connections between mental illness and homelessness are many. The downsizing of mental hospitals over 50 years ago began a process of deinstitutionalization, when many people were discharged without appropriate community services and programs in place. Many who experience mental illness face multiple barriers (such as stigma and lack of social support) to achieving high levels of education or full employment. Reductions in social assistance eligibility, fewer opportunities for unskilled work, the lack of affordable housing, and a propensity for substance abuse are also factors leading to poverty and homelessness. Estimates of the proportion of homeless people with a mental illness varies widely across Canada, but in various cities, they range from 23–75% (Mental Health Commission of Canada, 2012).

The NIMBY ("not in my backyard") syndrome is a common social attitude. Canadians want homeless people off the streets but reject having services and housing for them located in their own neighbourhoods.

Factors to bear in mind about homeless people with a mental illness:

- For some individuals, having a severe mental illness leads to being homeless; for others, the stress of being homeless leads to developing a mental illness.
- Homeless people with a mental illness are particularly vulnerable to being victimized in inner-city areas.
- Healthcare services for homeless people with a mental illness involve assertive outreach programs that provide medical and psychiatric care, social assistance, meals, temporary shelters and housing, vocational and life skills training, and advocacy.
- Respecting the dignity and rights of the client according to the five ethical principles in the CCPNR code of ethics guides practical nursing practice with homeless people with a mental illness.

Interpersonal Relationships with Mental Health Clients

Establishing a therapeutic relationship with a client with a mental health disorder obligates the practical nurse to act in both ethical and legal ways. People with a mental illness are very vulnerable; their relationships with healthcare providers are often lengthy and very important to them. Conscientious practical nurses establish and maintain caring relationships but stay within their professional boundaries. Practical nurses must also be very aware of their relative power in those relationships and avoid abusing that power, while trying to balance a client's rights and safety with the societal rights of others.

Privacy and Confidentiality

- The CCPNR code of ethics states that personal, family, and community information must be protected and kept confidential. The only exceptions occur (a) when the practical nurse is legally required to disclose information and (b) when revealing information could prevent serious harm to the client or to others. In such cases, the practical nurse should try (where possible) to avoid actually identifying the client and to minimize any resulting stigma.
- If a client refuses to share information with family members, an ethical dilemma may arise, particularly if the family member is the person's primary caregiver outside the hospital.
- In most provinces, a family member must legally be notified when a client is admitted to or discharged from the hospital or scheduled to appear before a review board. The client nominates a family member or a near-relative (someone who the client has identified as being equivalent to family) as the person who should be notified in these cases.

Clients' Rights

In Canada, unlike the United States, there is no *Client's Bill of Rights*. Clients with a mental illness, including those involuntarily admitted to hospital, are entitled to the same fundamental rights as all Canadians, under the *Canadian*

Charter of Rights and Freedoms. All provincial and territorial *Mental Health Acts* must comply with the Charter (Gray et al., 2008).

Voluntary Admission to Hospital

- Most clients with a psychiatric illness in Canada are admitted voluntarily, by their own consent, under the same processes as other hospital clients.
- Voluntary clients may discharge themselves from the hospital when they wish.
- In most parts of Canada, for clients who are incapable of giving consent (such as a child or an incapable adult), consent may be provided by a parent, legal guardian, or substitute decision maker nominated by the client while well. In such cases, clients may not discharge themselves without the consenting person's agreement.

Involuntary Admission to Hospital

Admission to a psychiatric facility without the client's consent is often called *commitment* and usually happens in response to a crisis or need for emergency care. Although admission without consent contradicts the ethical value of promoting and respecting informed decision making, a client may be admitted when all three of the following conditions are met:

- The person refuses to be admitted or is incapable of making that decision.
- The person appears to have a mental health disorder.
- The illness is likely to cause harm or danger to the person or to others.

A physician completes a medical certificate that allows the person to be apprehended, transported to a mental health facility, and admitted for a specified period that varies across Canada from 1 to 3 days. Involuntary clients can only be admitted to hospitals that are defined by that province's *Mental Health Act* as mental health facilities.

If an individual meets these three criteria but refuses to see a doctor, the police may apprehend the person and take her or him to a hospital emergency department. There, a physician examines the person and completes the first certificate, if necessary.

To keep the client longer than the legally limited initial period, another physician or psychiatrist must complete a second certificate. In New Brunswick, however, the admission decision is made by a tribunal; in Quebec, by a judge; and in the Northwest Territories (NWT) and Nunavut, by the Minister of Health. When the specified longer period of detention expires (between 2 and 4 weeks, depending on the jurisdiction), a renewal certificate must be completed or the client must be allowed to leave.

If a client who is involuntary admitted wishes to be discharged, he or she (or a substitute decision maker, if one is available) applies to a review panel. This board acts as a judge and can overrule the physician on the basis of evidence gathered. (In the NWT, this review takes place in court.) Review boards also meet at legally defined designated intervals for clients who are certified for long periods.

The Charter mandates that clients who are involuntary admitted must be informed of their legal rights upon admission. Some provincial and territorial *Mental Health Acts* require this notification to be repeated each time a certificate is renewed. Clients must be informed of the following:

- Why they were admitted
- That they have the right to contact a lawyer
- That they can apply to a review board for a legal ruling on the involuntary admission (Gray et al., 2008)

Informed Consent

For consent to be informed, a person must be provided with the following information to consider:

- Information about the condition
- Information about the proposed treatment
- The benefits to be expected from the treatment
- The risks and side effects of getting the treatment
- Any alternative treatments or courses of action
- The consequences to be expected from not receiving the treatment

Practical nurses value the right of people to make their own decisions about health care and services, without coercion, and to have sufficient information upon which to base those choices.

- The CCPNR code of ethics stipulates that practical nurses must assist people to obtain complete current knowledge of their condition and also must respect a client's decision (or that of a legally approved substitute decision maker), even if it differs from the practical nurse's own beliefs and opinions. This includes respecting the right to refuse consent or withdraw consent at any time.
- Further, a practical nurse is responsible for providing care that goes against his or her personal values, until a replacement care provider can be obtained.
- A person is considered incapable of providing consent if he or she cannot understand or appreciate the consequences of accepting or rejecting treatment.
- Involuntary admission does not necessarily mean that treatment can begin, although in some provinces or territories, the physician or facility director can authorize treatment. In others, a tribunal must meet to approve treatment, and this may mean a delay lasting a few days.
- If the client has requested a review, no treatment can begin until the review panel upholds the involuntary admission, even if a substitute decision maker has signed the consent for treatment.

Treatment in the Least Restrictive Setting

Aggressive behaviour is common with some mental illnesses. It is also important to assess the client's history of aggression or violence. Most of our reactions to stimuli come from our previous experiences; therefore, identifying clients' triggers is essential. Initial and ongoing assessment of the client can reveal problems before they escalate to anger and aggression. Such assessment also leads directly to the appropriate nursing diagnosis and intervention (Halter et al., 2019). When a mental illness is well controlled, however, there is no greater risk of violence than there would be from the general population. Violence is most common when the illness is poorly controlled, as in the case of a client who has stopped taking his or her medications.

Restraints and Seclusion

When a client or someone else is likely to be harmed or property may be destroyed, seclusion or restraint may be necessary. The following restraint principles must be followed:

- The client is always entitled to the least restrictive alternative that ensures safety.
- Restraints should be released and the client allowed out of seclusion as soon as he or she has calmed down.
- Restraints require a physician's order.
- Clients in restraints or seclusion must be closely monitored and all physical needs addressed, including safety, comfort, food, fluids, and elimination. Accurate and complete documentation is vital.
- Physical or chemical restraints (sedation) should not be used when a brief period of seclusion would suffice to calm the client and ease the situation.
- In most provinces and territories, the *Mental Health Act* provides legal protection for staff to give treatment or restrain individuals, if their health or safety is endangered or the safety of others would be compromised without that treatment or restraint (Gray et al., 2008).
- Restraints and seclusion should never be used as punishment or for staff convenience.
- Seclusion and restraints are contraindicated for people who are clearly suicidal and for those with delirium or dementia, for whom decreased stimulation is likely to increase agitation.

Managing Behavioural Crises

Behavioural crises can lead to client violence toward self or others and usually, but not always, escalate through fairly predictable stages. Staff in most mental health facilities practise crisis prevention and management techniques. Many general and psychiatric hospitals have special teams made up of nurses, psychiatric technicians, and other professionals who respond to psychiatric emergencies called codes. Each member of the team takes part in the team effort to defuse a crisis in its early stages. If preventive measures fail and imminent risk of harm to self or others persists, each member of the team participates in a rapid, organized plan to safely manage the situation. The nurse is most often this team's leader, not only organizing the plan but also timing the intervention and managing the concurrent use of prn medications (Halter et al., 2019).

Workplace violence toward nurses and other healthcare providers is an ongoing concern. Recommendations on how to deal with aggressive clients include creating a culture of safety, increasing the number of interventions, reporting incidents, and having skills on crisis intervention techniques (Halter et al., 2019). De-escalation techniques are described in Box 11.1.

BOX 11.1 De-escalation Techniques: Practice Principles

- Maintain the client's self-esteem and dignity.
- Maintain calmness (your own and the client's).
- Assess the client and the situation.
- Watch the client's body language (can indicate if client ready to hit or push).
- Identify stressors and stress indicators.
- Respond as early as possible.
- Use a calm, clear tone of voice.
- Invest time.
- Remain honest.
- Establish what the client considers to be his or her need.
- Be goal-oriented.
- Maintain a large personal space.
- Position yourself close to the door in case you have to escape quickly.
- Do not touch the client. Keep your hands free.
- Avoid verbal struggles.
- Give several options.
- Make the options clear.
- Utilize a nonaggressive posture.
- Use genuineness and empathy.
- Attempt to be confidently aware.
- Use verbal, non-verbal, and communication skills.
- Listen to the client. Restate what the client states in your own words.
- Be assertive (not aggressive).
- Assess for personal safety.
- Note location of call bells, alarms, and other security devices.
- If you are in the client's home, leave the house if you think you are in danger. Go to safe a place and call you supervisor. If cannot leave the house and feel threatened, call police 9-1-1.

Adapted from Halter, M. J., Pollard, C. L., & Jakubec, S. L. (2019). *Varcarolis's Canadian psychiatric mental health nursing: A clinical approach* (2nd Cdn. ed., Box 23-3, p. 519). Milton, ON: Elsevier Canada.

Duty to Report

People who are mentally ill are vulnerable to abuse. Practical nurses are legally and ethically obliged to report suspected or confirmed cases to the appropriate authorities in the following circumstances:

- Family abuse—Child abuse, elder abuse, and partner abuse are criminal acts and must be reported to the police for investigation.
- Abuse of clients—Staff who abuse clients should be reported to management, and criminal charges may be laid. Professional staff should be reported to their licensing bodies. Practical nurses have a duty to report any nursing colleague who abuses clients to the college or nursing association that registers nurses in their province or territory.

- Unsafe nursing practices—Practical nurses are also obligated to report unsafe nursing practices to management and to the body that registers nurses in their province or territory.

The Nursing Process in Mental Health Nursing

Stuart (2013) describes the nursing process in mental health nursing:

The nursing process is an interactive, problem-solving process and a systematic and individualized way to achieve the outcomes of nursing care. When used with psychiatric clients, the nursing process can present unique challenges. Mental health problems may be vague and elusive, not tangible or visible like many physiological illnesses. Many psychiatric clients may be unable to describe their problems. They may be withdrawn, highly anxious, or out of touch with reality. Their ability to participate in the problem-solving process also may be limited if they see themselves as powerless victims or if their illness impairs them from fully engaging in the treatment process. (p. 149)

The nursing process is a collaborative process that involves working with the client on developing client-centred, mutually agreed-upon goals and interventions.

SPECIFIC COMMUNICATION AND THERAPEUTIC APPROACHES WITH THE MENTAL HEALTH CLIENT

To fully understand mental health, mental illnesses, and therapeutic approaches in mental health nursing, we review the functions of the brain and central nervous system (CNS).

Brain Structure and Function

The structure and function of the brain are illustrated in Fig. 11.1.

Cerebrum. Two hemispheres are connected by the corpus callosum, where the pineal gland is located. The pineal gland regulates gonadal function and also produces melatonin, which influences the sleep cycle. Each hemisphere of the cerebrum contains the four lobes and other structures depicted in Fig. 11.1. The following points describe the function of the structures within the hemispheres:
- Right hemisphere—Regulates creativity and intuition and controls the left side of the body
- Left hemisphere—Regulates logical, analytic thinking and controls the right side of the body

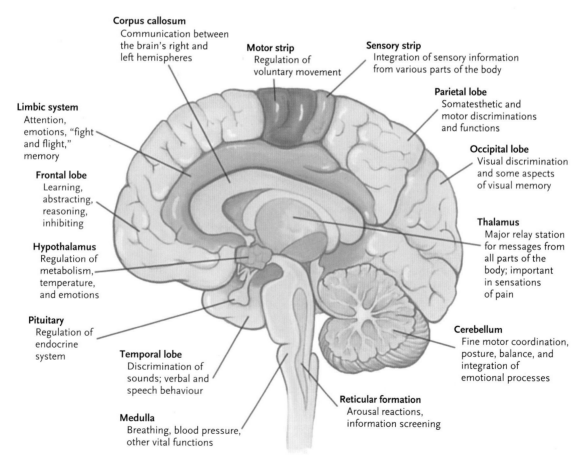

Fig. 11.1 Structure and function of the brain. (From Stuart, G. W. [2013]. *Principles and practice of psychiatric nursing* [10th ed. p. 71, Figure 5-5]. St. Louis: Mosby.)

- Frontal lobes—Integrate and organize complex thinking for solving problems, producing speech, planning and making decisions, regulating arousal, and focusing attention. Abnormalities in these lobes are found in schizophrenia, attention-deficit/hyperactivity disorder (ADHD), and dementia.
- Parietal lobes—Interpret taste and touch and help with spatial perceptions and balance
- Temporal lobes—Interpret hearing and smell and support memory, language comprehension, and the expression of emotions
- Occipital lobes—Help coordinate and interpret speech and vision

Cerebellum. The cerebellum coordinates movement and balance. Damage to the cerebellum is implicated in Parkinson's disease and dementia.

Brainstem. The brainstem structures control the following:
- Medulla oblongata—Controls cardiac and respiratory function
- Reticular activating system—Controls sleep and consciousness and relays motor neuron impulses
- Locus ceruleus—Is implicated in impulsive behaviour, related to stress and anxiety

Limbic system. The limbic system controls the following:
- Thalamus—Regulates mood, activity, and sensation
- Hypothalamus—Regulates temperature, appetite, hormones, and impulsive reactions, such as anger and excitement. The hypothalamus is involved in psychosomatic disorders and in stress response.
- Hippocampus and amygdala—Regulate emotions and memory

Psychopathology of the limbic system includes dementia, mania, and other psychoses.

Ventricles. These spaces between the hemispheres and other structures are filled with cerebrospinal fluid (CSF), which cushions and nourishes brain structures. In many psychiatric disorders, enlarged ventricles imply the destruction and atrophy of surrounding brain structures.

Neural Structure and Function

Fig. 11.2 illustrates the process of neurotransmission.

Neurotransmitters. Neurotransmission is the relaying of information in the synapse from neuron to neuron through electrical impulses and chemicals called neurotransmitters. Neurotransmitters and their function play an important role in many mental health conditions, as follows:
- Reuptake—After the message impulse is transmitted to the receptor cells, neurotransmitters return to the axon for storage or, alternatively, are inactivated and metabolized by enzymes, primarily monoamine oxidase (MAO).
- Psychiatric illnesses—They are characterized by abnormally high or low concentrations of certain neurotransmitters.
- Norepinephrine and epinephrine (noradrenaline and adrenalin)—Found mainly in the brainstem, these chemicals control the stress response ("fight or flight") and influence the brain's reward system. Norepinephrine also helps regulate mood.

- Dopamine—It has mainly an excitatory effect upon movement, emotions, motivation, and cognition. Dopamine is involved in movement disorders such as Parkinson's disease, as well as in schizophrenia and other psychotic illnesses.
- Serotonin—It has primarily an inhibitory effect. Serotonin is important in the regulation of sleep, appetite, and libido; therefore, serotonin-circuit dysfunction can result in sleep disturbances, decreased appetite, low sex drive, poor impulse control, and irritability (Halter et al., 2019). Serotonin also has been implicated in schizophrenia. It has a modulating effect on dopamine. The first-generation atypical antipsychotic drugs are combination serotonin/dopamine blocking agents, explaining their improved efficacy over the typical antipsychotics. Blocking serotonin in the limbic system increases frontal dopamine with a net effect of improving negative symptoms (Stuart, 2013).
- Acetylcholine—It may be excitatory or inhibitory, affecting sleep–wake cycles, and signalling muscular activity. People with Alzheimer's disease have low levels of acetylcholine.
- Glutamate—It opens the calcium ion channel to allow electrical impulses through the synapse. Excessively high levels (such as those found in stroke, hypoglycemia, and ischemia and as a result of taking drugs such as phencyclidine [PCP]) are toxic to brain cells.
- Gamma-aminobutyric acid (GABA)—It is an inhibitory neurotransmitter that helps regulate other neurotransmitters. Benzodiazepines increase GABA to reduce anxiety and promote sleep.
- Endorphins and enkephalins—They are the brain's natural opiates. They have an inhibitory effect, reducing pain and stimulating pleasure by affecting the brain's reward system.
- Histamine—In addition to moderating allergic responses and reducing gastric and cardiac stimulation, histamine controls alertness. People with depression have low levels of histamine.

Diagnostics Tools and Therapeutics Used in Mental Health Nursing
Diagnosis

Criteria for diagnosing all psychiatric disorders and illnesses are defined in the *Diagnostic and Statistical Manual of Mental Disorders*, fifth edition (DSM-5) (American Psychiatric Association [APA], 2013). This dimensional diagnostic system correlates with treatment planning by using the DSM and International Classification of Disease (ICD) as the standards to how mental diseases are diagnosed and treated. Section II of the DSM-5 contains 22 different diagnostic criteria and codes. It identifies disorders based on criteria in clinical settings such as inpatient, outpatient, partial hospitalization, consultation–liaison, clinics, private practice, primary care, and community populations.

The DSM-5 "organizes diagnoses for psychiatric disorders on a developmental hierarchy with disorders seen in infancy, childhood and adolescence appears in the first chapter and neurodevelopmental disorders and disorders that occur later in life, as neurocognitive disorders, are further down the list"

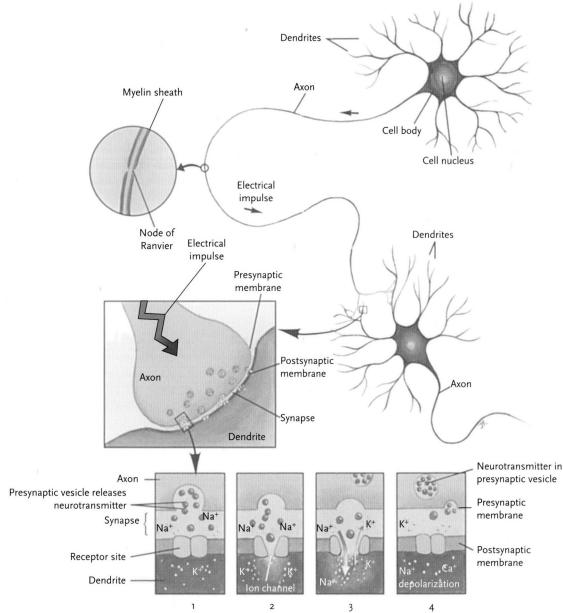

Fig. 11.2 Neurotransmission. (From Stuart, G. W. [2013]. *Principles and practice of psychiatric nursing* [10th ed., p. 75, Figure 5-7]. St. Louis: Mosby.)

(Halter et al., 2019, p. 11). The ICD "sets the global health information standard for mortality and morbidity statistics. Clinicians and researchers use this classification system to define diseases, study disease patterns, monitor outcomes, and subsequently allocate resources based on the prevalence of disease" (Halter et al., 2019, p. 11).

The DSM-5 enables mental healthcare providers to communicate using a common diagnostic tool. It helps to implement effective interventions in order to improve clinical outcomes. It helps practical nurses in their assessment findings and in communicating clinical information to other healthcare providers, families, and clients. The DSM classifies disorders, not people. In the DSM-5, experts have integrated issues related to culture and mental illness into the discussion

of each disorder. It is imperative to take the client's social and cultural influences into account during assessments and diagnoses. Frequently, when these illnesses are treated in culturally prescribed ways, the remedies are quite effective (Halter et al., 2019).

Psychological testing. Clinical psychologists administer many tests to measure intelligence and cognitive functioning, as well as aspects of personality, memory, impulse control, interpersonal behaviour, and self-concept. A common one is the Minnesota Multiphasic Personality Inventory (MMPI).

Electroencephalogram. Electroencephalograms (EEGs) are graphic tracings of the brain's electrical impulses, used to differentiate among neurological and psychiatric conditions and to evaluate various neurological symptoms, such as delirium, hallucinations, and altered states of consciousness.

Neuroimaging. Newer and more sophisticated technology for visualizing the brain includes the following:

- CT scans—Computed axial tomography uses X-rays and sometimes a contrast agent such as iodine is used to produce sharply defined images of a "slice" through body tissues.
- MRI scans—Magnetic resonance imaging uses magnetic energy to discriminate among different tissue densities. This technique is contraindicated in pregnancy and for people with metal in their bodies, including pacemakers, metal plates, and bone replacements.
    - CT and MRI scans detect structural abnormalities, such as tumours and hematomas.
- PET scans—Positron emission tomography helps investigate brain function by measuring glucose consumption, that is, metabolic activity, in brain cells. Blood flow and synaptic activity can be distinguished.

Common laboratory and diagnostic tests appear in Appendix D.

Pharmacotherapy

In general, medications used for psychiatric therapy regulate abnormal levels of specific neurotransmitters. Refer to Chapter 7 for medication action, side effects, and signs of overdose, with particular attention to the following classes of drugs:

- Antipsychotics—Typical and atypical
- Mood stabilizers—Lithium, antiepileptics
- Antidepressants—Tricyclic, selective serotonin reuptake inhibitors (SSRIs), MAO inhibitors (MAOIs), atypical antidepressants
- Antianxiety medications—Also called *anxiolytics*

The major interactions of psychotropic drugs and other substances are reviewed in Table 11.1.

TABLE 11.1   Interactions of Psychotropic Drugs and Other Substances

Psychotropic Category	Possible Interactions
Antianxiety Agents	
Benzodiazepines with:	
Central nervous system (CNS) depressants (alcohol, barbiturates, antipsychotics, antihistamines, cimetidine [Tagamet])	Potential additive CNS effects, especially sedation and decreased daytime performance
Selective serotonin reuptake inhibitors (SSRIs), disulfiram, estrogens	Increased benzodiazepine effects
Antacids, tobacco	Decreased benzodiazepine effects
Sedative–hypnotics with:	
CNS depressants (alcohol, antihistamines, antidepressants, narcotics, antipsychotics)	Enhancement of sedative effects; impairment of mental and physical performance; may result in lethargy, respiratory depression, coma, death
Anticoagulants (oral)*	Decreased warfarin plasma levels and effect; monitor and adjust dose of warfarin
Antidepressants	
Tricyclics (TCAs) with:	
Monoamine oxidase inhibitors (MAOIs)*	May cause hypertensive crisis
Alcohol and other CNS depressants	Additive CNS depression; decreased tricyclic antidepressant (TCA) effect
Antihypertensives* (guanethidine [Ismelin], methyldopa [Aldomet], clonidine [Catapres])	Antagonism of antihypertensive effect
Antipsychotics and anti-parkinsonians	Increased TCA effect; confusion, delirium, ileus
Anticholinergics	Additive anticholinergic effects
Antiarrhythmics (quinidine [Cardioquin], procainamide [Pronestyl], propranolol [Inderal])	Additive antiarrhythmic effects; myocardial depression
SSRIs*	Increased TCA serum level/toxicity through inhibition of cytochrome P-450 system
Anticonvulsants	Decreased TCA effect; seizures
Tobacco	Decreased TCA plasma levels
SSRIs with:	
Clomipramine (Anafranil), maprotiline (Ludiomil), bupropion (Wellbutrin), clozapine (Clozaril)	Increased risk of seizures
MAOIs*	Serotonin syndrome
Barbiturates, benzodiazepines, narcotics	Increased CNS depression

Continued

TABLE 11.1 Interactions of Psychotropic Drugs and Other Substances—cont'd	
Psychotropic Category	**Possible Interactions**
Carbamazepine (Tegretol)	Neurotoxicity: nausea, vomiting, vertigo, tinnitus, ataxia, lethargy, blurred vision
Aripiprazole (Abilify)	Fluoxetine and paroxetine lower levels
Risperidone (Risperdal)	Fluoxetine and paroxetine may increase risperidone to toxic levels
Selegiline* (Emsam)	Hypertensive crisis; increased serotoninergic effects; mania
St. John's wort, naratriptan, rizatriptan, sumatriptan, zolmitriptan, tramadol*	Serotonin syndrome
Haloperidol (Haldol)	Decreased effect of either drug
Calcium channel blockers	Neurotoxicity; dizziness, nausea, diplopia, headache
Valproate (valproic acid)	Decreased valproate serum concentration
Cimetidine (Tagamet), erythromycin (Erythrocin), isoniazid (Nydrazid), fluconazole (Diflucan)	Somnolence, lethargy, dizziness, blurred vision, ataxia, nausea, increased carbamazepine levels
Clozapine* (Clozaril)	Avoid due to increased risk of agranulocytosis
Aripiprazole (Abilify)	Increased blood levels of aripiprazole
Rifampin (Rifadin)	Decreased carbamazepine levels
Antipsychotics with:	
Antacids, tea, coffee, milk, fruit juice	Decreased phenothiazine effect
CNS depressants (narcotics, antianxiety drugs, alcohol, antihistamines, barbiturates)	Additive CNS depression
Anticholinergic agents (levodopa [Sinemet])*	Additive atropinelike side effects and increased anti-Parkinson effects
SSRIs	Increased neuroleptic serum level and extrapyramidal side effects (EPS)
Antipsychotics Clozapine (Clozaril) with:	
Carbamazepine* (Tegretol)	Additive bone marrow suppression
Benzodiazepines*	Circulatory collapse, respiratory arrest
SSRIs*	Increased risk of seizures

*Potentially clinically significant
Adapted from Stuart, G. W. (2013). *Principles and practice of psychiatric nursing* (10th ed., pp. 528–529, Table 26.1). St. Louis: Mosby.

Common Psychiatric Treatments

Psychotherapy refers to various approaches to the psychological treatment of mental or emotional disorders, aimed at changing people's attitudes, feelings, and behaviour. These approaches are conducted by trained therapists.

"Talk therapy" approaches.

- Psychoanalysis: Based on Freudian theory, this is a lengthy process of years of individual therapy aimed at uncovering repressed memories and other unconscious influences on thinking, behaviour, and relationships.
- Psychodynamic therapy: Also based on Freudian concepts but shorter in duration, this type of therapy can last weeks or months. The focus is on developing insight on particular issues thought to be causing the client's distress.
- Interpersonal therapy: This type of therapy is used to examine past relationship patterns to reveal ways of achieving more positive personal and interpersonal interactions.

Behaviour-oriented therapy. Various techniques of behaviour modification focus on changing clients' behaviour patterns. Overall, positive behaviours are positively rewarded and negative behaviours are negatively rewarded. Examples include the following:

- Assertiveness training—Clients learn to express their wishes in a matter-of-fact way and to say no to unreasonable expectations without feeling guilty.
- Positive conditioning—Clients learn to associate desirable behaviours and the sources of any phobias with pleasurable outcomes and relaxation.
- Aversion therapy—Undesirable behaviours are associated with painful or negative stimuli.
- Desensitization—Clients are gradually exposed to situations that they fear.
- Thought stopping and thought switching—Clients practise controlling fears by stopping the negative thoughts (e.g. by using a verbal reminder) or switching to more positive ones.
- Token economy—Good behaviour is rewarded with tokens that clients can trade for privileges or desired objects.

Group therapy. Small groups of people with similar problems meet together, facilitated by a therapist, to discuss and work through their concerns. In community settings, many groups focus on self-help, with members helping one another along with the guidance and support of a professional facilitator.

Cognitive therapy and cognitive–behavioural therapy.

- Cognitive therapy: It focuses on changing "irrational beliefs, faulty reasoning, and negative self-statements that underlie behavioral problems" (Stuart, 2013, p. 564). Therapists help clients change their self-concept and coping skills by altering their thought patterns and behaviour.
- Cognitive–behavioural therapy: It uses techniques similar to those of behaviour modification, along with strategies for cognitive restructuring and reducing anxiety (relaxation training, biofeedback, role-playing). Clients have homework assignments for practising between sessions.

Communication Techniques

Therapeutic communication is the heart of mental health nursing. While practical nurses may focus on developing therapeutic verbal communication techniques, non-verbal communication is equally important. Practical nurses need to be aware of a client's non-verbal signals, just as clients are sure to be aware of the practical nurse's. Clients know when a practical nurse is being genuine, honest, and sincere. They can sense a practical nurse's respect and empathy (and they sense the opposite responses just as easily).

Managing therapeutic communication implies that practical nurses monitor all aspects of their own and their client's communication, such as movement, gestures, posture, facial expression, and body language. Be aware of vocal tone, pitch, and volume, as well as nervous habits, such as coughing or giggling. We also communicate a great deal about ourselves and our regard for clients through touch. Always remember that cultural patterns of communication may be different, especially with regard to boundaries of personal space and touching.

When it is necessary to confront a client about undesirable behaviour or attitudes, be assertive, but not aggressive or angry. Point out discrepancies in a matter-of-fact way between a client's self-interpretation of behaviour and how others may view those same actions. In Table 11.2, you will find a summary of therapeutic communication techniques. Refer to pages 14–15, for more ideas on how to develop therapeutic communication techniques and interviewing skills.

Assessing Mental Status

Evaluating the client's mental status is an important aspect of clinical assessment. Combining what the client can tell you with your own observations, the mental state assessment evaluates the client's current mental functioning, not his or her psychiatric history. Most organizations have a structured form to help the practical nurse recall the range

TABLE 11.2 Selected Therapeutic Communication Techniques

Technique	Definition	Example
Listening	An active process of receiving information, showing interest and acceptance	Maintain eye contact and convey positive non-verbal responses.
Broad openings	Asking questions that allow the client to select topics for discussion	"What are you thinking about?"
Restating	Repeating the client's main thought to have him or her validate what you heard and to emphasize important points	"You say that your mother left you when you were 5 years old."
Clarification	Asking the client to explain what he or she means, to help the client examine issues in more detail	"I'm not sure that I fully understand. Could you tell me about that again?"
Reflection	Directing back the client's ideas, feelings, questions, and content to signify empathy and validate the practical nurse's understanding	"You're feeling anxious, and it's related to your conversation with your husband last night."
Informing	Providing information for health teaching and self-care	"It's important for you to know how this medication works."
Focusing	Questions or statements that help the client expand on the topic, keeping the communication goal-directed	"I think we should talk more about your relationship with your father."
Sharing perceptions	Asking the client to verify your understanding of his or her thoughts or feelings, to clear up confusion	"You're smiling, but I sense that you are really very angry with me."
Identifying themes	Identifying issues or problems that the client repeatedly refers to in conversation, aimed at helping the client understand and explore important problems	"I've noticed that you have spoken often of being hurt or rejected by men with whom you have formed relationships."
Silence	Intentionally not initiating verbal communication, to allow time for thinking and reflection and to encourage the client to initiate communication	Sit with the client to non-verbally communicate support and interest.
Suggesting	Presenting alternative ideas for the client to consider in problem solving, to increase possibilities and choices	"Have you thought about responding differently to your boss when he raises that issue with you? For example, you could ask him whether a specific problem has occurred."

Adapted from Stuart, G. W. (2013). *Principles and practice of psychiatric nursing* (10th ed., p. 30, Box 2.7). St. Louis: Mosby.

of questions to ask and observations to make, to ensure that sufficient and appropriate information is collected. In general, assessing mental status includes describing the following characteristics:

- Appearance, speech, activity, and interaction in the interview
- Emotions, mood, and affect
- His or her perceptions of personal experiences
- Thought content and thinking processes, including ability to concentrate
- Level of consciousness
- Memory
- Level of intelligence
- Evidence of judgement and insight

Further details on mental health assessment and neurological physical assessment appear in Chapter 4.

Milieu Therapy

Practical nurses help create a therapeutic community or milieu on the inpatient unit, in which clients become part of a community where they can learn new social skills, improve their coping mechanisms, and develop healthy interpersonal relationships. Establishing this type of environment to aid in social rehabilitation is more difficult in today's context of relatively brief hospital stays; in outpatient settings, such as group homes, a therapeutic community is more easily established.

Family Therapy

Family nursing is important in mental health practice. Families are both the context within which the client lives and may be in need of nursing care themselves. Often the family serves as caregiver and case manager for clients outside the hospital. Families need education about the client's illness and help with learning new patterns of interacting with the client. Different types of groups can help provide support to these families:

- Psychoeducational groups for families—They provide support to families coping with a member who has a severe mental illness. Families are taught about the signs and symptoms of the illness, medications, other options for therapy, sources of community help, and how to recognize signs of a relapse. In these groups, family members can share their experiences and successful strategies for managing the client at home.
- Self-help groups for families—They can be accessed through voluntary organizations, such as the Schizophrenia Society of Canada and the Canadian Mental Health Association. Such mutual aid groups empower families, reduce their isolation, and help them learn coping skills.

Community Mental Health Nursing

Because most people with a mental illness are treated outside the hospital, roles for community mental health nurses are expanding. Community treatment focuses clients on recovery, with a goal of helping clients learn to manage their illness and incorporate any limitations into a satisfying life. Social and functional-living skills (and, where possible, employment skills) enable clients to cope while living as independently as possible.

As members of interdisciplinary teams, practical nurses may work in a variety of models for community mental health services. Community outreach programs aim to assist clients where they live. Other services are provided in offices where clients must make and keep appointments. Many programs are a combination. Outreach programs may provide specific services for mentally ill clients and their families, or they may refer clients to other programs in the community. Examples of these services include the following:

- Assertive Community Treatment (ACT)—A specific interdisciplinary team model for intensive community support. Community programs and services may include client identification, mental health care and counselling, medical care, dental care, crisis response, social assistance, financial management, community education and advocacy, rehabilitation, housing, family support, and case management.
- Case management—Case managers develop caring and supportive therapeutic relationships with complex clients. They may be attached to an ACT team or a hospital outpatient service.
- Supported housing—This type pf housing varies from apartments with a resident manager who has some mental health knowledge to group homes. Some group homes follow the club house model, where residents are members and collaborate with staff in running the house and its programs.
- Community Mental Health Centres (CMHCs)—They provide outpatient clinics, mental health programs, and support services.
- Public health—In rural areas, the public health nurse may be the only source of community mental health outreach. In more urban areas, public health nurses are more likely to focus on prevention, such as stress management and parenting classes, school programming, or screening for depression. They make referrals to mental health programs and agencies.
- Addiction services—Street nurses may be the first point of contact for those with a mental illness and substance disorder.

MOOD DISORDERS: DEPRESSION AND BIPOLAR DISORDER

Mood disorders are also called *affective disorders*, "affect" meaning the expression of a person's mood. Emotional ups and downs are normal features of living; severe or prolonged changes in a person's mood may not be.

Abnormal mood ranges between two emotional extremes: depression and mania. Mania is an abnormally and persistently elevated mood state marked by hyperactivity, delusions, and lack of judgement. Depression is described in the next section.

Usually, hospitalized clients have either a severe depression or a bipolar illness, in which their mood swings between depression and mania.

Depression

Depression is one of the most common psychiatric illness in Canada, with one in eight adults (11.3%) identifying with symptoms that meet the criteria for depression (Public Health Agency of Canada, 2016). All age groups can be clinically depressed—even children. According to the 2012 Canadian Community Health Survey, 15- to 24-year-olds had the highest rates of mood and anxiety disorders of all age groups (Findlay, 2017).

Pathophysiology

Neurological, genetic, and psycho-social factors interact in complex ways to produce depression:

- Neurological factors—These include low levels of monoamines, such as serotonin and norepinephrine. Other neurotransmitters that are poorly regulated include dopamine, acetylcholine, GABA, and serotonin (5-HT). Serotonin also affects levels of growth hormone, cortisol, and prolactin, all of which are poorly regulated in people with depression.
- Brain—Brain scans can show decreased metabolic activity in the frontal and temporal lobes and increased blood flow to the amygdala.
- Genetic factors—People with a family history of depression have an increased incidence of depression. Genetic factors predispose people to develop depression when faced with environmental factors such as stressful life events.
- Endocrinology—Depression is commonly associated with Addison's disease, Cushing's syndrome, thyroid diseases, and abnormal estrogen levels. These hormonal imbalances disrupt the regulatory functions of the hypothalamus and pituitary glands. As well, the specifier for "with seasonal pattern" for major depression (previously called *seasonal affective disorder* [SAD]) may be linked to abnormalities in the hypothalamic control of circadian rhythms.
- Electrolytes—High levels of calcium, sodium bicarbonate, and either high or low levels of potassium are common with depression.
- Psycho-social factors—Factors such as multiple stressors or negative social interactions (criticism, anger, or bullying) are also risk factors for depression. By contrast, participation in physical activity and positive social support may offer some protection.

Clinical Manifestations

Depression is expressed as intense feelings of sadness, despair, and powerlessness, often as a consequence of loss. Depression can be brief and transient in the normal response to everyday disappointments or more prolonged, ranging through mild to moderate to severe chronic depression known as *depressive disorders*. Depressive disorders are severe enough to cause distress or impairment in the client's ability to function.

These disorders include major depressive disorder, persistent depressive disorder, premenstrual dysphoric disorder, substance/medication-induced depressive disorder, and depressive disorder due to another medical condition. Moderate depression (dysthymic disorder) and severe depression (major depressive disorder) tend not to resolve without professional help.

People with depression share a number of common characteristics. They will tell you that they feel empty and extremely sad, with no hope for the future. Their pain is both emotional and physical, with diffuse aches and pains throughout their bodies. Previously enjoyable activities now provide no pleasure, and, not surprisingly, they can be irritable and socially withdrawn.

Normally, grief for a loved one is experienced as depression, with many of the same symptoms.

Overwhelming sadness and hopelessness are manifested in sleep disturbances, changes in appetite and weight, and inability to concentrate or carry out usual activities. Unlike those experiencing chronic depression, grieving people recognize the reason for their feelings. Gradually, acceptance develops, the depressive symptoms resolve, and normal coping mechanisms resurface.

Depression is a common response with major loss, including the loss of health experienced with a chronic illness. Other risk factors include stressful life events, poor social support, substance disorder, and having a history of depression. Several specific depressive disorders are described next.

Major depressive disorder. Major depressive disorder (MDD; also called *major depression*) is persistent and devastating. MDD can occur in a single episode, more frequently as recurrent relapses or as a chronic condition lasting longer than 2 years. It can be characterized by a continuous depressed mood lasting for a minimum of 2 weeks (Halter et al., 2019). In some, the symptoms are severe enough to cause psychosis (a psychotic break from reality) with delusions, hallucinations, and psychomotor impairment to the point of catatonia. Almost 15% of untreated people with major depression commit suicide. MDD is characterized by the following symptoms:

- Feelings of sadness and emptiness, with crying
- Anhedonia, or no interest in activities that were previously enjoyed
- Appetite changes accompanied by either weight loss or weight gain
- Sleep pattern changes (insomnia, or sleeping during the day)
- Lack of energy, extreme fatigue
- Feelings of worthlessness or inappropriate and excessive guilt
- Psychomotor agitation (restlessness) or impairment (slowed movement)
- Inability to concentrate or make decisions, difficulty thinking
- Recurrent thoughts of suicide or death (Halter et al., 2019)

Dysthymic disorder. Persistent depressive disorder (dysthymia), less prevalent than major depression, is a chronic moderate level of depression. The somewhat milder symptoms are similar to major depression but chronic, persisting for at least 2 years. (For children and adolescents, the diagnosis may be made after 1 year.) Individuals feel depressed most of the time. When they are depressed, they also exhibit at least two of the other symptoms listed for major depression. Social and occupational impairment are significant.

Postpartum depression. Some degree of depression affects more than half of all new mothers. Postpartum depression is classified in the DSM-5 as Bipolar Disorder or Depression with Peripartum Onset. A person suffering from postpartum depression has to meet the symptoms of a major depressive episode. Postpartum depression is diagnosed when the depressive episode occurs before or after the birth of the person's child. "Fifty percent of postpartum major depression episodes actually begin prior to delivery. Thus, these episodes are referred to collectively as *peripartum episodes.* Women with peripartum major depressive episodes often have severe anxiety and even panic attacks" (APA, 2013, p. 186). Although most mothers experience "baby blues" in the week or two after the birth, postpartum depression is more severe and lasts longer. Women with limited social support, previous episodes of depression, or perinatal complications are most at risk.

Postpartum depression greatly reduces a woman's ability to care for her child, with negative consequences for both the mother's health and that of her baby. In severe cases, the mother can experience psychosis and may have thoughts of harming herself or her child. "Infanticide is more often associated with postpartum psychotic episodes that are characterized by command hallucinations to kill the infant or delusions that the infant is possessed but psychotic symptoms can occur in severe postpartum mood episodes without such specific delusions or hallucinations" (APA, 2013, p. 187).

Seasonal affective disorder. Seasonal affect disorder (SAD) is now classified in the DSM-5 as a specifier called "with seasonal pattern" for major depression disorders. In this disorder, changes in mood occur in response to a reduced exposure to daylight. In fall and winter, people with this disorder become clinically depressed. Depression generally resolves in the spring. Less commonly, there may be recurrent summer depressive episodes. The DSM-5 criteria for diagnosing depression with a seasonal pattern includes having these episodes for at least the last 2 years:

- "There has been a regular temporal relationship between the onset of major depressive episodes in major depressive disorder and a particular time of the year" (APA, 2013, p. 187).
- "Full remission (or a change from major depression to mania or hypomania) also occur at a characteristic time of the year" (APA, 2013, p. 187).
- "In the last 2 years, two major depressive episodes have occurred that demonstrate the temporal seasonal relationships defined above and no nonseasonal major depressive episodes have occurred during the same period" (APA, 2013, p. 187).

- "SAD (as described above) substantially outnumber the nonseasonal major depressive episodes that may have occurred over the individual's lifetime" (APA, 2013, p. 187).

Diagnostics

Along with a full history and physical examination to identify symptoms and comorbid illnesses, several rating scales are available to assess depression. Four of the most common rating scales are as follows:

- Beck Depression Inventory (BDI)—A self-rating scale that clients complete
- Zung Self-Rating Depression Scale (ZSRD)—Another self-report scale
- Hamilton Rating Scale for Depression (HAM-D)—Completed by clinicians
- Geriatric Depression Scale (GDS)—A self-reporting assessment scale for the older adult

Therapeutics

Pharmacotherapy is the predominant mode of treatment for mood disorders. Remember that medications may take several weeks to be effective. See Chapter 7, page 128, for more details about antidepressants, including drug classifications, actions, and side effects. Chapter 7 also includes nursing implications for these drugs.

Medications for depression.

- Tricyclic antidepressants (TCAs)—Side effects are significant; therefore, these are used less frequently now.
- Selective serotonin reuptake inhibitors (SSRIs)—They are considered first-line medications.
- Serotonin-norepinephrine reuptake inhibitors (SNIRs)—They are often considered the next medication of choice after trying SSRIs.
- Norepinephrine-dopamine reuptake inhibitor (NDRI)—A high dose may increase seizure risk.
- Monoamine oxidase inhibitors (MAOIs)—They are usually reserved for hard-to-treat MDD clients due to their severe side effects.

Nursing Considerations

Nursing assessment. Practical nurses working in all healthcare, occupational, and community settings should be attentive to signs of mood disorders. When a disorder is first suspected, the client may be asked to complete a self-assessment scale.

Assessment of depression. To assess for depression, the practical nurse determines whether the client has experienced the following:

- Previous history of depression or familial history
- Medical conditions that may increase risk of depression (hypothyroidism, Parkinson's)
- Recent life changes (divorce, unemployment, situational stressors)
- Misuse or overuse of alcohol, medications, or other drugs (marijuana, nicotine)
- Mental health problems that may contribute to depression

The practical nurse also assesses whether the client is at risk of harming himself or herself or other people (see the section "Psychiatric Emergencies: Crisis, Suicide, Violence" in this chapter).

If the client has a history of depression, find out what worked then and what did not. Discuss with the client his or her level of knowledge about depression and whether supportive family or friends are available. Finally, assess whether the client needs referral to a primary care provider (physician or nurse practitioner).

The nurse–client relationship. The cornerstone of connecting with clients with mood disorders is spending time with the person to reinforce reality and provide support. Use a calm approach and moderate tone of voice—neither overly cheerful nor too serious—and active listening. Establishing rapport and communicating with people at either end of the mood spectrum present additional and different challenges, as follows:

- Be kind and compassionate—Just sitting with an isolated person is comforting and supportive.
- Use simple, direct language—Doing so can counteract slowed thinking processes.
- Be patient—Allow extra time for the person to follow directions and respond.
- Offer observations—Instead of questioning an individual who is not talkative, point out characteristics of the person and the immediate environment, for example, "Your blue dress matches your eyes" or "Your son brought you some fruit."
- Avoid common expressions that can discount a client's feelings, such as "Oh, things will be better soon; it just takes time."

Pharmacotherapy

Be aware of and monitor for side effects, adverse reactions, and interactions of major medications used for mood disorders. Clients with mood disorders may object to taking medications; be sure to supervise as they swallow oral medications.

Antidepressants. Nursing implications for antidepressant drug side effects are discussed in Table 11.3.

Preventing hypertensive crisis associated with MAOIs. MAOIs increase levels of serotonin, epinephrine, and norepinephrine in the brain. These medications can cause severe interactions with certain medications and foods.

Medications. Over-the-counter cold medications interact with MAOIs, producing a hypertensive crisis, a life-threatening condition manifested by tachycardia, sudden increase in blood pressure, severe headache and nosebleeds, stiff neck, nausea and vomiting, and cold, clammy skin. Clients can develop chest pains or a stroke and die. Emergency treatment for hypertensive crisis involves the following:

- Discontinue MAOI.
- Keep the client's head elevated.
- Reduce fever by external methods, such as fans, tepid baths, or ice packs.
- Administer a calcium channel blocker (such as nifedipine [Adalat]) sublingually, intramuscularly (IM).

- Administer chlorpromazine (Thorazine) (it blocks norepinephrine).

Other contraindicated drugs for people taking MAOIs include narcotics, tricyclic antidepressants, antihypertensives, sedatives, including alcohol, and legal or illegal stimulants, such as amphetamines and cocaine.

Foods. In order to prevent a hypertensive crisis, which is rare but potentially fatal, the client also needs to avoid certain foods, particularly those with high levels of tyramine.

- Instruct the client *not to eat* any of the following foods: aged cheeses (cream cheese and cottage cheese are safe); red wine, sherry, and liqueurs; over-ripe fruit; sauerkraut; pickled or smoked fish; beef and chicken liver; fava beans; brewer's yeast; monosodium glutamate; and all fermented products.
- Instruct the client *to consume moderate amounts only* of alcohol, beer, and white wine; beverages with caffeine; ripe avocado, yogourt, soy sauce, figs, raisins, ripe bananas, chocolate, and meat tenderizers.

Complementary and alternative medications. St. John's wort is a herbal product with proven effects against mild to moderate depression, SAD, and sleep disturbance. Melatonin supports circadian rhythm equilibrium, thus improving sleep. Many people explore natural remedies and self-medicate for the management of mood disorders. Client's using alternative or complementary medications should be encouraged to discuss this with their physician, nurse practitioner, or pharmacist as interactions can either reduce or increase the action of prescribed medications, potentially causing toxic effects.

Nursing Interventions

- Maintain client safety—Observe closely for self-harm or suicidal thoughts. Remove belongings that could be used for self-harm.
- Maintain nutrition—Give small, frequent meals, taking preferences into account.
- Maintain elimination—Add high-fibre foods and ensure adequate hydration to counteract constipation.
- Assist with personal hygiene—Encourage the client to gradually resume self-care.
- Encourage social interaction—Provide reassurance and positive reinforcement for gradually joining group activities.

Bipolar Disorder and Related Disorders

According to Statistics Canada (2013), 1.5% of Canadians over 15 years of age and older experienced bipolar disorder in the previous year. Bipolar disorders are less common than depressive disorders. There are different types of bipolar disorders. All of them involve changes in mood, energy and activity levels. An older name for bipolar illness that you may still hear is *manic depression* (Halter et al., 2019).

Pathophysiology

A complex interplay of underlying biological factors can lead to the development of mania:

TABLE 11.3 Nursing Considerations for Antidepressant Drug Side Effects

Side Effect	Nursing Care and Teaching Considerations
Anticholinergic Side Effects	
Blurred vision	Temporary; avoid hazardous tasks
Dry mouth	Encourage fluids, frequent rinses, sugar-free hard candy and gums; check for mouth sores
Constipation	Increase fluids, dietary fibre and roughage, exercise; monitor bowel habits; use stool softeners and laxatives only if necessary
Tachycardia	Temporary, usually not significant (except with coronary artery disease), but can be frightening; eliminate caffeine; ß-blockers might help; provide supportive therapy
Urinary retention	Encourage fluids and frequent voiding; monitor voiding patterns; bethanechol; catheterize
Cognitive dysfunction	Temporary; avoid hazardous tasks; adjust lifestyle; provide supportive therapy
Cytochrome P-450 inhibition*	SSRIs inhibit the liver isoenzyme cytochrome P-450, which is instrumental in the metabolism of a variety of drugs (TCAs, trazodone, barbiturates, most benzodiazepines, carbamazepine, narcotics, neuroleptics, phenytoin, valproate, verapamil). This effect can be potentially life-threatening because it increases serum concentrations as well as therapeutic and toxic effects of these drugs.
Dizziness/ lightheadedness	Have client dangle the feet; provide adequate hydration, elastic stockings; protect from falls
ECG changes	Obtain complete cardiac history; obtain pre-treatment ECG for clients over 40 and children; ST segment depression, T wave flattened or inverted, QRS prolongation; worsening of intraventricular conduction problems; do not use if recent myocardial infarction or bundle-branch block
Ejaculatory dysfunction	Dose after sexual intercourse, not immediately before
GI disturbances (nausea, diarrhea)	Take with meals or at HS; adjust diet if indicated
Hallucinations, delusions, activation of schizophrenic or manic psychosis	Change to another antidepressant class of drug; initiate antipsychotics or mood stabilizers if appropriate
Hypertensive crisis*	See the discussion of MAOIs in the section "Preventing Hypertensive Crisis Associated with MAOIs."
Hypotension	Obtain frequent BP; hydrate; provide elastic stockings; may need to change drug. For postural hypotension: obtain lying and standing BP, encourage gradual change of positions, protect from falls.
Insomnia	Dose as early in the day as possible; promote sleep hygiene; decrease evening activities; eliminate caffeine, relaxation techniques; sedative–hypnotic therapy
Memory dysfunction	Temporary; encourage concentration, make lists, provide social support, adjust lifestyle
Perspiration (excessive)	Suggest frequent changes of clothes, cotton or linen clothing, good hygiene; increase fluids
Priapism	Change dose, change drug
Psychomotor activation	Take drug in morning rather than HS; adjust lifestyle
Sedation/drowsiness	Administer drug at HS; avoid hazardous tasks
Serotonin syndrome (SS)*	SS is a life-threatening emergency resulting from excess central nervous system 5-HT caused by combining 5-HT-enhancing drugs or administering SSRIs too close to the discontinuation of MAOIs. Symptoms are confusion, disorientation, mania, restlessness/agitation, myoclonus, hyper-reflexia, diaphoresis, shivering, tremor, diarrhea, nausea, ataxia, headache. Discontinue all serotoninergic drugs immediately; anticonvulsants for seizures; serotonin antagonist drugs may help; clonazepam for myoclonus, lorazepam for restlessness or agitation, other symptomatic care as indicated; do not reintroduce serotonin drugs
Sexual dysfunction	Dose after sexual intercourse; use lubricant if vaginal dryness is present; antidotes such as sildenafil, bupropion, or bethanechol
Tachycardia	See anticholinergic side effects
TCA withdrawal syndrome	Symptoms: malaise, muscle aches, chills, nausea, dizziness, coryza; when discontinuing drug, taper over several days or weeks
Tremors	Temporary; adjust lifestyle as indicated
Weight gain	Increase exercise; reduced-calorie diet if indicated; may need to change class of drug

*Potentially life-threatening.

NOTE: Always educate the client and use the techniques in this table. Consider decreasing or dividing drug dose. Change drug only if necessary.

BP, blood pressure; *ECG*, electrocardiogram; *GI*, gastro-intestinal; *HS*, at bedtime; *5-HT*, serotonin; *MAOIs*, monoamine oxidase inhibitors; *SSRIs*, selective serotonin reuptake inhibitors; *TCAs*, tricyclic antidepressants.

Adapted from Stuart, G. W. (2013). *Principles and practice of psychiatric nursing* (10th ed., p. 542, Table 26.11). St. Louis: Mosby.

- Neurological factors—Neurotransmitter abnormalities, that is, high plasma levels of epinephrine and norepinephrine, can lead to mania.
- Brain—Brain scans show abnormalities in the white matter (fatty sheaths surrounding neurons), particularly in those areas of the brain responsible for emotions.
- Genetic factors—As with depression, higher rates of mania are found among first-degree relatives.
- Endocrinology—The biological clock is located in the hypothalamus. In mania, circadian rhythms are disrupted; sleep deprivation is common. Hypothyroidism is linked to bipolar illness.

Clinical Manifestations

A mood change between mania and depression is called *rapid cycling*. The episode may vary in length. Clients may also vary in how frequently and quickly they cycle from the mood episodes of mania and depression. The person may have experienced four or more mood episodes in a 12-month period. "The cycling can also occur within the course of a month or even a 24-hour period. Rapid cycling is seen with more severe symptoms, such as poorer global functioning, high recurrence risk, and resistance to conventional somatic treatments" (Halter et al., 2019, p. 278).

A manic episode is a distinct period of abnormally and persistent elevated, expansive, or irritable mood that may include the following:
- Being overly talkative (pressured speech)
- Inflated self-esteem or grandiosity
- An increase in goal-related activity (either socially, at work, school, or sexually)
- Psychomotor agitation (purposeless, non–goal-directed activity)
- Rapid, often confusing, speech patterns; "pressured speech" or "flights of ideas" or person feels their thoughts are racing
- Disturbed sleep patterns and seemingly needing very little sleep
- Over involvement in activities that have a high potential for painful consequences (e.g. engagement in money-making schemes or irresponsible spending, sexual indiscretions, or foolish business investments)

A major depressive episode manifests when five or more of the following symptoms have been present during the same 2-week period and at least one of the symptoms is either depressed mood or significant decrease in interest or pleasure:
- Depressed mood most of the day, nearly every day, as reported by the person (sad, empty, hopeless) or through observations made by others (tearful)
- Significant decrease in interest or pleasure in most activities most of the day, nearly every day
- Weight loss when not dieting or weight gain (change of more of 5% of body weight in 1 month) or decrease in appetite most days
- Insomnia or hypersomnia most days
- Psychomotor agitation or impairment most days
- Fatigue or loss of energy most days
- Feelings of worthlessness or excessive or inappropriate guilt (may be delusional)
- Decreased ability to think, concentrate, or make decisions nearly every day
- Recurrent thoughts of death, suicidal ideation without a specific plan, or a suicide attempt or a specific plan for committing suicide

Diagnostics

Refer to the preceding symptoms in manic episode and major depressive episode.

Along with a full history and physical examination to identify symptoms and comorbid illnesses, several rating scales are available to assess depression (see the rating scales listed under "Diagnostics" in the section "Depression," page 402).

The symptoms of bipolar and related disorders usually happen in three phases: the acute phase (during an intense manic, hypomanic, or depressive episode), the continuation phase (when symptoms are controlled but the client's mental health status is still fragile), and the maintenance phase (when acute symptoms have subsided and the focus is on preventing relapse and limiting the severity and length of future episodes) (Halter et al., 2019, pp. 284, 285).

Medications for bipolar and related disorders.
- Lithium carbonate
- Anticonvulsants, such as carbamazepine (Tegretol), valproic acid
- Anxiolytics
- Antipsychotics—Typical and atypical
  See Chapter 7, page 128, for more details in the "Mood Stabilizers" section. Chapter 7 also includes drug classifications, actions, adverse effects, and nursing implications for these drugs.

Nursing Considerations

Nursing assessment of bipolar disorders.
To assess for manic episodes, the practical nurse determines whether the client:
- Is a danger to himself or herself (exhaustion in severe mania can lead to death) or others (due to poor impulse control) and needs to be hospitalized
- Is spending money uncontrollably and engaging in overly risky behaviours
- Has comorbid medical conditions
- Misuses or overuses alcohol, medications, or other drugs (marijuana, nicotine)
- Requires information about bipolar disorder, medications, and support groups for the client or family

Communication during manic episodes
- Try to maintain a calm, nonstimulating atmosphere on the unit.
- Convey self-confidence when setting limits on the client's behaviour.
- Guard against being manipulated and ensure consistency with the rest of the team in your response to manipulative behaviour or acting out.

- Provide brief and concise explanations and statements since their comprehension is limited due to a short attention span.

Pharmacotherapy

In the case of bipolar disorder, the medication dosage must be delicately balanced. Monitor clients' responses carefully; antidepressants can induce manic symptoms, and mood stabilizers may cause depression.

Lithium carbonate. Because achieving an adequate level of lithium in the body takes weeks or months, other mood stabilizers, antidepressants, or atypical antipsychotics may also be used for manic episodes until the therapeutic level of lithium is reached. Lithium toxicity is an abnormally high serum level of lithium. It can result from non-steroidal anti-inflammatory drugs (NSAIDs), diuretics, vomiting, diarrhea, and other causes of fluid and electrolyte imbalance or from an overdose.

- Monitor clients for early signs of lithium toxicity: anorexia, nausea, diarrhea, drowsiness, muscle weakness, tremors, unsteadiness, and lack of coordination.
- If toxicity is suspected, monitor vital signs and level of consciousness. Push fluids.
- Be aware that more severe signs—fever, decreased urine, low blood pressure, electrocardiogram (ECG) changes, irregular heartbeat, seizures, and loss of consciousness—can cause death.
- To prevent lithium toxicity, encourage fluid intake of 2–3 L daily and replace any fluid loss from exercise, vomiting, or diarrhea. Ensure a balanced diet with adequate salt intake. If a dose is forgotten or late, skip that dose and resume with the next scheduled dose.

Anticonvulsants.

- Action—These drugs stabilize mood by boosting the inhibitory effect of GABA on the stress response. Without inhibition due to GABA, high levels of epinephrine and norepinephrine heighten neural synapse activity.
- Kindling—This refers to the neurochemical sensitization of the brain due to stress, resulting in "automatic" initiation of the stress response, without a precipitating stressful event. Kindling also may result from reduced GABA inhibition.
- Serious side effects—Carbamazepine can cause agranulocytosis. Divalproex (a valproic acid derivative) can cause thrombocytopenia. Overdoses can be lethal.

It is important to monitor blood test results and observe the client for evidence of bruising and bleeding.

Nursing Interventions

- Maintain client's safety and that of other clients. Lock up sharp and hazardous possessions.
- Use seclusion if necessary when the client is argumentative and disruptive to other clients. Maintain close supervision and spend time with the client after he or she calms down, discussing his or her feelings and suggesting strategies to prevent future escalation of behaviour.
- Give emotional support and encourage rest periods.

- Set realistic limits on behaviour and reinforce socially appropriate conduct. For example, it may be necessary to impose controls on spending to prevent bankruptcy.
- Maintain nutrition and hydration—High energy levels require increased calories. Manic clients need reminders to eat and drink. Provide high-calorie finger foods between mealtimes and, if the client is on lithium, salty snacks.
- Assist with personal hygiene; promote self-care.
- Suggest activities that suit the client's short attention span.

Electroconvulsive Therapy

Electroconvulsive therapy (ECT) involves passing electrical current through the brain, producing a tonic–clonic seizure lasting about 30–60 seconds. Researchers have been unable to pinpoint exactly how ECT works, but the current speculation is that it improves brain chemistry in a manner similar to that of mood-disorder drug treatments. Muscle relaxants confine most seizure activity to the brain, almost completely eliminating contractions elsewhere in the body (unlike the depictions of ECT in the media). ECT remains the treatment of choice for a major depression that does not respond to antidepressants and for an acutely suicidal depressed client. Similarly, ECT can be used for acute mania, if lithium or other mood stabilizers have proven ineffective, or if the mania has escalated to dangerous behaviour or exhaustion, which are life-threatening.

ECT has risks, especially for those with cardiovascular disease. Most memory loss is temporary, although permanent loss can occur. The electrodes are now commonly placed unilaterally rather than bilaterally, thus reducing the level of memory loss that clients experience.

Commonly, a series of three treatments weekly is given for 2–4 weeks. Reassurance, empathy, and teaching are necessary to allay a client's fears. Nursing care, before and after the procedure, is similar to that required by any client undergoing a general anaesthetic. Nursing considerations for clients receiving ECT therapy include the following:

- Before ECT, educate the client and family about the procedure and effects and encourage them to express any concerns. Allow nothing by mouth for several hours prior to the treatment. Remove valuables and dentures. Client should wear comfortable, loose fitting clothing. Clients should urinate before the procedure.
- During the procedure, assist with monitoring vital signs and the electroencephalography.
- After ECT, monitor vital signs and maintain the client's airway until fully awake. Assist with ambulation and reorientation. Give analgesics and antiemetics as necessary. Reinforce teaching and ensure that family members understand the client's initial confusion or memory loss.

Transcranial Magnetic Stimulation

Transcranial magnetic stimulation (TMS) is a noninvasive procedure in which a changing magnetic field is introduced into the brain to influence the brain's activity. The field is generated by passing a large electrical current through a wire stimulation coil over a brief period. It is used frequently for mood disorders. When administered daily at the left prefrontal cortex, it has shown to be effective treatment for nonpsychotic depression. It may not be as effective as ECT for treatment resistant depression. Some clients may not be candidates for the treatment due to the strong magnetic fields involved. For example, clients with metal objects such as screws, plates, pacemakers, or other implants can prevent a client from receiving TMS (Stuart, 2013).

Therapies as Adjuncts to Medication

Therapies that are used as an adjunct to medications for treating clients with depression and bipolar disorders include the following:

- Individual psychotherapy—It is aimed at improved social functioning; therapy may focus on a client's interpersonal relationships, developmental problems, and role transitions.
- Group therapy—It provides peer support and education after clients are no longer acutely ill. Groups may be facilitated by professionals or peers. Peer-led groups are usually in community settings, often through voluntary agencies, such as the Mood Disorders Society of Canada.
- Family therapy or marital therapy—It is aimed at education and at restoring adaptive and functional family relationships.
- Cognitive therapy—It is aimed at guiding clients to examine the validity of their thinking and at modifying any distorted perceptions.
- Milieu therapy—The nurse may need to provide seclusion for highly manic bipolar clients.
- Phototherapy or light therapy for SAD—Regular exposure to broad-spectrum fluorescent lighting (which is of a higher intensity than normal indoor lighting) improves symptoms for most sufferers of SAD.

Teaching and Learning

For mood disorders, client and family teaching comes after ensuring the client's safety and addressing social needs. It is important to wait until the client is ready and able to learn.

Topics for the Family and Client Education

It is important for the practical nurse to educate the client and the family on the following topics:

- The illness, including the nature, causes, and symptoms of depression or bipolar disorder
- Medications, including the management of side effects and which side effects to report to the doctor
  - Emphasize the length of time required for medications to become fully effective, taking medications correctly and regularly, and diet restrictions for those on MAOIs.
  - For people on lithium, highlight having regular blood tests and reinforce the symptoms of lithium toxicity.
- Techniques for stress management, assertiveness (for depression), and anger management (for bipolar disorder)
- Available support services, including support groups, suicide hotline, and legal and financial assistance

ANXIETY DISORDERS, OBSESSIVE–COMPULSIVE DISORDER, AND POST-TRAUMATIC STRESS DISORDER

Anxiety and fear are normal stress responses to threatening situations. When anxiety is mild or moderate, people may have adaptive coping abilities to alleviate their concerns and overcome or avoid stressors. In contrast, with severe anxiety or panic, individuals experience considerable distress, the perceptive field narrows, and reactions are quite likely to be maladaptive and disorganized. In the DSM-5, obsessive–compulsive disorder (OCD) and post-traumatic stress disorder (PTSD) have been moved from the "Anxiety Disorders" section to new sections to emphasize their differences from other anxiety disorders. Anxiety and fear are still a major part of these two mental illnesses.

Anxiety that is without a specific source or higher than expected for a given threat indicates an anxiety disorder. People with this disorder suffer excessive levels of anxiety, fear, or worry, causing them to avoid situations. The symptoms must last at least 6 months for all ages according to the DSM-5 (APA, 2013). Many develop physical symptoms. In Canada, anxiety disorders are one the most common of all mental health problems. It is estimated that 12.2% of Canadians aged 12 and older reported that they had been diagnosed with either a mood disorder (such as depression, bipolar disorder, mania, or dysthymia) or an anxiety disorder (such as phobia or a panic disorder) by a healthcare provider. A higher percentage of females (15.3%) than males (9.1%) reported having a diagnosed mood or anxiety disorder. Most can be treated successfully in primary healthcare settings (Statistics Canada, 2017).

Anxiety Disorders
Pathophysiology

The normal autonomic stress response is called "fight or flight" or the "general adaptation syndrome." It consists of three stages:

1. Alarm—The body prepares for defence or escape. The hypothalamus stimulates the adrenal glands to release adrenalin and norepinephrine for fuel and the liver to convert glycogen to glucose for cellular nutrition.
2. Resistance—The body adapts for survival, either by "fight or flight." The pupils dilate. Breathing and heartbeat accelerate, shunting highly oxygenated blood to the muscles. Once the person is out of danger, body responses relax.
3. Exhaustion—Unless resolved by adaptation during the resistance stage, emotional arousal continues until the body is depleted of stored energy, which will eventually cause death.

Anxiety disorders cause a prolonged and exaggerated stress response. Neurotransmitters of the limbic system (epinephrine, norepinephrine, dopamine, serotonin, and GABA) regulate anxiety. The biological mechanisms include the following:

- Excessive secretion of norepinephrine—It stimulates the cerebral cortex, the limbic system (especially the right temporal lobe), brainstem, and spinal cord, even without a source of fear.

- Low levels of GABA—GABA inhibits the excitatory neurotransmitters norepinephrine and dopamine, thus lessening emotional arousal and preventing disorganized responses.
- Abnormal serotonin functioning and glucose metabolism are also implicated.
- Genetics—Anxiety disorders cluster in families, indicating a genetic component.
- Neuroimaging shows anatomical brain changes contributing to (or resulting from) chronic stress. These include smaller frontal and temporal lobes and abnormalities of the amygdala (which regulates fear, memory, and emotion) and the hippocampus (the site of emotion and memory storage).

Clinical Manifestations

- All age groups are affected. In children, separation anxiety consists of an intense fear of losing their primary caregiver. Symptoms include refusing to attend school, fear of the dark and of going to sleep, stomach aches, headaches, nausea, and feeling faint. Other common anxiety disorders in children are social phobias and generalized anxiety syndrome.
- Older adults: There is a high prevalence of anxiety disorders in older adults, although the incidence is slightly less than in other age groups.
  Examples of anxiety disorders.
- Panic disorder: It is characterized by recurrent unexpected panic attacks. A panic attack is an abrupt surge of intense fear or apprehensive with palpitations, diaphoresis, shakiness, hyperventilating, nausea, chest pain, feelings of choking, distorted perceptions of reality, and fear of death (Halter et al., 2019).
- Agoraphobia: "Individuals with agoraphobia are fearful and anxious about two (or more) of the following situations: using public transportation; being in open spaces; being in enclosed places, standing in line or being in a crowd; or being outside of the home alone in other situations. The individual fears these situations because of thoughts that escape might be difficult or help may not be availbale in the event of developing panic-like symptoms or other incapacitating or embarrassing symptoms" (APA, 2013, p. 190).
- Generalized anxiety disorder: It is characterized by persistent and distorted apprehension and fear. The individual has excessive anxiety in many situations with the inability to concentrate, fatigue, irritability, tension, restlessness, and sleep disturbances (Halter et al., 2019).
- Social anxiety (social phobia): It is characterized by marked anxiety or fear provoked by exposure to a social or performance situation (fear of being scrutinized or saying something foolish, performing on stage or public speaking, etc.). The individual goes to extremes to avoid the situation. Social anxiety is more than shyness (Halter et al., 2019).
- Substance-induced anxiety disorder: It involves symptoms of anxiety, panic attacks, obsessions, and compulsions that develop with the use of a substance or withdrawal

of the substance. Diagnosis of this disorder involves a comprehensive review of the client's history and physical examination, and laboratory values indicating use of a psychoactive substance (e.g. cocaine, alcohol, heroin, hallucinogens) (Halter et al., 2019).

Defence Mechanisms Related to Anxiety Disorders

People use defence mechanisms to cope with anxiety. For the most part, defence mechanisms are employed unconsciously to preserve emotional stability and a sense of self. Sometimes, however, defence mechanisms are overused, or they promote reality distortion and self-deception, hindering the person's ability to cope realistically and practically. Practical nurses can help clients learn appropriate problem-solving and more effective coping strategies. Some common defence mechanisms include the following:

- Repression—Unconsciously blocking awareness of anxiety-provoking or painful perceptions
- Suppression—Similar to forgetting. It may be conscious or unconscious.
- Denial—Rejecting the reality of threatening situations, even with confirming evidence
- Projection—Attributing one's emotions, thoughts, and impulses to another person
- Introjection—Adopting the values and attitudes of others without questioning them
- Reaction formation—Stating the opposite of what one actually feels and thinks
- Displacement—Directing negative responses, such as anger, toward someone who is usually less threatening than the person who triggered the response
- Regression—Behaviour that characterizes an earlier developmental stage when the person may have felt more secure
- Withdrawal—Becoming passive and emotionally uninvolved

Diagnostics and Therapeutics

Diagnosis. Clients suffering from anxiety often present with the following concerns:

- They feel that they are doomed and likely to die.
- They have difficulties with problem solving and concentration.
- Their vital signs are indicative of the stress response: perspiring; increased blood pressure (BP), heart rate, and respirations; muscle tension; and dilated pupils.
- They exhibit somatic symptoms, for example, nausea, palpitations, frequent voiding or urgency, throat tightening, or a shaky voice.
- They complain of feeling tired and being short-tempered, disorganized, and unable to sleep.

While the above complaints clearly indicate anxiety, before concluding that it is a mental health problem, it is important to rule out whether the apprehension and worries stem from an underlying medical ailment. Medical illnesses causing anxiety may require urgent treatment. For example:

- Respiratory diseases such as chronic obstructive pulmonary disease (COPD), asthma, pulmonary edema, pulmonary embolism

- Cardiovascular diseases such as angina, heart failure, hypertension, hypotension, arrhythmias
- Endocrine diseases such as hyperthyroidism and hypoglycemia
- Neurological diseases such as delirium, Parkinson's disease, post-concussion syndrome
- Metabolic diseases such as hypercalcemia, hyperkalemia, hyponatremia

Treatment. First, treat any comorbid medical conditions. Then consider the following:

- Cognitive–behavioural therapy (CBT), including psycho-education and cognitive restructuring
- Behavioural therapy, including relaxation, desensitization, response prevention, and thought stopping
- Psychotherapy, to help the client develop insight
- Pharmacotherapy, including anxiolytics (especially benzodiazepines), antidepressants, beta blockers, and antihistamines

The most common form of treatment is a combination of drug therapy and CBT.

Nursing Considerations

Nursing assessment. Begin with a full health history and physical assessment to ascertain whether there are concurrent medical conditions associated with the heightened anxiety. Ask about social activities and any worries, fears, or feelings of nervousness, tension, or insecurity. Does the person talk about a past traumatic experience?

- Several rating scales for anxiety are available, for example, the Hamilton Anxiety Rating Scale.
- Check vital signs (pulse, BP, respiratory rate, etc.), changes in appetite or weight, and other physiological symptoms, such as gastro-intestinal (GI) upsets, fatigue, diaphoresis, and insomnia.
- Assess the risk of self-harm or suicide (see the section "Psychiatric Emergencies: Crisis, Suicide, Violence").
- Inquire about cognitive capacity (ability to concentrate, disorientation, illogical thinking, narrowed perceptual field, etc.).
- Probe for any reasons for heightened anxiety.

The nurse–client relationship. Clients in any healthcare setting experience some level of anxiety. Reducing their anxiety to tolerable levels depends on a practical nurse's skill and patience in developing a trusting relationship. Be patient. There may not be much improvement for weeks or even months.

When communicating with clients with anxiety:

- Show respect by addressing your client using his or her preferred name.
- Use a calm, warmly accepting, and quiet approach.
- Encourage the client to talk about feelings and emotions.
- Convey compassion, empathy, and honesty.
- Speak slowly, wait patiently while your client responds, and then listen carefully.

Nursing Interventions

- Maintain a restful, nonstimulating environment or move the client to a quiet place and always stay with any person who is experiencing high levels of anxiety.

- Speak slowly in clear, simple language, repeating as necessary.
- Reinforce reality where there are distortions in the client's perception and understanding.
- Listen for themes in the client's communication.
- Monitor and encourage self-care activities for those clients with ritualistic and obsessive behaviours. Phobias and intense concentration on rituals can interfere with a client's personal hygiene and grooming, adequate nutrition and fluid intake, elimination, and sleep.
- Ensure client safety and protection from impulsive and destructive reactions based on fear.

Teaching and Learning

Teach relaxation techniques, either individually or in groups. Some examples of these techniques include the following:

- Deep muscle relaxation—Have the client lie down and tense and relax voluntary muscles, progressing from the toes upward and focusing attention on each area in turn.
- Controlled breathing or meditation or both
- Guided imagery of places and situations that the person has previously experienced as peaceful and restful
- Systematic desensitization of anxiety-causing situations, either through visualization, role-play, or repeated real exposure, while also engaging in controlled breathing or deep muscle relaxation techniques

Teach the client about anxiety and the client's specific diagnosis. Also provide information on the following:

- Support services—Provide resources on available community programs and services, such as support groups, crisis hotlines, and sources for individual psychotherapy.
- Medications—Teach clients and their families about medications and their side effects:
  - Clients should avoid working with dangerous equipment.
  - Clients should avoid both alcoholic and caffeinated beverages. Alcohol can enhance the effect of the medication, and caffeine can reduce it.
  - Women should avoid pregnancy and breastfeeding when taking benzodiazepines.
  - Clients should be taught dietary restrictions for MAOIs.
  - Clients should be warned that stopping the medications abruptly may cause withdrawal symptoms, such as tremors, convulsions, confusion, insomnia, irritability, and nervousness.

Obsessive–Compulsive and Related Disorders
Clinical Manifestations

Obsessions refer to persistent, reoccurring thoughts, impulses, or images that cannot be let go from the mind. Examples include perfectionism, fear of losing control, fear of being responsible for the harm of others, concern with getting a disease, and fear of germs or contamination.

Compulsions are ritualistic behaviours or thoughts that people feel compelled to perform in an attempt to reduce their anxiety. The gain achieved by the ritual is only temporary, so the compulsive act must be repeated over and over again. Examples include washing and cleaning, repeatedly checking on things, or counting.

Obsessions and compulsions can occur independently from one another, but they often accompany one another (Halter et al., 2019).

Other Obsessive–Compulsive and Related Disorders

- Hoarding disorder: It is "characterized by persistent difficulty discarding or parting with possessions, regardless of their actual value, as a result of a strong perceived need to save the items and to distress associated with discarding them" (APA, 2013, p. 236). Hoarding disorder is not the same as collecting. Collectors look for certain items they may want to organize or display. Individuals with hoarding disorder randomly save items and store them all over the place. They excessively store, buy, or steal items not needed or have no area to store them in. Leading to clutter that accumulates dust, mold, and other health and safety concerns. The consequences of clutter can cause fire hazards, tripping hazards, and strained relationships with family members.
  - Hoarding disorder can also involve anxiety associated with parting with animals. Individuals can be deeply attached to their pets and find it difficult to let them go. Health issues may result from overcrowding living conditions with the animals, animal excrement, fleas and ticks, and animalborne illnesses.
- Trichotillomania (hair pulling) disorder: It is the impulse to pull out their hair resulting in hair loss. Individuals may pull out their hair when distressed as a way to decrease their anxiety. The hair pulling can lead to significant distress in social situations and functional impairment.
- Body dysmorphic disorder: It is "preoccupation with one or more perceived defects or flaws in physical appearance that are not observable or appear only slight to others, and by repetitive behaviours (mirror checking, excessive grooming, skin picking, reassurance seeking) or mental acts (of comparing one's appearance with that of other people) in response to the appearance concerns" (APA, 2013, p. 236).
- Excoriation (skin-picking) disorder: It is the urge to recurrently pick at one's own skin that can lead to skin lesions. The skin picking can cause severe distress or functional impairment.
- Substance/medication-induced obsessive–compulsive and related disorder: It "consist[s] of symptoms that are due to substance intoxication or withdrawal or to a medication" (APA, 2013, p. 236).

Treatment and Therapies for Obsessive–Compulsive Disorders

Medications, psychotherapy, or a combination of the two are used to treat obsessive–compulsive disorders. Refer to the "Treatment" section under "Anxiety Disorders" for treatments and therapies.

Nursing Interventions

Refer to the "Nursing Interventions" section under "Anxiety Disorders."

Post-traumatic Stress Disorder
Clinical Manifestations

PTSD is triggered by a terrifying event or situation that a person has either experienced or witnessed. It involves exposure to trauma involving serious injury, threat of death or death, or sexual violence. Symptoms include flashbacks, nightmares, severe anxiety, or uncontrollable thoughts or feelings of being unsafe in the world as if experiencing the event in the present. Individuals may avoid triggers that remind them of the situation or event. They may experience symptoms of feeling very nervous all the time, irritability, and exaggerated startle. They may feel very numb or detached from others. They may have difficulty concentrating or sleeping. These symptoms can interfere with a person's normal daily tasks or create problems in social situations and relationships. Individuals with PTSD often have issues with developing trust (Halter et al., 2019).

Nursing Considerations

Nursing Assessment. Assessment involves screening tools and PTSD checklists. Comprehensive assessments are done if they screen positive for PTSD. Detailed history is assessed regarding onset, frequency, course, severity, level of distress, and the degree of functional impairment. Further assessment is made for suicidal or violent ideation, family and social supports, insomnia, social withdrawal, functional impairment, current life stressors, medication, and past medical and psychiatric history. A mental status examination is also performed (Halter et al., 2019).

The Nurse–Client Relationship

- The practical nurse should establish a therapeutic relationship through nonjudgemental acceptance and empathy.
- The practical nurse should interact with the client on regular intervals to display an opening, caring attitude that will allow the client the opportunity to talk. This will help develop a trusting relationship with the client.
- Using silence and listening communication techniques can encourage the client to express his or her feelings.
- One of the most helpful things a practical nurse can do is gently suggest to the client that he or she was not responsible for what happened (Halter et al., 2019).

Nursing Interventions

- Initial education should include reassurance that reactions to trauma are common and that these reactions do not indicate personal failure or weakness.
- Strategies to improve coping, enhance self-care, and facilitate recognition of problems are essential.
- Relaxation techniques are helpful.
- The client should avoid caffeine and alcohol (Halter et al., 2019).

Treatments

- All clients should be informed of effective treatment options for PTSD and referred to an experienced licensed mental health practitioner.

- Treatments include group therapy, psychotherapy, imagery, and hypnosis.

Initial medication may include an SSRI such as fluoxetine (Prozac), paroxetine (Paxil), or sertraline (Zoloft), or an SNRI such as venlafaxine (Effexor) to decrease anxiety and decrease depressive symptoms (Halter et al., 2019).

ADJUSTMENT DISORDERS

Adjustment disorders are classified under "Trauma and Stressor-Related Disorders" in the DSM-5. The DSM-5 diagnostic criteria for adjustment disorder appear in Box 11.2.

All ages can be affected, often at times of major life transitions, such as starting school, adolescence, family breakup, loss of a job, financial problems, menopause, retirement, or the death of a spouse. People with poorly developed social skills or coping strategies or lacking supportive social networks may be particularly vulnerable. If the stressor is ongoing, however, the adjustment disorder may also persist, accompanied by worsening financial problems or difficult relationships. Adjustment disorders are usually resolved with community treatment and seldom warrant hospitalization.

Pathophysiology

No clearly defined biological causes or physiological changes are correlated with adjustment disorders, although when people exhibit depressive or anxiety-related behaviours, the expected pathophysiological changes for those conditions would be present. Theorists suggest that genetic factors may be implicated, at least for those persons with cognitive disorders or developmental challenges who respond poorly to stressful situations.

BOX 11.2 DSM-5 Diagnostic Criteria for Adjustment Disorder

- The development of an emotional or behavioural symptoms in response to an identifiable stressor(s) occurring within 3 months of the onset of the stressor(s).
- These symptoms or behaviours are clinically significant, as evident by one or both of the following:
  1. Marked distress that is out of proportion to the severity or intensity of the stressor, taking into account the external context and the cultural factors that might influence symptom severity and presentation.
  2. Significant impairment in social, occupational, or other important areas of functioning.
- The stress-related disturbance does not meet the criteria for another mental disorder and is not merely an exacerbation of a pre-existing mental disorder.
- The symptoms do not represent normal bereavement.
- Once the stressor or its consequences have terminated, the symptoms do not persist for more than additional 6 months.

From American Psychiatric Association. (2013). *Diagnostic and statistical manual of mental disorders* (5th ed., p. 287). Washington, DC: Author.

Clinical Manifestations

The behavioural and emotional symptoms of adjustment disorders can negatively affect functioning at work or school, and clients typically use a variety of defence mechanisms. Six subtypes of adjustment disorders are identified:

- Adjustment disorder with depressed mood—This is the most common adjustment disorder. Depressed mood, crying spells, and feelings of hopelessness are characteristic symptoms of a mood disorder; however, they are less severe than major depression.
- Adjustment disorder with anxiety—Some people who have an adjustment disorder also display nervousness, worry, and anxious feelings and behaviour.
- Adjustment disorder with mixed anxiety and depressed mood—Here, both anxiety and depression affect the person's ability to adapt to stressful events.
- Adjustment disorder with disturbance of conduct—Acting out inappropriately defines this type. Adolescents with a history of skipping school, fighting, vandalism, rebelling against all forms of authority, and getting into trouble with the law are often diagnosed with this disorder.
- Adjustment disorder with mixed disturbance of emotions and conduct—As the name implies, this is a mixture of the above types.
- Adjustment disorder unspecified—People with this disorder do not display the above symptoms but may withdraw socially or develop physical symptoms.

Diagnostics and Therapeutics
Diagnosis

Diagnosing adjustment disorders requires a thorough personal history that shows a stressful event or social situation followed by the development of symptoms. These symptoms are more intense and last longer than usual, and all underlying physical or mental health disorders have been ruled out. Risk factors include social and environmental variables such as overprotective or abusive parents, frequent moves as a child, living in poverty, and being witness to wars and violence. Sometimes delayed or prolonged grief is classified as an adjustment disorder.

Treatment

- Individual psychotherapy
- Family therapy
- Behavioural therapy
- Self-help groups
- Pharmacotherapy with antidepressants and anxiolytics

Nursing Considerations
Nursing Assessment

- Assess the level of anxiety or depression.
- Assess the client's support system, including family dynamics.
- Examine how the client perceives the problem or problems.

The Nurse–Client Relationship

- Convey empathy and support.
- Avoid minimizing the client's struggle with empty reassurances, such as "You'll be fine" and "Everything will work out."
- Encourage the person to recognize that a problem exists and that it is important to talk together about his or her emotional reactions.
- Provide positive reinforcement for desirable behaviour. This helps increase self-esteem.

Nursing Interventions

- Have the client describe his or her life and lifestyle prior to the stressful event.
- Listen when the client expresses anger, fear, and other negative emotions.
- Encourage healthy self-care and lifestyle, such as eating well, adequate sleep, regular exercise, and enjoyable hobbies.
- Assist with problem solving, providing alternatives for the client to consider.
- Assist the client to identify family members and friends who can provide support.
- Encourage family and friends to provide strong support.

Teaching and Learning

- Teach stress management techniques.
- Involve family and friends in teaching and learning opportunities.
  Caring for persons with unresolved prolonged grief. Explain to clients and families the following stages of grief:
- Numbness and shock—This stage is characterized by an inability to feel anything, sometimes alternating with extreme emotional outbursts.
- Yearning and searching—Expressions of anger, intense sorrow, and weeping as the reality of the loss sets in. There are often moments of imagining that the loved one will reappear.
- Despair and disorganization—This stage is characterized by emotions of hopelessness and acute loneliness, depression, and apathy.
- Reorganization and acceptance—Finally, there is gradual restoring of the self and a return to regular activities. Memories of the loved one become more comforting and less painful.
  Practical nursing responsibilities in assisting a person who is grieving include the following:
- Help the client identify his or her current stage of grief.
- Be accepting of expressions of anger. Accompany the client to a private and quiet area and stay with him or her.
- Try to engage the person in activities (keeping busy).
- Assess a client's spirituality and make a referral to a chaplain or minister, if that is desired.
- Refer the person to a grief support group.

SCHIZOPHRENIA SPECTRUM AND OTHER PSYCHOTIC DISORDERS

Schizophrenia spectrum and other psychotic disorders "are potentially devastating brain disorders that affect a person's thinking, language, emotions, social behaviour, and ability to perceive reality accurately" (Halter et al., 2019, p. 301).

Schizophrenia spectrum disorder is a disorder with a lifetime prevalence of 1%, both in Canada and worldwide. The mortality rate for people with schizophrenia spectrum disorder is twice that of the general population, and life expectancy is 20% shorter. Estimates of attempted suicide among people with schizophrenia spectrum disorder is about 40%. Ten percent of those with schizophrenia spectrum disorder commit suicide (Statistics Canada, 2015c). Thus, for a substantial proportion of clients, schizophrenia spectrum disorder is a terminal illness.

The DSM-5 includes a number of disorders in the category "Schizophrenia Spectrum and Other Psychotic Disorders," including schizophreniform disorder, schizoaffective disorder, delusional disorder, brief psychotic disorder, and substance/medication-induced psychotic disorder. Although some people (and often the media) confuse dissociative identity disorder (DID) (previously referred to as *multiple personality disorder*) with schizophrenia, the two are distinctly different psychiatric illnesses, and DID is a much rarer condition.

Pathophysiology

Causation is complicated and involves many factors. Evidence is clear, however, that brain structure, balancing of neurochemical transmitters, and disrupted neural circuits underlie the development of schizophrenia. Although social and environmental factors may trigger the onset or exacerbation of schizophrenia symptoms, the psycho-social theories blaming dysfunctional families and parenting are both outdated and harmful. Some key factors include the following:

- Brain abnormalities—At the time of diagnosis, larger cerebral ventricles, atrophy of the cerebellum or frontal lobe, and a variety of other structural abnormalities can be seen; for example, the hippocampus may be smaller than normal. As the illness progresses, further degeneration is minimal. Abnormalities of the prefrontal cortex are associated with reductions in higher cognitive functions.
- Neurochemical transmitters—There is excessive dopamine activity. Serotonin, glutamate, and other neurotransmitters are also poorly regulated.
- Genetics—Decades of studies on twins provide ample evidence that inheritance is a factor. People with a parent or sibling with schizophrenia are at higher risk of developing schizophrenia. If both parents have schizophrenia, a child has almost a 50% risk of developing the disorder.
- Substances—Illegal drug use and substance misuse do not cause schizophrenia; however, when a person is genetically predisposed to schizophrenia, drugs and substances may initiate symptoms earlier and with more severity than would occur otherwise.

Clinical Manifestations

Schizophrenia affects men and women in equal numbers, although, on average, males are usually diagnosed in their late teens or early twenties, while women are often diagnosed during their mid-twenties. Males also tend to display more severe symptoms and more negative symptoms and be less responsive to pharmacological treatment, thus suffering a poorer outcome. Females, in contrast, are more likely to have a family history of schizophrenia but have less severe symptoms and cognitive impairment. Late onset, after the age of 40, occurs infrequently. Women and those with later onset tend to have better outcomes. Comorbid mental health conditions are common, especially depression and anxiety. As well, many people abuse substances, trying to relieve their symptoms through self-medication.

Schizophrenia is a lifelong illness for at least 95% of sufferers. Some people will have one severe episode for which they receive treatment but are then well stabilized on medications that they take for the remainder of their lives. A few are eventually able to function without antipsychotics. For many, however, the illness is marked by hospitalization during psychotic episodes interspersed with periods of community treatment. Over many years, the psychotic episodes may become further apart. A minority do not respond to antipsychotic medications and remain in psychiatric hospitals long term.

Diagnosis and Symptoms of Schizophrenia Spectrum Disorders and Psychotic Disorders

Many symptoms are visible to others and become a source of stigma against the disease, the people affected, and their families. Clients are often withdrawn and socially isolated, either to hide their illness or in an attempt to feel safe. Social isolation also is brought about by the ridicule and rejection that they experience, stemming from the stigma surrounding the illness and misunderstanding on the part of the public.

Positive symptoms. Positive symptoms are characterized by the exaggeration or distortion of normal functions. Sometimes positive symptoms are subdivided into psychotic and disorganized dimensions.

Psychotic symptoms

- Hallucinations: Distorted perceptions involving any of the five senses. Auditory hallucinations, in which the voices that clients hear are unusually threatening or disapproving, are particularly prevalent.
- Delusions: Unrealistic and unfounded beliefs. Common delusions are of grandeur, of being persecuted, of being controlled, or of having one's mind read.

Disorganized or catatonic behaviour

- When psychotic, the person's behaviour may be catatonic. Catatonia is defined as "a stuporous state in which the patient may require complete physical nursing care, similar to that for a comatose patient, sometimes with unpredictable outbursts of aggressive behavior or strange posturing" (Stuart, 2013, p. 353). Examples of catatonic behaviour include robotlike activity, complete immobility, or holding a position for long periods of time (waxy flexibility).

- Hostility and aggression may be present most often in response to paranoid and persecutory delusions. People who become violent while experiencing delusions are often trying to defend themselves.
- Cognitive disturbances are problems in processing information. Clients are often bombarded so rapidly with ideas that focusing on anything or sorting out what is relevant from what is not becomes impossible. Thoughts are illogical and disconnected. Terms used for cognitive disturbances include "thought disturbance," "loose associations," and "flight of ideas."
- Incoherent speech patterns reflect the disturbed thoughts and may be rapid, jumping from one topic to another. This is sometimes referred to as "word salad."

Negative symptoms.

- Inappropriate affect: Emotions that are inconsistent with the occasion
- Flattened affect: Emotions or emotional responses that are diminished
- Alogia: A lack of speech or inadequate communication caused by an interruption in the thought processes
- Poor attention span: Inattentiveness and impaired concentration
- Anhedonia: An inability to experience pleasure from activities or social relationships
- Apathy: Physical inertia
- Avolition: An inability to persist with activities, including grooming and hygiene

A summary of the signs and symptoms of schizophrenia appears in Fig. 11.3.

Phases of Schizophrenia

Schizophrenia usually progresses through predictable phases, although the presenting symptoms during a given phase and the length of the phase can vary widely. These phases tend to occur in sequence and appear in cycles throughout the course of the illness.

Phase I: Acute—Onset or exacerbation is characterized by florid, disruptive, symptoms such as delusions, hallucinations, marked distortion in thinking, apathy, withdrawal, and disorganized speech. The person exhibits disturbances in behaviours and feelings. Symptoms may progress to the point where the person requires hospitalization for acute care and treatment. Their functional ability may be severely impaired, and the person can be at risk of harming themselves and others (Halter et al., 2019).

Phase II: Stabilization—The person's symptoms diminish and are less severe than in the acute phase. The person is maintaining or improving, returning to the previous level of functioning. Day hospitalization, or care in a residential crisis centre or supervised group home, may be required (Halter et al., 2019).

Phase III: Maintenance—The symptoms are absent or diminished, and the person is nearing his or her baseline functioning. The person's level of functioning allows him or her to live in the community. The treatment goal is to maintain or improve functioning, improve quality of life,

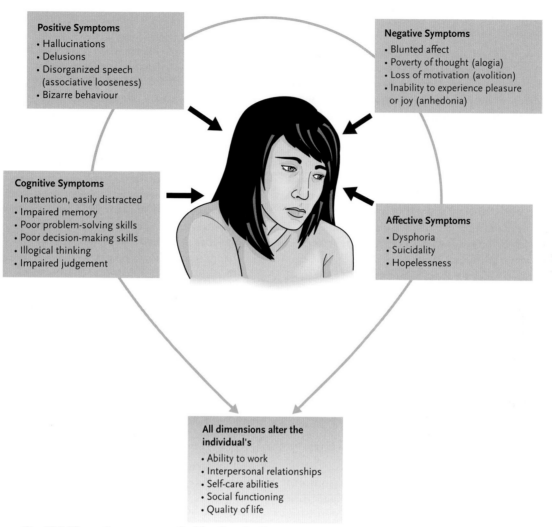

Positive Symptoms
- Hallucinations
- Delusions
- Disorganized speech (associative looseness)
- Bizarre behaviour

Negative Symptoms
- Blunted affect
- Poverty of thought (alogia)
- Loss of motivation (avolition)
- Inability to experience pleasure or joy (anhedonia)

Cognitive Symptoms
- Inattention, easily distracted
- Impaired memory
- Poor problem-solving skills
- Poor decision-making skills
- Illogical thinking
- Impaired judgement

Affective Symptoms
- Dysphoria
- Suicidality
- Hopelessness

All dimensions alter the individual's
- Ability to work
- Interpersonal relationships
- Self-care abilities
- Social functioning
- Quality of life

Fig. 11.3 **The main symptoms of schizophrenia.** (From Halter, M. J., Pollard, C. L., & Jakubec, S. L. [2019]. *Varcarolis's Canadian psychiatric health nursing: A clinical approach* [2nd Cdn. ed., p. 308, Figure 15-1]. Milton, ON: Elsevier Canada.)

and facilitate personal recovery. There may be setbacks and struggles in the recovery phase; therefore, ongoing assessment and monitoring is required to accommodate any new problems or demands that arise (Halter et al., 2019).

Types of Disorders

Schizophreniform disorder. A person with schizophreniform disorder has the symptoms of schizophrenia but for less than 6 months, during which there are periods of functional social and occupational activity.

Schizoaffective disorder. A person with schizoaffective disorder has schizophrenic symptoms and a concurrent major depressive or bipolar disorder, but no concurrent general medical disorder or substance abuse.

Delusional disorder. A person with delusional disorder experiences delusions for at least a month that contain either bizarre content (i.e. the person is not bizarre) or occur in real life, such as jealousy, persecution, delusions of grandeur, or having an infection or a somatic illness. The person can function

socially and at work. There are specify type of delusions based on the predominant delusional theme: erotomanic, grandiose, jealous, persecutory, somatic, mixed, and unspecified types.

Brief psychotic disorder. Following a very stressful life event, a person suddenly experiences psychotic and disorganized symptoms. These symptoms last for 1 day to a month, after which the person returns to his or her usual functioning.

Substance/medication-induced psychotic disorder. Psychosis may be caused by substances such as drugs of abuse, medications, alcohol, or toxins. The person may experience hallucinations or delusions (Halter et al., 2019).

Psychosis or catatonia associated with another medical condition or another mental disorder. According to Halter et al. (2019), "psychoses may also be caused by a medical condition (delirium, neurological or metabolic conditions, hepatic or renal diseases, and many others) as well as by mental illness such as post-traumatic stress disorder ... or depression, particularly with coexisting victimization from sexual violence of bullying. ... Medical conditions and substance abuse must always be ruled out before a diagnosis of schizophrenia or other psychotic disorder can be made" (p. 303).

Diagnostics and Therapeutics
Diagnosis

Diagnosing schizophrenia is complex for a number of reasons. Clients suffer from different combinations of symptoms, and none of the symptoms are completely confined to schizophrenia. In addition, most of the time, clients are at least partly in touch with reality and may be able to hide their symptoms to avoid stigma or admission to the hospital. As well, there is no single test for schizophrenia (Schizophrenia Society of Canada, 2018).

Commonly, schizophrenia is diagnosed once the person has experienced the following:

> at least one psychotic symptom such as delusions, hallucinations, disorganized thinking, speech or behaviour. The person experiences extreme difficulty with or an inability to function in family, social, or occupational realms and frequently neglects basic needs such as nutrition or hygiene. Over a period of 6 months, there may be times when the psychotic symptoms are absent, and in their place, the person may experience apathy or depression. (Halter et al., 2019, p. 302)

Schizophrenia spectrum and other psychotic disorders are complex mental health disorders that affect a person's language, thinking, emotion, social behaviours, and ability to perceive reality correctly. These disorders are identified by symptoms of psychosis. Psychosis is defined as a psychological break from reality. Associated behaviours include altered cognition and perception, great difficulty in functioning adequately, reduced level of awareness, and gross impairment in reality testing (Halter et al., 2019). Schizophrenia may be difficult to identify in the adolescent years since some of the early symptoms may be blamed on adolescent rebellion and immaturity. The DSM-5 diagnostic criteria for schizophrenia appear in Box 11.3.

Neuroimaging. CT, MRI, and PET scans may be used to narrow down the diagnosis.

Treatment

Antipsychotic medications. Antipsychotics are also called *neuroleptics* and *major tranquilizers*. There are two groups: the older typical antipsychotics and the newer atypicals (also called *novel antipsychotics*).

Typical antipsychotics
- Action: They block dopamine postsynaptic receptors in the hypothalamus, limbic system, brainstem, basal ganglia, and medulla.
- Effect: They provide some relief, primarily for the positive symptoms of schizophrenia.
  - Major side effects include neuromalignant syndrome and movement disorders (extrapyramidal symptoms [EPS]).
- Examples include chlorpromazine (Thorazine), thioridazine (Mellaril), trifluoperazine (Stelazine), thiothixene (Navane), loxapine (Loxitane), molindone (Moban),

mesoridazine (Serentil), perphenazine (Trilafon), fluphenazine (Prolixin), and haloperidol (Haldol).

Atypical antipsychotics
- Action: They block dopamine, serotonin, and other neurotransmitter receptors.
- Effect: They ease both the positive and negative symptoms, thus markedly enhancing quality of life for people with schizophrenia.
- Examples include clozapine (Clozaril), olanzapine (Zyprexa or Zydis), quetiapine (Seroquel), aripiprazole (Abilify), Ziprasidone (Geodon), and risperidone (Risperdal).

Other medical treatments.
- Additional drugs for symptoms of schizophrenia include antidepressants, antimania agents, and benzodiazepines.
- ECT is used for psychotic depression and for people who do not respond to antipsychotics.

Nursing Considerations
Nursing Assessment

Nursing assessment for psychosis is complex, but before focusing on the symptoms, try to rule out whether a medical condition or substance use is implicated, and think "safety first."

- Hallucinations: Assess especially if the person is hearing voices that order self-harm or harming others. If so, are the voices accepted as real, and is there intent to follow the commands?
- Delusions: Are there firm beliefs that are not reality based? Again, determine whether these could result in self-harm or harm to others and institute precautions if necessary.
- Co-occurring mental health disorders: These might include depression, suicidal thoughts, anxiety, substance abuse, or violent acts in the past.
- Medications: Has the individual been on any medications? If so, are they still being taken?
- Family: Is the family involved? In what way? Are they caring? Overprotective? Hostile? Suspicious? Does the family understand psychosis, the need for medication, and about support or respite services?

The Nurse–Client Relationship

Particular challenges in caring for someone who is psychotic involve communicating when a person is out of touch with reality. Mastering the following suggested communication skills will help the practical nurse establish a relationship of trust with these clients (Halter et al., 2019).

Communicating with a client experiencing delusions or hallucinations.
- To overcome suspicion and gain trust, be present, straightforward, honest, and reliable.
- Ask directly about delusions and hallucinations. For example, "Are you hearing voices?" "What are you hearing?" "Tell me more about someone trying to hurt you."
- Observe for cues, such as the client's eyes searching around or staring at a particular empty space, and for events that appear to generate the delusions. Try to discuss these observations with the client.

BOX 11.3   DSM-5 Diagnostic Criteria for Schizophrenia

A. Two or more of the following, each present for a significant portion of time during a 1-month period (or less if successfully treated). At least one of these must be (1), (2), or (3):
 1. Delusions.
 2. Hallucinations.
 3. Disorganized speech (e.g. frequent derailment or incoherence).
 4. Grossly disorganized or catatonic behavior.
 5. Negative symptoms (i.e. diminished emotional expression or avolition).

B. For a significant portion of the time since the onset of the disturbance, level of functioning in one or more major areas, such as work, interpersonal relations, or self-care, is markedly below the level achieved before the onset (or when the onset is in childhood or adolescence, there is failure to achieve expected level of interpersonal, academic, or occupational functioning).

C. Continuous signs of the disturbance persist for at least 6 months. This 6-month period must include at least 1 month of symptoms (or less if successfully treated) that meet Criterion A (i.e. active-phase symptoms) and may include periods of prodromal or residual symptoms. During these prodromal or residual periods, the signs of the disturbance may be manifested by only negative symptoms or by two or more symptoms listed in Criterion A present in an attenuated form (e.g. odd beliefs, unusual perceptual experiences).

D. Schizoaffective disorder and depressive or bipolar disorder with psychotic features have been ruled out because either (1) no major depressive or manic episodes have occurred concurrently with the active-phase symptoms, or (2) if mood episodes have occurred during active-phase symptoms, they have been present for a minority of the total duration of the active and residual periods of the illness.

E. The disturbance is not attributable to the physiological effects of a substance (e.g. a drug of abuse, a medication) or another medical condition.

F. If there is a history of autism spectrum disorder or a communication disorder of childhood onset, the additional diagnosis of schizophrenia is made only if prominent delusions or hallucinations, in addition to the other required symptoms of schizophrenia, are also present for at least 1 month (or less if successfully treated).

Specify if: The following course specifiers are only to be used after a 1-year duration of the disorder and if they are not in contradiction to the diagnostic course criteria.

First episode, currently in acute episode: First manifestation of the disorder meeting the defining diagnostic symptom and time criteria. An *acute episode* is a time period in which the symptom criteria are fulfilled.

First episode, currently in partial remission: *Partial remission* is a period of time during which an improvement after a previous episode is maintained and in which the defining criteria of the disorder are only partially fulfilled.

First episode, currently in full remission: *Full remission* is a period of time after a previous episode during which no disorder-specific symptoms are present.

Multiple episodes, currently in acute episode: Multiple episodes may be determined after a minimum of two episodes (i.e. after a first episode, a remission, and a minimum of one relapse).

Multiple episodes, currently in partial remission

Multiple episodes, currently in full remission

Continuous: Symptoms fulfilling the diagnostic symptom criteria of the disorder are remaining for the majority of the illness course with subthreshold symptom periods being very brief relative to the overall course.

Unspecified

Specify if: **With catatonia**

Specify current severity: Severity is rated by a quantitative assessment of the primary symptoms of psychosis, including delusions, hallucinations, disorganized speech, abnormal psychomotor behavior, and negative symptoms. Each of these symptoms may be rated for its current severity (most severe in the last 7 days) on a 5-point scale ranging from 0 (not present) to 4 (present and severe).

From Halter, M. (2018). *Varcarolis' foundations of psychiatric mental health nursing. A clinical approach* (8th ed. p. 193). St. Louis: Elsevier. Based on American Psychiatric Association. (2013). *Diagnostic and statistical manual of mental disorders* (5th ed.). Washington, DC: Author.

- Do not argue with the voices and beliefs or react as though they are real. Instead, provide your own observations and encourage the client to talk about feelings. For example, "I can't see what you do, but it seems to be upsetting you," or "It must be frightening to think that people are against you."
- Focus on reality-based, "here-and-now" activities such as conversations or simple projects. Tell the client, "The voice you hear is part of your illness; it cannot hurt you. Try to listen to me and the others you can see around you."
- If some aspect of the delusion or hallucination is real, validate that part, such as, "Yes, I heard Mr. Green talking on the phone, but he was discussing a movie he had seen. He didn't refer to you."
- Be alert to signs of anxiety in the client, which may indicate that hallucinations are increasing.
- Encourage the use of competing auditory stimuli such as listening to music through headphones.
- Address any underlying emotion, need, or theme that seems to be indicated by the hallucination, such as fear with menacing voices or guilt with accusing voices.
- Focus on the feelings or theme that underlie or flow from the delusions. For example, "You seem to wish you could be more powerful" or "It must feel frightening to think others want to hurt you" (Halter et al., 2019).

Interventions

Nursing interventions for schizophrenia vary depending on the stage of the client's illness. The focus for treatment and professional collaboration varies during each phase of schizophrenia. Interventions include crisis interventions, inpatient treatment teams, group therapies, social, vocational and self-care skills, medication maintenance education, psychoeducational interventions with families, community treatment agencies, and social support services.

Pharmacotherapy

Serious and sometimes permanent side effects occur with antipsychotic medications. In Table 11.4 nursing considerations for antipsychotic drug effects are described.

Drug interactions. Be aware of potential interactions with other medications. Note the following examples:

- Cimetidine (Tagamet), which is for acid indigestion, promotes liver detoxification of antipsychotics and thus decreases their effect.
- Other common antacids reduce absorption of oral antipsychotics. They should be taken 4 hours before or after the antipsychotic.

- Anticonvulsants lower the blood levels of antipsychotics, interfering with their efficacy.
- Epinephrine can produce severe hypotension if given with chlorpromazine.
- Lithium occasionally can produce neurological impairment when combined with antipsychotics. Clients should be monitored closely for neurological signs and symptoms.
- Some cardiac drugs reduce the effectiveness of antipsychotics, increasing psychosis.

    For more information on these drugs, see Chapter 7.

Engaging with Families

Having a family member with schizophrenia is emotionally painful, exhausting, and frightening. Relatives, often the main caregivers when the client is not in hospital, should be

TABLE 11.4 Nursing Considerations for Antipsychotic Drug Effects

CNS Side Effects	Nursing Care and Teaching Considerations
Extrapyramidal symptoms (EPS)	General treatment principles: • Tolerance usually develops by the third month. • Decrease dose of drug. • Add a drug to treat EPS, then taper after 3 months on the antipsychotic. • Use a drug with a lower EPS profile. • Give client education and support.
Acute dystonic reactions: oculogyric crisis, torticollis	Spasms of major muscle groups of neck, back, and eyes; occur suddenly; frightening; painful; parenteral medication works faster than PO; have respiratory support available; more common in children and young males and with high-potency drugs. Taper dose gradually when discontinuing antipsychotic drugs to avoid withdrawal dyskinesia.
Akathisia	Cannot remain still; pacing, inner restlessness, leg aches are relieved by movement; rule out anxiety or agitation; medicate.
Parkinson's syndrome: akinesia, cogwheel rigidity, fine tremor	More common in males and older adults; tolerance may not develop; medicate with DA antagonist amantadine (must have good renal function).
Tardive dyskinesia (TD)	Can occur after use (usually long term) of conventional antipsychotics; stereotyped involuntary movements (tongue protrusion, lip smacking, chewing, blinking, grimacing, choreiform movements of limbs and trunk, foot tapping); if using typical antipsychotics, use preventive measures and assess often; consider changing to an atypical antipsychotic drug; there is no treatment at present for TD.
Neuroleptic malignant syndrome (NMS)*	Potentially fatal: Fever, tachycardia, sweating, muscle rigidity, tremor, incontinence, stupor, leukocytosis, elevated creatine phosphokinase (CPK), renal failure; more common with high-potency drugs and in dehydrated clients; discontinue all drugs; supportive symptomatic care (hydration, renal dialysis, ventilation, and fever reduction as appropriate); can treat with dantrolene or promocriptine; antipsychotic drugs can be cautiously reintroduced eventually.
Seizures*	Potentially life-threatening: Seizures occur in approximately 1% of people taking these drugs; clozapine has a 5% rate (in clients on 600 to 900 mg/day); may have to discontinue clozapine.
Side effects on other systems **Agranulocytosis***	This is an emergency: It develops abruptly with fever, malaise, ulcerative sore throat, and leukopenia. High incidence (1–2%) is associated with clozapine; must do weekly CBC and prescribe only 1 week of drug at a time; discontinue drug immediately; may need reverse isolation and antibiotics.
Photosensitivity	Use sunscreen and sunglasses; cover body with clothing.
Anticholinergic effects	Symptoms: constipation, dry mouth, blurred vision, orthostatic hypotension, tachycardia, urinary retention, nasal congestion; see Table 11.3 for nursing care.
Weight gain	See Table 11.3 for nursing care.

*Potentially life-threatening.

CBC, complete blood count; *CNS,* central nervous system; *DA,* dopamine; *PO,* oral tablet or capsule.

Adapted from Stuart, G.W. (2013). *Principles and practice of psychiatric nursing* (10th ed., p. 554, Table 26.18). St. Louis: Mosby.

TABLE 11.5   Family Education Plan: Understanding Psychosis

Content	Instructional Activities	Evaluation
Describe psychosis	Introduce participants and leaders State purpose of group Define terminology associated with psychosis	The participant will describe the characteristics of psychosis
Identify the causes of psychotic disorders	Present theories of psychotic disorders Use audiovisual aids to explain brain anatomy, brain biochemistry, and major neurotransmitters	The participant will discuss the relationship between brain anatomy, brain biochemistry, major neurotransmitters, and the development of psychosis
Define schizophrenia according to symptoms and diagnostic criteria	Lead a discussion of the diagnostic criteria for schizophrenia Show a film on schizophrenia	The participant will describe the symptoms and diagnostic criteria for schizophrenia
Describe the relationship between anxiety and psychotic disorders	Present types and stages of anxiety Discuss steps in reducing and resolving anxiety	The participant will identify and describe the stages of anxiety and ways to reduce or resolve it
Analyze the impact of living with hallucinations	Describe the characteristics of hallucinations Demonstrate ways to communicate with someone who is hallucinating	The participant will demonstrate effective ways to communicate with a person who has hallucinations
Analyze the impact of living with delusions	Describe types of delusions Demonstrate ways to communicate with someone who has delusions Discuss interventions for delusions	The participant will demonstrate effective ways to communicate with a person who has delusions
Discuss the use of psychotropic medications	Provide and explain handouts describing the characteristics of psychotropic medications that are prescribed for schizophrenia	The participant will identify and describe the characteristics of medications prescribed for self or family member
Describe the characteristics of relapse and the role of adherence to the therapeutic regimen	Help the participants describe their own experiences with relapse Discuss symptom management techniques and the importance of complying with the therapeutic regimen	The participant will describe behaviours that indicate an impending relapse and discuss the importance of symptom management and adherence to the therapeutic regimen
Analyze behaviours that promote wellness	Discuss the components of wellness Relate wellness to the elements of symptom management	The participant will analyze the effect of maintaining wellness on the occurrence of symptoms
Discuss ways to cope adaptively with psychosis	Lead a group discussion focused on coping behaviours and the daily problems in living with psychosis Propose ways to create a low-stress environment	The participant will describe ways to modify his or her lifestyle to create a low-stress environment

From Stuart, G. W. (2013). *Principles and practice of psychiatric nursing* (10th ed., p.371, Table 20.8). St. Louis: Mosby.

consulted in treatment planning and decision making. Family caregivers generally know the client best.

When a client is first diagnosed, however, education for relatives is essential. A family educational plan for understanding psychoses appears in Table 11.5.

Community supports. Practical nurses should know what community resources and services are available and should assist families in accessing these services. The following two major community agencies provide comprehensive programs.

Schizophrenia Society of Canada. Provincial and local chapters are located across the country. Services and programs may include the following:

- Support groups and counselling services for family members; peer support for clients
- Monthly educational meetings and periodic conferences for family members
- Education programs for parents, siblings, and children of people with schizophrenia

- Public education programs for schools and other community agencies and service providers

Canadian Mental Health Association (CMHA). Services and programs may vary by location but may include the following:

- Educational programs for parents and families
- Community education programs
- Recreation and leisure opportunities for people with a mental health challenge
- Peer options for connecting people with a mental illness and reducing their isolation
- Supported housing
- Bereavement counselling

PERSONALITY DISORDERS

Personality "is an individual's characteristic pattern of relatively permanent thoughts, feelings, and behaviours that define his or her quality of experiences and relationships" (Halter et al., 2019, p. 452). Each person develops unique personality traits from his or her biological constitution, psycho-social experiences, and environment. Personality traits become deeply engrained and stable, exerting control over a person's attitudes and behaviour.

When a person's character and behaviour deviate markedly from social and cultural expectations, causing functional impairment and distress, the person may have a personality disorder (PD). PDs vary from mild to severe, and people can function quite well when symptoms are mild or intermittent. In fact, most people occasionally display maladaptive characteristics identified with a PD, and some people are clearly eccentric. Healthcare providers need to take a person's cultural, ethical, and social background into account to prevent the risk of overdiagnosis of a personality disorder (Halter et al., 2019). Box 11.4 presents the DSM-5 categories for personality disorders.

The DSM-5 also include two other groups of personality disorders: "Personality change due to another medical condition and other specified personality disorder and unspecified personality disorder" (APA, 2013, p. 645).

PDs affect between 6 and 15% of the Canadian population. The most common type of PD is obsessive–compulsive personality disorder (which is distinct from OCD). PDs typically become recognizable by adolescence or early adulthood, although some individuals may not seek clinical attention until much later. It is possible for a PD to become exacerbated after the loss of a significant supporting person or situation. The course of PD is relatively stable over time (Statistic Canada, 2015b).

Pathophysiology

Some evidence exists for neurobiological abnormalities, but as for most psychiatric disorders, no clear-cut cause for PDs has been identified. A complex interaction of the following factors correlate with PD:

- Genetics—Some evidence exists for a genetic link for antisocial and criminal personality traits, as well as for schizotypal and paranoid PD.
- EEG evidence—Research evidence is mixed. Some studies show a relationship between PD and abnormal temporal and frontal lobe waves, but others do not.
- Neurotransmitters—Low dopamine and serotonin levels are found in aggressive and impulsive behaviours, as well as in suicidality.
- Autonomic nervous system (ANS)—Dominance of parasympathetic over sympathetic impulses may amplify or jumble neural impulses, resulting in cognitive or affective problems.
- Limbic system—Because of controlling emotions, the limbic system (amygdala, hippocampus) and its connections to the thalamus and hypothalamus are also implicated in PD.
- Psycho-social development—Strong attachments to supportive family, peer, and community networks may protect people from PD by enhancing coping skills and personal growth. Conversely, a history of abuse or neglect in childhood puts people at increased risk.

Clinical Manifestations

PDs usually arise in adolescence and early adulthood. Thus, if there is a biological predisposition, the social and developmental challenges of this life stage, related to gaining independence and separation from family, may trigger a PD.

PDs share features of other mental illnesses, but no single illness completely explains the long-standing maladaptive thinking and behavioural patterns of PD, some of which are as follows:

- Inappropriate emotions, with poor impulse and emotional control
- Disturbed self-concept and inappropriate perceptions of others and the environment
- Unhealthy or very limited personal relationships

BOX 11.4 DSM-5 Categorization of Personality Disorders

According to the American Psychiatric Association, there are 10 personality disorders. These 10 disorders are grouped into three clusters of similar behaviour patterns and personality traits. These clusters are:

Cluster A: Individuals with these disorders share characteristics of eccentric behaviours, such as social isolation and detachment. They may also display perception distortions, unusual levels of suspiciousness, magical thinking, and cognitive impairment.
- Paranoid personality disorder
- Schizoid personality disorder
- Schizotypal personality disorder

Cluster B: People living with cluster B personality disorders show patterns of responding to life demands with dramatic, emotional, or erratic behaviour. Problems with impulse control, emotion processing and regulation, and interpersonal difficulties characterize this cluster of disorders. Insight into these issues is generally limited. To get their needs met, individuals with cluster B personality disorders may resort to behaviours that are considered desperate or entitled, including acting out, committing antisocial acts, or manipulating people and circumstances.
- Borderline personality disorder
- Narcissistic personality disorder
- Histrionic personality disorder
- Antisocial personality disorder

Cluster C: An individual with these types of personality disorders will demonstrate a consistent patterns of anxious and fearful behaviours, rigid patterns of social shyness, hypersensitivity, need for orderliness, and relationship dependency.
- Avoidant personality disorder
- Dependent personality disorder
- Obsessive–compulsive personality disorder

From Halter, M. J., Pollard, C. L., & Jacubec, S. L. (2019). *Varcarolis's Canadian psychiatric mental health nursing: A clinical approach* (2nd Cdn. ed., p. 433). Milton, ON: Elsevier. Based on American Psychiatric Association. (2013). *Diagnostic and statistical manual of mental disorders* (5th ed. Rev.). Washington, DC: Author.

- School or employment difficulties
- Often an associated depression or substance abuse, or both

PDs are classified into the three groups, or clusters, which are discussed next. Two additional groups exist as well. The first one is called "*personality change due to another medical condition*. It is a persistent personality disturbance that is judged to be due to the direct physiological effects of a medical condition. The other group is called *other specified personality disorder and unspecified personality disorder*. It is a category provided for two situations:

1. The individual's personality pattern meets the general criteria for a personal disorder, and traits of several personality disorders are present, but the criteria for any specific disorder is not met; or
2. The individual's personality pattern meets the general criteria for a personality disorder, but the individual is considered to have a personality disorder that is not included in the DSM-5 classification (e.g. passive-aggressive personality disorder)" (APA, 2013, pp. 645–646, emphasis added).

Cluster A: Odd and Eccentric

Odd and eccentric behaviour patterns are characteristic of three personality disorders, in which people tend toward social and emotional withdrawal. Descriptions of these three disorders follow.

Paranoid personality disorder. Symptoms include the following:

- Being suspicious and distrustful, misinterpreting others' motives as threatening, exploitive, or deceiving; often bears grudges
- Detachment and social isolation
- Overreaction to threats, even with no actual evidence of malice; has hostile outbursts often
- Fear of becoming close to others or confiding in anyone
- Hypervigilance and hyperactivity; is unable to relax
- Hypersensitivity and irritability; is often angry and jealous

Schizoid personality disorder. Symptoms include the following:

- Being a loner; is detached from social and family relationships
- Emotional detachment; prefers solitary activities, although the person may be lonely
- Avoidance of intimacy; is indifferent to the feelings or reactions of others
- Flattened affect, emotional coldness

Schizotypal personality disorder. Symptoms include the following:

- Acute discomfort in social relationships
- Eccentric and odd behaviour and appearance
- Strange beliefs or magical thinking (superstitions, clairvoyance, telepathy, distorted cognition, fantasies, and preoccupations) that is outside cultural norms
- Unusual patterns of speech (metaphorical, vague, very elaborate and flowery), unusual perceptual experiences, including bodily illusions
- Having suspicious or paranoid ideation

Cluster B: Dramatic and Emotional

These four PDs are distinguished by behaviour that is overly emotional, dramatic, and erratic.

Borderline personality disorder. Symptoms include the following:

- Instability of mood, interpersonal relationships, and self-image
- Impulsive, reckless behaviour that is often self-damaging, such as substance abuse, spending binges, heightened sexuality, or binge eating
- Uncontrolled, inappropriate, or frequent anger episodes
- Fear of rejection and being alone; feels empty; frantically tries to avoid being abandoned
- Transient, stress-related paranoid ideation or severe dissociative symptoms
- Common threats of self-injury and suicide

Narcissistic personality disorder. Symptoms include the following:

- Feelings of superiority; is rude and arrogant
- Attention-seeking; requires constant admiration and special treatment
- Envy of those with high status; pursues friendships with them
- Lacking in empathy for others—It's all about me!
- Manipulative; is driven to succeed; takes advantage of others to achieve personal goals

Histrionic personality disorder. Symptoms include the following:

- Desire to be the centre of attention; craves excitement and instant gratification
- Consistent use of physical appearance to draw attention to self
- Speech that is excessively impressionistic and lacking in detail
- Rapid shifting and shallow expression of emotions—and exaggerated expression of emotions—overly sensitive to criticism; reacts with anger
- Provocative and sexually inappropriate behaviour
- Suggestibility (easily influenced by others)
- Belief that relationships are more intimate than they actually are

Antisocial personality disorder. Symptoms include the following:

- Persistent disregard for the rights of safety for self and others; shows contempt for other's feelings and rights
- Disregard for the law; has had frequent arrests
- Lack of remorse
- Impulsiveness and irresponsibility
- Irritability and aggressiveness; is involved in repeated fights or assaults
- Deceitful; chronically lies and misrepresents self but can appear very charming
- Evidence of conduct disorder with onset before 15 years old
- Being at least 18 years old

Older diagnostic terms for this disorder are *psychopath* and *sociopath*, referring to a lack of social conscience.

Cluster C: Anxiety and Fear

The defining features of cluster C are anxious and fearful behaviour.

Obsessive–compulsive personality disorder. Avoid confusing obsessive–compulsive PD with OCD and related disorders. A person with OCD and related disorders exhibits considerable anxiety and distress. A person with obsessive–compulsive PD desires perfection and order. The true obsessions and compulsions of a person with OCD are more intense and compelling.

Symptoms of obsessive–compulsive PD include the following:

- Rigid desire for perfection and control, coupled with ruthless self-criticism
- Overattention to rules and regulations, schedules, and discipline
- Indecisiveness and inability to complete tasks; is afraid of making a mistake
- Inflexibility with ethics, thriftiness, and moral values, but not necessarily religious
- Diligent work habits and difficulty delegating work; is a "workaholic"

Avoidant personality disorder. Symptoms include the following:

- Low self-esteem; has feelings of inadequacy and of being a failure
- Being socially withdrawn; shows restraint within intimate relationships because of fear of being shamed or ridiculed
- Sensitivity to criticism and rejection
- Avoidance of personal risks, new activities, or relationships

Dependent personality disorder. Symptoms include the following:

- Clinging behaviour; has pervasive need to be taken care of; fears separation
- Indecisiveness; requires excessive advice and reassurance; defers major responsibilities to others
- Craving approval and support; therefore, unable to disagree with others
- Low self-confidence; is unable to initiate activities
- Craving relationships; desperately seeks a new relationship when one has ended

Diagnostics and Therapeutics

Diagnosis

Enduring but distressing behaviour patterns that deviate from cultural norms and that affect social and occupational functioning in a broad range of activities and social situations are identified. Diagnosis is challenging because of overlapping symptoms and the tendency for some people to have more than one PD. Initially, one must rule out other mental or medical disorders and treatment or medication side effects. PDs affect at least two of the following:

- Faulty cognitive schema—Misperceptions and interpretations of self, others, and social situations that lead to dysfunctional responses
- Inappropriate emotions—Abnormal range, intensity, and emotionally labile responses
- Poor interpersonal functioning—Maladaptive behaviours, being hard to get along with
- Poor impulse control

Treatment

Many PDs are difficult to treat because of the client's self-denial. Common treatments include intensive psychotherapy or group psychotherapy, along with psychopharmacology:

- Antipsychotics—For severe agitation or delusional thinking in paranoid, schizotypal, and borderline PD
- SSRIs, other antidepressants—For obsessive thoughts, anger, irritability, and unstable mood
- Anxiolytics—For cluster C disorders
- MAOIs—To decrease self-harm and impulsive acts
- Lithium carbonate, propranolol—For antisocial PD with violent episodes

Nursing Considerations

Individuals with a PD have a significant and persistent impairment in their interpersonal relationships and other aspects of functioning.

The following are three key features of PDs:

1. The individual has an inflexible and maladaptive approach to relationships and the environment.
2. The individual's needs, perceptions, and behaviour tend to foster cycles that promote unhelpful patterns and provoke negative reactions from others.
3. The individual's coping skills are unstable and fragile, and there is a lack of resilience when faced with stressful situations (Stuart, 2013).

The Nurse–Client Relationship

Practical nurses encounter PDs wherever they work, and establishing a therapeutic alliance challenges even very experienced nurses. These clients know just which "buttons to push." Pay special attention to professional boundaries and set realistic limits on the client's behaviour and your availability. Keep your communication clear and unambiguous, giving simple directions. Avoid power struggles or arguments, showing confidence in your abilities and decisions. Remember that for such enduring patterns of behaviour, improvement takes time.

Splitting behaviour, that is, setting staff members against one another, is common. Thus, professional teamwork is vital. Staff must support each other and be consistent with the client.

Nursing Interventions

Nursing care of people with PD involves providing them with structure and clear expectations for their behaviour. A contract may be helpful for encouraging specific behaviours. Communicate respect for the person. The behaviour is the problem, not the client. Set mutually agreed-upon goals and stick to them. Help clients identify and voice their emotions. Some specific considerations for specific PDs follow.

Paranoid personality disorder.

- Involve the client in planning care, thus helping the person feel in control.
- Teach clients to delay responding to others until they have validated their perceptions and assumptions. This helps them avoid acting on paranoid ideas.

Schizoid personality disorder.

- Support the client's ability to function in the community (e.g. provide a referral to social services to arrange supportive housing).
- Be aware that these clients are likely to require case management, either a professional case manager or at least a family member who can arrange for services and assistance.

Schizotypal personality disorder.

- Assist with development of self-care and social skills.
- Perform a detailed assessment to detect any other medical or psychological symptoms that may require intervention (suicidal thoughts).

Borderline personality disorder.

- Ensure safety; negotiate a no self-harm contract with the client. The client agrees not to engage in injurious actions and to inform a nurse if he or she is losing control.
- Help the client identify moods, emotions, and situations that trigger self-harm activities and explore more effective coping strategies for those triggers.
- Provide structured daily activities that include health-promoting activities.

Narcissistic personality disorder.

- Use a matter-of-fact approach as you try to gain the person's co-operation with treatment.
- Promote milieu therapy—Engage the individual in community activities (either the therapeutic community in the hospital or the larger community outside). Reinforce appropriate behaviour.

Histrionic personality disorder.

- Provide social skills training, with factual feedback about his or her behaviour.
- Understand that seductive behaviour is a response to distress. Nursing interventions should display this understanding.

Antisocial personality disorder.

- Teach effective problem-solving and anger management techniques.
- Confront the client when he or she oversteps acceptable limits on behaviour.

Obsessive–compulsive personality disorder.

- Engage in cognitive restructuring—Explore and encourage the client to accept outcomes that are "good enough" or "satisfactory."
- Assist the client with decision making and completing tasks.

Avoidant personality disorder.

- Promote self-esteem by providing support and reassurance.

- Cognitive restructuring—Try positive self-talk, reframing situations, and decatastrophizing (e.g. ask, "What is the worst thing that could happen?" "How likely is that?").

Dependent personality disorder.

- Encourage autonomy and self-reliance.
- Teach problem-solving and decision making skills.

SUBSTANCE-RELATED AND ADDICTIVE DISORDERS

Substance-related and addictive disorders refer to the consumption and excess consumption (by any route) of drugs and alcohol. Nurses often forget that the overuse of legally approved medications, both over-the-counter and prescription, also constitutes a substance disorder.

Many Canadians use alcohol, some use illicit drugs, some use both, and many abuse these substances. Three-quarters of Canadians over 12 years consume alcohol. In 2015, 19.2% admitted to heavy drinking (five or more drinks on one occasion) at least once a year; and half of those did so at least monthly (Statistics Canada, 2015a). The prevalence of past year cannabis (marijuana) use among Canadians aged 15 years and older was 10%. Risk factors for dependence on drugs, alcohol, or both include youth, low income, less education, and being male (Health Canada, 2012).

The comorbidity of mental illness and substance abuse (also called *dual diagnosis*) is common. Some people use substances to ease their psychiatric symptoms; for others, substance use and abuse may promote the development or severity of a mental illness. For this reason, many health authorities combine mental health and addiction services into one department.

Pathophysiology and Clinical Manifestations

Addictive substances either depress or stimulate the CNS. Marijuana seems to do both. All interfere with neurotransmission and the limbic system, altering emotions and the brain's reward system.

Central Nervous System Depressants

Drugs that depress the CNS produce drowsiness and sedation. They include alcohol, opioids, sedatives, anxiolytics, and probably inhalants. Alcohol, accepted in many cultures, is also the most commonly abused drug. People overuse these drugs because of the pleasant sensations of relaxation, euphoria, and reduced inhibition, commonly called being "high." Tolerance develops, such that higher and higher doses are required to produce the same effects, and eventually the person cannot function without the drug, experiencing cravings and physical dependence or addiction. Overdose can lead to respiratory or cardiovascular depression, coma, convulsions, and death.

Alcohol.

- Alcohol, soluble in fat and water, is absorbed from the stomach and small intestine. It is quickly disbursed throughout the body and metabolized by the liver at the rate of one drink (one beer, 5 oz. of wine, or 1 oz. of hard liquor) per hour.

- Alcohol initially stimulates the release of naturally produced opioids (endorphins and enkephalins) and dopamine (the reward centres of the limbic system), producing feelings of pleasure. In higher concentrations, alcohol is toxic to nerve cells, producing poor emotional control, reduced muscle coordination, and then mental confusion and loss of consciousness. At very high concentrations, it produces coma, respiratory depression, and eventual death.
- Chronic alcoholism produces general body damage. Complications are dementia, hepatitis and cirrhosis, cardiomyopathy, gastritis, peptic ulcers, pancreatitis, and peripheral neuropathy.
- Withdrawal produces neural excitation, with tremors, agitation and anxiety, irritability, insomnia, and sometimes delirium tremens (DTs) with hallucinations, seizures, and delirium. This is a medical emergency and, without treatment, can cause death. Symptoms include high fever, hypertension, tachycardia, and seizures.

Opioids.

- Opium derivatives are narcotics. Many are legally controlled, but heroin is illegal.
- Taken intravenously (IV) or nasally (snorting), they act on the reward centres of the brain, reducing neuron excitability, especially of the pain neurotransmitters, and producing analgesia and euphoria (a "rush"). Other effects include respiratory depression, constricted pupils, and constipation.

Sedative–hypnotics and anxiolytics.

- These include the benzodiazepines and barbiturates, taken orally or intravenously.
- Tolerance, dependence, and withdrawal usually do not develop if taken for under a month.
- Withdrawal symptoms can be avoided by gradually tapering the dosage under medical supervision.

Inhalants.

- These volatile substances are inhaled and include fuels, solvents, thinners, propellants, and nitrates.
- Inhalants produce a cheap "high" and are mostly used by youth. However, side effects from high doses or prolonged use are serious, damaging the brain, liver, kidneys, heart, and lungs.

Date rape drugs.

- These are given to unsuspecting victims prior to rape.
- They include rohypnol (roofies), GHB (gamma-hydroxybutyrate), and ketamine (vitamin K).
- Effects are reduced inhibition and sedation, often enhanced by mixing with alcohol. Overdose depresses respirations or causes seizures, coma, and death.
- Rohypnol also produces amnesia.

Central Nervous System Stimulants

Stimulants produce alertness, excitation, and aggressiveness and reduce fatigue. Metabolism is increased, and appetite is suppressed. They include caffeine, nicotine, amphetamines, cocaine, and hallucinogens. The stronger drugs produce restlessness, overtalkativeness, anxiety, irritability, suspicion, paranoia, and hallucinations. Tolerance and dependence occur. Withdrawal symptoms, however, are less physiologically dangerous than those of alcohol or opiates. Withdrawal brings depressed mood, sleep disturbance, fatigue, and anhedonia (inability to experience pleasure).

Caffeine and nicotine.

- Caffeine (coffee, cola soft drinks) can cause nervousness, anxiety, and difficulty sleeping.
- Nicotine (tobacco) is highly addictive. It became less socially acceptable with the recognition of the negative health effects, particularly for bystanders exposed to second-hand smoke. Effects include relaxation, excitement, and decreased appetite. Quitting smoking is very difficult, producing withdrawal (mood changes, anxiety, irritability, restlessness, and hunger).

Amphetamines and cocaine.

- The initial effect is stimulation, but CNS depression follows. Both drugs produce marked euphoria, but dangerous cardiovascular effects (tachycardia, arrhythmias, hypertension, vasoconstriction) that can cause heart failure, myocardial infarction, strokes, and renal complications can occur. First-time cocaine users have died. Continued use leads, however, to tolerance and some decrease in cardiovascular side effects.
- These drugs are absorbed directly into the bloodstream from direct injection into a vein and through mucous membranes (oral, nasal [snorted or smoked], or buccal membranes). Cocaine is the most addictive of all abused substances.
- Long-term sniffing causes ulcers in the nose and perforations of the septum; long-term smoking damages the throat, upper GI tract, and lungs.
- Crack cocaine is a purified, crystallized form. It is easily available and inexpensive, with an immediate but very short effect (5–7 minutes) followed by profound depression, and there is a strong drive to relieve the depression with another "hit." The result is that crack is extremely addictive.

Hallucinogens.

- These include LSD (acid), MDMA (Ecstasy), and mescaline.
- Effects are alterations in perception, including hallucinations with euphoria (a "trip") or frightening and depressing perceptions (a "bad trip"). People report awareness of themselves and surroundings but altered sensory perceptions of colours, time, arousal, body image, hearing, and so on.
- Sympathetic nervous system stimulation causes palpitations, increased BP, blurred vision, dilated pupils, and sweating. A bad trip may induce dizziness, anxiety, and panic.
- Flashbacks occur, perhaps more often if hallucinogens are combined with other substances.

PCP (Angel dust).
Effects include hyperactivity, aggressiveness, impulsivity, unpredictable behaviour, feeling superhuman, and sometimes psychosis. Dangerous respiratory and cardiovascular side effects can lead to seizures, coma, and death.

Marijuana.

- Also called cannabis, hashish, THC (tetrahydrocannabinol), pot, weed, grass, or Mary Jane.
- Marijuana has both CNS stimulant and CNS depressant effects, through its influence on a variety of neurotransmitters and neurochemicals.
- Common effects are euphoria, relaxation, drowsiness, heightened or altered sensory perceptions, reduced coordination, dry mouth, tachycardia, red eyes, disorientation, and appetite stimulation.
- "Canada plans to legalize recreational use of cannabis in 2018, which will lead to increased use if the pattern follows other jurisdictions. This in turn will likely produce increased health and social issues, including greater rates of impaired driving; child and some adult poisonings, primarily from edibles; increased criminal charges for public intoxication; increased rates of mental health issues such as anxiety and panic attacks, especially among adolescent users; marijuana-associated cyclic vomiting syndrome; and an increase in hospitalizations for burns resulting primarily from flash fires that occur when a user is trying to extract THC and other active marijuana constituents using butane" (Halter et al., 2019, p. 409).

Diagnostics and Therapeutics

Diagnosis

During a complete history and physical examination, special attention is paid to the manifestations noted earlier. The clinician may note needle tracks and bruising along arm and leg veins, signs of malnourishment, teary and reddened eyes, a runny nose, or frequent swallowing, indicating a postnasal drip. Laboratory tests may include toxicology urine screening, blood alcohol levels, or both, in addition to a full work-up for suspected complications. Denial is common with substance abusers, making history-taking challenging.

Substance use disorder is recurrent substance use, leading to the following:

- Unsatisfactory performance at home, work, or school
- Impairment in hazardous situations (such as driving)
- Frequent legal issues or being arrested
- Ongoing social and interpersonal problems

Physical dependence on substances is diagnosed with evidence of the following:

- Tolerance—Needing increased amounts to achieve intoxication
- Withdrawal symptoms when the substance is stopped or unavailable
- Failing attempts to quit or cut down substance use. People often continue to use, while at the same time recognizing the problems being created.
- Avoiding social, occupational, or recreational activities in favour of substance use
- Increased time, effort, and money spent on substances or on recovering from intoxication

Treatment

Treatment depends on the severity of the client's condition. First, treat an overdose and then address withdrawal symptoms. Only after stabilization can one begin to address addiction. Pharmacotherapy for treating chemical dependency varies according to the particular substance being abused. Some of the major pharmacological treatments follow.

Alcohol.

- Benzodiazepines for alcohol withdrawal
- Naltrexone (ReVia) and Antabuse (disulfiram) to help maintain abstinence
- Thiamine to help prevent major brain damage complications (Wernicke-Korsakoff syndrome) for long-term alcoholics

Other central nervous system depressants.

- Phenobarbital is given for withdrawal from sedative–hypnotics, benzodiazepines, and barbiturates.
- Methadone and clonidine are used to manage withdrawal from opiates. They reduce the severity of withdrawal symptoms by binding with opioid receptors.

Central nervous system stimulants.

- Nicotine gum and nicotine patches replace smoking, with gradual tapering over time.
- Bupropion (Zyban, Wellbutrin) aids withdrawal from smoking by reducing cravings.
- Benzodiazepines and antipsychotics lessen psychotic reactions from hallucinogens and PCP.
- Naloxone hydrochloride (Narcan), an opioid antagonist, is used for narcotic overdose.
- Buprenorphine (Buprenex), an opioid analgesic, is used for withdrawal from narcotics. It is less addicting than other narcotics.
- Currently, no specific medications are available for cocaine withdrawal or addiction, although antidepressants may ease mood changes due to abstinence; sedatives help with insomnia; and anxiolytics reduce symptoms of anxiety. Antabuse is used to discourage cocaine use.

Treatment for chemical addiction is multifaceted and may include the following:

- Psychotherapy and counselling
- Education
- Cognitive–behavioural therapy
- Behaviour modification
- Motivational therapy
- Group therapy—Peer support groups in the community, for example, Alcoholics Anonymous (AA). Newer programs, often modelled on the AA 12-step program, have been developed for other addictions and may be accessed, depending on community availability.

For dual diagnosis, successful treatment of the comorbid psychiatric diagnosis often reduces the individual's addictive behaviour.

Harm Reduction

Harm reduction is a relatively new and increasingly common approach to drug addiction, although it is not without political controversy. The first harm-reduction programs were methadone maintenance programs in the 1960s and 1970s. Recognizing the compulsion underlying dependence and that abstinence is difficult to achieve, the goal of these programs is to minimize the damage of addiction to the individual and to society (Pauly, Gray, Perkin, et al., 2016). By providing such things as clean equipment and education about safe practices, they aim to achieve the following:

- Decrease overdoses, infections, hepatitis B and C, tuberculosis, other diseases, such as HIV/AIDS, and deaths for injection drug users
- Reduce the violence and crime associated with the drug culture
- Reduce the use of impure street drugs that lack any quality control
- Provide access to community outreach, public health programs, education, detoxification programs, and other treatment
- Promote trust among drug users, their families, and health providers

Some examples include needle-exchange programs, methadone replacement, safe injection sites, heroin-assisted treatments, controlled drinking, managed alcohol programs, overdose prevention and education programs, and equipping automobiles with breathalyzer equipment that prevents ignition unless the driver "blows" below a specified alcohol level.

It is important to "create a substance-use care system that is built on harm reduction and continually moving people toward a path of recovery. The care provided must be integrated, because these approaches are stronger when used in combination rather than alone" (Johnson, 2017, p. 36).

Nursing Considerations
Nursing Assessment

Practical nurses should supplement their assessment of a client's physical and mental health with screening for substance use, dependence, and abuse. Ask clients about their pattern of substance use and experiences of withdrawal. At the very least, determine the amount and frequency of alcohol or drugs used by clients. Some suggested questions include the following:

- "Are you interested in stopping the use of a substance?"
- "Do you have any physical complications from addiction?" Examples include AIDS, hepatitis, abscesses, tachycardia.
- "Do you know what community resources are available for safe detoxification, treatment, and client and family support? Do you know how to access them?"
- A common, easily remembered assessment tool for alcoholism that all nurses should know and use is the CAGE Questionnaire. If a client answers "yes" to two of the following four questions, it is an indication for further assessment of probable alcoholism:
  - Cut down—"Have you ever been told you should cut down on your drinking?"
  - Annoyed—"Has anyone annoyed you by criticizing your drinking?"
  - Guilt—"Have you ever felt guilty or bad about your drinking?"
  - Eye-opener—"Have you ever had a drink first thing in the morning to get over a hangover?"

The Nurse–Client Relationship

In order to develop an effective therapeutic relationship with a client who is a substance user, the practical nurse must examine his or her personal beliefs and overcome any prejudice toward the client. Otherwise, the practical nurse should refer the client to another staff member who can accept the client more openly and with whom the client will feel safe to communicate openly and honestly. Interacting with substance users requires patience, honesty, persistence, and acceptance of the potential for relapses. Principles underlying interacting with substance users include the following:

- Abstinence—Negotiate a contract with the client to abstain from substance use.
- Individualized treatment and goals—Negotiate a plan addressing the client's personal issues.
- Set appropriate limits—Include in your contract the conditions under which you will work together. Outline behaviour that is acceptable and unacceptable.
- Anticipate defensive reactions—Address the client by identifying or redirecting the behaviour and supporting appropriate responses.
- Patience—Acknowledge that recovery occurs in stages and that each stage takes time.
- Sharpen the focus—Focus on the benefits of giving up substance use that make abstinence worthwhile.

Nursing Interventions

When clients are ready for psycho-social interventions, that is, at the point at which overdose or withdrawal symptoms are stabilized, attention turns to overcoming addiction and maintaining abstinence.

Individual interventions. Use all opportunities with the client to engage in brief interventions, aimed at motivating change and supporting healthy behaviours. A helpful acronym for recalling the elements of these encounters is FRAMES:

- Feedback—Give personal feedback about client progress, including liver enzyme values.
- Responsibility—Emphasize that change is the client's responsibility, no one else's.
- Advice—Clearly provide supportive advice on the need to change. Avoid being judgemental.
- Menu—Allow clients to choose from a menu of addiction treatment options and programs.
- Empathy—Communicate warmth, respect, understanding, and support.
- Self-efficacy—Reinforce with the client that he or she has the ability to be successful (Stuart, 2013).

Group therapy. Encourage the client to attend group therapy, where available, but be available afterward to discuss and reinforce what clients learn about their addiction and themselves. Advantages of group therapy include mutual support and sharing of strategies for success. Interacting with other addicts who have maintained sobriety reduces isolation and encourages learning new social skills. Groups also offer opportunities for socializing that are not dependent on substance use.

Self-help groups. Alcoholics Anonymous (AA) is the model for many other self-help groups that use the 12-step approach. Other groups are Narcotics Anonymous, Al-Anon for adult family members or friends of an alcoholic or chemically dependent person, and Alateen for teenage family members. (Some large urban centres also have Nar-Anon, a group specifically for families of those addicted to chemical substances.) Twelve-step programs require that members do the following:

- Admit to their powerlessness over the addictive substance and that they are unable to quit on their own, but require help from a power greater than themselves
- Accept responsibility for their own recovery
- Admit that no one and nothing else can be blamed for their addiction

In response to objections to the semi-religious nature of AA, the organization has altered references to God to either "a power greater than ourselves" or "God, as we understand Him."

Teaching and Learning

In addition to information about the types of substances abused, education for families and clients may include concepts such as tolerance, dependence, intoxication, withdrawal, flashbacks, dual diagnosis, co-dependency, and the social and physical complications of substance abuse. Even more important may be education on managing recovery. Some examples for topics are healthy nutrition, techniques for relaxation, stress relief, and problem solving, as well as the availability of community supports, including financial and legal assistance.

Relapse prevention. Avoid becoming discouraged when a client succumbs to temptation and relapses. Most clients will relapse, even when they are determined to succeed with abstinence. You can help clients prevent relapses using the following strategies (Halter, et al., 2019):

- Keep the program simple at first. Providing prompts and instructions for the client to review may help. Encouraging the use of the notebook to write important schedules, appointments, and quick review of information provided.
- Discuss difficult situations that the client has been able to handle relatively successfully.
- Discuss situations that the client has had little success in handling and rehearse some possible management strategies.
- Help the client recognize role models among his or her acquaintances.
- Help the client prepare for the possibility of a relapse through the following:
  - Identifying potential triggers to substance use
  - Learning skills to regain abstinence in the event of use
  - Adopting healthy coping, identity, and stress management skills to address triggers before they threaten sobriety

Engaging with Families

"Everyone in the family suffers, not just the client. Some problems that families experience include guilt, shame, resentment, insecurity, delinquency, financial troubles, isolation, fear, and violence" (Stuart, 2013, p. 466). Substance abuse can cause family breakup or become a self-sustaining pattern. Spouses and partners, if not already substance users, may become so, and many children learn patterns of addiction early. Many families, however, recognize the problems caused by substance abuse and seek education and help, whether or not the substance abuser wants to overcome the addiction.

Co-dependency. Sometimes family dynamics evolve to enable the alcoholic or drug abuser to continue using. Family members try to preserve the peace, hoping that unconditional support will help the substance user become strong enough to quit. They may cover up dysfunctions to preserve the individual's or family's reputation and financial integrity. Two unintended consequences are as follows:

- Co-dependence—The family member's own needs for self-actualization and fulfillment are blocked in favour of catering to the needs and desires of the substance user.
- Enabling—Inadvertently, co-dependency reinforces substance abuse by protecting the addicted person from the consequences of his or her behaviour. Family members who assist a loved one to maintain an addiction need help to understand their own enabling behaviour patterns and to face the reality that the addict, alone, must assume responsibility for quitting.

Self-help groups for partners and families. Practical nurses must be aware of self-help organizations so they can refer family members. Most communities have local chapters of Al-Anon and Alateen for families of alcoholics. Where self-help groups for drug addiction are located, such as Narcotics Anonymous and Cocaine Anonymous, associated programs for family members are also usually available.

SOMATIC SYMPTOM AND RELATED DISORDERS: CONVERSION DISORDER AND ILLNESS ANXIETY DISORDER

Most practical nurses agree that the connection between the mind and body is strong. Emotional stress often results in psychosomatic symptoms, producing or intensifying a physical illness. Conversely, having a disease or illness increases stress resulting in a wide variety of emotional responses. The expected conversion of mental states and experiences into physical symptoms is called *somatization*. People have a somatic symptom disorder if:

- Physical symptoms cannot be confirmed by laboratory tests or other medical evidence
- They have significant psychological issues or conflicts
- They are consciously unable to control the illness symptoms

Pathophysiology

Stressful psychophysiological responses were identified by Hans Selye as the *general adaptation syndrome* (GAS), or *stress response* (see the section "Anxiety Disorders"). The physiological results of stress can be confirmed by pathological changes; for example, chronic stress is implicated in heart disease. Without confirming pathology, however, the symptoms are presumed to be due to a mental health disorder. Nevertheless, healthcare providers must guard against this assumption until after a completed physical work-up as true somatoform disorders are relatively rare.

Clinical Manifestations

- Somatic symptom disorder: This disorder is characterized by a combination of multiple symptoms such as pain, fatigue, and neurological, GI, and sexual complaints to the point of excessive concern, preoccupation, and fear. These clients suffer from pain that seems to be related to their psychological state and that cannot be relieved by analgesics.
- Conversion disorder: The client suddenly loses sensory or motor functions, resulting in paralysis or blindness. Often the client seems less concerned than one would expect (termed *la belle indifférence*). In such cases, the deficit actually brings relief by preventing the client from participating in an anxiety-provoking activity. Neurological testing is negative.
- Illness anxiety disorder (previously known as *hypochondriasis*): Clients become obsessed with the fear that they have a serious disease, often when they have misinterpreted minor symptoms.
- Factitious disorder: A person with *factitious disorder imposed on self* intentionally creates symptoms in order to gain attention. He or she may even inflict a self-injury. "Perhaps the best known factitious disorder is Munchausen syndrome, in which clients make up symptoms to gain hospital admission and emotional attention over and over again" (Stuart, 2013, p. 248). When a person harms someone else or causes another person to be sick (so that he or she can be rewarded for caring for or saving the other person), the disorder is called *factitious disorder imposed on another* (previously known as *Munchausen's by proxy*). In the DSM-5, this illness now appears in the category "Somatic Symptom and Related Disorders."
  - Malingering is a differential diagnosis classified under "Factitious Disorder" in the DSM-5. It occurs when people fabricate physical symptoms for secondary gain. Either they want something (drugs, insurance payments), or they want to avoid something, such as going to work. The symptoms tend to dissipate after those hopes have been satisfied. This process of getting what they want is called *receiving a secondary gain.*

Diagnostics and Therapeutics
Diagnosis

Initially, a complete diagnostic work-up is done to rule out medical conditions, reactions to substances, or other mental health disorders (such as an anxiety disorder) that may be suspected from the client's symptoms. An in-depth medical and social history may help rule out malingering. After a somatic symptom disorder has been diagnosed, healthcare providers must continue to observe for ongoing and new symptoms. There is a real danger of discounting legitimate medical conditions that the person may later develop and that require treatment.

Treatment

- Individual psychotherapy is aimed at helping the client gain insight into their stress and learn more adaptive coping strategies. The client can be encouraged to discuss feelings and conflicts rather than repress them.
- Periodic physical examination is an opportunity to provide verbal reassurance of the client's positive state of health.
- Cognitive therapy helps the client appraise stressful situations realistically and reduce attention on distorted body sensations and perceptions.

Nursing Considerations
Nursing Assessment

A thorough physical and psychological assessment is required. Because the client perceives the symptoms as real, carefully evaluate his or her daily living patterns. Some fabricated symptoms will interfere with basic needs, for example, nutrition, exercise, hygiene, rest, and so on. Evaluate how well clients are able to express their feelings. Estimate their level of stress and any opportunities for secondary gain through a full psycho-social assessment, including the following:

- Income
- Work
- Other daily activities
- Living arrangements
- Social support
- Self-care
- Stressful events

Addressing the client's health concerns at an early stage may prevent repeated consultations, multiple trails of medication and medical examinations (Halter et al., 2019, p.210).

The Nurse–Client Relationship

Caring for clients with somatoform ailments requires patience and understanding, to allow a trusting relationship to develop in which a client will be able to discuss his or her feelings and fears. Provide positive feedback when clients are able to express their feelings to others. Emphasize that you want to know your client as a person and not just about any physical symptoms. Acknowledge physical complaints, but do not allow the person to dwell on them. Instead, try to promote insight by encouraging the person to tell you what causes stress in his or her life. Then together problem solve some ways of dealing with those stresses. Try to focus the conversation on positive aspects of the client's life and sources of satisfaction.

Nursing Interventions

- Give physical nursing care and explain all procedures fully, until physical illness has been ruled out by laboratory tests and other diagnostic investigation.
- Once a somatic symptom diagnosis has been confirmed, reduce opportunities for the client to achieve benefits from sick behaviour; for example, persuade the client to get out of bed and dress for the day, eat in the dining area, interact with others, perform self-care activities, and so on.

- Journal—Encourage the client to keep a diary, describing activities and interactions, occurrences that cause stress, and when symptoms appear. Help the client reflect on the relationship between stresses and symptoms. Explore other ways of achieving comfort and relieving symptoms rather than relying on medications and medical treatments.
- Encourage activities and exercise, both for promoting health and giving the client something to think about besides his or her complaints.
- Document any new physical complaints and report them to the medical staff for investigation.

Teaching and Learning

Client education focuses on learning about stress and about more adaptive coping strategies, including stress management techniques and establishing a healthy lifestyle. A client education plan (Halter et al., 2019) may cover the following:

- Define and describe stress, having the client share associated feelings and behaviours.
- Ask the client to describe and role-play stressful situations. Talk about the behaviours that you observe. What are some of the adaptive and maladaptive coping mechanisms observed?
- Provide alternative coping strategies. Teach stress reduction techniques such as relaxation, meditation, and mild physical exercise.
- Talk about events and experiences that are common stressors in everyday life. Try to have the client identify the elements in those experiences that heighten stress. Reinforce the client's strengths and problem-solving abilities. Help the client realize that needs can be met without resorting to somatic symptoms.
- Ask the client to choose one adaptive coping mechanism to practise for a day or a week and then review how it went at the end of the period and provide feedback.
- Teach assertive communication. Provide the client with a positive means of getting his or her needs met. This reduces the feelings of helplessness and need for manipulation.

Engaging with Families

Family education is essential. Once family members understand the reasons behind the client's symptoms, they can understand the importance of giving attention to the person when the client is not complaining of illness and reducing attention to their behaviour in the role of a sick person. Families and clients together can plan strategies for avoiding stress in the client's life and for reducing unavoidable stress. Family members may also need to learn the importance of expressing their feelings as repressing emotions may be a long-standing family dynamic that the client has learned.

COGNITIVE DISORDERS: DELIRIUM AND DEMENTIAS, INCLUDING ALZHEIMER'S DISEASE

Cognition "is the act or process of knowing. It involves awareness and judgement that allows the brain to process information in a way that provides accuracy, storage, and retrieval" (Stuart, 2013, p. 347). Cognitive ability is, for many people, synonymous with their sense of self. Two major classifications of cognitive impairment are dementia and delirium. Both of these conditions occur most often, although not exclusively, in older adults. With Canada's aging population, cognitive disorders will constitute an increasing proportion of nursing practice.

The greatest known risk for factor for dementia is increasing age, but not all older people will develop dementia. Most practical nurses recognize this to be an ageist attitude. In older adults, although physiological changes in the brain result in some cognitive decline, general intellectual capacity remains intact. Older adults retain their ability to learn, although processing new information and retrieving memories may take a little longer. Some older adults are more easily distracted. Thus, for older adults, cognitive functioning varies, just as it does for younger people. Only where significant cognitive deficits are noted should the practical nurse suspect a cognitive disorder.

Pathophysiology
Delirium

Although intellect is not markedly affected by age, the brain becomes less resistant to harm from factors such as electrolyte imbalance, medications, ischemia, hypoglycemia, and infections. The resulting cognitive impairment, called *delirium*, is also associated with many mental and physical illnesses, but, in general, the cognitive difficulties improve once the primary illness is resolved. Practical nurses on medical–surgical units frequently encounter delirium, especially following surgery or resulting from various other pathophysiological conditions that upset the biochemical balance of the CNS. In children and adolescents, the major causes are infection with a high fever, head trauma, drug toxicity, and brain tumours.

Dementias

In contrast, dementias involve progressive memory loss that is not reversible. Medications can slow the progression of the disease for a period of time but not reverse the symptoms. Alzheimer's disease is the most common form of dementia followed by vascular dementia, which occurs after a stroke. The third most common form of dementia is Lewy body dementia, which is type of progressive dementia that affects a decline in thinking, reasoning, and independent movements. Symptoms affecting independent movement are displaying a hunched back, rigid muscles and shuffling gait, and trouble initiating movements (Alzheimer's Association, 2018).

In 2016, 564 000 Canadians were living with Alzheimer's and other dementias. More than 65% of those diagnosed with dementia over the age of 65 were women (Alzheimer Society of Canada, 2018). There are many other conditions that can cause symptoms of dementia, including some that are reversible, such as thyroid problems and vitamin deficiencies. While most changes in the brain that cause dementia are permanent and worsen over time, thinking and memory problems caused by the following conditions may improve when the condition is treated or addressed: depression, medication side effects, excess alcohol, thyroid problems, and vitamin deficiencies (Alzheimer's Association, 2018). The cerebral atrophy and deterioration of Alzheimer's disease are caused by the following:

- Amyloid plaques, which are microscopic deposits composed of degenerated neuron cells
- Neurofibrillary tangles of the hippocampus that affect the memory and emotions
- Low acetylcholine levels resulting from insufficient levels of the enzyme necessary to produce acetylcholine, a major neurotransmitter
- A genetic defect involving at least four identified genes

Clinical Manifestations
Delirium

Symptoms of acute confusion and disorientation with bizarre behaviour patterns develop quickly, often at night. The person may be highly agitated or dazed, with hallucinations and aggressive behaviour (anger and lashing out). Speech may become incomprehensible. Over a 24-hour period, symptoms may fluctuate in intensity.

Dementias

Dementias are chronic and progressive. Onset is slow, with gradual deterioration of the cognitive and physical neurological systems. In the early stages, symptoms are often attributed to aging, stress, or mild depression. Symptoms may include forgetting, difficulty concentrating, limited problem-solving ability, apathy or irritability, and some language disturbance, such as searching for words. Over time, cognitive abilities decline and individuals become increasingly distressed, depressed, and debilitated, needing progressively more physical care, support, and supervision. The eventual outcome is death.

In Alzheimer's disease, the course of the illness is about 8–12 years, divided into three stages. Diagnosis usually is made between 40 and 65 years, and, in general, the younger the person at diagnosis, the faster the deterioration. The stages are outlined in Box 11.5.

Diagnostics and Therapeutics
Diagnosis

Diagnosing delirium usually involves diagnosing the underlying medical condition and identifying contributing factors, such as medications and substance abuse. Diagnosing dementia involves ruling out other illnesses and distinguishing among the various dementias. In addition to Alzheimer's disease, other dementia diagnoses include Lewy body dementia, Creutzfeldt-Jakob disease, Pick's disease, Huntington's disease, and vascular dementia. Dementia also occurs with advanced AIDS and Parkinson's disease.

Although delirium and dementias develop at different rates, symptoms overlap, and, not uncommonly, they are confounded. Postsurgical confusion is common in older adults, and too often, delirium goes unrecognized, and the confusion is blamed on dementia. Untreated, the delirium can result in permanent damage. As well, depression

---

> ### BOX 11.5 Three Stages of Alzheimer's Disease
>
> **Stage I: Mild—2 to 4 Average Years' Duration**
> - Repeats words or action
> - Has trouble remembering names and common objects
> - Gets lost easily
> - Loses things
> - Beginning problems in activities of daily living (ADLs)
> - Subtle personality changes
> - Shows lack of interest in usual activities
>
> **Stage II: Moderate—2 to 10 Average Years' Duration**
> - Obvious memory problems
> - Gets confused about recent events
> - Decreased ability to perform ADLs
> - Argues easily
> - Seems anxious and depressed
> - Paces
> - Noticeable behavioural difficulties
> - Close supervision needed
>
> **Stage III: Severe—1 to 3 Average Years' Duration**
> - Fragmented memory
> - No recognition of familiar people
> - No recognition of self in mirror
> - Uses words improperly
> - Depends on others for basic ADLs
> - Reduced mobility

Adapted from Stuart, G. (2013). *Principles and practice of psychiatric nursing* (10th ed., p. 408, Box 22-3). St. Louis: Mosby.

(common in both delirium and dementia) is also very common for older adults. Thus, diagnosing cognitive disorders can be tricky. Table 11.6 provides a comparison of the three Ds: delirium, dementia, and depression.

Diagnostic tests. No single test provides a definitive diagnosis for delirium or dementia, but laboratory findings can help ascertain the cause of delirium, guide treatment decisions, and rule out other diagnoses. Neuropsychological testing may be used for either delirium or dementias to assess mental status.

The following laboratory results may be indicative of delirium:

- Serum electrolyte levels—Low calcium, low potassium, abnormal sodium
- High blood urea nitrogen (BUN), high creatinine, protein in the urine—To assess renal function and fluid levels
- Elevated prothrombin time, low hematocrit, abnormal blood gases—To assess for anoxia and poor circulation
- Urinary tract infections—Elevated leukocyte Esterase, presence of nitrates in urine, increased white blood cells levels, positive urine culture and sensitivity samples
- Blood glucose, elevated aspartate transaminase (AST), and serum glutamic-oxaloacetic transaminase (SGOT)—To assess metabolism

Physicians will order many laboratory tests when ruling out other medical conditions before settling on the diagnosis

TABLE 11.6 Comparison of Delirium, Dementia, and Depression

	Delirium	Dementia	Depression
Onset	Sudden	Slowly over months	May have been gradual, with exacerbation during the crisis or stress
Causes or contributing factors	Hypoglycemia, fever, dehydration, hypotension, infection, other conditions that disrupt body's homeostasis, adverse drug reaction, head injury, change in environment (e.g. hospitalization), pain, emotional stress	Alzheimer's disease, vascular disease, human immunodeficiency virus infection, neurological disease, chronic alcoholism, head trauma	Lifelong history of losses, loneliness, crises, declining health, medical conditions
Cognition	Impaired memory, judgement, calculations, attention span, can fluctuate through the day	Impaired memory, judgement, calculations, attention span, abstract thinking, agnosia	Difficulty concentrating, forgetfulness, inattention
Level of consciousness	Altered	Not altered	Not altered
Activity level	Can be increased or reduced; restlessness; behaviours may worsen in evening (sundowning); sleep–wake cycle may be reversed	Not altered: behaviours may worsen in evening (sundowning)	Usually decreased; lethargy, fatigue, lack of motivation, may sleep poorly and awaken in early morning
Emotional state	Rapid swings; can be fearful, anxious, suspicious, aggressive, have hallucinations and /or delusions	Flat; agitation	Extreme sadness, apathy, irritability, anxiety, paranoid ideation
Speech and language	Rapid, inappropriate, incoherent, rambling	Incoherent, slow (sometimes due to effort to find the right word), inappropriate, rambling, repetitious	Slow, flat, low
Prognosis	Reversible with proper and timely treatment	Not reversible; progressive	Reversible with proper and timely treatment

Adapted from Halter, M. J., Pollard, C. L., & Jakubec, S. L. (2019). *Varcarolis's Canadian psychiatric mental health nursing: A clinical approach* (2nd Cdn. ed., p. 364, Table 17.1). Milton, ON: Elsevier Canada.

of dementia, including electrolytes, vitamin B_{12} level, thyroid function tests, EEG, ECG, HIV testing, and vision and hearing evaluation.

The diagnosis of dementia is usually confirmed through neuroimaging with CT scans, PET scans, an MRI, or some combination of these.

Treatment

Medical treatment of the underlying condition usually reverses delirium. All medication use in older adults should be carefully monitored for signs of overdose and side effects. This is vitally important to prevent both of the following:

- Drug interactions due to the high number of medications that many older persons routinely take (polypharmacy)
- Accumulation of toxic drug levels in the body due to less efficient and effective metabolism and excretion in older adults

Cholinesterase inhibitors (Aricept is a common one) are effective against some of the symptoms of Alzheimer's disease, slowing down the functional deterioration. By reducing the rate of acetylcholine metabolism, they may help preserve memory and learning and reduce anxiety. Other medications help ease behavioural symptoms, such as agitation (beta blockers, estrogen, anticonvulsants, SSRIs), anxiety (anti-depressants, benzodiazepines), aggression (anticonvulsants),

depression (antidepressants), and psychotic symptoms (SSRIs). Atypical antipsychotics are not recommended for older adult clients with BSPD (behavioural and psychotic symptoms of dementia). The decision to use an antipsychotic drug needs to be considered with extreme caution. Research has shown that these drugs are associated with increased risk of stroke and death in older adults with dementia. The U.S. Food and Drug Administration (FDA) has ordered manufacturers to label such drugs with a "black box" warning about their risks and a reminder that they are not approved to treat dementia symptoms (U.S. Food and Drug Administration, 2008, 2016).

Nursing Considerations
Nursing Assessment

A number of assessment tools for evaluating a person's mental status are available. In many centres, practical nurses use the Mini-Mental State Examination. Refer to Chapter 4, page 33, for more information on mental status and neurological assessment.

Because of the acuity of most delirium and the temporary duration, assessment focuses primarily on the client's medical and mental condition. Monitor neurological status for fluctuating levels of consciousness. Ask the family about the client's normal cognitive status and whether there is a history of periods of confusion. Be alert for changes in medical signs and symptoms, monitoring vital signs, edema, intake and output, signs of jaundice, and pain level.

In contrast, much of the practical nurse's assessment for dementia is directed toward the client and family together. Determine the client's present cognitive functioning level, what medications are regularly taken, and the family's understanding of dementia. Discuss with family caregivers their concerns, coping abilities, safety issues in the home environment, and their knowledge of and access to community resources.

The Nurse–Client Relationship

Mental confusion is frightening to clients. Person-centred care is a philosophy of care built around the needs of the individual and contingent upon knowing the person through an interpersonal relationship (Fazio, Pace, Flinner, et al., 2018). Interaction, while challenging for the practical nurse, can be extremely frustrating for clients, who may search for words to communicate but often speak incomprehensibly. The practical nurse should approach clients calmly, speaking slowly and using simple language. Always introduce yourself at each contact and call the client by name, making certain that he or she can see your face. Ensure that clients who have hearing aids and glasses use them. Encourage them to tell you about themselves, their families, and their lives. Avoid arguing about their misperceptions and delusions; instead, reinforce what is real and gently try to change the subject. Distraction can help defuse anger and frustration, but always acknowledge the person's feelings. Above all, respect clients' humanity and never address them like children.

Nursing Interventions

Person-centred care is essential to good dementia care and is the underlying philosophy of the Alzheimer's Association Dementia Care Practice Recommendations (Fazio, Pace, Maslow, et al., 2018).

Addressing fundamental areas in quality dementia care involves assessment, communication and understanding behaviour, social needs and activities, proper nutrition, reducing pain, falls, wandering, restraint-free care, and end-of-life care. Key components of person-centred dementia care include (a) holistic or person-centred care, (b) respect and value, (c) choice, (d) dignity, (e) self-determination, and (f) purposeful living. In all, it is clear that there is a shift in focus away from the traditional biomedical model in favour of embracing personal choice and autonomy (Fazio, Pace, Flinner, et al., 2018). Practice recommendations for a person-centred approach to caring for people with dementia and Alzheimer's disease appear in Box 11.6.

Restraints. Restraints are used to control a person's physical movement or behaviour and can be physical, environmental, and chemical (Potter, Perry, Stockert, et al., 2019). Use restraints as an absolute last resort. Restraints can cause emotional harm and serious physical injury. Confused persons react to restraints with agitation and anxiety, both of which provoke unsafe behaviour. You must have a physician's order to use a physical or chemical restraint after consultation

with the client's family (Sorrentino, Remmert, & Wilk, 2018). Safety measures for using restraints are presented in Box 11.7.

Caring for clients with challenging behaviours.

- Clients with dementia often display behaviours that may make it difficult for the practical nurse to manage when providing care and can be disturbing for other clients around them. These challenging behaviours may develop from a reaction to a symptom from an infection, illness, or some form of physical discomfort. (Sorrentino et al.,

---

BOX 11.6 Dementia Care Practice Recommendations

1. **Know the person living with dementia.**

   The individual living with dementia is more than a diagnosis. It is important to know the unique and complete person, including his/her values, beliefs, interests, abilities, likes and dislikes—both past and present. This information should inform every interaction and experience.

2. **Recognize and accept the person's reality.**

   It is important to see the world from the perspective of the individual living with dementia. Doing so recognizes behaviour as a form of communication, thereby promoting effective and empathetic communication that validates feelings and connects with the individual in his/her reality.

3. **Identify and support ongoing opportunities for meaningful engagement.**

   Every experience and interaction can be seen as an opportunity for engagement. Engagement should be meaningful to, and purposeful for, the individual living with dementia. It should support interests and preferences, allow for choice and success, and recognize that even when the dementia is most severe, the person can experience joy, comfort, and meaning in life.

4. **Build and nurture authentic, caring relationships.**

   Persons living with dementia should be part of relationships that treat them with dignity and respect, and where their individuality is always supported. This type of caring relationship is about being present and concentrating on the interaction, rather than the task. It is about "doing with" rather than "doing for," as part of a supportive and mutually beneficial relationship.

5. **Create and maintain a supportive community for individuals, families, and staff.**

   A supportive community allows for comfort and creates opportunities for success. It is a community that values each person and respects individual differences, celebrates accomplishments and occasions, and provides access to and opportunities for autonomy, engagement, and shared experiences.

6. **Evaluate care practices regularly and make appropriate changes.**

   Several tools are available to assess person-centered care practices for people living with dementia. It is important to regularly evaluate practices and models, share findings, and make changes to interactions, programs, and practices as needed.

From Fazio, S., Pace, D., Maslow, K., et al. (2018). Alzheimer's Association dementia care practice recommendations. *The Gerontologist, 58*(Suppl. 1), S1–S9.

BOX 11.7 Safety Measures for Using Restraints

- Use the restraint specified in the care plan. The least restrictive device is used.
- Follow employer policies and procedures.
- Use only restraints that have manufacturer instructions and warning labels.
- Follow the manufacturer's instructions for snug fitting and for specific use. Some restraints are safe for use with beds, chairs, and wheelchairs, whereas others are used only with certain equipment.
- Do not use sheets, towels, tape, rope, straps, bandages, or other items to restrain a client.
- Use only intact restraints. Check for tears, cuts, or frayed fabric or straps.
- Do not use restraints to position a client on furniture that does not allow for the correct application.
- Position the client in good body alignment before applying the restraint.
- If mitt restraints are applied, you should be able to slide one or two fingers under the restraint. Check the client's circulation every 15 minutes. You should feel a pulse at a pulse site below the restraint. The client should have good circulation and movement. Remove the restraint if you cannot feel a pulse; the client's fingers are cool to touch or pale and blue; or the client complains of pain, numbness, and tingling in the restrained hand.
- Use a belt restraint with chairs and wheelchairs. Position the client in the chair so that hips are well back of the chair. Apply a belt restraint at a 45-degree angle over the hips. If a belt restraint is used, check the client at least every 15 minutes. The client should be able to breathe easily. Clients have slipped down in wheelchairs and choked or strangled themselves with a belt restraint.
- Bedrails are one type of environmental restraint. Use them only as indicated in the care plan. Check the care plan for instructions on when to lower or raise bed rails. According to the care plan, use bed rail covers or gap protectors, which prevent the client from getting trapped between the rails or the bed rail bars.
- Check the client at least every 15 minutes for safety and comfort.
- Remove the restraint and reposition the client every 2 hours. Meet the client's basic needs during this time, and whenever necessary, do the following:
  - Meet the client's elimination needs.
  - Give skin care.
  - Perform range-of-motion exercises or help the client ambulate. Follow the care plan.
  - Offer food and fluids.
  - Record what was done, the care given, your observations, and the time and details of what you reported. Follow your employer policy for reporting.
  - Keep the call bell within the client's reach.

Based on Sorrentino, S., Remmert, L., & Wilk, M. (2018). *Mosby's Canadian textbook for the support worker* (4th ed., pp. 394–395). Toronto: Elsevier.

2018). The practical nurse's responsibility is to try and understand the reason for the challenging behaviour to help relieve the client's distress. Refer to Fig. 11.4, the cycle of challenging behaviours.

Involving Families

For disoriented people, a familiar face can be soothing and help the individual to feel safe. If possible, a family member should stay while the client is in hospital to assist with the following:

- Reducing fear—Unfamiliar surroundings and strangers increase anxiety and agitation.
- Reducing disorientation—Even if the client is unable to recognize the family member, structuring the client's care in terms of personal preferences and routines is less disorienting. Informal caregivers know a person's idiosyncrasies and can help with care planning. Request that the family bring in some familiar objects from home.
- Safety—Constant supervision helps maintain safety and avoids the use of restraints. Caring for the families and caregivers of confused people is integral to nursing care in cognitive disorders.

Additional considerations:

- Be honest with family members about the diagnosis and future outcomes.
- Invite family caregivers to talk with you about their fears and emotions.
- If the client rejects family members, compassionately explain that it is not intentional.
- Assist families who may need help with financial and legal affairs and accessing community resources.
- Know that families want to be helpful, but practical nurses must also remember that hospitalizing the client with dementia can provide respite for the primary caregiver. Encourage other family members to stay with the client to allow the primary caregiver frequent breaks and opportunities for rest.
- Help families identify and access community resources; for example, the Alzheimer Society of Canada and its local branches, the Caregiver Network, the CMHA, home care nursing services, home support services, respite care, Meals on Wheels, accessible transportation for disabled persons, and support groups for caregivers. Consult with the community health liaison nurse, if your hospital has one.
- Express appreciation to family caregivers for their devotion and assistance.

SEXUAL DYSFUNCTION, PARAPHILIC DISORDERS, AND GENDER DYSPHORIA

Sexuality and identity are important sources of personality. Sexuality, sexual health, and reproduction contribute significantly to health and well-being throughout life. Nurses recognize that normal sexuality includes the curiosity and experimentation of children, as well as the need and desires for sexual relationships among older adults and people who are disabled, either cognitively or physically.

A Preventing and Managing Resistive Responsive Behaviours When Attending to Activities of Daily Living (ADLs)

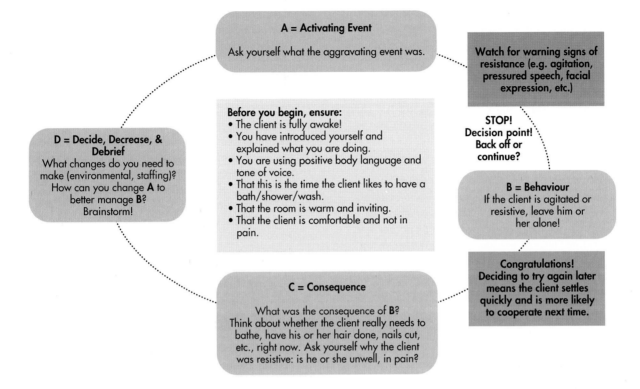

B Preventing and Managing Aggressive Responsive Behaviours

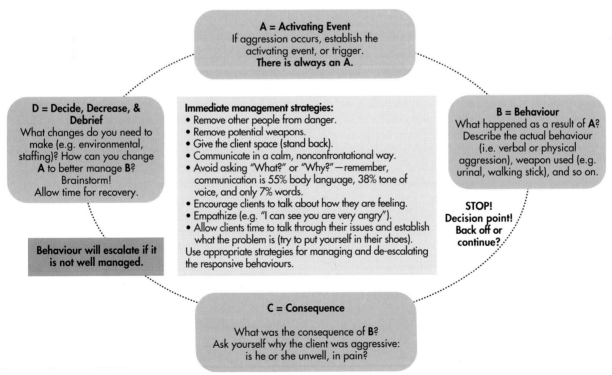

Fig. 11.4 The cycle of challenging behaviours. A, Preventing and managing resistance when attending to activities of daily living (ADLS). **B,** Preventing and managing aggression. (From Sorrentino, S., Remmert, L., & Wilk, M. [2018]. *Mosby's Canadian textbook for the support worker* [4th ed. p. 836, Fig. 36.6]. Toronto: Elsevier. Source: Regional Dementia Management Strategy Document Library. [2001]. Bendigo Health Care Group. Bendigo, Australia. Retrieved from http://www.bendigohealth.org.au/Regional-Dementia-Management/Library.html. Reprinted by permission of the Centre for Rural Rehabilitation & Aged Care.)

Sexual orientation includes heterosexuality (being straight), homosexuality (gay or lesbian), and bisexual attraction to both males and females. In the not too distant past, cultural and moral standards limited acceptable sexual behaviour to heterosexual relations, preferably within marriage. Now, variations in sexual orientation and behaviour are considered to be mental health disorders only if a client defines them as such or wants to change, or if the client's sexual behaviour impinges on the rights of another.

"Sexual response has requisite biological underpinning, yet it is usually experienced in an interpersonal, interpersonal, and cultural context. Thus, sexual function involves a complex interaction among biological, socio-cultural, and psychological factors. Nonetheless, a sexual dysfunction diagnosis requiring ruling out problems that are better explained by a non-sexual mental disorder, by the effects of a substance (e.g. drug or medication), by a medical condition (e.g. due to pelvic nerve damage), or by severe relationship distress, partner violence, or other stressors." (APA, 2013, p. 423)

In general, disorders of sexuality and identity can be divided into three categories:
- Sexual dysfunction
- Paraphilic disorders
- Gender dysphoria

Pathophysiology

Sexual identity is largely determined genetically and manifested as male or female anatomy and physiology, although psycho-social factors (i.e. how people perceive of themselves and behave in a sexual role) also influence gender. Another biological influence on sexual expression is hormonal, as evidenced by puberty and the fact that for both men and women, libido is related to testosterone levels or high serum prolactin. In addition, high levels of androgens are found in people who exhibit inappropriate sexual arousal and hypersexual behaviour.

Sexual function, or the sexual response cycle, consists of four stages: desire, excitement, orgasm, and resolution. Disturbance at any stage can result in a sexual dysfunction, as can pain experienced with sexual intercourse. Sexual functioning can also be affected by comorbid illness, physical injury, or the medications taken to contend with these.
- Depression, hypothyroidism, atherosclerosis, diabetes mellitus, and some urological infections and disorders, as well as neurological diseases such as epilepsy, multiple sclerosis, and Parkinson's disease, can negatively affect sexual functioning.
- Antihypertensives, antipsychotics, anxiolytics, anticonvulsants, antidepressants, and chronic alcohol or cocaine use may reduce levels of sexual desire and arousal.

Clinical Manifestations
Sexual Dysfunction

Sexual dysfunctions are a heterogeneous group of disorders that are typically characterized by a clinical disturbance in a person's ability to respond sexually or to experience sexual pleasure.

According to the DSM-5, the following four subtypes of sexual dysfunction describes the onset of the difficulty:
- *"Lifelong* refers to a sexual problem that has been present from first sexual experiences.
- *Acquired* refers to sexual disorders that develop after a period of relatively normal sexual function.
- *Generalized* refers to sexual difficulties that are not limited to certain types of stimulation, situations, or partners.
- *Situational* refers to sexual difficulties that only occur with certain types of stimulation, situations, or partners.

In many individuals with sexual dysfunctions, the time of onset may indicate different etiologies and interventions" (APA, 2013, p. 423).

A few of the various sexual dysfunctions are described next.

Female sexual interest/arousal disorders. It is characterized by emotional distress caused by absent or reduced interest in sexual fantasies, sexual activity, pleasure, and arousal. Some women experience these symptoms their whole lives, while others may gradually become less interested in sexual activities.

Erectile dysfunction. It is characterized by an inability to obtain and maintain an erection sufficient for sexual activity, or it is considered a disorder if it happens on 75% of sexual occasions and the condition has persisted for at least 6 months (Halter, 2018).

Female orgasmic disorders. It is having difficulty experiencing orgasm or the inhibition of female orgasm. It is characterized wit h marked reduced intensity of the orgasmic sensation.

For the recognition of a clinically significant problem, it must persist for at least 6 months and must occur during the majority of sexual encounters (Halter, 2018).

Genito-pelvic pain/penetration disorder. The following two disorders have been combined to describe Genito-pelvic pain/penetration disorder. It interferes with penile insertion during intercourse.
- Dyspareunia is recurrent or persistent pain during or after intercourse; it affects women. This disorder may be caused by infection, irritation, vaginal dryness, or common skin disorders such as eczema.
- Vaginismus is the involuntary constriction of the vagina, preventing penetration and intercourse.

Individuals experiencing these problems become fearful that pain and spasms will occur during the next encounter. This fear enhances the problem further by increasing anxiety and muscle tension (Halter, 2018).

Paraphilic Disorders

Paraphilias are characterized by sexual arousal resulting from fantasies and behaviours. Often the fantasies involve nonhuman objects, painful or humiliating sexual activity, or sex without mutual consent. Generally, such fantasies and behaviours lead to arousal and orgasm, often assisted by masturbation. Paraphilias include exhibitionism, fetishism, frotteurism, pedophilia, sexual sadism, sexual masochism, voyeurism, transvestic disorder, and paraphilic disorders not otherwise specified. People engage in paraphilias secretly to avoid social sanctions, with the result that they are likely underdiagnosed. As with many mental health disorders, paraphilias may intensify when a person experiences stress.

Gender Dysphoria

Gender identity relates to a person's awareness of being male or female. Gender dysphoria disorder occurs when biological sex and gender identity differ. From the outset, children with the disorder prefer opposite-gender playmates. With maturation, they become increasingly less comfortable with their assigned gender role. Individuals experiencing gender dysphoria disorder may face disapproval and rejection, which can lead to low self-esteem and impaired family and social interactions. As adults, wearing clothes of the opposite sex often helps decrease anxiety and depression and may or may not be accompanied by sexual excitement. These individuals do not usually consider themselves to be homosexual. The biological male who falls in love with a man believes himself actually to be a woman who loves that man (Halter, 2018).

An extreme version of gender dysphoria disorder is trans-sexualism. Often depressed and anxious from pressure to conform to their assigned sex role, people with trans-sexualism may feel disgust toward their own bodies. Biological males may cross-dress and live as transvestites. Females who adopt masculine dress have become more accepted as a result of feminism. Trans-sexualism is characterized by a person wishing to change his or her anatomical sexual characteristics to those of the opposite sex. The person often enters the mental health system requesting sexual reassignment.

Diagnostics and Therapeutics

Diagnosis of sexual dysfunction, gender dysphoria, and paraphilic disorders requires a detailed general and sexual history and complete physical examination. The therapist probes for predisposing and developmental factors, as well as family and social history.

Treatment

Treatment for sexual dysfunction, paraphilic disorders and gender dysphoria includes the following:
- Individual or group psychotherapy
- Couple therapy
- Behaviour modification
- Pharmacotherapy with antianxiety medications or antidepressants, as necessary

More specific treatments differ depending on the classification of the disorder.

Sexual dysfunction.
- Pharmacotherapy—Antidepressants, including SSRIs, have been successful against rapid ejaculation. Sildenafil (Viagra) and tadalafil (Cialis) are used for erectile dysfunction.
- Medications for female sexual disorders are less available, although studies with Viagra have shown some success when there is no history of sexual abuse.

Paraphilic disorder.
- Cognitive–behavioural therapy may be used as treatment.
- Medications to lower testosterone levels, such as methoxyprogesterone, may be effective.

Gender dysphoria.
- Hormone therapy for the development of opposite-sex secondary sexual characteristics may be used as treatment.
- Clients may undergo sex-change surgery, after intensive psychotherapy, hormone therapy, and living as a member of the opposite sex for a significant period, usually at least 2 years.

Nursing Considerations
Nursing Assessment

Prior to asking questions related to sexual history or sexuality, it is important for the practical nurse to develop a trusting, nonjudgemental, safe atmosphere. Clients with traumatic sexual histories or who may have faced previous discrimination and stigma may be reluctant to share information. Begin with a full health history, family history, and physical examination. Include questions about sexual activity, number and sex of sexual partners, birth control, concern regarding HIV and other sexually transmitted infections (STIs), and whether there are any concerns about sexual functioning. Once you have established a relationship, you can ask more specific questions. The Public Health Agency of Canada offers suggestions on a variety of topics to include in a comprehensive assessment:
- Sexual knowledge, family attitudes, and sexual experience during childhood and adolescence
- Cultural and religious beliefs regarding sexuality
- The client's concerns and depth of understanding of his or her sexuality
- Does the client have any concerns about sexual or relationship violence or abuse
- Sexual patterns within or outside marriage
- Self-esteem
- Anxiety and level of stress
- Social interaction
- Coping strategies (Government of Canada, 2013)

The Nurse–Client Relationship

Culture, family background, societal values, the media—all contribute to the taboos surrounding sexual conduct and what is considered to be "normal." Assumptions and inferences about a client's sexual health may prove inaccurate and damaging to the nurse–client relationship. Practical nurses need to examine their own attitudes and values regarding sexual expression and sexual behaviour to minimize anxiety when discussing sexual matters. Awareness of one's personal attitudes, beliefs, and knowledge regarding sexuality is necessary before the practical nurse can set those issues aside to allow for an open and sensitive discussion, communicating warmth, acceptance, and positive regard. Because sexuality is one of the most private and personal aspects of our lives, few people will volunteer information, leaving it to the practical nurse to introduce the topic and guide the conversation.

Nursing Interventions

Sexual therapy is not within the scope of practice for a newly qualified practical nurse. For intensive therapy, the practical nurse should make a referral to a qualified sex therapist. The practical nurse's role includes assessment, education, and support to a client being treated for a sexual disorder. Some basic approaches that are helpful to clients with sexual problems include the following:

- Active listening, allowing the client to explore sexual values and beliefs
- Helping the client set realistic goals
- Setting limits on the client's sexual behaviour, if included in the plan of care
- Relaxation techniques for stress and anxiety reduction
- Assisting with the behaviour modification plan by implementing the agreed-upon consequences for maladaptive behaviour

Teaching and Learning

If the client has a stable sexual relationship, include the partner in client education. Explore whether there are differences in their sexual beliefs and expectations as these can lead to conflict and misunderstanding. For example, the client's dissatisfaction with sexual desire and arousal may be less a matter of his or her personal lack of response than it is of not being able to match his or her partner's expectations.

Nursing Interventions Classification (NIC) interventions for sexual counselling appear in Box 11.8.

BOX 11.8   NIC Interventions for Sexual Counselling

Definition of *sexual counselling:* Use of an interactive helping process focusing on the need to make adjustments in sexual practice or to enhance coping with a sexual event or disorder

Activities*:

- Establish a therapeutic relationship based on trust and respect.
- Provide privacy and ensure confidentiality.
- Discuss the effects of changes in sexuality on significant others.
- Discuss the knowledge level of the patient about sexuality in general.
- Encourage the patient to verbalize fears and ask questions.
- Provide reassurance and permission to experiment with alternative forms of sexual expression, as appropriate.
- Provide referral or consultation with other members of the health care team, as appropriate.

From Halter, M. J., Pollard, C. L., & Jacubec, S. L. (2019). *Varcarolis's Canadian psychiatric mental health nursing: A clinical approach* (2nd Cdn. ed., p. 583). Milton, ON: Elsevier. Data from Bulechek, G. M., Butcher, H. K., Dochterman, J. M., et al. (Eds.). (2013). *Nursing Interventions Classification (NIC)* (6th ed.). Toronto: Elsevier.
*Partial list.

Responding to a Client's Sexual Advances

One very difficult aspect of caring for clients with paraphilic disorder is dealing with seductive advances and comments directed at the practical nurse. Sexually inappropriate behaviour toward practical nurses is not restricted to mental health settings but can be found in any healthcare environment. Inappropriate touching, asking for dates or personal contact information, and making explicit passes at the practical nurse cannot be tolerated, and the client must be so informed. The most professional response is to respond firmly and set clear limits.

FEEDING AND EATING DISORDERS: ANOREXIA NERVOSA AND BULIMIA NERVOSA

Eating disorders are appetite disturbances. The continuum ranges from eating too little (anorexia nervosa), through disordered eating with binging and purging (bulimia nervosa), to chronic overeating causing obesity (binge eating disorder). Other disorders include pica, rumination disorder, and avoidant/restrictive food intake disorder. In our culture, however, obesity is not always considered a mental health problem, and most treatment consists of diet therapy only. Binge eating disorder often goes unrecognized. Anorexia and bulimia often overlap, with about half of people with anorexia displaying bulimic behaviours at times or developing bulimia later in their lives. Eating disorders are primarily identified in women (85–90%). However, the prevalence of bulimia in men may be underestimated because of their reluctance to seek treatment.

Pathophysiology

Normal appetite regulation is a function of the hypothalamus, through several mechanisms that produce sensations of either hunger or satiety (feeling full). Hunger is experienced when the hypothalamus is stimulated by the following:

- low blood glucose levels,
- contractions of an empty stomach (and possibly stimulation of the vagus nerve), and
- high levels of neurotransmitters, such as serotonin.

Satiety is felt when the hypothalamus is suppressed. This occurs due to the following:

- high levels of fat and amino acids in the blood,
- slow emptying of the stomach and distension of the GI tract, and
- high cortisol levels (a physiological reaction to stress).

Clinical Manifestations

Eating disorders are closely related to body image and low self-esteem. Where thinness is admired and celebrated in all forms of the media, dissatisfaction with one's shape and size is widespread. Weight loss is big business, and some people engage in extreme measures to control their weight. Behaviours associated with eating disorders include the following:

- Binge eating—Consuming large amounts of food and excessive calories. The frequency of binging varies from occasionally to several times weekly or even many times each day.
- Dieting—Restricting food intake below what is necessary to maintain weight
- Fasting—Refusing to eat
- Purging—Inducing vomiting to lose weight or using over-the-counter laxatives or diuretics to stimulate fluid and waste excretion

Anorexia Nervosa and Bulimia

Individuals with anorexia nervosa refuse to maintain a normal body weight for their height and develop persistent behaviours that interfere with weight gain. Anorexia nervosa is a life-threatening condition. Symptoms include restriction of food intake, intense fear of gaining weight, and body image disturbance. The physiological effects of anorexia nervosa include constipation, cold intolerance, lanugo, lethargy, electrolyte imbalance, amenorrhea in females, and emaciation (Halter et al., 2019).

Bulimia nervosa is an eating disorder characterized by "recurrent episodes of binge eating and engage in inappropriate behaviours to avoid weight gain (e.g. self-induced vomiting), and are overly concerned with body shape and weight. However, unlike individuals with anorexia nervosa, binge eating/purging type, individuals with bulimia nervosa maintain body weight at or above a minimally normal level" (APA, 2013, p. 344). Clients who use recurrent vomiting to compensate for binge eating often experience changes to their teeth and oral mucosa, such as damage to tooth enamel and unexpected dental caries. Some clients may use laxatives or excessive exercise to avoid weight gain.

Complications of Eating Disorders

Without treatment, eating disorders cause medical complications in many body systems. Serious complications of starvation and dehydration include hypokalemia and hypoalbuminemia leading to hypotension, cardiac arrhythmias, and heart and renal failure, which are life-threatening. Frequent vomiting can cause stomach and esophageal ulcers, GI bleeding, tooth decay, and gum erosion. Amenorrhea is related to estrogen deficiencies that may result in calcium deficiency and osteoporosis. Deaths from eating disorders are tragic and much too frequent!

Diagnostics and Therapeutics
Predisposing Factors

There is no known specific cause for eating disorders. A number of risk factors have been identified such as biological factors (genetics, obesity), developmental factors (development of autonomy and control), and familial and social influences (lack of emotional support, child adversity, media influences). Criticism or teasing about one's weight from parents or peers can damage self-esteem, as can other family dysfunctions and a history of sexual or physical abuse.

Treatment

Unless there is a medical crisis, clients can be cared for as outpatients in community clinics, day treatment, or partial hospitalization. Selection of treatment setting is based on the severity of the illness as well as extent of comorbidities such as depression or life-threatening complications. Where possible, community care tends to be the best option, allowing clients to maintain autonomy while learning healthy self-control and a balanced lifestyle. Immediate medical intervention and possible hospitalization are required if the client presents with severe dehydration, cardiac damage, low blood glucose, and electrolyte imbalance, or if the client becomes psychotic, suicidal, or severely depressed. Sometimes people with an eating disorder may self-identify and ask to be admitted to the hospital.

Once in hospital, medical treatment to stabilize physiological health is the first priority, followed by behaviourally oriented interventions. Treatment may include the following:

- A healthy diet, possibly with liquid supplements
- Vitamin and mineral supplements
- Pharmacotherapy with anxiolytics (helpful for those with obsessive–compulsive features), tricyclics, and SSRIs (to decrease mood swings, depression, irritability, and food and fat obsessions). Sometimes appetite suppressants are used for bulimia, but only until new eating patterns have been established.
- Individual or group psychotherapy
- Cognitive–behavioural therapy
- Behaviour modification therapy
- Family therapy
- Stress management and self-monitoring

Nursing Considerations
Nursing Assessment

Assessment of eating disorders begins with two simple screening questions:

- "Are you satisfied with your eating patterns?" People with anorexia usually say "yes," but those with bulimia do not.
- "Do you ever eat in secret?" People with either anorexia or bulimia generally answer "yes" (Stuart, 2013, p. 480).

Continue your assessment with a full health history, family history, and physical examination, placing emphasis on the following:

- Nutritional status and diet history, including food preferences, eating behaviours, and purging episodes
- Weight history, height and weight measurement
- Signs of fluid and electrolyte imbalance
- Menstrual history, especially amenorrhea
- Frequency, type, and amount of exercise
- Mood and emotional state, for example, depression, anxiety, distress
- Evidence of obsession or compulsion, especially regarding food
- Evidence of disturbed body image, low self-esteem, self-criticism
- Risk of suicide

- Frequency, type, and amount of exercise
- History of dysfunctional family relationships
- Level of insight and motivation for treatment

The Nurse–Client Relationship

People with an eating disorder tend to be suspicious. The suspicion and mistrust is often a symptom of anxiety and fear. It is important for the practical nurse to develop a trusting, therapeutic relationship with the client. Focusing on identifying areas of strength not related to food or body image, assist in setting realistic goals and avoid power struggles over food intake.

Nursing Interventions

The practical nurse encourages healthy eating by negotiating agreement on a target weight and a mutually determined recovery plan that includes the following:

- Adequate food intake
- Structured, time-limited meal times (e.g. three small meals a day)
- Food preferences
- Nutritious snacks between meals
  Monitor the client's eating and weight in an accepting and nonpunitive way.
- Stay with the client during meals and for an hour after to reduce opportunities for purging (in anorexia and bulimia) or stashing food (in bulimia and obesity).
- Ensure a pleasant and social atmosphere at mealtimes, discussing topics other than food.
- Encourage use of a food diary.
- Offer small amounts of food and drink frequently.
- Weigh the client daily in the morning, in the same clothing, after first voiding, and on the same scale. Be vigilant for attempts to artificially increase her weight, such as stuffing items into pockets or under clothes.
- Record intake and output.
- Assess for signs of dehydration, such as skin turgor, colour, and moistness of oral mucous membranes.
- Encourage rest times and appropriate exercise with supervision.

Teaching and Learning

Provide information about normal nutrition and balanced diet nutrients, such as teaching about normal growth and body development and that cutting out all fat is unhealthy. Discuss the nature of the illness (symptoms, causes, effects on the body) and the importance of expressing emotions and fears rather than holding them inside. What emotions and beliefs does the client associate with eating? Help people with anorexia set attainable goals. Setting unrealistic goals can result in feelings of failure and frustration. Regularly review the client's food journal and diet plan with her or him and explain how better nutrition will improve symptoms and prevent complications. Review the action, dose, and possible adverse effects of any mediation that the client is taking. Additional important components of teaching for clients with anorexia nervosa include the following:

- The physiologically damaging effects of dieting
- The identification and avoidance of triggers
- Techniques for self-monitoring
- Community resources
  Additional important components of teaching for clients with bulimia include the following:
- The effects on the body of the binging and purging cycle
- Adequate hydration
- Self-monitoring and the avoidance of cues
- Learning to set limits and appropriate boundaries
- Assertiveness (Stuart, 2013)

Psycho-social Interventions

Behaviour modification.

- Use a nurse–client contract to ensure that the client understands the illness and treatment involved and is committed to participating in making informed decisions to benefit his or her health.
  - Agreed-upon consequences for not adhering to the contract terms, such as loss of privileges, should be imposed consistently and in a matter-of-fact manner and voice tone.
  - Provide encouragement and positive reinforcement for adherence to the contract.
- Help the client identify any cues that stimulate harmful eating behaviour and explore ways of avoiding those situations or changing to a more adaptive response.

Body image perception.

- Encourage the client to share his or her thoughts and feelings about body shape and weight.
- Avoid contradicting the client, but present alternative ideas and interpretations.
- Help the client reflect on and consider those alternative perceptions and explanations.
- Promote self-acceptance. Draw attention to positive physical characteristics.
- Encourage the client to use imagery and relaxation, which may reduce body-related anxiety.

Low self-esteem.

- Explore the client's desire for perfection and encourage acceptance of what is good enough.
- Explore family and relationship history and the impacts upon self-esteem and self-acceptance.
- Emphasize positive attributes and behaviours.

Interactions with families.

- Include families in treatment team meetings and in planning care, in both the hospital and community phases of treatment.
- Be emotionally supportive but also candid about the client's state of health.
- Advise families to make their visits social occasions and to talk about topics other than eating.
- Encourage families to become informed about nutrition and about eating disorders.

In addition, there are self-help groups for treating eating disorders. Two mutual-help groups that focus on people with an eating disorder and offer face-to-face, on-line, and telephone meetings are as follows: Overeaters Anonymous (OA), which is based on the 12-step model, and Eating Disorders Anonymous (EDA), which is appropriate for anyone with an eating disorder (Stuart, 2013).

PSYCHIATRIC EMERGENCIES: CRISIS, SUICIDE, VIOLENCE

In a highly stressful event or when confronted with a perceived threat for which the usual coping strategies are ineffective, people experience high levels of anxiety. This may escalate to a state of crisis. Crises may be developmental (such as adolescence, marriage, moving away from home to attend college) or situational (such as divorce or sudden unemployment). Extreme situational crises are sometimes called *adventitious*, indicating that the event is totally outside the person's control. Some examples include natural disasters, wars, or being the victim of a crime.

With no resolution of the crisis, behavioural reactions may continue to escalate. The most serious behavioural reactions include suicide and violence, neither of which are rare events. Although suicide deaths affect almost all ages, 2009 Statistics Canada data indicate that middle-aged people (40–59 years old) have the highest rates of suicide. Suicide is the second leading cause of death for young people between 15 and 34 years of age. The suicide death rate for men is three times as high as that for women. More than 90% of people who commit suicide have a mental health or addictive disorder. The most common psychiatric disorders associated with suicide are mood disorders, substance abuse, schizophrenia, and anxiety disorders (Navaneelan, 2017). The suicide rate is growing among the older adult population, and specifically among older adult men. In Canada, about 31 of every 100 000 older adults, especially those over 85 years, commit suicide. Most are white males, and most die through violent means (Sorrentino et al., 2018). The reasons for suicide include loneliness, loss of independence, deteriorating health, and wanting to avoid becoming a burden to families (Sorrentino et al., 2018).

Pathophysiology

For a description of the stress response, refer to the section "Anxiety Disorders."
- The limbic system is responsible for regulating emotions and aggression. The amygdala is involved in distinguishing between aversive and rewarding stimuli. Rage can be activated in animals by stimulating the amygdala.
- There is a correlation between low levels of serotonin and aggressive behaviour.
- Abnormalities in the temporal lobe may be related to aggressive responses.
- Some people are prone to aggressive behaviour after a traumatic brain injury.

Clinical Manifestations

Clients in crisis are overwhelmed by emotional pain and anxiety. After having attempted a number of solutions without success, they may reach the point of being "at their wit's end" and in a state of complete disorganization. Although people react to crises differently, common maladaptive behaviours include anger, apathy, somatic complaints, emotional outbursts, insomnia, fear, flashbacks, shock, hopelessness, helplessness, or substance abuse.

Diagnostics and Therapeutics
Diagnosis

Diagnosis is initially based on the client's behaviour and inability to control the source of extreme and intense anxiety. First, determine whether the person is suicidal or violent and initiate steps to ensure safety. Once safety is ensured, the practical nurse should try to identify the precipitating event or events. In psychiatric and community settings, the exacerbation of a mental illness often occurs when clients reject treatment. Apprehension under the *Mental Health Act* and certification for admission or treatment or both may be necessary (see the section "Legal, Ethical, and Interpersonal Considerations for Mental Health Nursing").

Practical nurses should know what services are locally available for crisis intervention and how to contact them. Some are as follows:
- "Crisis lines or Internet crisis services-telephone support by trained volunteers (for first aid or support) or professional (for assessment, triage, and referral).
- Mobile crisis outreach-outreach crisis response services often provided by collaborative teams, including police and other first responders.
- Urgent or walk-in-crisis care-services where people can present their crisis needs to professionals for assessment, intervention and referral.
- Psychiatric emergency care-services such as emergency mental health care in hospital triage; assessment; crisis counselling; emergency medical treatment, often for brief-stay admissions" (Halter et al., 2019, p. 487).

Treatment

Treatment varies depending on the root cause of the crisis. Treatment goals are to preserve the safety of the client and all those who could be exposed to danger, to prevent the client's anxiety from escalating, and to return the client to a pre-crisis state of being.

Psychopharmacology. Common medications for those prone to high levels of anxiety and impulsive behaviour include the following:
- Anxiolytics and sedative–hypnotics to manage agitation
- Antidepressants, especially SSRIs, to balance levels of serotonin
- Mood stabilizers to reduce aggressive behaviour
- Antipsychotics—The quick action of IM haloperidol combined with lorazepam (Ativan) is often used to calm people with escalating agitation. Atypical antipsychotics are given to reduce the incidence of violence in people at risk.

Nursing Considerations

Nursing Assessment

Assessment focuses on identifying the precipitating event, the client's interpretation of it, the client's coping resources, and the support systems available. Does the person in crisis require emergency psychiatric treatment or hospitalization? Whether you are a community nurse or in a hospital setting, your assessment will include several elements:

- Try to ascertain whether the person clearly understands the event that precipitated the crisis.
- What coping mechanisms may be helpful in this situation? Has the client used these coping strategies in the past?
- What or who are the client's current situational supports?
- Are there any cultural or religious beliefs or traditions that need to be taken into consideration?
- What is the appropriate level of intervention in this situation?
  - Primary intervention, such as education, changes in the environment, or new coping skills
  - Secondary, or crisis, intervention
  - Tertiary intervention, such as rehabilitation (Halter et al., 2019)

Suicide. Thoughts of suicide or suicide attempts should be suspected when clients appear alienated, disconnected, or in despair. In a kind but straightforward way, ask distressed clients if they are experiencing suicidal thoughts. If the answer is "Yes," ask whether the client has developed a plan. If so, evaluate whether the person has the ability and opportunity to carry it out.

Risk factors for suicide vary depending on the population group:

- Depressed adolescents with a family history of suicide and a personal history of legal trouble and substance abuse are at high risk.
- For older adults, high risk factors include a family member's death or having a serious or terminal illness.
- For depressed clients, times of greatest danger occur in the first few days following either admission to or discharge from the hospital. Clients are at high risk for suicide for the first few days following initiation of treatment with antidepressants or ECT. Psychomotor delay improves before mood improves. Thus, early in treatment, the client remains severely depressed but now has regained the motivation necessary to follow through with suicidal thoughts. Following discharge, some clients are more at risk of suicide when they return home to find that the things that initially caused their depression have not changed.
- People with schizophrenia are at less risk for suicide when they are psychotic than when they begin to recover and may feel little hope for a satisfying life.
- Psychiatric clients who are at high risk for suicide are those who engage in self-directed harm, including self-mutilation to relieve tension, and those who stop taking their medications or otherwise do not adhere to treatment.
- People who misuse substances are at high risk, as are those who have been recently separated, divorced, or bereaved.

- Be especially wary of a severely disturbed client who suddenly becomes calm and rational. When people see suicide as the only escape from an intolerable existence, and when they have thought through a plan and have the means to carry it out, they may feel comforted by knowing their struggles are nearly over.

Violence. Practical nurses should be able to distinguish between assertive and aggressive behaviour.

Assertive behaviour: People who are assertive are direct, persuasive, and self-assured in their communications and interactions with other people. They convey respect for others.

Aggressive behaviour: People who are aggressive exert their own rights at the expense of the rights of others. They tend to express anger. They fight to get what they want and expect others to approach interactions in the same way. Aggressive behaviour can escalate to violence, and practical nurses should be aware that setting limits on clients' behaviour is sometimes an antecedent of aggressive behaviour by hospitalized clients. On the one hand, aggression is more common in psychiatric clients with active psychosis and in those who abuse substances. On the other hand, people with schizophrenia and mania are no more violent than ordinary citizens as long as they are well controlled on their medications. The best predictor of a person becoming violent is past violent behaviour.

The Nurse–Client Relationship

Connecting with violent and aggressive clients is challenging. Some practical nurses worry that their own behaviour could trigger a client's angry response. If a client is verbally abusive, the practical nurse's first response should be to leave the room. Of course, it is always best to prevent angry outbursts if at all possible. For clients with a history of violence or who are otherwise deemed to be at risk for violence, reward appropriate behaviour by giving time and attention to the person.

Identify stressors and ways to avoid them and learn to recognize indicators that the client is becoming stressed. If so, the practical nurse draws on interpersonal skills for de-escalating the situation. Speak calmly and find out what the client needs or wants. If appropriate, help the client attain those wants. If not, then clearly state other more appropriate options from which the client might choose.

Be assertive and confident but also genuine and empathetic. Allow ample personal space between yourself and the client, continually assess for personal safety, and be certain that you have other nursing or security staff close by. Use medications for chemical restraint only when absolutely necessary and when less restrictive methods have been tried without success.

Nursing Interventions

Relieving acute stress involves helping the client process the traumatic event, emotionally and cognitively, and improve coping mechanisms. Ensuring the client's safety in a supportive environment always takes precedence. When a client feels safe, his or her anxiety should diminish, enabling the person to engage with the practical nurse, reflect on the experience, and explore alternative, more adaptive responses.

Suicide precautions. When suicide risk is high, toxic substances and sharp objects should be removed from the client's environment. No belts, neckties, or other articles of clothing that could be used for self-destruction should be worn, and the client should be monitored closely, one to one. Communicate a caring presence and provide reassurance that you will help the client stay safe. Some clients will agree to a no self-harm contract, which is one way of helping clients begin to re-establish personal control. Encourage the client to express feelings and discuss ways for the client to manage those feelings and keep safe. If at all possible, provide for continuity of care as establishing an emotional bond with someone could be a turning point toward suicide prevention.

Violence precautions. With violent clients, practical nurses must be hypervigilant of their own safety. A rule of thumb is to stay between the client and a door for escape. Call security to assist with violent episodes. Some behavioural strategies used with aggressive clients include the following:

- Setting limits—The practical nurse defines for the client acceptable behaviour patterns and the consequences of unacceptable behaviour. All staff must agree to monitor the behaviour and apply the agreed-upon consequences consistently.
- Behaviour contracts—The practical nurse and client negotiate and sign a contract outlining rewards for acceptable behaviour and the consequences of unacceptable behaviour.
- Time-outs—Socially unacceptable behaviour results in a time-out, removing the client from an overstimulating environment to a quiet area or the client's room. If the client agrees to this and goes voluntarily when reminded by the practical nurse, it is not considered to be the same as seclusion.
- Token economy—The client can earn tokens or points that can be used to barter for privileges. The client loses tokens for unacceptable behaviour.

Teaching and Learning

Here are some ideas for teaching clients about anger and how it can be used appropriately.

- Focus on non-verbal expressions of anger, role-playing, and talking about angry feelings in the client's own words, allowing the client to demonstrate angry body language and facial expressions.
- Talk about situations where it is okay to feel angry and role-play those types of situations.
- Help the client identify real situations that cause anger. Role-play confronting the object or person that generates the anger. Give feedback on appropriate verbal and non-verbal responses.
- Give permission for the client to confront the real object of his or her anger. Provide a supportive presence if needed and debrief with the client afterward.

Families and Violence

Interpersonal violence and abuse in family contexts can affect all generations: children, intimate partners, and older adults. Each form of abuse is an instance of the abuser exerting control or power over the abused person (Halter et al., 2019).

- Forms of family abuse include physical abuse or neglect, forced sexual activity (including rape), psychological intimidation and threats, emotional maltreatment, and financial exploitation.
- Alcohol and drug abuse often underlie violence and neglect within families.
- Practical nurses are ethically and legally responsible for reporting evidence of all types of abuse involving vulnerable people and child abuse to the appropriate legal authorities.

Intimate-partner abuse.

- "The cycle of violence" refers to the pattern of three phases of intimate-partner violence. In phase one, tension builds. In phase two, the actual incident of battering takes place. In phase three, the couple reconciles; this phase is also called "the honeymoon phase." The perpetrator vows that it will not happen again, with gifts and kindnesses to the victim as proof of love. Then the cycle begins again.
- Intimate-partner abuse is the most common form of family violence. Battered spouses tend to return and reconcile with their violent partner three times before they are able to leave permanently. Feminist theory suggests that patriarchy and sexual inequality make it difficult for women to maintain themselves independently, thus explaining the return to a dangerous home situation.
- Abusive partners are frequently pathologically jealous and prone to blame others for their own inadequacies.
- Victims suffer low self-esteem and feelings of helplessness and hopelessness and need help to make future plans. Practical nurses can teach victims of family violence strategies for ensuring their safety. A safety plan for victims of domestic violence may include the following:
  - Posting emergency numbers and teaching children to call 9-1-1
  - Making a plan for at least two different places the client can go to be safe and storing extra clothes, cash, and copies of important documents there, even if the client hopes that the violence is over. Shelters and safe houses are available in many communities and are open 24 hours through hotline crisis information and shelter numbers.
  - Providing a neighbour with a signal that will indicate he or she should call police
  - If there is a restraining order, keeping it with the client at all times and giving a copy to a child's school or daycare
  - Connecting with a support group and with old friends

Child abuse.

- Abusive parents often were abused as children. They have poor impulse control and ineffective coping and parenting skills.

- Sexual abuse may be suspected when children display the following dysfunctional behaviour patterns: excessive aggression, sexual activity that is inappropriate for their developmental stage, social withdrawal, poor performance at school, sleep disturbances, and low self-esteem.

See pages 331–332, for more details on pediatric abuse.

Elder abuse. Older adults are prone to abuse as their physical and/or mental health deteriorates and they become dependent on their relatives. The types of elder abuse are as follows:

- Emotional abuse
- Financial Exploitation
- Physical abuse
- Sexual abuse
- Neglect
- Violation of individual rights is another form of abuse involving failure to maintain clients' privacy or not allowing them to use the phone in private (Sorrentino et al., 2018).

Caregiver stress can lead to abuse in families that are dysfunctional in other ways or when caregivers are also at risk for mental health issues. Some of the types of abuse are harder to pinpoint but are prevalent and must be reported to the appropriate legal authorities.

Recognizing signs of family violence. Although the guidelines that follow refer specifically to clients who present in the emergency department, community nurses often will discover evidence of abuse during home visits or in ambulatory settings such as public health clinics. In any setting, signs of family stress could manifest as emotional and behavioural problems, including increased aggression, inability to sleep, trouble in school, or being accident-prone. Pregnancy is a particularly vulnerable time for women. Abuse may be suspected when people present to the emergency department with internal injuries, multiple contusions (especially facial or head and neck), burns (especially from cigarettes) and scalds, perforated eardrums, or miscarriage. There is often evidence of bruising at various stages of healing and a history of multiple emergency department or clinic visits with diffuse and varied complaints. Psychological trauma, anxiety, depression, and severe stress may be evident, and often the explanations fall short of matching the extent or seriousness of the injury. The type of abuse or neglect may be physical, sexual, emotional, or even financial (Sorrentino et al., 2018)

Interviewing victims of violence. Feelings of shame, fear, and worries of how to survive outside the family may make it difficult for victims of abuse to admit truthfully to the causes of their injuries. A healthcare provider who suspects abuse of a vulnerable client is obligated to report it and to validate the concerns to the greatest extent possible. Discuss issues of abuse with the client in a nonthreatening way in private; convey concern and understanding; reassure the client that he or she is not at fault; and encourage the client to tell the story by using open-ended questions. It is not within the scope of the entry-level practical nurse to gather in-depth information on the possible abuse. If the suspected abuse involves an adult, the practical nurse should share information on supports and resources. The practical nurse must understand that he or she cannot disclose client information without the client's consent. If the suspicions of abuse involve a child, dependent adult, or person in care (hospital, facility, etc.), the practical nurse is responsible for documenting the observations factually and accurately and reporting the abuse to the appropriate agency either independently or in collaboration with another healthcare provider.

PRACTICE QUESTIONS

Case 1

Jason Beames, age 17 years, was brought to the emergency department by the police. His mother called the police after Jason violently attacked his father with no provocation. Jason is admitted to the psychiatric unit for investigation of his psychosis, with a provisional diagnosis of schizophrenia.

Questions 1–5 refer to this case.

1. What is the definition of *psychosis*?
   1. A psychological break from reality
   2. A group of mental health disorders characterized by various anxiety symptoms
   3. A disturbance of consciousness and change in cognition
   4. Another term for schizophrenia
2. The emergency department physician completes a certificate designating Jason an involuntary client because Jason would not consent to admission. Which of the following should the practical nurse tell Jason concerning his rights as an involuntary client?
   1. The physician is not legally permitted to admit Jason without his consent.
   2. Since Jason is only 17 years old, he does not have the same rights as an adult.
   3. Jason can apply to a review board for a legal ruling on his involuntary admission.
   4. Jason has no legal rights since he has been certified as an involuntary psychiatric client.
3. Because of his violent behaviour, Jason is administered a chemical restraint. Which of the following statements is true with regard to using restraints in a psychiatric setting?
   1. Chemical restraints are preferable to other interventions for calming a psychotic client.
   2. Physical restraints are generally more effective than chemical restraints for psychotic episodes.
   3. Guidelines for the use of restraints apply to both chemical and physical restraints.
   4. A physician order for chemical restraints is generally not required in an emergency department setting.

4. Jason tells the practical nurse that the voices are yelling at him. What would be the most helpful response?
   1. "I don't hear the voices that you hear."
   2. "What are the voices yelling at you?"
   3. "You realize there are really no voices yelling at you."
   4. "Why do you think you are hearing voices?"
5. Jason's parents come to visit Jason. His mother asks the practical nurse if Jason has schizophrenia and will he will have to be in the hospital for the rest of his life. What might the practical nurse respond to Jason's mother?
   1. "I can refer you to the local Canadian Schizophrenia Society. They will provide education for you about Jason's disease."
   2. "Because Jason is young, he will likely not have any further serious psychotic episodes."
   3. "I don't really know. We will have to wait to see how Jason responds to his medications."
   4. "Schizophrenia is a lifelong disorder, but antipsychotic medications allow most people to live and be treated outside the hospital."

Case 2

Marty Steele, age 42, has been diagnosed with borderline personality disorder. He is admitted to a psychiatric unit.
   Questions 6 and 7 refer to this case.
6. Mr. Steele tells the practical nurse, Jeremy, that one of the other nurses, Sarah, is lazy and is not as good a nurse as Jeremy. What is this called?
   1. Narcissistic behaviour
   2. Schizoid behaviour
   3. Splitting behaviour
   4. Dependent behaviour
7. What is the priority assessment for the practical nurse to conduct with Mr. Steele?
   1. Potential for harm to himself or others
   2. Hallucinations
   3. History of child abuse
   4. Sexual orientation

Case 3

Tiffany Scolfield, age 15, comes to see the school practical nurse because she stopped menstruating several months ago. The practical nurse suspects an eating disorder.
   Questions 8–12 refer to this case.
8. Which of the following statements about eating disorders is true?
   1. People can die from anorexia but not from bulimia.
   2. Men can suffer from bulimia but not from anorexia.
   3. Women who recover from anorexia often develop bulimia later.
   4. People with bulimia deny feelings of hunger.
9. The practical nurse assesses Tiffany for medical complications associated with her eating disorder. Which of the following physical assessments would it be most important to perform while Tiffany was in her office?
   1. Complete skin survey for breakdown
   2. Abdominal palpation for constipation
   3. Oral examination for dental caries
   4. Blood pressure monitoring for hypotension
10. Tiffany talks to the practical nurse about her feelings. The practical nurse uses clarification as a form of therapeutic communication. Which of the following responses is an example of clarification?
    1. "I'm not sure what you mean. Could you tell me about that again?"
    2. "Can you tell me more about what is bothering you?"
    3. "What do you think is causing you to feel this way?"
    4. "You've mentioned many things. Let's go back to how eating makes you feel."
11. The practical nurse arranges for Tiffany to come to the health office at regular intervals to monitor her weight. What would the practical nurse be aware of regarding the process of weighing Tiffany?
    1. Tiffany may drink excessive fluids to increase her recorded weight.
    2. Tiffany will probably refuse to be weighed.
    3. Tiffany should be weighed wearing her street clothes and shoes.
    4. Tiffany's parents must be informed about the monitoring of her weight.
12. Tiffany's weight decreases, and she is admitted to an eating disorders unit at a local pediatric hospital. What should be included in her care plan?
    1. Large meals at frequent intervals to improve her nutritional status
    2. Accurate input and output to monitor fluid status
    3. Leisurely meals to promote decreased stress while eating
    4. Segregation from other adolescents with eating disorders

Case 4

Nandini Balkan, age 48, is admitted to an inpatient psychiatric facility due to acute depression with suicidal ideation.
   Questions 13–15 refer to this case.
13. With clients who have suicidal ideation, when is the person least likely to act on their suicidal impulses?
    1. On admission to a psychiatric facility
    2. On discharge from a psychiatric facility
    3. When symptoms of the depression are most severe
    4. As the symptoms, motivation, and energy begin to improve
14. The practical nurse finds Ms. Balkan curled in a fetal position, crying. Through her tears, she says to the practical nurse, "I really can't go on. I just want to end it all. Please, won't you help me die?" What is the most appropriate response by the practical nurse?
    1. "I am sorry you are feeling so badly today. Perhaps you will feel better tomorrow."
    2. "I see that you are terribly unhappy today. But you know I cannot help you to die."
    3. "You are feeling very badly today. Would you like to tell me about it?"
    4. "This feeling is just temporary. Why would you want to die?"

15. Ms. Balkan is prescribed fluoxetine hydrochloride (Prozac). The practical nurse would advise Ms. Balkan of which of the following about this medication?
    1. It may take up to 4 weeks to notice any improvement.
    2. There is increased risk of suicide after therapy is well established.
    3. Anxiety and nervousness will likely decrease in about 2 weeks.
    4. Herbal preparations are safe to take with his medication.

Independent Questions

Questions 16–25 do not refer to a particular case.

16. Mr. Fraser is receiving high doses of haloperidol (Haldol). What adverse effects would require the practical nurse to consult with the physician about stopping the drug?
    1. Mr. Fraser complains he feels sleepy and tired.
    2. Mr. Fraser's skin and eye conjunctiva display a yellowish tinge.
    3. Mr. Fraser states he is dizzy when he stands.
    4. Mr. Fraser displays extrapyramidal symptoms.

17. Which of the following individuals is at the highest risk of suicide?
    1. Mrs. Hardacre, age 42, who has a history of alcohol abuse
    2. Mrs. Blatchfor, age 49, who is distressed because her children have moved away from home
    3. Mr. Tyrell, age 19, who is upset that his girlfriend has broken off their relationship
    4. Mr. Grimes, age 82, who is lonely after the death of his wife

18. A newly graduated practical nurse obtains employment at a psychiatric outpatient clinic. A young client in distress confides to the practical nurse that he has a gender identity disorder. He feels he is a female trapped in the body of a man. What is the most effective action taken by the practical nurse?
    1. Provide him with relaxation exercises to decrease the anxiety associated with his distress.
    2. Refer him to a qualified sexual therapist.
    3. Enroll him in the clinic's sexual disorders psychotherapy group.
    4. Perform a complete physical examination to determine any contributing physical problems.

19. Which statement best supports a practical nurse providing advocacy during a multidisciplinary team meeting?
    1. Symptoms of mental illnesses are not influenced by a person's culture.
    2. Obsessive–compulsive disorder and hoarding have similar cultural issues.
    3. Cultural healing therapies will have little affect a person's mental illness.
    4. Assessment findings in mental illness are reflective of the persons cultural background.

20. Which form of substance abuse is most common in Canada?

1. Narcotics
2. Alcohol
3. Marijuana
4. Inhalants

21. Which of the following is an important consideration when conducting a culturally sensitive mental health assessment?
    1. Practical nurses must treat clients according to the established beliefs of their specific culture.
    2. Some cultures are not accepting of mental illnesses among their population.
    3. Practical nurses must facilitate verbal expressions of feelings in cultures in which this is not a common practice.
    4. Regardless of culture, all people react to adverse stressors with similar behaviours.

22. The practical nurse is unsure if Henry Picard, age 87, is manifesting symptoms of delirium or dementia. What question might he ask Mr. Picard's family?
    1. "Do you think Mr. Picard has Alzheimer's disease?"
    2. "How long has Mr. Picard shown confused thinking?"
    3. "Does Mr. Picard have any family members with a history of dementia?"
    4. "Has Mr. Picard ever been violent?"

23. Alex Carolis has been diagnosed with antisocial personality disorder. Which of the following comments by Mr. Carolis would be most typical of this disorder?
    1. "I am feeling very anxious."
    2. "I am going to buy myself a new top-of-the-line car today."
    3. "I have learned never to cheat on an exam again."
    4. "I have a responsibility to care for my younger brother."

24. Chandra Wasson, age 27 years, is an inpatient at a psychiatric facility. Her practical nurse, Sanjay, age 29 years, accompanies her to a local restaurant for coffee. Is this an appropriate behaviour for Sanjay?
    1. It is appropriate if it is part of the care plan.
    2. It is appropriate if the friendship is mutual and nonsexual.
    3. It is not appropriate as Ms. Wasson is a client with a mental health diagnosis.
    4. It is not appropriate as it is never ethical for a registered practical nurse to be in a social situation with a client.

25. The practical nurse is unhappy and stressed with her work situation in a busy medical unit. She manifests these feelings with passive–aggressive behaviour. Which of the following might be an example of the practical nurse's passive–aggressive behaviour?
    1. Yelling at clients
    2. Written complaints to the unit manager about the work environment
    3. Being chronically late for shifts
    4. Readily agreeing to work overtime

REFERENCES

Alzheimer Society of Canada. (2018). Dementia numbers in Canada. Retrieved from http://alzheimer.ca/en/Home/About-dementia/What-is-dementia/Dementia-numbers.

Alzheimer's Association. (2018). What is Alzheimer's and dementia? Treatments. Retrieved from https://www.alz.org/alzheimers-dementia/what-is-alzheimers.

American Psychiatric Association. (2013). *Diagnostic and statistical manual of mental disorders* (5th ed.). Washington, DC: Author.

Bulechek, G. M., Butcher, H. K., & Dochterman, J. M. (Eds.), (2013). *Nursing interventions classification (NIC)* (6th ed.). Toronto: Elsevier.

Canadian Council for Practical Nurse Regulators. (2013). Code of ethics for licensed practical nurses in Canada. Retrieved from http://www.clpna.com/wp-content/uploads/2013/02/doc_CCPNR_CLPNA_Code_of_Ethics.pdf.

Canadian Institute for Health Information. (2017). *Community mental health and addiction information: A snapshot of data collection and reporting in Canada*. Ottawa, ON. Retrieved from https://secure.cihi.ca/free_products/CIHI-comm-mental-health-en-web.pdf.

DeAngelis, T. (2010). Found in translation. *Monitor on Psychology*, 41(2), 52.

Fazio, S., Pace, D., Flinner, J., et al. (2018). The fundamentals of patient-centered care for individuals with dementia. *The Gerontologist*, 58(S1), S10–S19. Retrieved from https://doi.org/10.1093/geront/gnx122.

Fazio, S., Pace, D., Maslow, K., et al. (2018). Alzheimer's association dementia care practice recommendations. *The Gerontologist*, 58(S1), S1–S9. Retrieved from https://doi.org/10.1093/geront/gnx122.

Findlay, L. (2017). *Health reports: Depression and suicidal ideation among Canadians aged* (pp. 15–24). Ottawa: Statistics Canada. Retrieved from http://www.statcan.gc.ca/pub/82-003-x/2017001/article/14697-eng.htm.

Government of Canada. (2013). Section 2: Canadian guidelines on sexually transmitted infections—Primary care and sexually transmitted infections. Retrieved from https://www.canada.ca/en/public-health/services/infectious-diseases/sexual-health-sexually-transmitted-infections/canadian-guidelines/sexually-transmitted-infections/canadian-guidelines-sexually-transmitted-infections-17.html#a1.

Gray, J. E., Shone, M. A., & Liddle, P. F. (2008). *Canadian mental health law and policy* (2nd ed.). Markham, ON: LexisNexis Canada.

Halter, M. J. (2018). *Varcarolis' foundations of psychiatric mental health nursing: A clinical approach* (8th ed.). St. Louis: Elsevier/Saunders.

Halter, M. J., Pollard, C. L., & Jakubec, S. L. (2019). *Varcarolis's Canadian psychiatric mental health nursing: A clinical approach* (2nd ed.). Milton, ON: Elsevier Canada.

Hartrick Doane, G., & Varcoe, C. (2015). *How to nurse: Relational inquiry with individuals and families in changing health and health care contexts*. Philadelphia: Wolters Kluwer.

Health Canada. (2012). Canadian alcohol and drug use monitoring survey: Summary of results for 2012. Retrieved from https://www.canada.ca/en/health-canada/services/health-concerns/drug-prevention-treatment/drug-alcohol-use-statistics/canadian-alcohol-drug-use-monitoring-survey-summary-results-2012.html#s1.

Johnson, C. (2017). Harm reduction in the addiction continuum of care. *The Canadian Nurse*, 113(3), 36.

Mental Health Commission of Canada. (2012). The mental health strategy for Canada. Retrieved from http://strategy.mentalhealthcommission.ca/the-facts/.

Navaneelan, T. (2017). Health at a glance: Suicide rates: An overview. Retrieved from http://www.statcan.gc.ca/pub/82-624-x/2012001/article/11696-eng.htm#cvsd.

Pauly, B., Gray, E., Perkin, K., et al. (2016). Finding safety: A pilot of managed alcohol participants' perceptions of housing and quality of life. *Harm Reduction Journal*, 13(15), 2–11. Retrieved from https://harmreductionjournal.biomedcentral.com/track/pdf/10.1186/s12954-016-0102-5?site=harmreductionjournal.biomedcentral.com, https://doi.org/10.1186/s12954-016-0102-5.

Potter, P., Perry, A., Stockert, P., et al. (2019). *Canadian fundamentals of nursing* (6th ed.). Milton, ON: Elsevier.

Public Health Agency of Canada. (2016). What is depression? Retrieved from https://www.canada.ca/en/public-health/services/chronic-diseases/mental-illness/what-depression.html.

Schizophrenia Society of Canada. (2018). A reason to hope, the means to cope. Retrieved from http://www.schizophrenia.ca/learn_more_about_schizophrenia.php#2.

Shen, Z. (2015). Cultural competence models and cultural competence assessment instruments in nursing: A literature review. *Journal of Transcultural Nursing*, 26(3), 308–321. doi:10.1177/1043659614524790.

Sorrentino, S. A., Remmert, L. N., & Wilk, M. J. (2018). *Mosby's Canadian textbook for the support worker* (4th ed.). Toronto: Elsevier.

Statistics Canada. (2013). Canadian Community Health Survey: Mental health 2012. Retrieved from http://www.statcan.gc.ca/daily-quotidien/130918/dq130918a-eng.htm.

Statistics Canada. (2015a). Healthy fact Sheets. Heavy drinking, 2015. Retrieved from http://www.statcan.gc.ca/pub/82-625-x/2017001/article/14765-eng.htm.

Statistics Canada. (2015b). Section F—Personality disorders. Retrieved from http://www.statcan.gc.ca/pub/82-619-m/2012004/sections/sectionf-eng.htm.

Statistics Canada. (2015c). Section G—Schizophrenia. Retrieved from http://www.statcan.gc.ca/pub/82-619-m/2012004/sections/sectiong-eng.htm.

Statistics Canada. (2017). Canadian Community Health Survey, 2015. Retrieved from http://statcan.gc.ca/daily-quotidien/170322/dq170322a-eng.htm.

Stuart, G. W. (2013). *Principles and practice of psychiatric nursing* (10th ed.). St. Louis: Mosby.

U.S. Food and Drug Administration. (2008). FDA expands morality warnings on antipsychotic drugs [Press release]. Retrieved from https://www.fdanews.com/articles/107752-fda-expands-mortality-warnings-on-antipsychotic-drugs.

U.S. Food and Drug Administration. (2016). Atypical antipsychotic drugs information. Retrieved from https://www.fdanews.com/articles/107752-fda-expands-mortality-warnings-on-antipsychotic-drugs.

WEB SITES

- **Canadian Coalition of Alternative Mental Health Resources** (http://www.ccamhr.ca): This site contains resources about mental health services and organizations, including alternative treatment programs. It has a sections on mental health news and research.

- **Canadian Mental Health Association (CMHA)** (http://www.cmha.ca): This site provides information on many specific mental health conditions and explores ways in which to promote good mental health. CMHA has offices across Canada and national mental health programs.
- **Code of Ethics for Licensed Practical Nurses in Canada (CCPNR)** (https://www.ccpnr.ca/wp-content/uploads/2013/09/IJLPN-CE-Final.pdf): This document describes the code of ethics and ethical obligations of all licensed/registered practical nurses. The Canadian Council for Practical Nurse Regulators (CCPNR) is a federation of provincial and territorial members who are identified in legislation, and responsible for the safety of the public through the regulation of licensed/registered practical nurses.
- **eMentalHealth.ca** (http://www.ementalhealth.ca/site/ontario/index.php?m=1&ID=26): This Canadian mental health site provides a resource directory and event calendar with information relevant to both consumers and care providers.

The site is an anonymous and confidential source of mental health information.
- **Mental Health Commission of Canada** (http://www.mentalhealthcommission.ca): This organization's goal is to integrate mental health services in Canada. The site follows the progress of the commission in terms of its projects and policies.
- **Mood Disorders Society of Canada** (https://mdsc.ca): This site describes different mood and anxiety disorders and their diagnosis and treatment. It is primarily designed for clients and their families and links to resources that may be useful for healthcare providers.
- **Public Health Agency of Canada: Mental Health** (https://www.canada.ca/en/public-health/services/health-promotion/mental-health.html): This site provides information on mental health issues encountered by Canadians. It also provides access to a range of materials on mental health promotion relevant to both consumers and service providers.

INTRODUCTION TO PRACTICE EXAMS

The following practice examinations are designed to be similar to those you will encounter in the Canadian Practical Nurse Registration Examination (CPNRE). The exam is organized into two books that contain 130 multiple-choice questions each, for a total of 260 questions. You may want to write the practice exam in a group with fellow students to help replicate an actual exam situation.

Instructions

Read each question carefully and then choose the answer that you think is the best of the four options presented. If you cannot decide on an answer to a question, proceed to the next one and return to this question later if you have time. Try to answer all the questions. Marks are not subtracted for wrong answers. If you are unsure of an answer, it will be to your advantage to guess. Allow yourself 3 hours for each book.

When you have completed both practice exam books, tally your scores and calculate your percentage for the total examination. See Chapter 2 for more details on test-taking skills.

PRACTICE QUESTIONS

Case 1

Nada Wasson delivered a healthy, 3 600-g baby boy, Sandu, a week ago. She attends the newborn infant clinic at her local hospital, where the practical nurse examines Sandu.

Questions 1–5 refer to this case.

1. The practical nurse takes Sandu's vital signs. Which of the following would be normal for a 1-week-old infant?
   1. Heart rate 100 bpm, respirations 26 breaths per minute, blood pressure 44 mm Hg systolic
   2. Heart rate 165 bpm, respirations 65 breaths per minute, blood pressure 94 mm Hg systolic
   3. Heart rate 140 bpm, respirations 40 breaths per minute, blood pressure 70 mm Hg systolic
   4. Heart rate 130 bpm, respirations 32 breaths per minute, blood pressure 100 mm Hg systolic
2. The practical nurse tests Sandu's Babinski reflex. What is the expected response by Sandu to the Babinski test?
   1. Dorsiflexion of the big toe
   2. Flexion and extension of the leg
   3. Flexion of the fingers
   4. Extension and adduction of extremities

3. The practical nurse obtains a weight of 3 450 g for Sandu. Mrs. Wasson is concerned about the weight loss, telling the practical nurse that she is probably not producing enough milk. What would be the best response by the practical nurse?
   1. "This weight loss is normal in the first week. Continue breastfeeding at frequent intervals."
   2. "Although most newborns lose weight in the first week, you should probably supplement him with formula for the next few days."
   3. "This is not a significant weight loss, so don't be concerned."
   4. "To prevent further weight loss, you can increase your milk supply by drinking more liquids during the day."
4. Mrs. Wasson complains that her nipples are sore. What should the practical nurse suggest for care of the breasts?
   1. Air the nipples as much as possible.
   2. Use a lanolin-based cream after every feeding.
   3. Use plastic-lined breast pads.
   4. Begin nursing with the breast that is most painful.
5. Mrs. Wasson plans to express breast milk for use when she has a babysitter. She asks the practical nurse how she should instruct the babysitter to warm the bottle. What should be the practical nurse's response?
   1. Place the bottle in a pot of water and heat slowly on top of the stove.
   2. Place the bottle in a microwave oven and heat at a low temperature.
   3. Place the bottle in a bowl of lukewarm water.
   4. Warming is not necessary, as the bottle can be used directly from the refrigerator.

Case 2

Edgar is a 14-year-old boy who was diagnosed with type 1 diabetes at age 4 years. His blood sugar control has been poorly maintained for the past 2 months. It is suspected that the lack of control is related to an adolescent growth spurt and possible poor adherence to blood glucose monitoring, nutrition, and insulin administration. Edgar has been admitted to a short-stay unit in hospital for stabilization.

Questions 6–10 refer to this case.

6. When Edgar was diagnosed at age 4, he exhibited the cardinal symptoms of the three "polys." What are these manifestations?

1. Polycythemia, polyuria, polymyositis
2. Polydipsia, polyelectrolyte, polyneuropathy
3. Polyopia, polyarthritis, polyphagia
4. Polyphagia, polydipsia, polyuria

7. The practical nurse reviews insulin action, dosage, and administration with Edgar. What is the optimum insulin regimen for most children with diabetes?
   1. Twice-daily injections of rapid-acting and intermediate-acting insulins
   2. Multiple daily injections of rapid- and long-acting insulins
   3. Total dosage and percentage of regular- to intermediate-acting insulins determined individually
   4. Ratio and dose determined by weight in kilograms

8. Edgar admits to the practical nurse he has been experimenting with alcohol and binge drinking on the weekends. He states that his parents are "heavy drinkers" and are not aware of his behaviour. What is the most critical issue concerning Edgar's drinking of alcohol?
   1. Alcohol causes a rise in blood sugar, leading to a sustained period of hyperglycemia.
   2. Binge drinking can lead to inappropriate and dangerous behaviour.
   3. Alcohol causes a drop in blood sugar that could lead to severe hypoglycemia.
   4. Because Edgar's parents are "heavy drinkers," he is more likely to develop a dependency on alcohol.

9. Edgar injects seven units of regular (Humulin R) insulin at 1600 hours. When should the practical nurse caution him to be alert for a possible hypoglycemic episode?
   1. 1830 hours
   2. 2030 hours
   3. 2230 hours
   4. 2400 hours

10. The practical nurse assesses that Edgar has been non-adherent to his diabetes management. What is the most appropriate nursing action to address Edgar's non-adherence?
    1. Ask Edgar's parents to supervise him more closely.
    2. Provide education to Edgar and his family about the potential dangers of poorly controlled diabetes.
    3. In private, explore Edgar's feelings about diabetes and the treatment regimen.
    4. Suggest to Edgar that he join an adolescent diabetes support group.

Case 3

A practical nurse works on an orthopaedic surgery unit of a hospital. Many of the clients are older adults with increased risk for hospital-acquired infections.

Questions 11–15 refer to this case.

11. Which of the following is the most important step for the practical nurse to protect her clients from hospital-acquired infections?
    1. Identify clients who are at risk.
    2. Review hygiene practices with all clients.

3. Restrict visitors.
4. Lobby for the use of alcohol-based hand sanitizers.

12. Mr. Carolis, age 81, has just had a total hip replacement. He has a history of poor nutrition. Postoperatively, he has an in-dwelling urinary catheter. Which of these factors puts Mr. Carolis most at risk for developing an infection?
    1. Age
    2. Poor nutrition
    3. Surgery
    4. In-dwelling urinary catheter

13. Mr. Carolis develops manifestations of an infection. Which of the following abnormal findings indicates that Mr. Carolis may have an infection?
    1. Leukocytosis
    2. Neutropenia
    3. Thrombocytosis
    4. Leukopenia

14. Mr. Carolis is ordered to have urine cultures and then is started on intravenous antibiotics. What action should the practical nurse take with regard to the specimen collection and antibiotic administration?
    1. Commence the antibiotics as soon as the medication is received from the pharmacy department.
    2. Ask the physician for the correct order for specimen collection and medication administration.
    3. Take the urine sample from the in-dwelling catheter, and then commence the medication.
    4. Administer the antibiotics, and then collect the urine sample from the urinary collection bag.

15. The practical nurse discovers that she has administered twice the ordered dose of a medication to Mr. Carolis. What is the most important initial action for the practical nurse to perform?
    1. Complete an incident report.
    2. Notify the ordering physician.
    3. Assess Mr. Carolis for adverse effects of the overdose.
    4. Report the error to the nurse administrator.

Case 4

Mr. Kassam has chronic renal failure, secondary to type 2 diabetes. He has been attending an outpatient renal clinic for several years, and recently his condition has deteriorated. The practical nurse sees Mr. Kassam in the clinic.

Questions 16–21 refer to this case.

16. Which of the following laboratory blood test results would be of most concern to the practical nurse?
    1. Potassium: 7 mmol/L
    2. pH: 7.37
    3. Sodium: 142 mmol/L
    4. Blood urea nitrogen (BUN): 6.8 mmol/L

17. Mr. Kassam is on erythropoietin therapy. What is the rationale for this therapy?
    1. To treat the associated anemia
    2. To control hypertension
    3. To correct the acid–base balance
    4. To increase perfusion in the kidney

18. An important component of conservative treatment for chronic renal failure is diet therapy. Which of the following would be an appropriate lunch menu for Mr. Kassam?
   1. A 100-g cheese sandwich on whole wheat bread, a banana, and 200 mL of milk
   2. Canned tomato soup, 250 mL, saltine crackers, and 400 mL of orange juice
   3. Turkey, 60 g, on white bread with mayonnaise, an apple, and 250 mL of ginger ale
   4. Grilled beefsteak, 300 g, a baked potato, cooked spinach, and chocolate milk

19. Following several months of dialysis, Mr. Kassam exclaims to the practical nurse, "I just can't do this anymore. I'd rather be dead!" What is the most therapeutic response by the practical nurse?
   1. "You'd rather be dead?"
   2. "This is very difficult treatment. Tell me about what is bothering you the most."
   3. "Just hang on until we can get you a kidney transplant."
   4. "Are you depressed?"

20. Mr. Kassam reveals to the practical nurse he has found an Internet site that provides kidney transplant surgery in another country for a significant amount of money. What is the practical nurse's professional responsibility in response to Mr. Kassam?
   1. Tell Mr. Kassam it is illegal to buy or sell organs in Canada.
   2. Tell Mr. Kassam he must wait until he can receive a kidney in Canada.
   3. Ask Mr. Kassam for more details about the Internet site and details of the transplant service.
   4. Inform Mr. Kassam that he should not waste his money.

21. Mr. Kassam's condition is deteriorating, and he decides to no longer take dialysis. He tells the practical nurse he just wants to die. He is considering medical assistance in dying (MAID). Which of the following does *not* meet the criteria for MAID?
   1. The client is at least 18 years of age and capable of making decisions with respect to his or her health.
   2. The client has a grievous and terminal medical condition.
   3. The client has been encouraged by the physician and family members to request MAID to end his or her suffering.
   4. The client gave informed consent to receive MAID after having been informed of the palliative care.

Case 5

Mrs. Dhillon, age 58, is suspected of having ovarian cancer. She has been referred by her family physician to an oncologist. The practical nurse consults with cancer clients in the physician's office.

Questions 22–26 refer to this case.

22. What are the early manifestations of ovarian cancer?
   1. Vague or mild symptoms of abdominal pressure and digestive problems
   2. Painful menstrual periods with increased bleeding
   3. Sharp pain and swelling in the area of the affected ovary
   4. Swollen inguinal lymph nodes

23. The oncologist plans a biopsy via laparoscopy. Mrs. Dhillon asks the practical nurse about this test. What should the practical nurse explain to Mrs. Dhillon?
   1. "A laparoscopy is the insertion of a large needle through the abdomen into the ovary to collect cells for biopsy."
   2. "A laparoscopy is an operation done through a surgical incision in the abdomen and can be used to take a biopsy of ovarian tissue or to remove any visible cancer."
   3. "A laparoscopy is the insertion of a flexible tube through a small cut in the abdomen, through which small biopsy samples can be taken."
   4. "A laparoscopy is the insertion of air into the fallopian tubes to enable ovarian cells to be withdrawn via the tubes."

24. The results of the biopsy determine that Mrs. Dhillon has stage 3, grade 2 ovarian cancer. The practical nurse explains that these results help determine which treatment will be most effective for her. Which of the following is the correct interpretation of stage 3, grade 2?
   1. The cancer has spread to tissues in the pelvis but is slow-growing.
   2. The cancer has spread to organs of the abdomen and lymph nodes but is spreading at a moderate rate.
   3. The cancer is confined to the ovaries but is highly likely to spread.
   4. The cancer has spread outside the abdomen to distant parts of the body and is growing quickly.

25. The oncologist recommends surgery followed by chemotherapy to treat the cancer. Mrs. Dhillon telephones the practical nurse 2 days later, saying, "Surgery is too drastic, and the chemotherapy is poison that will destroy my body." She will, instead, try some special herbs she has heard about from a friend. What is the best response by the practical nurse to Mrs. Dhillon?
   1. "These herbs have not likely been tested for safety or effectiveness, so it is not known whether they will harm you or be effective for your cancer."
   2. "This is not recommended and will probably cause you to die sooner."
   3. "At this stage, you are in denial, so call us back when you change your mind."
   4. "You are right about the toxins in the chemotherapy, so it is a good idea to try the herbs first."

26. Mrs. Dhillon is experiencing difficulty deciding on a course of treatment for her cancer. She says to the practical nurse, "I am just so depressed. It doesn't matter

what treatment I have; I'll die anyway." What is the most appropriate response by the practical nurse?

1. "Why do you feel this way?"
2. "Everyone diagnosed with cancer feels this way just after they receive their diagnosis."
3. "Everything will be fine as soon as you start your treatment."
4. "Let's talk about your prognosis and treatment options."

Case 6

A practical nurse works at a fitness centre. She has been employed to perform health assessments, health counselling, and first aid as necessary.

Questions 27–32 refer to this case.

27. Reza Morhudi, age 32 years, has just run 10 km on a treadmill and asks the practical nurse to take his blood pressure (BP). The practical nurse obtains a reading of 146/90 mm Hg in Mr. Morhudi's right arm. What is the appropriate nursing action in response to this BP reading?
    1. Tell Mr. Morhudi to rest for 20 minutes and reassess the BP.
    2. Obtain a second BP reading in his left arm.
    3. Ask Mr. Morhudi if he has any history of hypertension.
    4. Tell Mr. Morhudi this is a normal reading for a man of his age and fitness level.

28. The practical nurse is called to see Valerya Dove, who is on the floor of the gym, crying and saying she has "twisted" her ankle. What interventions should the practical nurse perform while waiting for the doctor to assess Ms. Dove's ankle?
    1. Heat, passive range of motion (ROM), analgesics
    2. Rest, ice, compression, elevation
    3. Cool compresses, partial weight-bearing, maintaining joint in flexion
    4. Immobilization of the joint, then sending Ms. Dove to the emergency department for an X-ray

29. Mr. Lackraj introduces himself to the practical nurse as a new client to the fitness centre. He is 54, obese, and flushed and appears short of breath. What should be the practical nurse's initial assessment question?
    1. "What has been your past pattern of exercise?"
    2. "What is your personal goal for an exercise plan?"
    3. "Have you consulted your physician about an exercise plan?"
    4. "Are you anticipating exercise will help you lose weight?"

30. The practical nurse is concerned about transmission of pathogens among the clients of the fitness centre, as many people use the equipment during the day. What would be the most effective action to reduce the potential of transmission of communicable diseases?
    1. Terminal cleaning of all equipment at the end of the day
    2. Screening all clients for symptoms prior to use of equipment

3. Creating a poster board with information about communicable diseases
4. Installation of alcohol gel dispensers for client hand hygiene between uses of equipment

31. What additional advice might the practical nurse provide to her clients regarding "gym hygiene"?
    1. Place a towel on any surfaces you will be touching with bare skin.
    2. Bring your own towel and launder it once every five visits.
    3. Do not use the showers at the gym.
    4. Dress in pants and long-sleeved clothing rather than shorts and sleeveless tops.

32. The practical nurse has noticed that one of her adolescent clients, Bart Matthews, has developed acne and reduced body fat, with increased muscle size and strength. She suspects that he is using anabolic steroids to improve his sports performance. What would be the most appropriate approach for the practical nurse to initiate a discussion about the possible use of steroids?
    1. "I've noticed that your muscle size has increased quite a bit and you have developed acne."
    2. "Are you aware of the dangers of taking anabolic steroids?"
    3. "Did you know that using anabolic steroids would disqualify you from sports competitions?"
    4. "Are you taking any supplements to improve your performance?"

Case 7

Raize Manche is a 59-year-old woman who has been admitted to an inpatient psychiatric unit following a suicide attempt. She appears unkempt, lethargic, and tearful. She tells her primary practical nurse, "I'm no use to anyone. There's no point in me going on." Her diagnosis is dysthymia with suicidal ideation.

Questions 33–36 refer to this case.

33. During an interaction, Ms. Manche tells the practical nurse that no one cares about her, but she does love her grandchildren. What would be the most therapeutic response by the practical nurse?
    1. "Tell me more about your grandchildren."
    2. "I am sure that your family does care about you."
    3. "If you talk about your feelings, you will feel better and enjoy your grandchildren more."
    4. "Your grandchildren would be very upset if you harmed yourself."

34. Ms. Manche has not been eating during her depression and tells the practical nurse she "just isn't hungry." What would be an appropriate intervention by the practical nurse to encourage adequate nutrition?
    1. Have Ms. Manche's family bring in food from home.
    2. Consult with a dietitian about the most appropriate menu for Ms. Manche's anorexia.
    3. Offer Ms. Manche bland, high-protein foods.
    4. Ask Ms. Manche what foods and drinks she likes to eat.

35. After being on the unit for several days, Ms. Manche is asked to join a patient discussion group. Ms. Manche states that she does not want to go because she has "nothing to say." How should the practical nurse respond to Ms. Manche?
    1. "You must go to the group, but you don't have to talk."
    2. "Perhaps you could participate by talking about your grandchildren."
    3. "You feel you have nothing to say?"
    4. "The group will be very therapeutic for you."

36. Ms. Manche's physician orders a selective serotonin reuptake inhibitor, sertraline (Zoloft). Ms. Manche tells the practical nurse she doesn't want to take any drugs because they "won't fix anything." How should the practical nurse respond?
    1. "No one likes to take drugs, but these might help you."
    2. "Zoloft helps correct the flaw in brain chemistry in depression and should relieve many of your symptoms."
    3. "You should speak with your psychiatrist about whether you can participate in psychotherapy without taking medications."
    4. "Zoloft is one of the newer antidepressants and does not have many side effects."

Case 8

A practical nurse works in a long-term care facility, Sunset Acres. The clients are primarily adults over 80 years of age, with physical and cognitive disabilities.

Questions 37–40 refer to this case.

37. The practical nurse finds Ms. Abetiu, a client with Alzheimer's disease and dementia, on the floor by her bed. The practical nurse examines Ms Abetiu and finds no injuries. Throughout the day when she asks Ms. Abetiu if she has pain, Ms. Abetiu answers "No." The practical nurse documents the incident but takes no further action. The following day, the practical nurse notices Ms. Abetiu grimacing and occasionally crying out as if in pain. What is the most appropriate nursing action?
    1. Contact the facility physician.
    2. Call an ambulance to transport Ms. Abetiu to the hospital.
    3. Ask Ms. Abetiu if she is experiencing any pain.
    4. Contact Ms. Abetiu's family to report the incident and present manifestations.

38. Mrs. Ensoy is a newly admitted client with dementia. One morning, the practical nurse observes Mrs. Ensoy to be very agitated and aggressive. What action by the practical nurse may be of immediate help to manage Mrs. Ensoy's agitation?
    1. Sit and talk with Mrs. Ensoy to find out what is bothering her.
    2. Orient Mrs. Ensoy to the reality of her new environment.
    3. Hand Mrs. Ensoy a cloth and ask her to dust the furniture.

    4. Administer the ordered medication, risperidone (Risperdal).

39. Many of the clients at Sunset Acres have urinary incontinence. Evidence-informed practice suggests that which of the following is most effective in reducing urinary incontinence in people with dementia?
    1. Medication with cholinesterase inhibitors
    2. Reducing total fluid intake, especially in the evening
    3. Use of adult incontinence products, such as Attends or Depends
    4. Scheduled toileting and prompted voiding

40. The practical nurse is aware that her clients are at high risk for skin breakdown. Which of the following clients would be most at risk for a sacral pressure ulcer?
    1. Mr. Boston, age 92, who is fully ambulatory but has moderate dementia
    2. Mrs. Colorado, age 85, who is on bed rest and limited ambulation following total hip replacement
    3. Mrs. Carys, age 95, who has a fractured radius
    4. Mr. Cleveland, age 75, who has paraplegia and uses a wheelchair

Case 9

Anusha Satgun immigrated to Canada from Southeast Asia yesterday after a 12-hour flight. She felt unwell during the night, and her worried family took her to the local walk-in clinic the following day. The practical nurse sees Mrs. Satgun in the clinic.

Questions 41–44 refer to this case.

41. Mrs. Satgun does not have private insurance, nor is she eligible for care through the *Canada Health Act*. What is the necessary action by the practical nurse?
    1. She should refer to agency policies regarding provision of treatment to uninsured individuals.
    2. She should provide care based on professional humanitarian principles.
    3. She should advise Mrs. Satgun to arrange for health-care insurance, after which care will be provided.
    4. She should refer Mrs. Satgun to the local community clinic that provides care for recent immigrants to Canada.

42. The practical nurse conducts an initial health screening with Mrs. Satgun. What would be the most important question to ask Mrs. Satgun?
    1. "What is your previous medical history?"
    2. "Have you had any coughs, colds, or fever in the past week?"
    3. "What medications are you presently taking?"
    4. "Have you consulted a physician in the past year?"

43. Mrs. Satgun is assessed by the practical nurse and then referred to a physician due to a possible immobility-induced deep vein thrombosis (DVT). What symptoms is Mrs. Satgun likely to have manifested?
    1. Severe, stretching-type pain in the inguinal area
    2. Pain, swelling, and erythema in the affected calf
    3. A dull ache and feeling of coolness in the affected thigh

4. A line of erythema stretching from the popliteal area to the groin

44. What is the most serious complication of DVT?
    1. Gangrene in the affected limb
    2. Pulmonary embolism
    3. Varicose veins
    4. Cerebral thrombosis

Case 10

Matthew is a 5-month-old infant who was born with a large ventricular septal defect (VSD). He has a co-diagnosis of failure to thrive related to the heart defect. He is admitted to hospital for evaluation and treatment of his symptoms.

Questions 45–49 refer to this case.

45. What is a VSD?
    1. An area of scar tissue in the left ventricle of the heart
    2. Failure of the aorta to develop, causing a stricture of blood flow in the ventricles
    3. Right ventricular hypertrophy
    4. An abnormal opening between the two ventricles of the heart

46. Nursing considerations during hospitalization of an infant include:
    1. Do not allow the parents to participate in the child care if the infant has an IV and monitoring devices.
    2. Provide soft stuffed toys in the crib.
    3. Instruct parents that they need to keep the crib rails up only when they leave the room, otherwise the rails can be left down.
    4. Encourage the parents to voice their concerns and address them as much as possible.

47. Matthew has a cardiac catheterization to help determine the extent of his VSD. During the procedure, cardiac output is determined. What is cardiac output?
    1. The peak pressure in the left ventricle during systole
    2. The amount of blood present in the left ventricle at the end of diastole
    3. The amount of blood ejected from the heart in one contraction
    4. The amount of blood ejected by the heart in 1 minute

48. Matthew returns to the unit after his cardiac catheterization. What assessment will be a priority for the practical nurse?
    1. Level of consciousness
    2. Pulses in both extremities
    3. Pain
    4. Temperature

49. Matthew's parents, Mai Kassaye and Jerome Dime, are both 15 years old. They are in a common-law relationship and live with Jerome's parents. Who may legally provide consent for Matthew's care?
    1. Both Mai and Jerome
    2. Jerome
    3. Jerome's parents
    4. Mai

Case 11

A practical nurse works in a hospice for people who are terminally ill with HIV/AIDS. One of her clients is Georgia Wilcyska, an Indigenous woman who became HIV-positive many years ago as a result of intravenous heroin use. She was nonadherent to her antiretroviral therapy and is now receiving palliative care for late chronic infection and AIDS.

Questions 50–54 refer to this case.

50. Ms. Wilcyska talks to the practical nurse about the days when she was "turned on" to heroin by a male friend. What feeling would Ms. Wilcyska describe as a result of injecting heroin?
    1. Increased alertness
    2. Euphoria
    3. Insomnia
    4. Increased sexual drive

51. Prior to being a heroin addict, Ms. Wilcyska was married with children and had a job. She states she "lost everything" because of her addiction. What is the most likely reason Ms. Wilcyska continued to take heroin in spite of the effects on her family life?
    1. Neurophysical dependence
    2. Uncomfortable withdrawal symptoms
    3. Peer influence
    4. Cultural factors

52. The practical nurse is aware that scientific evidence has shown that the practice of harm-reduction reduces the financial and human costs of substance abuse. What might be included in harm-reduction strategies?
    1. Education targeted to abstinence from chemical substances
    2. "Tough on crime" law enforcement approach to drug dealers and users
    3. Supervised injection of illicit drugs in designated environments
    4. Segregated hostels for people addicted to harmful street drugs

53. Ms. Wilcyska has two children who were taken into care by child welfare authorities many years ago due to her heroin addiction, neglect, and physical abuse. Ms. Wilcyska tells the practical nurse she regrets she was not a better mother. How should the practical nurse respond?
    1. "I'm sure your children know you tried your best."
    2. "You must feel your life has been wasted."
    3. "Would you like me to help you write a letter to them?"
    4. "Do they have problems now due to the abuse and neglect?"

54. The practical nurse is trained in therapeutic touch, which she uses as therapy for Ms. Wilcyska. What is therapeutic touch?
    1. Rebalancing of energy through the hands of the practitioner to the person
    2. A group of therapeutic procedures that help the client redirect physiological responses

3. A type of therapeutic massage that increases blood flow and decreases tension

4. Directed attention to a single unchanging, repetitive stimulus to invoke relaxation

Case 12

Gabrielle French and her partner Jennifer Philips have conceived via in vitro fertilization. Ms. French has experienced an uneventful pregnancy and is now at 36 weeks' gestation. Ms. French and Ms. Philips plan to deliver their child at home with the assistance of a midwife and support from a doula.

Questions 55–60 refer to this case.

55. Ms. French's membranes spontaneously rupture at 36 weeks. After 12 hours, there are no contractions, and she becomes concerned. She contacts the midwife, who makes a home visit. Which classification of medication will the midwife most likely give her?
    1. An antibiotic
    2. An analgesic
    3. An antipyretic
    4. An oxytocic

56. Although Ms. French and Ms. Philips wish to stay at home, the midwife decides to admit Ms. French to the hospital as a precaution. Shortly afterward, Ms. French commences labour. On the antenatal unit, Ms. French has electronic fetal heart monitoring. The nurse performing the monitoring notes a pattern of early decelerations. What is this most likely caused by?
    1. Head compression
    2. Cord compression
    3. Placental insufficiency
    4. Uterine contractions

57. Gabrielle French is anxious, apprehensive, and upset that she will not be able to have a home delivery. Ms. Philips says to the nurse, "I don't seem to be able to help Gabrielle as well as the nurses. Do you think I should leave?" What would be the best response by the nurse?
    1. "As a woman, you should understand that Gabrielle needs you very much now."
    2. "This is difficult for you. Let me help you to support her."
    3. "Yes, you should leave if you are feeling unsure of the situation. Why don't you relax in the waiting room and come back when you are feeling better?"
    4. "It's probably best for you to take a break because you will transmit your anxiety to Gabrielle."

58. As a precaution, an intravenous (IV) infusion is inserted in Ms. French's left arm. What is the most appropriate method of helping her to put on a hospital gown with the IV in situ?
    1. Disconnect the IV, quickly put on the gown, and reconnect the IV.
    2. Apply the gown through her right arm and drape the other sleeve over her right shoulder.
    3. Insert the IV bag through the sleeve from the inside of the gown.

4. Apply the gown sleeves over both arms, keeping the tubing inside the gown.

59. Gabrielle French delivers a 36-week male infant with a 1-minute Apgar score of 3. Which of the following manifestations would be most likely to be observed in the baby?
    1. Muscle tone flaccid
    2. Heart rate 126 bpm
    3. Respirations 42 breaths per minute
    4. Blood pressure 60 mm Hg systolic

60. Ms. French is transferred to the postpartum unit 2 hours after the delivery. During the admission, Ms Philips returns from visiting their newborn in the special care nursery. She reports that their infant's breathing sounded "grunty." The practical nurse explains that grunting respirations are a premature newborn's attempt to do which of the following?
    1. Remove fluid from the lungs
    2. Trap carbon dioxide in the lungs
    3. Decrease mucus obstruction
    4. Open the alveoli

Case 13

A practical nurse works in a palliative care hospice. One of his clients is Mr. Morrissey, who has terminal pancreatic cancer. Mr. Morrissey is weak and has been unable to move from his bed for several days. He has stopped eating and is not able to drink more than a few sips of water every few hours.

Questions 61–65 refer to this case.

61. What is the most important factor for the practical nurse to consider when developing end-of-life care for Mr. Morrissey?
    1. Cultural
    2. Spiritual
    3. Religious
    4. Individual uniqueness

62. Mr. Morrissey has not completed an advance directive. When he is no longer able to make decisions regarding his care, who should be the substitute decision maker (SDM)?
    1. Mr. Morrissey's former spouse
    2. Mr. Morrissey's eldest son
    3. Mr. Morrissey's adult children
    4. Mr. Morrissey's sister

63. Mr. Morrissey develops pain that is not adequately controlled by morphine. He moans and cries out. His family demands additional and more frequent doses of morphine. What is the most appropriate information for the practical nurse to communicate in this situation?
    1. "I understand your distress. Let's discuss this."
    2. "I will arrange a meeting with the pain team for us to find a solution."
    3. "I will speak with the physician to ask him what to do."
    4. "I am not allowed, as a registered practical nurse, to administer increased doses of medication that will cause him to die more quickly."

64. Mr. Morrissey develops constipation. In consultation with the physician, what should be the practical nurse's initial intervention?
    1. Administer a cleansing enema.
    2. Remove fecal impactions.
    3. Administer a bulk-forming agent, such as Metamucil.
    4. Administer a stool-softening suppository.

65. In the last few days of his life, Mr. Morrissey becomes dehydrated. What should the practical nurse do?
    1. Apply lubricant to his lips and oral mucous membranes.
    2. Arrange for intravenous fluid replacement.
    3. Obtain an order for fluids via hypodermoclysis.
    4. Insert a nasogastric tube to administer fluids.

Case 14

During November, 5-month-old Sean is brought to the after-hours pediatric walk-in clinic by his parents. They do not have a vehicle, and the clinic was closer for the parents to seek out medical assistance than the children's hospital. He appears to be in respiratory distress, with dyspnea, chest retractions, and nasal flaring. He has a nonproductive, paroxysmal cough. His oxygen saturation is 94%. His parents report that he has had a "cold" with a runny nose for the past few days. The practical nurse performs a chest assessment and hears wheezing, crackles, and decreased breath sounds.

Questions 66–69 refer to this case.

66. Based on his signs and symptoms, the practical nurse should suspect that Sean has which of the following infectious viral conditions?
    1. Pharyngitis
    2. Croup
    3. Bronchiolitis
    4. Epiglottitis

67. The pediatrician indicates that Sean needs to go to the children's hospital. The practical nurse explains to the parents that Sean requires which of the following?
    1. Antiviral agents
    2. Humidified oxygen
    3. Cough suppressants
    4. Antibiotic agents

68. The practical nurse calls an ambulance to transport the infant to the hospital. Where is the most appropriate location for Sean and his parents to wait for the ambulance?
    1. In the waiting room to watch other children play
    2. In an office at the back of the clinic to maintain airborne precautions
    3. With adults in the waiting room
    4. In an examining room close by the nursing station to monitor Sean's respiratory status

69. Sean's parents are upset concerning Sean's illness and tell the practical nurse they would like to stay at the hospital with their son. What is the practical nurse's best response to this request?
    1. "It is best for Sean if you take a break, go home, and get some rest."
    2. "The children's hospital practises family-centred care, and parents are encouraged to stay."
    3. "It will help if you do stay at the hospital because there is a nursing shortage."
    4. "The pediatrician can write a prescription requesting that the children's hospital allow you to stay."

Independent Questions

Questions 70–125 do not refer to a particular case.

70. The practical nurse assists the physician to insert a peripherally inserted central catheter (PICC) line at the bedside of Mr. Blazevic. Immediately after the insertion, what should be the priority assessment?
    1. Hemorrhage at the insertion site
    2. Blood pressure monitoring
    3. Circulation distal to the insertion site
    4. Ability to withdraw blood from the catheter

71. The practical nurse teaches colostomy care to Mr. Singh following his colon resection surgery. Mr. Singh asks why he has to irrigate the colostomy. What should the practical nurse explain to him?
    1. Similar to colonic irrigations, irrigating a colostomy removes toxins from the gastro-intestinal tract.
    2. Irrigation helps regulate the evacuation of feces.
    3. Colostomy irrigations are necessary postsurgery to cleanse the surgical site.
    4. Routine irrigation prevents constipation.

72. Post–Caesarean section, Ms. Urquhart has her urinary catheter removed. Six hours later, she has not voided. What should be the practical nurse's first action?
    1. Provide her with a bedpan and provide privacy.
    2. Assess her for abdominal distension.
    3. Re-catheterize her for residual urine.
    4. Assist her to the bathroom and encourage her to void.

73. Mrs. Scales is experiencing a loss of peripheral vision. This is likely to be caused by which of the following eye conditions?
    1. Glaucoma
    2. Cataracts
    3. Macular degeneration
    4. Detached retina

74. Ms. Kyrios buys a home pregnancy test kit 1 week after her first missed menstrual period. What hormone will the kit test for to determine if she is pregnant?
    1. Human chorionic gonadotropin (HCG)
    2. Estrogen
    3. Progesterone
    4. Follicle-stimulating hormone (FSH)

75. A client in the thoracic unit pulls out his right-side chest tube. What is the immediate action by the practical nurse?
    1. Place an occlusive dressing over the puncture site.
    2. Call for the on-site physician.
    3. Position the client on his right side.
    4. Place a saline dressing over the exit site.

76. Mr. Gupta has a Mantoux skin test at a physician's office. The practical nurse reading the test obtains a result of 7 mm induration. What should be the next action by the practical nurse?
    1. No action is required, as this is a normal finding.
    2. The practical nurse should refer Mr. Gupta to a physician for further investigation.
    3. The practical nurse should inform Mr. Gupta that he requires prophylactic medications that will be ordered by a physician.
    4. The practical nurse should repeat the test, as the result is inconclusive.

77. The practical nurse finds a client, Lindsay Breakwell, covered in blood after slashing her wrists in a suicide attempt. What should be the immediate action to manage the bleeding?
    1. Apply pressure to the laceration.
    2. Apply a tourniquet distal to the laceration.
    3. Determine whether the bleeding is arterial blood.
    4. Elevate the arm.

78. The practical nurse is about to administer vitamin K by intramuscular (IM) injection to newborn Jeremy. Which site should the practical nurse choose for the IM injection?
    1. Vastus lateralis
    2. Dorsogluteal
    3. Deltoid
    4. Rectus femoris

79. A practical nurse is concerned about the morbidity of tuberculosis in her city. Which of the following best defines the morbidity of tuberculosis?
    1. The rate of tuberculosis infection in a population
    2. The effect of tuberculosis on a defined group of individuals
    3. The death rate from tuberculosis
    4. The extent of communicability of tuberculosis within a community

80. Mr. Broadshaw has experienced an episode of renal calculi. The practical nurse teaches him dietary strategies to help prevent another attack. Which of the following should the practical nurse include in health teaching for this client?
    1. To increase his intake of clear fluids
    2. To increase his intake of dairy products
    3. To increase his intake of tea and chocolate
    4. To use antacids for indigestion and nausea

81. Matthew, age 2 years, has chronic otitis media and has been on antibiotics eight times in the past year. What would the practical nurse be concerned about regarding the antibiotics?
    1. He may develop antibiotic resistant micro-organisms.
    2. He may develop chronic diarrhea.
    3. He will develop a hearing loss.
    4. His immune system will become dependent on the antibiotics.

82. Mr. Shafikhani, age 25 years, has been recently diagnosed with epilepsy. The practical nurse speaks with him just after his physician tells him that he is no longer allowed to drive a motor vehicle. What is the most therapeutic statement to make to Mr. Shafikhani?
    1. "Would you like a referral to the local Epilepsy Association?"
    2. "How will not being able to drive affect your life?"
    3. "I know this is difficult for you, but it is the safest option."
    4. "Do you understand why you are not allowed to drive?"

83. Ms. Aubrey Gans, gravida 1, para 0, has a spontaneous abortion (miscarriage) at 10 weeks' gestation. Of the following, which is the most important question for the practical nurse to ask?
    1. "Did you want this pregnancy?"
    2. "Do you know if you are Rh-negative or Rh-positive?"
    3. "Did you have difficulty becoming pregnant?"
    4. "Did you take any medications while you were pregnant?"

84. The practical nurse is performing oropharyngeal suctioning on Mr. Abernethy. Which of the following would be a nursing consideration during the suctioning?
    1. Encourage Mr. Abernethy to cough out secretions during suctioning.
    2. Maintain sterile technique.
    3. Measure the catheter from the mouth to the ear to the xiphoid process.
    4. Moisten the catheter tip with a petroleum jelly lubricant.

85. An agency practical nurse is working his first shift in a long-term care facility where he is to administer evening medications to the residents. Residents do not wear identification armbands. It is not possible to identify residents from pictures in the medication record as the pictures are of poor quality. What is the initial action by the practical nurse to ensure safe administration of medications?
    1. Ask residents their name and have them sign for the medication.
    2. Refuse to administer the medications as it is not safe.
    3. Contact the director of care for advice and directives.
    4. Use a combination of the picture, clothing identification labels, and resident self-identification.

86. The practical nurse must instill mineral oil eardrops bilaterally to Mr. Lewis every 8 hours. She directs him to lie in a side-lying position. What action should the practical nurse take to ensure successful instillation?
    1. Instill the drops in the right ear, insert a cotton swab, reposition him, and then instill drops in the left ear.
    2. Instill the drops in the right ear, and then 8 hours later, instill drops in the left ear.
    3. Instill the drops in the right ear, have Mr. Lewis sit upright, and then instill drops in the left ear.
    4. Instill the drops in the right ear, wait 10 minutes, and have him turn to the other side for the left eardrop instillation.

87. Ms. Samms has fatty liver disease, with resulting ascites. Which position would be best to assist her breathing?
    1. Prone
    2. Semi-Fowler's
    3. Sims'
    4. Supine

88. Harriet, a practical nurse, discovers her nursing colleague, Angie, smoking in the stairwell of the psychiatric facility where they work the night shift. Angie tells Harriet that she cannot last an entire shift without a cigarette, and it is too cold for her to go outside. What should Harriet do?
    1. Remind Angie that smoking is against agency policies and that unless Angie stops this behaviour, she will have to report this to nursing management.
    2. Understand that if Angie is on a scheduled break, Harriet has no responsibility to interfere with Angie's smoking.
    3. Caution Angie about the dangers of smoking in an unapproved area and the potential dangers to the clients of second-hand smoke.
    4. Discuss with Angie her addiction to cigarettes and provide support to establish a strategy that may assist her to quit smoking.

89. A practical nurse suspects one of her colleagues has falsified her credentials as a registered practical nurse. What should the practical nurse do?
    1. Talk with the colleague and ask to see her registration.
    2. Report her suspicion, with rationale, to the nurse manager.
    3. Report her suspicion to the provincial registration body.
    4. Intervene to stop the colleague from performing nursing care.

90. Mrs. Verde experiences frequent urinary tract infections (UTIs). What should the practical nurse advise to decrease the incidence of these infections?
    1. Drink orange juice daily.
    2. Do not wear cotton underpants.
    3. Use a lubricant and a condom during sexual intercourse.
    4. Treat vaginal yeast disorders promptly.

91. Mrs. Brankston has had colon resection surgery due to Crohn's disease. Physician orders include "NPO until bowel sounds are heard." What is the rationale for this order?
    1. There is a risk of emesis following gastro-intestinal surgery.
    2. Bowel sounds are an indication that peristalsis has resumed.
    3. Eating any food will disturb the operative site.
    4. It is intended to prevent nausea associated with anaesthetic administration.

92. On the postpartum unit, it is the practical nurse's responsibility to weigh the newborn prior to discharge and compare this weight to the birth weight. The parents ask why the second weight is required. The practical nurses best response is as follows:
    1. It is required to double check the birth weight for accuracy that will be used on the newborns growth chart.
    2. Weight loss of greater than 10% requires closer monitoring.
    3. Weight gain of greater than 10% indicates the infant is being overfed.
    4. The amount of weight gain or loss will determine whether to supplement a breastfed baby's diet with formula.

93. Ms. MacLeod has received 760 mL of IV fluid and has had 140 mL of tea. She has voided 540 mL of urine and vomited 110 mL. What is Ms. MacLeod's fluid balance?
    1. +900 mL
    2. +250 mL
    3. −650 mL
    4. −110 mL

94. Which of the following is an example of the defence mechanism "displacement"?
    1. Ms. Colm repeatedly tells her practical nurse, Reena, how much she admires her, when in fact Ms. Colm does not like Reena.
    2. Ms. Henry yells at the practical nurse after the physician is rude to Ms. Henry.
    3. Mr. Patrick forgets to make an appointment with his physician when he feels a lump on his testicle.
    4. Mrs. Miyagi refuses to believe that her sister has a diagnosis of terminal lung cancer.

95. Mrs. Townsend is 20 weeks pregnant. She tells the practical nurse that she has twin girls at home but had a miscarriage prior to this pregnancy. What is her pregnancy classification?
    1. Gravida 4, para 2
    2. Gravida 3, para 3
    3. Gravida 3, para 2
    4. Gravida 2, para 1

96. What supplement is recommended for women to take during their reproductive years to help decrease the risk of neural tube defects in newborns?
    1. Iron
    2. Folate
    3. Vitamin A
    4. Calcium with Vitamin D

97. Mr. Brendan asks the occupational health practical nurse why he always looks pale when he is cold. What should the practical nurse explain to Mr. Brendan?
    1. When you are cold, you have less melatonin.
    2. In a cold environment, blood vessels in your skin constrict to save heat.
    3. If your skin looks pink in warm weather, it is likely because you have mild sunburn.
    4. In cold weather, surface capillaries dilate and make the skin appear whitish.

98. A child at the Tiny Tots daycare centre has been diagnosed with impetigo. What advice should the practical

nurse working at the daycare provide to the centre's child-care workers?

1. Place the daycare centre under quarantine.
2. Close the daycare until complete cleaning has been performed.
3. No special precautions are required.
4. Suspend attendance for the infected child for 48 hours.

99. Which of the following behaviours would be considered to be a boundary violation of the nurse–client relationship in a mental health setting?
    1. Asking the client about his sexual history
    2. Sharing coffee and cookies with the client during a therapeutic session
    3. Nodding and smiling at the client
    4. Honouring a request by the client to keep a secret from the healthcare team

100. Brad Shaw tells the practical nurse he has been finding bright red blood on the toilet paper when he has a bowel movement. What should be the practical nurse's first response to Mr. Shaw?
    1. "Do you have abdominal bloating or cramping?"
    2. "We need to book you for a colonoscopy."
    3. "I will give you a test kit for fecal occult blood."
    4. "Are your stools hard, or are you constipated?"

101. A first-year practical nursing student about to enter her first clinical practice experience has artificial nails. Her nursing professor tells her the policy states she must have the nails removed. What is the most appropriate rationale for this policy?
    1. Artificial nails are too long and may injure the client.
    2. Artificial nails may accidentally be ripped off during client care, injuring the nurse.
    3. Artificial nails are not professional looking.
    4. Artificial nails may harbour micro-organisms.

102. Troy, age 16, tells the school practical nurse that he frequently feels tired during the day and sometimes falls asleep during his classes. What would be the most appropriate initial question for the practical nurse to ask Troy?
    1. "Are you taking any medications that would make you drowsy?"
    2. "How often do you exercise?"
    3. "When was the last time you had a complete physical exam?"
    4. "How much sleep do you get at night?"

103. Ms. Alexandra has 20/40 vision on the Snellen eye chart. She will most likely need which of the following assistive devices or services?
    1. Large-print books
    2. Instruction in Braille
    3. Referral to an ophthalmologist
    4. Corrective lenses

104. Which of the following is the most widespread sexually transmitted infection (STI) in Canada?
    1. Gonorrhea
    2. HIV/AIDS
    3. Non-gonococcal urethritis (NGU)
    4. Chlamydia

105. Mr. Schloss, a client with heart failure, is ambulating in the hall when he suddenly collapses. What is the priority assessment by the practical nurse?
    1. Check for injuries caused by the fall.
    2. Take an apical pulse to assess cardiac status.
    3. Assess for breathing.
    4. Observe for or establish a patent airway.

106. A physician has written the following order for pain relief for Mr. Madrigan: "meperidine (morphine), 10 mg, oral, q3–4h, prn." What is the appropriate practical nursing action?
    1. Administer the meperidine after completing the five rights.
    2. Perform a pain assessment on Mr. Madrigan.
    3. Calculate that this is an appropriate dose of meperidine for Mr. Madrigan.
    4. Contact the physician for clarification of the drug.

107. Jennie, age 18 months, is brought by her parents to the emergency department of her local community hospital. Jennie has bilateral otitis externa with enlarged tonsils and adenoids. She is mouth breathing and diaphoretic and appears febrile. What method should the practical nurse choose to take Jennie's temperature?
    1. Tympanic
    2. Axillary
    3. Oral
    4. Rectal

108. Mr. Rivers asks the practical nurse why he is being discharged home with community nursing care only 3 days after an uncomplicated appendectomy. What would be the practical nurse's best response?
    1. "You do not require acute care facilities."
    2. "Your condition is stable, so, with support, it is better to recover at home."
    3. "It is too expensive to have people stay in hospital to recover after surgery."
    4. "The trend in health care is to discharge clients as soon as possible."

109. The practical nurse tells Mr. Bartholomew, age 65, that his temperature is 36.6 degrees Celsius. He responds: "I only know Fahrenheit. Is 36.6 degrees Celsius the same as 98.6 degrees Fahrenheit? Is it normal?" What should the practical nurse tell Mr. Bartholomew?
    1. "Yes, it is the same as 98.6 degrees Fahrenheit."
    2. "It is about 98, almost the same as 98.6 degrees Fahrenheit, and is normal."
    3. "No, it is 99.7 degrees Fahrenheit and is slightly elevated."
    4. "It is quite a bit lower than 98.6 degrees Fahrenheit and shows you are cold."

110. Mr. Constant, a client in a psychiatric unit, tells the practical nurse: "The voices are saying bad things about me." What would be an appropriate response?
    1. "I do not hear the voices."
    2. "I understand you are frightened by the voices, and I will stay with you."

3. "Why don't you sit with the other clients and watch TV?"

4. "Don't listen to what the voices tell you."

111. Prior to the infusion of antibiotics for cellulitis, Mrs. Collins tells the practical nurse she is allergic to penicillin. What should be the practical nurse's first action?

1. Place an allergy band on Mrs. Collins's wrist.
2. Notify the prescribing physician of the allergy.
3. Check that the ordered antibiotics do not contain penicillin.
4. Ask Mrs. Collins what happens when she has penicillin.

112. Teklie, age 2 years, has had two episodes of watery diarrhea. What should the practical nurse recommend to Teklie's parents?

1. Encourage constipating foods such as cheese.
2. Administer an over-the-counter antidiarrhea medicine.
3. Offer clear fluids, ice pops, and crackers.
4. Continue with Teklie's normal diet.

113. Mrs. Bennett requires transfer from her wheelchair to the commode. She tells the practical nurse that usually two people perform this lift. The practical nurse has not previously cared for Mrs. Bennett, but assesses she can do the lift by herself. What should the practical nurse do?

1. Use a mechanical lift so she does not require two people.
2. Ask Mrs. Bennett for more details about why two people are required for the lift.
3. Find another co-worker to assist with the lift.
4. Begin the lift to see how difficult she thinks it will be.

114. Mrs. Sheyer, age 87 years, is brought to the walk in clinic by her family because she has had a fever for several days. The physician feels Mrs. Sheyer may be exhibiting early signs of delirium. What would be the most important step of data collection for the practical nurse to apply to help determine the possible cause of the delirium?

1. Review Mrs. Sheyer's medication profile.
2. Interview the family to determine cognitive function prior to admission.
3. Assess Mrs. Sheyer's level of hydration.
4. Take Mrs. Sheyer's temperature.

115. A practical nurse in a community mental health clinic is in the midst of a counselling session with Mr. Olan. Ms. Isabelle approaches the practical nurse and asks to speak with her. How should the practical nurse respond to this situation?

1. "What can I help you with, Ms. Isabelle?"
2. "Excuse me, Mr. Olan, I need to speak with Ms. Isabelle."
3. "Ms Isabelle, I am with Mr. Olan until 10. I will see you directly afterward."
4. "Ms. Isabelle, you should not interrupt Mr. Olan and me."

116. A practical nurse is grocery shopping when she observes a young toddler experience a tonic–clonic seizure.

What is the practical nurse's first responsibility in this situation?

1. Call 9-1-1.
2. Insert any safe object in the child's mouth to maintain an airway.
3. Observe the seizure and protect the child from injury.
4. Reassure the parents.

117. Ten-year-old Nicholas has just been diagnosed with a brain tumour. His parents tell the practical nurse Nicholas is not to be informed about the tumour. What is the practical nurse's most appropriate response to this request?

1. "At Nicholas's age, he is not able to understand the diagnosis, so this is a wise decision."
2. "Let's talk about the reasons why you don't think he should be told."
3. "The policy of this hospital is that children have a right to age-appropriate information."
4. "Children are very intuitive, and Nicholas probably already knows about the tumour."

118. The charge nurse on a busy surgical unit must assign care for Mr. Michener, age 27, who is 3 days postsurgery from an appendectomy. Mr. Michener's vital signs are stable, and the wound is approximated and shows no signs of infection. Mr. Michener is to be discharged the following day and requires health teaching. What category of healthcare worker is the most appropriate and cost-effective to be assigned to Mr. Michener?

1. Registered nurse (RN)
2. Registered practical nurse/licensed practical nurse (RPN/LPN)
3. Expanded role nurse/nurse practitioner/clinical nurse specialist
4. support worker

119. Mrs. Fraser, a pale-skinned woman of European descent, age 59 years, comes to the clinic. What is the most important observation by the practical nurse when performing a skin assessment on Mrs. Fraser?

1. Areas of dry, flaky skin
2. A reduction in skin elasticity
3. A change in a mole or lesion
4. Senile lentigines

120. The practical nurse obtains a thermometer reading of 39.6 degrees Celsius on Nick, age 4 years. His previous temperature 2 hours ago was 36.3 degrees Celsius, he does not feel hot, and he states that he feels well. What is the appropriate nursing action?

1. Take the temperature again in another hour.
2. Take a rectal temperature to obtain a core temperature.
3. Administer the ordered antipyretic.
4. Use a different thermometer to retake the temperature.

121. Mrs. Ginger has an amputation of her left leg. The afternoon following surgery, the practical nurse finds Mrs. Ginger lying in bed, in a fetal position, crying. What is the most appropriate documentation of this event?

1. "Lying in a fetal position, crying"
2. "Displaying manifestations of postsurgical depression"

3. "Grieving observed due to loss of leg"
4. "Client upset, manifesting sadness related to amputation"

122. Andre, age 6 years, is about to have an injected immunization. He is very tearful and apprehensive about how much the needle will hurt him. Which of the following would be the most effective method to reduce the pain of an injection for Andre?
1. Using a topical anaesthetic cream
2. Distracting Andre during the injection
3. Having the parent hold Andre during the injection
4. Providing postinjection analgesics, such as acetaminophen (Tylenol)

123. A nurse manager is concerned about the incidence of work-related accidents on the unit, causing many staff nurses to be on long-term disability. What is the first action the manager should take to address these problems?
1. Compile a list of all data on staff accidents for the past 2 years.
2. Tour the unit to observe hazardous workplace habits or environments.
3. Interview all staff on long-term disability to find out how they were injured.
4. Interview all staff for their opinions and observations about workplace hazards.

124. What part of the SBAR report does the following information fall under? Mrs. Rose's pain in the left lower leg is increasing for the past 1 hour. She has hypertension and type 2 diabetes. She is on metformin hydrochloride 500 mg bid. She is allergic to sulpha drugs.
1. Situation
2. Background
3. Assessment
4. Recommendation

125. During the influenza season, how should the practical nurse in a community walk-in health clinic best prevent transmission of the influenza virus to clients?
1. Place all clients with respiratory symptoms in a separate area and have them wear masks and wash their hands.
2. Immunize all clients with the influenza vaccine as they arrive.
3. Post a sign in the window of the clinic refusing care to people with symptoms of influenza.
4. Keep all clients at least half a metre apart in the waiting room.

ANSWERS AND RATIONALES FOR BOOK ONE

The correct answer is set off in boldface.
1. **C: Foundations of Practice T: Knowledge**
   1. These values are all low. See choice 3.
   2. These values are too high. See choice 3.
   3. **Normal vital signs for a 1-week-old infant are heart rate 120–160 bpm, respirations 30–60 breaths per minute, and median blood pressure generally** 65–80 mm Hg by Doppler (but can increase during crying or agitation).
   4. Heart rate and respirations are within normal ranges, but blood pressure is too high.

2. **C: Foundations of Practice T: Knowledge**
   1. **The Babinski reflex is elicited by stroking the outer sole of the foot upward from the heel across the ball of the foot, causing dorsiflexion of the big toe and fanning of the toes.**
   2. This is the response from the dance, or step, reflex.
   3. This is the expected response from the grasp reflex.
   4. This is the part of the expected response from the Moro, or startle, reflex.

3. **C: Professional, Ethical, and Legal Practice T: Application**
   1. **This response best addresses Mrs. Wasson's concerns. A weight loss of up to 10% is expected 3–4 days after birth. Adequate breast milk supply is best facilitated by frequent feedings.**
   2. It is well established that the use of supplemental formula feedings before breastfeeding is to be avoided.
   3. This is true but does not answer Mrs. Wasson's concerns about milk production.
   4. Increased fluids have not been proven to increase milk supply.

4. **C: Foundations of Practice T: Application**
   1. **Airing the nipples as much as possible, and using heat, will help dry the nipples and decrease discomfort.**
   2. Creams and oils are to be avoided.
   3. Plastic-lined breast pads may trap moisture, increasing the risk of skin breakdown.
   4. Nursing should start with the least affected breast.

5. **C: Foundations of Practice T: Application**
   1. Breast milk or infant formula does not need to be heated.
   2. It is unsafe and unnecessary to warm milk in the microwave because the heat is not evenly distributed. The bottle may remain at a cooler temperature than the liquid, and the liquid may burn the baby.
   3. **Warming a bottle in lukewarm water is sufficient to bring it to room temperature.**
   4. Infants are used to body temperature milk from the breast and may not adjust to cold milk.

6. **C: Foundations of Practice T: Knowledge**
   1. Polycythemia (an increase in red blood cells) and polymyositis (an inflammation of many muscles) are not manifestations of diabetes.
   2. Polyelectrolyte (many charged electrolytes) and polyneuropathy (a disorder of the peripheral nerves) are not manifestations of diabetes.
   3. Polyopia (a defect in sight) and polyarthritis (an inflammation of more than one joint) are not manifestations of diabetes.
   4. **Polyphagia (excessive hunger and eating), polydipsia (excessive thirst), and polyuria (excessive urination) are cardinal manifestations of type 1 diabetes.**

7. C: Foundations of Practice T: Application
   1. This is the conventional regimen and involves insulin administration in the morning before breakfast and before the evening meal. It may not suit all people with diabetes, particularly during illness, stress, growth spurts, and so on.
   2. Some children require more frequent administration of insulin, with multiple injections during the day. After individual assessment, this may be the optimum regimen.
   3. **The precise dose of insulin and optimum regimen cannot be predicted and need to be individualized for every child. Insulin requirements do not remain constant, changing with growth, activity, and pubertal status.**
   4. Although many pediatric medication dosages are calculated per kilogram, insulin dosages are not.

8. C: Foundations of Practice T: Application
   1. Alcohol causes a drop, not an increase, in blood sugar.
   2. This could be a serious problem, but more significant is an immediate and severe drop in blood glucose.
   3. **Alcohol causes hypoglycemia. The manifestations of slurred speech and antisocial combative behaviour are similar to those of being intoxicated; thus, Edgar may not receive appropriate life-saving treatment.**
   4. There is a family pattern to alcohol dependence, but this is not the most critical issue at this time.

9. C: Foundations of Practice T: Application
   1. **The peak action for regular insulin is 2–4 hours after administration; therefore, a hypoglycemic episode may occur between 1800 and 2000 hours.**
   2. This is past the time of peak action.
   3. The insulin would likely not be in the bloodstream at this time.
   4. There should be no effects from the insulin at this time.

10. C: Collaborative Practice T: Application
    1. This may need to occur but is not the best initial approach.
    2. Both Edgar and his parents may require more education, but an assessment of Edgar's needs and particular reasons for nonadherence must be explored first.
    3. **Prior to implementing interventions, the practical nurse must be aware of the reasons for Edgar's nonadherence. The practical nurse should discuss this with him in private, as he may speak more freely when his parents are not present.**
    4. This may be appropriate but does not address Edgar's individual needs with his present nonadherence.

11. C: Professional, Ethical, and Legal Practice T: Critical Thinking
    1. **Clients who are at high risk, for example, those who are immunosuppressed, need to be identified in order to implement appropriate precautions.**
    2. This may not be necessary with all clients.

3. In some facilities and in some situations, this may be necessary, but it does not need to be generally implemented.
4. Alcohol-based hand sanitizers are as effective as soap and water and aid in increasing the frequency of hand hygiene by healthcare workers but are not as important a step as the identification of at-risk clients.

12. C: Foundations of Practice T: Critical Thinking
    1. Age is a risk factor, as older adults generally have a decreased immune system; however, it is not as great a risk as a urinary catheter.
    2. Poor nutrition may lead to poor immunity, but this is not as great a risk as a urinary catheter.
    3. Surgery is a risk; however, the surgery should have taken place under strict sterile techniques.
    4. **An in-dwelling urinary catheter, even though it is a closed system, places Mr. Carolis at risk for a urinary tract infection and should be discontinued at the earliest opportunity.**

13. C: Foundations of Practice T: Application
    1. **Leukocytosis is an abnormal increase in white blood cells and is indicative of an infection.**
    2. Neutropenia is an abnormal decrease in neutrophils. During an infection, there is an increase in neutrophils.
    3. Thrombocytosis is an abnormal increase in platelets and may be indicative of malignancies or blood disorders.
    4. Leukopenia is an abnormal decrease in white blood cells and may indicate bone marrow suppression.

14. C: Foundations of Practice T: Application
    1. Antibiotics may interfere with accurate results from cultures.
    2. It is not necessary to consult with the physician. This is nursing judgement.
    3. **This is the correct sequence. Culture specimens can be inaccurate if taken after antibiotics are given.**
    4. Sterile urine specimens must be taken from the catheter port, not the collection bag. The specimen must be taken before the antibiotics are administered.

15. C: Professional, Ethical, and Legal Practice T: Critical Thinking
    1. Incident reports are specific agency documents. They are important for quality assurance purposes for the institution but are not the most important initial action for Mr. Carolis.
    2. This must be done but is not the first action.
    3. **The immediate action must be to address client safety. Administration of medication that is twice the ordered dose could have severe effects, particularly in an older client, and the nurse's first responsibility must be to assess Mr. Carolis.**
    4. This must be done but is not the first action.

16. C: Foundations of Practice T: Knowledge
    1. **Hyperkalemia, caused by decreased excretion by the kidney, is the most serious electrolyte disorder**

associated with kidney disease. A level of 7 mmol/L could result in a fatal arrhythmia.
2. This is a normal value.
3. This is a normal value.
4. This is a normal value.

17. **C: Foundations of Practice T: Knowledge**
   1. **Administration of erythropoietin intravenously or subcutaneously is effective in treating the anemia that results from the decrease in erythropoietin production occurring with kidney failure.**
   2. An adverse effect of erythropoietin may be hypertension.
   3. Erythropoietin will not affect the acid–base balance.
   4. Erythropoietin will not increase perfusion in the kidney.

18. **C: Foundations of Practice T: Critical Thinking**
   1. Cheese has high sodium and high protein. Banana and milk are high-potassium foods. Sodium, protein, and potassium are restricted in renal failure.
   2. Canned soups are high in sodium, as are saltine crackers. Orange juice is high in potassium. Fluids are restricted: 400 mL is too much fluid at one meal.
   3. **Nutrition therapy in renal failure is complex. It requires the expert determination by a nutritionist of menus that comply with guidelines of low sodium, protein, and phosphorus; restricted fluids; and unlimited carbohydrates and fats to ensure sufficient calories. Turkey, mayonnaise, bread, an apple, and ginger ale comply with these guidelines.**
   4. The beefsteak provides too much protein, and the baked potato, cooked spinach, and chocolate milk are high in potassium.

19. **C: Collaborative Practice T: Application**
   1. This reply does not necessarily allow Mr. Kassam to discuss his feelings.
   2. **This open-ended response confirms Mr. Kassam's feelings and invites him to share them.**
   3. This response closes the conversation and does nothing to help develop coping strategies. Kidney transplant may not yet have been discussed with him.
   4. This is not a therapeutic response and does not allow for Mr. Kassam to discuss his feelings.

20. **C: Professional, Ethical, and Legal Practice T: Critical Thinking**
   1. Although this is true, it is not pertinent, as the transplant surgery is being offered in another country.
   2. It is neither the ethical nor the professional responsibility of the practical nurse to tell the client what he must do.
   3. **This response provides the practical nurse with more information about a potentially dangerous, illegal, or unethical situation. It allows for a respectful discussion between the practical nurse and Mr. Kassam.**
   4. As in choice 2.

21. **C: Foundations of Practice T: Knowledge**
   1. This meets the criteria for MAID.
   2. This meets the criteria standard for MAID.
   3. **This is not a criteria for MAID. Clients must voluntarily request MAID with no external pressure.**
   4. This meets the criteria for MAID.

22. **C: Foundations of Practice T: Knowledge**
   1. **Ovarian cancer in its early stages may not cause symptoms, or they may include mild pressure in the abdomen, pelvis, or back of the legs. There may be abdominal swelling or gastro-intestinal symptoms, such as indigestion, nausea, and bloating.**
   2. This is not a manifestation of ovarian cancer but more likely of uterine cancer. At age 58, Mrs. Dhillon would likely be postmenopausal and thus not menstruating.
   3. This is not a manifestation of ovarian cancer.
   4. This is not a manifestation of early ovarian cancer.

23. **C: Foundations of Practice T: Application**
   1. This is a needle biopsy.
   2. This is a laparotomy.
   3. **This is the correct definition of laparoscopy. It may be preferable to laparotomy as it is less invasive, is less painful, and only requires a local anaesthetic.**
   4. This is not the definition of laparoscopy.

24. **C: Foundations of Practice T: Application**
   1. This is grade 2, stage 1.
   2. **This is the correct interpretation of grade 3, stage 2.**
   3. This is grade 1, stage 3.
   4. This is grade 4, stage 4.

25. **C: Collaborative Practice T: Application**
   1. **This is factual information that will assist Mrs. Dhillon to make an informed decision about her treatment.**
   2. The herbs are probably not recommended, but it is not a therapeutic response to tell Mrs. Dhillon that they will cause her to die sooner, especially as Mrs. Dhillon may not be aware of the possibility of a terminal diagnosis.
   3. This is not a therapeutic response. It presumes she is in denial and presumes that she will change her mind. It does not provide information to assist her in making her decision.
   4. This is an incorrect and potentially life-threatening response.

26. **C: Collaborative Practice T: Application**
   1. Mrs. Dhillon has a type of cancer that has a very poor prognosis. It is evident why she is depressed.
   2. This is patronizing and does not address Mrs. Dhillon as an individual. It ends the conversation.
   3. This is probably not true and would not encourage further discussion.
   4. **This is an open-ended response that invites further discussion with Mrs. Dhillon about her cancer and her feelings about the situation.**

27. C: Foundations of Practice T: Application
    1. **Physical activity increases the cardiac output and thus increases the BP. Twenty to 30 minutes of rest following exercise is indicated before a resting BP can be considered reliable.**
    2. This is not necessary. A BP in the left arm is likely to be the same as in the right arm.
    3. This action would be indicated if, after resting, Mr. Morhudi's BP remained elevated.
    4. A normal BP for Mr. Morhudi would be 120/80 mm Hg.

28. C: Foundations of Practice T: Application
    1. Ice, not heat, is recommended for a muscle sprain. Heat may be applied after 24 hours. The ankle should be rested initially. Analgesics may be required once the RICE therapy has been initiated.
    2. **This is RICE treatment. Movement should be limited, cold is applied to produce hypothermia, compression with an elastic bandage limits swelling, and the limb is elevated to impede edema formation.**
    3. Ice is more effective than a cool compress. Ms. Dove will be encouraged to move the ankle joint once it is supported with a bandage. There is no rationale for maintaining the joint in flexion.
    4. This is not necessary unless the practical nurse assesses there has been a possible fracture.

29. C: Professional, Ethical, and Legal Practice T: Application
    1. This is an appropriate question but is not the most important initial data collection.
    2. As in choice 1.
    3. **Mr. Lackraj appears to have risk factors for cardiovascular disease. All clients should consult with their physician prior to initiating an exercise plan.**
    4. As in choice 1.

30. C: Foundations of Practice T: Critical Thinking
    1. This is neither practical nor possible.
    2. This may help; however, many people are not symptomatic in the initial stages of many infections. It would be difficult for the practical nurse to screen all clients.
    3. This may help, but people may not read the poster.
    4. **Hand hygiene is the most effective action to reduce the transmission of infectious diseases.**

31. C: Foundations of Practice T: Critical Thinking
    1. **Placing a towel on common surfaces will protect the skin from bacteria that may be on the bench. Do not use the underside of the towel after it has been placed on the bench.**
    2. It is safer for clients to bring their own towels, but they should be laundered after each visit.
    3. There is no need to avoid the showers at the gym provided that plastic "flip-flops," or other waterproof barriers, protect feet. In fact, it is important to get out of sweaty clothes and shower after a workout.
    4. Clients are less likely to contract a skin rash if they are wearing long sleeves; however, this is not practical advice.

32. C: Collaborative Practice T: Application
    1. **This initial answer is a statement of facts and does not accuse Mr. Matthews. It will likely lead to a discussion of the causes of his muscle bulk and acne.**
    2. This accuses Mr. Matthews without any proof and will cause him to feel defensive.
    3. As in choice 2.
    4. This approach calls for a yes or no answer, is accusing, and is not likely to lead to a meaningful discussion.

33. C: Collaborative Practice T: Application
    1. **The depressed client often has difficulty acknowledging any positive aspects of his or her life. By asking about the grandchildren that Ms. Manche loves, the practical nurse is reinforcing that she has worthwhile relationships.**
    2. This ignores Ms. Manche's feelings and closes off the discussion.
    3. This provides false reassurance and applies pressure on Ms. Manche to talk.
    4. This answer is not therapeutic, as it may cause Ms. Manche to feel guilty.

34. C: Collaborative Practice T: Application
    1. This may be appropriate but does not consider Ms. Manche's preferences. She did not eat at home when these foods were available.
    2. There is no need to consult with a dietitian at this time. When Ms. Manche's food preferences have been established, a dietitian may be consulted.
    3. This does not consider Ms. Manche's preferences.
    4. **Ms. Manche is more likely to eat foods that she prefers.**

35. C: Collaborative Practice T: Application
    1. While this reassures Ms. Manche that she does not have to talk, it does not lead to a therapeutic discussion.
    2. This is a helpful response but may not lead to Ms. Manche exploring her feelings.
    3. **This allows the practical nurse to further explore Ms. Manche's feelings of low self-worth and may lead to a discussion about the therapeutic effects of the group discussion.**
    4. This response is autocratic, gives advice, and does not allow Ms. Manche to explore her feelings.

36. C: Foundations of Practice T: Critical Thinking
    1. Ms. Manche has not said that she does not like to take drugs. This response makes the use of antidepressants appear to be of limited effectiveness.
    2. **Antidepressant therapy benefits about 65 to 80% of people with depression. This response is factual and explains that depression is a chemical problem.**
    3. The antidepressant is a first-line agent in the treatment of depression and should be combined with psychotherapy. This response negates the role of the practical nurse.
    4. Ms. Manche has not asked about side effects; she has said she doubts the drugs will work.

37. **C: Foundations of Practice T: Critical Thinking**
    1. **Ms. Abetiu is manifesting symptoms of pain and needs to be assessed by a physician for any possible injury that could have occurred due to the fall.**
    2. The initial action is to contact the agency physician, if available, who should examine Ms. Abetiu. If there were no agency physician, the appropriate action would be to call for an ambulance for transport to a hospital.
    3. People with dementia have difficulty communicating symptoms of health problems or pain. While the practical nurse could ask Ms. Abetiu if she is experiencing pain, it is not likely that Ms. Abetiu would be able to provide accurate information, especially considering that she had previously denied pain. Healthcare staff must take the responsibility for assessment and diagnosis.
    4. This will be necessary but is not the most appropriate action at this time.

38. **C: Foundations of Practice T: Application**
    1. This is not likely to calm Mrs. Ensoy's agitation. In an agitated phase, logical discussions about feelings and cause and effect are not likely to be successful.
    2. While reality orientation is helpful with clients who have dementia, in the agitated state, this would not be effective.
    3. **Redirection is often helpful when dealing with difficult behaviour. Performing an activity such as dusting, which would be a familiar activity to Mrs. Ensoy, may calm her.**
    4. Risperidone is helpful in managing disruptive behaviour; however, nonpharmacological therapies should be attempted initially.

39. **C: Foundations of Practice T: Application**
    1. These drugs do not affect urination or continence.
    2. This practice is dangerous with older adults. It is necessary to ensure that older adults have sufficient fluid intake.
    3. Use of these products helps manage urinary incontinence but does not reduce incontinence.
    4. **Evidence-informed practice has determined that behaviour modification, in the form of routine toileting and prompting the client to void, reduces urinary incontinence in people with dementia.**

40. **C: Foundations of Practice T: Application**
    1. People who are ambulatory have a low risk for pressure ulcers.
    2. Mrs. Colorado is still able to change positions and ambulate.
    3. A fractured radius will not lead to a pressure ulcer in the sacral area.
    4. **With paraplegia, there is decreased sensation and immobility, both of which are risk factors for pressure ulcers.**

41. **C: Professional, Ethical, and Practice T: Critical Thinking**
    1. **The most appropriate action is to refer to agency policies. There is likelys to be an appropriate policy that will address ethical, financial, and legal implications of provision of treatment for nonresidents.**
    2. If Mrs. Satgun's condition were life-threatening, the humanitarian principle would be to provide emergency care.
    3. Mrs. Satgun may not be able financially to obtain the necessary medical insurance. Her condition could potentially deteriorate during the time it takes to obtain the insurance.
    4. This may ultimately be the solution; however, it is dependent on the policies of the agency.

42. **C: Foundations of Practice T: Critical Thinking**
    1. This is important but is not the most immediate concern.
    2. **This is the most important question, particularly as Mrs. Satgun has recently arrived in Canada from a foreign country. This question helps screen for recent communicable diseases, which may be a hazard to the rest of the clients, community, and staff in the clinic and may require specific isolation precautions.**
    3. This is important to develop a profile of Mrs. Satgun's health status but is not the most important question.
    4. This is important as it may reveal underlying conditions that are important for Mrs. Satgun's subsequent treatment; however, it is not as important as knowing her recent communicable disease status.

43. **C: Foundations of Practice T: Knowledge**
    1. DVT, particularly after a long air flight in a confined space, is most likely to occur in the calf.
    2. **In this type of DVT, the inflammatory response causes pain in the calf and swelling, and the area feels warm.**
    3. Mrs. Satgun may feel a dull pain but is likely to feel warmth rather than coolness, and it is not likely to be in the thigh.
    4. The swelling and erythema of DVT are generally not linear and are generally not in the popliteal–groin area.

44. **C: Foundations of Practice T: Knowledge**
    1. If untreated, the DVT could lead to necrosis and gangrene, but this is neither the most likely nor the most serious complication.
    2. **Pulmonary embolism is a life-threatening complication of DVT.**
    3. Varicose veins are not caused by DVT and are not as serious as pulmonary emboli.
    4. Cerebral thrombosis is serious and life-threatening; however, if the thrombus in the leg were to enter the venous circulation, it would first travel to the lungs.

45. **C: Foundations of Practice T: Knowledge**
    1. This is not the definition of VSD. It is not scar tissue.
    2. Coarctation of the aorta is failure of the aorta to develop, causing reduced systemic blood flow below the level of the defect.

3. A large VSD may cause right ventricular hypertrophy but is not the actual defect.

4. **This is the definition of a VSD.**

46. **C: Foundations of Practice T: Application**
    1. It is important to have parents actively participate in their child's care. Client- and family-centred care is a beneficial partnership that engages family as essential members of the healthcare team. It promotes health teaching and information sharing.
    2. Stuffed toys in an infant's crib are a suffocation risk.
    3. Crib rails need to be up when an infant is in the crib. They should never be left down when not attending to the infant. Infants can easily roll off beds. It is important to keep one hand on the infant at all times when giving care and the crib rails are down.
    4. **Parent collaboration helps parents feel in control, safe, and more comfortable caring for their child.**

47. **C: Foundations of Practice T: Knowledge**
    1. This is the definition of systolic left ventricular pressure.
    2. This is the end-diastolic volume.
    3. This is stroke volume.
    4. **This is the definition of cardiac output.**

48. **C: Foundations of Practice T: Critical Thinking**
    1. Matthew may need to be sedated for the procedure and may be sleepy, but this is not the priority assessment.
    2. **The catheter is inserted into either the femoral vein or the femoral artery. There is risk of vasospasm or thrombus formation, which could interfere with blood flow to the extremities. Thus, assessment of pulses is the priority assessment.**
    3. Matthew may be experiencing pain, but this is not the priority assessment.
    4. Matthew may be somewhat hypothermic if the temperature in the catheterization laboratory is reduced. It is not, however, the priority assessment.

49. **C: Professional, Ethical, and Legal Practice T: Application**
    1. **Both parents have equal rights and are considered emancipated minors because they have a child.**
    2. Jerome has no greater rights to provide consent than Mai. Both are emancipated minors.
    3. Jerome and Mai are emancipated minors and may provide consent for treatment for their son.
    4. Mai does not have greater rights than Jerome.

50. **C: Foundations of Practice T: Knowledge**
    1. Injection of heroin is more likely to cause detachment from the environment.
    2. **After injection of heroin, users feel a strong sense of euphoria.**
    3. Following the euphoria, users are more likely to feel drowsiness than insomnia.
    4. Heroin users often have a decreased libido.

51. **C: Foundations of Practice T: Critical Thinking**
    1. **Current research shows that addictive drugs appear to increase the availability of dopamine in the pleasure area of the brain. Without the substance,** the individual experiences depression, anxiety, irritability, and an intense craving for the drug. To feel "normal," the individual must take increasingly large doses of heroin.
    2. While the withdrawal symptoms (such as nausea, pain, vomiting, and so on) are unpleasant, the physical addiction is the primary difficulty.
    3. Peer influence is a documented influencing factor associated with drug abuse but is not as direct a factor as the physical addiction.
    4. Cultural factors affect the incidence of substance abuse and are a documented health problem with Indigenous people. However, culture is not as direct a factor as physical addiction.

52. **C: Foundations of Practice T: Application**
    1. Abstinence is not part of a harm-reduction strategy.
    2. This is a societal view that seeks to punish those who use illicit drugs.
    3. **This is a part of a continuum of strategies that aims to reduce the adverse health and social effects of problematic drug use.**
    4. This is repressive.

53. **C: Collaborative Practice T: Application**
    1. This is patronizing and is unlikely to help Ms. Wilcyska.
    2. This confirms to Ms. Wilcyska that she was a poor mother, and it is not therapeutic.
    3. **Reaching out to her estranged children may help Ms. Wilcyska. Writing letters to her children may bring the comfort of knowing that something of her may survive after her death.**
    4. This further emphasizes to Ms. Wilcyska that she was a poor mother and is not therapeutic.

54. **C: Foundations of Practice T: Knowledge**
    1. **With the hands of the practitioner either on the body or close to the body, energy flow is redirected and brings the person back into energy balance. It may be of value to reduce anxiety and pain.**
    2. This is biofeedback.
    3. Therapeutic touch is not a type of massage.
    4. This is meditation.

55. **C: Foundations of Practice T: Knowledge**
    1. **With ruptured membranes, there is a risk of ascending infection, particularly B *Streptococcus*. If the infant is not delivered, the risk of infection increases relative to the time that has passed since the membranes ruptured; therefore, antibiotics are given to the mother.**
    2. This is not indicated.
    3. This is not indicated.
    4. Labour will likely not be induced unless the infant is in distress.

56. **C: Foundations of Practice T: Knowledge**
    1. **Head compression may cause early decelerations.**
    2. Cord compression may cause variable decelerations.
    3. Placental insufficiency will cause late decelerations.
    4. Uterine contractions may cause fetal tachycardia.

57. **C: Collaborative Practice T: Application**
   1. This statement is judgemental and patronizing.
   2. **This acknowledges the fears of Ms. Philips. Both parents require additional support from the nurse at this time.**
   3. Ms. French needs the support of her partner at this time. Generally, partners will not be asked to leave unless they are in the way during the emergency.
   4. This does not help Ms. Philips fulfill her role in supporting Ms. French and may make Ms. Philips feel that she is failing her partner.

58. **C: Foundations of Practice T: Application**
   1. This is not safe, as there is potential for introducing pathogens into the IV.
   2. This would be uncomfortable for Ms. French.
   3. **This ensures that the bag and tubing are safely put through the arm of the gown, with no unsafe breaks in the system or tension applied to the tubing.**
   4. This would place the IV tubing inside the gown, where it is not in view, it may become kinked, and it may create tension on the insertion site.

59. **C: Foundations of Practice T: Knowledge**
   1. **An Apgar score of 3 indicates severe distress. Of the listed manifestations, this is the only abnormal finding. It is given a score of 1 on the Apgar.**
   2. This is normal. With an Apgar score of 3, the heart rate would likely be lower.
   3. This is normal and would likely be associated with an Apgar score of 7 to 10.
   4. Blood pressure is not a component of the Apgar score.

60. **C: Foundations of Practice T: Application**
   1. There may be fluid in the lungs, but it is not removed by grunting.
   2. The lungs require oxygen, not carbon dioxide.
   3. There is no mucus obstruction in neonatal respiratory distress.
   4. **With neonatal respiratory distress, the alveoli collapse due to insufficient surfactant. Grunting is an attempt by the body to open up the alveoli.**

61. **C: Professional, Ethical, and Legal Practice T: Critical Thinking**
   1. Cultural, spiritual, and religious factors will influence end-of-life care; however, each person is a unique individual.
   2. As in choice 1.
   3. As in choice 1.
   4. **Although a person's cultural, spiritual, and religious background must be included in end-of-life care, assumptions cannot be based on these factors. All people are unique.**

62. **C: Professional, Ethical, and Legal Practice T: Application**
   1. If they are no longer legally married, the former spouse cannot be the SDM unless Mr. Morrissey has designated her as the SDM.

   2. There is no provision in the legislation that states that the eldest child, whether male or female, should be the SDM.
   3. **The adult children are the legal next of kin and will be the SDMs. The children should agree upon decisions, and in practice, the child who has been most involved with the parent may have more influence.**
   4. The sister is not the next of kin, unless she has been designated as the SDM.

63. **C: Collaborative Practice T: Application**
   1. This is a patronizing answer and does not find a solution to the pain-management problem.
   2. **This is an action-oriented response. It is the role of the palliative care team to appropriately manage pain and the ethics of increased morphine.**
   3. This implies that the practical nurse does not have a professional role in pain management.
   4. Depending on the specifics of the situation, this may or may not be true. However, it does not solve the problem of Mr. Morrissey's pain management.

64. **C: Collaborative Practice T: Application**
   1. This should not be the initial action as it may be unpleasant for Mr. Morrissey and may not be necessary.
   2. This may be necessary depending on a thorough assessment of the constipation. It would be a last resort for impacted feces that did not respond to a suppository.
   3. Bulk-forming agents require the person to ingest larger amounts of fluids, which Mr. Morrissey is not able to do. They also require time to achieve results.
   4. **This is the most appropriate and comfortable initial action. The suppository may soften the stool so that Mr. Morrissey will be able to pass it with limited effort.**

65. **C: Foundations of Practice T: Application**
   1. **Skin dryness can lead to discomfort. Lubricating the lips and mucous membranes is soothing.**
   2. This is likely not appropriate close to death, unless he has requested an IV.
   3. Injections of saline under the skin are not appropriate to maintain hydration, unless he or the family has requested it.
   4. This is not appropriate unless requested.

66. **C: Foundations of Practice: Application**
   1. Clients with pharyngitis usually present with sore throat ranging in severity from "scratchy" to severe pain that makes swallowing painful. The pharynx is red and edematous, with or without patchy exudates.
   2. Symptoms of croup include a barky cough with low-grade fever. The voice may be harsh, but the client is able to speak and swallow.
   3. **Bronchiolitis, most often caused by the respiratory syncytial virus (RSV), is common in infants during**

the fall and winter. It often begins with an upper respiratory infection. Symptoms include dyspnea, paroxysmal nonproductive cough, tachypnea with retractions and nasal flaring, and wheezing.

4. Epiglottitis is most commonly found in children between the ages of 2 and 5 years. Signs and symptoms include sudden onset of high fever, difficulty breathing, severe sore throat, difficulty swallowing, drooling, and muffled voice, but no cough.

67. **C: Foundations of Practice T: Knowledge**
   1. Antivirals are not used with this condition.
   2. **Mist therapy is generally combined with oxygen to alleviate the dyspnea and hypoxia.**
   3. Cough suppressants are not recommended for children.
   4. Antibiotics are of no use with viral illnesses.

68. **C: Foundations of Practice T: Application**
   1. Respiratory syncytial virus (RSV) is very contagious, and Sean should not be with other infants.
   2. Sean does require isolation to prevent transmission to others, but also needs to be monitored by the nurse.
   3. Although adults are not as severely affected by RSV, being in the waiting room will not guarantee he will be isolated from children.
   4. **The nurse will need to monitor Sean's condition by having him close by and isolate him from the other children in the clinic.**

69. **C: Foundations of Practice T: Knowledge**
   1. This is not the philosophy of family-centred care. It is not the practical nurse's role to tell the parents it is best for them to leave their son.
   2. **This is the appropriate response and validates family-centred care and the role of his parents in Sean's care.**
   3. The practical nurse should not imply the hospital nursing staff would not be able to adequately look after Sean if they do not stay. This will not promote trust in the hospital's nursing care.
   4. The pediatrician does not need to write a prescription for the parents to stay at Sean's bedside.

70. **C: Foundations of Practice T: Critical Thinking**
   1. **This is the priority assessment. As with any invasive procedure, bleeding from an arterial access device carries considerable risk and could be life-threatening.**
   2. This is important but not a priority postprocedure. Blood pressure should be taken on the arm opposite the insertion site.
   3. This is an important observation postinsertion and will need to be assessed at all times while the device is in situ. Immediately postprocedure, it is not the priority assessment.
   4. This must be determined by the physician at the time of insertion and monitored thereafter by the practical nurse, but it is not the most critical assessment postprocedure.

71. **C: Foundations of Practice T: Application**
   1. This is not true, either for colonic irrigations or colostomy irrigations.
   2. **The primary purpose of irrigating a colostomy is to promote regular bowel movements.**
   3. It is not necessary to cleanse the anastomosis site.
   4. Constipation is not a common occurrence with a colostomy. Regular irrigation may help prevent constipation, but it does so by promoting regular bowel movements.

72. **C: Foundations of Practice T: Critical Thinking**
   1. The inability to void may be due to residual effects from an anaesthetic. As well, voiding into a bedpan is not easy for many clients, so this would not be the optimal strategy, unless Ms. Urquhart is unable to ambulate.
   2. **This should be the first action. If Ms. Urquhart has a full bladder, further and more immediate action will be required. If the bladder is not distended, the situation is less urgent.**
   3. This may happen but is not necessary until the bladder is assessed for distension.
   4. This should be done after Ms. Urquhart is assessed for bladder distension.

73. **C: Foundations of Practice T: Knowledge**
   1. **Glaucoma is manifested by loss of peripheral vision, producing "tunnel vision" and halos around lights.**
   2. With cataracts, vision loss is generally progressive blurring or haziness.
   3. With macular degeneration, close vision tasks become difficult.
   4. A detached retina may cause loss of vision in the affected area, blurring, or spots and flashes of light.

74. **C: Foundations of Practice T: Knowledge**
   1. **This hormone is produced by the chorionic villi of the developing embryo and is present in the blood and urine of a pregnant woman.**
   2. Estrogen prepares the uterus for pregnancy. An elevation in estrogen occurs later in pregnancy and does not necessarily indicate pregnancy.
   3. Progesterone helps maintain the pregnancy and prepare the breasts for lactation but is not the hormone detected in pregnancy tests.
   4. Follicle-stimulating hormone (FSH) helps mature follicles but is not the hormone detected in pregnancy tests.

75. **C: Foundations of Practice T: Critical Thinking**
   1. **An occlusive dressing is needed to prevent air from entering the pleural space.**
   2. The physician will need to be notified to reintroduce the tube; however, the initial action must be to occlude the puncture site.
   3. This will not be as effective as the occlusive dressing.
   4. This will not prevent air from entering the pleural space.

76. **C: Collaborative Practice T: Application**
   1. Five to 10 mm of induration may be significant. This is not normal.
   2. **This is the appropriate action as it is the physician's responsibility to further interpret the results and decide on further diagnostics.**
   3. This is not a definitively positive test. It is presumptive to tell Mr. Gupta that he requires prophylactic treatment.
   4. Although the protocol on repeating inconclusive tests varies among agencies, in this situation, it is not apparent that the practical nurse has the authority to repeat the test without consulting the physician.

77. **C: Foundations of Practice T: Critical Thinking**
   1. **This is the correct emergency action. Pressure to the site of bleeding will help control the bleeding.**
   2. This should not be done as it may compromise arterial blood flow.
   3. This is important, but the priority is to control the bleeding.
   4. Elevating the arm will help control the hemorrhage but is not as important as pressure at the site.

78. **C: Foundations of Practice T: Application**
   1. **The vastus lateralis is the best-developed muscle in infants and is the safest for IM injections.**
   2. This is not a well-developed muscle in the infant.
   3. As in choice 2.
   4. As in choice 2.

79. **C: Foundations of Practice T: Knowledge**
   1. **Morbidity refers to the incidence of disease within a defined population.**
   2. Morbidity does not refer to disease effects.
   3. This is the definition of mortality.
   4. This refers to the ability of an infectious disease to spread within a population.

80. **C: Foundations of Practice T: Application**
   1. **Calculi are more likely to form when the urine is concentrated. Increased fluids help dilute the urine.**
   2. Dairy products should be decreased as they contain calcium. Most kidney stones are calcium oxalate.
   3. Tea and chocolate have high levels of oxalate and should be reduced in the diet.
   4. Use of antacids is to be avoided as they contain calcium.

81. **C: Foundations of Practice T: Critical Thinking**
   1. **A concern about overuse of antibiotics is that they will lose their effectiveness and create drug-resistant strains.**
   2. Some antibiotics cause diarrhea, but they will not cause chronic diarrhea.
   3. Hearing loss may occur due to the chronic otitis media, but not due to the family of antibiotics used for otitis.
   4. Antibiotics do not cause dependence.

82. **C: Collaborative Practice T: Application**
   1. While a referral is a good option for Mr. Shafikhani, this does not address the immediate concern of not being able to drive.
   2. **This open-ended question deals practically and emotionally with the issue of a young male no longer being able to drive.**
   3. The practical nurse does not know Mr. Shafikhani's feelings. This sounds patronizing and does not invite therapeutic communication.
   4. This is a closed question. The practical nurse may only get a yes or no answer. He may infer that she thinks he is not intelligent enough to understand.

83. **C: Foundations of Practice T: Critical Thinking**
   1. Emotional reactions to the pregnancy loss must be explored, but this question is inappropriate and insensitive.
   2. **Aubrey's Rh status must be identified. If she is Rh-negative, she will require administration of RhoGAM within 72 hours of the miscarriage to prevent antibody formation in future pregnancies.**
   3. This is an appropriate question but is not as important as determination of the mother's Rh status.
   4. This may be an important question if Aubrey requires a D&C (dilation and curettage), but it is not important at this stage and may imply that Aubrey was at fault for the miscarriage.

84. **C: Foundations of Practice T: Application**
   1. **Coughing moves secretions from the lower airway into the mouth and upper airway and may decrease the amount of suctioning required.**
   2. Oral suctioning does not require sterile technique.
   3. This is a measurement for a nasogastric tube.
   4. Oil-based lubricants are not to be used as they are not water soluble and may be aspirated.

85. **C: Professional, Ethical, and Legal Practice T: Critical Thinking**
   1. This is not a safe option, as some residents may answer to any name.
   2. This is not a professional option.
   3. **The director of care is responsible for policies and care in the agency and needs to be consulted regarding the safest option. This may involve the director administering the medications.**
   4. This may be safer than the photos or self-reporting alone, but does not necessarily guarantee the correct resident would receive the medication.

86. **C: Foundations of Practice T: Critical Thinking**
   1. Cotton may be ordered post–eardrop instillation, but it will not prevent the mineral oil from flowing back out of the right ear during immediate instillation in the left ear.
   2. This would be a medication error, as the drops must be instilled in both ears every 8 hours.
   3. This will not prevent the drops from flowing back out of the right ear.

4. **This is the correct procedure. Mr. Lewis must remain in the side-lying position for at least 10 minutes in order for the drops to effectively be delivered to deeper ear structures.**

87. **C: Foundations of Practice T: Application**
    1. This may compromise her breathing.
    2. **The semi-Fowler's position reduces the pressure of the enlarged abdomen on the diaphragm.**
    3. This will assist breathing somewhat but is not the most effective.
    4. This may compromise breathing.

88. **C: Professional, Ethical, and Legal Practice T: Application**
    1. **Angie's behaviour is unprofessional: smoking on healthcare premises is contrary to agency policies and most municipal bylaws. As well, Angie is placing the clients at risk from second-hand smoke. Harriet must report Angie's disregard of policies, the law, and client safety.**
    2. Angie is on agency property; whether she is on a scheduled break is not pertinent.
    3. It is likely that Angie is already aware of agency policies and the dangers of second-hand smoke. This does not address her unprofessional behaviour.
    4. This discussion may be held at a different time. The professional responsibility for Harriet is to stop and report the behaviour.

89. **C: Professional, Ethical, and Legal Practice T: Critical Thinking**
    1. This is potential fraud and needs to be reported.
    2. **This is the appropriate chain of command. The nurse manager will investigate.**
    3. This will be done by the nurse manager.
    4. This could be done, but only if the practical nurse views unsafe practice.

90. **C: Foundations of Practice T: Application**
    1. Cranberry and blueberry juices, not orange juice, will help prevent UTIs.
    2. Cotton, not synthetic, underpants are recommended.
    3. **Sexual intercourse can "milk" bacteria from the vagina and perineum into the urethra. Use of a lubricant will decrease the incidence of skin breakdown in the urethral area, and use of a condom may prevent the transmission of bacteria from her partner(s).**
    4. Vaginal yeast disorders do not predispose clients to UTIs, unless related itching causes skin breakdown.

91. **C: Foundations of Practice T: Critical Thinking**
    1. There may be a risk of vomiting, but this is not the primary rationale. The answer must provide a rationale for both the NPO and the detection of bowel sounds.
    2. **Anaesthesia slows peristalsis. Hearing bowel sounds is an indication that peristalsis has returned. If Mrs. Brankston is fed when the bowel is not moving, the food would remain in the upper GI system, possibly leading to vomiting, obstruction, discomfort, and potential aspiration.**

3. Unless there is peristalsis, it is not likely that any food will reach the operative site.
4. A side effect of anaesthesia is nausea; however, this is not a postoperative rationale for NPO until bowel sounds are heard.

92. **C: Foundations of Practice T: Critical Thinking**
    1. The weight of the infant 24 hours postdelivery will be less than the birth weight and should not be substituted.
    2. **Weight loss up to 10% is expected. More than 10% indicates feeding has not been well established. Possible delay in discharge may occur to assist the parents in feeding.**
    3. Weight gain within the first 24 hours is unusual. It is not the reason for taking a discharge weight.
    4. It is not recommended to use formula as a supplement. More frequent breastfeeding will accomplish the same outcome.

93. **C: Foundations of Practice T: Application**
    1. +900 mL: incorrect calculation
    2. **+250 mL: 760 mL + 140 mL = 900 mL; total intake 540 mL + 110 mL = 650 mL total output. For fluid balance, subtract output from intake: 900 mL − 650 mL = 250 mL positive balance**
    3. −650 mL: incorrect calculation
    4. −110 mL: incorrect calculation

94. **C: Foundations of Practice T: Knowledge**
    1. This is reaction formation.
    2. **This is the definition of displacement. Ms. Henry is displacing her anger at the physician toward the practical nurse.**
    3. This is repression.
    4. This is denial.

95. **C: Foundations of Practice T: Application**
    1. This would indicate four pregnancies, but Mrs. Townsend has been pregnant only three times.
    2. This would denote three pregnancies, which is correct, but also three living children. Mrs. Townsend has only two living children.
    3. **Gravida 3 is correct: the present pregnancy, the pregnancy that resulted in twin births, and the previous miscarriage. Para 2 is correct: Mrs. Townsend has two living twin children.**
    4. This would indicate two pregnancies and one living child.

96. **C: Foundations of Practice T: Knowledge**
    1. Iron is recommended to support and increase maternal red blood cell production.
    2. **Folate (folic acid) supplements decrease the risk for neural tube defects in the newborn. Folate is recommended before and during pregnancy to prevent some major birth defects that can happen in the first few weeks of pregnancy, often before a woman finds out she is pregnant (400 mcg of folic acid is recommended daily). A woman should start taking folic acid as soon as she plans to become pregnant.**

3. This is not recommended. Vitamin A increases the risk for birth defects at intakes of 10 000 IU daily.

4. Calcium and Vitamin D are necessary for the development and maintenance of bone mass both prior to and during pregnancy. Adequate intake is required for fetal development.

97. **C: Foundations of Practice T: Application**

1. This is not necessarily true. Melatonin is increased in response to sun exposure, not when someone feels hot or cold. Also, people vary in the amount of melatonin they have naturally.

2. **This is a physiological response to cold. The constriction of the blood vessels to conserve heat means that there is not as much blood close to the skin surface, with the result that the skin appears a paler colour.**

3. This may occur, but this is not what Mr. Brendan asked.

4. This is the opposite of what occurs.

98. **C: Foundations of Practice T: Application**

1. This is an extreme measure and not necessary.

2. Although thorough cleaning is necessary at any daycare, in this situation, it is not necessary for the daycare to close. Transmission is most likely via contact with the infected child.

3. This is not true. See choice 4.

4. **Impetigo is an infection of the skin caused by *Streptococcus* or *Staphylococcus* bacteria and is transmissible to other children. The child with impetigo must be isolated from other children until 24–48 hours after treatment has started.**

99. **C: Professional, Ethical, and Legal Practice T: Application**

1. This may be an important part of the client assessment, depending on the situation and client problem.

2. This may help put the client at ease.

3. This is a therapeutic response.

4. **This is crossing a boundary. It implies a special relationship between the client and the practical nurse. The practical nurse must inform the client that all relevant information must be shared with other members of the healthcare team.**

100. **C: Foundations of Practice T: Application**

1. These are manifestations of irritable bowel disease, which does not cause rectal bleeding.

2. This may be necessary once hemorrhoids or constipation is ruled out as a cause for the bleeding.

3. This is not a necessary test, as Brad has said the blood is visible.

4. **The most common cause of minor rectal bleeding is tearing of the rectal mucosa due to constipation and hard stool.**

101. **C: Professional, Ethical, and Legal Practice T: Critical Thinking**

1. Artificial nails may be trimmed to an appropriate length that would not scratch or injure a client.

2. This is possible, but not likely, and would not be the most appropriate reason for the policy.

3. Artificial nails, if kept well-trimmed and without polish, may be professional in appearance.

4. **Studies have shown that artificial nails, especially if not well maintained, may have crevices that enable micro-organisms to flourish.**

102. **C: Foundations of Practice T: Critical Thinking**

1. This question could be asked as some prescription and nonprescription drugs cause drowsiness as a side effect. However, medications are not the most frequent cause of adolescent fatigue.

2. Lack of exercise may lead to fatigue during the day but is not the most common cause of adolescent fatigue.

3. This may be important information to obtain but should not be the initial question.

4. **The most common cause of daytime fatigue at all ages is inadequate sleep. Most teenagers do not know they need approximately 9 hours of sleep each night.**

103. **C: Foundations of Practice T: Application**

1. Large-print books are needed for people who have severe vision problems.

2. Instruction in Braille is not necessary. Vision of 20/40 is mild vision loss.

3. While an ophthalmologist can prescribe corrective lenses, generally, for simple near-sightedness, referral is not required.

4. **A score of 20/40 indicates vision that will likely respond well to corrective lenses, either glasses or contact lenses.**

104. **C: Foundations of Practice T: Application**

1. This is a common STI in both sexes but is not the most prevalent.

2. This is not the most prevalent STI in Canada.

3. This is the most common STI in males but not in the general population.

4. **Chlamydia is the most widespread STI in Canada.**

105. **C: Foundations of Practice T: Critical Thinking**

1. Injuries occurring from the fall will need to be assessed, treated, and documented, but this is not the most important initial action.

2. Circulation is not the first priority.

3. Breathing is assessed after assessing for a patent airway.

4. **The priority of assessment is according to the ABCs: airway, breathing, and circulation. A clear airway is necessary for breathing and must be the initial assessment.**

106. **C: Professional, Ethical, and Legal Practice T: Critical Thinking**

1. Meperidine should not be administered, as there is confusion concerning the correct drug.

2. This should not be done until the correct drug is clarified.

3. This could be done once the drug is clarified.

4. Meperidine is the generic name for Demerol, not morphine. The ordered dose is within the normal dosing range for morphine. The medication order must be clarified with the prescriber prior to any other action.

107. **C: Foundations of Practice T: Critical Thinking**
   1. Tympanic thermometers should not be used with clients who have ear infections or ear pain.
   2. An axillary temperature is not as accurate as tympanic, oral, or rectal temperature, but in this situation, it is the most appropriate approach. The thermometer should be kept under the axilla for 5 minutes.
   3. Oral thermometers should not be used with an 18-month-old child. In addition, a child who is mouth breathing may not be able to keep his or her mouth closed for the required time, and this may lead to an inaccurate reading.
   4. Rectal temperatures should not generally be used with children due to the risk of rectal injury and the discomfort and distress related to the procedure.

108. **C: Collaborative Practice T: Application**
   1. This does not answer Mr. Rivers's question.
   2. This reassures Mr. Rivers that he is well enough to be discharged, he will have support by nurses in his home, and this is better for him.
   3. This may be true but will not be reassuring for Mr. Rivers.
   4. This is true but does not answer Mr. Rivers's question or reassure him.

109. **C: Foundations of Practice T: Application**
   1. It is not exactly the same, and the practical nurse has not answered that it is a normal temperature.
   2. The conversion of 36.6 degrees Celsius to Fahrenheit is 97.9, or 98 degrees.

$$\frac{36.6 \times 9}{5} + 32 = 97.9$$

This is considered a normal temperature. Many clients who were not educated in the metric system prefer to use the Fahrenheit scale.
   3. This is an incorrect conversion and is not elevated.
   4. It is lower, but not significantly, and is still considered to be a normal temperature.

110. **C: Collaborative Practice T: Application**
   1. The voices are real to Mr. Constant, so this is not therapeutic.
   2. The voices are real and frightening to Mr. Constant. Acknowledging this, and staying with him, demonstrates concern and may reduce his fears.
   3. Mr. Constant will not be able to concentrate on the TV because of his fears.
   4. Mr. Constant is not able to separate the voices from reality.

111. **C: Professional, Ethical, and Legal Practice T: Critical Thinking**
   1. This will need to be done once the practical nurse assesses the type of allergic reaction.
   2. As in choice 1.
   3. This is important, but the practical nurse initially needs more information about the allergy.
   4. It is important to first obtain more information from Mrs. Collins about the allergy. Some clients have a sensitivity reaction; with others, it may be anaphylactic.

112. **C: Foundations of Practice T: Application**
   1. Milk-based foods are likely to irritate the gut and cause further diarrhea.
   2. This is not appropriate for a child.
   3. With mild diarrhea, clear fluids will maintain hydration and will not irritate the gut. Crackers are also appropriate and will decrease Teklie's hunger.
   4. A normal diet may be resumed once the diarrhea has stopped.

113. **C: Professional, Ethical, and Legal Practice T: Critical Thinking**
   1. This may help, but generally two people are required for a mechanical lift.
   2. The practical nurse needs more data, as what the client is telling her is different from her assessment.
   3. The practical nurse will probably have to obtain assistance, but it is best to find out first from Mrs. Bennett more information about the lift.
   4. This could potentially be dangerous for both Mrs. Bennett and the practical nurse.

114. **C: Foundations of Practice T: Critical Thinking**
   1. Medications can trigger delirium, but this is not the most important step in the data collection.
   2. All of these responses are important when assessing the cause of Mrs. Sheyer's delirium. By obtaining a baseline understanding of Mrs. Sheyer's cognitive function, it can be better determined how, or if, her behaviour has changed and what particular triggers may have been involved.
   3. Dehydration can cause delirium in an older adult but is not the most important step in the data collection.
   4. Fever or infection may trigger delirium, but this is not the most important step in the data collection.

115. **C: Collaborative Practice T: Application**
   1. This allows Ms. Isabelle to continue with inappropriate behaviour and is not therapeutic toward Mr. Olan.
   2. As in choice 1.
   3. This response is clear, provides exact information without appearing punitive toward Ms. Isabelle, and demonstrates respect for both clients.
   4. This response is punitive.

116. **C: Professional, Ethical, and Legal Practice T: Critical Thinking**
    1. This is important; however, the practical nurse's expertise is needed with the toddler. It is more appropriate for the practical nurse to delegate another to call 9-1-1.
    2. The practical nurse should observe for a patent airway, but this is not a safe option. It may cause damage to the mouth and teeth.
    3. **The safest option with a child is to observe the seizure, make sure the child is not injuring him- or herself, and ensure that they are maintaining a patent airway and not to actively intervene or attempt to restrain the child. These observations will be helpful when emergency medical personnel arrive at the scene.**
    4. This is not the priority action. It may be appropriate once the seizure is over.

117. **C: Collaborative Practice T: Critical Thinking**
    1. This is not true. At age 10 years, Nicholas would have an understanding of the diagnosis.
    2. **This response opens up communication with the parents.**
    3. This may be true but closes communication.
    4. This may be true but may upset the parents and may not encourage communication.

118. **C: Professional, Ethical, and Legal Practice T: Critical Thinking**
    1. This category of nurse is appropriate; however, the knowledge and skills of an RN would be more appropriately used for a more acutely ill, unstable client.
    2. **The RPN or LPN is the most appropriate caregiver as the practical nurse provides care to clients such as Mr. Michener, whose conditions are stable and whose outcomes are predictable. The practical nurse has the competency to perform discharge health teaching, and assigning this task to him or her is more cost-effective than assigning it to an RN.**
    3. While this category of nurse is certainly competent to provide care, his or her knowledge and skills would be more appropriately used for an acutely ill or complex client; therefore, this is not the most cost-effective option.
    4. The support worker would be appropriate to provide some basic care for Mr. Michener but would not have the knowledge to provide discharge health teaching or wound assessment.

119. **C: Foundations of Practice T: Application**
    1. This is a normal finding in the skin of a 59-year-old woman.
    2. As in choice 1.
    3. **This could be a possible finding of skin cancer and should be further investigated.**
    4. These are more commonly known as "age spots" or "liver spots" and may be seen in adults starting in their late 40s or 50s.

120. **C: Foundations of Practice T: Critical Thinking**
    1. There is no reason to wait an hour. The elevated temperature must be confirmed as soon as possible as temperatures in children can rise rapidly.
    2. It is neither appropriate nor necessary to obtain a rectal temperature. The use of a rectal thermometer would be very upsetting and intrusive for a 4-year-old.
    3. This action should not be taken until the temperature is confirmed. Other evidence suggests that Nick may not have a fever.
    4. **The second step of the nursing process is validation of data collected. Nick does not display manifestations of a fever; therefore, it is possible that the thermometer is malfunctioning or requires recalibration. The temperature should be confirmed using another thermometer.**

121. **C: Foundations of Practice T: Application**
    1. **This is factual documentation of observed behaviour.**
    2. This is an assumption and interpretation of behaviour. Documentation requires the inclusion only of observable facts.
    3. As in choice 2.
    4. As in choice 2.

122. **C: Foundations of Practice T: Critical Thinking**
    1. **Topical anaesthetic creams are effective in preventing pain from immunization and may help prevent future fear of needles.**
    2. Distraction techniques may help decrease stress and minimize pain, but they are not as effective as the anaesthetic cream.
    3. As in choice 2.
    4. Postinjection analgesics are often prescribed but are most useful with children who develop swelling and fever postimmunization. They do not prevent the pain of injections but treat it after the fact.

123. **C: Professional, Ethical, and Legal Practice T: Critical Thinking**
    1. **All responses could be correct. This is the first action, as the manager needs objective data: the number of accidents and types of accidents on the unit.**
    2. This is a good action but is not as important as the actual accident statistics.
    3. The manager should know this information. Not all accidents may cause staff to be on long-term disability.
    4. As in Choice 2.

124. **C: Foundations of Practice T: Knowledge**
    1. The situation describes what is going on with the client. It is a concise statement of the problem.
    2. **The information provided is the background report of a SBAR. This information is the clinical background. It describes the information and history that is relevant to the situation.**

3. Assessment describes what you find and considerations of options. It includes a physical assessment of the client along with the vital signs and lab reports.
4. Recommendation is what action is needed to correct the problem or what you want.

125. **C: Foundations of Practice T: Critical Thinking**
    1. **Influenza is communicated primarily by droplet and contact transmission. Having symptomatic clients segregated, wearing masks, and performing hand hygiene will decrease the incidence of viral particles coming in contact with other clients.**
    2. This is not practical, and the vaccine requires up to 2 weeks to provide immunity.
    3. This is not ethical. As well, people with influenza may be infectious before they have symptoms.
    4. Droplet transmission is possible up to 2 m from an infected person.

Practice Exam: Book Two

PRACTICE QUESTIONS

Case 1

A practical nurse is employed by a hospital-based palliative care team that includes a physician, a pharmacist, and a social worker. The practical nurse is supporting the family of Mrs. Haliburton, who is terminally ill with stomach cancer and has chosen to die at home.

Questions 1–5 refer to this case.

1. The family asks the practical nurse how they will know Mrs. Haliburton's death is imminent. What should the nurse respond?
   1. Her skin may become mottled.
   2. Her respirations will become slow and deep.
   3. Her pulse will increase.
   4. Her temperature will decrease.

2. One morning when the practical nurse visits, he finds the family sitting around Mrs. Haliburton's bed, crying. They tell him that she stopped breathing 30 minutes ago. The practical nurse examines Mrs. Haliburton and finds no respirations, no heart rate, and no pupillary reaction, and her body is cooling. What should be the first action by the nurse?
   1. Confirm to the family that Mrs. Haliburton has died.
   2. Pronounce death and document it in the health record.
   3. Call the physician so that he or she can complete a death certificate.
   4. Notify the funeral home.

3. Mrs. Haliburton's health record had been kept in her home during her palliative care. What should the practical nurse do with Mrs. Haliburton's health record after her death?
   1. Leave it with the family.
   2. Put it in a sealed envelope for the physician.
   3. Take it to the agency that employs the palliative care team.
   4. Destroy the record, as it is no longer needed.

4. Several days later, the family calls the practical nurse to ask him what to do with Mrs. Haliburton's left-over morphine. What should the practical nurse say to them?
   1. "Take it to your pharmacy."
   2. "I will pick it up."
   3. "Dispose of it in the biohazard container I left."
   4. "Keep it just in case another family member requires morphine."

5. The practical nurse has been working in palliative care for several years and is surprised when he feels tremendous sadness at Mrs. Haliburton's death. What should the practical nurse initially do to cope with these emotions?
   1. Examine his patterns of dealing with grief.
   2. Arrange for time off or a vacation.
   3. Reflect on the need to change to another specialty in nursing.
   4. Make an appointment with a psychiatrist who specializes in palliative care.

Case 2

Jean Cetaine, age 68, is golfing with his friends when he develops severe chest pain and shortness of breath. His friends call an ambulance, and he is transported to hospital, where he is diagnosed with unstable angina.

Questions 6–9 refer to this case.

6. Upon Mr. Cetaine's arrival in the emergency department, which of the following is a "first-line" medication he will likely receive?
   1. Nitroglycerine (Nitrolingual)
   2. Propranolol (Inderal)
   3. Tissue plasminogen activator (t-PA)
   4. Captopril (Capoten)

7. Which of the following tests will best evaluate the extent of Mr. Cetaine's coronary artery disease?
   1. Chest X-ray
   2. Cardiac ultrasonography
   3. Electrocardiography (ECG)
   4. Angiography

8. It is decided that Mr. Cetaine requires coronary artery bypass graft (CABG) surgery. What is the purpose of CABG surgery?
   1. To provide a new circuit for blood flow to get to the heart muscle
   2. To repair damage to the heart muscle
   3. To provide new vessels bringing blood to the right atrium
   4. To provide a route for blood to flow past obstructions in the ascending aorta

9. Nursing care within the first 3 days postsurgery for Mr. Cetaine would include which of the following?
   1. Complete bed rest
   2. Care for two surgical sites
   3. Administration of oxygen via nasal cannula at 3 L/min
   4. Prn analgesia

Case 3

A nurse educator provides an orientation session about documentation to recently hired nurses.

Questions 10–13 refer to this case.

10. The nurse educator reviews the purpose of documentation. Of the following, which is the most important reason for client documentation?
    1. To facilitate communication concerning the client
    2. To demonstrate nursing accountability and professional practice
    3. To provide a source of data for evidence-informed practice
    4. To identify the type and amount of care clients require

11. The nurse educator presents a case scenario about a client who requests information from his health record. When care is provided through an agency, who owns and has access to the health record?
    1. The agency owns the health record, and the client has access only in exceptional circumstances.
    2. The client owns the health record and must provide consent to agency staff for its use for purposes related to care.
    3. The agency and the client co-own the health record, and both have equal access to the information.
    4. The agency owns the health record, but the client has legal access to the information according to agency policies.

12. The nurse educator cautions the nurses to only record care they personally provide. When is it acceptable to document care provided by another nurse?
    1. When the other nurse is not registered/licensed
    2. During an emergency when more than one nurse is involved
    3. When two or more nurses care for a client, only one nurse is required to document
    4. There are no exceptions to the practice of never documenting for another

13. The nurse educator presents another case scenario to the group. A postmastectomy client, Ms. Scharfe, has been crying, refuses to eat, and will not speak to her husband. The nurse educator asks the group to record this behaviour. What is the best documentation of this client situation?
    1. "Ms. Scharfe shows manifestations of depression."
    2. "Ms. Scharfe is upset due to her mastectomy."
    3. "Ms. Scharfe is crying, refuses food, will not talk to her husband."

4. "Ms. Scharfe experienced an emotional postop day, with periods of weeping and anorexia due to pain and anaesthetic, and was ignoring her husband."

Case 4

Glen Martin has a history of alcohol dependence with a high daily intake of alcohol for 15 years. He has made several attempts to stop drinking, has attended Alcoholics Anonymous and private counselling, and has told his wife that he no longer drinks. She arrives home one day to find him confused, smelling of alcohol, and with hand tremors. She takes him to the local emergency department.

Questions 14–19 refer to this case.

14. The healthcare team tell Mrs. Martin that her husband is experiencing acute alcohol withdrawal and must be admitted to hospital. What is the most important reason alcohol-dependent people need to be monitored carefully while withdrawing from alcohol?
    1. Cardiac failure
    2. Acute organ failure
    3. Seizures
    4. Risk of suicide

15. Mrs. Martin says that she can't understand why her husband was drinking because he had promised her he had stopped. What should the practical nurse respond to Mrs. Martin?
    1. "Because of the effects of alcohol on the brain, he likely did not know what he was doing."
    2. "Why do you think he was lying to you?"
    3. "Your husband is trying to change a long-term habit, and lapses are sometimes to be expected."
    4. "He probably can't help himself."

16. After Mr. Martin's successful detoxification, the healthcare team notices that he has jaundice. Tests are ordered to confirm a diagnosis of cirrhosis of the liver. Which test should be ordered to confirm the level of jaundice?
    1. Alkaline phosphatase
    2. Serum bilirubin
    3. Alanine aminotransferase (ALT)
    4. Prothrombin time (PT)

17. Mrs. Martin asks the practical nurse why her husband is yellow. What would be the most appropriate answer by the nurse?
    1. "Your husband has jaundice."
    2. "There is inadequate hepatodetoxification of cellular metabolites resulting from scleroses related to alcohol."
    3. "The effects of alcohol on the liver have interfered with the ability to remove a yellow pigment that is released when red blood cells break down."
    4. "Pressure of the liver on the kidneys prevents them from filtering urine effectively, so it builds up in his system, causing the yellow colour."

18. The practical nurse teaches Mr. and Mrs. Martin about therapeutic nutrition related to cirrhosis. Which of the following breakfast menus should the nurse recommend?

1. Toast, margarine, and banana
2. Cheese omelette
3. Bagel and peanut butter
4. Ham, eggs, and hash brown potatoes

19. Mr. Martin is ready to be discharged home, with a referral to an outpatient alcohol rehabilitation program. He has refused alcohol aversion medications. Mrs. Martin is concerned that he will start drinking again. She states that she will consent to giving him disulfiram (Antabuse) but tell him that it is a vitamin. How should the practical nurse respond?
    1. "Can you arrange to be made his substitute decision maker so that you can consent to the Antabuse?"
    2. "Mr. Martin cannot be given Antabuse without his consent."
    3. "That would be helpful, but I don't think you would be allowed to consent for him."
    4. "Perhaps you can get the doctor to order it for you and then give it to your husband."

Case 5

Mr. Ian Lewis is an 83-year-old man who has been referred to the respiratory clinic. He has chronic obstructive pulmonary disease (COPD) and asthma, with poor symptom control for the past few months. Mr. Lewis is frail but lives alone and independently.

Questions 20–23 refer to this case.

20. The practical nurse reviews Mr. Lewis's health history. She asks him about his use of over-the-counter (OTC) medications. What medication would be of most concern to the nurse?
    1. Aspirin (ASA)
    2. Acetaminophen (Tylenol)
    3. Ibuprofen (Advil, Motrin)
    4. Loratadine (Claritin)

21. Mr. Lewis reports that he takes a combination inhaler that contains a long-acting beta$_2$-agonist as well as a steroid. What is the therapeutic action of these two medications?
    1. The medications act in combination to decrease airway inflammation.
    2. They work in combination to decrease airway bronchoconstriction.
    3. They provide bronchodilation and reduced airway inflammation.
    4. The two medications potentiate each other and provide longer-acting symptom control.

22. The practical nurse asks Mr. Lewis to demonstrate the use of his aerosol metered-dose inhaler (MDI) and observes that he has difficulty using the MDI effectively. What should the practical nurse recommend to Mr. Lewis?
    1. He should consult with the pharmacist about taking his medications in a form other than the inhaled route.
    2. There are oral forms of the medications that are just as effective and easier for him to take.

3. A spacer used with the MDI is easier to use and will provide better delivery of medication to his airway.
4. He will need to be re-educated in the use of inhaled medications.

23. Mr. Lewis tells the practical nurse he becomes quite frightened when he has a "bad attack" of asthma. He becomes very short of breath, wheezes, and feels as if he is drowning. What should the practical nurse teach him about the first thing he should do for a serious acute episode of shortness of breath?
    1. Take his combination inhaled drugs to relieve the bronchoconstriction.
    2. Call 9-1-1 to take him to the hospital for emergency respiratory therapy.
    3. Breathe cool, humidified air to liquefy secretions and open the airways.
    4. Use his "rescue inhaler" and wait for about 10 minutes to assess if it restores normal breathing.

Case 6

A practical nurse provides primary nursing care to clients at a busy family practice clinic.

Questions 24–27 refer to this case.

24. Ryan Fraser is a new client to the clinic. He brings his health record from his previous doctor and asks the practical nurse who will have access to his health record at this clinic. What should the practical nurse tell Mr. Fraser?
    1. "Only the doctor has access to your record."
    2. "Any of the staff working in the clinic may see your record."
    3. "The doctor, clerical staff, and myself are able to view your health record."
    4. "You may keep your record if you are concerned about confidentiality."

25. The practical nurse facilitates booking screening tests for clients. Which of the following clients should have priority in scheduling for a screening colonoscopy?
    1. Nonie Masseur, age 48, who has a sister recently diagnosed with colon cancer
    2. Norma Williams, age 36, who has hemorrhoids
    3. Nancy Morgan, age 42, who has irritable bowel syndrome
    4. Anne Daniels, age 29, who has tested positive for the *BRCA1* gene mutation

26. Miss Shannon has had disabling knee pain for several months and is booked to have magnetic resonance imaging (MRI) in several months. Miss Shannon does not want to wait this long and asks the practical nurse how she can get the test done earlier. What should the nurse respond?
    1. "Only clients with life-threatening illnesses can have immediate MRI scans."
    2. "You could call the MRI clinic to ask to be put on the cancellation list."
    3. "In Canada, there are not sufficient MRI machines, so you will have to wait until one is available."

4. "It is not likely that your knee pain is serious, so be reassured that waiting will not contribute to a worsening of your condition."

27. The practical nurse performs an intramuscular injection on Mr. Gold. Mr. Gold says to the practical nurse, "Why did you pull back on the syringe before you pushed the plunger?" What would be the best response by the nurse?
    1. "Because that is how we were taught to perform injections."
    2. "Because best practice guidelines state the nurse should aspirate before injecting."
    3. "Because I want to make sure the plunger slides smoothly in the syringe."
    4. "Because I need to ensure the needle has not hit a blood vessel."

Case 7

Tom Rutlege, 63 years old, has had surgery for a ruptured aortic aneurysm. The repair was successful, and after stabilization in the Critical Care Unit, he is transferred to a cardiovascular surgical unit.

Questions 28–32 refer to this case.

28. The practical nurse takes and records Mr. Rutlege's vital signs on admission to the unit: temperature 36.4°C; blood pressure 100/60 mm Hg; pulse 90 beats/minute; respirations 20 breaths/minute; oxygen saturation 96%. What should be the practical nurse's action in response to Mr. Rutlege's vital signs?
    1. Cover him with a warm blanket.
    2. Increase the oxygen, within medical directives.
    3. Continue to monitor the vital signs.
    4. Call the surgeon.

29. Which of the following would be of concern to the practical nurse when providing postoperative care to Mr. Rutlege?
    1. Urinary output of less than 30 mL per hour
    2. Absent bowel sounds
    3. Pain from the incision site
    4. Scant serosanguinous drainage from the incision

30. Mr. Rutlege has chest tubes attached to a Pleur-evac chest drainage system. The practical nurse is aware that care of this type of chest tube drainage system includes which of the following?
    1. Ensuring continuous bubbling in the water seal chamber
    2. Taping the connection between the chest tube and drainage system
    3. Adding sterile water to the suction control chamber every 8 hours
    4. Maintaining the system above waist level

31. Mr. Rutlege is ordered a type and cross-match prior to a blood transfusion. What is the purpose of the type and cross-match test?
    1. To determine whether Rh agglutinins are present
    2. To determine whether there is ABO incompatibility
    3. To determine the presence of A or O antigens

4. To determine the compatibility of his blood with donor blood

32. Mr. Rutlege recovers from surgery and is to be discharged home. He will be caring for his incision himself. How should the practical nurse best evaluate his ability to perform incision care?
    1. Have him explain how to care for the incision.
    2. Have him demonstrate how to care for the incision.
    3. Ask him questions based on the instructional DVD he has viewed.
    4. Ask him if he has any questions about the care of his incision.

Case 8

Four-year-old Sam has fallen out of a tree. His mother calls a neighbour, who is a practical nurse, for help. The practical nurse observes Sam lying on the ground, moaning and crying. He has several abrasions and a 1-cm cut on his forehead.

Questions 33–37 refer to this case.

33. The practical nurse assesses Sam for injuries. What is the priority assessment?
    1. Signs of head injury
    2. Evidence of limb fracture
    3. Sam's pulse
    4. Other injuries that may not be visible

34. The practical nurse needs to examine Sam's left leg. What would be the most appropriate initial action to determine whether there is a fracture?
    1. Ask Sam to stand on his left leg.
    2. Rotate the leg and ankle.
    3. Ask Sam to point to where his leg hurts.
    4. Apply pressure to the injured area to assess for bone integrity.

35. The practical nurse determines that Sam probably has a fracture close to or at the ankle. What is the most appropriate first aid to apply before transporting him to the hospital?
    1. Wrap the leg in a soft blanket.
    2. Immobilize the foot, ankle, and lower leg in a rolled magazine.
    3. Splint the left leg against the right leg.
    4. Apply ice to the fracture site.

36. At the hospital, Sam is seen by a nurse practitioner who orders tests to determine whether Sam has a fractured bone in his leg. What test will the nurse practitioner most likely order?
    1. X-ray
    2. Bone scan
    3. Bone densitometry
    4. Computed tomography (CT) scan

37. It is determined that Sam has a fracture, and his leg is encased in a plaster of Paris cast. Which of the following should be instructions to Sam's parents regarding cast care in the first 24 hours?
    1. Wrap the cast in a plastic bag to prevent it from getting wet or dirty.
    2. Expose the cast to air until dry.

3. Lift and support the wet cast with the fingertips.
4. Use a hair dryer to speed the drying process.

Case 9

Roberta Wilmot, age 54 years, has osteoarthritis. Ms. Wilmot, who admits to being overweight, is a postal worker who walks a route to deliver mail. She is the single mother of a disabled adult son and must work to maintain health benefits.

Questions 38–41 refer to this case.

38. Which of the following manifestations of osteoarthritis is Ms. Wilmot most likely to experience?
    1. Pain in her knees
    2. Sudden onset of pain in most joints
    3. Swelling and erythema in her feet
    4. Paraesthesia in her fingers

39. The practical nurse counselling Ms. Wilmot discusses lifestyle changes to help with the osteoarthritis. Which of the following should the practical nurse most appropriately recommend to Ms. Wilmot?
    1. Change of job
    2. Weight loss
    3. Assistance with her disabled son
    4. More exercise

40. Which of the following medications will be of greatest help to alleviate the symptoms of osteoarthritis?
    1. Muscle relaxants
    2. Nonsteroidal anti-inflammatory drugs (NSAIDs)
    3. Antibiotics
    4. Acetaminophen (Tylenol)

41. An interprofessional team works with Ms. Wilmot to manage her osteoarthritis. In addition to the nurse and physician, which of the following healthcare workers would be most important to include on the team?
    1. Pharmacist
    2. Naturopath
    3. Social worker
    4. Physiotherapist

Case 10

Meredith Marshall is a 42-year-old woman who is 22 weeks pregnant with her fifth child. She attends the antenatal clinic for her prenatal care.

Questions 42–44 refer to this case.

42. What is the most important assessment for the practical nurse at this visit?
    1. Mrs. Marshall's blood pressure
    2. Presence of ketones in Mrs. Marshall's urine
    3. Estimate of fetal growth
    4. Weight gain or loss

43. It is determined that Mrs. Marshall has pre-eclampsia. What is the recommended treatment for mild pre-eclampsia?
    1. Complete bed rest in hospital
    2. Restricted activity at home
    3. Sodium-restricted diet
    4. Administration of magnesium sulphate

44. Which of the following questions related to pre-eclampsia should the practical nurse ask Mrs. Marshall?
    1. "Do you have headaches or visual disturbances?"
    2. "Are you constipated or bloated?"
    3. "Have you experienced any vaginal bleeding or mucus discharge?"
    4. "Have you felt any mild contractions or tightening in your abdomen?"

Case 11

Ross is a 14-year-old adolescent in foster care. Ross was diagnosed as HIV-positive when he was an infant. He has been generally well, except for occasional acute infections that have required hospitalization. Ross is adherent to his antiretroviral therapy. He attends the HIV clinic every 2 months. The clinic practical nurse notes that Ross's CD4 counts have been dropping (below 500 cells) over the past few months.

Questions 45–49 refer to this case.

45. When Ross has his appointment at the clinic, which of the following initial actions, specific to his HIV status, should the practical nurse implement?
    1. Performing hand hygiene
    2. Gloving when she examines Ross
    3. Placing him in a room separate from infectious clients
    4. Asking him if he has been taking his medications

46. The practical nurse weighs Ross and notes that he has lost 2 kg since his last appointment. What would be an appropriate initial comment to Ross about his weight loss?
    1. "What has your appetite been like in the past 2 months?"
    2. "Have you had any episodes of diarrhea?"
    3. "This may be a sign that your condition is getting worse."
    4. "It's good to see you are not one of these obese children we've been reading about."

47. Which of the following is an appropriate topic for the practical nurse to discuss with Ross at this clinic visit?
    1. Feelings and concerns about sexuality
    2. Pain management
    3. Education regarding transmission of HIV
    4. Stress-management techniques

48. Which of the following is a principle of drug therapy for HIV infection?
    1. Clients with chronic HIV do not require treatment if they are asymptomatic.
    2. Treatment regimens should be individualized depending on CD4 counts.
    3. It is preferable to begin treatment with single-drug therapy.
    4. Pediatric treatment is limited due to fewer antiretrovirals that are safe for children.

49. The physician in the clinic discusses starting a new research medication with Ross. The practical nurse is not sure whether Ross is able to consent to the research

drug because he is 14 and in foster care. What knowledge should the practical nurse have in this situation?

1. Ross is an emancipated minor and may provide his own consent for the research drug.
2. Foster parents are legally able to provide consent for minors.
3. Agency policies for consent guidelines regarding age and research drug protocols
4. An assessment of Ross's understanding of the proposed treatment

Case 12

Mr. Red Ford has been seriously burned in an industrial fire. His condition is stabilized in hospital, but he is only able to manage small sips of fluid by mouth and is not able to maintain adequate nutrition. The physician orders total parenteral nutrition (TPN) of protein electrolyte, vitamin, trace elements, and fat emulsion via a peripherally inserted central catheter (PICC).

Questions 50–56 refer to this case.

50. The nurse practitioner inserts the single-lumen PICC line at Mr. Ford's bedside. What precautions are necessary for this procedure?
    1. A tourniquet placed around his upper arm
    2. Sterile conditions
    3. Intravenous infusion of midazolam (Versed) for light anaesthesia
    4. Mr. Ford positioned with his head to the side to facilitate subclavian access

51. What must be done by the practical nurse prior to the first infusion of the TPN solution?
    1. Ensure correct catheter placement is verified by chest X-ray.
    2. Educate Mr. Ford about the PICC line and TPN.
    3. Warm the solution for a minimum of 3 hours.
    4. Add ordered electrolytes and trace elements to the solution.

52. Mr. Ford is ordered an intravenous antibiotic. How should the practical nurse administer this medication?
    1. Add the antibiotic to the protein and electrolyte solution.
    2. Administer it in the fat emulsion solution.
    3. Administer it via Y-tubing to the PICC line.
    4. Commence an additional peripheral intravenous line in a separate vein.

53. The practical nurse is aware that she needs to observe many safety measures related to Mr. Ford's PICC line and the TPN infusion. Which of the following is a nursing action related to client safety?
    1. Change all TPN tubing lines every 24 hours.
    2. Label the tubing and filter with the date and time they were changed.
    3. Change the dressing at the catheter insertion site once per shift.
    4. Send the tubing for culture once per week.

54. How should the practical nurse best evaluate Mr. Ford's tolerance of the TPN?

1. Daily weights
2. Positive balance for intake and output
3. Improved healing of his burns
4. Laboratory values

55. Several days later, Mr. Ford tells the practical nurse he still doesn't really understand the PICC line and where it is in his body. What would be the most appropriate response by the nurse?
    1. "Let me draw you some pictures of where the PICC line is in your body."
    2. "The PICC line is a flexible catheter that sits inside the large vein leading to your heart."
    3. "The manufacturer's monograph provides most of the information you need."
    4. "The nurse practitioner who inserted the line will explain it to you."

56. Mr. Ford's TPN solution is stopped one day because he is off the unit for tests. He is behind a total of 500 mL of solution. The solution is running at 200 mL per hour. What should the practical nurse do, in accordance with agency policies, in this situation?
    1. Do not make up the 500 mL.
    2. Increase the ordered flow to 220 mL until the 500 mL is made up.
    3. Take the solution off the infusion pump and increase the rate to 300 mL per hour.
    4. Offer Mr. Ford increased fluids by mouth.

Case 13

Jennifer and Ronald Buxton are clients at a family practice clinic. Mr. and Mrs. Buxton have lived together in a "stormy" relationship for 10 years. A practical nurse at the clinic has often suspected intimate-partner violence and has spoken with Mrs. Buxton about it, but Mrs. Buxton has denied any abuse.

Questions 57–61 refer to this case.

57. One day, the practical nurse receives a phone call from Mrs. Buxton, who is hysterical and crying, saying, "Ronnie is beating me up." What should be the practical nurse's first response to Mrs. Buxton?
    1. "How long has he been abusing you?"
    2. "You need to come to the doctor's office right away."
    3. "How badly has he beaten you up?"
    4. "Are you in a safe place?"

58. Mr. Buxton is arrested by the police and subsequently convicted of assault. His sentencing requires him to have mandatory counselling. During the first session with the counsellor, who is a mental health nurse, what is the nurse's most important initial therapeutic goal?
    1. Establishing trust between himself and Mr. Buxton
    2. Determining the causative factors involved in the abuse of Mrs. Buxton
    3. Developing healthy and open patterns of communication
    4. Ensuring that Mr. Buxton understands that counselling is mandatory

59. Mr. Buxton tells the mental health nurse that he has absolutely no memory of hitting Mrs. Buxton. What defence mechanism is this an example of?
    1. Splitting
    2. Repression
    3. Introjection
    4. Compensation

60. Mr. Buxton eventually admits to abusing Mrs. Buxton. He tells the mental health nurse that it is all because she "nags" him. What would be a therapeutic response by the mental health nurse?
    1. "That is no excuse to hit Mrs. Buxton."
    2. "Does hitting Mrs. Buxton make her stop nagging?"
    3. "I'm not sure what you mean; please explain that to me again."
    4. "Why does Mrs. Buxton nag you?"

61. As the mental health nurse learns more about Mr. Buxton, he finds that Mr. Buxton has some typical characteristics of abusers. Which of the following is most characteristic of perpetrators of abuse?
    1. A history of alcohol abuse
    2. Low socio-economic status
    3. Cultural factors
    4. A family history of abuse and authoritarianism

Case 14

Aubrey Hudson and her partner, Christof Peters, are a couple in their 30s who have experienced fertility problems. After taking clomiphene (Clomid) for several months, Ms. Hudson becomes pregnant. An ultrasonogram at 8 weeks' gestation confirms that Ms. Hudson is expecting twins. Ms. Hudson attends a health clinic routinely for prenatal care and counselling.

Questions 62–69 refer to this case.

62. Ms. Hudson is likely expecting fraternal twins. Which of the following is a characteristic of fraternal twins?
    1. A single ovum has divided into two embryos.
    2. They will be the same sex.
    3. They are more likely to occur in younger women.
    4. There are two placentas.

63. During her second trimester, Ms. Hudson asks the practical nurse what to do about constipation. What should be the first action the practical nurse recommends?
    1. Increase fluids, fresh fruits, and vegetables in her diet.
    2. Increase exercise.
    3. Use a natural laxative.
    4. Take a stool softener, such as docusate sodium (Colace).

64. Ms. Hudson will be monitored carefully during the pregnancy because of the previous fertility problems and multiple gestation. She will deliver in hospital rather than the birthing centre. Which of the following is a significant risk for women with fraternal twin pregnancy?
    1. Preterm labour
    2. Twin to twin transfusion

3. Conjoined twins
4. Oligohydramnios

65. During the latter half of the second trimester, situations in the third trimester that require immediately notifying the physician are reviewed with the client. Which of the following would be a danger sign during a pregnancy?
    1. Dyspnea
    2. A weight gain of 0.5–0.75 kg in the third trimester
    3. Leg cramps
    4. Fewer than 10 fetal movements in 12 hours

66. Ms. Hudson has brown eyes, and her partner, Mr. Peters, has blue eyes. Ms. Hudson asks the practical nurse what colour the babies' eyes will be. What should be the practical nurse's response?
    1. Both babies will likely have blue eyes.
    2. Both babies will most likely, but not certainly, have brown eyes.
    3. One baby will have brown eyes, and the other will have blue eyes.
    4. Eye colour is genetically random, and it is not possible to predict.

67. As the pregnancy progresses, Ms. Hudson develops edema in her ankles. What should the practical nurse recommend to reduce the edema?
    1. Fluid restriction
    2. Keeping her legs uncrossed
    3. Elevating her legs
    4. Range-of-motion exercises

68. Ms. Hudson tells the practical nurse that although she is happy to have twins, she is disappointed because she will not be able to breastfeed two infants. What should the nurse respond?
    1. "You could breastfeed one and formula-feed the other."
    2. "Perhaps if you are able to get pregnant again, you could breastfeed the next baby."
    3. "It is very difficult to breastfeed twins, and most women are not successful."
    4. "With planning and extra nourishment, you may be able to breastfeed both infants."

69. At 36 weeks, Ms. Hudson delivers twins by Caesarean section. Each twin has a separate healthcare team in the delivery room. What is the first assessment each nurse would perform with the infants?
    1. Heart rate
    2. Temperature
    3. Respirations
    4. Blood pressure

Case 15

A nursing teacher is assisting student practical nurses who are conducting a blood pressure clinic at a local shopping mall.

Questions 70–72 refer to this case.

70. The nursing teacher instructs a student practical nurse how to correctly perform blood pressure monitoring by auscultation. Which of the following should the teacher demonstrate as the proper technique?

1. Have the client lie down with the arm extended.
2. Use a cuff width that is 80% of the length of the client's upper arm.
3. Quickly inflate the cuff to 10% above the client's expected blood pressure.
4. Place the bell of the stethoscope over the brachial artery.

71. The nursing teacher instructs a student how to perform self–blood pressure monitoring using an electronic device. What would be the most effective evaluation of the teaching?
    1. The student is able to correctly perform blood pressure monitoring on another student.
    2. The student is able to verbalize the correct procedure for blood pressure monitoring.
    3. The student is able to state normal blood pressure values.
    4. The student is able to demonstrate the technique on himself.

72. One of the students takes Mr. Brown's blood pressure using the portable electronic blood pressure monitor and obtains a reading of 186/110 mm Hg. He retakes the blood pressure but obtains the same result. Mr. Brown tells the teacher and the student that although he takes antihypertensives, to his knowledge, his blood pressure has previously been within normal limits. What should be the nursing teacher's first action?
    1. Retake the blood pressure with a manual device.
    2. Ask Mr. Brown to lie down and relax and then take the blood pressure again.
    3. Find out from Mr. Brown which antihypertensive medication he takes.
    4. Replace the batteries in the electronic monitor.

Independent Questions

Questions 73–128 do not refer to a particular case.

73. Which of the following drugs may depress a client's immune system?
    1. Meperidine (Demerol)
    2. Cefazolin (Ancef)
    3. Prednisone (Apo-Prednisone)
    4. Salbutamol (Ventolin)

74. What is the primary reason why practical nurses should be involved in social justice issues?
    1. Socio-economic and political issues have an impact on health.
    2. Social justice will improve the working conditions of practical nurses.
    3. Advocacy is part of the role of the practical nurse.
    4. Politicians will change laws based on nursing input.

75. Ms. Hope, mother of 5-month-old Isabelle, asks the nurse when Isabelle will be able to pull herself to a standing position. What should the practical nurse tell her?
    1. "It should be any time now."
    2. "Infants generally pull themselves up onto furniture at about 6 to 7 months."

3. "Isabelle will probably stand holding onto a table by about 8 to 10 months."
4. "I don't think you should expect Isabelle to stand until about 11 to 12 months."

76. When are antilipidemic medications such as atorvastatin (Lipitor) most appropriately ordered?
    1. In people over 65 years of age
    2. In people who do not exercise sufficiently
    3. In people for whom dietary measures have not lowered cholesterol
    4. In people who have elevated cholesterol for over 2 months

77. Health Canada recommends that all women of child-bearing years take a folic acid supplement. What is the reason for this recommendation?
    1. It helps prevent neural tube defects in the fetus, should the woman become pregnant.
    2. It maximizes the nutritional status of the woman prior to becoming pregnant.
    3. It prevents the occurrence of cleft lip and palate, which occurs early in pregnancy.
    4. It is necessary for the adequate formation of estrogen and progesterone.

78. A community practical nurse is concerned because many of her chronically ill clients do not have a primary care provider. What short-term solution should the practical nurse suggest to the clients?
    1. Advise them to go to the local community walk-in clinic as necessary.
    2. Provide them with a list of all the community physicians for them to call.
    3. Advise them to call the provincial telephone health information line for advice.
    4. Provide the clients with comprehensive health care to the best of her ability.

79. Manifestations of sickle cell disease may include which of the following?
    1. Anemia
    2. Fever
    3. Vomiting
    4. Bradycardia

80. Ms. Blatchberg has leukopenia. Which of the following should the nurse include in client teaching?
    1. Her gums may bleed when she brushes her teeth.
    2. She should try to eat green leafy vegetables.
    3. She should ensure she receives the influenza vaccine.
    4. She should avoid people with communicable diseases.

81. Mr. Skinner has sustained a C6 spinal cord injury and has developed autonomic dysreflexia. Which of the following is the most common precipitating cause of autonomic dysreflexia?
    1. Distended bladder or rectum
    2. Nasal congestion
    3. High dietary fibre
    4. Low blood pressure

82. Ms. Benjamin, age 52 years, is scheduled for an elective hysterectomy. She has a prosthetic mitral valve and was

advised by her physician to discontinue her daily dose of Aspirin (ASA) prior to surgery. What property of Aspirin forms the rationale for this action?

1. Analgesic
2. Antipyretic
3. Anti-inflammatory
4. Antiplatelet

83. A practical nurse reviews client data when she arrives on shift. She notes that one of her clients, Mr. Barry, routinely takes Advair, which is a combined inhaled steroid and bronchodilator. Which of the following would be a priority assessment for the nurse to perform on Mr. Barry?

1. Cardiovascular
2. Gastro-intestinal
3. Neurological
4. Respiratory

84. Which of the following would be the correct procedure when taking the blood pressure of a hypertensive client who is monitored at the clinic once a week?

1. Ensure that the client has not had caffeine within the last 5 hours.
2. Allow the client to rest for 5 minutes prior to taking the blood pressure.
3. Use manual rather than electronic blood pressure devices.
4. Alternate arms for each visit.

85. Ms. Brette is voluntarily admitted, on a short-term basis, to a psychiatric unit for management of her anxiety disorder. She experiences a severe anxiety attack while she is in the client lounge. What should the practical nurse do?

1. Comfort Ms. Brette by holding and hugging her.
2. Move Ms. Brette closer to other clients.
3. Administer her ordered prn lorazepam (Ativan).
4. Take her to her room.

86. A practical nurse is on an airplane flight and is asked to come to the aid of a fellow passenger. The practical nurse assesses a man who is approximately in his 60s, diaphoretic, and complaining of severe pain in his chest. What should be the nurse's first action?

1. Tell airline staff the passenger may be having a heart attack.
2. Ask the man if he has any history of heart disease.
3. Take the man's vital signs with equipment provided by the airline.
4. Administer oxygen via passenger mask.

87. A practical nurse receives a telephone call from her neighbour Mrs. Dunlop, who tells the practical nurse that her husband is experiencing chest pain and is sweating. Which of the following should the practical nurse recommend?

1. Call 9-1-1.
2. Call 9-1-1 and give her husband an Aspirin (ASA) if available.
3. Call 9-1-1 and place her husband in a knee-chest position.
4. Call 9-1-1 and cover her husband with a blanket.

88. Dina Shpak, age 54, has chronic stable angina pectoris. Her physician orders nitroglycerine in the form of a spray (Nitrolingual sublingual spray). The practical nurse teaches Mrs. Shpak about the use of the spray. Which of the following should she include in teaching?

1. The aerosol should be inhaled as she takes a deep breath.
2. If she experiences headache, she should immediately notify the physician.
3. She will experience pain relief in approximately 30 minutes.
4. The spray should be taken before exercise or stressful physical activity.

89. Mrs. Wiesenthal, a client on a chronic care rehabilitation unit, has a positive test for *Clostridium difficile* (*C. difficile*). What organism-specific manifestation is she most likely to experience?

1. Fever
2. Vomiting
3. Chills
4. Diarrhea

90. After many years of symptoms and diagnostic tests, Ms. Drummond has been diagnosed with fibromyalgia. Which of the following is characteristic of this condition?

1. It is primarily a psychiatric diagnosis.
2. There is no effective treatment.
3. There are neither manifestations nor diagnostics specific to the disease.
4. Pain and fatigue become progressively worse.

91. A practical nurse wishes to join an organization to protest social and economic inequality. Another nurse asks what this has to do with health. What is the practical nurse's best response?

1. Economics is a social determinant of health.
2. People at the lower end of the socio-economic scale have proven poorer health than those at the upper end.
3. Health care must be equal and available to all.
4. Nurses have an obligation to be advocates for all levels of society.

92. Mr. Hardacre has just returned to the surgical unit following tracheotomy surgery. What is the priority nursing action?

1. Observing for hemorrhage
2. Maintaining a patent airway
3. Performing frequent suctioning
4. Taking vital signs

93. Mr. Scott is diagnosed with hepatitis A after returning from a tropical vacation. He asks the practical nurse how he got the virus. What should the practical nurse respond?

1. "Did you have any sexual encounters when you were on vacation?"
2. "Because of the air circulation in planes, it is likely you got the virus on the flight."
3. "Hepatitis A is endemic to tropical countries."

4. "You most likely ingested contaminated food or water."

94. A practical nurse finds that she has difficulty sleeping after working a 12-hour night shift and feels chronically sleep-deprived. Which of the following may be a recommendation to help her obtain more sleep?
    1. Eat a main meal consisting of high protein and low fat toward the end of the night shift.
    2. Wear dark sunglasses before leaving work after her night shift.
    3. Perform aerobic exercise for 30 minutes after working the night shift.
    4. Advocate for a minimum of 12 hours off between rotating from night to day shift.

95. Mrs. Bedford, the mother of 4-month-old Garth, asks the practical nurse, "Which of my son's teeth are going to come in first?" What should the practical nurse respond?
    1. The upper two teeth, the frontal incisors
    2. The bottom two teeth, the central incisors
    3. The two "eye teeth," or canine teeth
    4. His primary molars

96. The practical nurse notes that Mr. Varcoe's nasogastric tube has not drained for several hours, and his abdomen appears distended. What should be the practical nurse's first action?
    1. Irrigate the tube.
    2. Instill saline in the tube.
    3. Remove the tube.
    4. Notify the physician.

97. Ms. Bacci is 10 weeks' gestation with her third pregnancy. She tells the practical nurse, "I make big babies. My other two were over 10 pounds when they were born." What screening test, related to this statement, would be most appropriate for Ms. Bacci?
    1. Fasting blood glucose
    2. Amniocentesis
    3. Maternal nutrition analysis
    4. Pelvimetry

98. A family visits the child health clinic. The father tells the practical nurse, "I have read on several Web sites that there is scientific evidence vaccines are not effective, so I will not consent to immunizing my child." What would be the best response by the practical nurse?
    1. "Has your child, or any child you know, ever had a serious adverse effect after an immunization?"
    2. "Do you have any cultural, religious, or personal beliefs regarding immunization?"
    3. "Which vaccines have you read about that are not effective?"
    4. "I agree there is much conflicting information. Can you tell me more about what you read?"

99. Ann Atkins's mother died several years ago of ovarian cancer at age 48. Ann is now 25 years old. Although she is healthy and is manifesting no symptoms of cancer, what screening test should she be advised to have?

1. Transvaginal ultrasonography
2. Mammography and clinical breast examination
3. Chest X-ray
4. Blood test for tumour marker CA-125

100. A pregnant woman has just received results indicating that she is HIV-positive. She says to the practical nurse, "How am I going to tell my boyfriend that I have AIDS?" What is the most appropriate response by the practical nurse?
    1. "Is there a chance you got HIV from your boyfriend?"
    2. "You do not have AIDS; let's talk about being HIV-positive."
    3. "It is more important at this time to think about protecting your baby from HIV."
    4. "He will have to know you are HIV-positive; let's talk about how to tell him."

101. A practical nurse works in a multilingual environment. In many instances, he cannot communicate with his clients and knows he is not providing optimal care. What is the practical nurse's best action for a long-term solution to this problem?
    1. Communicate to all clients to bring a family member to interpret.
    2. Advocate for the purchase of English translation dictionaries for the most common languages.
    3. As part of his reflective practice, enroll in classes to learn the most common languages.
    4. Speak with the agency representative regarding purchase of an on-site telephone or video link interpreter service.

102. A practical nurse who works in a corrections facility has been called as a witness for an inquest into the death of an inmate. What is the purpose of a medical inquest?
    1. To determine criminal liability in an unexpected medical event
    2. To determine civil liability in a suspicious death
    3. To prosecute persons or agencies suspected of neglect with regard to their clients
    4. To make recommendations to improve the healthcare system in the future

103. Which of the following people, according to their body shape and body mass index (BMI), have the highest risk of cardiovascular disease (CVD) and type 2 diabetes?
    1. Mark: apple shape, BMI 24
    2. Consuelo: apple shape, BMI 31
    3. Pedro: pear shape, BMI 27
    4. Christa: pear shape, BMI 18

104. Aisha has anorexia nervosa. She has severely restricted fat in her diet. If Aisha were to eat 12 g of fat and a total of 1 100 kcal per day, what percentage of her daily intake would be from fat?
    1. 8%
    2. 10%
    3. 12%
    4. 15%

105. Mrs. Carnegy is hospitalized for pneumonia. She tells the practical nurse that she would like to continue to take peppermint, an herbal preparation, which she finds is effective for her irritable bowel syndrome (IBS). What should the nurse do?
    1. Consult with the healthcare team to see if they agree to include peppermint in the plan of care.
    2. Tell Mrs. Carnegy that herbal preparations cannot be administered while she is in hospital.
    3. Agree to provide Mrs. Carnegy with peppermint, as it is a recognized complementary therapy.
    4. Recommend that Mrs. Carnegy consult with her physician about other prescription medications that may be more effective than peppermint.

106. A practical nurse visits an older adults' residence in northern Saskatchewan. What would be an important safety precaution the practical nurse should suggest to the residents?
    1. Stay inside during icy winter days.
    2. Place area rugs on bare floors.
    3. Use a stove to warm food rather than microwave ovens.
    4. Take over-the-counter cough preparations at the first sign of a chest cold.

107. What is the most conclusive screening test for colorectal cancer?
    1. Fecal occult blood
    2. Sigmoidoscopy
    3. Colonoscopy
    4. Barium enema

108. A 2-year-old child in respiratory distress has the following physician order: "Give oxygen by face mask to keep the O_2 saturation above 95%." The nurse notes that the oxygen saturation has fallen to 80%. What should be the initial action by the practical nurse?
    1. Double-check the order with the physician.
    2. Administer additional oxygen.
    3. Arrange for arterial blood gases to confirm the O_2 saturation reading.
    4. Perform a chest assessment.

109. Mr. Patrick has had seasonal allergies for many years. Recently he has found his usual over-the-counter allergy medication is not working as effectively. He asks the nurse what he should do. What would the practical nurse initially suggest?
    1. Speak with his pharmacist.
    2. Make an appointment with the nurse practitioner.
    3. Arrange for allergy testing with a medical allergist.
    4. Discuss environmental controls with a respiratory therapist.

110. Mr. Price is admitted to hospital for investigation of abdominal pain. The practical nurse notes that one of Mr. Price's medications is clozapine (Clozaril), an antipsychotic. What action should the nurse take prior to administration of the Clozaril?
    1. Ask Mr. Price why he is taking an antipsychotic medication.
    2. Look in the chart for information related to why he is on an antipsychotic drug.
    3. Perform an orientation to reality assessment on Mr. Price.
    4. Ensure that safety measures are in place prior to entering his room with the medication.

111. What is a frequent complaint of older adults who are beginning to experience age-related hearing loss?
    1. Ringing in the ears
    2. Other people mumbling when they talk
    3. Not being able to hear men's voices
    4. Not being able to hear themselves speaking

112. Mr. Braham has been on the rehabilitation unit for 2 days. He has been identified by the nurses as being a "demanding" client. He rings the call bell frequently for what are felt to be minor concerns and complains he is not receiving enough attention. When Mr. Braham calls for his nurse the fourth time within 1 hour, what is the best intervention by the nurse?
    1. Tell Mr. Braham that he is not allowed to ring the call bell more often than once an hour, unless it is an emergency.
    2. Sit with Mr. Braham and ask him to describe his feelings and concerns.
    3. Alternate care with the other nurse on duty so that he feels he is receiving more attention.
    4. Set limits by telling Mr. Braham his physical condition does not require the attention he is demanding and his behaviour is not appropriate.

113. Mr. Hill is a caregiver for his wife, Verna, who has dementia. He expresses frustration to the nurse because of difficulties communicating with Verna. What communication technique would be most effective for the practical nurse to suggest to Mr. Hill?
    1. Speak slowly and loudly.
    2. Use written rather than verbal communication.
    3. Speak in short, simple sentences.
    4. Repeat phrases several times.

114. Ms. Enright, a client newly admitted to a mental health facility, says to the practical nurse, "Do you have a boyfriend?" What is the most appropriate response by the nurse?
    1. "Let's talk about you. Do you have a boyfriend?"
    2. "I am not allowed to tell you about my personal life."
    3. "Yes I do. We have been together for three wonderful years."
    4. "This interview is about you, not me."

115. Mr. Dovgan has just been admitted to the neurology unit. Mr. Dovgan is recovering from a brain injury and also has unstable bipolar disorder. When the practical nurse enters the room to assess Mr. Dovgan, he says to her, "Get out of here or I am going to kill you." What should be the primary action by the practical nurse?
    1. Document and report to the nurse in charge the facts of the verbal abuse and threat.
    2. Recognize that the behaviour is related to Mr. Dovgan's diagnosis and not take the abuse personally.

3. Implement safety strategies to protect herself.

4. Obtain support from nursing colleagues who are involved in Mr. Dovgan's care.

116. A practical nurse works at a suicide prevention telephone hotline. Which of the following callers would the practical nurse consider to be most at risk for suicide?

1. Lindsay, age 16, who says she is going to buy razor blades to cut her wrists

2. Ahmet, age 21, who tells the nurse he is going to use his gun to shoot himself

3. Florence, a 40-year-old woman who expresses the desire to overdose on antidepressants but has agreed to go to the hospital

4. Fred, an older adult who is recently widowed and says he no longer wants to live

117. Mrs. Scales is a resident of a long-term care facility. She has advanced dementia, no spontaneous mobility, and severe contractures of her hands. The family asks how often splints are applied to her hands. What is the most appropriate response by the practical nurse to their question?

1. The splints are ordered to be applied for 4 hours a day.

2. The physiotherapist has recommended the splints be applied 4 hours a day.

3. I have just assessed Mrs. Scales, and she has the splints on.

4. The practical nurse's documentation shows the splints are applied 4 hours a day from 8 in the morning to noon.

118. The practical nurse is planning a teaching session about nutrition with a group of children. What must the practical nurse initially assess prior to the teaching session?

1. What the children know about nutrition

2. What the children normally eat

3. What the developmental level of the children is

4. What the learning outcomes should be from the session

119. Douglas, age 3, has recently been diagnosed with autism. What is a priority goal for Douglas's development?

1. Provision of appropriate pharmacological treatment

2. Intensive early intervention and education therapy

3. Referral to a pediatric psychiatrist

4. Safety assessment of the home

120. Antonia Chaley, age 6, experiences frequent epistaxis, particularly in cold, dry weather. What should the practical nurse advise Antonia and her parents for first aid treatment?

1. Pinch both nostrils closed just below the nasal bone and hold for 10 to 15 minutes.

2. Tilt the head back and hold the bridge of the nose.

3. Blow the nose gently and repeatedly until the bleeding stops.

4. Pack the nose with tissue or cotton balls.

121. Martina is a preceptor for a practical nursing student in her final clinical placement. The student has difficulty finishing her work before the end of the shift and has not been able to accurately assess client acuity. Martina has never been a preceptor before. What should be her initial action to address the situation with the student?

1. Discuss with the student her learning goals, present performance, and past experience.

2. Consult with the faculty advisor concerning the expected level of performance for students in the final clinical placement.

3. Discuss the student's performance with the unit nurse educator.

4. Refer to written material, provided by the nursing school, concerning student and preceptor expectations.

122. Ms. San explains to Ms. Ryerson, a practical nurse at a health clinic, that she has always taken ibuprofen (Advil) for aches, pains, and mild headaches but now finds that it bothers her stomach. Which of the following medications could be considered as an alternative?

1. Naproxen (Aleve)

2. Celecoxib (Celebrex)

3. Acetaminophen (Tylenol)

4. Acetylsalicylic Acid (Aspirin)

123. Liam Douglas is receiving intravenous (IV) fluids of 0.9% sodium chloride at 40 mL per hour. His practical nurse must hang a 2-L bag of IV fluid as no smaller bags are available. The practical nurse is not certain how long he can safely leave the bag hanging before he changes it. What is the most appropriate action by the nurse?

1. Change the bag of IV solution after 24 hours.

2. Label the date and time of hanging the bag.

3. Consult agency policies regarding IV solution "hang times."

4. Change the bag when it is empty.

124. A moderately active female requires 18 kcal per 0.45 kg to maintain an ideal weight. How many kilocalories would a 56.7 kg woman require per day?

1. 1 021 kcal

2. 1 936 kcal

3. 2 268　kcal

4. 2 420 kcal

125. Following hip replacement surgery, Ms. Cakebread, age 92, develops pneumonia. She is receiving intravenous antibiotics and oxygen via a nasal cannula. Which of the following manifestations would be of most concern to her practical nurse?

1. Respiratory rate of 20 breaths per minute

2. Productive cough

3. Restlessness

4. Arterial pO_2 of 90 mm Hg

ANSWERS AND RATIONALES FOR BOOK TWO

The correct answer is set off in boldface.

1. **C: Foundations of Practice T: Application**

1. **As death approaches, the skin becomes cool, clammy, and mottled due to diminished circulation.**

2. Respirations are often rapid and shallow, progressing to Cheyne-Stokes respirations.

3. The pulse becomes weak, but the rate does not increase.

4. Although the skin feels cool to the touch, body temperature often increases prior to death.

2. **C: Professional, Ethical, and Legal Practice T: Critical Thinking**

1. **The practical nurse will need to perform all the listed actions. Because the family is right there, the first action is to confirm for them that Mrs. Haliburton has passed away. It would be inappropriate to document or make calls before speaking with the family. He can offer them time alone with the body while he performs other duties.**

2. The practical nurse must do this after speaking with the family.

3. As in choice 2.

4. As in choice 2.

3. **C: Professional, Ethical, and Legal Practice T: Critical Thinking**

1. The health record does not belong to the family.

2. The physician is part of the palliative care team. He does not own the health record.

3. **The healthcare record belongs to the agency, in this case, the agency that employs the palliative care team. The practical nurse must take the record to the agency for legally specified storage.**

4. This is not legal. Records must be maintained by the agency for a length of time as specified in legislation.

4. **C: Professional, Ethical, and Legal Practice T: Application**

1. **The morphine is the legal property of the Haliburtons. They have no means to dispose of it safely. Pharmacies will safely dispose of unused medications.**

2. The practical nurse should not be transporting narcotics. This is not a practical nursing responsibility.

3. It is not optimum for a narcotic to be disposed of in a biohazard container.

4. This is not safe advice. One person should not use medications prescribed for someone else.

5. **C: Professional, Ethical, and Legal Practice T: Application**

1. **The practical nurse's initial action should be to reflect on his coping mechanisms for grief and whether they have been effective in the past. Once he has analyzed his reactions, he may choose one of the other options.**

2. This may be an option after self-reflection.

3. Reflection may determine a need to change to another specialty.

4. This is not likely to be necessary at this stage, only if the practical nurse experiences further emotional difficulties.

6. **C: Foundations of Practice T: Application**

1. **Nitrates are first-line therapy for treatment of acute anginal symptoms. They will dilate peripheral blood vessels and coronary arteries, increasing blood flow to the heart.**

2. Beta adrenergic blockers reduce the heart rate and contractility and reduce afterload. They are not first-line drugs in emergency angina care.

3. This would be given only if the presence of thrombi were confirmed.

4. Angiotensin-converting enzyme inhibitors are useful with heart failure, tachycardia, myocardial infarction, and hypertension. They are not first-line drugs for stable angina.

7. **C: Foundations of Practice T: Critical Thinking**

1. A chest X-ray will be taken to assess cardiac enlargement, cardiac calcification, and pulmonary congestion. It does not allow for visualization of the coronary arteries.

2. Cardiac ultrasonography is not of significant use with angina.

3. An ECG is obtained to determine abnormalities of electrical function in the heart. In Mr. Cetaine's case, it will likely be used to rule out myocardial infarction but does not confirm the extent of angina.

4. **Coronary angiography allows visualization of the coronary arteries and helps determine appropriate treatment.**

8. **C: Foundations of Practice T: Knowledge**

1. **The construction of new conduits beyond the coronary obstruction restores blood flow to the myocardium.**

2. CABG cannot repair damage to the myocardium but can help prevent further damage.

3. CABG provides new blood vessels to the myocardium, not the right atrium.

4. The obstruction is in the coronary artery, not the aorta.

9. **C: Foundations of Practice T: Application**

1. Complete bed rest is rarely indicated postsurgery as it is likely to increase postoperative complications. Mr. Cetaine likely would be permitted to gradually resume a limited degree of activity.

2. **CABG requires a graft from another site, most often the saphenous vein, internal mammary artery, or radial artery; thus, there would be a chest and a graft site.**

3. Oxygen will be ordered according to oxygen saturations. It may not necessarily be required.

4. Pain management is important, particularly if there is a thoracotomy. Narcotics are used; however, they are administered around the clock, not prn.

10. **C: Professional, Ethical, and Legal Practice T: Critical Thinking**

1. **The primary purpose of documentation is to communicate client information among care providers.**

Documentation is communication that reflects the client's health and well-being, the care provided, the effect of care, and the continuity of care. All healthcare providers need ongoing access to client information to provide safe and effective care and treatment.

2. Documentation does demonstrate nursing accountability and gives credit to nurses for their professional practice. However, the primary purpose is to communicate information about the client.

3. Health records can be a valuable source of data for research and quality assurance purposes; however, this is not the primary purpose.

4. Data from nursing documentation can identify the care and services provided to clients and the efficiency of the care. However, this is not the primary purpose of documentation.

11. **C: Professional, Ethical, and Legal Practice T: Application**
    1. The agency does own the health record, but the client has the right of access to the information, not just in exceptional circumstances.
    2. The client does not own the record. Consent for disclosure to agency staff for purposes related to care is implied upon admission.
    3. Only the agency owns the record.
    4. **When care is provided by an agency, the actual record belongs to that agency. With very few exceptions, clients have right of access to their own records. Agencies generally have policies about what to do if clients ask for their charts.**

12. **C: Professional, Ethical, and Legal Practice T: Application**
    1. The term *nurse* is applied only to registered/licensed individuals. Although student nurses are not yet registered/licensed, and there may be others who have not yet received confirmation of registration/licence, those people must document the care they provide.
    2. **This is the exception. The nurse who documents the care provided by another nurse in such situations would have been involved and have had personal knowledge of the situation. This most frequently occurs in emergency or "code" situations, in which one nurse may be designated as the recorder.**
    3. This is not true. Both nurses are required to document the care they provided.
    4. There is an exception, as noted in choice 2.

13. **C: Professional, Ethical, and Legal Practice T: Application**
    1. This is a judgement and not fact.
    2. As in choice 1.
    3. **This is an accurate description of the facts concerning Ms. Scharfe's behaviour. Information should be recorded concisely and accurately and focus on facts rather than assumptions.**
    4. This entry is too wordy and makes assumptions.

14. **C: Foundations of Practice T: Critical Thinking**
    1. **Alcohol withdrawal delirium, or delirium tremens (DTs), may lead to death caused by hyperthermia, peripheral vascular collapse, and cardiac failure.**
    2. This does not occur in alcohol withdrawal.
    3. Seizures may occur but are not as serious as cardiac failure.
    4. The client in alcohol withdrawal is unlikely to be able to commit suicide.

15. **C: Foundations of Practice T: Application**
    1. This is not likely. He would be aware of his drinking.
    2. This is not a therapeutic response.
    3. **This is a factual response. It may help Mrs. Martin understand the disease and that support, although not acceptance, will be most helpful to her husband's recovery.**
    4. Alcohol is a strong addiction; however, if Mr. Martin wishes to stop drinking, he has the ability to help himself.

16. **C: Foundations of Practice T: Knowledge**
    1. This is a test for liver enzymes.
    2. **Bilirubin metabolism abnormalities with cirrhosis are responsible for the deposit of yellow pigment in the skin (jaundice).**
    3. As in choice 1.
    4. Prothrombin time is a reflection of clotting factors.

17. **C: Foundations of Practice T: Critical Thinking**
    1. This does not explain why Mr. Martin is yellow.
    2. This is too complex an answer for Mrs. Martin.
    3. **This is the correct physiological rationale for the jaundice and is at a level that Mrs. Martin can understand.**
    4. This is not physiologically correct.

18. **C: Foundations of Practice T: Application**
    1. **Cirrhosis interferes with the liver's ability to eliminate ammonia. Protein is converted to ammonia; therefore, Mr. Martin requires a low-protein diet. This breakfast is low in protein.**
    2. This is a high-protein meal.
    3. This is a high-protein meal.
    4. This is a high-protein meal.

19. **C: Foundations of Practice T: Application**
    1. There is no reason to assume that Mr. Martin is not cognitively able to make his own treatment decisions.
    2. **This is a factual answer. Giving Mr. Martin Antabuse without his consent is unethical.**
    3. This implies that an unethical practice is condoned and that the nurse is not sure of the legal and ethical implications.
    4. This is an unprofessional and unethical response.

20. **C: Foundations of Practice T: Application**
    1. **Aspirin can trigger asthma attacks in 20% of adults.**
    2. There are no contraindications for the use of acetaminophen in clients with asthma.
    3. There are no contraindications for the use of ibuprofen in clients with asthma.

4. Many people with asthma have seasonal allergies and use antihistamines such as loratadine for symptom control. These drugs are not contraindicated except during an acute attack.

21. **C: Foundations of Practice T: Application**
    1. Beta$_2$-agonists do not decrease airway inflammation.
    2. Inhaled steroids do not decrease bronchoconstriction.
    3. **The long-acting beta2-agonist provides bronchodilation for up to 12 hours. The inhaled steroid decreases inflammation. Combining the two medications provides a convenient dosing regimen for the client.**
    4. The medications do not potentiate each other, nor is it necessary to combine the drugs in one inhaler to provide longer-acting symptom control.

22. **C: Foundations of Practice T: Application**
    1. Inhaled medications are the preferred therapy for asthma. Other forms are not as effective and may have increased side effects.
    2. As in choice 1.
    3. **Many people have difficulty using the MDI properly. A spacer is a tube that attaches to the MDI. Drugs are inhaled from the tube, resulting in better delivery of the medications into the airway.**
    4. This is a possibility; however, the use of a spacer is easier for Mr. Lewis and is most likely to be successful.

23. **C: Foundations of Practice T: Critical Thinking**
    1. The combination drugs need to be taken to stabilize and control chronic symptoms. They are not effective during an acute attack.
    2. Mr. Lewis may need to do this if the rescue inhaler is not effective.
    3. This is of value in croup but will not produce the bronchodilation necessary during an asthma attack.
    4. **Short-acting bronchodilators (also known as "rescue" medications) provide temporary relief of bronchospasm and should help restore normal breathing within 10 to 15 minutes. Another puff may be taken if optimum breathing does not resume.**

24. **C: Professional, Ethical, and Legal Practice T: Application**
    1. Any healthcare worker who provides care to Mr. Fraser has access to the record.
    2. Only healthcare providers who are caring for Mr. Fraser have access to his record.
    3. **These people are legally entitled to view the health record. While clerical staff may not be considered healthcare workers, they must view the chart in order to insert and maintain the information.**
    4. This is unrealistic. The family practice clinic is responsible for initiating and maintaining relevant information and maintaining confidentiality. Mr. Fraser may have copies if he wishes.

25. **C: Foundations of Practice T: Critical Thinking**
    1. **There is a familial risk for close relatives of people who have been diagnosed with colorectal cancer. Ms. Masseur should have a screening colonoscopy to rule out tumours and identify colon polyps.**

2. Hemorrhoids are not a risk for colorectal cancer. Screening colonoscopies are recommended for people age 50 and older.
3. Irritable bowel syndrome has manifestations similar to colorectal cancer but has not been shown to be a risk for developing cancer.
4. This gene mutation contributes primarily to the development of breast and ovarian cancers. There is an increased incidence of familial colorectal cancer and breast or ovarian cancer, but Ms. Daniels will likely not require a colonoscopy screening as yet.

26. **C: Foundations of Practice T: Application**
    1. While this is true, it does not answer Miss Shannon's question.
    2. **If Miss Shannon asks the clinic to put her on the cancellation list, she may be able to take a spot that opens up, allowing her to have the scan earlier.**
    3. This is true, but Miss Shannon may be able to have the test earlier if she accesses the cancellation list.
    4. This may not be true and does not advocate for Miss Shannon to be involved with her plan of care.

27. **C: Professional, Ethical, and Legal Practice T: Critical Thinking**
    1. This is correct but does not answer Mr. Gold's question.
    2. Although practical nurses should follow best practice guidelines, this does not answer Mr. Gold's question.
    3. This is partially correct, but this should have been assessed prior to injecting Mr. Gold.
    4. **This answers Mr. Gold's question and provides a rationale for action.**

28. **C: Foundations of Practice T: Application**
    1. Mr. Rutlege's temperature is within normal limits. A blanket may be used for comfort if he wishes but is not necessary.
    2. The oxygen saturation is within normal limits. There is no reason to increase the oxygen.
    3. **The vital signs are within normal limits for a postoperative client and should be monitored as per protocol.**
    4. There is no reason to contact the physician.

29. **C: Foundations of Practice T: Application**
    1. **An adult's urinary output should be a minimum of 30 mL per hour. Urinary output below this level may indicate inadequate perfusion of the kidneys, or urinary retention.**
    2. This is normal following abdominal surgery.
    3. This is a normal finding postsurgery.
    4. This is a normal finding.

30. **C: Foundations of Practice T: Application**
    1. There should not be any bubbling in the chamber. This indicates a leak.
    2. **Taping connections prevents accidental disconnection.**
    3. Sterile water is added only as necessary to replace evaporation.
    4. The system should be maintained below waist level.

31. **C: Foundations of Practice T: Knowledge**
    1. Type and cross-matching determines more than Rh information.
    2. Type and cross-matching determines more than ABO information.
    3. Type and cross-matching determines more than ABO information.
    4. **Type and cross-matching provides a complete blood profile to determine the compatibility with donor blood.**

32. **C: Foundations of Practice T: Critical Thinking**
    1. He may be able to explain the care but not able to actually perform care.
    2. **This is the most appropriate method to evaluate his ability to care for the incision.**
    3. This does not demonstrate competence.
    4. This does not demonstrate competence. Most clients will not want to admit that they do not understand instructions and so may tell the practical nurse they do not have questions.

33. **C: Foundations of Practice T: Critical Thinking**
    1. **With a fall from a height, there is the danger of head injury. In view of the fact that Sam is moaning, and therefore can breathe, and there is no evidence of critical hemorrhaging from the small cut, the most important assessment is for signs of head injury.**
    2. This assessment would be made after assessing for head injury.
    3. Because Sam is crying, this is evidence that he has an adequate, although likely elevated, pulse. The pulse should be taken, but it is not the priority.
    4. These should be assessed after the level of consciousness.

34. **C: Foundations of Practice T: Critical Thinking**
    1. This is not appropriate if there is a fracture as it may cause further injury.
    2. The injured limb should be moved as little as possible.
    3. **The initial practical nursing efforts are directed at calming the child. It is best not to touch children initially but to ask them to point to the painful area.**
    4. Sam will be frightened and upset. Applying pressure to the area will cause unnecessary pain and make the remainder of the assessment difficult.

35. **C: Foundations of Practice T: Critical Thinking**
    1. It is better to immobilize the limb and joint in a rigid rather than a soft splint.
    2. **A rolled magazine may be used for a young child to form a rigid splint to keep the ankle in alignment and prevent further injury, especially to soft tissues.**
    3. This can be done if no splint is available.
    4. This can be done, but it is more important to immobilize the area of fracture.

36. **C: Foundations of Practice T: Knowledge**
    1. **In this situation, the diagnosis can be easily and most cost-effectively determined with an X-ray.**

    2. A bone scan is isotope imaging and is not required for what is believed to be a simple fracture.
    3. Bone densitometry is used to determine osteoporosis.
    4. A CT scan is not necessary for a fractured limb.

37. **C: Foundations of Practice T: Application**
    1. This will slow the drying process. The cast may be put in plastic after it is dry for purposes of bathing the child.
    2. **A plaster of Paris cast does not fully dry for up to 72 hours. Until then, it must be left exposed to the air to speed the drying process.**
    3. The cast should be handled with the palms of the hands rather than the fingers to prevent indentations.
    4. Dryers are not to be used because they may cause the cast to dry on the outside but remain wet on the inside, thus becoming mouldy.

38. **C: Foundations of Practice T: Knowledge**
    1. **Osteoarthritis is a joint disorder primarily affecting weight-bearing joints such as the knees.**
    2. The onset of osteoarthritis is more gradual.
    3. This occurs with osteomyelitis.
    4. Paraesthesia, or a "pins and needles" feeling, occurs more often in rheumatoid arthritis.

39. **C: Foundations of Practice T: Critical Thinking**
    1. Ms. Wilmot may not be able to change her job as she needs the health insurance benefits.
    2. **A modifiable factor in Ms. Wilmot's osteoarthritis is reducing the weight on her knees.**
    3. There is no evidence that Ms. Wilmot needs assistance in caring for her son.
    4. Ms. Wilmot obtains exercise by walking her postal route. She more likely may need rest during a period of acute inflammation.

40. **C: Foundations of Practice T: Application**
    1. These are used for muscle spasms, not osteoarthritis.
    2. **NSAIDs have been shown to provide greater relief than acetaminophen (Tylenol) in clients with knee pain from osteoarthritis.**
    3. Antibiotics are not useful in osteoarthritis.
    4. NSAIDs provide greater pain relief than does acetaminophen (Tylenol).

41. **C: Collaborative Practice T: Critical Thinking**
    1. Unless Ms. Wilmot experiences difficulties or lack of therapeutic effect with her medications, there is no need for a pharmacist.
    2. A naturopath would not necessarily be part of the team unless requested by Ms. Wilmot.
    3. There is no evidence that at present Ms. Wilmot requires the services of a social worker.
    4. **Physiotherapy is useful in planning appropriate exercise programs and recommending necessary assistive devices.**

42. **C: Foundations of Practice T: Critical Thinking**
    1. **Pregnancy-induced hypertension occurs after 20 weeks' gestation, more frequently in high-risk pregnancies. It can result in pre-eclampsia and eclampsia, which are dangerous to the mother and the fetus.**

2. This is an indication of diabetes that is not controlled. The practical nurse would be testing for protein in the urine, a sign of pre-eclampsia.

3. This is important but not as vital as the blood pressure determination.

4. This may be important as an indication of fetal well-being but is not as important as the blood pressure.

43. **C: Foundations of Practice T: Knowledge**

1. Hospitalization is not necessary. Bed rest has proven to be controversial and may have adverse physiological outcomes.

2. **Most women with mild pre-eclampsia may be managed at home with restricted activity and mild exercise.**

3. Because pregnant women with hypertension have lower plasma volume than do normotensive women, sodium restriction is not necessary.

4. Magnesium sulphate is used to prevent or control convulsions in women with eclampsia. It is not necessary in mild pre-eclampsia.

44. **C: Foundations of Practice T: Application**

1. **These are signs of more severe pre-eclampsia.**

2. Constipation is not related to pre-eclampsia.

3. This may be a sign of early labour, not pre-eclampsia.

4. These are signs of early labour, not pre-eclampsia.

45. **C: Foundations of Practice T: Critical Thinking**

1. This is mandatory prior to all client care, not specific to clients with HIV.

2. Gloves are not necessary unless the nurse is handling blood or body fluids.

3. **Ross is at risk of infection and thus must have restricted contact with persons who have infections.**

4. This may be an appropriate question later on during the appointment, particularly as adolescents are often nonadherent to taking medications. It is not important initially.

46. **C: Foundations of Practice T: Application**

1. **Weight loss and a decrease in growth are potential complications in children with HIV/AIDS. Weight loss may also be part of normal adolescence. The initial question for data collection should be to determine the reason for the weight loss.**

2. It may be that the weight loss is due to diarrhea, but this should not be the initial question.

3. This is insensitive and may not be true.

4. While a relatively high percentage of Canadian children are considered obese, this is not an appropriate comment to make with an HIV-positive client.

47. **C: Foundations of Practice T: Application**

1. **At Ross's age, he will have normal age-related concerns about sexuality. He needs to have anticipatory education about safe, healthy expressions of sexuality considering his HIV status.**

2. There is no indication that Ross is experiencing pain.

3. At age 14, if Ross has had HIV for his entire life, he is likely well aware of the modes of transmission.

4. This may be appropriate, but Ross has not indicated to the practical nurse that he is experiencing stress.

48. **C: Foundations of Practice T: Application**

1. Guidelines for the use of antiretroviral agents in HIV-infected adults and adolescents recommend that asymptomatic HIV-positive clients should be treated.

2. **Because rates of disease progression differ among individuals, treatment decisions should be individualized by the level of risk indicated by CD4 T-cell counts and plasma HIV RNA levels.**

3. The most effective means to suppress HIV replication is by combination antiretroviral therapy.

4. Many drugs are available for pediatric use.

49. **C: Professional Practice T: Application**

1. Ross is not an emancipated minor.

2. In many cases, foster parents are not legal guardians and may not provide consent.

3. **The nurse must know agency policies that will provide specific direction for investigational drugs and age of consent.**

4. The physician is recommending the treatment; thus, it is the doctor's responsibility to provide the necessary information.

50. **C: Foundations of Practice T: Application**

1. A tourniquet helps the nurse practitioner examine the antecubital fossa to select a suitable vein but is not necessary.

2. **Placement of a PICC line is performed under sterile conditions with preparation of the insertion site according to institution policy.**

3. There is no need for light anaesthesia. A topical anaesthetic cream is usually used at the insertion site.

4. A PICC line is not inserted in the subclavian vein.

51. **C: Foundations of Practice T: Application**

1. **An X-ray is necessary to confirm placement of the catheter in the superior vena cava prior to administration of the TPN.**

2. Education is appropriate before insertion of the PICC line, not after.

3. The solutions are to be refrigerated until 30 minutes before use. Leaving the solutions at room temperature for longer encourages microbial growth.

4. The solutions are prepared by the agency pharmacy, and nursing staff make no additions.

52. **C: Foundations of Practice T: Application**

1. Once established for TPN, a single-lumen catheter is not to be used for administration of blood or antibiotics or the drawing of blood samples.

2. As in choice 1.

3. As in choice 1. Use of Y-tubing will infuse the antibiotic into the PICC line.

4. **An additional intravenous line is required for the administration of antibiotics.**

53. **C: Foundations of Practice T: Application**
   1. This creates an unnecessary break in the system. Canadian Infection Control Guidelines recommend that all intravascular delivery system components up to the hub should be changed at 72-hour intervals and lipid emulsions every 24 hours.
   2. **This not only identifies the tubing but also is a reminder to other nursing staff when the tubing will need to be changed.**
   3. Dressing changes are per institution protocol and usually not more often than once every other day.
   4. This is not necessary. Only if there are signs of infection is the tubing cultured.

54. **C: Foundations of Practice T: Critical Thinking**
   1. Weight gain or loss may be an indication of fluid shift, edema, or diuresis and does not evaluate tolerance of the TPN.
   2. This evaluates his hydration status, not his tolerance of the TPN.
   3. This will be a result of the improved nutrition but is not an ongoing accurate assessment of tolerance of the TPN.
   4. **Blood glucose, electrolytes, urea nitrogen, complete blood count, and hepatic enzyme studies are performed at routine intervals. Assessment of these values will assist the practical nurse in evaluating Mr. Ford's tolerance of parenteral nutrition.**

55. **C: Foundations of Practice T: Critical Thinking**
   1. **Visuals, such as drawings and pictures, will increase Mr. Ford's understanding.**
   2. A picture, rather than a verbal description, would improve Mr. Ford's understanding.
   3. Manufacturers' monographs are written at a technical level not suitable for most clients.
   4. If the explanation were requested prior to insertion, the nurse practitioner would be responsible for the education in order to obtain informed consent. After insertion, the nurse has the knowledge to explain the PICC line.

56. **C: Foundations of Practice T: Critical Thinking**
   1. If possible, the 500 mL should be made up to maintain normal blood values and nutrition.
   2. **The flow of parenteral solutions can be increased by no more than 10%; thus, this is an appropriate option to make up the lost amount.**
   3. TPN solutions should never be taken off an infusion pump and, due to their hypertonicity, may not run any faster than at 10% above the ordered rate.
   4. Mr. Ford is not able to ingest sufficient fluids; therefore, this may not be possible.

57. **C: Foundations of Practice T: Critical Thinking**
   1. This is not the most important information at this time.
   2. Mrs. Buxton may not be able to come to the doctor's office. Other information needs to be determined first.

   3. This is an important question, but the nurse first needs to determine whether Mrs. Buxton is safe.
   4. **The initial priority is Mrs. Buxton's safety. The practical nurse needs to determine whether she is somewhere that Mr. Buxton can find her and continue the beating.**

58. **C: Foundations of Practice T: Critical Thinking**
   1. **Establishing trust is essential when counselling any client.**
   2. This may come out later on in the counselling but is not the most important initial goal.
   3. Communication is important, but it is an ongoing process and is likely to be facilitated by trust between the mental health nurse and Mr. Buxton.
   4. This puts the mental health nurse in an authoritative rather than a therapeutic relationship.

59. **C: Foundations of Practice T: Knowledge**
   1. Splitting is viewing people and situations as either all good or all bad.
   2. **Repression is the involuntary exclusion from awareness of a painful or conflictual thought, impulse, or memory. It is the primary ego defence. Mr. Buxton does not want to believe that he beats Mrs. Buxton.**
   3. Introjection is intense identification with another.
   4. Compensation is a process by which a person makes up for a perceived deficiency by strongly emphasizing a feature thought of as an asset.

60. **C: Foundations of Practice T: Application**
   1. This is a punitive response.
   2. This could be viewed as a sarcastic response.
   3. **This is the therapeutic communication technique called clarification. Attempting to put into words Mr. Buxton's unclear thoughts helps clarify his feelings, ideas, and perceptions.**
   4. This avoids the topic and is not therapeutic.

61. **C: Foundations of Practice T: Application**
   1. Some abusers blame their behaviour on alcohol, but this is a myth. Abuse is a learned behaviour, not the result of the loss of inhibitions.
   2. This may be a contributing factor, the hopelessness of poverty, but is not the most characteristic. Most people with a low socio-economic status are not abusive.
   3. While there are cultures that may appear to ignore or condone family violence, there are no specific cultural factors that are most characteristic of abusers.
   4. **This is the most frequent finding in perpetrators of family violence. There is a history of violence, neglect, or emotional deprivation. The role model is abusive.**

62. **C: Foundations of Practice T: Knowledge**
   1. Identical twins begin with a single ovum that has been fertilized with one sperm and divides into two embryos.
   2. Identical twins are the same sex. Fraternal twins may be the same or different sexes.
   3. Older women are more likely to release two ova.

4. Fraternals twins are two ova that have been fertilized by two sperm. They develop as two fetuses and will have two placentas.

63. C: Foundations of Practice T: Application

1. **Fluids and roughage in fruits and vegetables increase the fluids in stool, making them softer and more easily passed through the colon.**
2. Exercise does help constipation; however, because of the twin pregnancy, the physician should clear this. It would not be the first approach.
3. Laxatives, whether or not they are natural, should not be used without consulting the physician. They are not the first approach.
4. The first approach would not be taking a stool softener, and a physician must order it.

64. C: Foundations of Practice T: Application

1. **Women with a multiple gestation are at high risk for developing preterm labour.**
2. This is a rare complication of twin pregnancy but occurs in monozygotic twins.
3. This is a rare occurrence in monozygotic twins, when the division of the embryo occurs very late, causing incomplete cleavage.
4. With twin pregnancy, there is more likely to be hydramnios, or an excess of amniotic fluid. Oligohydramnios is a decrease in amniotic fluid and may be associated with fetal kidney disorders.

65. C: Foundations of Practice T: Application

1. Dyspnea is a common discomfort, particularly in the latter half of the third trimester and in multiple births. It is caused by pressure of the enlarged uterus on the diaphragm.
2. This is normal weight gain.
3. Leg cramps are a common discomfort of pregnancy, caused by a calcium–phosphorus imbalance.
4. **A decrease in fetal movement is an ominous sign that indicates a loss of vitality in one or both infants. In a twin pregnancy, this is a greater risk, and it may be difficult for the mother to determine whether one or both infants are not moving or are moving less.**

66. C: Foundations of Practice T: Application

1. Blue eyes are a recessive genetic trait; therefore, it is not as likely for both infants to have blue eyes.
2. **Brown eyes are a dominant trait; therefore, it is most likely that both infants will have brown eyes.**
3. This is possible, but not as likely as both infants having brown eyes.
4. Eye colour is not a random genetic trait. Brown eyes are dominant.

67. C: Foundations of Practice T: Application

1. Fluids should not be restricted in pregnancy.
2. Legs should be uncrossed as much as possible to help prevent varicosities, but this is not likely to be of benefit for ankle edema.
3. **Elevating the legs will help venous return and decrease ankle edema.**

4. Range-of-motion exercises may be of limited benefit but are not as helpful as elevating the legs.

68. C: Foundations of Practice T: Application

1. This is a possibility but is not necessary. Both infants can be breastfed.
2. With Ms. Hudson's fertility problems, this may not happen, and they may not want more than two children. She is able to breastfeed twins.
3. It is more difficult to breastfeed twins, but it is not true that most women are not successful.
4. **While breastfeeding twins does require planning and adaptation, mothers can successfully breastfeed twins, either simultaneously or one at a time.**

69. C: Foundations of Practice T: Critical Thinking

1. This would be the second assessment.
2. Because the infants are preterm, they have a greater risk for hypothermia. However, this is not the most important assessment just after birth.
3. **Respirations are the most important initial assessment. Adequate respiratory effort is necessary for transition to extrauterine life.**
4. Blood pressure is not a necessary assessment in the delivery room.

70. C: Foundations of Practice T: Application

1. It is not necessary for the client to lie down. He or she may sit, with the arm extended at heart level.
2. The cuff width should be at least 40% of the length of the client's upper arm.
3. The cuff should be inflated to 30% above the expected systolic pressure.
4. **The brachial artery is used for blood pressure determination. The teacher will demonstrate palpation of the brachial artery and place the bell of the stethoscope over the pulse point.**

71. C: Professional, Ethical, and Legal Practice T: Critical Thinking

1. This is a valuable step in learning how to manage the equipment, but being able to perform blood pressure monitoring on himself is more effective.
2. Verbalizing the procedure is not as effective as actually being able to demonstrate the skill.
3. This is important but is not an evaluation of the skill.
4. **This is the most effective evaluation as the nursing teacher will be able to determine whether the student can manipulate the equipment on himself.**

72. C: Professional Ethical, and Legal Practice T: Critical Thinking

1. **The second step of the nursing process is to validate data. The best way to validate the high reading, and reassure Mr. Brown, is to take the blood pressure again using a manual device that is not dependent on correct calibration.**
2. This would be the next step if the high blood pressure were confirmed by the manual method.
3. This question should be asked but is not the first step.

4. This is likely required, but it may be that the monitor requires recalibration. Also, this will not quickly reassure Mr. Brown.

73. **C: Foundations of Practice T: Knowledge**
   1. Meperidine, an analgesic, does not depress the immune system.
   2. Cefazolin, an antibiotic, will not depress the immune system.
   3. **Prednisone, a corticosteroid, has recognized immuno-suppressive effects.**
   4. Salbutamol, a bronchodilator, does not have immuno-suppressive effects.

74. **C: Foundations of Practice T: Critical Thinking**
   1. **Developing an awareness of social justice involves socio-economic and political issues that can contribute to poor health in disadvantaged populations.**
   2. This may occur but is not the primary reason.
   3. This is true but does not answer the question of why practical nurses should be social justice advocates.
   4. The purpose of advocacy in social justice is to improve conditions for all people. It does not necessarily involve changes in law. Practical nurses may influence politicians, but it is not a given that laws will be changed based on nursing input.

75. **C: Foundations of Practice T: Application**
   1. This is too early for an infant to pull himself or herself to a standing position.
   2. This is too early for most infants to pull themselves to a standing position.
   3. **While there is considerable variation among infants with regard to milestones, this is the approximate age at which an infant can pull himself or herself to a standing position holding onto furniture.**
   4. If a child is not able to pull himself or herself to a standing position by 11 to 12 months, he or she should be further evaluated.

76. **C: Foundations of Practice T: Application**
   1. Lipid-lowering medications are ordered depending on lipid levels, not age.
   2. Exercise is only one factor influencing lipid levels.
   3. **Generally, diet therapy is attempted prior to medications.**
   4. Only chronically elevated cholesterol levels with failure of conservative lifestyle measures require medications.

77. **C: Foundations of Practice T: Application**
   1. **Folic acid is recommended to prevent neural tube defects during pregnancy. Women should take it prior to becoming pregnant as it is necessary from the early stages, when the woman may not be aware she is pregnant.**
   2. This is not the role of folic acid.
   3. As in choice 2.
   4. As in choice 2.

78. **C: Professional, Ethical, and Legal Practice T: Critical Thinking**
   1. **The clinic will have healthcare providers who can manage chronic health problems.**
   2. This may take a long time and may not be successful.
   3. The practical nurse will have better information on availability of physicians in the community.
   4. The client may have needs beyond the scope of practice of the practical nurse.

79. **C: Foundations of Practice T: Knowledge**
   1. **Sickle cell disease, often termed sickle cell anemia, is a chronic inherited condition that results in abnormally shaped hemoglobin, resulting in anemia.**
   2. Fever is not a manifestation of sickle cell disease.
   3. Vomiting is not a manifestation of sickle cell disease.
   4. Children with sickle cell disease are more likely to be tachycardic, in response to red blood cell destruction and anemia.

80. **C: Foundations of Practice T: Application**
   1. Thrombocytopenia, not leukopenia, causes gums to bleed.
   2. There is no particular reason to eat these foods with leukopenia.
   3. Clients with leukopenia should not be immunized except on the judgement of their physician.
   4. **Leukopenia is reduced white blood cells (WBCs). With fewer WBCs, the immune system is depressed, causing the client to be at risk for communicable diseases.**

81. **C: Foundations of Practice T: Critical Thinking**
   1. **This is the most common cause of autonomic dysreflexia.**
   2. Nasal congestion is a symptom of autonomic dysreflexia.
   3. A high fibre diet may decrease the risk of occurrence of autonomic dysreflexia by reducing risk of constipation.
   4. Low blood pressure does not cause autonomic dysreflexia.

82. **C: Foundations of Practice T: Application**
   1. There would be no rationale for discontinuing an analgesic prior to surgery.
   2. There would be no rationale for discontinuing an antipyretic prior to surgery. If she did have a fever, surgery would likely be cancelled.
   3. There is no rationale for discontinuing an anti-inflammatory drug prior to surgery.
   4. **People with prosthetic heart valves are at risk for thrombus formation. Aspirin decreases platelet aggregation, preventing formation of thrombi. However, during surgery, there is an increased risk of hemorrhage if the client is taking an antiplatelet medication; thus, the medication should be stopped prior to surgery.**

83. **C: Foundations of Practice T: Critical Thinking**
   1. Although the bronchodilator has cardiovascular side effects, the priority assessment is respiratory.

2. These are respiratory drugs.

3. As in choice 2.

4. **Advair, which is a combination of fluticasone (an inhaled steroid) and salmeterol (an inhaled bronchodilator), is commonly used on clients with asthma. A respiratory assessment would be a priority to form a baseline and to assess the therapeutic effects of the drugs.**

84. C: Foundations of Practice T: Application

1. Caffeine can cause false elevations in blood pressure lasting up to 3 hours. There should be no effect after 5 hours.

2. **Relaxation facilitates a more accurate blood pressure reading.**

3. Electronic monitoring devices, if properly calibrated, are as reliable as manual devices. Care should be taken if interchanging the devices or if the electronic reading shows significant variance in comparison with previous readings.

4. The same arm should be used at each visit.

85. C: Foundations of Practice T: Application

1. This is an invasion of Ms. Brette's personal space and not an appropriate therapeutic technique.

2. This may prove to be too stimulating for Ms. Brette. She requires a calm, quiet environment.

3. **Antianxiety medications are commonly used to bring the anxiety to a manageable level.**

4. Ms. Brette may view this as punishment, unless she initiates moving to her room.

86. C: Foundations of Practice T: Critical Thinking

1. Airline staff will need to know this information so a decision can be made regarding landing at the closest airport or obtaining on-ground medical advice. It is not, however, the priority action.

2. This is an important question, but it can be asked after oxygen is administered.

3. As in choice 2.

4. **If the man is experiencing a myocardial infarction, the heart muscle is being deprived of oxygen. The oxygen supply to the heart must be increased immediately to prevent heart damage.**

87. C: Foundations of Practice T: Critical Thinking

1. Mr. Dunlop is displaying manifestations of myocardial infarction (MI); thus, 9-1-1 must be called. This is not the most complete answer.

2. **This is the most complete answer. ASA is a fibrinolytic that may help break up thrombi that contribute to MIs. It is recognized to be part of appropriate first aid treatment if myocardial infarction is suspected.**

3. There is no need to put Mr. Dunlop in a knee-chest position.

4. A blanket may provide increased comfort for Mr. Dunlop, but administration of ASA is more important.

88. C: Foundations of Practice T: Application

1. The spray is directed under the tongue, not inhaled.

2. Headache is an expected side effect.

3. Pain relief should be within 2 minutes. If there is no significant relief within 15 minutes, she should notify her physician.

4. **Exercise creates cardiovascular demand. Administration of nitroglycerine prior to physical activity will increase blood flow to the heart, increasing tolerance for the activity.**

89. C: Foundations of Practice T: Application

1. Fever is likely to be manifested, but it is not the classic symptom of *C. difficile* infection.

2. Vomiting sometimes, but not always, accompanies a *C. difficile* infection.

3. Chills often accompany the fever, but are not specific to *C. difficile*.

4. **Overgrowth of *C. difficile* in the colon causes diarrhea that is usually watery and voluminous.**

90. C: Foundations of Practice T: Knowledge

1. Fibromyalgia is not a psychiatric disorder. Depression and anxiety may be involved, possibly due to living with chronic pain and fatigue.

2. While fibromyalgia cannot be cured, there are treatments, including antidepressants, physiotherapy, rest, and analgesics.

3. **A definitive diagnosis of fibromyalgia is difficult to establish as there are no specific diagnostic tests. Often the diagnosis is achieved by ruling out other conditions. Manifestations may be similar to many other conditions.**

4. The pain and fatigue are not progressive.

91. C: Professional, Ethical, and Legal Practice T: Critical Thinking

1. True, but this does not answer the question.

2. **This explains why nurses support political advocacy for social determinants of health.**

3. This is part of the *Canada Health Act* but does not answer the question.

4. This is true but does not answer the question.

92. C: Foundations of Practice T: Critical Thinking

1. This is an important nursing action but not the priority.

2. **Maintaining a patent airway is the priority action based on the type of surgery and the ABC principles of care.**

3. This is one action that will assist in maintaining the patent airway.

4. As in choice 1.

93. C: Foundations of Practice T: Application

1. Hepatitis A is not transmitted by blood or body fluids.

2. Hepatitis A is not an airborne virus.

3. This does not explain the mode of transmission. While there may be more cases of hepatitis A in tropical countries, it is not necessarily considered endemic.

4. **Hepatitis A is transmitted by the fecal–oral route, most commonly in contaminated food and water. It may be more prevalent in countries where there is a warmer climate and poor sanitation practices.**

94. **C: Professional, Ethical, and Legal Practice T: Application**
    1. This meal should be eaten around 0100 of the night shift. Large meals eaten shortly before going to bed after a night shift do not facilitate sleepiness.
    2. **This may help prevent the circadian rhythm from being triggered by the morning light.**
    3. Because of its potentially stimulating effects, shift workers are advised to avoid strenuous activity just before bedtime.
    4. A 24-hour time period is recommended between shifts for those who rotate shifts.

95. **C: Foundations of Practice T: Application**
    1. These are generally the second set of teeth to erupt.
    2. **The lower central incisors are generally the first teeth to erupt, at about 6 to 8 months of age.**
    3. The canine teeth do not generally erupt until about 20 months.
    4. The first molar does not generally erupt until 14–18 months.

96. **C: Foundations of Practice T: Critical Thinking**
    1. **The tube must be assessed for patency. Irrigating can be done by instilling, and then withdrawing, saline.**
    2. Instillation may not determine patency and may add to the residuals in the stomach.
    3. The tube should not be removed as this may not be necessary and should not be done without a physician's order.
    4. The physician does not need to be notified until the patency of the tube has been determined.

97. **C: Foundations of Practice T: Application**
    1. **Women with gestational diabetes often deliver large infants. It is important to determine the maternal baseline blood sugar level as early as possible.**
    2. Amniocentesis is not indicated for large infants unless there had been previous anomalies with the infants.
    3. Maternal diet can be related to the size of the infant at term but is not the most important test at this time.
    4. Pelvimetry will be important later in the pregnancy to determine whether Ms. Bacci will be able to deliver a large baby vaginally.

98. **C: Foundations of Practice T: Critical Thinking**
    1. This is important to know, but the nurse requires more information about what the father has read.
    2. As in choice 1.
    3. As in choice 2.
    4. **This response validates the father's findings and invites him to discuss with the practical nurse what he has read.**

99. **C: Foundations of Practice T: Application**
    1. This test is done to diagnose or stage ovarian cancer and is not a screening test.
    2. **Women with close relatives, a mother or a sister, who have had ovarian cancer are at greater risk for breast, uterine, ovarian, and colorectal cancer. They should be screened at an earlier age than women with no familial history.**
    3. Chest X-ray may be used to diagnose or screen for other cancers, primarily lung cancer. There is no reported increase in lung cancer with a family history of ovarian cancer.
    4. This test is performed when there are indications of ovarian cancer and is generally not a screening test.

100. **C: Foundations of Practice T: Application**
    1. This avoids the question and puts the blame on the boyfriend.
    2. While this is true, the woman has expressed concern about telling her boyfriend, and this is the subject that needs to be discussed.
    3. As in choice 2.
    4. **This introduces the legal and ethical implications of telling the boyfriend and encourages communication about how to approach the discussion.**

101. **C: Foundations of Practice T: Critical Thinking**
    1. This may help in the short term, but it is best not to use family.
    2. This may help, but there are too many languages and staff may not be able to effectively use a written dictionary.
    3. The practical nurse may want to learn the most common languages, but it is not reasonable to be fluent in all.
    4. **This is the best long-term option. Telephone and video link call centres with healthcare interpreters are available around the clock.**

102. **C: Professional, Ethical, and Legal Practice T: Knowledge**
    1. Inquests are not held to determine criminal liability, although evidence provided may lead to formal charges.
    2. Inquests are not held to determine civil liability.
    3. Inquests are not held to prosecute persons or agencies.
    4. **Inquests are held to provide recommendations that may be used to improve systems or practices in health care. They must answer how the person died and the manner of death.**

103. **C: Foundations of Practice T: Application**
    1. A person with an apple body shape carries weight around the waist, which creates a higher risk of developing CVD and type 2 diabetes. However, Mark's BMI is within the normal range.
    2. **An apple-shaped person carries weight around the waist, which creates a higher risk of developing CVD and type 2 diabetes. A BMI above 25 indicates that Consuelo is overweight.**
    3. A pear shape indicates that the person carries weight around the hips and thighs and is not as unhealthy as someone who carries weight around the waist. The BMI indicates that Pedro is only slightly overweight.

4. Christa has a pear shape, but her BMI indicates that she is slightly underweight, which may not be a risk factor for CVD and type 2 diabetes.

104. **C: Foundations of Practice T: Application**
1. This is an incorrect calculation.
2. **The correct calculation is 12 grams × 9 kcal/gram = 108 kcal. 1 100 kcal divided by 108 kcal = 10.1, or 10%.**
3. This is an incorrect calculation.
4. This is an incorrect calculation.

105. **C: Foundations of Practice T: Application**
1. **Practical nurses should consult with the healthcare team before starting a complementary therapy. If the team agrees, the peppermint may be added to the plan of care.**
2. This is not true.
3. The practical nurse needs to consult with the healthcare team prior to providing Mrs. Carnegy with the peppermint.
4. Mrs. Carnegy has found the peppermint to be effective, so there may be no need to consult with the physician about an alternative medication.

106. **C: Foundations of Practice T: Application**
1. **Falls are the leading cause of injury in older adults. In icy winter conditions, there is a greater risk of falls with severe injuries.**
2. Area rugs may be a safety hazard. Bare floors decrease the likelihood of tripping, falling, and slipping due to rugs that may not be firmly attached to the floors.
3. An open element on a stove is more dangerous than a microwave, provided that the microwave is properly used.
4. Over-the-counter cough medications are not recommended for children or older adults. These clients should, more appropriately, drink fluids and take acetaminophen (Tylenol) for discomfort. The practical nurse or physician should assess them if their symptoms worsen.

107. **C: Foundations of Practice T: Critical Thinking**
1. This is a useful screening test and is recommended for people over the age of 50. However, it is not as conclusive as a colonoscopy.
2. A sigmoidoscopy looks only at the sigmoid colon.
3. **A colonoscopy is direct visualization of the entire colon from rectum to cecum. Because polyps and cancerous growths actually can be seen, colonoscopy is the recommended screening test.**
4. A barium enema is an X-ray of the lower bowel following the insertion of barium contrast medium. It can be used to see areas of obstruction; however, it is not as conclusive as the colonoscopy.

108. **C: Foundations of Practice T: Critical Thinking**
1. This is not necessary as the order is clear to provide oxygen. The practical nurse may want to further consult with the physician regarding the child's decreasing O_2 saturation.

2. **This is the first action as it is has been ordered by the physician, and the child is in need of supplemental oxygen.**
3. This may occur but is not the initial action.
4. This should occur and will be ongoing; however, the first action is to provide additional oxygen.

109. **C: Professional, Ethical, and Legal Practice T: Critical Thinking**
1. **The pharmacist has the specific scope of practice to best recommend effective over-the-counter antihistamines to Mr. Patrick.**
2. The nurse practitioner may be able to recommend effective therapies, but the pharmacist would be the most appropriate first choice.
3. This may be an alternative, but it would be better for Mr. Patrick to first consult with a pharmacist concerning effective medications.
4. A respiratory therapist might be an appropriate referral if Mr. Patrick were experiencing breathing difficulties.

110. **C: Professional, Ethical, and Legal Practice T: Application**
1. Although, in some situations, it is appropriate to discuss with the client his or her medication regimen, the professional practical nurse must display knowledge of the rationale for the medications being administered. Having to ask Mr. Price may create a lack of trust in the nurse's knowledge.
2. **This is the appropriate resource to determine the rationale for the antipsychotic. The practical nurse must have this knowledge prior to administration of the medication.**
3. This may be part of the psychiatric assessment but is not the first action.
4. Because Mr. Price is receiving an antipsychotic medication, this is not a reason to assume that he will be violent or that the practical nurse will need safety measures when performing care.

111. **C: Foundations of Practice T: Application**
1. This is not a manifestation of presbycusis.
2. **With age-related hearing loss, the ability to hear high-pitched consonants decreases, and sound becomes muffled. It seems to the person that others are not speaking clearly.**
3. The higher-pitched sounds of women's voices are lost initially.
4. People are able to hear their own speech.

112. **C: Foundations of Practice T: Application**
1. This is setting limits to behaviour, and in this case, it may make Mr. Braham more anxious. Demanding behaviour is often an attempt to decrease anxiety.
2. **All behaviour has meaning. The practical nurse needs to determine what is causing Mr. Braham's demanding behaviour. By sitting with him and asking open-ended questions, she may be able to determine the underlying problems.**

3. Maintaining continuity of care with one nurse is optimum to developing a trusting relationship between Mr. Braham and the nurse.

4. This is confrontational and will likely escalate the demanding behaviour. It is not a therapeutic response.

113. **C: Foundations of Practice T: Application**

1. The person with dementia is not necessarily deaf, and Mr. Hill does not have to speak loudly.

2. The person with dementia will not understand written communication any better than verbal communication.

3. **The person with dementia has lost some ability to interpret complex language. Short, simple sentences may enable the client with dementia to comprehend the spoken word.**

4. Repeating the communication will not aid in comprehension of what has been spoken.

114. **C: Professional, Ethical, and Legal Practice T: Application**

1. **A practical nurse may or may not decide to answer a question that may be a natural conversational question for a client. If the practical nurse chooses to respond, it should be a brief answer. The most appropriate response, however, is to refocus the conversation to the client. In this scenario, Ms. Enright may be using the question to open the topic of her boyfriend.**

2. This response indicates that rules rather than professional judgement direct her practice.

3. This response provides too much personal information about the practical nurse. It may be considered a boundary crossing.

4. This response may sound harsh and punitive to the client. There are better words to redirect the client.

115. **C: Professional, Ethical, and Legal Practice T: Critical Thinking**

1. This is necessary, as most threats against healthcare workers are under-reported. It is not, however, the primary action.

2. This is true; however, it is not the primary action or consideration.

3. **The practical nurse must first protect herself from verbal abuse that may turn to physical abuse. Once safeguards are in place, she may address documentation, support, communication with colleagues, and methods to provide care to Mr. Dovgan.**

4. This is important to obtain support and assistance in devising methods for caring for Mr. Dovgan. It is not, however, the primary action.

116. **C: Foundations of Practice T: Critical Thinking**

1. Lindsay is asking for help, but she does not actually have the razor blades, so the suicide risk is not imminent.

2. **Young men have a high risk of suicide, often by violent means. Ahmet has the gun and is able to act on his impulse immediately.**

3. Florence has agreed to treatment.

4. Older adults are at risk for suicide, but Fred may be feeling a grief reaction that will improve. He has not formed a plan.

117. **C: Foundations of Practice T: Critical Thinking**

1. This is the order, not what might be actually occurring.

2. This is the recommendation by the physiotherapist, but not what might be actually happening.

3. This is current, but may not be what occurs all the time.

4. **Only this response specifically answers the family's question.**

118. **C: Foundations of Practice T: Critical Thinking**

1. This is an important assessment, but the developmental stage must first be determined.

2. As in choice 1.

3. **Developmental level is essential in assessing children's ability and level of understanding. It must be determined prior to a teaching plan.**

4. As in choice 1.

119. **C: Foundations of Practice T: Critical Thinking**

1. Autism is not treated with medications, although some drugs appear to alleviate particular symptoms in individuals.

2. **This is the cornerstone of treatment for autism and assists clients to achieve their potential.**

3. Autism is not considered to be a psychiatric disease and cannot be helped with psychiatric treatment. In the past, it was viewed to be maladaptive parenting, which may have responded to psychiatric treatment.

4. While a safety assessment is important, it does not help achieve developmental goals.

120. **C: Foundations of Practice T: Application**

1. **This is the most effective method for stopping a nosebleed.**

2. The head should not be tilted back as the blood may flow down the back of the throat. Holding the bridge of the nose is ineffective.

3. This may increase the bleeding.

4. This is a last resort, and cotton balls should not be used.

121. **C: Professional, Ethical, and Legal Practice T: Application**

1. **The initial step in any type of conflict is to discuss the situation with the people involved. By discussing the student's performance with her, it provides an opportunity to clarify both appropriate roles and expectations.**

2. This is a correct action but should occur after the discussion with the student.

3. The nurse educator may be a valuable resource, but the initial action is for Martina to speak with the student.

4. Martina should have read this information prior to the beginning of the preceptorship.

122. **C: Foundations of Practice T: Application**
  1. Naproxen may cause stomach irritation.
  2. Celecoxib is used for pain related to arthritis.
  3. **Acetaminophen is generally considered to be a safe analgesic and is appropriate for mild aches, pyrexia, and headache.**
  4. Aspirin may cause stomach irritation.

123. **C: Professional, Ethical, and Legal Practice T: Application**
  1. This is not necessary.
  2. This is an expected nursing action but does not answer when the bag will need to be replaced.
  3. **There are no recommendations by the Centers for Disease Control and Prevention for the "hang time" of IV fluids. It is the responsibility of each agency to develop policies, which the nurse will need to consult.**
  4. The bag will not be empty for several days. This may be contrary to agency policies.

124. **C: Foundations of Practice T: Application**
  1. This is an incorrect calculation.
  2. This is an incorrect calculation.
  3. **Correct calculation: 56.7 kg / 0.45 kg = 126 × 18 kcal = 2268 kcal.**
  4. This is an incorrect calculation.

125. **C: Foundations of Practice T: Critical Thinking**
  1. This is a slightly elevated respiratory rate and should be monitored.
  2. A productive cough is expected and aids the lungs in clearing mucus.
  3. **Restlessness is a cerebral manifestation of hypoxia.**
  4. This may be normal in an older adult but should be monitored.

The CPNRE Competencies

ASSUMPTIONS

The following assumptions were made in developing the competencies for the Canadian Practical Nurse Registration Examination (CPNRE):

1. Entry-level practical nurses are beginning practitioners whose level of practice, autonomy, and proficiency will be enhanced through reflective practice, evidence-informed knowledge, collaboration, mentoring, and support from colleagues.
2. The foundation of practical nursing is defined by legislation, regulation, scope of practice, standards of practice, professional ethics, and entry-level competencies.
3. The competencies represent the combined nursing knowledge, skills, behaviours, and attitudes required by entry-level practical nurses across Canada.
4. Practical nurses provide, facilitate, and promote safe, competent, compassionate, and ethical care for clients throughout the lifespan in a variety of settings.
5. Practical nurses are active participants in health promotion, illness prevention, reduction of harm, quality improvement, and risk management activities.
6. Practical nurses use critical inquiry, critical thinking, and clinical judgments when applying the nursing process.
7. Practical nurses are self-regulated and accountable for their decisions and actions, and are committed to putting the public interest over their self-interest.
8. Practical nurses engage in self-reflection and continuous learning to maintain and enhance competence.
9. Practical nurses demonstrate leadership and professionalism.
10. Practical nurses provide client-centred care for individuals, families, groups, and communities.
11. Practical nurses practise collaboratively, while respecting the shared and unique competencies of a diverse healthcare team.
12. Practical nurses advocate for and facilitate change reflecting evidence-informed practice.
13. Practical nurses are knowledgeable about trends and issues that impact health and healthcare delivery, and contribute to the body of knowledge of the profession.
14. Practical nurses articulate their scope, role, and contribution to health care.

PROFESSIONAL, ETHICAL, AND LEGAL PRACTICE

Practical nurses are responsible for providing safe, competent, compassionate, and ethical nursing care while developing and maintaining a therapeutic nurse–client relationship. Professional standards and ethics provide direction for practical nurses to uphold the highest quality of care. The practical nurse maintains autonomy and is accountable to the public, the client, the employer, the profession, colleagues, and one's self.

Competency 1: Professional, Ethical, and Legal Practice
Professional
Competent entry-level practical nurses:
   PR-1 are responsible and accountable for their own decisions and actions.
a. practise autonomously within legislated scope of practice.
b. determine when to seek assistance and guidance.
c. engage in critical inquiry, critical thinking, and clinical judgment for decision-making.
   PR-2 develop the therapeutic nurse-client relationship.
a. initiate, maintain, and terminate the therapeutic nurse-client relationship.
b. provide client care without bias.
c. respect client's right to self-determination.
   PR-3 demonstrate leadership in all aspects of practice.
a. assess and develop professional competence.
b. advocate for best practices.
c. advocate for client, self, and others.
   PR-4 demonstrate and model professional behaviour.
a. adhere to standards of practice and ethics.
b. assess and maintain own fitness to practise.
c. respond to inappropriate behaviour and communication.
d. respond to incidents of unsafe practice.
e. respond to incidents of professional misconduct.

Ethical
Competent entry-level practical nurses:
   PR-5 apply an ethical framework to nursing practice.
a. establish and maintain respect, empathy, trust, and integrity in interactions with clients and others.

b. recognize and respect the values, opinions, needs, and beliefs of clients, self, and others.

c. accommodate client diversity.

d. recognize and adhere to the duty to provide care.

e. identify and address situations involving moral and ethical challenges.

PR-6 advocate for clients' rights and responsibilities.

a. ensure that implied and/or informed consent is obtained.

b. maintain client's confidentiality, privacy, and dignity.

Legal

Competent entry-level practical nurses:

PR-7 adhere to legal requirements of practice.

a. practise within the confines of established policies, procedures, and standards.

b. recognize and respond to questionable orders, actions, or decisions.

c. adhere to relevant abuse, communicable disease, and mental health legislation.

PR-8 adhere to legal requirements regarding personal information.

a. maintain confidentiality in all forms of communication.

b. respond to the client's right to information.

c. disclose relevant information to appropriate individuals.

PR-9 adhere to legal requirements regarding documentation.

a. document according to established policies, procedures, and standards.

b. initiate contact and receive, transcribe, and verify orders.

c. complete occurrence reports as require.

FOUNDATIONS OF PRACTICE

As a member of the healthcare team, practical nurses are integral in the assessment, nursing diagnosis, planning, implementation, evaluation, and documentation of nursing care. Using critical inquiry, practical nurses formulate clinical decisions based on evidence. Practical nurses promote, support, and advocate for client self-determination to achieve optimum health outcomes.

Competency 2: Foundations of Practice
Assessment

Competent entry-level practical nurses:

FP-1 complete comprehensive assessments.

a. conduct individualized health assessments.

b. perform physical assessments using observation, inspection, auscultation, and palpation.

c. perform psychological, spiritual, and sociocultural assessments.

d. collect clinical data using appropriate methodology.

e. analyze and integrate relevant clinical data.

f. recognize determinants of health in individuals, groups, and communities.

Planning and Implementation

Competent entry-level practical nurses:

FP-2 formulate decisions consistent with client needs and priorities.

a. organize and manage multiple priorities.

b. respond appropriately to changing situations.

c. develop individualized nursing interventions.

d. set priorities that reflect individual client needs.

FP-3 plan and implement interventions based on assessment and desired outcomes.

a. determine nursing diagnosis.

b. identify health goals and outcomes in collaboration with the client.

c. engage client in developing and prioritizing the plan of care.

d. implement the plan of care.

FP-4 promote client self-care.

a. assess client health literacy and health knowledge.

b. support clients to assume responsibility for their health.

c. support access to available resources and information.

d. participate in discharge planning.

FP-5 facilitate health education.

a. provide health education in collaboration with the client.

b. plan and implement strategies to enhance client learning.

c. evaluate client learning and revise strategies as necessary.

d. evaluate the quality of health-related resources.

FP-6 apply principles of safety.

a. implement routine practices (standard precautions).

b. assess needs and implement strategies related to risk management and reduction of harm.

c. assess needs and implement strategies to enhance infection prevention and control of communicable diseases.

d. apply knowledge of principles and implications of immunization.

e. promote psychological health and safety.

FP-7 engage in safe medication practices.

a. analyze clinical data.

b. apply principles of medication administration and pharmacology when preparing and administering medications (excluding intravenous push).

c. implement strategies to optimize medication safety.

d. evaluate and document client's response to medication.

FP-8 engage in safe infusion therapy practices.

a. analyze clinical data.

b. apply principles of infusion therapy when preparing and administering peripheral and subcutaneous infusions.

c. apply principles of infusion therapy to assess and monitor central venous catheters.

d. apply knowledge of pain management systems (e.g. patient-controlled analgesia, epidural).

e. apply standards and principles when administering blood and blood products.

f. implement strategies to optimize infusion therapy safety.

g. evaluate and document client's response to infusion therapy.

Evaluation

Competent entry-level practical nurses:

FP-9 perform ongoing evaluation throughout delivery of care.

a.   evaluate the effectiveness of nursing interventions.
b.   compare actual outcomes to expected outcomes.
c.   review and revise the plan of care.

COLLABORATIVE PRACTICE

Practical nurses work collaboratively while maintaining autonomy within their legislated scope of practice and individual competence. They recognize that collaborative practice is guided by shared values and accountability, a common purpose, care outcomes, mutual respect, and effective communication (CCPNR, 2013). The practical nurse demonstrates leadership while fostering continued growth of self and others to meet the challenges of the evolving healthcare system.

Competency 3: Collaborative Practice

Competent entry-level practical nurses:

CP-1 Develop and Maintain Collaborative Relationships.

a.   develop partnerships based on trust and respect.
b.   promote quality, healthy work environments.
c.   apply conflict management skills.

CP-2 Communicate Collaboratively.

a.   demonstrate effective communication techniques.
b.   communicate in a respectful, timely, open, and honest manner.
c.   communicate relevant information to the appropriate person or agency.

CP-3 Demonstrate Leadership in Collaborative Practice.

a.   practise collaboratively with the healthcare team.
b.   engage others to support effective teamwork.
c.   lead, direct, assign, or supervise unregulated health workers and others.
d.   seek, provide, and reflect on constructive feedback.
e.   collaborate with the healthcare team to coordinate the actions of others in emergency situations.
f.   integrate best evidence in collaboration with the healthcare team.
g.   participate in quality improvement and risk management activities.
h.   promote a culture of safety.

BIBLIOGRAPHY

Assessment Strategies Inc. (2017). *Canadian Practical Nurse Registration examination blueprint (Appendix C)*. Ottawa: Author pp. 19–23).

Terminology

An understanding of the distinct language used in the health sciences is of critical importance for safe nursing practice. Medical terminology can be simplified and better understood by analyzing the structural characteristics of the words.

Understanding the meaning of the basic prefixes and suffixes, and the definition of the root word, will allow you to derive the meaning of specific terms and greatly enhance your vocabulary.

ROOT WORD: The foundation word; directs us to the general, fundamental meaning of the word; e.g. cardio (pertaining to the heart) = cardiology (the study of the heart)

PREFIX: Added to the beginning of a word to specify a particular meaning of the root word; e.g. endo (within or inside) = endocardium (inner lining of the heart)

SUFFIX: Added to the end of a word to specify a particular meaning of the root word; e.g. itis (inflammation of) = endocarditis (inflammation of the inner lining of the heart)

Commonly Used PREFIXES in Medical Terminology

Prefix	Meaning	Example
a-	without/not	**a**pnea: absence of breathing
ab-	away from	**ab**duction (of arm): moving arm away from the centre of the body
ad-	toward	**ad**duction (of arm): bringing arm toward the centre of the body
ante-	before	**ante**natal: before birth
anti-	against	**anti**histamine: against (opposes) histamine
auto-	self	**auto**graft: grafting tissue from one part of the body to another part
brady-	slow	**brady**cardia: slow heart rate
contra-	against	**contra**ceptive: against conception
dorsi-	back	**dorsi**flexion: flexing a joint backward
dys-	faulty/difficult	**dys**pnea: difficulty in breathing
ecto-	outside	**ecto**pic pregnancy: embryo growing outside the uterus
endo-	inside	**endo**cardium: inner lining of the heart
exo-	outside	**exo**crine gland: gland that secretes onto an outside surface
eu-	normal	**eu**pnea: normal breathing
hemi-	half	**hemi**plegia: paralysis of half the body
hyper-	above/excessive	**hyper**tension: abnormally high blood pressure
hypo-	below/deficient	**hypo**thermia: below normal body temperature
infra-	below/beneath	**infra**mandibular: below the jaw
inter-	between	**inter**cellular: between the cells
intra-	inside	**intra**venous: inside the veins
macro-	large	**macro**cyte: an enlarged erythrocyte
mal-	bad	**mal**absorption: faulty absorption
micro-	small	**micro**cytic: small blood cell
neo-	new	**neo**plasm: new tumour growth
noct-	night	**noct**uria: urination during the night
para-	beside, near, resembling	**para**plegia: paralysis of the lower half of the body
peri-	around	**peri**cardium: around (outer layer of) the heart
pneum-	breathing	**pneum**onia: condition of abnormal breathing due to infection of the lungs
poly-	many	**poly**uria: excessive urine

Continued

Commonly Used PREFIXES in Medical Terminology—cont'd

Prefix	Meaning	Example
post-	after	**post**operative: after surgery
pre-	before	**pre**ganglionic: before a ganglion
pro-	in front of, before	**pro**dromal: beginning, initial stages
retro-	behind	**retro**peritoneal: behind the peritoneum
sub-	below	**sub**chondral: below the cartilage
super-	above/excess	**super**sensitive: extra sensitivity
supra-	above	**supra**pubic: above the pubic region
tachy-	fast	**tachy**cardia: fast heart rate
trans-	across/through	**trans**membrane: across a membrane

Commonly Used SUFFIXES in Medical Terminology

Suffix	Meaning	Example
-ac	pertaining/relating to	cardi**ac**: pertaining to the heart
-al	"	abdomin**al**: pertaining to the abdomen
-ar	"	ventricul**ar**: pertaining to a ventricle
-eal	"	perin**eal**: pertaining to the perineum
-ic	"	opt**ic**: pertaining to the eye
-ose	"	adip**ose**: pertaining to fatty tissue
-ous	"	cutane**ous**: pertaining to skin
-algia	pain	neur**algia**: neural pain
-cele	sac/pouch/hernia	cysto**cele**: herniation of the bladder
-centesis	puncture into a cavity	thora**centesis**: puncture wound into thorax to remove fluid
-clasia	breaking up, division	osteo**clasia**: intentional fracture of a bone to correct abnormality
-ectomy	removal of	append**ectomy**: removal of appendix
-emia	condition of the blood	leuk**emia**: cancer of the white blood cells (WBCs)
-genic	begin/generate/produce	patho**genic**: producing disease
-gram	a drawing or recording	cardio**gram**: a recording of the electrical activity of the heart
-graph	recording instrument	cardio**graph**: recording device that registers the electrical activity of the heart
-graphy	recording process	cardio**graphy**: recording and study of the electrical activity of the heart
-ia	condition/abnormal state	anem**ia**: condition of reduced red blood cells (RBCs)
-ian/ist	specialist in field of study	pediatric**ian**: physician who specializes in the care of children
-iasis	formation/condition of	nephrolith**iasis**: formation of calculi (stones) in the kidney
-ism	condition of	alcohol**ism**: condition of excess alcohol intake
-itis	inflammation of	dermat**itis**: inflammation of the skin
-logist	specialist in area of study	patho**logist**: physician who specializes in the study of disease
-logy	study of	cyto**logy**: the study of cells
-lysis	breaking down	hemo**lysis**: breaking down of blood cells
-megaly	enlargement	cardio**megaly**: enlargement of the cells
-oma	neoplasm or tumour	sarc**oma**: cancerous tumour of connective tissue
-parous	bearing or giving birth to	multi**parous**: pertaining to multiple births
-pathy	disease	nephro**pathy**: disease of the kidney
-penia	pathological reduction/reduced amount	erythrocyto**penia**: abnormal decrease in the number of RBCs
-phile, -philia	an attraction to or abnormal tendency toward	lipo**philic**: attracted to fats
-phobia	fear of	hydro**phobia**: fear of water
-plasia	formation	hyper**plasia**: excessive formation of new cells
-plasm	a material that forms cells	neo**plasm**: new growth/tumour
-plasty	repair of/reconstruction	rhino**plasty**: reconstruction of the nose
-pnea	breathing	ortho**pnea**: difficulty breathing in recumbent position
-poiesis	formation of	erythro**poiesis**: formation of RBCs
-scope	instrument for visual examination	broncho**scope**: instrument that visualizes the bronchial tree
-scopy	examination using a scope	cysto**scopy**: procedure that uses a cystoscope to visualize the urinary bladder

Commonly Used SUFFIXES in Medical Terminology—cont'd

Suffix	Meaning	Example
-stasis	constancy, stillness, or stagnation	hemo**stasis**: arrested or halted blood flow
-stenosis	narrowing	pyloric **stenosis**: narrowing of the pyloric valve
-stomy	creation of artificial opening	colo**stomy**: an opening from the colon to the surface of the body
-therapy	treatment	cryo**therapy**: treatment of diseased body tissues by using extreme cold
-trophy	development; a certain type of growth	hyper**trophy**: increase in the size of a body structure or organ
-uria	condition of the urine	olig**uria**: abnormally low urine output

Commonly Used ROOT WORDS in Medical Terminology

Root Word	Meaning	Example
amnio-	amnion	**amnio**centesis: aspiration of fluid from the amniotic sac
angi-	vessel	**angi**ogram: X-ray of blood vessel
arter-	artery	**arter**iosclerosis: hardening of the arteries
arth-	joint	**arth**rectomy: removal of a joint
ather-	fatty material/plaque	**ather**osclerosis: fatty deposit causing hardening of an artery
audi-	hearing	**audi**ogram: a graphic recording of hearing
bronch-	bronchus	**bronch**oscopy: examination of the bronchi
carcin-	cancer	**carcin**ogen: cancer-producing substance
cardi-	heart	**cardi**ologist: heart specialist
cephal-	head	**cephal**opathy: disease involving the brain
cerebr-	brain	**cerebr**ovascular: blood vessel of brain
cervic-	neck of body or uterus	**cervic**itis: inflammation of uterine cervix
chem-	chemical	**chem**otherapy: drug therapy (for cancer)
cholecyst-	gallbladder	**cholecyst**ectomy: removal of gallbladder
chondr-	cartilage	**chondr**oma: tumour of cartilage
col-	colon	**col**onoscopy: examination of the colon
crani-	skull	**crani**otomy: opening in cranium
cutane-	skin	**cutane**ous: pertaining to the skin
cyst-	bladder	**cyst**ectomy: removal of the bladder
cyt-	cell	**cyt**ology: study of cells
derm-	skin	**derm**atitis: inflammation of the skin
dipl-	double	**dipl**opia: double vision
encephal-	brain	**encephal**opathy: disease of the brain
enter-	intestines	**enter**itis: inflammation of small intestine
erythr-	red	**erythr**ocyte: red blood cell
esophag-	esophagus	**esophag**itis: inflamed esophagus
gastr-	stomach	**gastr**ectomy: removal of stomach
gloss-	tongue	**gloss**itis: inflammation of the tongue
gly-	sugar	**gly**cosuria: sugar in the urine
gynec-	woman	**gynec**ology: study of diseases of women
hem-	blood	**hem**atoma: blood clot
hepat-	liver	**hepat**omegaly: enlarged liver
hydr-	water	**hydr**ophobia: fear of water
hyster-	uterus	**hyster**ectomy: removal of uterus
lapar-	abdomen	**lapar**oscopy: endoscopic examination of abdomen
laryng-	larynx	**laryng**itis: inflammation of larynx
leuk(c)-	white	**leuk**ocytosis: increased number of WBCs
lingu-	tongue	**lingu**al: pertaining to the tongue
mamm-	breast	**mamm**ogram: X-ray of the breasts
muc-	mucus	**muc**olytic: substance that breaks down mucus
my-	muscle	**my**opathy: muscle disease
myel-	spinal cord	**myel**ogram: X-ray of spinal cord
necr-	death	**necr**osis: tissue death
nephr-	kidney	**nephr**itis: inflammation of the kidney
neur-	nerve	**neur**ectomy: removal of a nerve
onc-	tumour	**onc**ology: study of tumours

Continued

Commonly Used ROOT WORDS in Medical Terminology—cont'd

Root Word	Meaning	Example
ophthalm-	eye	**ophthalm**ologist: eye specialist
oste-	bone	**oste**oporosis: loss of calcium from the bones
ot-	ear	**ot**ic: pertaining to the ear
path-	disease	**path**ogen: disease-causing organism
p(a)ed-	child	**ped**iatrics: study of medical care and treatment of children
periton-	peritoneum	**periton**itis: inflammation of the peritoneum
pleur-	pleura	**pleur**al: pertaining to the pleura
pneum-	air, lungs	**pneum**onia: infection of the lungs
proct-	anus, rectum	**proct**itis: inflammation of the rectum
pulmon-	lung	**pulmon**ary artery: blood vessel leading to the lungs
ren-	kidney	**ren**al: pertaining to the kidneys
rhin-	nose	**rhin**oplasty: plastic surgery on the nose
seps-	infection	a**seps**is: absence of infection
thorac-	thorax	**thorac**otomy: surgical opening into the thorax
thromb-	clot	**thromb**us: blood clot attached to side of blood vessel obstructing blood flow
tox-	toxin	**tox**icology: study of poisons (toxins)
trache-	trachea	**trache**otomy: surgical opening into the trachea
ur-	urine	**ur**ology: study of the urinary system
ven-	vein	intra**ven**ous: into a vein

Common Directional Terms and Body Positions Relating to Medical Terminology

Term	Meaning
abduction	moving a body part away from the midline of the body
adduction	moving a body part toward the midline of the body
anterior	toward the front of the body
bilateral	both sides of the body
coronal (frontal)	lengthwise plane of the body; dividing the body into front and back halves
deep	interior of the body
distal	away from the centre of the body
dorsal recumbent	lying supine with knees bent
eversion	turning a body part outward
extension	straightening out a joint
flexion	bending a joint
inferior	lower; toward the feet
inversion	turning inward
lateral	to the side of the body
medial	toward the midline of the body
palmar	relating to the palm of the hand
plantar	relating to the sole of the foot
posterior	toward the back of the body
prone	lying on the stomach with legs extended
proximal	close to the centre of the body
sagittal	lengthwise plane dividing the body into front and back halves
Sims' position	lying on left side, left arm extended along back, chest forward, left knee slightly flexed, right knee highly flexed
superficial	on or near the surface of the body
superior	toward the head
supine	lying on the back, with legs extended
transverse (horizontal)	cross-section of body dividing it into upper and lower parts
Trendelenburg position	lying supine with the head lower than the feet
unilateral	applying to one side of the body

BIBLIOGRAPHY

Chabner, D. (2015). *Medical terminology—A short course* (7th ed.). St. Louis: Saunders.

Approved List of Abbreviations

Abbreviation	Meaning	Abbreviation	Meaning
BP	blood pressure	kg	kilogram(s)
BUN	blood urea nitrogen	kJ	kilojoule(s)
°C	degrees Celsius	L	litre(s)
cc	cubic centimetre	mcg	microgram
cm	centimetre(s)	mEq	milliequivalent
ECG	electrocardiogram	mg	milligram(s)
EEG	electroencephalogram	min	minute(s)
EENT	ear, eye, nose, throat	mL	millilitre(s)
h	hour	mmol/L	millimoles per litre
Hgb	hemoglobin	mm Hg	millimetres of mercury
HIV	human immunodeficiency virus	pH	Hydrogen ion concentration; potential of hydrogen
HR	heart rate (beats/min)		
HR	pulse	prn	as needed
IM	intramuscular	stat.	immediately
IV	intravenous	T	temperature
g	gram		

BIBLIOGRAPHY

Adapted from Assessment Strategies Inc. (2016). *The Canadian Practical Nurse Registration Examination (CPNRE) prep guide* (5th ed., p. 127). Ottawa: Author. Appendix A.

$\mathbf{D}$ APPENDIX

Common Laboratory and Diagnostic Tests

Laboratory Values Abbreviations

Abbreviation	Meaning	Abbreviation	Meaning	Abbreviation	Meaning
<	less than	kPa	kilopascal	mm	millimetre
>	greater than	L	litre	mm Hg	millimetres of mercury
≤	less than or equal to	mcg	microgram	mmol	millimole
≥	greater than or equal to	mcL	microlitre	mOsm	milliosmole
dL	decilitre	mcmol	micromole	ng	nanogram
EU	Ehrlich unit	microU	microunit	nmol	nanomole
fL	femtolitre	mEq	milliequivalent	pg	picogram
g	gram	mg	milligram	pmol	picomole
IU	international unit	mL	millilitre	U/L	units per litre

Hematology

- Involves tests on whole blood
- Tests focus on the examination of the blood cells

Test	Normal Value	Interpretation
Complete Blood Count and Differential (CBC and diff.)	Screening of all blood cells, including Hgb, Hct, platelets, and breakdown of white blood cells (WBCs)	
Erythrocyte Count (red blood cell [RBC])	Male: $4.7–6.1 \times 10^{12}$/L Female: $4.2–5.4 \times 10^{12}$/L	• The number of circulating RBCs
Hematocrit (Hct)	Male: 42–52% Female: 37–47%	• Percentage of RBCs to whole blood
Hemoglobin (Hgb)	Male: 140–180 g/L Female: 120–160 g/L	• Measures hemoglobin on RBC of venous blood

Test	Normal Value	Interpretation
Red Blood Cell (RBC) Indices		
• Mean Corpuscular Volume (MCV)	80–95 mm^3	• Average size of RBC
• Mean Corpuscular Hemoglobin (MCH)	27–31 pg	• Average Hgb weight of RBC
• Mean Corpuscular Hemoglobin Concentration (MCHC)	32–36%	• % of Hgb on RBC
• Erythrocyte Sedimentation Rate (ESR)	Male: ≤15 mm/hr Female: <20 mm/hr	• Measures the time it takes RBC to settle out on standing • Indicative of systemic inflammatory disease
White Blood Cell (WBC) Count	5 000–10 000 mm^3	• WBCs in venous blood

Test	Normal Value	Interpretation
Differential WBC Count		
• Neutrophils	62–68%	• Bacterial infections
• Monocytes	2–8%	• Infection, inflammation
• Eosinophils	1–4%	• Allergic reactions, parasites
• Basophils	0.5–1%	• Inflammation
• Lymphocytes	1 000–4 000/mm^3	• Immune response

Test	Normal Value	Interpretation
Coagulation Tests		
Prothrombin Time (PT)	11–12.5 sec	• Used to measure degree of anticoagulation, therapeutic level: 2–3 min
International Normalization Ratio (INR)	0.81–1.2 min	• Standardized PT for clients on coumarin
Activated Partial Thromboplastin Time (aPTT)	30–40 sec	• Used for clients on heparin to measure degree of anticoagulation
Partial Thromboplastin Time (PTT)	60–70 sec	• Therapeutic level: 46–76 sec
Platelets (Thrombocytes)	150 000–400 000 × 10^9	• Necessary for normal clotting of blood in the early stages of the clotting process

Blood Chemistry

• Measures noncellular components of the blood

Test	Normal Value	Interpretation
Arterial Blood Gases (ABGs)		
• Arterial pH	7.35–7.45	• Evaluates respiratory, cardiac, and renal functioning and determines acid–base balance
• Arterial PaO$_2$	80–100 mm Hg	
• Arterial PaCO$_2$	35–45 mm Hg	
• Bicarbonate (HCO$_3^-$)	21–28 mmol/L	
• O$_2$ Saturation	95–100%	
Cardiac Markers		
Cholesterol	<5 mmol/L	↑ Risk of coronary artery disease (CAD)
High-Density Lipoproteins (HDL)	>1.55 mmol/L	"Good cholesterol"
Low-Density Lipoproteins (LDL)	<2.59 mmol/L	"Bad cholesterol"
Triglycerides	Male: 0.45–1.81 mmol/L	• Storage form of lipids
	Female: 0.40–1.52 mmol/L	• ↑ Risk of CAD
Transaminases		
• Aspartate Aminotransferase (AST)	0–35 IU/L	• ↑ Liver disease, pulmonary and myocardial infarctions
• Alanine Aminotransferase (ALT)	<4–36 IU/L	• ↑ Liver disease, shock
• Troponin T (TnT)	<0.1 mcg/L	• Cardiac damage, renal failure
• Troponin I (TnI)	<0.35 mcg/L	• ↑ 3 hours following damage
• Creatine Kinase (CK)	Male: 55–170/mcL	• ↑ Cardiac muscle, skeletal muscle, brain damage
	Female: 30–135 mcL	• ↑ 6 hours following damage
Lactic Dehydrogenase (LDH)	100–190 U/L	• Tissue damage, heart failure, myocardial infarction (MI), liver disease, muscle damage
Gamma-Glutamyl Transpeptidase (GGT)	Male: 8–38 U/L	• ↑ MI; liver disease, pancreatic disease, cytomegalovirus infections
	Female: 5–27 U/L	
Folic Acid	11–57 mmol/L	• ↑ Pernicious anemia, vegan diet
		• ↓ Alcoholism, deficiency, malnutrition, renal disease
Diabetic Markers		
• Fasting Blood Glucose (FBG)	4–6 mmol/L	• ↑ Indicates hyperglycemia (diabetes mellitus)

Test	Normal Value	Interpretation
Two-Hour Oral Glucose Tolerance Test (OGTT)		
• After 1 hour postintake	<11.1 mmol/L	• Evaluates absorption of glucose into cells, assesses for diabetes mellitus or excess insulin secretion
• After 2 hours postintake	<7.8 mmol/L	
Glycosylated Hemoglobin (HbA$_{1c}$)	HbA$_{1c}$: <6%	• Measures the average blood glucose levels over approx. 2 months. A high value indicates blood glucose level fluctuations (unbalanced diet).
• Glycohemoglobin		
Electrolytes		
• Sodium (Na$^+$)	135–145 mmol/L	• Required for normal fluid and electrolyte balance, acid–base balance, nerve impulse conduction, muscle contraction
• Potassium (K$^+$)	3.5–5 mmol/L	
• Chloride (Cl$^-$)	98–106 mmol/L	
• CO$_2$ content	21–28 mmol/L	
Calcium		
• Total Calcium	2.25–2.755 mmol/L	• Osteoporosis, hypo- and hyperparathyroidism
• Ionized Calcium	1.05–1.30 mmol/L	
Serum Magnesium	0.74–1.07 mmol/L	• Required for adenosine triphosphate (ATP) production, neuromuscular functioning
		• ↓ Malnutrition, alcoholism
		• ↑ Mg^{++} antacids, renal disease
Serum Phosphorus	Adult: 0.97–1.45 mmol/L	• ↑ P = ↓ Ca^{++}
		• ↓ Hypercalcemia; chronic P-containing antacids, low dietary intake, alcoholism
		• ↑ Renal and liver failure, hypocalcemia, bone cancer
Iron		
• Serum Iron	Male: 14–32 mcmol/L	• ↓ Inadequate dietary intake, malabsorption, blood loss, neoplasms
	Female: 11–29 pmol/L	
• TIBC (total iron-binding capacity)	45–82 mcmol/L	
• Ferritin	Male: 26–674 pmol/L	• ↑ Liver disease, hemochromocytosis, hemolytic anemias
	Female: 22–337 pmol/L	

Test	Normal Value	Interpretation
Liver and Renal Disease Markers		
Protein		
• Total	64–83 g/L	• Malnutrition, renal disease, liver disease, burns
• Albumin	35–50 g/L	
• Globulin	23–34 g/L	
Bilirubin		
• Total	5.1–17 mcmol/L	• Elevated with impaired liver functioning
• Indirect	3.4–12 mcmol/L	
• Direct	1.7–5.1 mcmol/L	
Blood Urea Nitrogen (BUN)	3.6–7.1 mmol/L	• Liver and renal disease, protein catabolism
Creatinine	15.3–76.3 mcmol/L	• Secreted by kidneys, result of creatine metabolism

Test	Normal Value	Interpretation
Uric Acid	Male: 240–501 mcmol/L	• End product of purine metabolism
	Female: 160–430 mcmol/L	• High-protein diet, alcoholism, tissue destruction
Serum Amylase	100–300 U/L	• Assess for pancreatitis
		• ↑ Bowel obstruction and perforation, mumps
Thyroxine (T$_4$) Free	10–36 pmol/L	• Diagnosis of hypo- or hyperthyroidism
Triiodothyronine (T$_3$)	1.7–5.2 pmol/L	
Viral Testing for AIDS		
Enzyme Immunoassay Assay (EIA)	Negative	• Identifies antibodies to HIV, not viral antigens; usually takes 2–12 weeks to develop
Western Blot Test	Negative	• Used to verify positive EIA test, presence of viral genetic material in blood, viral load of less than 500 copies/mL is indicative of effective treatment
Viral Load	Undetected	
Polymerase Chain Reaction (PCR)	Negative	• Detects presence of virus

Urine Chemistry

- Measures components of the urine
- General characteristics: clear, amber yellow, aromatic odour

Test	Normal Value	Interpretation
pH	4.6–8	• Alkaline urine: vegetarian diet, renal failure • Acidic urine: acidosis, starvation, diarrhea, fever
Specific Gravity (SG)	1.005–1.030	• ↑ (meaning a high specific gravity, above the high range given): dehydration, glycosuria, syndrome of inappropriate antidiuretic hormone (SIADH) • ↓ (meaning a low specific gravity, below the low range given): overhydration, diabetes insipidus
Bilirubin	5.1–16 mcmol/L	• Presence indicative of liver disease
Catecholamines		
• Epinephrine	<109 nmol/day	• ↑ Indicative of heart failure, pheochromocytoma
• Norepinephrine	<590 nmol/day	• 24-hour specimen
Chloride (Cl⁻)	110–250 mmol/L	• 24-hour specimen • ↑ Addison's disease • ↓ Dehydration, perspiration, burns, vomiting

Test	Normal Value	Interpretation
Creatinine	Male: 53–106 mcmol/L Female: 44–97 mcmol/L	• 24-hour specimen • ↓ Renal disease • ↑ Anemia, leukemia, atrophy
Creatinine Clearance	1.42–2.25 mL/sec	• 24-hour specimen • ↓ Renal disease
Glucose	Negative	• Presence indicative of diabetes mellitus, stress, infection; low renal threshold for reabsorption of glucose
Ketone Bodies	Negative	• Presence indicative of diabetes mellitus, excess protein in diet, starvation
Protein (Single Specimen)	Negative	• Presence indicative of heart disease, stress, renal disease
Protein (24-hr Specimen)	<0.15 g/day	• Renal disease
Sodium (Na⁺)	40–250 mmol/day	• 24-hour specimen • ↑ Renal disease • ↓ Hyponatremia
Vitamin B$_{12}$	8–40% of radioactive vitamin B$_{12}$ in urine in 24 hours	• Measured dose of vitamin B$_{12}$ administered followed by 24-hour urine specimen • Identifies vitamin B$_{12}$ deficiency • Lack of B$_{12}$ in urine indicates malabsorption; lack of intrinsic factor
Uric Acid	1.48–4.43 mmol/day	• 24-hour specimen • ↑ Gout, leukemia • ↓ Renal inflammation
Urobilinogen	0.5–4 mmol/day	• 24-hour specimen • ↑ Liver disease, hemolytic disease • ↓ Biliary obstruction
Microscopic Examination		
• Red blood cells	0–2	• Presence indicative of infection, renal disease, trauma
• White blood cells	0–4	• ↑ Indicative of infection
• Casts	Negative	• ↑ Glomerulonephritis
• Crystals	Negative	• ↑ Infections, renal calculi
• Bacteria	Negative	• ↑ Infections

Stool

Test	Normal Value	Interpretation
Occult Blood	Negative	• Intestinal bleeding that cannot be visualized directly • May indicate tumours, diverticulitis, ulcers, inflammatory bowel disease, oral or nasopharyngeal bleeding
Ova and Parasites	Presence of pathogenic organisms	• Intestines normally contain bacteria (e.g. *Escherichia coli, Staphylococcus aureus, Clostridium*) • Overgrowth due to imbalance may cause disease • Ova = parasitic eggs

Miscellaneous

Test	Normal Value	Interpretation
Cerebrospinal Fluid (CSF)	Clear, colourless RBC: negative WBC: 0–5 cells/L (adult) Organisms: negative Pressure: <20 cm H_2O	• Change → infection, tumour, hemorrhage, trauma
Sweat Chloride Test	<50 mmol/L	• ↑ Used to diagnose cystic fibrosis

Diagnostic Procedures

Abdominal Paracentesis

This is a sterile procedure in which accumulated fluid from within the abdominal cavity is removed for client comfort or for analysis. The client first voids to avoid bladder injury and is then, in most instances, placed in a supine position for the procedure. A large-bore needle is inserted into the peritoneal cavity, and fluid is withdrawn into a syringe or drained into a vacuum bottle. Following the procedure, pressure to the inserting site is applied for several minutes, followed by a sterile dressing.

Amniocentesis

This sterile test involves the insertion of a needle trans-abdominally to remove a sample of amniotic fluid from the amniotic sac. The woman voids and is placed in a supine position with a towel under the right buttock to displace the uterus. A fetal monitor assesses the fetus during the procedure, and a sonogram is used to direct the needle. The test is used to detect certain defects, such as chromosomal abnormalities, ABO and Rh incompatibilities, and disorders such as fetal anemia.

Angiography

An angiogram is an X-ray of blood vessels following the injection of a radio-opaque contrast medium. The contrast medium is injected via a percutaneous catheter. Images of the area being examined are visualized on a monitor and may be recorded on film. The contrast medium will outline abnormalities and obstructions.

Arthroscopy

This test is an invasive surgical procedure involving the insertion of a fibre-optic arthroscope into a joint space for the purpose of directly visualizing the internal structures of the joint. Abnormalities caused by injury or disease can be identified. In addition, boney debris can be removed and specimens obtained for laboratory examination.

Barium Enema

This test is an X-ray of the lower bowel following the insertion of a radio-opaque barium contrast medium enema. Preparation of the bowel with laxatives or enemas is required on the day prior to the examination to ensure that the lower bowel is clear of stool. The examination identifies any gross abnormalities, such as growths or obstructions.

Barium Swallow

X-rays are taken as the client swallows a radio-opaque contrast barium drink. X-rays can identify abnormalities of structure and motility in the pharynx, esophagus, and stomach. The client needs to be on nil per os (NPO) 8 hours prior to the test, and all metal objects must be removed. To promote excretion of the barium, the client is encouraged to drink plenty of fluids following the test.

Bone Marrow Aspiration

This sterile test involves the removal of bone marrow cells from sites such as the iliac crest or sternum, for laboratory examination. Bone marrow cells are responsible for the production of blood cells (hematopoiesis), and, consequently, laboratory examination can identify defects in the cells and their formation. Specimens may be taken for the diagnosis of such conditions as anemias, blood carcinomas, lymphomas, and effects of chemotherapy.

Colposcopy

This procedure is used to locate suspicious areas of the cervix requiring biopsy. A colposcope is a microscope containing a light source and magnifying glass that allows the physician to see abnormal areas of the cervix that would not be visible to the naked eye. It directs the physician more accurately to areas of tissue that need to be biopsied. After the specimen for cytological examination has been obtained, the cervix is cleansed with 3% acetic acid to remove cellular debris. Changes in epithelial tissues can more clearly be observed. Following the procedure, the client should be advised that a small amount of bleeding may occur if a biopsy was taken. Abstinence from intercourse is recommended until biopsy results have been obtained.

Bone Mineral Density (BMD)

The dual-energy X-ray absorptiometry (DEXA) procedure measures the mass of bone density per unit volume. Two X-rays of different energy levels measure the density of the bones being examined. The procedure measures the density of the bone in the specific areas of the hips, spine, and forearm. This test is commonly done on menopausal women to assess for osteoporosis.

Bone Scan

A bone scan is a nuclear medicine procedure used in the examination of bones. A radioactive contrast medium is injected, and then a scanner visualizes the condition of the bone. The procedure is used in the diagnosis of metastatic bone disease.

Bronchoscopy

Direct visualization of the upper respiratory passageways (tracheobronchial tree) is done through the use of a bronchoscope. The bronchoscope may be rigid or flexible. Specimens may be taken during the procedure for laboratory examination. The procedure may also be used for therapeutic purposes, such as removal of foreign bodies or obstructions. The client requires sedation and local anaesthesia to prevent activation of the choking reflex.

Cardiac Catheterization

This test is a sterile, invasive procedure that involves the insertion of a catheter through a vein or artery that is then passed into the heart chambers. Following injection of a radio-opaque dye through the catheter, X-ray images of the gross cardiac structures and coronary arteries can be visualized. For right-sided catheterization, the catheter is inserted into the femoral, brachial, or subclavian vein and passed into the structures of the right side of the heart. For left-sided heart catheterization, the catheter is inserted into the right

femoral or brachial artery and then passed into the aorta and left heart chambers.

Cardiac catheterization is used to determine pressures within the heart structures, narrowing of coronary arteries, congenital abnormalities, and ventricular aneurysms and to perform angioplasty surgery. Clients require sedation and should be NPO for at least 8 hours. An intravenous line is inserted for access should medications be required during the procedure. The client should void prior to the procedure.

Following the procedure, the client remains on bed rest for 8 hours; a pressure dressing is applied to the catheter insertion site and monitored carefully for hemorrhage; the affected extremity remains extended and immobilized to ensure effective clotting at the catheter insertion site; and vital signs are monitored carefully.

Cardiac Exercise Stress Test

This noninvasive test is used to evaluate cardiac functioning under physical stress. The client undertakes controlled exercise on a stationary bicycle or treadmill while an electrocardiography (ECG, EKG), the heart rate, blood pressure, and development of chest pain are monitored. At regular intervals, the intensity of the exercise is increased in order to identify any abnormal changes that may occur as the exercise increases. The degree of intensity of the exercise is predetermined by the cardiologist based on the client's health, physical condition, and age. Abnormal changes in the ECG, heart rate, blood pressure, and development of pain indicate the inability of the coronary arteries to meet the demands of the heart, as in coronary artery disease. Stress testing is contraindicated in clients suffering from conditions such as unstable angina, severe congestive heart failure, recent MI, certain chronic lung diseases, and so on.

Colonoscopy

Direct visualization of the colon is observed through the use of an endoscope. The endoscope is long and flexible and is inserted through the rectum, back through the colon to the cecum. The physician is able to visualize the lining of the colon for abnormalities and growths. On the day prior to the test, complete cleansing of the bowel is required through the prescription of strong cleansing laxatives or enemas. The client is also restricted to clear fluids. This ensures that the bowel can be visualized clearly.

Computed Tomography Scan (CT Scan)

A CT scan is a noninvasive, specialized computerized scanner that X-rays the body from different angles, providing a three-dimensional picture of the specific body part to identify abnormalities. The procedure uses ionized radiation as an energy source.

Cystoscopy

Direct visualization of the urethra and inner lining of the urinary bladder is observed through the use of a cystoscope. The procedure is usually performed with the use of a local anaesthetic. Abnormalities in the urethra, prostate, and bladder lining can be identified.

Biopsy

A biopsy involves the removal of a small sample of tissue for macroscopic and microscopic pathological examination. Biopsies may be taken by a needle inserted into the tissue and withdrawing a sample, excision of a small piece of tissue, a scraping from a surface of the tissue to be biopsied, or a punch that when placed on top of the tissue excises a sample. In some instances, local anaesthesia may be used to reduce discomfort. Tissue for biopsy is also commonly taken during surgical procedures under general anaesthetic.

Echocardiogram (Heart Sonogram)

This noninvasive ultrasound test uses sound waves to assess the structures of the heart and how they function. A transducer is moved over the chest wall emitting high-frequency sound waves that reflect off the heart structures and back to the transducer. The waves are then displayed on an oscilloscope, allowing for direct visualization of the heart shape, size, and thickness; activity of the heart valves; and related structures. Structural and functional abnormalities can be identified, such as atrial septal defects, valve disease, and aortic stenosis.

Electrocardiogram (ECG, EKG)

This noninvasive test provides a graphic recording of the cardiac cycle during depolarization and repolarization of the heart. Electrodes (leads) are placed on each of the client's limbs and at specific regions of the chest. The electrodes detect the activity of the heart from a variety of regions and can detect abnormalities in the electrical conduction of the intrinsic cardiac conducting system, such as cardiac arrhythmias or damage to myocardial tissue. An individual ECG using 12 leads provides a comprehensive recording of myocardial currents in two different planes. ECG monitoring may be continuous at the bedside, allowing for constant monitoring of cardiac activity, as in critical care units. In this situation, either three or five leads are usually applied to the chest.

Electroencephalography (EEG)

This test is a noninvasive electrophysiological procedure that evaluates the electrical activity within the brain. With the client in a sitting or supine position, approximately 10 electrodes are placed in specific positions around the head. Electrical records are then taken and produced on paper for analysis. Specific wave patterns indicate certain disorders, such as seizure activity, the presence of lesions, effects of certain toxic substances, inflammation, increased intracranial pressure, and the determination of death.

Endoscopy

The direct visualization of a hollow organ or a tubular structure within the body is achieved using a flexible fibre-optic scope or an inflexible scope. Endoscopy can be used to examine the bronchi, esophagus, stomach, colon, bladder, and so on. See the sections on bronchoscopy, gastroscopy, and cystoscopy

Endoscopic Retrograde Cholangiopancreatography (ERCP)

This test uses a fibre-optic endoscope to provide direct visualization of the pancreatic and biliary ducts. Injection of radio-opaque dye into the area allows for X-ray visualization of the pancreatic, common bile, and hepatic ducts. With the client sedated, the endoscope is inserted down the esophagus, through the stomach, and into the duodenum for examination of the area.

The endoscopic procedure also allows for gallstones to be removed from the common bile duct, drainage of bile in jaundiced clients, insertion of stents in areas that have become narrowed, and widening of the bile duct. Specimens of tissue may also be taken for pathological examination.

The client is on NPO from midnight of the day before and is administered sedation just prior to the procedure. Following the procedure, the client remains on NPO until the gag reflex returns.

Gastroscopy

Direct visualization of the lining of the stomach is observed through the use of an endoscope. The esophagus is also visualized during the procedure. Sedation is required to prevent choking.

Intravenous Pyelogram (IVP)

Following the intravenous injection of a radio-opaque contrast medium, a series of X-rays are taken as the dye is excreted in the urine, passing through the kidneys, ureters, and bladder. Obstructions and abnormalities can be identified. Care needs to be taken when using the dye as clients may have adverse reactions. The dye can also be nephrotoxic to the kidneys.

Laparoscopy

This procedure involves the insertion of a scope into the abdomen to directly observe the abdominal and pelvic organs. It is used to identify pathological conditions that are manifested by acute and chronic abdominal pain, such as cancerous lesions. Certain surgical procedures may also be performed using a laparoscope, such as cholecystectomy, appendectomy, tubal ligation, and hernia repair.

This procedure is performed under general anaesthetic and requires all the pre- and postoperative care precautions and nursing care.

Lumbar Puncture

This invasive test involves the insertion of a cannular needle into the subarachnoid space of the spinal column at the 3–4 lumbar space. The client is side-lying, the back rounded and knees flexed toward the abdomen. The client should be directed to remain still during the procedure and, following completion of the procedure, remain flat for approximately 8 hours.

This test allows for measurement of cerebrospinal fluid (CSF) pressure by attaching a manometer to the needle. It also allows the removal of CSF for examination (colour, clarity, presence of RBCs, bacteria, malignant cells, protein, glucose, etc.). Medications can also be administered via this route, such as antimicrobials or anaesthetics.

Magnetic Resonance Imaging (MRI)

MRI is a noninvasive examination of a particular area of the body using magnetic and radio waves. A three-dimensional picture of the area is created, and abnormalities can then be identified. MRI does not use ionized radiation. All loose metal objects need to be removed from the client and procedure room.

Mammography

This test is a low-dose X-ray that reveals images and views of the breast from different angles. The breast is placed between two plastic plates that then gently compress and flatten the breast to provide a clearer image of the breast tissue. No preparation is required for this X-ray. Based on research, the Canadian Cancer Society suggests that under normal circumstances, women over the age of 40 have a yearly mammogram. Between the ages of 50–69, a mammogram every two years is suggested. The rationale for this change is based on the different types of breast cancer that develop in the different age groups.

Nuclear Scan

This test scans different areas of the body and involves the injection of a radionucleotide that is taken up by specific tissues. Gamma rays are emitted by the radionucleotide and detected by a scintillator. The scintillator converts the rays to an image of the body part.

Bone Scan

Abnormal bone tissue absorbs greater quantities of the radionucleotide, producing areas of concentration (hot spots). Bone scan is used in the diagnosis of such conditions as tumour growth, osteomyelitis, and arthritis.

Cardiac Scan

A radionucleotide identifies cardiac dysfunction, such as myocardial ischemia, myocardial infarction, myocardial dysfunction, and coronary artery perfusion.

Lung Scan

This test identifies changes in blood perfusion through the lungs, as well as pulmonary emboli.

Gallium Scan

Gallium is the radionucleotide used for scanning the entire body. The body is scanned at 24, 48, and 72 hours following the injection of the radionucleotide. Gallium scan is used to identify tumours (benign and malignant), inflammation, infection, and abscesses.

Positron Emission Tomography (PET) Scan

This type of scanning procedure is commonly used for evaluation of the brain and heart and in oncology. Radioactive chemicals are administered to the client that in turn become part of the normal metabolic processes of the particular organ.

Positrons are emitted from the radioactive chemicals and detected and converted by sensors and computed tomography to two- or three-dimensional images indicating a particular metabolic process at a particular site.

Pelvic Ultrasonography

A noninvasive procedure to confirm pregnancy and evaluate whether it is normal, abnormal, or multiple; the stage of development of the fetus; fetal position; or whether a tumour exists instead of a pregnancy.

A transducer is passed over the abdomen above the uterus, reflecting sound waves off the structures within the uterus back to the transducer. The waves are translated into pictures on an oscilloscope. Ectopic pregnancies, placenta previa, abruptio placentae, and tubal pregnancies can be identified.

Pulmonary Function Tests

These tests are prescribed to determine respiratory functioning: to assess for the presence and degree of lung disease, identify the type of lung disease, or assess for the effectiveness of therapeutic interventions for lung disease.

Tests include spirometry, lung volume and capacity, rates of airflow, and gas exchange. For the airflow rates and spirometry, the client breathes through a sterile mouthpiece, inhaling deeply and then forcibly exhaling several times. Calculations are made to assess for the following:

- Forced vital capacity (FVC)
- Forced expiratory volume in one second (FEV_1)
- Peak inspiratory and expiratory flow rates (PIFR/PEFR)
- Maximum mid-expiratory flow (MMEF)
- Maximal volume ventilation (MVV) is calculated by having the client breathe deeply and frequently for 15 seconds.
- Expiratory reserve volume (ERV) is calculated by having the client breathe normally into the spirometer and then exhale forcibly.
- Inspiratory capacity (IC) is calculated by having the client breathe normally into the spirometer and then inhale forcibly.
- Total lung capacity (TLC) is calculated by having the client breathe normally into the spirometer.
- Gas exchange of the lungs is usually evaluated by having the client inhale CO and then determining the difference between the amount of CO inhaled and exhaled.

For these tests to be successful, the cooperation of the client is important. Directions given to the client need to be clear. For 6 hours prior to the test, the client should refrain from taking any bronchodilators or smoking tobacco.

Thoracentesis

This sterile test involves the insertion of a needle into the pleural cavity for the purpose of removing fluid that has accumulated within the pleural space. With the client sitting upright, a large-bore needle is inserted into the pleural space and fluid is then aspirated.

Following removal of the needle, pressure is applied to the insertion site followed by a chest X-ray to check for pneumothorax.

Transcranial Magnetic Stimulation

This is noninvasive procedure in which a changing magnetic field is introduced into the brain to influence the brain's activity. The field is generated by passing a large electrical current through a wire stimulation coil over a brief period. After assessing a patient's resting motor threshold to determine dosing, an insulated coil is placed on or close to a specific area of the patient's head, allowing the magnetic field to pass through the skull and into target areas of the brain. Used in psychiatry for treatment of mood disorders.

Tuberculin Skin Testing

This test is used to identify a tuberculosis infection. It does not, however, detect whether the infection is active or dormant. An intradermal injection of purified protein derivative (PPD) of the tubercle bacillus is administered into the arm. An individual who is infected will produce a reaction at the injection site as lymphocytes that have been activated by the original infection will react to the PPD. A reaction (induration, not redness) at the injection site of greater than 5 mm in diameter read 48–72 hours following the injection indicates a positive result. A second injection may be administered to an individual who is suspected as having been infected but was negative for the first injection.

Individuals who received bacille Calmette-Guérin (BCG) vaccine in the past will show a positive result even though they have not been infected with the tubercle bacillus.

Ultrasonography

High-frequency sound waves are passed into the body, echo off body organs, and are then translated into a picture. Ultrasonography helps identify abnormalities. Depending on the area of the body being examined, certain preparation of the client may be required, such as NPO.

Ultrasonography can be performed on many areas of the body, such as the cardiac, abdominal, and pelvic regions, as well as the breast, to identify abnormalities in structure and function.

BIBLIOGRAPHY

Lewis, S. M., Bucher, L., Heitkemper, M. M., et al. (2019). *Medical-surgical nursing in Canada: Assessment and management of clinical problems* (4th Cdn. ed.). Milton, ON: Elsevier.
Pagana, K. D., Pagana, T. J., & Pike MacDonald, S. A. (2019). *Mosby's Canadian manual of diagnostic and laboratory tests* (2nd Cdn. ed.). St. Louis: Elsevier.
Potter, P., Perry, A., Stockert, P., et al. (2019). *Canadian fundamentals of nursing* (6th ed.). Milton, ON: Elsevier.
Stuart, G. (2013). *Principles and practices of psychiatric nursing* (10th ed.). St. Louis: Elsevier.

Mathematical Formulae Related to the Practice of Nursing

CALCULATION OF ORAL AND PARENTERAL DOSES OF MEDICATIONS

The **dosage ordered** refers to the dosage of the drug that has been prescribed for the client, for example, 500 mg, 2 g, or 30 UI. The **dosage available** is the dosage of the drug that is on hand, such as 250 mg or 0.5 g. The **drug form** is the form in which the available dosage is supplied, for example, tablets, capsules, or liquid.

Formula

$$\frac{\text{Dosage ordered}}{\text{Dosage available}} \times \text{Drug form}$$
$$= \text{Amount of drug to administer}$$

Example 1

Your client is ordered digoxin (Lanoxin) 0.125 mg by mouth daily. You have Lanoxin available in 0.25 mg tablets. How many tablets should you administer daily to your client?

$$\frac{0.125\,\text{mg}}{0.25\,\text{mg}} \times 1\,\text{tablet} = \textbf{0.5 tablet} \text{ of Lanoxin}$$

Example 2

Your client is ordered furosemide (Lasix) oral solution 40 mg daily for edema due to renal failure. The label on the container indicates 20 mg per 5 mL. How many millilitres should you administer daily to your client?

$$\frac{40\,\text{mg}}{20\,\text{mg}} \times 5\,\text{mL} = \textbf{10 mL} \text{ of Lasix}$$

CALCULATIONS FOR PEDIATRIC DOSAGES OF ORAL AND PARENTERAL MEDICATIONS

Medications prescribed for infants and children require adjustments in the dosages to accommodate the differences in their weights and body surface areas; gastro-intestinal, liver, and kidney functions; and metabolic activities. Much smaller doses of medications are required to avoid overdosage and toxicity. The child's weight and height are often used to calculate the correct dosage for a child. In addition, dosages for young children are usually ordered in liquid form.

Calculating Pediatric Dosage Based on Body Weight

Formula

$$\frac{\text{Drug dosage per}}{\text{kg of body weight}} \times \text{Weight of child (kg)}$$
$$= \text{Dosage to administer}$$

Example

A 2-month-old infant with septicemia is ordered ampicillin (Ampicin) 100 mg/kg/day every 8 hours intravenously. The infant weighs 4 kg. How many milligrams should be administered with each dose?

$$100\,\text{mg} \times 4\,\text{kg} = 400\,\text{mg of ampicillin daily (3 doses)}$$
$$400\,\text{mg} \div 3 = 133.3\,\text{mg per dose of ampicillin}$$

CALCULATIONS FOR INTRAVENOUS DRIP RATE

The **amount of solution to administer** is the quantity of fluid in millilitres that is to be administered during the shift. Intravenous tubing is selected according to the amount of fluid to be administered. The **drip factor** is the amount of fluid delivered by the specific tubing being used.

$$\frac{\text{Amount of solution to administer}}{\text{Time for infusion in hours}} \times \frac{\text{Drip factor of tubing}}{60\,\text{min}}$$
$$= \text{Drip rate (gtt/min)}$$

Example 1

The client is receiving 1 200 mL of 2/3 and 1/3 per 8-hr shift. At what rate should you set the drip rate if the intravenous tubing delivers 10 drops per minute?

$$\frac{1200\,\text{mL}}{8\,\text{hr}} \times \frac{10}{60\,\text{min}} = 25\,\text{gtt/min}$$

Example 2

The client is receiving 50 mL of 5% dextrose in water per hour. At what rate should you set the drip rate if the intravenous tubing delivers 60 drops per minute?

$$\frac{50\,mL}{1\,hr} \times \frac{60}{60\,min} = 50\,gtt/min$$

UNITS OF MEASUREMENT

Canada adopted the international system of units (called *Système Internationale d'Unités* in French and abbreviated as *SI*), or the metric system of measurement, in 1970. It is used by most countries of the world.

Although this system of measurement has been universally adopted throughout the healthcare system, the household system of measurement occasionally appears due to long-term habit. It is therefore important for the nurse to be aware of the more common equivalents.

Liquid Measure

3 teaspoons (tsp)	=	1 tablespoon (tbsp)
2 tablespoons (tbsp)	=	1 fluid ounce (fl oz)
8 fluid ounces (fl oz)	=	1 cup (C)
2 cups (C)	=	1 pint
2 pints	=	1 quart
4 quarts	=	1 gallon (gal)

Mass Measure

16 ounces (oz)	=	1 pound (lb)

Linear Measure

12 inches (in)	=	1 foot (ft)
3 feet (ft)	=	1 yard (yd)

Conversion of Household Measure to SI Measure

Liquid Measure

1 teaspoon (tsp)	=	5 mL
1 tablespoon (tbsp)	=	15 mL
1 ounce (oz)	=	30 mL
1 cup (C)	=	240/250 mL
1 pint	=	500 mL
1 quart	=	1 000 mL (1 L)
1 gallon (gal)	=	4 000 mL

Mass Measure

2.2 pounds (lb)	=	1 kg

Linear Measure

1 inch	=	2.54 cm
39.4 inches	=	1 m

Measurement of Temperature

To Convert Celsius to Fahrenheit

°Celsius × 1.8 + 32	=	°F

To Convert Fahrenheit to Celsius

°Fahrenheit − 32 ÷ 1.8	=	°Celsius

ANSWERS AND RATIONALES FOR PRACTICE QUESTIONS

CHAPTER 3

The correct answer is set off in boldface.

1. **C: Professional, Ethical, and Legal Practice T: Application**
   1. Abbreviations must be approved by the organization or agency.
   2. The Canadian Nurses Association does not approve abbreviations for documentation.
   3. **Abbreviations must be approved by the organization or agency.**
   4. Abbreviations must be approved by the organization or agency, not the individual unit.

2. **C: Professional, Ethical, and Legal Practice T: Critical Thinking**
   1. The person most involved in the procedure must obtain client consent. Practical nurses do not obtain consent for procedures performed by others.
   2. **The person most involved in the procedure and the one who can explain the procedure fully should obtain client consent.**
   3. Verbal consent is acceptable for some procedures, but surgery usually requires written consent.
   4. Consent can be withdrawn at any time during investigation or treatment, even if a signed consent had previously been obtained.

3. **C: Professional, Ethical, and Legal Practice T: Application**
   1. **Verbal orders are not telephone orders and should not be utilized unless in an emergency situation.**
   2. Verbal orders are not equivalent to telephone orders.
   3. Verbal orders may need to be accepted in emergency situations.
   4. There are no regulations that define which kind of nurse can accept verbal orders.

4. **C: Professional, Ethical, and Legal Practice T: Application**
   1. The dose is not correct, and the frequency is not identified.
   2. **The dose is accurate, the route is identified, the frequency is identified, and the qualifier is identified.**
   3. The dose is not correct, and the frequency is not identified.
   4. The dose is not correct, and the route is not identified.

5. **C: Professional, Ethical, and Legal Practice T: Knowledge**
   1. Evidence-informed care does not relate to government funding.
   2. **Evidence-informed care is founded in the transfer of current research into practice.**
   3. Evidence-informed care is described after research has been completed.
   4. Not all evidence-informed care focuses on assessment skills.

6. **C: Professional, Ethical, and Legal Practice T: Knowledge**
   1. This is not correct.
   2. This is not correct.
   3. This is not correct.
   4. **A nurse practitioner is usually educated at the master's level.**

7. **C: Collaborative Practice T: Application**
   1. Different learning styles require different teaching approaches.
   2. Learning is easier when the material is connected to what the learner already knows.
   3. **Learning occurs best when the learner identifies a learning need.**
   4. It is best to offer a variety of options to learners because some individuals learn best in the morning, whereas others learn best in the afternoon or evening.

8. **C: Collaborative Practice T: Application**
   1. "I" statements should be utilized with clients and colleagues.
   2. **When genuineness and warmth are utilized, the communication is more effective.**
   3. Communication is better facilitated by open-ended questions.
   4. Self-disclosure should be utilized minimally and only to build a therapeutic nurse–client relationship, not to share the practical nurse's point of view.

9. **C: Collaborative Practice T: Critical Thinking**
   1. Differences may contribute to conflict, but the conflict must then be acknowledged and resolved rather than the differences suppressed.
   2. Team collaboration is the most effective method of conflict resolution, even more effective than introducing a third party.
   3. **Team collaboration is the most effective method of conflict resolution. The team is required to work together to resolve the conflict.**
   4. At times there must be imposed guidelines, but team collaboration is most effective.

10. **C: Professional, Ethical, and Legal Practice T: Critical Thinking**
    1. This may not be practical or applicable in every client situation.
    2. **This is the primary consideration prior to the decision to apply restraints.**
    3. This is not a consideration.
    4. Consent may be required, but it may be verbal, or it may be from a substitute decision maker. It does not necessarily have to be a signed consent.

11. **C: Professional, Ethical, and Legal Practice T: Application**
    1. This is an assumption rather than factual documentation and does not note the exact time.
    2. As in choice 1.

3. **This is factual documentation.**
4. As in choice 1.

12. C: **Professional, Ethical, and Legal Practice T: Critical Thinking**
    1. Standards may help the practical nurse identify learning gaps, but this is not the most important purpose.
    2. **Standards of nursing practice define the expectation for practical nurses in various practice settings and situations and generally guide nursing practice.**
    3. While standards of nursing practice focus on defining expectations for acceptable practice, they do not focus on malpractice.
    4. The primary purpose of nursing practice and health professions acts, and thereby standards of nursing practice, is to protect the public's (not the nurse's) health, safety, and welfare.

13. C: **Professional, Ethical, and Legal Practice T: Knowledge**
    1. **The primary mandate of a health regulatory organization is protection of the public.**
    2. Labour organizations have the mandate of protecting practical nurses.
    3. The employer has a responsibility to serve the clients to whom they provide service.
    4. The nursing regulatory body protects the public from unsafe, unethical nursing care—it cannot be generalized to any other regulated profession.

14. C: **Professional, Ethical, and Legal Practice T: Application**
    1. Analysis and grouping of data is part of the nursing process, not the Best Practice Guidelines.
    2. Advance directives are individualized to specific clients; they cannot be generalized as best practice for whole groups.
    3. **Evidence-informed guidelines are tools that improve client, practical nurse, and organizational outcomes. They involve care that is based on actual observed and proven outcomes, not tradition-based care.**
    4. A code of ethics provides guidelines for compassionate care, educates about ethical responsibilities, and informs about moral commitments.

15. C: **Professional, Ethical, and Legal Practice T: Critical Thinking**
    1. This is a generally accepted interpretation but is not the most correct answer as the healthcare team has the responsibility to determine the client's exact wishes.
    2. Do Not Resuscitate may be open to interpretation and not involve only cardiac compressions.
    3. This is too vague an interpretation.
    4. **The client or substitute decision maker must decide what, if any, resuscitation is desired. The practical nurse has the responsibility to comply with the stated wishes of the capable client, whether they are written as a DNR or not.**

16. C: **Collaborative Practice: T: Knowledge**
    1. The physiotherapist helps people to restore, maintain, or maximize their physical strength, and improve their balance, muscle control, and walking.

2. **The speech-language pathologist helps people improve their speech and learn different strategies and ways to communicate. The speech-language pathologist also assists people with swallowing problems.**
3. The dietitian helps people plan health meals to make lifestyle changes for controlling their cholesterol levels and weight.
4. The social worker helps people cope with challenges faced in their lives after the disorder and assists with community services, finances, and work and discharge plans.

17. C: **Collaborative Practice T: Application**
    1. The nurse does not have Meaghan's consent to call her physician.
    2. The nurse does not have consent from Meaghan to call her parents.
    3. **The nurse requires consent from Meaghan to contact the physician or parents.**
    4. If the nurse suspects potential abuse or neglect, she must involve the Children's Aid Society immediately rather than wait until after the birth.

18. C: **Collaborative Practice T: Application**
    1. This does not ensure that client care is provided. The practical nurse has an ethical obligation to provide the required client care or find a substitute to provide the care.
    2. **The practical nurse has an ethical obligation to provide client care since no one else is available to provide the care.**
    3. The practical nurse must first provide the care (the referral to the gynecologist) or find a substitute to provide the care.
    4. The client's care cannot be deferred until next week. The practical nurse has an ethical obligation to provide the required care.

19. C: **Professional, Ethical, and Legal Practice T: Critical Thinking**
    1. The resident may not accurately recall what was said or may be afraid to discuss the event for fear of reprisal from the unregulated care provider.
    2. This action does not deal with the issue of verbal abuse. Situations of abuse must be addressed as close to the time of the incident as possible.
    3. **It is the professional responsibility of the practical nurse to stop the abuse immediately and notify the manager in order to ensure resident safety.**
    4. This action does not deal with the issue of verbal abuse.

20. C: **Professional, Ethical, and Legal Practice T: Application**
    1. The practical nurse is not accountable for the actions of the unregulated care provider (UCP); the UCP is accountable for her own actions.
    2. The practical nurse is not accountable for the actions of the UCP despite being on her lunch break.
    3. The practical nurse is not accountable for the actions of the UCP despite being the only registered/licensed staff on duty at the time of the fall.

4. UCPs are accountable for their care, including any actions or inactions taken that relate to the resident falling.

21. **C: Professional, Ethical, and Legal Practice T: Application**
   1. The practical nurse's decision to work the additional hours is his choice.
   2. The practical nurse's involvement of the labour union is separate from the practical nurse's accountability to provide safe and effective care.
   3. Payment of overtime is not the primary concern for the practical nurse; he must be competent to provide care.
   4. **The practical nurse's first priority is to provide high-quality client care. He must determine if he is too tired to provide competent care.**

22. **C: Professional, Ethical, and Legal Practice T: Application**
   1. **Inserting an intravenous line (with a physician or a nurse practitioner [NP] order) that is used to administer medication that will cause death of a client is within the scope of practice for the practical nurse when assisting with medical assistance in dying (MAID).**
   2. The law only allows NPs or physicians to administer medication to cause the death of a client who is receiving MAID. No other persons are legally permitted to administer medication for MAID.
   3. Practical nurses who provide information to clients about the lawful provision of MAID must ensure that they do not encourage the client to choose MAID. It remains a crime for anyone to encourage, counsel, advise, recommend, or in any way influence a person to end his or her life.
   4. The practical nurse can provide post-mortem care and bereavement care to families of clients who received MAID.

23. **C: Professional, Ethical, and Legal Practice T: Critical Thinking**
   1. **The student practical nurse is responsible for her knowledge and actions.**
   2. The staff nurse working with the student practical nurse is not responsible for the student practical nurse's actions.
   3. The student practical nurse is accountable for her knowledge and actions, not the clinical instructor.
   4. The student practical nurse is responsible for her knowledge and actions.

24. **C: Professional, Ethical, and Legal Practice T: Critical Thinking**
   1. **Aspirin is contraindicated for clients who are receiving Coumadin. The practical nurse must clarify the order with the physician.**
   2. The client may not have accurate knowledge of his medications.
   3. The pharmacist cannot change the prescribed drug order.
   4. The practical nurse does not need to consult with colleagues.

25. **C: Professional, Ethical, and Legal Practice T: Knowledge**
   1. Chemical restraints include medications.
   2. Physical restraints include side rails, Posey vests, etc.
   3. **"Hazardous" is not a restraint category.**
   4. Environmental restraints include a locked ward or room.

26. **C: Professional, Ethical, and Legal Practice T: Application**
   1. Passwords should never be shared, even if client care is provided.
   2. The student practical nurse who provided the care should document the care.
   3. **Passwords should not be shared. Anyone who will be documenting client care should be provided with a password.**
   4. The student practical nurse should take responsibility for retrieving a forgotten password.

27. **C: Professional, Ethical, and Legal Practice T: Application**
   1. **The client has withdrawn consent; the practical nurse cannot force treatment.**
   2. The client has expressed her wishes. This does not require intervention from the charge nurse.
   3. The diagnosis of depression does not mean the client is unable to provide informed consent for treatments.
   4. It is not ethical nor therapeutic for the practical nurse to insist that the client take the medication.

28. **C: Professional, Ethical, and Legal Practice T: Critical Thinking**
   1. **Checking the client's identification bracelet is the safest method to ensure the "right client."**
   2. Clients may have similar names.
   3. Some clients may not have access to their health card or hospital identification card.
   4. Clients may not be in the correct bed.

29. **C: Professional, Ethical, and Legal Practice T: Application**
   1. The client may not have accurate knowledge of the obstetrician's orders for postpartum pain relief.
   2. **Practical nurses must have the original prescriber clarify the order.**
   3. Clarification must be obtained from the prescriber, not other healthcare providers.
   4. As in choice 2.

30. **C: Professional, Ethical, and Legal Practice T: Application**
   1. Codes of ethics provide general guidelines about practice and behaviour and would not include specific details as to how to reposition a client.
   2. **Confidentiality and privacy are included in ethical behaviour.**
   3. Negotiation related to use of skills is not part of a code of ethics and depends on the workplace.
   4. As in choice 3.

CHAPTER 4

The correct answer is set off in boldface.

1. **C: Professional, Ethical, and Legal Practice T: Application**
   1. Practical nurses should always address the person by the last name, as some older adults may resent being called by their first names by younger persons.

2. If Mrs. Sloane was hard of hearing, it is best for the practical nurse to face her directly so that her mouth and face are visible. Speaking loudly or shouting may distort speech.

3. **It is important to adjust the pace of the interview to allow older adults sufficient time to report background historical information. Also, it may take the older adult a greater amount of response time to interpret the question and process the answer.**

4. Touch is a non-verbal skill that is very important to older people. Touch communicates empathy and understanding of their problems.

2. **C: Foundations of Practice T: Critical Thinking**

1. Older adults do lose muscle mass as they age, but this is not the cause of shortened stature.

2. **With age, the intervertebral discs become thinner, thus shortening the spinal column and leading to shortened stature.**

3. Many older adults develop osteoporosis leading to decreased height, but this is not the primary reason.

4. Kyphosis mostly occurs as a result of osteoporosis.

3. **C: Foundations of Practice T: Knowledge**

1. Systolic, but not diastolic, pressures tend to increase.

2. As in choice 1.

3. Blood pressure does not become variable due to age.

4. **As the heart pumps against a stiffer aorta, the systolic pressure increases, leading to a widened pulse pressure.**

4. **C: Foundations of Practice T: Knowledge**

1. **Skin tags are overgrowths of normal skin that form a stalk and are polyplike. They occur frequently on the eyelids, cheeks, neck, axillae, and trunk of the older adult.**

2. Edema is an abnormal finding and may indicate a circulatory or cardiac problem.

3. There is often increased hair on the chin, upper lip, and eyebrows of older females due to unopposed androgens.

4. Older adults have thinner skin on the backs of their hands, forearms, lower legs, and dorsa of feet and over bony prominences.

5. **C: Foundations of Practice T: Application**

1. This greyish-white arc is called *arcus senilis*. It is not related to cataracts.

2. **Arcus senilis is commonly seen around the cornea and is due to deposition of lipid material. Although the cornea may appear thickened and raised, it does not affect vision.**

3. Although arcus senilis may cause the cornea to look thickened, it does not affect vision.

4. Xanthelasma are soft raised yellow plaques occurring on the lids at the inner canthus and are more frequent in women. They are found with both high and normal blood levels of cholesterol.

6. **C: Foundations of Practice T: Application**

1. **Impacted cerumen ("ear wax") is a common but reversible cause of hearing loss in older people. Ear canal irrigation can remove the impacted cerumen and will be performed more easily if the cerumen is softened. Application of a cotton ball will help to seal the oil in the ear canal and soften the cerumen.**

2. Although coarse ear hairs may increase the accumulation of cerumen, application of a cotton ball is the appropriate action.

3. This is not necessary unless the cerumen cannot be removed by irrigation.

4. It is likely that use of a cotton swab will push the cerumen farther into the ear canal and could cause damage to the canal and eardrum.

7. **C: Foundations of Practice T: Critical Thinking**

1. It is normal for many older adults to temporarily forget the day of the week, especially due to the lack of structure or routine of not going out to a job. While a person may not provide the precise date, Mrs. Sloane would be considered oriented if she knew generally the present period of time and place.

2. Scores of 24–27 indicate no cognitive impairment. A slight decline to 25 may be a normal variable.

3. Most people temporarily misplace articles. It would be of concern if Mrs. Sloane were placing her belongings in inappropriate places, such as putting her hearing aid in the refrigerator.

4. **This indicates confusion, loss of orientation, and impairment of short-term memory and is an indication of dementia.**

8. **C: Foundations of Practice T: Critical Thinking**

1. This would be the second assessment.

2. This would be done early in the assessment provided that the infant was not crying.

3. This would disturb the infant and should be left until after the general assessment, heart rate, and respirations.

4. **Prior to the practical nurse disturbing the infant, she should develop an overall impression: body symmetry, spontaneous position, flexion of limbs, spontaneous movement, and any obvious facial abnormalities.**

9. **C: Foundations of Practice T: Application**

1. Although the baby needs to be examined while naked, there may be concerns about heat regulation if the environment is not warm. In addition, particularly for male babies, the diaper should be left on until the genitalia and anus are examined.

2. The parents should be present so they may be reassured by the examination, so they may learn about the normal growth and development of their infant, and so the infant is calmed by their presence.

3. **The baby responds to a soft, soothing tone of voice.**

4. The exam should be scheduled 1–2 hours after feeding, when the baby is not hungry or drowsy.

10. **C: Foundations of Practice T: Application**

1. **An infant's respirations are primarily diaphragmatic rather than thoracic; thus, the abdomen is watched to count and evaluate respirations.**

2. The normal respiratory rate for a newborn is 30–60 breaths per minute. A rate of 70 is tachypnea.

3. Infants display a respiratory pattern that is irregular, from rapid breaths to short periods of apnea.

4. Young infants are obligatory nose-breathers up to the age of 3 months, at which point they become nose- and mouth-breathers, so mouth-breathing would be an abnormal finding.

11. **C: Foundations of Practice T: Application**
    1. This may be visually assessed and is rarely clinically important.
    2. Head circumference is not part of the Apgar score.
    3. **The newborn's head measures about 32–38 cm and is about 2 cm larger than the chest. The measurement is plotted on a standard growth chart. An enlarged head circumference may be an indication of increased intracranial pressure, such as in hydrocephalus. A smaller than normal head circumference is an indication of microcephaly resulting from genetic or congenital problems.**
    4. Fontanelles are assessed visually and by palpation.

12. **C: Foundations of Practice T: Critical Thinking**
    1. **This is the most reliable and least invasive determination of a patent rectum and anus. It guarantees that the intestine is sufficiently patent to allow the passage of stool.**
    2. This is the anal reflex and is used to check sphincter tone.
    3. This is not a recommended practice as there is danger of harming the rectal mucosa.
    4. This should not be necessary, and even the fifth finger may be too large for the size of the newborn rectum.

13. **C: Foundations of Practice T: Knowledge**
    1. This elicits the Babinski reflex.
    2. **This will elicit the Moro reflex, as will placing the infant on a flat surface and hitting the surface sharply.**
    3. This will elicit the startle reflex.
    4. This will elicit the stepping reflex.

14. **C: Collaborative Practice T: Application**
    1. Depending on the age of the teenager, it may not be appropriate to involve the parents. Most adolescents need to feel in control of their bodies and their lives and may not want parents involved unless a serious problem is identified.
    2. Adolescents may not respond positively to authority, particularly in a health assessment situation. It is more important for the practical nurse to obtain their trust.
    3. **With this approach, the practical nurse will be able to gain the trust of the adolescent.**
    4. Future health problems will not be of interest or concern to the adolescent.

15. **C: Foundations of Practice T: Application**
    1. Alcohol has no effect on menstruation.
    2. Family history of ovarian cancer has no relation to the onset of menstruation.
    3. **Because Hilary is thin, she may have anorexia and be malnourished. Onset of menstruation is affected by nutritional status.**
    4. Sleep has no effect on menstruation.

16. **C: Collaborative Practice T: Critical Thinking**
    1. This does nothing to reassure Bradley and may sound patronizing.
    2. It is normal for boys of Bradley's age to be short prior to a growth spurt at puberty. Evaluation by a physician is necessary only if Bradley is extremely short.
    3. While some exercises may help to increase muscle size, they will not affect Bradley's height. It is more important to reassure him that this will occur at puberty.
    4. **This is a factual answer that will reassure Bradley that he is normal and that he will grow and be more like his friends when he reaches puberty.**

17. **C: Foundations of Practice T: Application**
    1. **This is called the forward bend test. The spine should appear vertical. If there is unequal height of scapulae, shoulders, or iliac crests, scoliosis is suspected.**
    2. Kyphosis is common during adolescence because of chronic poor posture. This is not a test for scoliosis.
    3. This will not identify scoliosis.
    4. This will not help to identify a curvature of the spine seen in scoliosis.

18. **C: Foundations of Practice T: Application**
    1. This question may solicit information about the parent–child relationship but is not the most important safety-related question.
    2. This question is directed at finding information concerning Sheldon's ability to manage the stress of balancing sports and school demands, but it is not the most important safety-related question.
    3. This question may lead to an assessment of Sheldon's goals and aspirations for his future but is not the most important safety-related question at this time.
    4. **Adolescents playing football are at particular risk of injury. The practical nurse needs to obtain information regarding protective equipment.**

19. **C: Foundations of Practice T: Critical Thinking**
    1. This obtains information about his cognitive function and compliance with academic expectations, not thought processes.
    2. This is a question that may obtain information about mood and affect.
    3. This is a test of a person's ability to remember new learning. It is more useful in assessing for dementia.
    4. **Paranoia and auditory and visual hallucinations occur with psychiatric and organic brain disease and with psychedelic drugs.**

20. **C: Foundations of Practice T: Knowledge**
    1. This is a common inflammatory condition of the skin but is not the most common skin condition in adolescence.
    2. **All teens have some form of acne, although with some, it is in the milder form of open comedones (blackheads).**
    3. Eczema is a type of dermatitis with various forms. It is not specific to the adolescent.
    4. Rosacea is a type of acne found primarily in adults.

21. **C: Foundations of Practice T: Critical Thinking**
    1. **A third heart sound is an abnormal finding.**
    2. Palpation of the apical pulse is a normal finding.
    3. Capillary refill less than 3 seconds is a normal finding.
    4. Calf circumferences within 1 cm is a normal finding.
22. **C: Foundations of Practice T: Application**
    1. **This is the correct sequence, as auscultation must precede palpation in order not to increase peristalsis.**
    2. Palpation may increase peristalsis and yield incorrect information.
    3. Light palpation may increase peristalsis.
    4. Auscultation must precede palpation to obtain accurate data.
23. **C: Foundations of Practice T: Application**
    1. This is a normal heart rate for a 2-month-old infant.
    2. This is a normal heart rate for a child this age after exercise.
    3. Although lower than the textbook normal heart rate, 50 is not abnormal in a young, well-conditioned athlete.
    4. **This is bradycardia in a 5-day-old infant. Although there are wide variations published as normal neonatal heart rates that range from approximately 100–160, this rate, especially after crying, is below normal.**
24. **C: Foundations of Practice T: Critical Thinking**
    1. This is a common but not ominous sign in a client who has had a head injury.
    2. **This is of concern as it implies that there has been some injury to the brain with loss of memory and cognitive function.**
    3. This is a normal finding postinjury and implies superficial rather than brain injury.
    4. The blood pressure presently remains within normal limits. It may become elevated due to pain, or there may be later deviations indicative of shock or brain swelling.
25. **C: Foundations of Practice T: Knowledge**
    1. Renal failure has no effect on the colour of stool.
    2. Intestinal polyps do not alter the colour of stool.
    3. **Gallbladder disease causing limited bile to be released may cause the stools to lighten in colour.**
    4. Celiac disease is a condition of gluten intolerance. While stools may change in consistency, there are no colour changes as indicated by Mrs. Sandoz.
26. **C: Foundations of Practice T: Application**
    1. This tests abstract reasoning, not judgement and decision making.
    2. This is a test of cognitive function and does not evaluate judgement.
    3. **This requires Mr. Robin to apply judgement and decision-making abilities to develop a wise course of action.**
    4. This tests abstract reasoning.
27. **C: Foundations of Practice T: Knowledge**
    1. **PERRLA is the acronym for Pupils Equal, Round, React to Light, and Accommodation. It is an evaluation of function of the pupil in the eyes.**
    2. PERRLA does not relate to this body part.

3. As in choice 2.
4. As in choice 2.
28. **C: Foundations of Practice T: Knowledge**
    1. A goitre is an enlarged thyroid. The thyroid is located in the neck area, not the scapulae.
    2. The thyroid is not located in the face.
    3. **This is the correct position for assessing the thyroid, which can be palpated to assess for enlargement or goitre.**
    4. This is located in the sternum, not the neck.
29. **C: Foundations of Practice T: Critical Thinking**
    1. **The suicide rates in Indigenous communities are three to five times greater than the national rates. Suicide is a particular risk in the young male population.**
    2. The prevalence of type 2 diabetes in this population is three to five times greater than the national rate. Although it occurs at a younger age, it is still not common in adolescence.
    3. There are higher rates of cardiac disease with this population but not specifically in this age group.
    4. People of Indigenous descent have a rate of tuberculosis almost seven times higher than that of the rest of Canada. However, the numbers still do not compare with the number of suicides in the adolescent age group.
30. **C: Collaborative Practice T: Critical Thinking**
    1. This is a question that would be asked as part of an abuse assessment screening but is not an appropriate introduction to the topic.
    2. As in choice 1.
    3. This introduction implies that the practical nurse is asking about abuse only because of clinic policy.
    4. **This introduction alerts the woman that questions will be asked about domestic violence and ensures that she is aware that she is not being singled out.**

CHAPTER 5

The correct answer is set off in boldface.
1. **C: Health and Wellness T: Foundations of Practice**
    1. **The health sector uses a significant amount of electrical energy by burning nonrenewable fossil fuels. This process produces greenhouse gases and significantly contributes to global climate change. Hospital waste and incineration practices contribute emissions of dioxins, mercury, and other heavy metals, which are toxic to human health.**
    2. Although hospital practices often lead to waste that could otherwise be recycled or avoided, any landfill runoff is not directly associated with hospital practices.
    3. The energy used and the waste produced affect the quality of the outdoor environment—the air, food, soil, and water.
    4. Although wind energy may be an alternative source of energy, it is not the result of the energy used and the waste produced by the health sector.

2. **C: Health and Wellness T: Collaborative Practice**
   1. This assumes that there is a conflict, which may not be true.
   2. **For effective and sustainable change, it is critical to build a community of people within the organization who understand and are motivated to work on the issues.**
   3. Focus groups may be used to facilitate discussion and input on the issues but are only mechanisms for the advocacy process and community building.
   4. Community promotion is not an actual process.

3. **C: Health and Wellness T: Collaborative Practice**
   1. Administrators are not likely to support policy changes without first understanding the rationale for and significance of the problem.
   2. Assessing clients for exposure to environmental contaminants would not increase awareness of environmentally responsible behaviours within the organization.
   3. **Implementing educational sessions on environmentally responsible health care would help to increase awareness of the issues among staff and administrators.**
   4. Promoting environmentally friendly products in the hospital gift store would not be the most effective strategy for increasing awareness of environmentally responsible behaviours in the health sector.

4. **C: Health and Wellness T: Foundations of Practice**
   1. Calorie-rich foods provide energy but often lack other essential nutrients.
   2. **Nutrient-rich foods are best to correct and prevent malnutrition-related diseases.**
   3. Inexpensive foods may not necessarily provide the nutrients required for a population that is malnourished.
   4. Some canned foods are nutrient-rich, but canned foods are not the only source of nutrient-rich foods.

5. **C: Health and Wellness T: Foundations of Practice**
   1. This improves health but is a long-term goal that may not be achieved.
   2. **Studies have shown that stable housing is the most important determinant for homeless clients to improve their socio-economic status and health.**
   3. This is a long-term goal but is unlikely to be achieved if there is no stable housing.
   4. This will improve general health, but stable housing has a greater influence.

6. **C: Health and Wellness T: Foundations of Practice**
   1. Most cases of tuberculosis may be treated in the community. Unless the person is a danger to others due to the communicability of the tuberculosis, the client cannot be forced into hospital.
   2. **Directly observed therapy is recommended for clients, such as those at a shelter for the homeless, known to be at risk for noncompliance.**
   3. The medications do not come in sustained-release formulations.

4. This may improve compliance but is not the best method to ensure treatment. Drugs that have the fewest side effects may not be the most effective for the particular strain of tuberculosis.

7. **C: Health and Wellness T: Foundations of Practice**
   1. While it is true that homeless people are more likely to be reinjured on the streets, if they are adequately nourished, the injuries would not likely become chronic.
   2. This may cause skin breakdown and injuries; however, with adequate nutrition, the lesions would not necessarily be chronic.
   3. Communicability of pathogens is possible; however, improved nutrition would strengthen the immune system to fight the pathogens.
   4. **Major complications of protein–calorie malnutrition are delayed wound healing and increased susceptibility to infection from a compromised immune system.**

8. **C: Health and Wellness T: Professional, Ethical, and Legal Practice**
   1. Complementary therapies may be controversial, but fully informed clients may request them, and practical nurses can become trained and certified.
   2. **Reiki is a complementary therapy. Such therapies may be integrated into the scope of professional practice provided that the practitioners have the requisite knowledge, skill, and competency; the client has made an informed decision, and it is sanctioned by agency policies and procedures.**
   3. The practical nurse does not need to schedule Reiki treatments outside of her scheduled shift.
   4. Olga is asking for Reiki treatment now, not after discharge.

9. **C: Health and Wellness T: Foundations of Practice**
   1. **Complementary therapies are those therapies used in addition to and in conjunction with conventional, or traditional, Western medicine.**
   2. Therapies that are used instead of traditional or conventional medicine are called *alternative therapies*. Many of the same interventions can be complementary and alternative therapies.
   3. Homeopathic remedies are a type of alternative or complementary therapy.
   4. Most complementary therapies are considered to be natural; however, this is not the definition.

10. **C: Health and Wellness T: Foundations of Practice**
    1. Mrs. Broadfoot has not stated that this is how she wishes to be treated. This is not individualized care.
    2. **This is client-centred, individualized care.**
    3. Mrs. Broadfoot—not the family—should be providing information about her plan of care.
    4. Clients should not all be treated the same. They should be treated as individuals.

11. **C: Nurse–Client Partnership T: Foundations of Practice**
    1. While there are many Indigenous dialects, most Indigenous people speak and understand English.
    2. There is no indication from her admission diagnosis that she would be too weak to talk.

3. There is no indication that she is in denial.
4. **Use of silence is a common communication phenomenon among members of Indigenous communities.**

12. **C: Health and Wellness T: Foundations of Practice**
    1. **Red meats have high iron content that is well absorbed by the body. There is no indication that Mrs. Broadfoot is vegetarian and will not eat a meat-containing diet.**
    2. Plant sources of iron are not as well absorbed as those in meat.
    3. As in choice 2.
    4. As in choice 2.

13. **C: Health and Wellness T: Professional, Ethical, and Legal Practice**
    1. This may be neither practical nor possible as it is not known how long it will take the family to arrive. Also, it is not known if they wish to view the body.
    2. There will likely be an autopsy as this is an unexpected death, but consent is not required.
    3. There is no indication that this is necessary. If it were, it would be included in specific cultural death rites.
    4. **This is the most inclusive answer. The practical nurse should obtain information by telephone from the family or consult other cultural resources.**

14. **C: Health and Wellness T: Foundations of Practice**
    1. **The Canadian Paediatric Society recommends that babies be positioned "back to sleep" to reduce the risk of sudden unexpected infant death (SUID).**
    2. Research has found associations between SUID and the prone position for sleep.
    3. There is controversy regarding co-sleeping. While some studies do suggest it is a factor in SUID, it is not as important as positioning infants on their backs.
    4. Hats and booties are required only when babies are exposed to cold.

15. **C: Health and Wellness T: Foundations of Practice**
    1. Early detection is secondary prevention.
    2. Megavitamin therapy is controversial and in this situation "postdiagnosis" of disease.
    3. Surgical treatment (appendectomy) is tertiary-level prevention.
    4. **Research has shown that remaining out of direct sunlight contributes to primary risk reduction of skin cancers.**

16. **C: Health and Wellness T: Foundations of Practice**
    1. Although cancer remains a serious life-threatening illness, the overall incidence of cancer in children is low, and survival rates among children with cancer have improved significantly in recent decades. It is not possible at this time to prevent most cancers.
    2. Asthma is common but not a common cause of death. Some asthma attacks can be prevented, but the disease cannot be prevented.
    3. **Injuries are by far the most common preventable cause of child death in Canada.**
    4. Although some children have congenital anomalies that are incompatible with life, most congenital anomalies are not preventable.

17. **C: Health and Wellness T: Foundations of Practice**
    1. **Research indicates that respiratory disease can be directly linked to contaminants in the environment.**
    2. The development of type 1 diabetes is not associated with exposure to environmental contaminants.
    3. Juvenile arthritis is not directly associated with exposure to environmental contaminants.
    4. Irritable bowel is not directly associated with exposure to environmental contaminants.

18. **C: Health and Wellness T: Professional, Ethical, and Legal Practice**
    1. Research has shown that good body mechanics alone are insufficient to prevent back injuries among practical nurses.
    2. This is not the safest way to move the client and could cause injury to personal support workers and the client.
    3. **Use of a mechanical lift is the only safe way to accomplish this transfer.**
    4. Explaining the procedure will not change his limited ability to stand even if using a support aid. Both client and nurse could sustain injuries.

19. **C: Health and Wellness T: Foundations of Practice**
    1. Some herbal remedies are safe, but pregnant women need full information.
    2. Ginger is known to have many medicinal properties.
    3. **Although knowledge about herbal remedies is incomplete, research about the pharmacology of ginger is available and can be shared with clients to enable their informed decision making.**
    4. The first trimester is a time of organogenesis; however, women need to be able to differentiate between benign, helpful, and harmful exposures.

20. **C: Nurse–Client Partnership T: Professional, Ethical, and Legal Practice**
    1. This statement assumes that the practical nurse knows what Mr. Drosinsky is feeling and may elicit an answer based on bravado.
    2. Initially, Mr. Drosinsky may not want to reveal information about his sexual relationships.
    3. **This sentence assures Mr. Drosinsky that he is not unique in his possible concerns and opens up the discussion about sexuality.**
    4. While nerve-sparing surgery is effective, this is not a conclusion that can be definite.

21. **C: Health and Wellness T: Foundations of Practice**
    1. This is a factor in childhood obesity, but it is not the major factor.
    2. As in choice 1.
    3. As in choice 1.
    4. **Childhood obesity is a multifactorial problem that is likely a combination of genetics and environment. She may have inherited a tendency to be overweight, combined with the role-modelling of her parents that led to their obesity.**

22. **C: Health and Wellness T: Foundations of Practice**
    1. Reducing fat alone does not cause weight loss unless total calories are restricted. It is difficult to sustain

a low-fat diet because many people feel unsatisfied and hungry. It is better to replace bad fats with good fats.

2. Complex carbohydrates are essential to good health. Restricting sources of fibre and phytochemicals has the potential to adversely impact health.

3. Low-calorie diets are most appropriate for clients who need to lose weight quickly. Very-low-calorie diets may be deficient in some nutrients. Choice is restricted and boredom is common, so the diet is difficult to sustain.

4. **By observing serving size from each food group, nutritional intake is balanced and calories are relatively controlled. This appears to be the optimal approach to achieving sustained weight loss.**

23. C: Health and Wellness T: Foundations of Practice
1. Because of Canada's geographical location, Ms. Blanche is not likely to obtain adequate vitamin D all year round. There is also the danger of skin cancer as a result of being exposed to direct sunlight.

2. Milk is a source of vitamin D, but it is not likely that Ms. Blanche will be able to drink enough to achieve 1 000 IU per day.

3. **Although in most cases it is best to achieve optimum nutrition through the diet, in the case of vitamin D, an intake of 1 000 IU can best be achieved by taking a supplement.**

4. Fortified cereals contain vitamin D, but it is not likely that Ms. Blanche will be able to eat a sufficient amount to achieve 1 000 IU per day.

24. C: Health and Wellness T: Collaborative Practice
1. **All people, regardless of age, handicap, or life choices, are sexual beings. Sexuality involves one's inner sense of being male, female, or some combination; gender role; and biological identity.**

2. Many parents would disagree with this statement, preferring that their children learn about sexuality in the home.

3. The purpose of teaching children about sexuality is not to prepare them for sexual intercourse. This may be what the parents are concerned about.

4. This is not necessarily a Canadian value. All cultures must be respected with discussions about sexuality.

25. C: Health and Wellness T: Foundations of Practice
1. **The practical nurse needs to first find out the total hours of sleep to determine if there is a sleep deficit. Adolescents and young adults frequently do not have sufficient sleep due to daytime responsibilities and extracurricular activities that do not fit with their circadian rhythms.**

2. This is important information, but the total number of hours of sleep is more pertinent.

3. As in choice 2.

4. This may be an underlying reason for Brendan's tiredness, but first the total number of hours of sleep must be determined.

26. C: Health and Wellness T: Foundations of Practice
1. There is no indication that the Waleses need assistance with walking.

2. **Older adults are at risk for falls in the bathtub and shower, where the water causes the surfaces to be slippery. Grab bars assist people to safely get in and out of the bath.**

3. These raise the height of the furniture to enable less difficulty rising from a sitting position. There is no indication that this is a problem for the Waleses.

4. This enables people to sit in the shower while holding the attachment to wash themselves. There is no indication that the Waleses are not able to stand in the shower.

27. C: Health and Wellness T: Foundations of Practice
1. Purchased chicken soup often has high levels of sodium, and most bagels are high in calories and have trans fats.

2. Delicatessen meat sandwiches have high levels of sodium. Caesar salad dressing is high in fat content.

3. Purchased bakery bran muffins often have high levels of trans fats. Cheddar cheese contains fat and is high in sodium.

4. **This menu provides low-calorie protein, vegetables, and fibre and is low in sodium.**

28. C: Health and Wellness T: Collaborative Practice
1. This is good advice, but people are not always symptomatic at the beginning of a communicable disease. It is not as important as handwashing.

2. **Hand hygiene is the single most effective action to stop the spread of communicable diseases.**

3. Young children are at increased risk of having and transmitting communicable diseases, but this is not the most important action.

4. It is now recommended that people cough or sneeze into their upper arm to redirect aerosol particles away from others. If a tissue is used, it must be disposed of appropriately, and the hands must be washed immediately afterward.

29. C: Health and Wellness T: Professional, Ethical, and legal Practice
1. **One way in which poverty adversely affects health is the inability to purchase needed medications. Asking an open-ended questions invites the person to share thoughts and feelings about the medication expense. The practical nurse needs to determine whether Ms. Price is able to buy Kyle's drugs. If not, the practical nurse may be able to access alternate means of obtaining the necessary medications.**

2. This is not a therapeutic approach, particularly if Ms. Price does not have the financial resources to purchase the medications.

3. It is not within the scope of practical nursing practice or ethical to tell a client which drugs are not important for Kyle.

4. It is not within the scope of practical nursing practice or legal to change a physician's prescription.

30. **C: Health and Wellness T: Foundations of Practice**
    1. The most effective teaching and learning is experiential. A computer game, while it may be a good supplement, is not as effective as actual practice.
    2. Rewards may work to reinforce learned behaviours but are not as effective as role-modelling as a teaching tool.
    3. Role-modelling and actual practice are more effective.
    4. **Children learn best from role-modelling and practice.**

31. **C: Professional Practice T: Professional, Ethical, and Legal Practice**
    1. This is not a practical solution, and it is unlikely that this is a police responsibility.
    2. This does not solve the initial problem of the contaminated needles and syringes and may encourage future use of the washroom as a place for the clients to inject.
    3. **The needles and syringes must be disposed of so they are not a hazard to others. The practical nurse has the knowledge to safely dispose of these articles.**
    4. This is not an ethical choice, particularly if the client was not the person who used the needles and syringes. The practical nurse may take the opportunity to later discuss the incident with this client.

CHAPTER 6

The correct answer is set off in boldface.

1. **C: Foundations of Practice T: Knowledge**
   1. An auscultatory gap is more common in older clients or clients with hypertension, but it does not always occur in these populations.
   2. Normal pulse pressure is 40 mm Hg.
   3. Orthostatic hypertension is measured by recording blood pressure (BP) and pulse with the client in three positions: supine, sitting, and standing.
   4. **This statement is correct. The nurse might make the mistake of recording the last sound at the beginning of the auscultatory gap as diastolic BP or the last sound at the end of the auscultatory gap as systolic BP.**

2. **C: Changes in Health Foundations of Practice T: Knowledge**
   1. **Rectal is the correct site for core temperatures.**
   2. Oral is only a surface temperature.
   3. Axillary is a surface temperature.
   4. Skin is only a surface temperature.

3. **C: Foundations of Practice T: Application**
   1. The pain and tingling is from poor circulation to the left foot because the elastic bandage is applied too tight. No blood flow is getting to the toes. The dressing will need to be removed.
   2. Administration of the analgesia will not decrease the pain if the poor circulation is result of the elastic bandage being too tight.
   3. **First the practical nurse needs to assess the circulation, sensation, and movement of the toes and foot to help determine if the dressing is too tight and affecting the blood flow to the foot. Then the practical nurse**

can remove the dressing once he or she has made the appropriate assessment.
   4. Elevation will not decrease the pain and tingling in the foot if the elastic bandage is on too tight.

4. **C: Foundations of Practice T: Application**
   1. Giving the injection quickly may increase client discomfort, and putting it into the sharps container without using the safety shield needles could still cause a needle-stick injury.
   2. **Safety-engineered needles retract after the injection is given and reduce the risk of needle-stick injuries.**
   3. This is not appropriate in this case.
   4. Wearing gloves prevents the practical nurse from coming in contact with any blood that oozes from the injection site. It does not prevent needle-stick injuries. It might prevent the needle from entering the practical nurse's skin as deeply or decrease the amount of blood entering the practical nurse's skin from the needle tip.

5. **C: Foundations of Practice T: Application**
   1. It is not correct to slow down the intravenous (IV) line if the practical nurse needs it to finish within the 8-hour time limit.
   2. It is not correct to slow down the IV line if the practical nurse needs it to finish within the 8-hour time limit.
   3. The IV line would normally be running at 125 mL/hr, but that rate must be increased slightly as there is 100 mL extra in the IV bag at 1500 hours.
   4. **The IV line is 100 mL behind schedule, and there is 600 mL to be infused over the next 4 hours. To calculate the new rate, divide the volume remaining over the time remaining: 600 mL ÷ 4 hr = 150 mL/hr. Although agency policies should be consulted, it is acceptable to increase the IV rate (25 mL/hr over the ordered rate) in this situation as the client is not an older adult, has no apparent cardiac history, is not at risk for fluid overload, and does require the fluid volume as ordered.**

6. **C: Foundations of Practice T: Application**
   1. Transdermal patches or discs should not be applied to hairy areas. They do not stick well to hairy areas, and that could affect the amount of medication absorbed.
   2. Transdermal medications can stay in place from 1 to 7 days, depending on what drug is being used.
   3. All old patches and discs of the same medication must be removed prior to applying a new transdermal medication or an overdose could occur.
   4. **The practical nurse should wear gloves when applying transdermal medications as they can be absorbed through the skin during application.**

7. **C: Foundations of Practice T: Critical Thinking**
   1. **Mrs. Gupta may have a baseline blood pressure of 90/60. The practical nurse needs to check the health record for previous baseline vital signs. If Mrs. Gupta is feeling faint or lightheaded, she could be symptomatic from the hypotension and needs treatment. The other vital signs are all within the normal range.**

2. The practical nurse needs more information before calling the doctor. The doctor will want to know the baseline vital signs, and the practical nurse will want to recheck the client's blood pressure prior to calling the doctor.

3. Dehydration or decreased circulating blood volume can cause the blood pressure to be lower, but that cannot be assumed before checking the urine output, asking the client how she feels, and looking at the baseline vital signs.

4. Modified Trendelenburg is a position in which the legs are elevated to promote venous return to the heart and thus increase cardiac output and blood pressure. That is not necessary unless Mrs. Gupta is going into shock, which her vital signs do not indicate.

8. **C: Foundations of Practice T: Application**
   1. Porridge is only allowed on a full fluid diet. Broth and apple juice would be permitted on a clear fluid diet.
   2. None of these foods are part of a clear fluid diet but can be eaten with a full fluid diet.
   3. Broth and Popsicles are part of a clear fluid diet, but orange juice would only be permitted on a full fluid diet.
   4. **All these foods would be allowed on a clear fluid diet.**

9. **C: Foundations of Practice T: Application**
   1. Limited mobility and exercise can be contributing factors, but they are not the cause of paralytic ileus in this situation.
   2. Eating too much too soon after surgery is much more likely to contribute to paralytic ileus. In a postoperative client, it is advised to wait until bowel sounds return after surgery before advancing to the postoperative diet.
   3. **Paralytic ileus in a postoperative client is most often caused by the action of narcotics and anaesthetics, delayed gastric emptying, slowed peristalsis resulting from the handling of the bowel during surgery, and resumption of the oral intake too soon after surgery.**
   4. Mrs. Gupta might need a rectal suppository (often on postoperative day 2 or later) to stimulate peristalsis and expulsion of the flatus; however, not giving it on postoperative day 1 would not have caused a paralytic ileus.

10. **C: Foundations of Practice T: Critical Thinking**
    1. **The practical nurse's first priority is to do a further assessment, which should include looking for redness or swelling in the calf area, measuring calf circumference in both legs, asking Mrs. Gupta if she has any pain in that area, and possibly gently palpating the area.**
    2. It is possible that Mrs. Gupta has a clot in her leg (thrombophlebitis), so it is best not to put the TED stocking back on until the medical team does a further assessment. It is appropriate to place the leg on a pillow to promote venous return to the heart.
    3. The calf circumference should be measured, but both legs should be measured to compare results. This is done after the area is assessed for redness and pain and

the client is asked about the history of the present swelling. The doctor would be notified after the practical nurse has done her assessment.

4. The practical nurse should not wash the client's leg or encourage her to exercise the leg until she is sure that there is no clot in her leg. Clots from the leg can travel to the lungs and cause a pulmonary embolism.

11. **C: Foundations of Practice T: Application**
    1. Measuring from the tip of the nose to the earlobe to the xiphoid process is the correct measurement to determine length of insertion.
    2. The client should not have too much water as this may cause aspiration. The client can dry swallow or sip on water (if allowed) while the nurse advances the tube. The client swallows to the predetermined length.
    3. Radiography is the most reliable way to check placement of nasogastric tubes. Many healthcare settings only insist on radiography to check the placement of small-bore feeding tubes prior to the start of enteral feeds. Some agencies may require X-ray confirmation of the placement of all nasogastric tubes prior to enteral feeds. In this scenario, a placement X-ray is not necessary as the tube is being used for decompression.
    4. **As the nasogastric tube is to be used for decompression, assessing tube placement by aspirating gastric contents and testing pH is reliable. Gastric pH should be less than 4.**

12. **C: Foundations of Practice T: Application**
    1. This is the hourly flow rate for the replacement intravenous line (IV) (640 mL ÷ 8 hr = 80 mL/hr).
    2. This is the hourly flow rate for the main IV.
    3. **This rate is correct, using the following formula:**

$$\frac{80 \text{ mL} \times 15 \text{ gtt/mL}}{60 \text{ min}} = 20 \text{ gtt/min}$$

    4. This is using an hourly flow rate of 100 mL/hr for the calculations rather than 80 mL.

13. **C: Foundations of Practice T: Application**
    1. All intravascular delivery system components up to the hub are changed every 24–72 hours, according to agency policy, to prevent infection.
    2. When total parenteral nutrition (TPN) infusions are started, serum glucose levels are checked frequently at the bedside as some elevation of blood glucose is expected. Weights are taken daily to monitor the client's hydration status and weight gain with therapy.
    3. More frequent monitoring of the temperature is required as infection is the most common TPN complication. At least monitor the temperature every 4 hours, not daily.
    4. **Speeding up the rate can cause hyperglycemia and slowing the rate can cause hypoglycemia. TPN is almost always managed with an infusion pump.**

14. **C: Collaborate Practice T: Critical Thinking**
    1. It is not necessary to isolate a client for a catheter-related infection and septicemia.

2. **A blood culture will determine if the infection is from the total parenteral nutrition (TPN) site. Other common sources of infection are the bladder or lung, thus the urine and sputum tests.**

3. The TPN is not held. If the blood cultures are positive, the central line might be removed and a new one started elsewhere. Antibiotics would be prescribed, but TPN would not be stopped abruptly.

4. There is no reason to stop the TPN and run dextrose 10%. The central line might need to be relocated, however, if it is thought to be the cause of the infection.

15. C: Foundations of Practice T: Application
1. This does not interfere with sterile technique as the saline has already been poured.
2. This is correct procedure and does not compromise sterile technique.
3. This is medical asepsis and correct procedure prior to doing a dressing change.
4. **This compromises sterile technique. If the normal saline was already open and not labelled, the practical nurse cannot assume that it is still sterile. It is considered sterile for only 24 hours after opening.**

16. C: Foundations of Practice T: Critical Thinking
1. Overuse of antibiotics predisposes clients to healthcare–associated infections (HAIs) such as MRSA (methicillin-resistant *Staphylococcus aureus*), although this is not likely to be the most significant factor with Mr. Roustas.
2. Spinal cord injury could lead to skin breakdown and the decubitus ulcer, but the actual skin breakdown is the most significant factor.
3. Mr. Roustas is only 42, which is generally not an age that predisposes him to decreased immunity, poorer nutrition, inadequate circulation, or skin breakdown.
4. **With skin breakdown, pathogens are able to enter the body, making this the most significant factor in the development of his HAI.**

17. C: Foundations of Practice T: Critical Thinking
1. A colonized or infected healthcare worker may disseminate the organism, but this is not the principal mode of transmission. The most frequently colonized site is the anterior nares.
2. **The principal mode of transmission is transfer from client to client on the hands of hospital personnel.**
3. Environmental contamination is uncommon.
4. Droplet transmission may occur during the care of a client with MRSA (methicillin-resistant *Staphylococcus aureus*) pneumonia, but this is not common.

18. C: Foundations of Practice T: Application
1. Slowing the rate will not help to correct the tissue irritation.
2. **These are signs that the vancomycin is irritating the intravenous (IV) site and it needs to be changed.**
3. It is not necessary to notify the physician.
4. The infusion will be stopped briefly while the IV site is changed.

19. C: Foundations of Practice T: Knowledge
1. Iodine should not be used on a wound bed as this solution is toxic to cells involved in wound healing.
2. **Moist, interactive wound healing promotes faster healing, better tissue quality, and less pain than other methods. Other methods, such as wet-to-dry dressings for pressure injury, are no longer recommended as they cause mechanical debridement that is not selective and can damage healthy tissue.**
3. Moist dressings often require more supplies than simple dry dressings.
4. There is no current research to indicate increased bacteria in a moist dressing.

20. C: Foundations of Practice T: Application
1. It is important to chart findings, but initially the practical nurse needs to respond and treat the hypoxia.
2. Deep breathing and coughing will not provide the oxygen the client needs first for hypoxia.
3. **Elevating the head of the bed and administering oxygen will relieve the client's symptoms of hypoxia.**
4. It is important to treat the client's breathing difficulties first, before calling the doctor.

21. C: Foundations of Practice T: Application
1. The practical nurse needs to perform an assessment prior to administering any analgesia and find out why the client is feeling prickling and itchiness sensations. Pain analgesia may not be the appropriate action.
2. **The practical nurse needs to perform a proper assessment. He or she must look at the incision to determine the cause of the prickling and itchiness sensations. They could be caused by the type of dressing used, infection, or other reasons.**
3. This is not a normal sensation to have at the incision site after surgery.
4. The practical nurse needs to perform a proper assessment before calling the physician.

22. C: Foundations of Practice T: Critical Thinking
1. To validate pain relief, the practical nurse needs to ask the client to rate the pain before and after administration of analgesics. The words "mild" and "severe" may not be specific enough.
2. Facial expressions do not always reflect the amount of pain that a client is experiencing.
3. Vital signs may or may not change when clients are in pain or after they receive analgesics. It is important to ask clients to rate their pain before and after analgesics as pain is subjective. Only the client knows the level of pain and pain relief.
4. **An effective way to rate pain relief in most adults is to use a numeric rating scale from 0–10 (0 being no pain; 10 being the most severe pain) before and after the administration of analgesics. For clients unable to respond to other pain intensity scales (such as children and older adults), a series of faces ranging from "smiling" to "crying" can be used. The rating scale has been shown to be ineffective in some studies, but it remains the most effective tool at present.**

23. **C: Foundations of Practice T: Application**
    1. People with diabetes should not soak their feet, as the skin can become macerated and more susceptible to injury and infection.
    2. **Nails should be filed straight across. Clippers or scissors should not be used on the toenails of diabetic clients.**
    3. The feet of diabetic clients should be inspected daily, as they have poor circulation.
    4. People with diabetes should not use a hot water bottle or heating pad on their feet, as they sometimes have loss of sensation in their lower limbs. They might suffer a burn without being aware of it.

24. **C: Foundations of Practice T: Application**
    1. If the client is coughing up the sputum, it is not necessary to suction. Suctioning is traumatic and should be used only when there are indications that the client cannot cough up the secretions without assistance.
    2. Sometimes the client is able to tell the practical nurse when to suction, but not always. Clients with a new tracheostomy or clients who are unconscious might not be able to communicate the need for suctioning.
    3. Suctioning is not a medical order. The practical nurse uses her clinical judgement in deciding when to suction a particular client.
    4. **The practical nurse uses clinical judgement to decide whether the client needs to be suctioned. Signs that the client needs to be suctioned may include one or more of the following: gurgling respirations, respiratory distress, low oxygen-saturation levels, and coarse crackles on auscultation.**

25. **C: Foundations of Practice T: Application**
    1. The client should not sit in a bathtub of warm water as she has just given birth and infection is a possibility.
    2. **The bladder needs to be emptied via catheterization. An intermittent catheterization carries less risk of infection.**
    3. The client should not go home until her bladder has been emptied. The full bladder would interfere with uterine contractions that are necessary to expel blood and any remaining uterine contents.
    4. An in-dwelling catheter is not necessary. It might be a source of a healthcare-associated infection (nosocomial infection).

26. **C: Foundations of Practice T: Application**
    1. Urinary catheterization is an example of surgical asepsis or sterile technique. This includes all procedures used to eliminate all micro-organisms from an area.
    2. Surgical asepsis or sterile technique is used to change a dressing on nonintact skin immediately postoperatively.
    3. **Cleaning the hospital environment and equipment routinely with approved solutions is used to reduce and prevent the spread of micro-organisms. This is called *medical asepsis* or *clean technique*.**

    4. An intramuscular injection is given using surgical asepsis. A sterile needle is used to perforate the client's skin.

27. **C: Foundations of Practice T: Application**
    1. This is true, but it is not the complete rationale for personal protective equipment (PPE).
    2. PPE will not necessarily prevent a healthcare-associated infection.
    3. It is true that it will protect the practical nurse from possible infection, but this is not the most correct answer.
    4. **The practical nurse assesses the risk for exposure and puts on the appropriate PPE to protect himself and his client. The nurse is using standard precautions/ routine practices, which are infection-control practices designed for the care of all clients all the time (regardless of their diagnosis or presumed infectiveness).**

28. **C: Foundations of Practice T: Application**
    1. Incorrect calculation.
    2. Incorrect calculation.
    3. **This is the correct calculation. The child's weight must first be converted from pounds to kilograms (1 kg = 2.2 pounds). Omotayo weighs 11 pounds, which is 11 lb. ÷ 2.2 lb. = 5 kg. The lowest dosage is 200 mg × 5 kg = 1 000 mg/day. The highest dosage is 400 mg × 5 kg = 2 000 mg/day.**
    4. This is not correct as it is for one dose only rather than the range for the day.

29. **C: Foundations of Practice T: Application**
    1. This is the method for giving an intramuscular injection. For a subcutaneous injection, the skin should be pinched before injection to elevate the skin and subcutaneous tissue above the muscle and ensure that the injection is given subcutaneously rather than intramuscularly.
    2. The site of a heparin injection should not be massaged, as this can cause bruising.
    3. It is not necessary to aspirate for subcutaneous injections, as adipose tissue is not very vascular and injection into a blood vessel is rare. It is particularly important not to aspirate heparin because it can cause bruising.
    4. **Aspiration for subcutaneous injections is not necessary, as adipose tissue is not very vascular and injection into a blood vessel is rare.**

30. **C: Professional, Ethical, and Legal Practice T: Critical Thinking**
    1. Restraints might possibly make him more agitated, but this is not the most appropriate explanation.
    2. Most healthcare facilities are either restraint-free or advocate minimum restraints. This statement makes the nurse appear to be basing action on rules rather than professional judgement.
    3. **Restraints should be a last resort. The presence of a family member may prevent him from trying to get out of bed. If a family member could be present around the clock, it might be a good short-term solution until Mr. Valencia's confusion clears.**

4. It is true that the doctor must order restraints, but this is not the best answer. It is better to use restraints as a last resort.

31. **C: Foundations of Practice T: Application**
    1. With stomatitis, it is important to continue gentle flossing and brushing with a soft toothbrush or toothette to keep the mouth, teeth, and gums clean and prevent infection.
    2. Commercial mouthwashes contain alcohol, which stings and dries mucous membranes. Commercial mouthwashes such as Listerine are not recommended.
    3. **Normal saline mouthwashes are recommended as often as every 2 hours if necessary for clients with stomatitis.**
    4. Regular oral hygiene is important for clients with stomatitis to prevent infections. It is recommended that the client use a mild analgesic if necessary for pain so that mouth care can be done.

32. **C: Professional, Ethical, and Legal Practice T: Application**
    1. Chest tubes can remove air and fluid from the pleural space, not the lungs.
    2. **Turning in bed or ambulating can shift the position of the chest tube in the pleural space slightly and promote drainage. Lying on the side of the unaffected lung can expand the affected lung more fully as well.**
    3. Chest tubes are not commonly clamped, as clamping can cause a tension pneumothorax. Air pressure builds up in the pleural space, collapsing the lung and creating a life-threatening emergency. Clamping chest tubes requires an order from the physician.
    4. The chest tube drainage system should remain below the chest to aid gravity by drainage and to prevent reflux of drainage back into the chest cavity.

33. **C: Foundations of Practice T: Application**
    1. Reactions most commonly occur during the first 15 minutes.
    2. **Before beginning the infusion, two nurses or a nurse and practical nurse (check agency policies) verify the blood type, Rh factor, client and blood numbers, and expiration date on the blood bag and the chart.**
    3. This is not frequent enough. The practical nurse needs pre- and postadministration vital signs but also continues to monitor the client throughout and obtains vital signs periodically during the transfusion as directed by agency policy.
    4. These are signs of an allergic reaction. Signs of a febrile reaction include shaking, headache, elevated temperature, back pain, confusion, and hematemesis.

34. **C: Professional, Ethical, and Legal Practice T: Critical Thinking**
    1. The practical nurse follows agency policy about disclosure, but this is not her first priority.
    2. The practical nurse informs the manager and prescriber (physician, extended role nurse, dentist, chiropractor), but that is not her first responsibility.

3. She must complete an incident report with the details after she makes sure the client is not in danger and has informed the appropriate agency personnel.
4. **The practical nurse's first responsibility is to assess the client and make sure he is not in immediate danger.**

35. **C: Professional, Ethical, and Legal Practice T: Application**
    1. This is not appropriate unless the practical nurse knows why the client is restrained and the cost of a sitter has been negotiated with the unit manager or family.
    2. Restraints should be tied with a quick-release tie rather than a knot for safety reasons.
    3. **Proper placement of the restraint, skin integrity, pulses, colour, and sensation of the restrained part should be assessed every hour or according to agency policy.**
    4. Reviewing the order for restraints should be done frequently but varies from agency to agency. Restraints may need to be reordered on a daily or weekly basis.

36. **C: Foundations of Practice T: Knowledge**
    1. Normal oral temperature for an older adult is 36°C.
    2. **Infections in older adults may not present typically as they tend to have lower body temperatures, decreased pain sensation, and less immune response to infection. Older adults can often have advanced infection before it is identified.**
    3. The older adult has decreased pain sensation.
    4. Constipation can be a common complaint in older persons due to a combination of many factors, such as impaired general health, use of medication, and decreased bowel motility and physical activity.

37. **C: Collaborative Practice T: Application**
    1. It is not possible, nor is there any reason, to restrain someone during a seizure.
    2. Nothing should be inserted into the mouth of someone having a seizure.
    3. Only put the client in a side-lying position if it is possible. This is usually possible only at the beginning of a seizure.
    4. **It is most important to protect the client from traumatic injury. They should make sure he is safe and protect him from injury by putting him on a flat surface and clearing the area of hazards.**

38. **C: Foundations of Practice T: Application**
    1. **The Braden Scale measures sensory perception, moisture, activity, mobility, nutrition, and friction and shear, in an attempt to identify clients most at risk for pressure injuries.**
    2. The Braden Scale is a risk-assessment tool and does not identify interventions.
    3. The Braden Scale does not only measure friction and shear. It also measures sensory perception, moisture, activity, mobility, and nutrition.
    4. The Braden Scale is a risk-assessment tool and does not identify preventive measures.

39. C: Foundations of Practice T: Application
    1. Incentive spirometry is used to prevent or treat atelectasis in the postoperative client and should be used hourly while awake.
    2. **Leg exercises, including foot circles, dorsiflexion and plantar flexion, quadriceps setting, and hip and knee exercises, should be performed at least every 2 hours for five successive times while awake.**
    3. All postoperative clients are encouraged to use controlled rather than vigorous coughing to loosen and expectorate mucus that will have collected during and postsurgery in their lungs. Vigorous coughing may disturb the surgical site.
    4. The client will likely have a chest tube but will probably not be on bed rest for long. Movement in bed as well as ambulation is encouraged to promote drainage from the pleural space and lung expansion.

40. C: Foundations of Practice T: Application
    1. **Palliative care is supportive treatment designed to relieve or reduce uncomfortable symptoms such as pain, nausea, and shortness of breath.**
    2. Palliative care should be supportive rather than curative. It should not postpone or delay death. Enteral feeds would postpone death.
    3. Both client and family needs are the focus of any interventions.
    4. The palliative care team offers bereavement support to families after the death of a client.

CHAPTER 7

The correct answer is set off in boldface.

1. C: **Foundations of Practice T: Application**
    1. It is not within the role of the practical nurse to make an adjustment to a drug dosage. Concerns need to be reported to the physician, who will make changes as necessary.
    2. It is the physician's role to decide whether medications are to be given. Practical nurses do not withhold medications unless an order is written or they have a concern. If there is a concern, practical nurses consult with the physician or prescriber of the medication.
    3. As a general rule, digoxin is withheld and reported if the heart rate is less than 60 beats per minute.
    4. **Withholding digoxin and reporting is the established procedure if the heart rate is less than 60 beats per minute. The physician will then determine whether the client is to receive the medication at that time.**

2. C: Foundations of Practice T: Application
    1. Furosemide will start to work within an hour, causing the client to awaken to void during the night and therefore to lose sleep.
    2. While doses of furosemide should be spaced to maintain therapeutic levels, the medication should be administered in the morning to avoid nocturnal diuresis.

    3. **This is the correct time to administer a diuretic in order for diuresis to take place during the day prior to bedtime. This permits a restful sleep.**
    4. It is not necessary to take furosemide with meals.

3. C: **Foundations of Practice T: Knowledge**
    1. **Diuretics remove electrolytes, including potassium, putting the client at risk of developing hypokalemia. Supplements prevent this from occurring.**
    2. Potassium supplements do not facilitate the action of diuretics.
    3. Although potassium plays a major role in the generation of a nerve impulse, potassium supplementation in this case is not for that purpose.
    4. Potassium supplementation plays no significant role in preventing the adverse effects of digoxin.

4. C: **Foundations of Practice T: Application**
    1. Patches should remain on the skin until a new dose is applied. The purpose of a dermal patch is to provide continuous, slow absorption of the medication throughout the day. Occasionally, patches may be removed overnight to reduce the development of tolerance.
    2. Skin areas should be rotated to avoid skin irritation. Absorption will naturally occur in all areas of skin.
    3. **The patch should be removed and the skin cleansed to remove medication left on the skin; then the new patch is applied to a different area. Leaving the skin uncleansed may produce added dosage of the drug when added to the new dosage, causing undesirable effects.**
    4. This is incorrect, as the patch is applied to provide slow, natural absorption. By massaging the site, absorption will occur more quickly, with the possibility of undesirable adverse effects.

5. C: **Foundations of Practice T: Application**
    1. Only a maximum of three sprays should be taken. If pain persists, medical attention should be obtained immediately as a myocardial infarction may be occurring.
    2. One spray may not be sufficient. Up to three sprays may be taken at 5-minute intervals. Sublingual forms of nitroglycerine are destroyed by gastric secretions and will not be absorbed.
    3. One spray may not be enough to relieve the pain. Up to three sprays may be administered. Patches are used as a preventive and have no effect on acute pain due to their slow absorption.
    4. **This is the correct method of using sublingual nitroglycerine sprays to relieve anginal pain. Three successive doses are acceptable, but persistent pain may indicate a myocardial infarction, and medical attention is required.**

6. C: **Foundations of Practice T: Application**
    1. At noon, regular insulin is at peak action, so no additional insulin is required.
    2. At mid-morning (about 1000 hours), regular insulin is near the peak level and NPH insulin is above the minimum effective concentration; therefore, no new dose is required.

3. At mid-afternoon (1500 hours), regular insulin has reached its minimum effective concentration level, but NPH insulin is at peak; therefore, no new dose is required.

4. **By bedtime (2100–2200 hours), NPH insulin is present but will fall below the MEC soon after midnight.**

7. **C: Foundations of Practice T: Application**

1. Between 0.5–1 hours and 2–3 hours after administering the insulins, the minimum effective concentration is reached for both types of insulin and blood levels are too low to cause adverse effects (hypoglycemia).

2. **Between 2–4 hours and 5–8 hours after administering the insulins, the peak is reached for both types of insulin and the adverse effects occur at these peak levels.**

3. Between 5–8 hours and 18 hours after administering the insulins, the minimum effective concentration is reached and adverse effects are unlikely.

4. After 18 hours, no adverse effect is likely because the MEC is passed.

8. **C: Foundations of Practice T: Knowledge**

1. H_2 receptor antagonists do not act as bases. Only bases neutralize acids.

2. **By blocking the receptor sites, H_2 receptor antagonists prevent histamine from binding to the surface of parietal cells, which prevents the cells from producing H^+. H^+ increases the stomach pH.**

3. H_2 receptor antagonists have no effect on digestive enzymes.

4. Acid plus base converts to salt and water, but H_2 receptor antagonists are not bases.

9. **C: Foundations of Practice T: Knowledge**

1. Stimulation of peristalsis is helpful in the presence of constipation, but it does not relieve gas.

2. **Simethicone changes the surface tension of gas bubbles in the gastro-intestinal tract, resulting in collection of one large gas bubble. This enables the individual to eructate or pass flatus.**

3. Simethicone is not an antidiarrheal medication. Although simethicone relieves gaseous distension, it has no effect on the intestinal lining to prevent diarrhea.

4. Simethicone is not an absorbent. It does not absorb excess HCl.

10. **C: Foundations of Practice T: Knowledge**

1. If an antimicrobial affects only bacteria, it is simply called an *antibiotic*.

2. The therapeutic index has to do with the safety of administration of a drug. A drug with a narrow therapeutic index means the therapeutic dose is very close to the toxic dose.

3. Spectrum is not related to toxicity.

4. **The spectrum of microbial activity is the range of distinctly different types of microbes affected by an antimicrobial drug. Narrow-spectrum antibiotics treat effectively only a limited number of types of bacteria.**

11. **C: Foundations of Practice T: Application**

1. Chlamydia is a bacteria that can be treated with antibiotics.

2. *E. coli* is a bacteria that can be treated with antibiotics.

3. Gonorrhea is caused by a bacteria and can be treated with antibiotics.

4. **Influenza A and B are viral infections. They are not susceptible to antibiotics but can be treated with antiviral drugs.**

12. **C: Foundations of Practice T: Application**

1. Mr. Simmons will possibly require lower doses of his medications, but it is not a nursing responsibility to independently change the dose.

2. He will likely need lower, not higher, doses.

3. **Due to the renal failure, there is likely to be reduced excretion of some of the medications. It is the responsibility of the physician and pharmacist to decide if altered doses are required, depending on the particular drug and Mr. Simmons's condition.**

4. It is not within the role of the practical nurse, in this situation, to independently withhold medications for Mr. Simmons.

13. **C: Foundations of Practice T: Application**

1. **Opioid analgesics are known to cause nausea and vomiting. Administration of antiemetics at the same time as administration of the morphine may prevent this side effect.**

2. With the severe pain of colon cancer, this is an inappropriate choice. If the morphine is ordered with a range of dosing, the amount given should be based on the pain as rated by Mr. Shafikhani and previous doses that have resulted in therapeutic effects.

3. While a history of previous abuse is a nursing consideration in many cases of morphine administration, this is neither an important nor necessary assessment with a client who has severe pain from terminal cancer.

4. The morphine may need to be held if Mr. Shafikhani has a respiratory rate of less than 10 respirations per minute.

14. **C: Foundations of Practice T: Knowledge**

1. **Warfarin suppresses vitamin K–dependent clotting factors, prolonging clotting time and leading to hemorrhage. This may be evidenced by excessive bruising and bleeding in the gums.**

2. Warfarin is given to prevent, not promote, thrombus formation.

3. If there is a therapeutic level of warfarin, mobilization of blood clots is not likely.

4. With a therapeutic level of warfarin, there should be no thrombosis mobilization.

15. **C: Foundations of Practice T: Knowledge**

1. **A high level of low-density lipoprotein (LDL) cholesterol is a major risk factor for cardiovascular disease (CVD); hence, the goal of therapy is to lower it to the normal physiological level.**

2. High-density lipoprotein (HDL) is the "good" cholesterol. High levels are not a risk factor for CVD.

3. The goal of antilipemic therapy is to lower serum LDL cholesterol levels.

4. HDL cannot be effectively raised by drug therapy alone. Fibric acids used to treat a high triglyceride level do increase HDL but only slightly.

16. **C: Foundations of Practice T: Application**

1. Mr. Michael's blood pressure (BP) may be normal only because it is being effectively controlled by Dixarit. The BP would likely increase as soon as the client is off the medication.

2. This is not a safe option, as the BP is likely being controlled by the Dixarit.

3. Exercise and salt restriction are used to help control high BP but may not be sufficient for many clients with stage I or stage II hypertension.

4. **The decision has to be made by the prescriber, who can diagnose and prescribe alternative therapy as the situation dictates.**

17. **C: Foundations of Practice T: Knowledge**

1. Renal insufficiency is not a contraindication for taking an opioid analgesic.

2. **Respiratory insufficiency, as in severe chronic obstructive pulmonary disease, would be a contraindication for giving an opioid analgesic due to the potential for respiratory depression.**

3. Liver disease is not a contraindication for taking an opioid analgesic.

4. Diabetes mellitus is not a contraindication for taking an opioid analgesic.

18. **C: Foundations of Practice T: Knowledge**

1. Cyclo-oxygenase-2 (COX-2) inhibitors are second-generation non-steroidal anti-inflammatories and are not considered to be safe in pregnancy.

2. COX-2 inhibitors may cause gastro-intestinal distress, but that is not the reason they should be avoided in pregnancy.

3. This is partly true but depends on the drug and the health problem. The risks for a pregnant woman taking particular medications must be determined by a physician.

4. **COX-2 inhibitors are in the U.S. Food and Drug Administration's pregnancy category D. This means that they pose a definite risk to the fetus and that the risk versus benefit must be assessed by a physician.**

19. **C: Foundations of Practice T: Knowledge**

1. Librium is an anxiolytic that is not usually administered to children under 6.

2. Lithium is used for treating bipolar disorder and is not indicated for attention-deficit/hyperactivity disorder (ADHD).

3. **Ritalin is the drug of choice to treat ADHD. Its mechanism of action is not clear, but it helps children with ADHD focus on one activity for a longer period of time.**

4. Phenobarbital is an antiepileptic drug not indicated for treatment of ADHD.

20. **C: Foundations of Practice T: Knowledge**

1. The rate of excretion may be decreased because drugs metabolized by the liver may not be water soluble and therefore cannot be excreted in the urine.

2. The duration of action of the drug will increase due to the failure of the medication to be metabolized for excretion.

3. Only antagonist drugs, not liver disease, block receptors to produce no response.

4. **When a drug is metabolized by the liver, inactive or active metabolites are produced. Inactive metabolites are usually removed by excretory organs, thus preventing drug accumulation. Active metabolites go to target cells and are subsequently inactive or excreted. If the drug is not metabolized by the liver because of cirrhosis, higher levels remain in the body for longer periods and produce actions and effects similar to a drug overdose.**

21. **C: Foundations of Practice T: Application**

1. Routine adult doses can cause toxicity, since liver metabolism and renal excretion decline with age.

2. The frequency of drug administration is dependent on the drug's half-life, not the age of the recipient.

3. **Body organs have fewer cells and reduced function with age; hence, the body requires a lower amount than the routine adult dose to produce the therapeutic effect.**

4. Oral administration is easier, safer, and more practical than parenteral administration.

22. **C: Foundations of Practice T: Knowledge**

1. Barbiturates promote drowsiness, which is not therapeutic for depression.

2. Antianxiolytics are used to treat anxiety, not depression.

3. **Depressive symptoms are related to insensitivity of receptors and low serotonin levels. Selective serotonin reuptake inhibitors work to promote the continued presence of serotonin in the synaptic cleft by inhibiting its uptake.**

4. Cholinergic agonists have no effect on serotonin receptors.

23. **C: Foundations of Practice T: Knowledge**

1. Although cortisone limits the activity of white blood cells (WBCs), it does not attract microbes.

2. **Higher than normal physiological levels of cortisone promote protein breakdown. Antibodies are composed of proteins. In addition, cortisone impairs the ability of antibodies to bind to cell surface receptors and so reduces cell-mediated response. The net result is lowering of the immune response.**

3. Cortisone has no direct or indirect antibiotic activity.

4. Cortisone reduces cellular factors that lead to vascular permeability.

24. **C: Foundations of Practice T: Knowledge**

1. **Raltegravir is an antiretroviral used in the treatment of HIV/AIDS.**

2. Valganciclovir is used to treat cytomegalovirus infection and is of no use as treatment for HIV/AIDS.

3. Amantadine is a dopamine agonist with antiviral activity that is used to treat influenza.
4. Acyclovir is used to treat herpes virus infection.

25. **C: Foundations of Practice T: Knowledge**
    1. B-complex vitamins produce orange-coloured urine. INH may cause vitamin B deficiency.
    2. **INH is hepatotoxic, and liver function must be monitored carefully. Alcohol is not permitted while on INH, a factor that causes nonadherence in many cases.**
    3. While INH is used to treat and prevent tuberculosis, monthly X-rays are not necessary. If the disease is active, the client will be monitored by collecting sputum cultures.
    4. Antacids interfere with the absorption of INH and should never be taken concurrently.

CHAPTER 8

The correct answer is set off in boldface.

1. **C: Foundations of Practice T: Critical Thinking**
   1. **The throat is a vascular area, and even with laser surgery, there is a recognized danger of hemorrhage. It may occur quickly and is the most immediately life-threatening postsurgical complication.**
   2. It is expected that the throat will be very sore after surgery. Around-the-clock analgesia with acetaminophen (Tylenol), rather than ASA (Aspirin), is administered. An ice collar may provide relief.
   3. This is a normal postoperative finding.
   4. Oral pharyngeal edema is a common postoperative complication from throat surgery resulting from trauma to the site. It may lead to a gradual increase in airway obstruction. The practical nurse must monitor Mr. Kingsley's airway status but, more immediately, must be alert for sudden signs of hemorrhage.

2. **C: Foundations of Practice T: Application**
   1. This position would encourage pooling of the secretions in the mouth and possibly cause choking, coughing, or aspiration.
   2. This position would not encourage drainage of secretions out of the mouth.
   3. **Positioning the client in a semi-Fowler's with the neck flexed helps prevent pooling of secretions in the mouth and allows easier breathing and less chance of choking, coughing, and aspirating. Clients often put themselves into the high Fowler's position for comfort and ease of breathing.**
   4. This position would be uncomfortable and impossible for the client to remain in for very long.

3. **C: Foundations of Practice T: Application**
   1. Clients are given cool, not warm, fluids once they are able to swallow. The coolness helps soothe the sore throat and decrease the chance of swelling. Coolness also reduces spasms in the muscles surrounding the throat.
   2. Aspirin or any other medication that alters bleeding time is not given to postoperative clients.

3. **Acetaminophen (Tylenol) elixir or pills is the analgesic of choice and should be given around the clock. Sometimes rinsing the mouth out with viscous lidocaine is effective to decrease pain in the throat.**
4. Ice collars rather than heating pads are used to help decrease swelling and pain. Heat may cause increased swelling and bleeding.

4. **C: Foundations of Practice T: Application**
   1. Active disease is diagnosed by sputum cultures for acid-fast bacilli. Three consecutive sputum specimens collected on different days are obtained and sent for smear and culture. Material obtained from gastric washing, cerebrospinal fluid, and pus from an abscess may also be examined.
   2. **This is a positive reaction. It indicates the presence of a tuberculosis (TB) infection but does not show whether the infection is active or dormant. People who have been vaccinated with bacille Calmette-Guérin will have positive skin tests due to exposure to the vaccine.**
   3. Further studies need to be done before treatment is started. The healthcare provider needs to know if, in fact, the client has TB before initiating treatment.
   4. Two-step testing is generally recommended only for initial testing for healthcare workers who require repeated testing and for those who have a decreased response to allergens. For these people, a second purified protein derivative (PPD) test later may cause an accelerated response (booster effect), misinterpreted as a new PPD conversion.

5. **C: Foundations of Practice T: Critical Thinking**
   1. Although the findings of a chest X-ray are important, it is not possible to make a diagnosis of tuberculosis (TB) solely on the basis of the X-ray. Other diseases can mimic the X-ray appearance of TB.
   2. **The demonstration of tubercle bacilli bacteriologically is essential for establishing a diagnosis.**
   3. This is a new rapid diagnostic test for TB that provides results within a few hours. It does not replace the routine sputum smears and cultures, but it offers a healthcare provider increased confidence in the diagnosis.
   4. Repeated Mantoux testing will only show that the person has either been vaccinated with bacille Calmette-Guérin or exposed to the mycobacterium. It does not mean that the person has contracted the disease.

6. **C: Foundations of Practice T: Application**
   1. Side effects of ethambutol include skin rash, gastrointestinal (GI) disturbances, malaise, peripheral neuritis, and optic neuritis.
   2. Side effects of isoniazid include peripheral neuritis, hepatotoxicity, skin rash, optic neuritis, and vitamin B_6 neuritis.
   3. Side effects of rifampin include hepatitis, GI disturbances, and peripheral neuritis.
   4. **Side effects of streptomycin include ototoxicity (affecting the eighth cranial nerve), nephrotoxicity, and hypersensitivity.**

7. **C: Foundations of Practice T: Application**
   1. This is too short a time.
   2. As in choice 1.
   3. As in choice 1.
   4. **A problem with adherence to therapy for tuberculosis has been the length of time medication must be taken. Six to 9 months of therapy have proven to be effective.**

8. **C: Foundations of Practice T: Knowledge**
   1. Primary hypertension may be managed by drugs, but lifestyle modifications will often be attempted initially to bring the pressure within normal range.
   2. **Primary hypertension has no identifiable cause.**
   3. This answer refers to secondary hypertension, in which an identifiable cause can be determined.
   4. Research has shown that blood pressure is related to obesity and that if Ms. Mathias were to decrease her weight, her blood pressure could be lowered.

9. **C: Foundations of Practice T: Knowledge**
   1. **HydroDIURIL may cause loss of potassium. Clients are encouraged to eat foods containing potassium, such as bananas, and monitor serum potassium levels.**
   2. While this is advised for clients who are hypertensive, it is not related to the HydroDIURIL.
   3. High-sodium diets are contraindicated.
   4. This may cause hypokalemia.

10. **C: Foundations of Practice T: Application**
    1. Calcium channel blockers may cause polyuria in some clients.
    2. Calcium channel blockers may cause skin rash, dermatitis, pruritus, and urticaria, but they do not cause hair loss.
    3. Calcium channel blockers may cause hypotension, not hypertension.
    4. **Cardiovascular effects from the use of calcium channel blockers may include peripheral edema, hypotension, palpitations, bradycardia, tachycardia, and arrhythmias that may induce orthostatic hypotension.**

11. **C: Foundations of Practice T: Application**
    1. **Clients with Cushing's syndrome may have thin, fragile skin, purplish red striae, petechial hemorrhages, bruises, facial plethora, acne, and poor wound healing.**
    2. There is usually increased axilla and pubic hair. Hirsutism is commonly found with Cushing's syndrome.
    3. Tachycardia and bulging eyes suggest hyperthyroid disease.
    4. Hypertension and hyperglycemia are found with Cushing's syndrome.

12. **C: Collaborative Practice T: Application**
    1. This statement is patronizing and ineffective.
    2. This statement does not address Ms. Hynes's concern.
    3. Her appearance will change after surgery, but it will take time for all the physical and mental changes to occur.
    4. **The statement addresses Ms. Hynes's concern and gives accurate information.**

13. **C: Foundations of Practice T: Application**
    1. Because the client is unable to open his or her mouth after surgery, the client must be closely monitored for airway obstruction and aspiration of vomitus. Lying on the stomach will not facilitate this.
    2. **Brian should be positioned on his side with his head slightly elevated to help drain secretions and prevent airway obstruction.**
    3. Lying on his back will not facilitate drainage of secretions and could result in airway obstruction.
    4. Having the head slightly below the chest will encourage secretions to drain into the mouth, causing a potential for aspiration and choking.

14. **C: Foundations of Practice T: Critical Thinking**
    1. Adequate nutrition is important but is not the priority postoperatively.
    2. The jaw is immobilized by wiring the jaws together during surgery; therefore, it is not the nursing priority.
    3. Oral hygiene is another important intervention but is not the priority immediately postoperatively.
    4. **Two major potential problems in the immediate postoperative period are airway obstruction and aspiration of vomitus. The practical nurse must observe for signs of respiratory distress.**

15. **C: Foundations of Practice T: Critical Thinking**
    1. Suctioning should be necessary only if the client vomits or chokes. The nasopharyngeal or oral route may be used, depending on the extent of injury and the type of repair. A nasogastric tube may be needed to remove fluids and gas from the stomach.
    2. This is one method of suctioning if needed.
    3. **Wire cutters or scissors (for rubber bands) must be taped to the head of the bed and sent with Brian on all appointments and examinations away from the bedside. These may be used to cut the wires and elastic bands in case of an emergency.**
    4. Oxygen is required only if Brian experiences any respiratory distress.

16. **C: Foundations of Practice T: Application**
    1. This is not necessary. Mrs. Cheng may use a slipper bedpan.
    2. **A trapeze suspended over Mrs. Cheng's bed will allow her to lift herself if she is uncomfortable or for use with the bedpan.**
    3. This would encourage a twisting motion, and the limb and joint must be maintained in alignment.
    4. Mrs. Cheng will not be allowed to sit in a chair until after surgery. Moving her into a chair would cause pain and would not keep the leg in alignment.

17. **C: Foundations of Practice T: Application**
    1. **Bisphosphonate medication, such as risedronate (Actonel), inhibits bone resorption and absorbs calcium–phosphate crystals in bone. Bisphosphonates are "front-line" drugs in the treatment of osteoporosis. Calcium supplements are required to increase available calcium to the bone.**

2. Weight-bearing exercises are recommended for osteoporosis as they help strengthen muscles around the bone and increase the strength of the bones.

3. Vitamin D is needed for regulation of calcium. Recommended levels for women of Mrs. Cheng's age are 1 000 IU or greater; 200 IU is not sufficient.

4. This is a premature recommendation. There is no indication that Mrs. Cheng may require any assistance with activities of daily living postrehabilitation.

18. **C: Foundations of Practice T: Application**

1. Symptoms for urinary tract infection may include dysuria, frequency of urination, urgency, and suprapubic discomfort or pressure.

2. Pyelonephritis may manifest with symptoms of cystitis, flank pain, fever, chills, vomiting, and malaise.

3. Nephrotic syndrome may manifest with peripheral edema, massive proteinuria, dyslipidemia, and hypoalbuminemia.

4. **Acute glomerulonephritis may present with a variety of signs and symptoms, including edema, hypertension, oliguria, hematuria, and proteinuria. Fluid retention is usually first found in the low-pressure tissues, such as those around the eyes. Acute post-streptococcal glomerulonephritis develops 5–21 days after an infection of the pharynx or skin by group A beta-hemolytic *Streptococcus*.**

19. **C: Foundations of Practice T: Application**

1. Management for acute glomerulonephritis focuses on symptomatic relief. If Ms. Procinski has a high potassium level, she will be instructed to eat foods low in potassium and to stay away from foods high in potassium. In some instances, the client will be given polystyrene sulfonate (Kayexalate) to remove potassium from the body.

2. **For all cases of glomerulonephritis, rest is recommended until the signs of the glomerular inflammation subside.**

3. If Ms. Procinski is hypertensive, she may be started on a short-term course of antihypertensives.

4. Glomerulonephritis is an antigen–antibody immune situation resulting from a previous infection. Antibiotics will not correct the glomerulonephritis, although some doctors do prescribe antibiotics prophylactically.

20. **C: Foundations of Practice T: Critical Thinking**

1. International normalized ratio is used to measure warfarin (Coumadin) action in the body.

2. **Partial thromboplastin time is used to measure heparin action in the body.**

3. Platelet function assay is used to detect platelet dysfunction.

4. Prothrombin time is used to measure Coumadin action in the body.

21. **C: Foundations of Practice T: Critical Thinking**

1. Heparin should not be stopped until a therapeutic level of Coumadin is attained.

2. As in choice 1.

3. Five milligrams of Coumadin is an appropriate dose.

4. **A therapeutic level of Coumadin must be attained before heparin is stopped to maintain anticoagulant blood levels.**

22. **C: Foundations of Practice T: Knowledge**

1. This refers to adduction.

2. **This is the definition of *abduction*.**

3. This refers to external rotation.

4. This refers to internal rotation.

23. **C: Foundations of Practice T: Application**

1. **Diminished or absent pedal, popliteal, or femoral pulses are frequently noted in clients with Peripheral arterial disease (PAD) due to obstruction of the artery.**

2. The foot will become pale on elevation. Clients with PAD will have reddened feet when they are in a dependent position.

3. Lower leg edema may be seen in venous, not arterial, obstruction.

4. Assessment requires more than just a blood pressure at the thigh. Segmental blood pressures are taken at the thigh, below the knee, and at ankle level while the client is supine. A fall-off in segmental pressure of more than 30 mm Hg indicates PAD.

24. **C: Foundations of Practice T: Application**

1. Heating devices should not be used on the feet of clients with vascular problems as the client may not be able to feel a burn injury.

2. Support stockings are used for venous problems.

3. **Walking promotes the development of collateral circulation.**

4. Feet should be inspected daily for redness.

25. **C: Foundations of Practice T: Knowledge**

1. These are manifestations of hypernatremia.

2. **Severe diarrhea can lead to excessive loss of potassium. Hypokalemia can lead to rapid arrhythmias, which, in turn, can lead to a cardiac arrest. Other symptoms include muscle fatigue and weakness, leg cramps, nausea and vomiting, polyuritis, and hyperglycemia.**

3. These are manifestations of hyperphosphatemia.

4. These are manifestations of hypocalcemia.

26. **C: Foundations of Practice T: Application**

1. The rectal packing helps stop bleeding in the perineal area. It should not be removed right after surgery unless it is saturated with serosanguinous drainage.

2. Feeding of any kind would not be established until peristalsis has returned and drainage appears in the ileostomy bag.

3. **In the first 24–48 hours after surgery, the amount of drainage from the stoma may be negligible. An ileostomy causes a loss of absorptive functions provided by the colon. Once peristalsis returns, there may be a period of high-volume bilious output, up to 1 200–1 800 mL per day. Fluid and electrolyte imbalance is a potential problem.**

4. The nasogastric tube would not be removed until peristalsis has returned.

27. C: Foundations of Practice T: Application
    1. **Clients are encouraged to cook fruits and vegetables and limit their amounts in the initial postoperative period, as there is the potential for these foods to cause obstruction.**
    2. Beans and legumes are gas forming.
    3. Eggs are odour producing.
    4. Strong cheese is gas forming.

28. C: Foundations of Practice T: Application
    1. There is no reason Mrs. O'Brien cannot have sharp utensils. The aide should help Mrs. O'Brien locate the utensils on the meal tray.
    2. Mrs. O'Brien does not require finger foods. She is able to use utensils. Finger foods would be more appropriate for the person who has dementia and experiences difficulty managing a knife and fork.
    3. **At mealtime, Mrs. O'Brien can be oriented to her meal by comparing her plate to a clock. This visual image will help her easily locate each item of food.**
    4. There is no indication that Mrs. O'Brien needs assistance with eating. She just needs assistance in finding food she cannot see.

29. C: Foundations of Practice T: Application
    1. **The practical nurse could offer a stool softener to prevent constipation. Straining at stool increases intraocular pressure and must be avoided post–cataract surgery.**
    2. There is no need to either increase or decrease fluids after cataract surgery.
    3. Some physicians may restrict showers after cataract surgery, but there is no contraindication to baths.
    4. Mrs. O'Brien's right eye will likely be patched, making watching TV or reading difficult. However, there are no contraindications to reading or watching TV provided that there are no rapid head or eye movements.

30. C: Foundations of Practice T: Application
    1. A prone position would encourage fluid buildup in the lungs, which is what is causing her shortness of breath.
    2. A semi-Fowler's position is not adequate to help decrease fluid buildup in the lungs. In this position, the legs are level with the sacrum and encourage fluid return from the lower limbs.
    3. This position would simply magnify the shortness of breath while encouraging fluid return from the extremities.
    4. **A high Fowler's position, sitting upright with legs dependent, promotes fluid retention in the legs, decreasing the fluid return to the heart and keeping the fluid in the bases of the lungs.**

31. C: Foundations of Practice T: Critical Thinking
    1. The electrolytes will need to be monitored but will not significantly change as quickly as the blood pressure (BP).
    2. **Although all assessments are important, the priority of care is BP. Once Mrs. Gardner starts to diurese**

volume from the intravascular space, BP can decrease drastically and result in hypotension.
    3. Hourly output tells the practical nurse how much volume the client is voiding, but the more important determination is the effect the decreased volume has on the lungs. The practical nurse would monitor lung sounds to evaluate the decrease in crackles, signifying the loss of fluid in the lungs.
    4. Monitoring the respiratory rate is important as a decreased rate will indicate improvement. Mrs. Gardner may have clear lung fields but be hypotensive; therefore, BP is the priority.

32. C: Foundations of Practice T: Knowledge
    1. This is a manifestation of left-sided heart failure.
    2. As in choice 1.
    3. As in choice 1.
    4. **Fluid in the lungs is symptomatic of left-sided heart failure.**

33. C: Foundations of Practice T: Application
    1. Clients with gout, not renal failure, are encouraged to limit purine in their diet. Purine is found in red meat, particularly organ meat and shellfish.
    2. **Failing kidneys do not excrete potassium efficiently; thus, a renal diet is low in potassium. Potatoes and citrus fruit such as oranges, grapefruit, and strawberries are high in potassium and should be avoided.**
    3. Cookies and cake are high in calories and low in nutritive value. Mrs. Gardner will be allowed to eat these but will be encouraged to include more complex carbohydrates.
    4. Mrs. Gardner may need to limit protein; however, protein is necessary for tissue repair and maintenance of the immune system.

34. C: Professional, Ethical, and Legal Practice T: Critical Thinking
    1. The nurse is not the most knowledgeable healthcare provider to teach about home oxygen therapy. It is also likely that Mr. Sharapov will require continual support when he is at home.
    2. This is an appropriate educational tool but is not as effective as a consultation with a respiratory therapist or technologist.
    3. **This is part of the role of the respiratory therapist or technologist. An in-home consultation will provide the best information and support for correct use of home oxygen therapy.**
    4. Mr. Sharapov will require follow-up pulse oximetry to determine if the supplemental oxygen is required and is being administered at the correct rate. It is not a strategy to assist Mr. Sharapov to manage the home oxygen.

35. C: Foundations of Practice T: Knowledge
    1. Prothrombin time, partial thromboplastin time, and international normalized ratio are all tests that evaluate clotting time, not heart damage.
    2. **Troponin I and cardiac troponin T are proteins in myocardial tissue. When cardiac muscle is damaged,**

this protein is released into the blood within an hour of injury. CK-MB is one of the three isoenzymes that can be separated for creatine kinase (CK). CK-MB is released into the blood when cardiac tissue has been damaged. LDH refers to lactate dehydrogenase, which is released into the blood when tissues are damaged.

3. Sodium and potassium levels are important in that abnormal levels may hinder conduction, but they do not detect heart muscle damage. CK-BB is an isoenzyme separated from CK and shows when brain tissue has been damaged.

4. Blood urea nitrogen and creatinine are kidney function tests. Elevated levels show that the kidneys are not functioning optimally. CK-MM is an isoenzyme separated from CK and shows when skeletal muscle tissue has been damaged.

36. **C: Foundations of Practice T: Critical Thinking**
   1. This is a good strategy to provide immobilization to the neck injury and can be done while the guest is still in the pool. However, breathing is the priority.
   2. This is a possibly appropriate first aid measure but is not as urgent as providing rescue breathing.
   3. This is appropriate as people who have sustained a spinal cord injury while swimming should not be lifted out of the pool until there is experienced help. Moving the guest may cause further damage. However, it is not as important as breathing.
   4. **Spinal cord injuries above C3 may cause respiratory paralysis. The priority action must be to provide rescue breathing until the paramedics arrive.**

37. **C: Collaborative Practice T: Critical Thinking**
   1. While this is true, it is in language that she may not understand.
   2. This is true, but it does not answer Minh's question.
   3. **This describes the action and the rationale in language that Minh will be able to understand.**
   4. This is true but does not answer Minh's question.

38. **C: Collaborative Practice T: Critical Thinking**
   1. This is an encouraging but not helpful comment. The practical nurse cannot predict how fast his Parkinson's disease will progress or whether drugs will be effective.
   2. **This is the first step of the nursing process: data collection. The practical nurse needs to find out, by using an open-ended question, what Mr. Sanders has been told by the physician and whether Mr. Sanders understands what was discussed. Once the practical nurse has this information, she may gauge his level of readiness for clarification of information and teaching about the disease.**
   3. This is true, but it is not the appropriate response at this time. It may downplay Mr. Sanders' worries and may not invite dialogue between Mr. Sanders and the practical nurse.
   4. While this may be an appropriate action in some situations, it is not likely to be helpful initially with Mr. Sanders. If Mr. Sanders indicates to the practical

nurse that he is neither able nor willing to talk at present, then the practical nurse might offer to sit with him quietly.

39. **C: Foundations of Practice T: Knowledge**
   1. Neurological symptoms do not develop until the anemia is severe. Then the client may experience headaches, vertigo, irritability, depression, or impaired thought processes.
   2. Bradycardia is not a manifestation of anemia. Tachycardia and palpitations occur even in mild anemia as the body attempts to compensate for the decrease in oxygen in the blood.
   3. The eyes and skin are not affected until the anemia is severe. Then the client may experience pallor, jaundice, pruritus, icteric conjunctiva and sclera, retinal hemorrhage, and blurred vision.
   4. **With anemia, the body must work hard to get what oxygen it has to all tissues. Clients frequently complain of weakness, malaise, and being unable to accomplish normal activities.**

40. **C: Foundations of Practice T: Knowledge**
   1. Hypermagnesemia usually occurs only in renal insufficiency or failure.
   2. Hypocalcemia can be caused by any condition that results in a decrease in the production of parathyroid hormone. Diarrhea does not cause hypocalcemia.
   3. **Hypokalemia, or low potassium, can result from abnormal losses of potassium due to a shift of potassium from extracellular fluid to intracellular fluid or, rarely, from a dietary deficiency of potassium. The most common causes of hypokalemia are abnormal losses via either the kidneys or the gastrointestinal tract.**
   4. Hypernatremia, or high sodium, can be caused by an increase in insensible water loss, such as in diabetes insipidus, or osmotic diuresis. Hypernatremia is not a result of diarrhea.

41. **C: Foundations of Practice T: Application**
   1. Swallowing difficulties, or dysphagia, are a manifestation of esophageal cancer. When difficulty swallowing occurs in clients who have had strokes or dementia, a therapist will evaluate the swallowing and recommend appropriate interventions.
   2. Pain in the epigastric area is a manifestation of peptic ulcer.
   3. **Pyrosis (heartburn) is the most common manifestation of gastroesophageal reflux disease (GERD) and can be soothed by antacid preparations prior to H_2 antagonist treatment.**
   4. Nausea and vomiting are not necessarily manifestations of GERD.

42. **C: Foundations of Practice T: Critical Thinking**
   1. This is a priority for bleeding from esophageal varices, not peptic ulcer disease.
   2. Establishing an intravenous line is important so the practical nurse has access to a vein if volume replacement is required. However, it is not the priority.

3. **A nasogastric tube will be established, followed by saline or water lavages until the returns are clear and the bleeding has stopped.**

4. In many situations, oxygen is the priority. However, in this situation, the priority is to stop the bleeding. There is no indication that Mr. Tibor is in respiratory distress.

43. C: Foundations of Practice T: Knowledge
    1. A high fever would be present only if perforation had occurred.
    2. Diverticulitis usually develops because of constipation rather than diarrhea.
    3. Abdominal pain is localized over the involved area of the colon, usually the sigmoid colon, not the epigastric area.
    4. **The cause of diverticulitis is related to the retention of stool and bacteria in the diverticulum, forming a hardened mass called a *fecalith*. This causes inflammation and possible small perforations that may become edematous. The majority of clients with diverticulitis do not have any symptoms. Diverticuli may occur at any point within the gastro-intestinal tract but are most commonly found in the sigmoid colon; thus, lower left quadrant pain would be present when pain is present.**

44. C: Foundations of Practice T: Application
    1. **Initially, pain is found around the periumbilical area. As appendicitis worsens, the pain becomes persistent and shifts to the right lower quadrant, localizing at McBurney's point. Coughing aggravates the pain.**
    2. Esophageal reflux is not symptomatic of appendicitis.
    3. Clients may or may not present with low-grade fever, not a high-grade fever.
    4. Clients may present with a positive Rovsing's sign when palpation of the left lower quadrant causes pain to the right lower quadrant.

45. C: Foundations of Practice T: Knowledge
    1. The liver does not store vitamin C or E, so these would not be affected by hepatitis.
    2. Potassium levels are not affected by hepatitis.
    3. **The liver may not be able to produce prothrombin and other factors essential for blood clotting. Therefore, the prothrombin time may be prolonged.**
    4. Calcium is not stored in the liver.

46. C: Foundations of Practice T: Application
    1. A high-fibre diet helps reduce fat absorption.
    2. A high-fibre diet helps decrease the risk of constipation.
    3. A high-fibre diet does not affect potassium absorption.
    4. **A high-fibre diet helps trap ammonia in the gut before it is absorbed into the bloodstream.**

47. C: Foundations of Practice T: Critical Thinking
    1. Postoperative pain should be expected.
    2. Low-grade fever is expected.
    3. **Stridor is a serious finding as it could indicate that inflammation is compressing the trachea. Mr. Hawkins should be placed in a semi-Fowler's position to decrease edema and limit tension on the suture line.**
    4. Serosanguinous drainage is expected initially.

48. C: Foundations of Practice T: Knowledge
    1. This is seen in Graves' disease or hyperthyroidism.
    2. These are manifestations of diabetes insipidus.
    3. These are manifestations of Cushing's syndrome.
    4. **These are manifestations of Addison's disease.**

49. C: Foundations of Practice T: Knowledge
    1. This describes tension-type headache.
    2. This describes migraine headache.
    3. This describes tension-type headache.
    4. **These are manifestations of cluster headaches.**

50. C: Foundations of Practice T: Critical Thinking
    1. He has recovered from the upper respiratory infection.
    2. **Guillain-Barré syndrome may cause respiratory paralysis.**
    3. This will be done but is not a priority.
    4. This is an aspect of care but is not the priority.

51. C: Foundations of Practice T: Knowledge
    1. Refers to receptive (Wernicke's) aphasia.
    2. **Refers to apraxia.**
    3. Refers to agnosia.
    4. Refers to expressive (Broca's) aphasia.

52. C: Collaborative Practice T: Application
    1. This statement does not value Mrs. Tetrault's feelings or concerns.
    2. This statement is not helping her grief or suggesting ways to help her. It may be interpreted as being patronizing.
    3. **This response acknowledges Mrs. Tetrault's concern and allows her to vent and question without being judged.**
    4. Although this statement acknowledges the concern, the practical nurse talks about herself, not focusing on the client.

53. C: Foundations of Practice T: Knowledge
    1. This refers to possible gastro-intestinal upset such as gastroesophageal reflux disease (GERD). People with abdominal aortic aneurysm (AAA) do not usually complain of pain.
    2. This refers to heartburn, experienced by clients with GERD.
    3. **Abdominal bruit is symptomatic of AAA.**
    4. This refers to a dissecting AAA.

54. C: Foundations of Practice T: Application
    1. Mrs. Olsen is extremely lethargic and will not be able to drink enough fluids to bring the sodium level to within normal limits.
    2. A 10% dextrose solution is a hypertonic solution that will draw fluid from the tissues and increase diuresis in an already dehydrated client.
    3. **Establishing an intravenous line of an isotonic solution will help rehydrate Mrs. Olsen and bring the hematocrit and sodium levels within their normal limits.**
    4. Inserting a nasogastric tube will not bring the sodium and hematocrit to within normal limits.

55. C: Foundations of Practice T: Knowledge
    1. Adenocarcinomas are malignant tumours arising from glandular organs.

2. **Basal cell carcinoma is the most common human cancer, a malignancy typically found on skin exposed to sun or other forms of ultraviolet light.**

3. Mr. Ulrinski is also at risk for malignant melanoma. Although the incidence is increasing, it is not as common as basal cell carcinoma.

4. Spongioblastoma is a glioma of the brain (a neoplasm or tumour composed of neuroglial cells) derived from spongioblasts.

56. **C: Foundations of Practice T: Critical Thinking**
   1. Papanicolaou tests will discover abnormal cells but will not prevent cancer of the cervix.
   2. Colposcopy will aid in diagnosis of cancer of the cervix but will not prevent it.
   3. **The human papilloma virus vaccine protects against human papilloma virus, which is considered to be the major causative factor in the development of cancer of the cervix.**
   4. Warts can be removed with lasers, but this is not preventive.

57. **C: Foundations of Practice T: Application**
   1. Weight-bearing exercises are recommended for osteoporosis. Swimming is not a weight-bearing exercise.
   2. **The best exercises for osteoporosis are weight-bearing ones. Ms. Blinker will be able to walk using her walker.**
   3. While aerobics are beneficial for older adults for increased muscle strength, coordination, and osteoporosis, it is unlikely that if Ms. Blinker requires a walker, she would be able to participate in aerobic exercise.
   4. This is not a weight-bearing exercise.

58. **C: Foundations of Practice T: Application**
   1. **Multiple sclerosis is a chronic, progressive, degenerative disorder of the central nervous system characterized by disseminated demyelination of nerve fibres of the brain and spinal cord. The initial manifestations are often vague and inconsistent but include sensory disturbances such as blurred vision and tinnitus.**
   2. This refers to Parkinson's disease.
   3. This refers to myasthenia gravis.
   4. This refers to restless legs syndrome.

59. **C: Foundations of Practice T: Application**
   1. This is a component of postsurgical care and is not directly related to the manifestations of abdominal pain and bladder distension.
   2. **Posttransurethral resection of the prostate with continuous bladder irrigation, it is common for blood clots to block the catheter, requiring the practical nurse to flush the catheter.**
   3. The catheter is likely blocked by clots. Decreasing the flow will not solve this problem.
   4. The physician does not need to be notified unless flushing does not solve the problem.

60. **C: Foundations of Practice T: Application**
   1. **As death approaches, the skin becomes cool, clammy, and mottled due to diminished circulation.**

2. Respirations are often rapid and shallow, progressing to Cheyne-Stokes respirations.

3. The pulse becomes weak, but the rate does not increase.

4. Although the skin feels cool to touch, body temperature often increases prior to death.

CHAPTER 9

1. **C: Foundations of Practice T: Application**
   1. Early postpartum hemorrhage is most often associated with failure of the uterus to remain contracted and poor uterine tone on palpation.
   2. There are no apparent signs of infection.
   3. **A full bladder will push the uterus higher in the abdomen and cause it to deviate away from the expected midline position. It is common for the bladder to become full in the first 24–48 hours postpartum due to swelling and trauma from birth and elimination of excess intravascular volume.**
   4. A normal uterine involution would mean that the top of the uterus could be found midline in the abdomen and about two fingerbreadths below the umbilicus.

2. **C: Foundations of Practice T: Application**
   1. Newborns will demand feed frequently every 2–3 hours in the first weeks of life, and frequent feedings are encouraged.
   2. **Six to eight wet diapers in 24 hours indicate adequate hydration and nourishment.**
   3. It is impractical and unreliable to weigh a newborn as a sign of adequate feeding and nutrition.
   4. Passage of stools for a breastfed or formula-fed infant is not a reliable or predictable indicator of adequate hydration.

3. **C: Foundations of Practice T: Application**
   1. **Breastfed infants need vitamin D supplementation of 400 IU/day, available in infant drops.**
   2. The breastfed newborn has adequate iron stores for the first 6 months of life.
   3. Vitamin A supplementation is not recommended or required.
   4. Breast milk contains all the necessary essential fatty acids.

4. **C: Foundations of Practice T: Application**
   1. While the partner might be tired, this answer ignores his question and does not provide useful information about the process of taking in the experience of labour and birth.
   2. Referral for counselling is not indicated in this situation.
   3. Attachment is a process that takes place over time. No one event or behaviour is essential. The term *bonding* is avoided as it implies a short-term process that may fail or succeed if feelings and behaviours are not quickly established.
   4. **Ms. Viraj's behaviour is a normal part of adaptation to parenting. Providing information to the partner**

about this expected behaviour would help address his concerns.

5. C: **Foundations of Practice T: Knowledge**
   1. Moulding is a temporary overlapping of the cranial bones. The head appears pointed and elongated in shape.
   2. **Caput succedaneum is soft scalp swelling commonly due to pressure on the head from the cervix. It is poorly defined and crosses the suture lines of the skull. It appears at or shortly after birth and resolves within a few days.**
   3. Cephalohematoma appears after 24 hours, is localized on one side of the head, and does not cross the suture lines of the skull. It is a collection of blood under the periosteum and takes several weeks to be reabsorbed.
   4. A Mongolian spot is a darkened pigmentation of the skin located over the lumbar spine area.

6. C: **Foundations of Practice T: Application**
   1. Circumcision is most often practised to comply with religious or cultural beliefs but may also be a personal preference and choice made by the parents.
   2. The practical nurse's responsibility is to provide current, evidence-informed information so the parents can make an informed decision.
   3. **Routine circumcision is not recommended (Canadian Paediatric Society, 2015).**
   4. The evidence supporting or refuting the need for circumcision is not absolute or definitive in supporting routine circumcision in infancy.

7. C: **Foundations of Practice T: Critical Thinking**
   1. Fetal well-being in this situation would be better assessed with the use of fetal heart monitoring.
   2. Detecting fetal abnormalities by ultrasound would be part of an ultrasound assessment early in the pregnancy and is not a priority in this situation.
   3. **Ultrasound would be used to locate and confirm the position of the placenta to determine whether it is implanted near the cervix.**
   4. These determinations are made in early ultrasonograms and would not be a priority in this situation.

8. C: **Foundations of Practice T: Application**
   1. **Placenta previa is manifested by painless red vaginal bleeding in the third trimester. Ms. Smitherman's advanced maternal age is also a known risk factor.**
   2. Placental abruption more often occurs during labour and is manifested by concealed or apparent vaginal bleeding and pain, with the uterus feeling hard, tense, and painful.
   3. Spontaneous abortion occurs prior to 20 weeks' gestation.
   4. Rh incompatibility is not indicated by these manifestations. The hemolytic process would affect the newborn only and does not result in painless vaginal bleeding in the third trimester.

9. C: **Foundations of Practice T: Application**
   1. Women have been able to give birth vaginally after having a Caesarean section.
   2. It is not possible to predict whether a vaginal birth will be an option with the next delivery.
   3. It takes longer to recover from a Caesarean surgery than a vaginal birth.
   4. **There are parameters the physician will use as a guide to help make the decision for a vaginal birth after Caesarean section (VBAC). It will be based on the next pregnancy and labour experience.**

10. C: **Foundations of Practice T: Critical Thinking**
    1. **The priority assessment is ensuring spontaneous respirations so that the infant may be adequately oxygenated. If the infant is not breathing adequately, the infant will require supplemental oxygen, bagging, and possibly intubation with mechanical ventilation.**
    2. This would be an important assessment, but breathing is the priority.
    3. Colour is part of the assessment related to breathing. A newborn at birth will likely be cyanosed, becoming pink centrally after spontaneous respirations or supplemental bagging is initiated.
    4. This is part of the neonatal assessment but is not the priority assessment.

11. C: **Foundations of Practice T: Application**
    1. **Pathological jaundice associated with liver damage would occur at birth or in the first 24 hours. Physiological jaundice in a full-term, otherwise healthy infant occurs after 24 hours, peaks within 3–4 days, and resolves within a week.**
    2. The bruising and blood from the cephalohematoma may have contributed to the elevated bilirubin levels but are not the cause. An immature liver and limited ability to conjugate bilirubin lead to physiological jaundice.
    3. Pathological hyperbilirubinemia occurs at birth or in the first 24 hours of life and requires investigation.
    4. A blood exchange transfusion is not always required, especially for physiological jaundice.

12. C: **Foundations of Practice T: Application**
    1. Fluid requirements increase by 10%, and more frequent breastfeeding should be supported.
    2. Stools become looser and more frequent.
    3. The baby will be drowsier and lethargic.
    4. **Skin exposure is important to maximize the benefit of the ultraviolet lights. Eyes must always be covered for protection.**

13. C: **Foundations of Practice T: Application**
    1. This is not a safe option. In many cases, the membranes do not rupture until shortly before delivery.
    2. **Regular contractions at 7 minutes apart indicate the end of the latent phase of labour. It is not known how quickly Ms. Cooke's labour will progress; therefore, she should be assessed by a nurse or physician at the hospital.**
    3. Suggesting the pregnant woman walk when she feels contractions is often advised to distinguish between true and false labour. Ms. Cooke has indicated that the contractions are regular, so it is not likely that this is false labour. She should be assessed at the hospital.

4. Contractions that are 4 minutes apart occur during the active phase of labour. As it is not known how quickly the labour will progress, Ms. Cooke should not delay being assessed.

14. **C: Professional, Ethical, and Legal Practice T: Knowledge**
   1. Infants do not possess the ability to shiver at birth.
   2. **Nonshivering thermogenesis uses the chemical breakdown of brown fat stores to generate heat.**
   3. Cold, stress, and heat production increase oxygen demands and consumption.
   4. An extended body posture increases heat loss.

15. **C: Professional, Ethical, and Legal Practice T: Knowledge**
   1. Weight is not used to assess gestational age as infants may be small, large, or average weight independent of their gestational age.
   2. Head circumference is not a reliable indicator of gestational age. A newborn may be small, large, or average in growth regardless of gestational age.
   3. **Absence of ear cartilage is seen in prematurity, while the presence of ear cartilage is a sign of full-term gestational maturity.**
   4. Body length is influenced by growth patterns, and infants may be average, below, or above average in length regardless of gestational age.

16. **C: Professional, Ethical, and Legal Practice T: Application**
   1. Increased oxygen levels cause the ductus arteriosus to constrict.
   2. Clamping of the umbilical cord closes the ductus venosus.
   3. **When the pulmonary vessels open, more blood flows into the left atrium, increasing pressure and volume. This pressure becomes greater than the pressure in the right atrium, and the foramen ovale functionally closes.**
   4. During transition, the pulmonary blood vessels dilate and pulmonary blood pressure decreases.

17. **C: Professional, Ethical, and Legal Practice T: Application**
   1. **Fetal well-being is indicated by heart rate variability of 6–25 bpm, with a normal baseline heart rate of 110–160 bpm and no periodic decelerations.**
   2. Head compression is associated with early decelerations during labour near the time of birth.
   3. Umbilical cord compression is associated with variable decelerations.
   4. Periodic late decelerations are associated with utero-placental insufficiency, which can occur when the placental supply of oxygen is reduced or interrupted, as in chronic hypertension.

18. **C: Foundations of Practice T: Application**
   1. WinRho is administered to Rh-negative mothers who give birth to an Rh-positive newborn. There will not be an immune response if the newborn is also Rh-negative; therefore, prophylaxis is not required.
   2. **WinRho is given in this situation in case the embryo or fetus was Rh-positive and isoimmunization has occurred.**

3. WinRho is administered to Rh-negative mothers who give birth to an Rh-positive newborn or in situations where the Rh factor of the embryo or newborn is unknown, including ectopic pregnancies and spontaneous or induced abortions. Blood type is not a consideration.
4. WinRho is not required in this situation as the incompatibility occurs with an O-positive mother who has anti-A and anti-B antibodies. WinRho will not affect blood type incompatibilities.

19. **C: Foundations of Practice T: Application**
   1. Bed sharing is not recommended by the Canadian Paediatric Society.
   2. **The incidence of sudden unexpected infant death (SUID) is lowered when these guidelines are followed.**
   3. These positions are not required to prevent aspiration and are linked to an increased risk of SUID.
   4. Extra clothing layers and blankets are not needed or recommended.

20. **C: Professional, Ethical, and Legal Practice T: Critical Thinking**
   1. **Infertility increases in women who delay pregnancy until after the age of 30. Aging is a major contributing factor in increased infertility.**
   2. Being in a same-sex relationship does not necessarily affect female fertility. Same-sex female couples may choose to use a sperm donor and conceive either through intercourse or artificial insemination.
   3. Sexually transmitted infections are known risk factors for infertility. Provided that safer sex with barrier methods was practised to prevent infections, more than five partners is not necessarily a risk for infertility.
   4. The onset of puberty and menarche does not affect fertility over a woman's reproductive lifespan.

21. **C: Professional, Ethical, and Legal Practice T: Knowledge**
   1. **There is an increased risk of hypoglycemia as maternal glucose supply stops at birth, the newborn's pancreas continues to produce large amounts of insulin, and the infant, particularly if the child is large for gestational age (LGA), uses up glucose stores quickly.**
   2. Infants of mothers with gestational diabetes are at risk of being LGA due to the additional maternal glucose supply. Small for gestational age is a risk for people with type 1 diabetes who may experience chronic urinary tract infections.
   3. There is an increased risk of hypoglycemia, not hyperglycemia. See rationale 1.
   4. The fetal pancreas responds to increased glucose from the mother by producing large amounts of insulin in the first few days of life, resulting in temporary hyperinsulinism, not insulin resistance.

22. **C: Professional, Ethical, and Legal Practice T: Knowledge**
   1. Blood from placenta previa would present as bright red in the fluid.
   2. The fetus kidneys are immature and do not produce concentrated urine. Uric acid is not green in colour.

3. **When a fetus is under stress, it will pass the meconium stool during labour.**
4. Chlamydia discharge can be yellowish green in colour but would have been present in the vaginal cavity prior to the ruptured membranes.

23. **C: Foundations of Practice T: Knowledge**
    1. Calcium requirements increase to 1 200–1 500 mg per day, depending on age.
    2. A supplement of 400 mcg daily in addition to dietary intake is recommended.
    3. Recommended iron intake increases from 13 to 18 mg in the second trimester and to 23 mg by the third trimester.
    4. **There is a known increased risk of birth defects at intakes of vitamin A of 10 000 IU daily. The recommended intake for vitamin A, 4 355 IU, is easily met through dietary means; supplementation is therefore not recommended.**

24. **C: Foundations of Practice T: Application**
    1. Systemic opioids are avoided if birth is anticipated within 2 hours and would therefore not be administered up to the second stage of labour.
    2. Narcan is administered to the newborn to reverse the opioid effect, not to the mother.
    3. **Systemic opioids do cross the placenta to the fetus and may cause central nervous system depression in the newborn. Narcan can be administered to the newborn to reverse the side effects.**
    4. Opioids are found in insignificant amounts in breast milk and will not cause adverse effects in the newborn. It is important to provide effective pain management for the mother so she is able to interact with and learn to care for her newborn.

25. **C: Foundations of Practice T: Application**
    1. **Human milk is the ideal food for preterm infants. Mothers of preterm infants should begin pumping their breasts with a hospital-grade electric pump as soon as possible after birth and should pump 10 times daily to establish milk flow.**
    2. The mother needs to start pumping her breasts as soon as possible. After several weeks, she may not be able to establish adequate milk flow.
    3. Breast milk is more beneficial than formula for all infants. Breast milk can be measured to provide exact volumes for the infant.
    4. Depending on the suck and swallow reflex, the behavioural readiness to take oral feedings, and the infant's physical condition, it is not known when the infant will be able to be put to breast.

CHAPTER 10

The correct answer is set off in boldface.
1. **C: Foundations of Practice T: Application**
   1. **The child adopts this position in an attempt to facilitate the use of accessory muscles of respiration. If the child is able to lie down, the asthma attack is not likely to be severe.**

2. This is a manifestation of laryngotracheobronchitis (croup).
3. Children with asthma try to breathe deeply. There are rarely periods of apnea, unless the child is progressing to respiratory arrest.
4. This is a manifestation of laryngotracheobronchitis (croup).

2. **C: Foundations of Practice T: Application**
   1. This is a recognized side effect of Ventolin. The inhalation should not be stopped.
   2. **Shaking is a recognized side effect of Ventolin and occurs especially with increased frequency of inhalations. Simon should be reassured that it is normal.**
   3. The shakes are not due to Simon being cold. A blanket will not help.
   4. Air flow does not influence the side effect of shaking with Ventolin.

3. **C: Foundations of Practice T: Application**
   1. Milk products tend to increase mucus secretions in the airways and so should be avoided in clients with respiratory distress.
   2. Solid foods are not recommended during respiratory distress as they may increase the risk of vomiting and aspiration.
   3. It is appropriate to have clear fluids, but a child would not be likely to choose beef soup.
   4. **Children with respiratory distress should have diets consisting of clear fluids. These are better tolerated, provide recommended fluids to help liquefy mucus secretions, and do not pose a risk for aspiration. Ice pops would be an attractive choice for a child.**

4. **C: Foundations of Practice T: Critical Thinking**
   1. **Research has shown that children who have developed a comprehensive plan for asthma management with their healthcare provider have the best management of symptoms and the fewest hospitalizations.**
   2. This may be true, but it is not the most helpful answer.
   3. This is true, but an asthma plan will help identify triggers.
   4. While this is true for some children with asthma, it is not known if Simon will require this level of medication.

5. **C: Foundations of Practice T: Critical Thinking**
   1. This may be necessary but would be distressing for Simon. Removal of pets should not be considered unless allergen testing proves Simon is allergic to dog dander.
   2. **Second-hand smoke is a definite trigger for asthma. Several Canadian provinces have enacted legislation preventing adults from smoking in cars with children.**
   3. This is a valuable strategy to help clean the air in Simon's home but is not the most important, immediate strategy.
   4. Wet dusting is necessary to remove dust accumulation but is not as important or immediate as not smoking in the car.

6. **C: Foundations of Practice T: Application**
   1. A visit to a physician for a "cold" is not necessary. She will need to see a physician if the fever continues for a week or if the illness becomes worse.

2. Aspirin should not be given to children due to the risk of Reye's syndrome.

3. **Pediatric acetaminophen and ibuprofen are appropriate analgesics and antipyretics for minor childhood conditions such as teething, colds, immunizations, and so on.**

4. These medications are not recommended for infants and children and in some cases have been removed from pharmacies.

7. **C: Foundations of Practice T: Application**
   1. Infant walkers are unsafe and not allowed for sale in Canada.
   2. A baby rattle is more appropriate for an infant of 1–3 months.
   3. Reading, while an excellent method of promoting bonding, literacy, and reading readiness, does not develop motor skills.
   4. **Manipulating these objects will assist in the development of fine motor skills.**

8. **C: Foundations of Practice T: Application**
   1. Provided that the finger foods are not hard and large (such as peanuts or carrots), finger foods are nutritious, help develop motor skills, and are well liked by older infants and toddlers.
   2. This is not necessary. If the sides of the crib are in the raised position, Leah will not fall.
   3. This is not realistic. Other closures such as zippers and snaps are safe.
   4. **Small movable parts may become dislodged from the toy and are a hazard to infants and toddlers.**

9. **C: Professional, Ethical, and Legal Practice T: Application**
   1. Leah is exhibiting stranger anxiety, which is developmentally normal at 9 months. Removing Leah from her father will frighten her.
   2. This should not be necessary if the right approach is taken and Leah is given time to get used to the practical nurse.
   3. **This is the recommended approach as the soft voice is comforting and meeting the child at eye level makes the stranger appear smaller.**
   4. This is intrusive and is likely to frighten Leah.

10. **C: Foundations of Practice T: Application**
    1. This is an appropriate developmental milestone for a 9-month-old infant.
    2. **This would be expected to be achieved by 7 months.**
    3. This becomes evident at 6 months of age.
    4. This is appropriate to a developmental age of 12 months.

11. **C: Foundations of Practice T: Critical Thinking**
    1. **Peanuts may be used in many ingredients that may not be evident. A ban on all homemade foods (such as cakes and ice cream) will prevent inadvertent sources of peanut by-products from being ingested by the children. Many daycare centres have enacted this practice.**
    2. This will communicate the peanut allergy problem to the parents but may not prevent food substances that contain peanuts from being available to the children. Parents may not be aware of which foods are likely to have traces of peanuts.

    3. This will help the staff identify children at risk but will do nothing to prevent foods containing peanuts from being in the daycare centre.
    4. All sources of peanut, for example, peanut oil, may not be easily identifiable.

12. **C: Foundations of Practice T: Critical Thinking**
    1. This is a safe practice but should be performed before changing diapers as well. It may not be effective in preventing airborne transmission of micro-organisms.
    2. Hand hygiene is the best infection control practice, but several times a day is not frequent enough to prevent transmission.
    3. This is not practical in most daycare settings.
    4. **Children with obvious signs of infection should be cared for at home. However, if they develop symptoms during the day, they should be isolated from the rest of the children.**

13. **C: Foundations of Practice T: Application**
    1. This is too frequent and will tire Jayden unnecessarily. There will not be sufficient rest time between feedings.
    2. **Feeding of the infant with heart failure is similar to exercise in an adult. The infant often tires and may need frequent rest periods.**
    3. Infants with a congenital heart defect require feedings with increased caloric density in the formula or breast milk.
    4. This may be necessary if it is found Jayden cannot tolerate bottle feedings. There may not be trained staff at the daycare centre to competently gavage-feed infants.

14. **C: Foundations of Practice T: Knowledge**
    1. **Varicella-zoster virus is the name of the herpes virus that causes the disease varicella, or chicken pox.**
    2. MMR is the vaccine that protects the child from measles, mumps, and rubella.
    3. Hib is the *Haemophilus influenzae* type b (Hib) vaccine and protects the child primarily against bacterial meningitis and epiglottitis.
    4. DTaP is a combination vaccine that provides immunity to diphtheria, tetanus, and pertussis.

15. **C: Foundations of Practice T: Application**
    1. This is a breach of confidential information. The child with pediculosis (lice) does not have to be specifically identified. Shobana may not be the only child with head lice.
    2. **This alerts the families to the problem and provides practical information to examine and treat their children. Treatment at home will prevent transmission of the head lice at the daycare centre.**
    3. It is not practical to examine the hair of every child on arrival and then to send the child home without prior notice to the parents. A useful alternative would be to screen all children early in the day, isolate those found to have lice, and then notify the families.

4. This is not the responsibility of the daycare centre. Treatment should be provided in the home.

16. **C: Foundations of Practice T: Application**
   1. **Wet skin, especially if contaminated with urine and fecal irritants, promotes dermatitis. Exposure to air helps dry the skin.**
   2. Use of a hair dryer or heat lamp is not recommended as it may cause burns.
   3. Overwashing, particularly with commercial wipes and perfumed soaps, may cause irritation.
   4. Cornstarch rather than talc is recommended as it is more effective in reducing friction and tends to cake less than talc. There is also a danger that infants may aspirate talc.

17. **C: Foundations of Practice T: Application**
   1. Blood glucose levels will need to be checked before each meal and at bedtime.
   2. **To prevent future long-term complications maintaining a blood glucose level, between 4 to 7 mmol/L is recommended.**
   3. There are no restrictions on sugar. It is recommended that a healthy diet is followed.
   4. A 6-year-old is too young to take on this responsibility.

18. **C: Foundations of Practice T: Application**
   1. **Infants with Down syndrome often have difficulty with feedings due to their large tongues and poor muscle control and coordination.**
   2. There can be decreased immunity with Down syndrome, but it is not a common finding.
   3. Down syndrome infants and children are very receptive to affection.
   4. There is a gradual increase, not deterioration, in developmental functioning.

19. **C: Foundations of Practice T: Application**
   1. The continuous infusion of opioids provides better pain relief than does intermittent therapy.
   2. **During a sickle cell crisis, increased fluids are required to prevent further sickling and to delay the vaso-occlusion and hypoxia–ischemia cycle. The kidneys are not able to concentrate urine. Strict monitoring of intake and output is required.**
   3. While most children can gauge their tolerance for exercise, and strict bed rest is not required, children in a vaso-occlusive crisis should limit exercise to avoid additional tissue oxygen needs.
   4. Cold compresses are not applied to the area because this may enhance vasoconstriction and occlusion.

20. **C: Foundations of Practice T: Critical Thinking**
   1. **This is the first step in the nursing process: data collection. The nurse needs more information about the diet and pattern of discomfort. The infant likely has colic, and the detailed history will assist the nurse to provide potential therapeutic measures to ease the infant's discomfort.**
   2. This is a possibility, but a thorough history is required initially.

3. Re-establishing breast milk may not be possible at this stage. Breastfed infants also develop colic.
4. This may be true, but in order to develop individualized and appropriate comfort measures, the practical nurse requires more information.

21. **C: Foundations of Practice T: Knowledge**
   1. **Leukemias are the most common form of childhood cancer in Canada, occurring at a rate of 32.2 cases per million children per year.**
   2. Lymphomas occur in children at a rate of 27.5 cases per million per year.
   3. Central nervous system tumours occur in children at a rate of 26.8 cases per million per year.
   4. Renal tumours occur in children at a rate of 6.8 cases per million per year.

22. **C: Foundations of Practice T: Knowledge**
   1. This explanation relates to cryptorchidism, or undescended testicles.
   2. This is epispadias.
   3. Hypospadias is not a small penis, although men with the defect may also have a small penis as a result of the defect.
   4. **Hypospadias is a condition in which the urethral opening is localized anywhere along the ventral surface of the penis. Depending on the severity, it can generally be surgically corrected to improve appearance, to enable the client to urinate while standing, and to preserve sexual function.**

23. **C: Professional, Ethical, and Legal practice T: Application**
   1. This is not true. There are a variety of pain rating scales and behavioural indicators that are useful for assessing pain in children. Children by the age of 4 can accurately point to the body area where they have pain.
   2. Narcotics can be successfully and safely used with children. They are no more dangerous for children than for adults.
   3. **Several research studies have examined the pattern of pain medication in children compared with adults and have found consistently that many children are not medicated appropriately for their degree of pain.**
   4. Children may not admit having pain to avoid an injection or may not ask for analgesia because they believe adults know how they feel.

24. **C: Foundations of Practice T: Application**
   1. **Having the parent assist may help calm the child and achieve compliance with taking the prednisone. The child is more likely to trust the parent than the practical nurse.**
   2. Prednisone does not come in suppository form. A suppository is inappropriate and invasive.
   3. Children should never be restrained unless there is a medical order. Restraints would be frightening for the child.
   4. This may sound like an attractive option, but the bitter taste of the prednisone would not be masked by the applesauce, and it is unlikely that the child would eat

a sufficient amount to receive all of the prednisone. The child may be offered applesauce or another favourite food after the prednisone to help clear the mouth of the bitter taste.

25. C: Collaborative Practice T: Critical Thinking
    1. **The family is included to collaborate with all levels of care. Family-centred care values the family as the spokespersons for their children during healthcare discussions and decisions.**
    2. The family will need guidance in understanding the lab values and how it will affect treatment. They will need this understanding in order to make informed decisions about the care of their child.
    3. Most facilities do have Internet access, which is used for a variety of reasons. Although resources for completing school work are often offered in pediatric care settings, they are not an integral part of family-centred care.
    4. It is encouraged that parents continue to follow bedtime routines that have been established at home rather than have the agency establish these routines.

CHAPTER 11

The correct answer is set off in boldface.
1. C: Foundations of Practice T: Knowledge
   1. **This is the definition of *psychosis*.**
   2. This is the definition of *neurosis*.
   3. This is the definition of *delirium*.
   4. Schizophrenia is a psychotic illness but is not synonymous with psychosis. Psychosis may also occur in manic phases of bipolar disorder, substance abuse, delirium, organic mental health disorders, post-traumatic stress disorder, and major depression.
2. C: Foundations of Practice T: Application
   1. Emergency involuntary admission is permitted when a person is deemed in need of psychiatric treatment, presents a danger to self or others, or is unable to meet his basic needs.
   2. Depending on the province or territory, there are different ages for consent. Many have an age of consent that is 16 years or younger. Regardless of his age or the age of consent of the jurisdiction, Jason has rights.
   3. **Under law, Jason may apply to a review board to review the involuntary admission.**
   4. Jason does have legal rights.
3. C: Professional, Ethical, and Legal Practice T: Application
   1. Quiet seclusion may help some clients. Chemical restraints may not always be preferable.
   2. In many cases, physical restraints increase violent behaviour and chemical restraints are preferable.
   3. **The policy of least restraint and guidelines for use of restraints apply equally to physical and chemical restraints.**
   4. The setting of an emergency department still requires a physician order for a chemical restraint as it is a medication.

4. C: Foundations of Practice T: Application
   1. **This is an honest and truthful response, which helps identify the voices as a unique experience for Jason but does not involve arguing reality with him.**
   2. Although it may be useful for the practical nurse to find out more about the hallucinations, it is not helpful to Jason to pretend to believe in them.
   3. It is not helpful to Jason to argue with him about reality. The voices are real to him.
   4. Hallucinations are a symptom of psychosis. It is neither helpful nor therapeutic to explore why Jason is hearing voices.
5. C: Foundations of Practice T: Application
   1. This is a good suggestion but does not answer Jason's mother's question.
   2. This may not be true.
   3. This is a vague response and implies that the practical nurse is not competent to provide an answer.
   4. **This is the most complete and most correct response to Jason's mother's question.**
6. C: Foundations of Practice T: Knowledge
   1. People who exhibit narcissistic behaviour feel superior to everyone else and lack empathy for others. This is evident in narcissistic behaviour disorder.
   2. People who exhibit schizoid behaviour, found in schizoid personality disorder, are loners. They display very little emotion and tend to be indifferent to the feelings of others.
   3. **Mr. Steele displays splitting behaviour, setting one person up against another. It is a type of manipulative behaviour common in people with borderline personality disorder and some other personality disorders.**
   4. People with dependent personality disorder are very dependent on others. They lack self-confidence and would be unlikely to say anything negative about Sarah or anyone else for fear of losing that person's support and approval.
7. C: Foundations of Practice T: Application
   1. **People with borderline personality disorder are impulsive. Self-injury and suicide threats are common with this disorder. The practical nurse must assess for suicidal or homicidal thoughts, as ensuring the safety of the client and others is a practical nurse's first priority.**
   2. Hallucinations are a sign of psychosis. Borderline personality disorder is not a psychotic illness.
   3. While personality disorders may develop from a socially disrupted childhood, the practical nurse would not probe for such information until he or she is confident that the client is safe and until a relationship has been established.
   4. Sexual orientation is unrelated to personality disorders, although some symptoms, such as low self-esteem, fear of rejection, and sensitivity to criticism, that are common in personality disorders may also be present in people if they are confused or not accepting of their sexual orientation.

8. C: **Foundations of Practice T: Application**
   1. People with both anorexia and bulimia suffer complications in many body systems. In extreme cases, death can result from cardiac, gastro-intestinal, metabolic, or central nervous system complications.
   2. Although eating disorders are much more common in women than men, men do suffer from both anorexia and bulimia.
   3. **About half the women with anorexia display bulimic behaviours or develop bulimia later in their lives.**
   4. People with bulimia may feel intense hunger and binge to satisfy this hunger.

9. C: **Foundations of Practice T: Critical Thinking**
   1. Skin breakdown may occur secondary to inadequate nutrition but is not as important as blood pressure.
   2. While constipation may occur with eating disorders, it is more logical to ask Tiffany about her bowel pattern rather than perform an abdominal palpation.
   3. People with an eating disorder often develop dental caries. While the practical nurse may examine Tiffany's mouth, it may not be possible to determine dental caries on inspection. It would be more efficient to refer Tiffany to a dentist or dental hygienist.
   4. **People with an eating disorder often have a lower than normal blood volume, leading to hypotension.**

10. C: **Professional, Ethical, and Legal Practice T: Application**
    1. **This is an example of clarification. It helps clients clarify their own thoughts and maximizes mutual understanding.**
    2. This is the therapeutic technique of exploring, which examines experiences more fully.
    3. This is reflecting, directing feelings and ideas back to the client.
    4. This is focusing, which concentrates attention on a single point.

11. C: **Foundations of Practice T: Application**
    1. **Young women with eating disorders, particularly anorexia, may attempt to mask their weight loss by drinking excessive water (water loading) or hiding articles within their clothing prior to weighing.**
    2. Generally, most young women with anorexia are superficially compliant with weight monitoring.
    3. It is more important that Tiffany be weighed wearing the same clothes at each occasion. It is preferable not to wear shoes or clothing where heavy articles may be hidden.
    4. Depending on the provincial law, there may be no legal imperative to inform Tiffany's parents. This needs to be discussed between Tiffany and the practical nurse, and parental involvement should be encouraged.

12. C: **Foundations of Practice T: Application**
    1. People with anorexia are not able to tolerate large meals. They should be offered small meals and frequent nutritious drinks and snacks, paying special attention to their likes and dislikes.
    2. **The practical nurse must record intake and output carefully as a measure of adequate hydration. Other indicators to be monitored are skin turgor and colour and moistness of oral mucous membranes.**
    3. Mealtimes should be time limited. To decrease stress while eating, ensure a pleasant atmosphere and conversation about topics other than food.
    4. Adolescents with eating disorders generally respond well to group therapy. In addition, isolating the client provides more opportunities for secretive purging.

13. C: **Foundations of Practice T: Application**
    1. Clients are at risk immediately on admission as medications are not effective yet.
    2. Clients are at risk on discharge when the reality that things are the same as before. They return home to find that things caused the depression have not changed.
    3. **As depression deepens, the client has less motivation and physical energy to follow through on suicidal action.**
    4. Clients are at high risk for suicide for the first few days following initiation of treatment. Energy levels and motivation have improved as now the person is less apathetic. Thus, early in treatment, the client is still severely depressed but may now have the energy necessary to follow through with suicidal thoughts

14. C: **Professional, Ethical, and Legal Practice T: Application**
    1. This is not a therapeutic response. It does not address Ms. Balkan's present feelings, and she may not feel better the next day.
    2. This is not a therapeutic response as it does not invite Ms. Balkan to discuss her feelings.
    3. **This recognizes Ms. Balkan's feelings and invites her to discuss these feelings.**
    4. This is not therapeutic as it may appear to belittle Ms. Balkan's feelings, and it may not be true that the feeling is temporary.

15. C: **Foundations of Practice T: Knowledge**
    1. **Therapeutic effects may take up to 4 weeks to be achieved.**
    2. Although there have been reports of an increase in suicide after starting Prozac (fluoxetine hydrochloride), there is not a large body of research to substantiate this. It is possible that in early treatment, there is an increased risk of suicide due to the fact that the clients are beginning to feel better.
    3. Anxiety and nervousness are side effects of Prozac and may increase.
    4. Herbal preparations (such as St. John's wort) may have an additive effect with Prozac and should not be taken.

16. C: **Collaborative Practice T: Application**
    1. This is a side effect that usually disappears after several weeks.
    2. **The yellow skin and conjunctiva indicate jaundice, which is a sign of liver damage. The drug should be stopped.**
    3. As in choice 1.
    4. Extrapyramidal signs usually indicate that the dose of Haldol should be reduced. The Haldol is not stopped

unless the extrapyramidal symptoms persist at the lower dose.

17. **C: Foundations of Practice T: Critical Thinking**
    1. Mrs. Hardacre is at increased risk of suicide due to her alcohol abuse, but she does not have the highest level of risk of the four individuals.
    2. Women attempt suicide more often than men, but more men are successful.
    3. While men have a higher rate of successful suicide, it is in the 40–59 age group. Mr. Tyrell would be at risk if he had a concrete plan for taking his life.
    4. **Mr. Grimes is at the highest risk of suicide. There is a higher incidence of suicide than previously thought in the older adult. Older men have a much higher suicide rate than older women.**

18. **C: Collaborative Practice T: Critical Thinking**
    1. This is within the scope of practice for this nurse and may be helpful, but it is not the most effective option.
    2. **Gender identity disorders are complex and beyond the scope of practice of a new nurse. They require the skills of a qualified sexual therapist.**
    3. This may be advised by the sexual therapist.
    4. This is best performed by the sexual therapist or physician.

19. **C: Collaborative Practice T: Critical Thinking**
    1. All mental illnesses are culturally determined.
    2. It is inaccurate and judgemental to associate certain mental illnesses with an individual cultural group.
    3. When mental illnesses are treated in culturally prescribed ways, remedies are quite effective.
    4. **Practical nurses who understand that the client's symptoms are influenced by culture will be able to advocate for the client. It is imperative to take the client's social and cultural influences into account during assessments.**

20. **C: Foundations of Practice T: Knowledge**
    1. A very small percentage of Canadians use illegal narcotics, such as heroin and cocaine. A small percentage of people prescribed narcotics for medical treatment of pain become addicted.
    2. **Alcohol is the most common type of substance abuse in Canada. In a 2015 study, 19.2% of Canadians aged 12 years and older reported alcohol consumption that classified them as a heavy drinker.**
    3. Cannabis, or marijuana, is used by approximately 10% of Canadians.
    4. Inhalants are hallucinogenic drugs. Altogether, 2% of Canadians abuse drugs such as cocaine, Ecstasy, heroin, speed, and solvents (inhalants).

21. **C: Foundations of Practice T: Application**
    1. Individual expressions of culture vary according to the persons characteristics and experiences. Clients should be first treated as individuals and then consider their culture preferences in order to provide culturally competent care.
    2. **In some cultures, mental health disorders are considered shameful or frightening.**
    3. In some cultures, a discussion of feelings is neither acceptable nor comfortable. The practical nurse must interview in accordance with the comfort level of the client.
    4. Manifestations of stress may vary from one culture to another.

22. **C: Foundations of Practice T: Application**
    1. It is not likely that Mr. Picard's family will be able to distinguish between dementia and delirium. This question will not elicit the most important information.
    2. **Delirium tends to be of short duration and may be triggered by a specific condition. Dementia is a progressive cognitive disorder, occurring gradually over a period of time.**
    3. This may be an important question if it is determined that Mr. Picard has dementia.
    4. Violent behaviour does not help distinguish between delirium and dementia.

23. **C: Foundations of Practice T: Application**
    1. People with antisocial personality disorder rarely feel anxious.
    2. **People with antisocial personality disorder tend to be impulsive with poor self-control.**
    3. People with this disorder tend not to learn from past mistakes or from punishment.
    4. People with this disorder are generally self-centred and do not display responsibility toward others.

24. **C: Professional, Ethical, and Legal Practice T: Application**
    1. **There are situations where the therapeutic plan includes monitoring and assistance in a social situation. If the outing is part of the agreed-upon care plan, it is appropriate. Sanjay must take care to keep the outing strictly professional.**
    2. It is not appropriate for a practical nurse to have a social relationship with a mental health client.
    3. It is appropriate if it is decided upon by the healthcare team and is part of the care plan.
    4. As in choice 3.

25. **C: Professional, Ethical, and Legal Practice T: Application**
    1. This is aggressive behaviour.
    2. This is focused, positive behaviour in response to stress.
    3. **A feature of passive–aggressive behaviour is resistance to meeting the demands of others. Instead of voicing her unhappiness and stress, and taking positive steps to correct the situation, the practical nurse responds passive–aggressively by arriving late for work.**
    4. This is passive behaviour.

Page numbers followed by "*f*" indicate figures, "*t*" indicate tables, and "*b*" indicate boxes.